MANUAL OF
# MEDICAL-SURGICAL NURSING CARE

**Nursing Interventions and Collaborative Management**

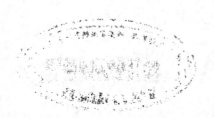

Manual of
# MEDICAL-SURGICAL NURSING CARE

Nursing Interventions and
Collaborative Management

**Pamela L. Swearingen, R.N.**
*Special Project Editor*

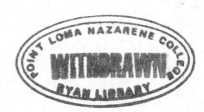

**Third Edition**

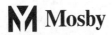 **Mosby**

St. Louis  Baltimore  Boston  Chicago  London  Madrid
Philadelphia  Sydney  Toronto

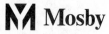
**Mosby**

Dedicated to Publishing Excellence

*Publisher:* Alison Miller
*Editor-in-Chief:* Nancy Coon
*Editor:* Robin Carter
*Associate Developmental Editor:* Jeanne Allison
*Project Manager:* Linda Clarke
*Production Editor:* Vicki Hoenigke
*Designer:* Betty Schulz
*Cover:* Renee Duenow

**THIRD EDITION**

Printed in the United States of America
Composition by the Clarinda Company
Printing/binding by R.R. Donnelley & Sons Company

Mosby–Year Book, Inc.
11830 Westline Industrial Drive
St. Louis, Missouri 63146

ISBN 0-8016-7694-0

95  96  97  98  /  9  8  7  6  5  4  3  2

# CONTRIBUTORS

**Lolita Adrien, RN, MS, CETN, CGRN**
Enterostomal Therapy Nurse
John Muir Medical Center
Walnut Creek, California

**Linda S. Baas, RN, MSN, PhD, CCRN**
Visiting Assistant Professor
Miami University,
Department of Nursing
Hamilton, Ohio

**Marianne S. Baird, RN, MN, CCRN**
Clinical Specialist, Critical Care
St. Joseph's Hospital
Atlanta, Georgia

**Mary E. Cooley, RN, CRNP, MSN, OCN**
Oncology Clinical Specialist/Adult Nurse Practitioner
Philadelphia Veteran's Affairs Medical Center
Philadelphia, Pennsylvania

**Barbara J. Deveau, RN, BA, MA**
Director, Outpatient Services
New England Baptist Hospital
Boston, Massachusetts

**Patricia Hall, RN, MSN**
Medical Cardiovascular
Clinical Nurse Specialist
St. Joseph's Hospital
Atlanta, Georgia

**Ellen L. Hellman, RN, MN, CFNP**
Nurse Practitioner
North Atlanta Endocrinology and Diabetes
Atlanta, Georgia

**Mima M. Horne, RN, MS**
Lecturer, School of Nursing
University of North Carolina–Wilmington
Wilmington, North Carolina

**Cheri Howard, RN, MSN**
Unit Director
Indiana University Hospitals
Indianapolis, Indiana

**Marguerite M. Jackson, RN, MS, CIC, FAAN**
Administrative Director
Medical Center Epidemiology Unit/Assistant Clinical Professor
Community and Family Medicine
University of California–San Diego
San Diego, California

**Patricia E.R. Jansen, RN, MSN**
Geriatric Nurse Specialist/Staff
 Development Instructor
El Camino Hospital
Mountain View, California

**Janet Hicks Keen, RN, MSN, CCRN, CEN**
Consultant and Educator
Emergency and Critical Care
 Nursing
St. Joseph's Hospital
Atlanta, Georgia

**Kenneth Miller, RN, MS, PhD**
Director, Clinical Nursing
 Research
National Naval Medical Center
 (US Navy)
Bethesda, Maryland

**Dennis G. Ross, RN, MSN, MAE, PhD**
Associate Professor of Nursing
University of Pittsburgh,
 School of Nursing
Pittsburgh, Pennsylvania

**Kathryn L. Schroeder, RN, BSN**
Clinical Services
 Facilitator/Staff Nurse
Indiana University Hospitals
Indianapolis, Indiana

**Barbara Tueller Steuble, RN, MS**
Education and Infection
 Control Coordinator
Amador Hospital
Jackson, California

**Nancy A. Stotts RN, MN, EdD**
Associate Professor
Department of Physiological
 Nursing
University of California–
 San Francisco
San Francisco, California

**Carol Monlux Swift, RN, BSN**
Clinical Nurse II, Transitional
 Care Unit
El Camino Hospital
Mountain View, California

**Diane Wind Wardell, RNC, PhD**
Assistant Professor
University of Texas Health
 Science Center at Houston
Houston, Texas

**Karen S. Webber, RN, MN**
Assistant Professor
School of Nursing
Memorial University of
 Newfoundland
St. Johns
Newfoundland, Canada

# CONSULTANTS

**Jan Barrett, RN, PhD**
Deaconess College of Nursing
St. Louis, Missouri

**Jacqueline J. Clibourn**
Manager, Clinical Research
  Program
Haemonetics, Inc.
Braintree, Massachusetts

**Robin Webb Corbett, RNC,
  MSN**
North Carolina Special Care
  Center
Wilson, North Carolina

**Patti Coughlin Dalleske, RN,
  MSN, CCRN**
Youngstown State University
Youngstown, Ohio
      and
Eastern Ohio Pulmonary
  Consultants
Boardman, Ohio

**Martha Davidson, RN, MN,
  CETN**
Emory University Hospital
Atlanta, Georgia

**Susan Donckers, RN, EdD**
Radford University
Radford, Virginia

**Carole Edelman, RN, MS**
Columbia University School of
  Nursing
New York, New York

**Patti Eisenberg, RN, MSN**
The Jewish Hospital of
  St. Louis
St. Louis, Missouri

**Karolyn Givens, RN, MS,
  EdD**
Radford University
Radford, Virginia

**Lorrie N. Hegstad, RN, PhD**
The University of Texas at
  Arlington School of Nursing
Arlington, Texas

**Mima M. Horne, RN, MS**
University of North Carolina at
  Wilmington and New
  Hanover Regional Medical
  Center
Wilmington, North Carolina

**Gay Howard, RN, CPHQ**
Independent Consultant
Agoura, California

**Mary Huch, RN, PhD**
University of Southern
  Mississippi
Hattiesburg, Mississippi

**Roxanne Hurley, RN, MS**
University of North Dakota
  College of Nursing
Grand Forks, North Dakota

**Marguerite M. Jackson, RN, MS, CIC, FAAN**
University of California at San Diego Medical Center
San Diego, California

**Carolyn Livingston, RN, PhD**
Seattle Sexual Health Center
Seattle, Washington

**Edwina McConnell, RN, PhD**
Texas Tech University Health Sciences Center
School of Nursing
Lubbock, Texas

**Linda Moore, RN, EdD**
University of North Carolina College of Nursing
Charlotte, North Carolina

**Jacquelin Neatherlin RN, MSN, CNRN**
Baylor University School of Nursing
Dallas, Texas

**Janice Nunnelee, RN, MSN**
Vascular and General Surgery
St. John's Mercy Medical Center
St. Louis, Missouri

**Cecilia Owens, RN, MSN**
Georgia Baptist School of Nursing
Atlanta, Georgia

**Demetrius J. Porche, RN, MN, CCRN**
Tulane University Medical Center
New Orleans, Louisiana

**Tracy Riley, RNC, MSN**
The University of Akron
Akron, Ohio

**Anna Louise Scandiffio, RN, MS**
Department of Veteran's Affairs Medical Center
Baltimore, Maryland

**Edna Schade, RN, MS**
Delaware Technical and Community College
Newark, Delaware

**Pamela Becker Weilitz, RN, MSN(R)**
Barnes Hospital at Washington University Medical Center
St. Louis, Missouri

**Mary Jo Wellhaven, RN, MS**
Winona State University
Rochester, Minnesota

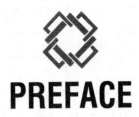

# PREFACE

**Manual of Medical-Surgical Nursing Care: Nursing Interventions and Collaborative Management** (titled **Manual of Nursing Therapeutics** in its first two editions) was designed to enable both staff and student nurses to plan and evaluate care of the adult medical-surgical patient. Focusing on NANDA-approved nursing diagnoses that are specific to each disorder, the manual provides a quick review of pathophysiology, physical assessment, diagnostic testing, collaborative management, and patient/family teaching and discharge planning data. The order of presentation of the information in each health alteration provides a hierarchy of data that enables the nurse to make nursing diagnoses and to plan interventions specific to each patient. More generic information can be found in the appendices, where nursing diagnoses and interventions for preoperative and postoperative patients, patients on prolonged bed rest, patients with cancer and other life-disrupting illnesses, and older adults are discussed.

Staff and student nurses can use this reference to obtain clinical information formerly found only in medical-surgical textbooks or large manuals. It is the first reference of its size to feature the application of nursing diagnoses and interventions to more than 165 health alterations. A new, consistent, easy-to-use format has been incorporated to enhance the quick-reference feature of this book.

This edition has been thoroughly revised and updated. The outcome criteria are specific, positive statements that facilitate evaluation of care. New to this edition, we have added timeframes to the outcome criteria, where appropriate, and they have been reviewed for accuracy by an expert in quality assurance. Timeframes are provided as guidelines—individual patients having their own, unique response times—and to serve as reminders that Medicare and other third-party payors monitor the fine line between quality, cost-effective care, and premature discharge, enabling nurses to set more realistic goals for nursing outcomes. This manual advocates use of the Body Substance Isolation (BSI) by Lynch, Jackson, et al, because it is a broad strategy that incorporates all the elements of Universal Precautions as well as reduces risks for patient and health-care workers of transmission of other than bloodborne organisms.

Also new to this edition are discussions of pulmonary tuberculosis, dysrhythmias and conduction disturbances, angioplasty, syndrome of inappropriate antidiuretic hormone, iron deficiency anemia, lymphomas, breast reduction, vulvar cancers, and cochlear implantation. The appendices have been expanded to include sections addressing topics of special interest in the 1990s, such as the latest information on pain control management based on the Clinical Practice guidelines from the U.S. Department of Health and Human Services. A new section on the care of the older adult also has been added, addressing the special needs of this evergrowing population. A new appendix is included called "Infection Prevention and Control," which discusses the various systems of infection control. In addition, we have added a section that lists normal values for the laboratory tests discussed in this manual.

Finally, a word about the health alterations we selected: we chose those that are either commonly seen as primary admission diagnoses or those that are seen frequently as secondary diagnoses in hospitalized patients. To control the number of pages and ensure a portable, handbook-sized reference, we did not include specific discussions of pediatric, critical care, mental health, or other specialized areas.

**Manual of Medical-Surgical Nursing Care** was designed to help students and staff nurses apply nursing diagnoses in the "real world" of the acute care hospital. Reviewers indicate that it achieves this objective. The ultimate judgment rests with those nurses who read and use the manual on a daily basis. We welcome comments on how we might enhance its usefulness in subsequent editions.

*Pamela L. Swearingen*

# Acknowledgments

The contributors and I want to thank the many individuals whose input was of value in the development of this manuscript. In particular, we wish to acknowledge the second edition contributions of Patricia Brown, RNC, PhD; Bertie Chuong, RN, MS, CCRN; Michelle M. Ferguson, RN, MSN, OCN; Donna Kershner, RN, MS; Carol E. Lang, RD, MS; Julie Klausen Moe, RN, MSN; and Andrea Walsh-Matz, RN, BSN, CD.

                                                                    P.L.S.

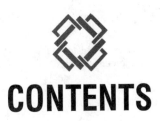

# CONTENTS

## 1 RESPIRATORY DISORDERS

### Cheri Howard

Section One   Acute Respiratory Disorders   1
  Atelectasis   1
  Pneumonia   3
  Pleural effusion   12
  Pulmonary embolus   13
  Pneumothorax/Hemothorax   19
  Pulmonary tuberculosis   24
Section Two   Acute Respiratory Failure   25
Section Three   Chronic Obstructive Pulmonary Disease   28
  Asthma   28
  Chronic bronchitis   32
  Emphysema   35
Section Four   Restrictive Pulmonary Disorders   37
  Pulmonary fibrosis   37
Section Five   Bronchogenic Carcinoma   39
Selected Bibliography   41

## 2 CARDIOVASCULAR DISORDERS

### Barbara Tueller Steuble

Section One   Degenerative Cardiovascular Disorders   44
  Pulmonary hypertension   44
  Cardiomyopathy   47
  Coronary artery disease   50
  Myocardial infarction   56
  Heart failure   60
Section Two   Inflammatory Heart Disorders   63
  Pericarditis   63
  Infective endocarditis   66

Section Three   Valvular Heart Disorders   69
   Mitral stenosis   69
   Mitral regurgitation   72
   Aortic stenosis   74
   Aortic regurgitation   75
Section Four   Cardiovascular Conditions Secondary to Other Disease
               Processes   76
   Cardiac and noncardiac shock (circulatory failure)   76
   Dysrhythmias and conduction disturbances   80
   Cardiac arrest   84
   Pulmonary edema   85
Section Five   Special Cardiac Procedures   88
   Pacemakers   88
   Cardiac catheterization and angioplasty   91
   Cardiac surgery   94
Section Six   Disorders of the Peripheral Vascular System   96
   Atherosclerotic arterial occlusive disease   96
   Aneurysms: abdominal, thoracic, and femoral   101
   Arterial embolism   103
   Venous thrombosis/Thrombophlebitis   104
   Varicose veins   107
Selected Bibliography   109

# 3 RENAL-URINARY DISORDERS

Section One   Renal Disorders   113
**Mima M. Horne**
   Glomerulonephritis   113
   Nephrotic syndrome   118
   Acute pyelonephritis   120
   Renal calculi   123
   Hydronephrosis   125
   Renal artery stenosis   127
Section Two   Renal Failure   129
**Mima M. Horne**
   Acute renal failure   129
   Chronic renal failure   135
Section Three   Care of the Renal Transplant Recipient   140
**Mima M. Horne**
Section Four   Renal Dialysis   142
**Mima M. Horne**
   Care of the patient undergoing peritoneal dialysis   143
   Care of the patient undergoing hemodialysis   145
Section Five   Disorders of the Urinary Tract   147
**Patti E.R. Jansen**
   Ureteral calculi   147
   Urinary tract obstruction   152
   Cancer of the bladder   154

Section Six   Urinary Disorders Secondary to Other Disease Processes   158
**Patti E.R. Jansen**
    Urinary incontinence   158
    Urinary retention   165
    Neurogenic bladder   167
Section Seven   Urinary Diversions   172
**Patti E.R. Jansen**
Selected Bibliography   178

# 4 NEUROLOGIC DISORDERS
### Carol Monlux Swift

Section One   Inflammatory Disorders of the Nervous System   181
    Multiple sclerosis   182
    Guillain-Barré syndrome   188
    Bacterial meningitis   194
    Encephalitis   199
Section Two   Degenerative Disorders of the Nervous System   202
    Parkinsonism   203
    Alzheimer's disease   213
Section Three   Traumatic Disorders of the Nervous System   224
    Intervertebral disk disease: Dennis G. Ross, contributor   224
    Spinal cord injury   232
    Head injury   247
Section Four   Nervous System Tumors   258
    Brain tumors   258
    Spinal cord tumors   266
Section Five   Vascular Disorders of the Nervous System   269
    Cerebral aneurysm   269
    Cerebrovascular accident   276
Section Six   Seizure Disorders   288
Section Seven   General Care of Patients with Neurologic Disorders   298
Selected Bibliography   316

# 5 ENDOCRINE DISORDERS

Section One   Disorders of the Thyroid Gland   319
**Ellen L. Hellman**
    Hyperthyroidism   319
    Hypothyroidism   324
Section Two   Disorders of the Parathyroid Glands   329
**Ellen L. Hellman**
    Hyperparathyroidism   329
    Hypoparathyroidism   334
Section Three   Disorders of the Adrenal Glands   336
**Ellen L. Hellman**
    Addison's disease   337
    Cushing's disease   340

Section Four    Disorders of the Pituitary Gland   342
**Marianne S. Baird**
  Diabetes insipidus   343
  Pituitary and hypothalamic tumors   347
  Syndrome of inappropriate antidiuretic hormone   351
Section Five   Diabetes Mellitus   353
**Marianne S. Baird**
  General discussion   353
  Diabetic ketoacidosis   363
  Hyperosmolar hyperglycemic nonketotic syndrome   371
  Hypoglycemia   373
Selected Bibliography   376

# 6 GASTROINTESTINAL DISORDERS

Section One    Disorders of the Mouth and Esophagus   379
**Kathryn L. Schroeder**
  Stomatitis   379
  Hiatal hernia and reflux esophagitis   382
  Achalasia   386
Section Two    Disorders of the Stomach and Intestines   389
  Peptic ulcers   389
**Janet Hicks Keen**
  Malabsorption/Maldigestion   394
**Janet Hicks Keen**
  Obstructive processes   398
**Janet Hicks Keen**
  Hernia   402
**Janet Hicks Keen**
  Peritonitis   404
**Kathryn L. Schroeder**
  Appendicitis   407
**Kathryn L. Schroeder**
  Hemorrhoids   411
**Kathryn L. Schroeder**
Section Three    Intestinal Neoplasms and Inflammatory Processes   414
**Lolita Adrien**
  Diverticulosis/Diverticulitis   414
  Colorectal cancer   417
  Polyps/Familial adenomatous polyposis   420
  Ulcerative colitis   421
  Crohn's disease   428
  Fecal diversions   434
Section Four    Abdominal Trauma   439
**Janet Hicks Keen**
Section Five   Hepatic and Biliary Disorders   449
**Janet Hicks Keen**
  Hepatitis   450
  Cirrhosis   457
  Cholelithiasis and cholecystitis   465

Section Six   Pancreatic Disorders   470
**Janet Hicks Keen**
  Pancreatitis   470
  Pancreatic tumors   476
Selected Bibliography   479

# 7 HEMATOLOGIC DISORDERS

### Barbara Tueller Steuble

Section One   Disorders of the Red Blood Cells   483
  Iron deficiency anemia   483
  Pernicious anemia   485
  Hemolytic anemia   488
  Hypoplastic (aplastic) anemia   491
  Polycythemia   497
Section Two   Disorders of Coagulation   499
  Thrombocytopenia   500
  Hemophilia   502
  Disseminated intravascular coagulation   504
Section Three   Neoplastic Disorders of the Hematopoietic System   508
  Lymphomas   508
  Acute leukemia   510
  Chronic leukemia   513
Selected Bibliography   514

# 8 MUSCULOSKELETAL DISORDERS

### Dennis G. Ross

Section One   Inflammatory Disorders   517
  Osteoarthritis   518
  Gouty arthritis   522
  Rheumatoid arthritis   525
Section Two   Muscular and Connective Tissue Disorders   529
  Ligamentous injuries   529
  Dislocation/Subluxation   532
  Meniscal injuries   535
  Torn anterior cruciate ligament   536
  Ischemic myositis (compartment syndrome)   538
Section Three   Skeletal Disorders   542
  Osteomyelitis   542
  Fractures   546
  Benign neoplasms   553
  Malignant neoplasms   555
  Osteoporosis   557
  Paget's disease (osteitis deformans)   560
Section Four   Musculoskeletal Surgical Procedures   562
  Bunionectomy   562

Amputation   564
Tendon transfer   569
Bone grafting   570
Repair of recurrent shoulder dislocation   571
Total hip arthroplasty   573
Total knee arthroplasty   577
Selected Bibliography   579

# 9 REPRODUCTIVE DISORDERS

Section One   Surgeries and Disorders of the Breast   583
**Diane Wind Wardell**
Breast reduction   583
Breast reconstruction   585
Benign breast disorders and conditions   588
Malignant breast disorders   590
Section Two   Neoplasms of the Female Pelvis   596
**Diane Wind Wardell**
Cancer of the cervix   596
Ovarian tumors   600
Endometrial cancer   602
Vulvar cancer   603
Section Three   Disorders of the Female Pelvis   605
**Diane Wind Wardell**
Endometriosis   605
Cystocele   607
Rectocele   608
Uterine prolapse   609
Section Four   Interruption of Pregnancy   610
**Diane Wind Wardell**
Spontaneous abortion   610
Ectopic pregnancy   613
Section Five   Disorders and Surgeries of the Male Pelvis   615
**Patti E.R. Jansen**
Benign prostatic hypertrophy   615
Prostatic neoplasm   622
Testicular neoplasm   626
Penile implants   629
Selected Bibliography   631

# 10 SENSORY DISORDERS

**Barbara J. Deveau**

Section One   Disorders and Surgeries of the Eye   633
Corneal ulceration/Trauma   633
Keratoplasty (corneal transplant)   638
Vitreous disorders/Vitrectomy   639
Glaucoma   641

Retinal detachment 644
Enucleation 646
Section Two   Disorders and Surgeries of the Ear 648
Otosclerosis (Otospongiosis) 648
Cochlear implantation 650
Selected Bibliography 652

# 11 PROVIDING CARE FOR PATIENTS WITH SPECIAL NEEDS

Section One   Caring for Individuals with Human Immunodeficiency Virus
Disease 653
**Kenneth Miller**
Section Two   Providing Nutritional Support 665
**Karen S. Webber**
Nutritional assessment 665
Nutritional support modalities 669
Section Three   Managing Wound Care 681
**Nancy A. Stotts**
Wounds closed by primary intention 681
Surgical or traumatic wounds healing by secondary intention 683
Pressure ulcers 686
Selected Bibliography 689

## APPENDICES

Appendix One   Patient Care 693
Section One   Caring for preoperative and postoperative patients 693
**Janet Hicks Keen**
Section Two   Caring for patients on prolonged bed rest 711
**Linda S. Baas and Dennis G. Ross**
Section Three   Caring for patients with cancer and other life-disrupting
illnesses 719
**Mary E. Cooley and Patricia Hall**
Section Four   Caring for older adults 767
**Patti E.R. Jansen**
Appendix Two   Infection Prevention and Control 777
**Marguerite M. Jackson**
Appendix Three   Heart and Breath Sounds 783
**Pamela L. Swearingen**
Appendix Four   Laboratory Tests Discussed in This Manual: Normal
Values 791
Appendix Five   Abbreviations Used in This Manual 795

MANUAL OF
# MEDICAL-SURGICAL NURSING CARE
## Nursing Interventions and Collaborative Management

# 1 RESPIRATORY DISORDERS

Section One   Acute Respiratory Disorders   1
   Atelectasis   1
   Pneumonia   3
   Pleural effusion   12
   Pulmonary embolus   13
   Pneumothorax/Hemothorax   19
   Pulmonary tuberculosis   24
Section Two   Acute Respiratory Failure   25
Section Three   Chronic Obstructive Pulmonary Disease   28
   Asthma   28
   Chronic bronchitis   32
   Emphysema   35
Section Four   Restrictive Pulmonary Disorders   37
   Pulmonary fibrosis   37
Section Five   Bronchogenic Carcinoma   39
Selected Bibliography   41

## Section One:   Acute Respiratory Disorders

Acute respiratory disorders are short-term diseases or acute complications of chronic conditions. They can occur once and respond to treatment or recur to further complicate an underlying disease process.

## Atelectasis

Atelectasis is a spontaneous collapse of alveolar lung tissue secondary to persistent hypoinflation. It is most commonly seen following major abdominal or thoracic surgery as a result of hypoventilation of dependent portions of the lungs or inadequate clearing of secretions. Atelectasis can be either an acute or chronic condition, and it occurs most frequently in individuals with chronic obstructive pulmonary disease (COPD). In the postoperative period atelectasis can be precipitated by the effects of anesthesia, sedation, and decreased mobility. Other precipitating factors include mucus plugs, foreign objects in the airways, pleural effusion, bronchogenic carcinoma, history of smoking, and obesity. Atelectasis can lead to pulmonary infection.

### ASSESSMENT
The clinical picture is determined by the site of collapse, rate of development, and size of the affected area.

1

**Signs and symptoms:**    Pleuritic chest pain, tachypnea, SOB, fever, dyspnea.
**Physical assessment:**    Decreased chest wall movement on affected side, dullness to percussion, decreased or absent breath sounds, crackles after deep inspiration or cough, restlessness, agitation, change in LOC, cyanosis.

## DIAGNOSTIC TESTS
**Chest x-ray:**    Reveals higher density in affected lung, elevation of the hemidiaphragm on affected side, and compensatory hyperinflation of adjacent lobes on the opposite side.
**ABG values:**    May reveal acute respiratory acidosis, with pH $<7.35$ and $Paco_2$ $>45$ mm Hg. $Pao_2$ may be $<80$ mm Hg, which is consistent with hypoxemia.

## COLLABORATIVE MANAGEMENT
Management is aimed at preventing this condition in all patients. If atelectasis occurs and is left untreated, the affected lung area may become infected, fibrotic, and functionless.
**Deep breathing and coughing exercises:**    To expand alveoli deep in the lungs and mobilize/clear secretions.
**Chest physiotherapy:**    To mobilize secretions.
**Hyperinflation therapy:**    For example, incentive spirometry to expand partially collapsed lung areas, thereby improving gas exchange.
**Analgesics:**    To reduce pain, thereby facilitating production of an effective cough.
**Bronchoscopy:**    Procedure in which patient is intubated and a fiberoptic scope is passed into the bronchi to visualize the area and remove mucus plugs, retained secretions, or foreign objects.
**Oxygen therapy:**    To maintain $Pao_2$ $>80$ mm Hg or within patient's normal baseline range.

## NURSING DIAGNOSES AND INTERVENTIONS
*For patients with atelectasis*
**Impaired gas exchange** related to altered oxygen supply or alveolar hypoventilation secondary to ventilation/perfusion mismatch occurring as a result of alveolar collapse.
*Desired outcomes:*    Following intervention/treatment, patient has adequate gas exchange as evidenced by normal skin color and orientation to person, place, and time. At a minimum of 24 h before hospital discharge, patient's ABG results are normal: $Pao_2$ $\geq80$ mm Hg, pH 7.35-7.45, $Paco_2$ $<45$ mm Hg (or ABG results consistent with patient's baseline parameters).
- Auscultate breath sounds at least q2h. Report any decrease in breath sounds or an increase in adventitious breath sounds.
- Monitor patient for signs and symptoms of hypoxia: restlessness, agitation, changes in LOC, and cyanosis. Report significant changes to physician.
- Maintain a patent airway and ensure removal of secretions at least q2h; suction as indicated/prescribed.
- Position patient for comfort and to promote optimal gas exchange (usually semi-Fowler's position).
- Monitor serial ABG values. Be alert to decreasing $Pao_2$ or increasing $Paco_2$, both of which can signal impending respiratory failure.

*For patients at risk for atelectasis*
**Ineffective breathing pattern** related to decreased lung expansion secondary to inactivity or omission of deep breathing.
*Desired outcome:*    Patient demonstrates deep breathing and effective coughing at least hourly and is eupneic (RR 12-20 breaths/min with normal depth and pattern) at all other times.

- Auscultate breath sounds at least q2h and during hyperinflation therapy. Report any decrease in breath sounds or presence of/increase in adventitious breath sounds.
- Instruct patient in the use of hyperinflation device. Ensure that patient inhales slowly and deeply 2× normal tidal volume and holds the breath at least 5 sec at the end of inspiration. Ten breaths per hour is recommended to maintain adequate alveolar inflation. Deep breathing expands the alveoli, while coughing mobilizes and clears the secretions. Monitor patient's progress and document in nurses' notes.
- Administer analgesics as prescribed to reduce pain, which may facilitate patient's ease with coughing and deep-breathing exercises.
- Encourage activity as prescribed to help mobilize secretions and promote effective airway clearance.

## PATIENT-FAMILY TEACHING AND DISCHARGE PLANNING

Give patient and significant others verbal and written instructions about the following:

- Use of hyperinflation device if patient is to continue this therapy at home. Conduct a predischarge check of patient's technique, and document assessment in the progress notes.
- Importance of maintaining activity level as prescribed to promote optimal lung expansion, mobilize secretions, and promote effective airway clearance.
- Medications, including name, purpose, dosage, schedule, precautions, and potential side effects.
- Precipitating factors in the development of atelectasis.
- Importance of notifying physician if signs and symptoms recur.
- Importance of medical follow-up. Review date and time of next appointment.

## Pneumonia

Pneumonia is an acute bacterial or viral infection that causes inflammation of the lung parenchyma (alveolar spaces and interstitial tissue). As a result of the inflammation the involved lung tissue becomes edematous and the air spaces fill with exudate (consolidation), gas exchange cannot occur, and nonoxygenated blood is shunted into the vascular system, causing hypoxemia. Bacterial pneumonias involve all or part of a lobe, whereas viral pneumonias appear diffusely throughout the lungs.

Pneumonias generally are classified into two groups: community-acquired and hospital-associated (nosocomial). A third type that occurs is pneumonia in the immunocompromised individual.

**Community-acquired:**  Individuals with this type of pneumonia generally do not require hospitalization unless an underlying medical condition, such as chronic obstructive pulmonary disease (COPD), cardiac disease, diabetes mellitus, or an immunocompromised state, complicates the illness.

**Hospital-associated (nosocomial):**  These pneumonias usually occur following aspiration of oropharyngeal flora in an individual whose resistance is altered or whose coughing mechanisms are impaired (e.g., a patient who has decreased LOC, dysphagia, diminished gag reflex, presence of gastric tube, or who has undergone thoracoabdominal surgery). Bacteria invade the lower respiratory tract *via* three routes: aspiration of oropharyngeal organisms (most common route), inhalation of aerosols that contain bacteria, or hematogenous spread to the lung from another site of infection (rare). Gram-negative pneumonias have a high mortality rate, even with appropriate antibiotic therapy. *Aspiration pneumonia* is a nonbacterial cause of hospital-associated pneumo-

*Text continued on p. 8.*

**TABLE 1-1  Assessment Guidelines by Pneumonia Type**

| Type/pathogen | Onset | Risk groups | Defining characteristics | Complications/comments |
|---|---|---|---|---|
| *Community-acquired* | | | | |
| Pneumococcal (*Pneumococcus pneumoniae, Streptococcus pneumoniae*) | Abrupt | Persons >40 yr, especially males; risk increased with alcoholism and debilitating diseases (e.g., COPD, CHF, multiple myeloma, sickle cell disease); often preceded by viral upper respiratory tract infections | Single shaking chill, fever, pleuritic chest pain, severe cough, SOB, rust-colored sputum, and diaphoresis. Many patients also have herpes labialis, abdominal pain and distention, and paralytic ileus | Pleural effusions, empyema, impaired liver function, bacteremia, and meningitis. Incidence of pneumococcal pneumonia peaks in winter and early spring. Mortality rate increases if more than one lobe is involved |
| Mycoplasma (*Mycoplasma pneumoniae*) | Gradual | School-aged children to young adult (5-30 yr); intrafamilial spread common | Cough, sore throat, fever, headache, chills, malaise, anorexia, nausea, vomiting, diarrhea. In children arthralgias involving the large joints are common | Rare. Persistent cough and sinusitis are possible. Pulse-temperature dissociation is common |
| Legionnaires' (*Legionella pneumophila*) | Abrupt | Middle-aged, elderly (males at increased risk) populations; smokers; individuals with malignancy, immunosuppression, or chronic renal failure; exposure to contaminated construction site | Malaise, headache within 24 hr, fever with normal HR, shaking chills, progressive dyspnea, cough that may become productive; GI symptoms, including anorexia, vomiting, diarrhea; arthralgias, myalgias | Respiratory failure, hypotension, shock, acute renal failure |

| | | | | |
|---|---|---|---|---|
| Viral influenza A | Elderly persons with chronic diseases (e.g., COPD, diabetes mellitus, CHF); pregnancy | 1 wk after onset of influenza symptoms | Severe dyspnea, cyanosis, scant sputum occasionally with blood, fever, persistent and dry cough | Rapid course leading frequently to acute respiratory failure; secondary bacterial pneumonia |
| *Haemophilus influenzae* | Adults (especially ≥50 yr of age) with chronic diseases (e.g., diabetes mellitus, COPD, chronic alcohol ingestion) | 2-6 wk after URI | Fever, chills, dyspnea, cough, nausea, vomiting, pain | Fever may be minimal or absent; HR and RR may be normal |
| ***Nosocomial*** | | | | |
| Klebsiella (*Klebsiella pneumoniae*); also may be acquired in the community | Males >40 yr, alcoholics; patients with diabetes mellitus, COPD, or heart disease; those previously treated with antibiotics or ET intubation | Abrupt | Chills, fever, productive cough (copious purulent green or "currant jelly" sputum), severe pleuritic chest pain, dyspnea, cyanosis, jaundice, vomiting, and diarrhea | Lung abscess and empyema, necrotizing pneumonitis with cavitation, acute respiratory failure. High mortality rate (~50%). Aspiration of oropharyngeal flora is responsible for nosocomial and community-acquired cases |
| *Pseudomonas* (also may be acquired in the community) | Patients neutropenic from chemotherapy or immunosuppressed secondary to cortisone therapy or other illnesses | Gradual | Fever, chills, confusion, delirium, bradycardia, purulent sputum (green, foul-smelling) | Rarely occurs in previously healthy adults; high mortality rate |

*Continued.*

CHF = congestive heart failure; URI = upper respiratory infection; ET = endotracheal; NG = nasogastric; AIDS = acquired immunodeficiency syndrome.

**T A B L E   1 - 1   Assessment Guidelines by Pneumonia Type—cont'd.**

| Type/pathogen | Risk groups | Onset | Defining characteristics | Complications/comments |
|---|---|---|---|---|
| **Nosocomial—cont'd** | | | | |
| *Proteus* | Older adults with debilitating underlying diseases | Abrupt | High fever, chills, pleuritic chest pain | Rare. Localizes to areas that are already damaged. Occurs as a mixed infection; has four pathogenic species with differing antibiotic susceptibilities |
| *Staphylococcus aureus* | Patients with debilitating diseases (e.g., diabetes mellitus, renal failure, liver disease, COPD); those with a prior viral or influenza infection; injecting drug users | Abrupt with community-acquired; insidious with hospital-associated | Cough, chills, high fever, pleuritic pain, progressive dyspnea, cyanosis, bloody sputum | Pulmonary abscesses, empyema, pleural effusions; slow response to antibiotics |
| Aspiration of gastric contents | Patients with impaired gag/cough reflexes; general anesthesia; presence of NG/ET tube | Gradual: latent period between aspiration and onset of symptoms | Fever, wheezes, crackles (rales), rhonchi, dyspnea, cyanosis | Physiologic response depends on pH of material aspirated: $\geq 2.5$, little necrosis occurs; $<2.5$, atelectasis, pulmonary edema, hemorrhage, and necrosis can occur |

NOTE: *Enterobacter* and *Serratia* are enteric organisms that cause pneumonia with the same clinical pattern as *Klebsiella* organisms.

**Immunocompromised patient**

| | | | | |
|---|---|---|---|---|
| Pneumocystis (*Pneumocystis carinii*) | Patients with AIDS or organ transplants | Insidious | Several weeks of fever, nonproductive cough, night sweats, dyspnea; hypoxemia with few auscultatory signs | Bronchoscopy with transbronchial biopsy usually required for diagnosis |
| Aspergillosis (*Aspergillus*) | Patients with AIDS, COPD, and transplants (especially autologous bone marrow transplant); also those receiving cytotoxic agents or steroids | Abrupt with immunosuppression; insidious with COPD | High fever; fungal ball within lung cyst or cavity; nonproductive cough; pleuritic chest pain | Cavitation frequently occurs; hematogenous spread common in immunocompromised patient |

CHF = congestive heart failure; URI = upper respiratory infection; ET = endotracheal; NG = nasogastric; AIDS = acquired immunodeficiency syndrome.

nia that occurs when gastric contents are aspirated. If the alveolar-capillary membrane is affected, adult respiratory distress syndrome (ARDS) may be seen.

**Pneumonia in the immunocompromised individual:**  Immunosuppression and neutropenia are predisposing factors in the development of nosocomial pneumonias, from both common and unusual pathogens. Severely immunocompromised patients are affected not only by bacteria but also by fungi *(Candida, Aspergillus)*, viruses (cytomegalovirus), and protozoa *(Pneumocystis carinii)*. Most commonly, *P. carinii* is seen in persons with HIV disease or in those who are immunosuppressed therapeutically following organ transplants.

## ASSESSMENT

Findings are influenced by the patient's age, extent of the disease process, underlying medical condition, and pathogen involved. Generally, any factor that alters the integrity of the lower airways, thereby inhibiting ciliary activity, increases the likelihood of developing pneumonia (Table 1-1).

**General signs and symptoms:**  Cough (productive and nonproductive); increased sputum (rust-colored, purulent, bloody, or mucoid) production; fever; pleuritic chest pain (more common in community-acquired bacterial pneumonias); dyspnea; chills; headache; myalgia. Elders may be confused or disoriented and run low-grade fevers but may present with few other signs and symptoms.

**General physical assessment findings:**  Restlessness; anxiety; decreased skin turgor and dry mucous membranes secondary to dehydration; presence of nasal flaring and expiratory grunt; use of accessory muscles of respiration (scalene, sternocleidomastoid, external intercostals); decreased chest expansion caused by pleuritic pain; dullness on percussion over affected (consolidated) areas; tachypnea (RR >20 breaths/min); tachycardia (HR >100 bpm); increased vocal fremitus; egophony ("e to a" change) over area of consolidation; decreased breath sounds; high-pitched and inspiratory crackles (increased by or heard only after coughing); low-pitched inspiratory crackles caused by airway secretions; and circumoral cyanosis (a late finding). **Note:** Findings may be normal, even with an abnormal chest x-ray.

## DIAGNOSTIC TESTS

**Chest x-ray:**  Confirms the presence of pneumonia (i.e., vague haziness to consolidation in the affected lung fields).

**Sputum for gram stain and culture and sensitivity tests:**  Sputum is obtained from the lower respiratory tract before initiation of antibiotic therapy in order to identify the causative organism. It can be obtained *via* expectoration, suctioning, transtracheal aspiration, bronchoscopy, or open-lung biopsy.

**WBC:**  Will be increased (>11,000/$\mu$l) in the presence of bacterial pneumonias. Normal or low WBC count may be seen with viral or mycoplasma pneumonias.

**Blood culture and sensitivity:**  To determine presence of bacteremia and aid in the identification of the causative organism.

**ABG values:**  May vary, depending on the presence of underlying pulmonary or other debilitating disease. Hypoxemia ($Pao_2$ <80 mm Hg) and hypocarbia ($Paco_2$ <35 mm Hg), with a resultant respiratory alkalosis (pH >7.45), will be seen in the absence of an underlying pulmonary disease.

**Serologic studies:**  Acute and convalescent titers are drawn to diagnose viral pneumonia. A relative rise in antibody titers is suggestive of a viral infection.

**Acid-fast stains and cultures:**  To rule out tuberculosis.

## COLLABORATIVE MANAGEMENT

**Oxygen therapy:** Administered when ABG results demonstrate presence of hypoxemia. Special consideration must be given to patients with chronic $CO_2$ retention. (Normally, the respiratory drive is stimulated by the presence of increasing $Paco_2$ levels. In patients with $CO_2$ retention the respiratory drive is paradoxically stimulated by decreasing $Pao_2$ levels. Therefore, in the presence of high concentrations of oxygen, the respiratory drive actually may be depressed in these patients.) Initially, oxygen is delivered in low concentrations, and ABG levels are watched closely. If $Pao_2$ does not rise to acceptable levels ($\geq 60$ mm Hg), $FIO_2$ is increased in small increments, with concomitant checks of ABG values.

**Antibiotic agents:** Prescribed empirically based on presenting signs and symptoms, clinical findings, and chest x-ray results until sputum or blood culture results are available. Erythromycin is the most commonly used antibiotic in community-acquired pneumonia. Many of the organisms responsible for nosocomial pneumonias are resistant to multiple antibiotics. Proper identification of the organism and determination of sensitivity to specific antibiotics are critical for appropriate therapy.

**Hydration:** IV fluids may be necessary to replace fluids lost from insensible sources (e.g., tachypnea, diaphoresis, fevers) and decreased oral intake.

**Percussion and postural drainage:** Indicated if deep breathing and coughing are ineffective in mobilizing secretions.

**Hyperinflation therapy:** Prescribed for patients with inadequate inspiratory effort.

**Antitussives:** Given in the absence of sputum production if coughing is continuous and exhausting to the patient.

**Antipyretics and analgesics:** Prescribed to reduce fever and provide relief from pleuritic pain or pain from coughing.

**Body substance isolation:** See discussion in Appendix Two, p. 777.

## NURSING DIAGNOSES AND INTERVENTIONS

*For patients with pneumonia*

**Impaired gas exchange** related to altered oxygen supply and alveolar-capillary membrane changes secondary to inflammatory process in the lungs

*Desired outcomes:* Following intervention/treatment, patient has adequate gas exchange as evidenced by RR 12-20 breaths/min with normal depth and pattern and absence of signs and symptoms of respiratory distress. At a minimum of 24 h before hospital discharge patient's $Pao_2$ is $\geq 80$ mm Hg, $Paco_2$ is 35-45 mm Hg, and pH is 7.35-7.45 (or values consistent with patient's baseline).

- Observe for signs and symptoms of respiratory distress (e.g., restlessness, anxiety, SOB, tachypnea, use of accessory muscles of respiration). Remember that cyanosis of the lips and nailbeds may be a late indicator of hypoxia.
- Monitor and document VS q2-4h. Be alert to a rising temperature and other changes in VS that may be indicative of infection (e.g., increased HR, increased RR).
- Auscultate breath sounds at least q2h. Monitor for decreased or adventitious sounds (e.g., crackles or wheezes).
- Monitor ABG results. A decreasing $Pao_2$ often is indicative of the need for oxygen therapy.
- Position patient for comfort (usually semi-Fowler's position) to promote diaphragmatic descent, maximize inhalation, and decrease WOB. In patients with unilateral pneumonia, positioning on the unaffected side (i.e., "good side down") will promote ventilation-perfusion matching.
- Deliver oxygen as prescribed; monitor $FIO_2$ to ensure that oxygen is within prescribed concentrations. Be aware that patients with COPD may not tol-

erate oxygen at a delivery of >2 L/min, which can suppress the centrally mediated respiratory drive.

• Provide periods of rest between care activities to decrease oxygen demand.

**Ineffective airway clearance** related to presence of tracheobronchial secretions secondary to infection or related to pain and fatigue secondary to lung consolidation

*Desired outcomes:*  Patient demonstrates effective cough. Following intervention, patient's airway is free of adventitious breath sounds.

• Maintain a patent airway and ensure that secretions are removed at least q2h. Suction as indicated/prescribed. Auscultate breath sounds q2–4h, and report changes in the patient's ability to clear pulmonary secretions.

• Inspect sputum for quantity, color, and consistency; document findings. As patient's condition worsens, the sputum can change in color from clear→white→yellow→green.

• Ensure that patient performs deep breathing with coughing exercises at least q2h. Assist patient into position of comfort, usually semi-Fowler's position, to facilitate effectiveness and ease of these exercises.

• Assess need for hyperinflation therapy (i.e., patient's inability to take deep breaths). Report complications of hyperinflation therapy to physician, including hyperventilation, gastric distention, headache, hypotension, and signs and symptoms of pneumothorax (SOB, sharp chest pain, dyspnea, cough).

• Teach patient to splint chest with pillow or crossed arms when coughing to reduce pain.

• Ensure that patient gets prescribed chest physiotherapy. Document patient's response to treatment.

• Assist patient with position changes q2h to help mobilize secretions. If the patient is ambulatory, encourage ambulation to patient's tolerance.

• Suction as prescribed and indicated.

**Fluid volume deficit** related to increased insensible loss secondary to tachypnea, fever, or diaphoresis

*Desired outcome:*  At a minimum of 24 h before hospital discharge, patient is normovolemic as evidenced by urine output ≥30 ml/h with specific gravity 1.010-1.030, stable weight, HR and BP within patient's normal limits, CVP >2 mm Hg (5 cm $H_2O$), moist mucous membranes, and normal skin turgor.

• Monitor I&O. Consider insensible losses if patient is diaphoretic and tachypneic. Be alert to urinary output <30 ml/h.

• Weigh patient daily, at the same time of day and on the same scale; record weight. Report weight decreases of 1-1.5 kg/day.

• Encourage fluid intake (at least 2-3 L/day in the unrestricted patient) to ensure adequate hydration.

• Maintain IV fluid therapy as prescribed.

• Promote oral hygiene, including lip and tongue care to moisten dried tissues and mucous membranes.

**Altered nutrition:**  Less than body requirements related to anorexia

*Desired outcome:*  At a minimum of 24 h before hospital discharge patient has adequate nutrition as evidenced by stable weight, balanced or positive N state per N studies, and serum albumin 3.5-5.5 g/dl.

• Provide small, frequent feedings of nutritious foods that are easy to consume. Monitor and record amount of nutrients consumed.

• Request dietitian consultation so that patient can verbalize food likes and dislikes.

• Request that physician prescribe dietary supplements if patient is unable to consume adequate diet.

• Discuss with patient and significant others the importance of good nutrition in the treatment of pneumonia.

• For other interventions, see "Providing Nutritional Support," p. 665.

*For patients at risk for developing pneumonia*

**High risk for infection** (nosocomial pneumonia) related to inadequate primary defenses (e.g., decreased ciliary action), invasive procedures (e.g., intubation), and/or chronic disease

***Desired outcome:*** Patient is free of infection as evidenced by normothermia, WBC count ≤11,000 μl, and sputum clear to whitish in color.

- Perform good handwashing technique before and after contact with patient (even though gloves were worn).
- Identify presurgical candidate who is at increased risk for nosocomial pneumonia because of the following: older adult (>70 years), obesity, COPD, history of smoking, abnormal pulmonary function tests (especially decreased forced expiratory flow rate), intubation, and upper abdominal/thoracic surgery.
- Provide preoperative teaching, explaining and demonstrating the following pulmonary exercises that will be used postoperatively to prevent respiratory infection: deep breathing, coughing, turning in bed, ambulation, and use of hyperinflation device. Make sure that patient verbalizes knowledge of the exercises and their rationale and *returns* the demonstrations appropriately. Encourage individuals who smoke to discontinue smoking, especially during preoperative and postoperative periods.
- Control pain, which interferes with lung expansion, by administering analgesics one-half hour before deep-breathing exercises. Support (splint) surgical wound with hands or pillows placed firmly across site of incision.
- Identify patients who are at increased risk for aspiration: individuals with a depressed LOC, dysphagia, or a nasogastric (NG) tube in place. Maintain HOB at 30-degree elevation, and turn patient onto side rather than back. When patient receives enteral alimentation, recommend continuous rather than bolus feedings.
- Recognize risk factors for patients with tracheostomy: presence of underlying lung disease or other serious illness, increased colonization of oropharynx or trachea by aerobic gram-negative bacteria, greater access of bacteria to lower respiratory tract, and cross-contamination due to manipulation of tracheostomy tube.
- Use "no-touch" technique or wear sterile gloves on both hands until tracheostomy wound has healed or formed granulation tissue around the tube.
- Suction on an as-needed rather than routine basis, because frequent suctioning increases risk of trauma and cross-contamination.
- Use sterile catheter for each suctioning procedure, and sterile solutions if secretions are tenacious and catheter flushing is necessary. Consider use of closed suction system to further minimize the risk of contamination.
- Always wear gloves on both hands to suction.
- Recognize the following ways in which nebulizer reservoirs can contaminate patient: introduction of nonsterile fluids or air, manipulation of nebulizer cup, or backflow of condensate from delivery tubing into reservoir or into patient when tubing is manipulated.
- Use only sterile fluids and dispense them aseptically.
- Replace (rather than replenish) solutions and equipment at frequent intervals. For example, empty reservoir completely and refill with sterile solution q8-24h, according to agency protocol.
- Change breathing circuits q48h or according to agency policy; if used for multiple patients, replace breathing circuit with sterilized or disinfected breathing circuit between patients.
- Fill fluid reservoirs immediately before use (not far in advance).
- Discard any fluid that has condensed in tubing; do not allow it to drain back into reservoir or into patient.

## PATIENT-FAMILY TEACHING AND DISCHARGE PLANNING

Give patient and significant others verbal and written information about the following:

- Techniques that promote gas exchange and minimize stasis of secretions (e.g., deep breathing, coughing, use of incentive spirometry, increasing activity level as appropriate for patient's medical condition, and percussion and postural drainage as necessary).
- Medications, including drug name, purpose, dosage, frequency, precautions, and potential side effects, particularly of antibiotics (see p. 544).
- Signs and symptoms of pneumonia and the importance of reporting them promptly to health professional should they recur. Teach patient's significant others that changes in sensorium may be the only indicator of pneumonia if patient is elderly.
- Importance of preventing fatigue by pacing activities and allowing for frequent rest periods.
- Importance of avoiding exposure to individuals known to have flu and colds. Recommend that patient get annual flu and pneumococcal vaccines.
- Minimizing factors that can cause reinfection, including close living conditions, poor nutrition, and poorly ventilated living quarters or work environment.

# Pleural effusion

A pleural effusion is an accumulation of fluid (blood, pus, chyle, serous fluid) in the pleural space. Generally, fluid gravitates to the most dependent area of the thorax, and the adjacent lung becomes compressed. Pleural effusion is rarely a disease in itself, but rather it is caused by a number of inflammatory, circulatory, or neoplastic diseases. *Transudate effusion* results from changes in hydrodynamic forces in the circulation and usually is caused by congestive heart failure or cirrhosis. *Exudate effusion* results from irritation of the pleural membranes secondary to inflammatory, infective, or malignant processes.

## ASSESSMENT

Clinical indicators of pleural effusion are related to the underlying disease. Dyspnea is present when there is a large effusion. With a small effusion the patient may be asymptomatic.

**Signs and symptoms:**   Pleuritic chest pain, diaphoresis, cough, fever.

**Physical assessment:**   Decreased breath sounds, dullness to percussion, decreased tactile fremitus, egophony ("e" to "a" change) above the infusion site, tracheal deviation away from affected side, pleural friction rub.

## DIAGNOSTIC TESTS

**Chest x-ray:**   Will show evidence of effusion if there is >300 ml of fluid in the pleural space. The costophrenic angle will be obliterated, and opacification of the hemithorax, as evidenced by shadiness on the x-ray, increases as the effusion increases. With a large effusion the x-ray may show mediastinal shift away from the affected lung.

**Thoracentesis:**   Removal of fluid from the pleural space for examination to provide the definitive diagnosis and determine type of effusion.

**Pleural biopsy:**   Aids in diagnosing cause of effusion. Tissue is removed *via* biopsy needle and sent to pathologist for examination.

## COLLABORATIVE MANAGEMENT

**Therapeutic thoracentesis:**   Removal of fluid, thereby allowing the lung to reexpand. The rate of recurrence and time span for return of symptoms is recorded.

**Chest tube insertion:** To provide continuous drainage of larger effusions through a 26-30 Fr catheter that is connected to a closed chest-drainage system.

**Sclerosing pleurodesis:** Instillation of sclerosing agent (tetracycline, bleomycin, or nitrogen mustard) *via* the chest tube to produce pleural fibrosis and symphysis (a line of fusion below the pleura and chest wall).

## NURSING DIAGNOSES AND INTERVENTIONS

**Ineffective breathing pattern** related to decreased lung expansion secondary to fluid accumulation in the pleural space

*Desired outcome:* Following intervention, patient's breathing pattern moves toward eupnea.

- Auscultate breath sounds q2-3h, monitoring for decreasing breath sounds or the presence of a pleural friction rub.
- Ensure patency of chest drainage system (see guidelines, p. 22, in "Pneumothorax/Hemothorax").
- Position patient for maximum chest expansion, generally semi-Fowler's position.
- If hyperinflation therapy is prescribed, instruct patient in its use. Reinforce teaching, and document patient's progress.
- For patients with gross pleural effusion, provide the following instructions for apical expansion breathing exercises:
  - Sit upright.
  - Position fingers just below the clavicles.
  - Inhale and attempt to push upper chest wall against the pressure of the fingers.
  - Hold breath for a few seconds, and then exhale passively.

When performed at frequent intervals, this exercise will help expand the involved lung tissues, minimize flattening of the upper chest, and mobilize secretions.

---

**Note:** Also see "Pneumonia" for **Impaired gas exchange,** p. 9, and **Altered nutrition** p. 10. See "Pneumothorax/Hemothorax" for **Pain,** p. 23.

---

## PATIENT-FAMILY TEACHING AND DISCHARGE PLANNING

Give patient and significant others verbal and written instructions about the following:

- Importance of smoking cessation. Provide patient with resources related to smoking cessation programs.
- Signs of respiratory distress, such as restlessness, agitation, changes in behavior, and complaints of SOB or dyspnea, and the importance of notifying physician if these signs occur.
- Use of equipment at home (e.g., hyperinflation device, nebulizer, oxygen).
- Medications, including drug name, dosage, purpose, schedule, precautions, and potential side effects.

# Pulmonary embolus

The most common pulmonary perfusion abnormality, a pulmonary embolus (PE) is caused by the passage of a foreign substance (blood clot, fat, air, or amniotic fluid) into the pulmonary artery or its branches, with resulting obstruction of the blood supply to lung tissue and subsequent collapse. The most common source is a dislodged blood clot from the systemic circulation, typically the deep veins of the legs or pelvis. Thrombus formation is the result of the following factors: blood stasis, alterations in clotting factors, and injury to vessel walls. A fat embolus is the most common nonthrombotic cause of pulmonary perfusion disorders. It is the result of the release of free fatty acids, causing a toxic vasculitis, followed by thrombosis and obstruction of small pulmonary arteries by fat.

Total obstruction leading to pulmonary infarction is rare because the pulmonary circulation has multiple sources of blood supply. Early diagnosis and appropriate treatment reduce mortality to under 10%. Although most pulmonary emboli resolve completely and leave no residual deficits, some patients may be left with chronic pulmonary hypertension.

## ASSESSMENT

Signs and symptoms often are nonspecific and variable, depending on the extent of the obstruction and whether or not the patient has infarction as a result of the obstruction.

**Pulmonary embolus:**   Sudden onset of dyspnea and sharp chest pain, restlessness, anxiety, nonproductive cough, palpitations, nausea, and syncope. With a large embolism, oppressive substernal chest discomfort will be present.

**Pulmonary infarction:**   Fever, pleuritic chest pain, and hemoptysis.

**Physical assessment:**   Tachypnea, tachycardia, hypotension, crackles (rales), decreased chest wall excursion secondary to splinting, $S_3$ and $S_4$ gallop rhythms, transient friction rub, jugular venous distention, diaphoresis, edema, and cyanosis. Temperature may be elevated if infarction has occurred.

**History and risk factors**

*Prolonged immobility:*   Especially significant when it coexists with surgical or nonsurgical trauma, carcinoma, or cardiopulmonary disease. Risk increases as duration of immobility increases.

*Cardiac disorders:*   Atrial fibrillation, congestive heart failure, myocardial infarction, rheumatic heart disease.

*Surgical intervention:*   Risk increases in postoperative period, especially for patients with pelvic, thoracic, and abdominal surgery, and for those with extensive burns or musculoskeletal injuries of the hip or knee.

*Pregnancy:*   Especially during the postpartum period.

*Chronic pulmonary disease.*

*Trauma:*   Especially fractures of the lower extremities and burns. The degree of risk is related to the severity, site, and extent of trauma.

*Carcinoma:*   Particularly neoplasms involving the breast, lung, pancreas, and genitourinary and alimentary tracts.

*Obesity:*   A 20% increase in ideal body weight is associated with an increased incidence of PE.

*Varicose veins or prior thromboembolic disease.*

*Age:*   Risk of thromboembolism is greatest between patients 55 and 65 years of age.

**Specific findings for fat embolus:**   Typically, patient is asymptomatic for a period lasting 12-24 h following embolization; this period ends with sudden cardiopulmonary and neurologic deterioration: restlessness, confusion, delirium, coma, and dyspnea.

**Physical assessment for fat embolus:**   Tachypnea, tachycardia, and hypertension; fever, petechiae, especially of the upper torso and axillae; inspiratory crowing; and expiratory wheezes.

**History and risk factors for fat embolus**

*Multiple long bone fractures:*   Especially fractures of the femur and pelvis.

*Trauma to adipose tissue or liver.*

*Burns.*

*Osteomyelitis.*

*Sickle cell crisis.*

## DIAGNOSTIC TESTS
### General findings for pulmonary emboli
**ABG values:**   Hypoxemia ($Pao_2$ <80 mm Hg), hypocarbia ($Paco_2$ <35 mm Hg), and respiratory alkalosis (pH >7.45) usually are present. A normal $Pao_2$ does not rule out the presence of pulmonary emboli.

**Chest x-ray:**   Initially, the chest x-ray is normal, or an elevated hemidiaphragm may be present. After 24 h the x-ray may reveal small infiltrates secondary to atelectasis that results from the decrease in surfactant. If pulmonary infarction is present, infiltrates and pleural effusions may be seen within 12-36 h.

**ECG:**   If PEs are extensive, signs of acute pulmonary hypertension may be present: right-shift QRS axes, tall and peaked P waves, ST-segment changes, and T-wave inversion in leads $V_1$-$V_4$.

**Pulmonary ventilation-perfusion scan:**   Used to detect presence of abnormalities of ventilation or perfusion in the pulmonary system. Radiopaque agents are inhaled and injected peripherally. Images of both agents' distribution throughout the lung are scanned. If the scan shows a mismatch of ventilation and perfusion (i.e., a pattern of normal ventilation with decreased perfusion), vascular obstruction is suggested.

**Pulmonary angiography:**   The definitive study for PE. It is an invasive procedure that involves right heart catheterization and injection of dye into the pulmonary artery (PA) to visualize pulmonary vessels. An abrupt vessel "cutoff" may be seen at the site of embolization. Usually, filling defects are seen. More specific findings are abnormal blood vessel diameters (i.e., obstruction of right pulmonary artery would cause dilatation of left pulmonary artery) and shapes (i.e., the affected blood vessel may taper to a sharp point and disappear).

### Findings specific for fat emboli
**ABG values:**   Hypoxemia ($Pao_2$ <80 mm Hg) and hypercarbia ($Paco_2$ >45 mm Hg) will be present with a respiratory acidosis (pH <7.35).

**Chest x-ray:**   A pattern similar to adult respiratory distress syndrome is seen: diffuse, extensive bilateral interstitial and alveolar infiltrates.

**CBC:**   May reveal decreased hemoglobin (Hgb) and hematocrit (Hct) secondary to hemorrhage into the lung, in addition to thrombocytopenia.

## COLLABORATIVE MANAGEMENT
The three goals of therapy are as follows: (1) prophylaxis for individuals at risk for development of PE; (2) treatment during the acute embolic event; and (3) prevention of future embolic events in the individual who has experienced a PE.

### General management of pulmonary emboli
**Oxygen therapy:**   Delivered at appropriate concentration to maintain a $Pao_2$ of >60 mm Hg.

**IV heparin therapy:**   Treatment of choice; it is started immediately in patients without bleeding or clotting disorders and in whom PEs are strongly suspected.

*Initial dose:*   IV bolus of 5,000-10,000 U.

*Maintenance dose:*   From 2-4 h after initial dose, either a continuous infusion of 1,000 U/h or 5,000-7,500 U IV q4h.

*Goals of therapy:*   To inhibit thrombus growth, promote resolution of the formed thrombus, and prevent further embolus formation. These goals are achieved by keeping partial thromboplastin time (PTT) at 1.5-2.5 × the normal. This test should be done just before each bolus and q4–6h thereafter.

*Protamine sulfate:*   Heparin antidote, which should be readily available during heparin therapy. Fatal hemorrhage occurs in 1%-2% of patients undergoing heparin therapy. Risk of bleeding is greatest in women who are >60 years of age.

**Oral anticoagulants (warfarin sodium):**   Started 48-72 h after initiation of heparin therapy. The two are given simultaneously for 6–7 days to allow time for warfarin to inhibit vitamin K–dependent clotting factors before heparin is discontinued.

***Prothrombin time (PT):***   Monitored daily, with the goal of $1.25-1.50 \times$ normal. Once the patient has stabilized and the heparin is discontinued, weekly monitoring of PT is acceptable. After hospital discharge, the PT should be monitored q2weeks for as long as the patient continues to take oral anticoagulants.

***Maintenance:***   Usually 10 mg/day continued for 3–6 months, based on the continued presence of risk factors. Certain tumors (e.g., Trousseau syndrome) necessitate lifetime therapy.

***Vitamin K:***   Reverses the effects of warfarin in 24–36 h. Fresh frozen plasma may be required in cases of serious bleeding.

---

**Caution:**   Warfarin crosses the placental barrier and can cause spontaneous abortion and birth defects.

---

**Thrombolytic therapy (i.e., streptokinase and urokinase):**   May be given in the first 24–72 h after PE to speed the process of clot lysis *via* conversion of plasminogen to plasma. After the first 24–72 h of thrombolytic therapy, heparin therapy is initiated. Thrombolytic therapy may be preferred for initial treatment of PE in patients with hemodynamic compromise, >30% occlusion of pulmonary vasculature, and in whom therapy has been initiated no later than 3 days after onset of PE.

***Streptokinase:***   Loading dose of 250,000 IU in normal saline or 5% dextrose in water ($D_5W$) given IV over a 30-min period. Maintenance dose is 100,000 IU/h given IV for 24–72 h.

***Urokinase:***   Loading dose of 4,400 IU/kg of body weight in 5 ml of solution given IV over a 10-min period. Maintenance dose is 4,400 IU/kg/h for 12 h.

***Thrombin time:***   Monitors therapy for both drugs. The test is repeated q4h during therapy to ensure adequate response, which should be between 2 and $5 \times$ normal. PTT can be used instead of thrombin time and should be $2-5 \times$ control. Once thrombolytic therapy is stopped, thrombin time or PTT should be checked frequently until values fall below $2 \times$ normal. When the values are below $2 \times$ normal, heparin is started and continued as described under IV heparin therapy, above.

***Contraindications:***   Active internal bleeding, cerebrovascular accident, or intracranial bleeding within 2 months of PE. Other contraindications include trauma or surgery within 15 days of PE, diastolic hypertension >100 mm Hg, recent cardiopulmonary resuscitation, pregnancy, and <10 days postpartum.

---

**Note:**   Up to 33% of patients receiving thrombolytic therapy have hemorrhagic complications. Discontinuing the drug and administering fresh frozen plasma are the appropriate treatments.

---

**Surgical interventions:**   Used only in select cases owing to the success rate of anticoagulant therapy.

***Vena caval interruption/ligation:***   Multiple methods that share the common purpose of interrupting passage of venous thrombi through the inferior vena cava.

***Pulmonary embolectomy:***   To remove clots from the pulmonary circulation. Generally, the use of thrombolytic agents eliminates the need for this procedure.

## Management of fat emboli

**Oxygen:**   Concentration of oxygen is based on clinical picture, ABG results, and patient's prior respiratory status. Intubation and mechanical ventilation may be required.

**Steroids:** Cortisone, 100 mg, or methylprednisone, 30 mg/kg, is used to decrease local injury to pulmonary tissue and pulmonary edema.

**Diuretics:** Approximately 30% of patients with fat emboli develop pulmonary edema, necessitating use of diuretics.

## NURSING DIAGNOSES AND INTERVENTIONS

**Impaired gas exchange** related to altered oxygen supply secondary to ventilation-perfusion mismatch occurring with PE

*Desired outcomes:* Following intervention/treatment, patient exhibits adequate gas exchange and ventilatory function as evidenced by RR 12-20 breaths/min with normal pattern and depth (eupnea) and orientation to person, place, and time. At a minimum of 24 h before hospital discharge patient has $Pao_2$ ≥80 mm Hg, $Paco_2$ 35-45 mm Hg, and pH 7.35-7.45 (or values consistent with patient's acceptable baseline parameters).

- Monitor patient for signs and symptoms of increasing respiratory distress: RR increased from baseline, increasing dyspnea, anxiety, restlessness, confusion, and cyanosis.
- Position patient for comfort and optimal gas exchange. Ensure that the area of the lung affected by the embolus is not dependent when patient is in the lateral decubitus position. Elevate HOB 30 degrees to improve ventilation.
- Avoid positioning patient with knees bent (i.e., gatching the bed) because this impedes venous return from the legs and can increase the risk of PE.
- Decrease metabolic demands for oxygen by limiting or pacing patient's activities and procedures.
- Ensure that patient performs deep-breathing and coughing exercises 3-5 times q2h.
- Ensure delivery of prescribed concentrations of oxygen.
- Monitor serial ABG values, assessing for the desired response to treatment. Report lack of response to treatment or worsening ABG values.

**Altered protection** related to risk of prolonged bleeding or hemorrhage secondary to anticoagulation therapy

*Desired outcome:* Patient is free of frank or occult bleeding; body secretions/excretions test negative for blood.

- Monitor VS for indicators of profuse bleeding or hemorrhage resulting from anticoagulant therapy: hypotension, tachycardia, and tachypnea.
- At least once a shift check stool, urine, sputum, and vomitus for occult blood, using agency-approved method for testing.
- At least once a shift inspect wounds, oral mucous membranes, any entry site of an invasive procedure, and nares for evidence of bleeding.
- At least once a shift inspect the torso and extremities for petechiae or ecchymoses.
- To prevent hematoma formation, avoid giving an IM injection unless it is unavoidable.
- Apply pressure to all venipuncture or arterial puncture sites until bleeding stops completely.
- Ensure easy access to antidotes for prescribed treatment.
  - *Protamine sulfate:* 1 mg counteracts 100 U of heparin. Usually, the initial dose is 50 mg.
  - *Vitamin K:* 20 mg given SC to counteract the effects of oral anticoagulants.
  - *E-aminocaproic acid* (e.g., Amicar): Administered *via* slow IV infusion of 5 g, it reverses the fibrinolytic condition related to thrombolytic therapy.
- If patient is on heparin therapy, monitor serial PTT (desired range is 1.5-2.5 × control). If patient is on warfarin (Coumadin) therapy, monitor serial PT. Desired range is 1.25-1.5 × control. Report values outside the desired range.

- To avoid negative interactions with anticoagulants or thrombolytic therapy, establish compatability of all drugs before administering them.
  - *Heparin:* Digitalis, tetracyclines, nicotine, and antihistamines decrease the effect of heparin therapy. Consult with pharmacist about compatability before infusing other IV drugs through heparin IV line.
  - *Warfarin sodium:* Numerous drugs result in a decrease or increase in response to treatment with warfarin. Consult with pharmacist to obtain specific information about patient's medication profile.
  - *Thrombolytic therapy (e.g., streptokinase, urokinase):* No specific drug interactions are noted. However, consult with pharmacist before infusing any other medication through the same IV line.
- Because aspirin and nonsteroidal antiinflammatory drugs (e.g., ibuprofen) are platelet aggregation inhibitors and can prolong episodes of bleeding, avoid use of *any* drug that contains these medications.
- Discuss with patient and significant others the importance of reporting promptly the presence of bleeding from any source.
- Teach patient the necessity of using sponge-tipped applicators and mouthwash for oral care to minimize the risk of gum bleeding. Instruct patient to shave with an electric rather than straight razor.
- If patient is restless and combative, provide a safe environment: Pad the side rails, restrain patient as necessary to prevent falls, and use extreme care when moving patient to avoid bumping of extremities into side rails.

**Knowledge deficit:**   Oral anticoagulant therapy, potential side effects, and foods and medications to avoid during therapy
*Desired outcome:*   Within the 24-h period before hospital discharge, patient verbalizes knowledge of the prescribed anticoagulant drug, the potential side effects, and foods and medications to avoid while on oral anticoagulant therapy.

- Determine patient's knowledge of oral anticoagulant therapy. As appropriate, discuss the drug name, purpose, dose, schedule, and side effects.
- Inform patient of the potential side effects/complications of anticoagulant therapy: easy bruising, prolonged bleeding from cuts, spontaneous nosebleeds, black and tarry stools, and blood in urine and sputum.
- Discuss with patient the importance of laboratory testing and follow-up visits with physician.
- Explain the importance of informing all health-care providers (e.g., dentists and other physicians) that patient is on anticoagulant therapy. Suggest that patient wear a Medic-Alert tag or other method of informing health-care providers about the anticoagulant therapy.
- Teach patient about foods high in vitamin K (e.g., fish, bananas, dark green vegetables, tomatoes, and cauliflower), which can interfere with anticoagulation.
- Caution patient that a soft-bristled, rather than hard-bristled, toothbrush and an electric, rather than straight, razor should be used during anticoagulant therapy to minimize the risk of injury that could cause bleeding.
- Instruct patient to consult with physician before taking over-the-counter (OTC) or prescribed drugs that were used before initiating anticoagulants. Aspirin, cimetidine, and trimethaphan are among the many drugs that enhance the response to warfarin. Drugs that decrease the response include antacids, diuretics, oral contraceptives, and barbiturates, among others.

---

**Note:**   Also, if appropriate, see Appendix One, "Caring for Preoperative and Postoperative Patients," p. 693, and "Caring for Patients on Prolonged Bed Rest," p. 711.

---

## PATIENT-FAMILY TEACHING AND DISCHARGE PLANNING

Give patient and significant others verbal and written instructions about the following:

- Risk factors related to the development of thrombi and embolization and preventive measures to reduce the risk.
- Signs and symptoms of *thrombophlebitis:* swelling of the calf, tenderness or warmth in the involved area, possible presence of pain in affected calf when ankle is flexed, slight fever, distention of veins in affected leg. Signs and symptoms of *pulmonary embolism:* sudden onset of dyspnea and anxiety, nonproductive cough, palpitations, nausea, syncope.
- Rationale and application procedure for antiembolism hose. Explain that patient should put them on in the morning before getting out of bed.
- Importance of preventing impairment of venous return from the lower extremities by avoiding prolonged sitting, crossing legs, and constrictive clothing.

---

**Note:** Rehabilitation and family teaching concepts for fat emboli are nonspecific.

---

# Pneumothorax/Hemothorax

*Pneumothorax* is an accumulation of air in the pleural space, which leads to increased intrapleural pressure. Risk factors include blunt or penetrating chest injury, chronic obstructive pulmonary disease (COPD), previous pneumothorax, and positive pressure ventilation. There are three types:

**Spontaneous:** Also referred to as closed pneumothorax because the chest wall remains intact with no leak to the atmosphere. It results from the rupture of a bleb or bulla on the visceral pleural surface, usually near the apex. Generally, the cause of the rupture is unknown, although it may result from a weakness related to a respiratory infection or from an underlying pulmonary disease (e.g., COPD, tuberculosis, malignant neoplasm). The affected individual is usually young (20-40 years), previously healthy, and male. Generally, onset of symptoms occurs at rest, rather than with vigorous exercise or coughing. Potential for recurrence is great, with the second pneumothorax occurring an average of 2-3 years after the first.

**Traumatic:** Can be open or closed. An open pneumothorax occurs when air enters the pleural space from the atmosphere through an opening in the chest wall, such as with a gunshot wound, stab wound, or invasive medical procedure (e.g., lung biopsy, thoracentesis, or placement of a central line into a subclavian vein). A sucking sound may be heard over the area of penetration during inspiration. A closed pneumothorax occurs when the visceral pleura is penetrated but the chest wall remains intact with no atmospheric leak. This usually occurs with blunt trauma that results in a fracture and dislocation of the ribs. It also may occur from the use of positive end-expiratory pressure (PEEP) or after cardiopulmonary resuscitation (CPR).

**Tension:** Generally occurs with closed pneumothorax; also can occur with open pneumothorax when pleural tissue acts as a one-way valve. Air enters the pleural space through the pleural tear when the individual inhales, and it continues to accumulate but cannot escape during expiration because the pleural flap closes. With tension pneumothorax, as the pressure in the thorax and mediastinum increases, it produces a shift in the affected lung and mediastinum toward the unaffected side, which further impairs ventilatory efforts. The increase in pressure also compresses the vena cava, which impedes venous return, leading to a decrease in cardiac output and, ultimately, to circulatory collapse if the condition is not diagnosed and treated quickly. Tension pneumothorax is a life-threatening medical emergency.

*Hemothorax* is an accumulation of blood in the pleural space. Hemothorax generally results from blunt trauma to the chest wall, but it can occur following thoracic surgery as a result of anticoagulant therapy, after the insertion of a central venous catheter, or following various thoracoabdominal organ biopsies. Mediastinal shift, ventilatory compromise, and lung collapse can occur, depending on the amount of blood accumulated.

## ASSESSMENT

Clinical presentation will vary, depending on the type and size of the pneumothorax or hemothorax (Table 1-2).

## DIAGNOSTIC TESTS

**Chest x-ray:**   Will reveal the presence of air or blood in the pleural space on the affected side, size of the pneumothorax/hemothorax, and any shift in the mediastinum.

**ABG values:**   Hypoxemia ($Pao_2$ <80 mm Hg) may be accompanied by hypercarbia ($Paco_2$ >45 mm Hg) with resultant respiratory acidosis (pH <7.35). Arterial oxygen saturation may be decreased initially but usually returns to normal within 24 h.

**CBC:**   May reveal decreased hemoglobin (Hgb) proportionate to the amount of blood lost in a hemothorax.

## COLLABORATIVE MANAGEMENT

Management is determined by the signs and symptoms. A small pneumothorax may heal itself *via* reabsorption of the free air, making invasive procedures unnecessary unless an underlying disease process or injury is present. A hemothorax nearly always requires intervention.

**Oxygen therapy:**   Administered when ABG values demonstrate the presence of hypoxemia, which usually occurs when the pneumothorax/hemothorax is large.

**Thoracentesis:**   For hemothorax to remove blood from the pleural space. For cases of tension pneumothorax, it is performed immediately to remove air from the pleural space. A large-bore needle is inserted in the second intercostal space, midclavicular line, which correlates to the superior portion of the anterior axillary lobe. A sudden rushing out of air confirms the diagnosis of tension pneumothorax. To decrease risk of further pleural laceration as the chest reexpands, a stylet introducer needle with a plastic sheath may be used. The needle is removed after penetration, and the plastic catheter sheath is left in place to allow decompression of the chest cavity. Following air aspiration, chest tubes are inserted.

**Chest tube placement:**   A chest tube (thoracic catheter) may be inserted in any patient who is symptomatic. During insertion the patient should be in an upright position so that the lung falls away from the chest wall. The position of the thoracic catheter will depend on whether the physician wants to drain air, fluid, or both. The thoracic catheter must be connected to an underwater-seal drainage system or a one-way flutter valve device. Usually, simple underwater-seal drainage is all that is necessary for 6-24 h. Suction may be used, depending on size of the pneumothorax or hemothorax, patient's condition, and amount of drainage. If drainage is minimal and no suction is required, a one-way flutter valve may be used instead of an underwater-seal drainage system. After chest tube insertion and removal of air or fluid from the pleural space, the lung begins to reexpand. A chest tube may produce inflammation of the pleura, causing pleuritic pain, slight temperature elevation, and pleural friction rub.

**Thoracotomy:**   Often indicated if patient has had two or more spontaneous pneumothoraces on one side, owing to the risk of continuous recurrence, or if

**TABLE 1-2 Assessment of the Patient with Pneumothorax or Hemothorax**

| | Spontaneous or traumatic pneumothorax | | Tension pneumothorax | Hemothorax |
| | Closed | Open | | |
| --- | --- | --- | --- | --- |
| *Signs and symptoms* | SOB, cough, chest tightness, chest pain | SOB, sharp chest pain | Dyspnea, chest pain | Dyspnea, chest pain |
| *Physical assessment* | Tachypnea, decreased thoracic movement, cyanosis, subcutaneous emphysema, hyperresonance over affected area, diminished breath sounds, paradoxical movement of chest wall (may signal flail chest), change in mental status | Agitation, restlessness, tachypnea, cyanosis, presence of chest wound, hyperresonance over affected area, sucking sound on inspiration, diminished breath sounds, change in mental status | Anxiety, tachycardia, cyanosis, jugular vein distention, tracheal deviation toward the unaffected side, absent breath sounds on affected side, distant heart sounds, hypotension, change in mental status | Tachypnea, pallor, cyanosis, dullness over affected side, tachycardia, hypotension, diminished or absent breath sounds, change in mental status |

resolution of the pneumothorax does not occur within 7 days. With a hemothorax a thoracotomy is performed to locate the source and control bleeding if blood loss exceeds 200 ml/h over 2 h. Thoracotomy may include mechanical abrasion of the pleural surfaces with a dry sterile sponge or chemical abrasion *via* an agent such as tetracycline solution or talc, which results in pleural adhesions that help prevent recurrence of pneumothorax. A partial pleurectomy may be performed instead of mechanical or chemical abrasion.

**IV therapy:**    If there is significant loss of fluids or blood.

**Analgesia:**    Provides relief of pain from the pneumothorax/hemothorax or its treatment.

## NURSING DIAGNOSES AND INTERVENTIONS

**Impaired gas exchange** related to altered oxygen supply secondary to ventilation-perfusion mismatch

*Desired outcomes:*    Following treatment/intervention, patient exhibits adequate gas exchange and ventilatory function as evidenced by RR $\leq$20 breaths/min with normal depth and pattern (eupnea) and orientation to person, place, and time. At a minimum of 24 h before hospital discharge, patient's ABG values are as follows: $Pao_2$ $\geq$80 mm Hg and $Paco_2$ 35-45 mm Hg (or values within patient's acceptable baseline parameters).

- Monitor serial ABG results to detect decreasing $Pao_2$ and increasing $Paco_2$, which can signal impending respiratory failure. Report significant findings to physician.
- Observe for indicators of hypoxia, including increased restlessness, anxiety, and changes in mental status. Cyanosis may be a late sign.
- Assess patient's VS and breath sounds q2h (patient will require checks q15min after thoracotomy until stable) for signs of respiratory distress: increased RR, diminished or absent movement of chest wall on affected side, paradoxical movement of the chest wall, increased WOB, use of accessory muscles of respiration, complaints of increased dyspnea, and cyanosis. Evaluate HR and BP for indications of shock (i.e., tachycardia and hypotension).
- Position patient to allow for full expansion of the unaffected lung. Semi-Fowler's position usually provides comfort and allows adequate expansion of chest wall and descent of diaphragm.
- Change patient's position q2h to promote drainage and lung reexpansion and facilitate alveolar perfusion.
- Encourage patient to take deep breaths, providing necessary analgesia to decrease discomfort during deep-breathing exercises. Deep breathing will promote full lung expansion and may decrease the risk of atelectasis. Coughing will facilitate mobilization of tracheobronchial secretions, if present.
- Deliver and monitor oxygen as indicated.

**Ineffective breathing pattern (or risk of same)** related to decreased lung expansion secondary to malfunction of chest drainage system

*Desired outcome:*    Following intervention, patient becomes eupneic.

- Monitor patient at frequent intervals (q2-4h, as appropriate) to assess breathing pattern while chest-drainage system is in place. Auscultate breath sounds, reporting a decrease; be alert to and report signs of respiratory distress, including restlessness, anxiety, and changes in mental status.
- Assess and maintain the closed chest-drainage system.
  - Tape all connections, and secure chest tube to thorax with tape.
  - Avoid all kinks in the tubing, and ensure that the bed and equipment are not compressing any component of the system.
  - Eliminate all dependent loops in tubing. These may impede removal of air and fluid from the pleural space.

- Maintain fluid in underwater-seal chamber and suction chamber at appropriate levels.
- Be aware that the suction apparatus does not regulate the amount of suction applied to the closed chest-drainage system. The amount of suction is determined by the water level in the suction control chamber. Minimal bubbling in this chamber is acceptable and desirable. **Note:** Suction aids in the reexpansion of the lung, but removing suction for short periods of time, such as for transporting, will not be detrimental or disrupt the closed chest-drainage system.
- Follow institution's policy about chest-tube stripping. Be aware that this mechanism for maintaining chest-tube patency is controversial and has been associated with creating high negative pressures in the pleural space, which can damage fragile lung tissue. Chest-tube stripping may be indicated when bloody drainage or clots are visible in the tubing. Squeezing alternately hand-over-hand along the drainage tube may generate sufficient pressure to move fluid along the tube.
- Be aware that fluctuations in the long tube of the underwater-seal chamber are characteristic of a patent chest tube. Fluctuations stop when either the lung has reexpanded or there is a kink or obstruction in the chest tube.
  - Bubbling in the underwater-seal chamber occurs on expiration and is a sign that air is leaving the pleural space.
  - Continuous bubbling in the underwater-seal chamber may be a signal that air is leaking into the drainage system. Locate and seal the system's air leak, if possible.
- Keep necessary emergency supplies at the bedside: petrolatum gauze pad to apply over insertion site if the chest tube becomes dislodged, and sterile water in which to submerge the chest tube if it becomes disconnected from the underwater-seal system. *Never* clamp a chest tube without a specific directive from the physician, inasmuch as clamping may lead to tension pneumothorax because air in the pleural space no longer can escape.

**Pain** related to impaired pleural integrity, inflammation, or presence of a chest tube
*Desired outcomes:* Within 1 h of intervention, patient's subjective perception of pain decreases, as documented by a pain scale. Objective indicators, such as grimacing, are absent or diminished.
- At frequent intervals, assess patient's degree of discomfort, using patient's verbal and nonverbal cues. Devise a pain scale with patient, rating pain from 0 (no pain) to 10 (worst pain). Medicate with analgesics as prescribed, using the pain scale to evaluate and document the effectiveness of the medication.
- Premedicate patient 30 min before initiating coughing, exercising, or repositioning.
- Teach patient to splint affected side when coughing, moving, or repositioning.
- Schedule activities to provide for 90-min periods of undisturbed rest, which may increase patient's pain threshold.
- Stabilize chest tube to reduce pull or drag on latex connector tubing. Tape chest tube securely to thorax.
- For additional interventions, see Appendix One, p. 694.

---

**Note:** See "Abdominal Trauma" for **Fluid volume deficit,** p. 444. Also see psychosocial nursing diagnoses and interventions in Appendix One, "Caring for Patients with Cancer and Other Life-Disrupting Illnesses," p. 753.

## PATIENT-FAMILY TEACHING AND DISCHARGE PLANNING

Give patient and significant others verbal and written instructions about the following:

- Purpose for chest-tube placement and maintenance.
- Potential for recurrence of spontaneous pneumothorax. Average time between occurrences is 2-3 years. Explain the importance of seeking medical care immediately if the symptoms recur (see Table 1-2).
- Medications, including drug name, purpose, dosage, schedule, precautions, and potential side effects.

# Pulmonary tuberculosis

Tuberculosis (TB) was a leading cause of death in the United States until the late 1940s and early 1950s, when antituberculosis drug therapy was introduced, resulting in a decline in the disease until the 1980s. Since 1986, however, case rates of TB have been increasing. Factors contributing to the rise include immigration of individuals to the United States from countries where TB is endemic, and increasing prevalence of individuals who are immunocompromised (i.e., those receiving immunosuppressive therapy or with a disease that impairs the immune response, such as HIV disease).

TB is a highly infectious disease spread by contact with respiratory droplets containing mycobacteria, generally the *Mycobacterium tuberculosis* bacillus in humans. The most common mode of transmission is inhalation of bacilli in airborne mucus droplets from sputum of persons with active disease. Less frequently, transmission may result from ingestion or skin penetration. When infection with tubercle bacilli occurs, lung parenchyma become inflamed. Natural body defenses attempt to counteract the infection, and lymph nodes in the hilar region of the lung may begin to filter drainage from the infected site. The inflammatory process and cellular reaction produce a small, firm white nodule called the primary tubercle, the center of which contains tubercle bacilli. Cells gather around the center, and the outer portion becomes fibrosed. As blood vessels become compressed, nutrition to the tubercle ceases and the center begins to necrose. The area is further walled off by fibrotic tissue, and the center becomes soft and cheesy in consistency, a process known as caseation. This fluid may calcify (calcium deposits) or liquefy (liquefaction necrosis). Most individuals (90%) infected with the tubercle bacillus do not progress to active disease, because the disease usually settles into the latency phase.

## ASSESSMENT

It is important to assess whether the patient was exposed to a person with active TB. Also, close contacts of the patient require identification so that they can undergo evaluation for the presence of infection.

**Signs and symptoms:**   Cough, afternoon temperature elevation, night sweats.

## DIAGNOSTIC TESTS

**Sputum culture:**   To ascertain presence of *M. tuberculosis;* will not be positive during latency period.

**Acid-fast stain:**   Culture of sputum positive for acid-fast bacilli (AFB) in the presence of active TB.

**Chest x-ray:**   While not diagnostically definitive, will reveal calcification at original site, enlargement of hilar lymph nodes, parenchymal infiltrate, pleural effusion, cavitation.

**Intradermal injection of antigen:**   purified protein derivative (PPD); old tuberculin (OT). Considered positive when an area of induration >10 mm is present within 48-72 h after injection. A positive test indicates past infection and presence of antibodies; it is not definitive of active disease.

**Gastric washings:**    May reveal presence of tubercle bacilli secondary to swallowed sputum.

## COLLABORATIVE MANAGEMENT

**AFB isolation:**    Until antimicrobial therapy is successful as indicated by AFB smears. AFB isolation (or "airborne precautions" in the nomenclature of body substance isolation) requires a private room with special ventilation that dilutes and removes airborne contaminants and controls the direction of air flow. High-efficiency masks (e.g., particulate respirators) designed to provide a tight face seal and filter particles in the 1-5 micron range are worn by all individuals entering the patient's room and by the patient if it is necessary to leave the room.

**Pharmacologic agents:**    A combination of antiinfective agents is recommended to prevent development of resistant strains of tubercle bacillus. The drug of choice, along with the dosage and duration of administration, depends on the stage of the infection or disease, presence of extrapulmonary disease, and sensitivity of the patient to the chemotherapeutic agent. The most common combination is isoniazid and rifampin, which is given for 6-12 months. Other drugs, which may added to this protocol if the organism shows resistance to the first-line drugs, include ethambutol, pyrazinamide, and streptomycin.

**Surgery:**    Resection for persistent cavitary lesions; surgical intervention for massive hemoptysis, spontaneous pneumothorax, abscess drainage, and other complications.

## NURSING DIAGNOSES AND INTERVENTIONS

**Knowledge deficit:**    The spread of TB and the procedure for AFB isolation
*Desired outcome:*    Following the instruction, patient and significant others verbalize how TB is spread and the measures necessary to prevent the spread.
- Teach patient about TB and the mechanism by which it is spread.
- Explain AFB isolation to patient and significant others. Post a notice of AFB isolation/airborne precautions on the patient's room door.
- Explain to staff and visitors the importance of wearing high-efficiency masks, including their proper fit and use. Provide masks at doorway or other convenient place.
- Teach patient the importance of covering mouth and nose with tissue when sneezing or coughing and disposing of used tissue in container suitable for biohazardous waste disposal.
- Stress the importance of good handwashing technique to reduce the risk of ingesting the organism.

## PATIENT-FAMILY TEACHING AND DISCHARGE PLANNING

Give patient and significant others verbal and written information about the following:
- Importance of good handwashing technique.
- Antituberculosis medications, including name, purpose, dosage, schedule, precautions, and potential side effects. Remind patient that medications are to be taken uninterruptedly for the prescribed period of time.
- Importance of periodic reculturing of sputum.

# Section Two:   Acute Respiratory Failure

Acute respiratory failure (ARF) develops when the lungs are unable to exchange $O_2$ and $CO_2$ adequately. Clinically, respiratory failure exists when $Pao_2$ is <50 mm Hg with the patient at rest and breathing room air. $Paco_2 \geq 50$

## T A B L E  1 - 3   Disease Processes Leading to the Development of Respiratory Failure

*Impaired alveolar ventilation*

Chronic obstructive pulmonary disease (emphysema, bronchitis, asthma, cystic fibrosis)

Restrictive pulmonary disease (interstitial fibrosis, pleural effusion, pneumothorax, kyphoscoliosis, obesity, diaphragmatic paralysis)

Neuromuscular defects (Guillain-Barré syndrome, myasthenia gravis, multiple sclerosis, muscular dystrophy)

Depression of respiratory control centers (drug-induced cerebral infarction, inappropriate use of high-dose $O_2$ therapy)

*Diffusion disturbances*

Pulmonary/interstitial fibrosis

Pulmonary edema

Adult respiratory distress syndrome

Anatomic loss of functioning lung tissue (tumor pneumonectomy)

*Ventilation or perfusion disturbances*

Pulmonary emboli

Atelectasis

Pneumonia

Emphysema

Chronic bronchitis

Bronchiolitis

Adult respiratory distress syndrome

*Right-to-left shunting*

Atelectasis

Pneumonia

Pulmonary edema

Pulmonary emboli

$O_2$ toxicity

From Howard C and Heitz UE. In Swearingen PL and Keen JH: *Manual of critical care: applying nursing diagnoses to adult critical illness*, ed 2, St Louis, Mosby-Year Book, 1991.

mm Hg or pH <7.35 is significant for respiratory acidosis, which is the common precursor to ARF.

While a variety of disease processes can lead to the development of respiratory failure (Table 1-3), four basic mechanisms are involved:

**Alveolar hypoventilation:**   Occurs secondary to reduction in alveolar minute ventilation. Because differential indicators (cyanosis and somnolence) occur late in the process, the condition may go unnoticed until tissue hypoxia is severe.

**Ventilation-perfusion mismatch:**   Considered the most common cause of hypoxemia. Normal alveolar ventilation occurs at a rate of 4 L/min, with normal pulmonary vascular blood flow occurring at a rate of 5 L/min. Normal ventilation/perfusion ratio is 0.8:1. Any disease process that interferes with either side of the equation upsets the physiologic balance and can lead to respiratory failure as a result of the reduction in arterial $O_2$ levels.

**Diffusion disturbances:**   Processes that physically impair gas exchange across the alveolar-capillary membrane. Diffusion is impaired owing to the increase in anatomic distance the gas must travel from alveoli to capillary and capillary to alveoli.

**Right-to-left shunt:**   Occurs when the above processes go untreated. Large amounts of blood pass from the right side of the heart to the left and out into the general circulation without adequate ventilation; therefore blood is poorly oxygenated. This mechanism occurs when alveoli are atelectatic or fluid-filled, inasmuch as these conditions interfere with gas exchange. Unlike the first three responses, hypoxemia secondary to right-to-left shunting does not improve with the administration of $O_2$, because the additional $FiO_2$ is unable to cross the alveolar-capillary membrane.

## ASSESSMENT

Clinical indicators of ARF vary according to the underlying disease process and severity of the failure. ARF is one of the most common causes of impaired LOC. Often it is misdiagnosed as congestive heart failure, pneumonia, or cerebrovascular accident. Sometimes the onset of ARF is so insidious that it is missed because the staff does not want to disturb the patient who appears to be sleeping.

**Early indicators:** Restlessness, anxiety, headache, fatigue, cool and dry skin, increased BP, tachycardia, and cardiac dysrhythmias.

**Intermediate indicators:** Confusion, lethargy, tachypnea, hypotension caused by vasodilatation, cardiac dysrhythmias.

**Late indicators:** Cyanosis, diaphoresis, coma, respiratory arrest.

## DIAGNOSTIC TESTS

**ABG analysis:** Assesses adequacy of oxygenation and effectiveness of ventilation and is the most important diagnostic tool. Typical results are $Pao_2 \leq 60$ mm Hg, $Paco_2 \geq 45$ mm Hg, and pH $<7.35$, which are consistent with severe respiratory acidosis.

**Chest x-ray:** Ascertains presence of underlying pathophysiology or disease process that may be contributing to the failure.

## COLLABORATIVE MANAGEMENT

Treatment is aimed at correcting the acid-base disturbance, while at the same time treating the underlying pathophysiology in an effort to prevent or correct ARF. Although the general rule is to bring the $Pao_2$ to $>60$ mm Hg and the $Paco_2$ to 35–45 mm Hg, patients with chronic obstructive pulmonary disease (COPD) may be clinically stable with a $Paco_2 >45$ mm Hg, so determination of pH is critical with these individuals. For example, the patient with a chronically high $Paco_2$ whose pH drops below baseline is at risk for development of respiratory failure.

**$O_2$ therapy:** As determined by ABG values. $O_2$ therapy at an $FiO_2$ of 0.50 or less and chest physiotherapy in conjunction with pharmacotherapy (e.g., bronchodilators, steroids, antibiotics) often improve ABGs sufficiently to get the patient out of danger. Persistent respiratory acidosis following medical intervention may be an indicator of the need for intubation and mechanical ventilation.

**IV aminophylline:** To treat bronchospasms. Therapeutic range is 10-20 μg/ml. Daily serum levels are drawn to evaluate the patient.

**Bronchodilator therapy:** Delivered *via* nebulizer or intermittent positive pressure breathing (IPPB) machine q2-4h to minimize $CO_2$ retention.

**Chest physiotherapy:** To assist in mobilization of secretions.

**Coughing/deep breathing exercises:** To mobilize secretions and promote full lung expansion. If the cough is ineffective, suctioning may be necessary to stimulate cough reflex and clear secretions.

**IV fluids:** To maintain fluid balance and prevent dehydration.

**Antibiotics:** If infection is present.

**Intubation and mechanical ventilation:** To prevent further airway collapse and tissue injury. The patient may require intubation and mechanical ventilation to provide adequate respiratory function and stabilize ABGs if ARF progresses. Mechanical support is used until the underlying cause of the failure can be corrected and the patient can resume ventilatory efforts independently.

## NURSING DIAGNOSES AND INTERVENTIONS

See "Pneumonia" for **Impaired gas exchange,** p. 9, and **Fluid volume deficit,** p. 10. Also see "Atelectasis," p. 1, "Pleural Effusion," p. 12, "Pulmonary Embolus," p. 13, "Pneumothorax/Hemothorax," p. 19, "Asthma," p. 28, "Chronic Bronchitis," p. 32, "Emphysema," p. 35, "Pulmonary

Fibrosis," p. 37, "Pulmonary Edema," p. 82, "Guillain-Barré Syndrome," p. 188, and "Multiple Sclerosis," p. 182, because these disorders may be precursors to ARF. For psychosocial nursing diagnoses and interventions, see Appendix One, "Caring for Patients with Cancer and Other Life-Disrupting Illnesses," p. 753.

## PATIENT-FAMILY TEACHING AND DISCHARGE PLANNING

ARF is an acute condition that is symptomatically treated during the patient's hospitalization. Discharge planning and teaching should be directed at educating the patient and significant others about the underlying pathophysiology and treatment specific for that process. See sections in this chapter that relate specifically to the underlying pathophysiology contributing to the development of ARF.

# Section Three:    Chronic Obstructive Pulmonary Disease

Chronic obstructive pulmonary disease (COPD) is the second leading cause of disability in the United States. It is a chronic respiratory condition that obstructs the flow of air to or from the bronchioles. Causative factors include smoking, allergens, and environmental and occupational pollutants. This section will discuss the following types of COPD: asthma, chronic bronchitis, and emphysema.

## Asthma

Asthma is a broad clinical syndrome in which there is recurrent, reversible obstruction of air flow in the bronchioles and smaller bronchi secondary to bronchospasm, mucosal edema, and excessive mucus production. It can occur in any age group, and its symptoms are intermittent and usually alleviated with treatment. *Extrinsic asthma* is precipitated by environmental allergens (pollens, dust, feathers, animal dander, foods, etc.). *Intrinsic asthma* occurs secondary to factors that cannot fully be defined, but it is believed to be caused by an infection in the upper or lower respiratory tract and occurs more frequently in individuals older than age 35 years.

An acute asthma attack is caused by an antigen-antibody reaction in which chemical mediators (histamine, a slow-releasing substance of anaphylaxis, and eosinophilic chemotactic factor of anaphylaxis) are released, causing constriction of the smooth muscle in the airways, resulting in bronchospasm, increased capillary permeability leading to mucosal edema, and increased mucous gland secretion with increased mucus production.

## ASSESSMENT

**Signs and symptoms:**   Coughing, chest tightness, increased sputum production, dyspnea.
**Physical assessment:**   Agitation, prolonged expiratory phase, use of accessory muscles of respiration, tachypnea, chest retractions, nasal flaring, expiratory wheezing.

---

**Note:**   If symptoms are untreated, the condition can progress to status asthmaticus (SA), a severe and unrelenting asthma attack. If SA is not reversed, death can ensue.

---

## DIAGNOSTIC TESTS

**ABG values:**  Reveal status of oxygenation and acid-base balance. Generally, acute respiratory acidosis is present during an acute asthma attack ($Paco_2$ >45 mm Hg and pH <7.35).

**Chest x-ray:**  The x-ray usually shows lung hyperinflation, due to air trapping, and a flat diaphragm related to increased intrathoracic volume.

**Sputum:**  Gross examination may reveal increased viscosity or actual mucus plugs. Culture and sensitivity may reveal microorganisms if infection was the precipitating event.

**CBC:**  Differential may show increased eosinophils (in patients not on corticosteroids), which is indicative of allergic response.

**Serum theophylline level:**  Important baseline indicator for patients who are on this therapy. Acceptable therapeutic range is 10-20 $\mu$g/ml. The therapeutic level is close to the toxic level, and the patient must be monitored for toxic side effects (e.g., nausea, central nervous system [CNS] stimulation, dysrhythmias). Serial levels are drawn at frequent intervals.

**Pulmonary function testing:**  To evaluate the degree of obstruction. Forced expiratory volume (FEV) is decreased during acute episodes because of severely narrowed airways, which prevent forceful exhalation of inspired volume (see Table 1-4).

**ECG:**  Presence of sinus tachycardia is an important baseline indicator because use of some bronchodilators (e.g., metaproterenol) may produce cardiac stimulant effects and dysrhythmias. Prominent P waves appear in chronic asthma.

## COLLABORATIVE MANAGEMENT

Primarily, management is directed toward decreasing bronchospasm and increasing pulmonary ventilation.

### Acute phase

**O$_2$ therapy:**  Generally, these patients experience mild to moderate hypoxemia. Low-flow (1-3 L/min) $O_2$ is delivered *via* nasal cannula with humidity.

**Pharmacotherapy:**  Initiated to relieve bronchospasm and continued until wheezing subsides and pulmonary function tests return to baseline.

*Bronchodilators:*  Dilate smooth muscles of the airways (Table 1-5).

*Corticosteroids:*  To inhibit the inflammatory response. Dosage varies according to severity of the episode and whether patient is currently taking steroids.

---

**Note:**  Acute adrenal insufficiency can develop in patients who take steroids routinely at home if these drugs are not given to the patient during hospitalization.

---

*Antibiotics:*  Given if infectious pulmonary process is present as evidenced by fever, purulent sputum, or leukocytosis.

**Fluid replacement:**  To maintain adequate hydration. Generally, crystalloid fluids (i.e., 5% dextrose in water or 5% dextrose in normal saline) are used.

**Chest physiotherapy:**  Generally contraindicated in acute phases owing to hyperreactive state of airways. The patient may benefit from the cautious use of percussion and postural drainage to help mobilize secretions.

### Chronic phase

**Aminophylline:**  Dosage is determined by blood levels of theophylline.

**Nebulizer/aerosolized bronchodilators:**  For short-term, acute exacerbations of symptoms.

**Steroids:**  May be prescribed, depending on severity of symptoms. Generally physicians try to wean patients completely off steroids, but some patients may require low-dose steroids indefinitely.

**T A B L E   1 - 4    Pulmonary Function Tests Used in Individuals with Asthma**

| Test | Description | Normal values | Parameters in asthma |
|---|---|---|---|
| FVC | Total amount of gas exhaled as forcefully and as rapidly as possible after maximal inspiration | ≥80% of predicted normal | Normal or slightly decreased due to air trapping |
| $FEV_1$ | Volume of gas exhaled over first second of FVC. ($FEV_2$ and $FEV_3$ may also be measured, at 2 and 3 sec, respectively) | ≥75% of predicted normal | Decreased due to airway obstruction; may return to normal after administration of aerosolized bronchodilator |
| FEF. Formerly this was called maximal mid-expiratory flow | Average rate of flow during middle half of FEV. It is an accurate estimate of airway resistance | ≥80% of predicted normal | Decreased due to small airways obstruction; may return to normal after administration of aerosolized bronchodilator |

FVC = forced vital capacity; $FEV_1$ = forced expiratory volume in 1 second; FEF = forced midexpiratory flow; $FEV_2$ = forced expiratory volume in 2 seconds; $FEV_3$ = forced expiratory volume in 3 seconds.

## T A B L E 1 - 5  Bronchodilators Used in The Treatment of Acute Asthma

| Medication | Usual dosage | Action | Side effects |
| --- | --- | --- | --- |
| epinephrine | 0.2–0.5 ml of 1:1000 solution given SC q15-30min | Immediate adrenergic effects; activates adrenergic sympathomimetic receptors; acts on $\alpha$, $\beta_1$, and $\beta_2$ receptors; relieves bronchospasm | Cardiac stimulation, palpitations, anxiety |
| terbutaline (Brethine) | 0.2–0.3 ml given SC q30min × 3 doses | Selective $\beta$-adrenergic; relaxes bronchial smooth muscle | Fewer than with epinephrine and usually transient; increased HR (>120 bpm), nervousness, tremor, palpitations, nausea, vomiting, headache |
| methylxanthines (theophylline) | *Loading dosage:* 6 mg/kg given as IV bolus. **Note:** Loading dose may be omitted if the patient is already taking oral methylxanthine and serum level is therapeutic. *Maintenance dosage:* 0.1-0.5 µg/kg/hr given *via* continuous IV infusion | Short-acting nonadrenergic; directly relaxes smooth muscle of bronchial airways and pulmonary vasculature | Nausea, vomiting, GI bleeding, gastric distress, HR > 120 bpm, decreased BP, restlessness. **Note:** Because toxic levels are close to therapeutic loads, serum levels should be monitored to ensure correct dosage adjustment; dysrhythmias may result from toxic levels of theophylline |

HR = heart rate; GI = gastrointestinal.
**Note:** Isoproterenol and isoetharine are two inhalants usually avoided during acute asthma because the patient's gas flow may be too minimal to provide adequate distribution of medication.

## NURSING DIAGNOSES AND INTERVENTIONS

**Impaired gas exchange** related to altered oxygen supply secondary to decreased alveolar ventilation as a result of narrowed airways

***Desired outcomes:*** Following treatment/intervention, patient has adequate gas exchange as evidenced by RR 12-20 breaths/min (or values consistent with patient's baseline). Before hospital discharge, patient's ABG values are as follows: $Pao_2$ $\geq$80 mm Hg, $Paco_2$ 35-45 mm Hg, and pH 7.35-7.45.

- Observe for signs and symptoms of hypoxia (e.g., agitation, restlessness, changes in LOC). Remember that cyanosis of the lips and nailbeds is a late indicator of hypoxia.
- Position patient for comfort and to promote optimal gas exchange. Usually this is accomplished using high-Fowler's position, with the patient leaning forward and elbows propped on the over-the-bed table to promote maximal chest expansion. Record patient's response to positioning.
- Auscultate breath sounds q2-4h. Monitor for decreased or adventitious sounds (e.g., crackles or wheezes).
- Monitor ABG results. Be alert to decreasing $Pao_2$ and increasing $Paco_2$, which can signal respiratory failure.
- Deliver and monitor $O_2$ as prescribed.

See "Chronic Bronchitis" for **Ineffective airway clearance,** p. 33. See "Emphysema" for **Ineffective breathing pattern,** p. 36. For anxiety, see Appendix One, p. 753. For other nursing diagnoses related to psychosocial interventions, see Appendix One, "Caring for Patients with Cancer and Other Life-Disrupting illnesses," p. 753.

## PATIENT-FAMILY TEACHING AND DISCHARGE PLANNING

Give patient and significant others verbal and written instructions about the following:

- Irritants that can precipitate an attack, and the importance of removing these irritants from patient's environment.
- Signs and symptoms of pulmonary infection (e.g., increased cough, increasing sputum production, change in color of sputum from clear white to yellow-green, fever) or bronchial irritation (e.g., dry, hacking cough).
- Medications, including name, route, purpose, dosage, precautions, and potential side effects. In addition, teach patient the proper use of metered-dose inhalers, documenting accurate return of demonstration before hospital discharge. Remind patient that over-the-counter (OTC) inhalers contain medications that can interfere with the prescribed therapy. Instruct patient to contact physician before taking any OTC medications.
- Importance of avoiding contact with infectious individuals, especially those with respiratory infections. Encourage patient to get yearly flu and pneumococcal vaccines.
- Importance of follow-up care. Confirm date and time of next appointment.

# Chronic bronchitis

Chronic bronchitis is the most common respiratory disease in the United States. It occurs in individuals who have smoked cigarettes for a long period of time or lived in areas of severe air pollution. The extent of the disease is somewhat dependent on the length of time the lungs have been exposed to these pollutants.

Lung changes that occur with this disease include airway inflammation, loss of ciliary action, hypertrophy of mucosal glands, hyperinflation of the alveoli, and edema of bronchial mucosa, all of which result in increased mucus production. When this occurs, mucus plugs develop in the stretched alveoli, causing obstruction of the bronchioles. As the disease progresses there is further destruction of the lungs, causing inadequate ventilation. Recurrent upper respiratory infections (URIs) with *Streptococcus pneumoniae* and *Hemophilus influenzae* are common in this population secondary to the inability to clear the bronchial tree of mucus. As the disease progresses, acute exacerbations of the disease increase in severity and duration. Respiratory failure and cardiac problems can develop.

## ASSESSMENT

**Chronic indicators:** Morning cough, clear and copious secretions, anorexia, cyanosis, dependent edema.
**Acute indicators (exacerbation):** Fever, dyspnea, thick and tenacious sputum.
**Physical assessment:** Use of accessory muscles of respiration, prolonged expiratory phase, digital clubbing, decreased thoracic expansion, dullness over areas of consolidation, adventitious breath sounds (especially coarse rhonchi and wheezing), ankle edema, distended neck veins, bloated appearance.

## DIAGNOSTIC TESTS

**Chest x-ray:** Will reveal normal A-P diameter, nearly normal diaphragm position, and increased peripheral lung markings.
**ABG values:** Will reveal hypoxemia ($Pao_2$ <60 mm Hg) and hypercapnia ($Paco_2$ >50-60 mm Hg) in most patients. Baseline pH may be 7.35-7.38, but during acute exacerbation, as the $Paco_2$ increases, pH may fall below 7.35.
**Sputum culture:** May reveal presence of infective organisms.
**CBC:** Will reveal chronically elevated hemoglobin (Hgb) in the presence of chronic hypoxemia and elevated WBC count in the presence of acute bacterial infection.
**Pulmonary function tests:** Will show reduced vital capacity, increased residual volume due to trapping of air, and increased expiratory reserve volume. For descriptions and normal values of these tests, see Table 1-4.

## COLLABORATIVE MANAGEMENT

**$O_2$ therapy:** To treat hypoxemia. It is used cautiously and at a low flow rate (1-2 L/min) in patients with chronic $CO_2$ retention for whom hypoxemia, rather than hypercapnia, stimulates the respiratory drive.
**Pharmacotherapy**
*Bronchodilators:* To open the airways by relaxing smooth muscles. The resultant increased air flow may help loosen mucus.
*Steroids (i.e., prednisone):* To decrease inflammation, thereby increasing air flow. **Note:** Acute adrenal insufficiency can develop in patients who take steroids routinely at home if these drugs are not given during hospitalization.
*Antibiotics:* Based on sensitivity studies from sputum cultures.
**Chest physiotherapy:** To help loosen and mobilize pulmonary secretions.
**IV or oral fluids:** To promote adequate hydration.
**Diuretics or sodium (Na) restriction:** To reduce fluid overload in the presence of cardiac complications, such as congestive heart failure (CHF).

## NURSING DIAGNOSES AND INTERVENTIONS

**Ineffective airway clearance** related to decreased energy, which results in ineffective cough, or related to presence of increased tracheobronchial secretions
*Desired outcome:* Following intervention, patient coughs appropriately and has effective airway clearance as evidenced by absence of adventitious breath sounds.
• Auscultate breath sounds q2-4h and after coughing. Be alert to and report changes in adventitious breath sounds.

---

**T A B L E  1 - 6   Recommended Calorie Sources for Patients with COPD**

| Foods high in fat | Foods to avoid |
|---|---|
| Whole milk | Cakes |
| Cream | Cookies |
| Evaporated milk | Jams |
| Cream soups | Pastries |
| Custards | Sugar-concentrated snacks |
| Cheese | |
| Salad and cooking oils | |
| Margarine | |
| Mayonnaise | |
| Nuts | |
| Meat | |
| Poultry | |
| Fish | |

---

- Teach patient the "double cough" technique:
  - Sit upright with upper body flexed forward slightly.
  - Take two to three breaths and exhale passively.
  - Inhale again, but only to the mid-inspiratory point.
  - Exhale by coughing quickly two to three times.
    This technique prevents small airway collapse, which can occur with force-ful coughing.
- Administer chest physiotherapy as prescribed to mobilize secretions.

**Altered nutrition:**   Less than body requirements, related to decreased intake secondary to fatigue and anorexia

*Desired outcome*:   For a minimum of the 24-h period before hospital discharge, patient has adequate nutrition as evidenced by stable weight, positive nitrogen (N) state on N studies, and serum albumin 3.5-5.5 µg/dl.

- Monitor patient's food and fluid intake. If indicated, obtain dietary consultation for calorie counts.
- Provide diet in small, frequent meals that are nutritious and easy to consume.
- Request a dietitian consultation so that patient can verbalize food likes and dislikes.
- Unless otherwise indicated, provide calories more from unsaturated fat sources (Table 1-6) than from carbohydrate sources. During the process of carbohydrate metabolism, the body uses $O_2$ and produces $CO_2$, which is then excreted by the lungs. The patient with chronic obstructive pulmonary disease (COPD) takes in less $O_2$ and retains $CO_2$. A high-fat diet minimizes this problem because fat generates the least amount of $CO_2$ for a given amount of $O_2$ used, while carbohydrates generate the most.
- Discuss with the patient and significant others the importance of good nutrition in the treatment of chronic bronchitis.

---

**Note:**   Also see "Asthma" for **Impaired gas exchange,** p. 32. See "Emphysema" for **Ineffective breathing pattern,** p. 36, and **Activity intolerance,** p. 36. See "Heart Failure" for **Fluid volume excess,** p. 61. In addition, see Appendix One, p. 753, for **Anxiety.**

---

## PATIENT-FAMILY TEACHING AND DISCHARGE PLANNING

Give patient and significant others verbal and written instructions about the following:

- Use of home $O_2$, including instructions for when to use it, importance of not increasing prescribed flow rate, precautions, and community resources for $O_2$ replacement when necessary. Request respiratory therapy consultation to assist with teaching related to $O_2$ therapy, if indicated.
- Medications, including name, route, purpose, dosage, schedule, precautions, and potential side effects.
- Signs and symptoms of CHF that necessitate medical attention: increased dyspnea; fatigue; increased coughing; changes in the amount, color, or consistency of sputum; swelling of the ankles and legs; fever; and sudden weight gain. Patients with COPD often have right-sided heart failure secondary to cardiac effects of the disease. For more information, see "Heart Failure," p. 60.
- Avoiding individuals who are known to be infectious, especially those with URIs.
- Review of Na-restricted diet (Table 3-2, p. 115) and other dietary considerations, as indicated.
- Importance of pacing activity level to conserve energy.
- Importance of yearly flu and pneumococcal vaccines.
- Follow-up appointment with physician; confirm date and time of next appointment.
- Introduction to local chapter of American Lung Association activities and pulmonary rehabilitation programs. Physical training programs may improve ventilation and cardiac muscle function, which may compensate for nonreversible lung disease.

## Emphysema

Pulmonary emphysema is a degenerative process characterized by enlargement of the air spaces distal to the terminal bronchioles accompanied by destruction of the alveolar walls. Because of the destruction of the alveoli, air becomes trapped, and distal airways become hyperinflated and may rupture or collapse. Emphysema is a progressive disease, and affected individuals can become totally disabled because they must use all available energy for breathing. In the later stages of the disease, pulmonary hypertension develops, leading to cor pulmonale, a condition that produces cardiac as well as respiratory problems.

## ASSESSMENT

**Chronic indicators:** Nonproductive cough (unless patient also has bronchitis), dyspnea on exertion.
**Acute indicators (exacerbation):** Increased dyspnea, productive cough, fever, peripheral edema, fatigue.
**Physical assessment:** Emaciation, increased A-P chest diameter, pursed-lip breathing, hypertrophy of accessory muscles of respiration, decreased fremitus over affected lung fields, decreased thoracic excursion, hyperresonance over affected lung fields, decreased breath sounds, and prolonged expiratory phase. Digital clubbing occurs late in the disease.

## DIAGNOSTIC TESTS

**Chest x-ray:** Will show hyperinflation of the lungs, an increased A-P diameter, lowered and flattened diaphragm, and a small cardiac silhouette.
**ABG values:** May reveal a slight decrease in $Pao_2$. As disease progresses, the $Pao_2$ will continue to decrease and $Paco_2$ may increase because of hypoventilation and $CO_2$ retention. Early in the disease process, however, the $Paco_2$

may be normal if the patient has good ventilation-perfusion matching. The pH will be low-normal once $CO_2$ retention begins.

**CBC:**   May reveal a chronically elevated RBC count (polycythemia) later in the disease process as a compensatory response to chronic hypoxemia.

**Pulmonary function tests:**   Will show an increased total lung capacity, increased residual volume, and decreased forced expiratory reserve volume. The vital capacity will be normal or slightly decreased. For descriptions and normal values of these tests, see Table 1-4.

**ECG:**   May reveal atrial and ventricular dysrhythmias. Most patients will have an atrial dysrhythmia as a result of atrial dilatation and right ventricular hypertrophy caused by pulmonary hypertension.

**Sputum culture:**   May be requested to determine presence of pulmonary infection.

## COLLABORATIVE MANAGEMENT
See "Chronic Bronchitis," p. 33.

## NURSING DIAGNOSES AND INTERVENTIONS

**Ineffective breathing pattern** related to decreased lung expansion secondary to chronic air flow limitations

*Desired outcome:*   Following treatment/intervention, patient's breathing pattern improves as evidenced by reduction in or absence of dyspnea and movement toward a state of eupnea.

- Assess patient's respiratory status q2-4h, being alert for indicators of respiratory distress (i.e., agitation, restlessness, decreased LOC, and use of accessory muscles of respiration). Auscultate breath sounds; report a decrease in breath sounds or an increase in adventitious breath sounds.
- Instruct patient in the use of pursed-lip breathing, which provides internal stability to the airways and may prevent airway collapse during expiration, as follows:
  - Sit upright with hands on thighs or lean forward with elbows propped on the over-the-bed table.
  - Inhale slowly through the nose with the mouth closed.
  - Form lips in an *O* shape as though whistling.
  - Exhale slowly through pursed lips. Exhalation should take twice as long as inhalation (e.g., count to five on inhalation; count to ten on exhalation).
    Record patient's response to breathing technique.
- Administer bronchodilator therapy as prescribed. Monitor patient for side effects, including tachycardia and dysrhythmias.
- Monitor patient's response to prescribed $O_2$ therapy. Be aware that high concentrations of $O_2$ can depress the respiratory drive in individuals with chronic $CO_2$ retention.
- Monitor serial ABG values. Patients with chronic $CO_2$ retention may have chronically compensated respiratory acidosis with a low-normal pH (7.35-7.38) and a $Paco_2$ >45 mm Hg.

**Activity intolerance** related to imbalance between oxygen supply and demand secondary to inefficient work of breathing

*Desired outcome:*   Patient reports decreasing dyspnea during activity or exercise and rates his or her perceived exertion at ≤3 on a 0-10 scale.

- Maintain prescribed activity levels and explain rationale to patient.
- Monitor patient's respiratory response to activity. Activity intolerance is indicated by excessively increased respiratory rate (e.g., >10 breaths/min above baseline) and depth, dyspnea, and use of accessory muscles of respiration. Ask patient to rate perceived exertion (see p. 711 for a description). If activity intolerance is noted, instruct patient to stop the activity and rest.
- Organize care so that periods of activity are interspersed with periods of at least 90 min of undisturbed rest.

- Assist patient with active ROM exercises to build stamina and prevent complications of decreased mobility. For more information, see **High risk for activity intolerance** in Appendix One, "Caring for Patients on Prolonged Bed Rest," p. 711.

---

**Note:**   See "Asthma" for **Impaired gas exchange,** p. 32. See "Chronic Bronchitis" for **Ineffective airway clearance,** p. 33, and **Altered nutrition:** Less than body requirements, p. 34. Also see psychosocial nursing diagnoses and interventions in Appendix One, "Caring for Patients with Cancer and Other Life-Disrupting Illnesses," p. 753.

---

PATIENT-FAMILY TEACHING AND DISCHARGE PLANNING
See "Chronic Bronchitis," p. 35.

# Section Four:   Restrictive Pulmonary Disorders

Restrictive lung disease is a category of pulmonary pathologies in which restricting alveolar inflation impairs lung function. Restrictive disorders are characterized by decreased vital capacity, reduced resting volumes, and normal airway resistance. Lung compliance (distensibility) decreases, and elastic recoil (deflating force) increases, resulting in an increase in the WOB. Physiologic consequences are similar for all restrictive processes and can be mildly, moderately, or severely debilitating for the patient. See Table 1-7 for some of the pathologies identified as causes of restrictive lung disease. This section discusses pulmonary fibrosis.

## Pulmonary fibrosis

The physiologic mechanisms in the development of pulmonary fibrosis are not clearly defined. It is theorized that pulmonary fibrosis occurs as a reaction to the inhalation of noxious materials or exposure to radiation. The fibrotic process is a continuous one and does not abate, even when the causative agent is no longer present. Fibrotic tissue forms as a natural process of tissue repair following infection, inflammation, or destruction of tissue. The fibrosis primarily affects the alveoli and causes an increase in the bronchial diameter in relation to lung volume. WOB is increased because of decreased lung compliance, and affected individuals adopt a rapid, shallow breathing pattern since it requires less energy. Cardiac complications can occur as a result of pulmonary hypertension.

### ASSESSMENT
The causative factors in pulmonary fibrosis are very difficult to uncover. A meticulous history of life-style, occupation, habits, and background can provide valuable information.
**Signs and symptoms:**   Dyspnea, cough.
**Physical assessment:**   Tachypnea, shallow respirations, cyanosis, digital clubbing, use of accessory muscles of respiration, and crackles.
**Risk factors:**   See Table 1-7.

### DIAGNOSTIC TESTS
**Chest x-ray:**   Reveals the extent of the fibrosis as evidenced by diffuse, mottled shadowing of the lung fields (honeycombing).
**Pulmonary function tests:**   Will demonstrate concentric reduction in lung volumes; normal airway resistance.

**T A B L E  1 - 7    Causative Factors in the Development of Restrictive Lung Disease**

| Extrapulmonary (involves respiratory muscles, pleura, and chest wall) | Intrapulmonary (involves lung parenchyma) |
|---|---|
| Bony deformities | Alveolar fibrosis, secondary to: |
|   Scoliosis |   Infection |
|   Ankylosing spondylitis |   Chronic aspiration |
| Neuromuscular disorders |   Inhalation of toxins |
|   Guillain-Barré syndrome |   Chemotherapy |
|   Amyotrophic lateral sclerosis |   Radiation therapy |
|   Myasthenia gravis |   Alveolar cell cancer |
|   Muscular dystrophy |   Goodpasture's syndrome |
| Pleural effusion |   Idiopathic |
| Pleural thickening | Pneumoconioses |
| Pneumothorax |   Asbestosis |
| Ascites |   Silicosis |
| Obesity |   Black lung |
| Pregnancy | Atelectasis |
| | Pulmonary edema |
| | Lung resection |

**ABG values:**   $Pao_2$ may be normal at rest but may decrease with exercise. $Paco_2$ may be within normal limits secondary to tachypnea but may increase in late stages of the disease.

**Lung biopsy:**   To determine cause and pathologic mechanism of the process.

## COLLABORATIVE MANAGEMENT

**Oxygen therapy:**   To correct the hypoxemia, which will relieve the dyspnea. Generally, low-flow (2-4 L/min) oxygen therapy is indicated.

**Corticosteroids:**   To decrease inflammation. Prednisone is usually given, at 1 mg/kg daily.

**Lung transplantation:**   Emerging as a therapy for patients who have a functional disability refractory to conventional therapies and a life expectancy of <18 months without transplantation.

## NURSING DIAGNOSES AND INTERVENTIONS

**Ineffective breathing pattern** related to decreased lung expansion secondary to fibrotic condition in the lungs

***Desired outcomes:***   Following treatment/intervention, patient verbalizes a subjective relief of dyspnea; patient moves toward a state of eupnea.

- Assess respiratory status q2-4h. Auscultate breath sounds and report increasing crackles or other adventitious sounds.
- Monitor patient's serial ABG values for decreasing $Pao_2$ and be alert to early signs of hypoxia (restlessness, anxiety, dyspnea), especially with activity.
- Assist patient in identifying ways to conserve energy during daily activities (e.g., planning frequent rest periods before and after activities as needed, stopping the activity and resting if dyspnea increases, and waiting for 1 h after eating before engaging in activities, because digestion draws blood and hence $O_2$ away from the muscles). As indicated, arrange for a consultation with occupational therapist or physical therapist.
- Deliver $O_2$ as prescribed. Remember that the $Pao_2$ may be normal at rest

but may decrease with exercise. The patient may require supplemental $O_2$ with activity.

---

**Note:** See "Chronic Bronchitis" for **Altered nutrition:** Less than body requirements, p. 34. See "Glomerulonephritis" for **Knowledge deficit:** Side effects of corticosteroids, p. 116. Also see psychosocial nursing diagnoses in Appendix One, "Caring for Patients with Cancer and Other Life-Disrupting Illnesses," p. 753.

---

### PATIENT-FAMILY TEACHING AND DISCHARGE PLANNING

Give patient and significant others verbal and written instructions about the following:
- Importance of pacing activities to tolerance and avoiding strenuous exercises that would increase cardiac and respiratory symptoms.
- Medications, including drug name, dosage, purpose, schedule, precautions, and potential side effects. It is likely that the patient will take corticosteroids while at home. Provide instructions accordingly to ensure that the patient takes the correct amount, particularly during the period in which the medication will be tapered.
- Use of $O_2$ and the necessary precautions if it is to be used at home.
- Avoiding exposure to individuals known to have pulmonary infections. Recommend annual flu and pneumococcal vaccines.
- Date and time of follow-up visit.

# Section Five:    Bronchogenic Carcinoma

In 1986 lung cancer became the number one cause of cancer deaths in American women. For over 40 years it has been the leading cancer killer in men. Of individuals diagnosed with lung cancer, 87% die in less than 5 years. The length of survival depends on the tumor histology and stage of the disease at the time treatment begins. Statistically, 80%-90% of lung cancer occurs among people who smoke tobacco. Environmental and occupational exposure to chemicals, toxins, and pollutants also may contribute to the development of this disease.

Lung cancer can be categorized as small-cell or nonsmall-cell cancer. *Small-cell lung cancer* (SCLC) is composed of classic or "oat" cells, intermediate cells, and mixed cells. SCLC accounts for 25%-30% of all lung cancers and has the following characteristics: (1) it arises from basal lining of bronchial mucosa; (2) shows rapid cell growth (is highly proliferative); (3) has propensity for widespread dissemination; and (4) is highly sensitive to cytotoxic drugs and radiation therapy. When first seen, approximately 60% of patients with SCLC have extensive disease and 40% have limited disease. The period of time between onset of symptoms and diagnosis is approximately 3-4 months, and a change in the character of a chronic cough is the typical presenting symptom. Tumors generally form in larger, central bronchi, causing obstruction, wheezing, coughing, and dyspnea. Hemoptysis occurs as cancers erode blood vessels and capillaries in the airways. The tumors can compress nerves, causing radiating chest pain.

*Nonsmall-cell lung cancer* (NSCLC) is composed of epidermoid (squamous cell), adenocarcinoma, and large-cell cancer. NSCLC accounts for approximately 70%-75% of all lung cancers and possesses the following characteristics: (1) it arises from large bronchi (squamous) or periphery of lung (adenocarcinoma); (2) it is slower growing (less proliferative); (3) squamous cell generally is less disseminated; (4) adenocarcinoma and large-cell often have distant metastases; (5) response to therapy is limited except for surgical excision (only form of treatment currently considered curative); and (6) it is generally not curable once metastasized outside the thoracic cavity.

Most patients have advanced disease at the time of diagnosis and receive multimodality therapy with minimal or partial response. Ultimately patients succumb to both local and distant disease with multiple complications. Tumors generally grow in the small peripheral bronchi and alveoli and may press against nerves in the pleural tissues. Typical presenting symptoms include shortness of breath and sharp chest pain on inspiration.

## ASSESSMENT

Patients often are asymptomatic in early stages of the disease process. When symptoms do occur they are likely to be vague and easily confused with other pulmonary conditions.

**Early indicators:**   Cough, dyspnea, SOB, change in character of sputum, hemoptysis, fatigue, dull chest pain, frequent respiratory infections.

**Advanced disease:**   Weakness, anorexia, dysphagia, hoarseness, weight loss.

**Physical assessment:**   Presence of adventitious breath sounds and pleural friction rub. In advanced disease, the patient may exhibit use of accessory muscles of respiration, nasal flaring, cyanosis, and severe muscle wasting.

## DIAGNOSTIC TESTS

**Sputum for cytology:**   Generally, a first morning specimen is obtained for 3 consecutive days. Sputum contains cells that shed from the tumor, which aids in identifying tumor type.

**Chest x-ray:**   To define tumor outline. X-ray may reveal presence of solitary nodules and possibly pleural effusion, atelectasis, and lymph node enlargement.

**Bronchoscopy:**   To visualize central tumor directly and take tissue samples for biopsy, along with bronchial washings.

**Fine-needle aspiration:**   Needle biopsy to obtain tissue samples from peripheral tumor for histologic exam.

**Lung tomogram:**   To locate tumor and determine depth and extent.

**Other tests:**   Once the cancer has metastasized from the primary site to nearby lymph nodes or distant organs, tests may include fluoroscopy, rib x-ray, abdominal and chest computerized axial tomography (CT) scan, bone studies, radionuclide studies, and bone marrow aspiration.

## COLLABORATIVE MANAGEMENT

The most effective intervention is prevention. Treatment of disease is planned according to histology, location, and extent of the disease.

**Surgery:**   To excise a tumor confined to lung tissue and remove involved lymph nodes.

**Radiation therapy:**   Use can be curative, adjuvant to chemotherapy/surgery, or palliative. It is used if the tumor has grown to adjacent tissues or if cancer has produced clearly defined secondary tumors elsewhere in the body. Usual dose is 2,500-6,000 cGy delivered over a 5-6 week period. This therapy generally shrinks tumors more often than eradicating them. Side effects include anorexia, esophagitis, dysphasia, radiation pneumonitis, and skin changes.

**Chemotherapy:**   Used when primary tumor extends beyond the lungs into surrounding tissues or metastasizes outside the lungs. It is also given to patients with SCLC whose disease has not yet spread beyond the lung. Treatment agents are generally used in combination. Drugs commonly used include cyclophosphamide, doxorubicin, methotrexate, procarbazine, mitomycin C, vinblastine, cisplatin, and bleomycin.

**Antiemetics:**   To control nausea and vomiting associated with chemotherapy. Generally, phenothiazines, metaclopramide, and steroids are used.

**Analgesics:**   To control pain.

**Sedatives:** Benzodiazepines are given for their amnesic effects, helping patients forget unpleasantness of the chemotherapy and thus promoting therapy continuation.

## NURSING DIAGNOSES AND INTERVENTIONS

**Pain** related to biologic and physiologic agents secondary to compression of nerves by the tumor

*Desired outcome:* Within 1 h of intervention, patient's subjective perception of pain decreases, as documented by a pain scale.

- Assess and document the following: location, description, onset, duration, and factors that precipitate and alleviate patient's pain. Devise a pain scale with the patient, rating pain from 0 (no pain) to 10 (worst pain).
- Offer prescribed analgesics. Encourage patient to ask for pain medication before pain becomes severe. If patient has more than one analgesic, confer with patient regarding which would be more beneficial for pain control. Document the amount of pain relief obtained using the pain scale.
- Position patient for comfort.
- Encourage patient to use relaxation techniques (e.g., deep breathing, imagery, meditation, and biofeedback) and diversional activities (e.g., television, books, radio, and crafts). For a description of an effective relaxation technique, see "Coronary Artery Disease" for **Health-seeking behaviors:** Relaxation technique effective for stress reduction, p. 54.
- For other effective pain interventions, see Appendix One, "Caring for Preoperative and Postoperative Patients," **Pain,** p. 694.

---

**Note:** See "Pulmonary Fibrosis" for **Ineffective breathing pattern** related to decreased lung expansion, p. 38. Also see Appendix One, "Caring for Preoperative and Postoperative Patients," p. 693, and "Caring for Patients with Cancer and other Life-Disrupting Illnesses," p. 719.

---

## PATIENT-FAMILY TEACHING AND DISCHARGE PLANNING

Give patient and significant others verbal and written instructions about the following:

- Signs and symptoms of respiratory complications that may necessitate medical attention: increased dyspnea, cyanosis, agitation.
- If surgery was performed, the indicators of wound infection: redness at wound site, local warmth, purulent drainage, pain, fever.
- Medications, including name, purpose, dosage, schedule, precautions, and potential side effects.
- Operation of all equipment that will be used at home, including $O_2$.
- Need for follow-up care with physician; confirm date and time of next appointment.
- Local American Cancer Society and American Lung Society programs. Provide available literature.

### Selected Bibliography

Anderson S: Six easy steps to interpreting blood gases, *Am J Nurs* 90(8):42-45, 1990.

Archibald C et al: Pulmonary alterations. In Thelan L et al: *Textbook of critical care nursing,* St Louis, 1990, Mosby–Year Book.

Conner P et al: Two stages of care for pleural effusion, *RN* 52:30-34, 1989.

Dettenmeier P et al: The respiratory system. In Beare P, Myers J, editors: *Principles and practices of adult health nursing,* St Louis, 1990, Mosby–Year Book.

DeVito AJ: Dyspnea during hospitalization for acute phase of illness as recalled by patients with chronic obstructive pulmonary disease, *Heart Lung* 19(2):186-191, 1990.

Ehrhardt B, Graham M: Pulse oximetry, *Nursing* 90(3):50-54, 1990.

Interqual: The ISD-A review system with adult ISD criteria, August 1992, Northhampton, NH, and Marlboro, MA, Interqual, Inc.

Fishman AP: *Pulmonary diseases and disorders,* ed 2, New York, 1988, McGraw-Hill Book Co.

Gerdes L: Recognizing the multisystem effects of embolism, *Nursing* 87(12):34-41, 1987.

Horne M, Heitz UE, Swearingen PL: *Fluid, electrolyte, and acid-base balance: a case study approach,* St Louis, 1991, Mosby–Year Book.

Howard C, Heitz UE: Respiratory dysfunctions. In Swearingen PL, Keen JH, editors: *Manual of critical care: applying nursing diagnoses to adult critical illness,* ed 2, St Louis, 1991, Mosby–Year Book.

How to use a metered dose inhaler, *Am J Nurs* 90(3):35-39, 1990.

Jackson MM: Infection control, *Lab Notes* 3(3):1-11, Fall 1992.

Kim MJ, McFarland GK, McLane AM: *Pocket guide to nursing diagnoses,* ed 5, St Louis, 1993, Mosby–Year Book.

Lancaster E: Tuberculosis in the OR, *Today's OR Nurse* 13(10):31-35, 1991.

Matus V, Glennon S: Pulmonary patient care problems. In Kinny M et al: *AACN's clinical reference for critical care nurses,* ed 2, New York, 1988, McGraw-Hill Book Co.

Roberts S: Pulmonary tissue perfusion, altered: emboli, *Heart Lung* 16(2):128-137, 1987.

Rostad M: Advances in nursing management of patients with lung cancer, *Nurs Clin North Am* 25(2):393-403, 1990.

Siskind MM: A standard of care for the nursing diagnosis of ineffective airway clearance, *Heart Lung* 18(5):477-482, 1989.

Thompson J: Respiratory system. In Thompson J et al: *Mosby's manual of clinical nursing,* ed 2, St Louis, 1989, Mosby–Year Book.

# 2 CARDIOVAS-CULAR DISORDERS

Section One   Degenerative Cardiovascular Disorders   44
   Pulmonary hypertension   44
   Cardiomyopathy   47
   Coronary artery disease   50
   Myocardial infarction   56
   Heart failure   60
Section Two   Inflammatory Heart Disorders   63
   Pericarditis   63
   Infective endocarditis   66
Section Three   Valvular Heart Disorders   69
   Mitral stenosis   69
   Mitral regurgitation   72
   Aortic stenosis   74
   Aortic regurgitation   75
Section Four   Cardiovascular Conditions Secondary to Other Disease
            Processes   76
   Cardiac and noncardiac shock (circulatory failure)   76
   Dysrhythmias and conduction disturbances   80
   Cardiac arrest   84
   Pulmonary edema   85
Section Five   Special Cardiac Procedures   88
   Pacemakers   88
   Cardiac catheterization and angioplasty   91
   Cardiac surgery   94
Section Six   Disorders of the Peripheral Vascular System   96
   Atherosclerotic arterial occlusive disease   96
   Aneurysms: abdominal, thoracic, and femoral   101
   Arterial embolism   103
   Venous thrombosis/Thrombophlebitis   104
   Varicose veins   107
Selected Bibliography   109

# Section One: Degenerative Cardiovascular Disorders

## Pulmonary hypertension

As blood passes through the pulmonary vasculature, it exchanges $CO_2$ and particulate matter for $O_2$. Normally the pulmonary vascular bed offers little resistance to blood flow, but when resistance occurs, pulmonary hypertension results. Pulmonary hypertension can be primary (rare), which has a poor prognosis and affects primarily young and middle-aged women, or it can be secondary (most common), which often responds to therapy and is found in a variety of medical conditions. Possible causes of secondary pulmonary hypertension include increased pulmonary blood flow from a ventricular or atrial shunt, left ventricular failure, chronic hypoxia related to chronic obstructive pulmonary disease (COPD), pulmonary embolus, pulmonary stenosis, or any physiologic occurrence that increases pulmonary vascular resistance or constriction of the vessels in the pulmonary tree.

### ASSESSMENT

**Acute indicators:** Exertional dyspnea, syncope, and precordial chest pain, all of which result from low cardiac output or hypoxia. Cough and palpitations can also occur.
**Chronic indicators:** Signs of right or left ventricular failure:
*Right ventricular failure:* Peripheral edema, increased venous pressure and pulsations, liver engorgement, distended neck veins.
*Left ventricular failure:* Dyspnea; SOB, particularly on exertion; decreased BP; oliguria; orthopnea; anorexia.
**Physical assessment:** Cyanosis from decreased cardiac output and subsequent systemic vasoconstriction, systolic murmur caused by tricuspid regurgitation or pulmonary stenosis, diastolic murmur due to pulmonary valvular incompetence, and accentuated $S_2$ heart sound.

### DIAGNOSTIC TESTS

**Chest x-ray:** Will show enlargement of the pulmonary artery and right atrium and ventricle.
**Echocardiography:** Often valuable for showing increased right ventricular dimension, thickened right ventricular wall, and possible tricuspid or pulmonary valve dysfunction.
**Radionuclide imaging:** For example, equilibrium-gated blood pool imaging and thallium imaging to assess function of the right ventricle.
**Cardiac catheterization with angiography:** Necessary to confirm pulmonary hypertension. Pulmonary vascular resistance will be very high, and pulmonary artery and right ventricular pressures can approach or equal systemic arterial pressures. (See "Cardiac Catheterization and Angioplasty," p. 91, for further detail.)
**Pulmonary perfusion scintigraphy** (perfusion scan): A noninvasive way to assess pulmonary blood flow. This study involves IV injection of serum albumin tagged with trace amounts of a radioisotope, most often technetium. The particles pass through the circulation and lodge in the pulmonary vascular bed. Subsequent scanning reveals concentrations of particles in areas of adequate pulmonary blood flow.
**ECG:** Will show evidence of right atrial enlargement and right ventricular enlargement (evidenced by right axis deviation and tall, peaked P waves) secondary to the increased pressure needed to force blood through the hypertensive pulmonary vascular bed.
**Pulmonary function test:** Results are usually normal, although some indi-

viduals will have increased residual volume, reduced maximum voluntary ventilation, and decreased vital capacity.

**ABG analysis:**  May show low $Paco_2$ and high pH, which occur with hyperventilation, or increased $Paco_2$ with decreased gas exchange.

**CBC:**  Polycythemia can occur in the presence of chronic hypoxemia due to compensation.

**Liver function tests:**  May be abnormal if venous congestion is significant. Examples include increased serum glutamic-oxaloacetic transaminase (SGOT), serum glutamic-pyruvic transaminase (SGPT), and bilirubin.

**Open lung biopsy:**  May be done to establish the type of disorder causing the hypertension.

## COLLABORATIVE MANAGEMENT

**$O_2$:**  Usually 2-5 L/min by nasal cannula. If hypoxia is severe, $O_2$ is administered by mask. **Caution:** Use care when administering $O_2$ to patients with a history of COPD.

**Diet:**  Low in Na (see Table 3-2, p. 115) if signs of heart failure are present.

**Pharmacotherapy**

*Diuretics:*  If indicators of right- or left-sided heart failure are present.

*Anticoagulants (warfarin sodium):*  Although prophylactic use is controversial, it may be administered if pulmonary emboli are present.

*Vasodilators and calcium antagonists:*  To decrease cardiac work load by vasodilatation.

*Bronchodilators (aminophylline):*  Have been shown to reduce pulmonary artery and right ventricular pressures in some cases.

*Beta-adrenergic agents such as terbutaline:*  To decrease pulmonary vascular resistance.

**Treatment of causative factor if possible:**  For example, by surgically closing arteriovenous shunts or replacing defective valves.

**Heart-lung transplantation:**  For advanced pulmonary vascular disease.

## NURSING DIAGNOSES AND INTERVENTIONS

**Impaired gas exchange** related to altered blood flow secondary to pulmonary capillary constriction

*Desired outcome:*  Patient has improved gas exchange by a minimum of the 24-h period before hospital discharge, as evidenced by $Pao_2$ $\geq$80 mm Hg.

- Monitor ABG results for evidence of hypoventilation: decreased $Pao_2$, increased $Paco_2$, and decreased pH; and for hyperventilation: low $Paco_2$ and high pH.
- Auscultate lung fields q4-8h to assess lung sounds. Note the presence of adventitious sounds, which can occur with fluid extravasation.
- Assess respiratory rate, pattern, and depth; chest excursion; and use of accessory muscles of respiration q4h.
- Observe for and document presence of cyanosis or skin color change, which can occur with decreased gas exchange.
- Teach patient to take slow, deep breaths to enhance gas exchange.
- Assist patient into Fowler's position, if possible, to decrease WOB and maximize chest excursion.
- Administer prescribed low-flow $O_2$ as indicated.

**Activity intolerance** related to generalized weakness and imbalance between oxygen supply and demand secondary to right and left ventricular failure

*Desired outcome:*  By a minimum of the 24-h period before hospital discharge, patient rates perceived exertion at $\leq$3 on a 0-10 scale and exhibits cardiac tolerance to activity as evidenced by RR $\leq$20 breaths/min, HR $\leq$20 bpm over resting HR, and systolic BP within 20 mm Hg of resting range.

- Monitor patient for evidence of activity intolerance and ask patient to rate perceived exertion (see Appendix One, p. 711, for a description).
- Observe for and document any changes in VS. Monitor BP at least q4h.

Report drops >10-20 mm Hg, which can signal decompensation of the cardiac muscle. Also be alert to other signs of left ventricular failure, including dyspnea, SOB, and crackles (rales).

- Measure and document I&O, as well as weight, reporting any steady gains or losses. Be alert to other signs of right ventricular failure, including peripheral edema, both pedal and sacral; ascites; distended neck veins; and increased CVP (>12 cm $H_2O$).
- Administer diuretics, vasodilators, and calcium channel blockers as prescribed.
- Provide periods of undisturbed rest; limit visitors as appropriate.
- Keep frequently used items within patient's reach so that exertion can be avoided as much as possible.
- Assist patient with maintaining prescribed activity level and progress as tolerated. If activity intolerance is observed, stop the activity and have patient rest.
- Assist patient with ROM exercises at frequent intervals. To help prevent complications caused by immobility, plan progressive ambulation and exercise based on patient's tolerance and prescribed activity restrictions (see Appendix One, "Caring for Patients on Prolonged Bed Rest," **High risk for activity intolerance,** p. 711, and **High risk for disuse syndrome,** p. 713).

**Knowledge deficit:**    Disease process and treatment
*Desired outcome:*    Within 24 h before hospital discharge, patient and significant others verbalize knowledge of the disease, its treatment, and measures that promote wellness.

- Assess the patient's level of knowledge of the disease process and its treatment.
- Discuss the purposes of the medications: to ease the work load of the heart (vasodilators); "relax" the heart (calcium antagonists); and prevent fluid accumulation (diuretics).
- Support patient in dealing with the concept of having a chronic disease.
- If the cause of pulmonary hypertension is known, reinforce explanations of the disease process, treatment, and the need for changing life-style, if appropriate.
- Explain the value of relaxation techniques, including tapes, soothing music, meditation, and biofeedback. See "Coronary Artery Disease," **Health-seeking behaviors:** Relaxation technique effective for stress reduction, p. 54.
- If the patient smokes, explain that smoking increases the work load of the heart by causing vasoconstriction. Provide materials that explain the benefits of quitting smoking, such as pamphlets prepared by the American Heart Association.
- Confer with physician about type of exercise program that will benefit the patient; provide patient teaching as indicated.
- If appropriate, involve the dietitian to assist patient with planning low-sodium meals.

---

**Note:**    See "Heart Failure" for **Fluid volume excess,** p. 61, **Knowledge deficit:** Precautions and side effects of diuretic therapy, p. 62, and **Knowledge deficit:** Precautions and side effects of vasodilators, p. 62. Also see psychosocial nursing diagnoses in Appendix One, "Caring for Patients with Cancer and Other Life-Disrupting Illnesses," p.753.

---

## PATIENT-FAMILY TEACHING AND DISCHARGE PLANNING

Give patient and significant others verbal and written information about the following:

- Indicators that necessitate medical attention: decreased exercise tolerance, increasing SOB or dyspnea, swelling of ankles and legs, steady weight gain.

- Medications, including drug name, purpose, dosage, schedule, precautions, and potential side effects.
- For additional information see **Knowledge deficit,** above.

# Cardiomyopathy

Cardiomyopathy is a disorder of the heart muscle, usually of unknown origin. It is classified according to abnormalities in structure and function. The disorder involves the heart muscle and usually results in heart failure.

**Dilated (or congestive) cardiomyopathy:**   Characterized by dilatation of all four of the heart chambers, especially the ventricles. Contractile dysfunction usually is the first sign, followed by congestive heart failure. There is progressive deterioration of cardiac muscle function caused by toxic (e.g., alcohol), metabolic (e.g., thyrotoxicosis), or infectious (bacterial, viral) agents. Pathophysiologic changes include loss of functioning myofibrils, decreased contractile strength, and dilatation followed by sympathetic nervous system stimulation, increased myocardial oxygen consumption, increased pulmonary pressures, increased venous pressures, and heart failure.

**Hypertrophic cardiomyopathy:**   Characterized by an abnormally hypertrophied left ventricle that is not accompanied by a concomitant increase in cavity size. Therefore, filling is restricted, and there is the potential for outflow obstruction. This causes increased left atrial and left ventricular pressures, resulting in increased work load and increased pulmonary pressures causing dyspnea. Cardiac function can remain normal for varying periods of time before decompensation occurs. Symptoms include increased diastolic BP, decreased cardiac output, pulmonary hypertension, and right ventricular failure. Although it is theorized that hypertrophic cardiomyopathy has a strong hereditary link, the etiology is unknown. Possible causes include increased circulating catecholamine levels, subendocardial ischemia, or abnormal conduction patterns that lead to abnormal ventricular contraction.

**Restrictive cardiomyopathy:**   Least common in Western countries, it is characterized by restrictive ventricular filling caused by fibrosis, infiltration, hypertrophy, and cardiac stiffness.

## ASSESSMENT

**Signs and symptoms:**   Dyspnea usually is the symptom that brings the patient to the physician. Decreased exercise tolerance, fatigue, weakness, syncope, peripheral edema, palpitations, right or left ventricular failure, and peripheral or pulmonary emboli also can occur. Chest pain may occur owing to ischemia of the hypertrophied muscle.

**Physical assessment:**   Presence of $S_3$ or $S_4$ heart sounds and valve murmurs, systolic murmur, prominent apical pulse, increased venous pressure and pulsations, crackles (rales), decreased BP, and increased HR and RR related to decreased cardiac output. In addition, hepatomegaly and mild to severe cardiomegaly may be present.

## DIAGNOSTIC TESTS

**Chest x-ray:**   To detect cardiac enlargement, particularly of the ventricle and left atrium. Pulmonary hypertension also may be seen.

**ECG results:**   Determined by the extent and location of myocardial involvement. ECG changes indicative of cardiomyopathy include left ventricular hypertrophy, conduction defects, nonspecific ST-segment changes, and Q waves that resemble those found with infarction.

**Echocardiography:**   Will identify thickened ventricular walls, septal thickening, and chamber dilatation or restriction, depending on the type of cardiomyopathy. Poor contractility also may be seen if myocardial muscle deterioration has progressed.

**Cardiac catheterization:**  Does not confirm cardiomyopathy, but it can be valuable for ruling out other disorders such as ischemic heart disease. Findings may include decreased cardiac output, decreased ventricular movement, increased filling pressures, and valvular regurgitation. See "Cardiac Catheterization and Angioplasty," p. 91, for further detail.

**Endomyocardial biopsy:**  Sometimes necessary to identify the type of pathologic agent; it can be done during the cardiac catheterization procedure.

**Radionuclide studies:**  May demonstrate contractile dysfunction.

## COLLABORATIVE MANAGEMENT

Medical management is aimed toward support, maintenance of normal function for as long as possible, and delaying disease progression.

**Controlling symptoms of heart failure:**  See "Heart Failure," p. 61.

**Limiting or restricting activity:**  To decrease $O_2$ demand. Activity is increased gradually.

**Prohibiting alcohol intake:**  Alcohol can worsen myopathy.

**Pharmacotherapy**

*Antiarrhythmic agents:*  To control dysrhythmias.

*Beta-blockers:*  To decrease outflow obstruction during exercise.

*Calcium antagonists:*  To produce arterial vasodilatation, decrease cardiac work load, and improve symptoms and exercise capacity.

*Anticoagulants (warfarin sodium):*  To prevent embolus formation.

*Diuretics:*  To decrease pulmonary congestion.

*Vasodilators:*  To decrease cardiac work load.

*Inotropic agents:*  To increase contractile strength.

**Surgical replacement of valves:**  See "Cardiac Surgery," p. 94.

**Cardiac transplant.**

## NURSING DIAGNOSES AND INTERVENTIONS

**Decreased cardiac output** related to negative inotropic changes in the heart (decreased cardiac contractility) secondary to cardiac muscle changes

*Desired outcomes:*  By a minimum of 24 h before hospital discharge, patient has adequate cardiac output as evidenced by systolic BP ≥90 mm Hg, HR ≤100 bpm, urinary output ≥30 ml/h, stable weight, eupnea, normal breath sounds, and edema ≤1+ on a 0-4+ scale. By a minimum of 48 h before hospital discharge, patient is free of new dysrhythmias. Patient remains oriented to person, place, and time.

- Assess for, document, and report evidence of decreased cardiac output, such as edema, jugular venous distention, adventitious breath sounds, SOB, decreased urinary output, extra heart sound such as $S_3$, changes in LOC, cool extremities, hypotension, tachycardia, and tachypnea.
- Keep accurate I&O records; weigh patient daily.
- Help minimize patient's cardiac work load by assisting with ADL and ensuring 90-min periods of undisturbed rest.
- Administer medications as prescribed, such as beta blockers, calcium channel blockers, and antiarrhythmics.
- Assist patient in position of comfort, usually semi-Fowler's position.

**Altered cardiopulmonary and peripheral tissue perfusion (or risk of same)** related to interrupted arterial or venous flow secondary to embolus formation

*Desired outcome:*  Within 1-2 h of treatment/intervention, patient's tissue perfusion is adequate as evidenced by eupnea, absence of chest pain, warm extremities, and peripheral pulses >2+ on a 0-4+ scale.

- Observe for and report indicators of pulmonary emboli (e.g., sudden onset of chest pain, dyspnea, SOB, and hemoptysis). For more information, see "Pulmonary Embolus," p. 13.
- Observe for and report indicators of peripheral emboli (e.g., decreased peripheral pulses and calf pain or tenderness).

- In the *absence* of decreased peripheral pulses and calf pain or tenderness, assess for a positive Homan's sign by flexing the knee 30 degrees and dorsiflexing the foot. Pain elicited in the calf signifies a positive Homan's sign, which occurs in the presence of deep-vein thrombosis. Report significant findings to physician. **Note:** For patients who are asymptomatic for embolization, see interventions for prevention of this disorder in **Altered peripheral tissue perfusion,** p. 715, in Appendix One.
- Administer prescribed anticoagulants (e.g., warfarin) to prevent embolus formation.

**Activity intolerance** related to imbalance between oxygen supply and demand secondary to decrease in cardiac muscle contractility

*Desired outcome:* During activity, patient rates perceived exertion at ≤3 on a 0-10 scale and exhibits cardiac tolerance to activity as evidenced by RR ≤20 breaths/min, systolic BP within 20 mm Hg of resting range, HR within 20 bpm of resting HR, and absence of chest pain and new dysrhythmias.

- Monitor patient's physiologic response to activity. Report chest pain, new dysrhythmias, increased SOB, HR increased >20 bpm over resting HR, and systolic BP >20 mm Hg over resting systolic BP. Ask patient to rate perceived exertion (see p. 711 for a description).
- Monitor BP and VS q4h, and report changes such as irregular HR, HR >100 bpm, or decreasing BP.
- Observe for and report signs of acute decreased cardiac output, including oliguria, decreasing BP, decreased mentation, and dizziness.
- Assess integrity of peripheral perfusion by monitoring peripheral pulses and urine output. Report changes such as decreased amplitude of pulses and decreased urinary output.
- In the presence of acute decreased cardiac output, ensure that the patient's needs are met so that activity can be avoided (e.g., by keeping water at the bedside and urinal or commode nearby, maintaining a quiet environment, and limiting visitors as necessary).
- Plan nursing care to allow for 90-min periods of undisturbed rest.
- Administer medications as prescribed.
- To help prevent complications caused by immobility, assist patient with passive and some active or assistive ROM and other exercises, depending on patient's tolerance and prescribed limitations. For discussion of a progressive in-bed exercise program, see Appendix One, "Caring for Patients on Prolonged Bed Rest," **High risk for activity intolerance,** p. 711, and **High risk for disuse syndrome,** p. 713.

---

**Note:** See "Pulmonary Embolus" for **Altered protection** related to risk of prolonged bleeding or hemorrhage secondary to anticoagulant therapy, p. 17. See "Pulmonary Hypertension" for **Activity intolerance,** p. 45. See "Coronary Artery Disease" for **Knowledge deficit:** Precautions and side effects of beta blockers, p. 54. See "Heart Failure" for **Knowledge deficit:** Precautions and side effects of diuretic therapy, p. 62, and **Knowledge deficit:** Precautions and side effects of vasodilators, p. 62, and **Fluid volume excess,** p. 62. Also see Appendix One, "Caring for Patients on Prolonged Bed Rest," p. 711, and psychosocial nursing diagnoses and interventions in "Caring for Patients with Cancer and Other Life-Disrupting Illnesses," p. 753.

---

## PATIENT-FAMILY TEACHING AND DISCHARGE PLANNING

Give patient and significant others verbal and written information about the following:

- Medications, including drug name, purpose, dosage, schedule, precautions, and potential side effects.
- Signs and symptoms that necessitate immediate medical attention: dyspnea,

decreased exercise tolerance, alterations in pulse rate/rhythm, loss of consciousness (caused by dysrhythmias or decreased cardiac output), and steady weight gain (caused by heart failure).
• Reinforcement that cardiomyopathy is a chronic disease requiring lifetime treatment.
• Importance of abstaining from alcohol, which increases cardiac muscle deterioration.
• Need for physical support from family and outside agencies as disease progresses.
• Availability of community and medical support such as American Heart Association.

# Coronary artery disease

The coronary arteries are the vessels that supply the myocardial muscle with $O_2$ and the nutrients necessary for optimal function. Atherosclerotic lesions within these arteries are a major cause of obstruction and subsequent ischemia, which ultimately can lead to myocardial infarction (MI). Other mechanisms include spasm, platelet aggregation, and thrombus formation. The most common symptom of coronary artery disease (CAD) is angina (Table 2-1), a result of decreasing blood flow and decreased $O_2$ supply through narrowed or obstructed arteries (ischemia). This often occurs during exercise, but it may occur at rest or during a condition of decreased perfusion, such as an episode of hypotension. Often, CAD is diagnosed only after the patient is seen for angina or MI. It is important to note that symptoms do not appear until approximately 75% of the artery is occluded.

## ASSESSMENT

**Chronic indicators:**   Stable or progressively worsening angina that occurs when myocardial demand for $O_2$ is more than the supply, such as during exercise. The pain usually is described as pressure or a crushing or burning substernal pain that radiates down one or both arms. It also can be felt in the neck, cheeks, and teeth. Usually it is relieved by discontinuation of exercise or administration of nitroglycerine (NTG).
**Acute indicators:**   CAD is considered unstable (acute) when angina becomes more frequent and is unrelieved by NTG and rest, when it occurs during sleep or rest, or when it occurs with progressively lower levels of exercise.
**Risk factors:**   Family history, race, increasing age, male gender, smoking, high serum and lipid levels, hypertension, obesity, abnormal glucose tolerance, sedentary and stressful life-style.

## DIAGNOSTIC TESTS

**ECG:**   Usually normal unless MI has occurred or the individual is experiencing angina at the time of the test. If performed during angina, characteristic changes include ST-segment depression in leads over the area of ischemia.
**Chest x-ray:**   Usually normal unless heart failure is present.
**Treadmill exercise test:**   To determine the amount of exercise that causes angina, as well as the degree of ischemia and the ECG changes produced. Significant findings can include 1 mm or more ST-segment depression or elevation and ventricular ectopic beats.
**Radionuclide studies**
  • Infarct imaging: Use of an imaging agent, usually technetium pyrophosphate, that concentrates in the infarcted zone.
  • Myocardial perfusion imaging: Use of an imaging agent, usually thallium, that concentrates in "normal" tissue.
  • Radionuclide ventriculography: Enables visualization of the ventricular muscle during the cardiac cycle.

**T A B L E  2 - 1  Classification of Angina**

**Stable:** Pattern of frequency, duration, and severity stable over several months.

**Unstable:** Pattern of frequency, duration, or severity changed or increased; associated with decreased exercise or exertion.

**Preinfarction (also called crescendo):** Unstable, with progression to MI possible (term sometimes used interchangably with *unstable*).

**Prinzmetal's (also called variant):** Often occurs at rest (unrelated to exercise) or during sleep; usually caused by coronary artery spasm.

**Intractable:** Continuous or frequent; unrelieved by therapy.

---

**Ambulatory monitoring:**  A 24-h ECG monitoring that can show activity-induced ST-segment changes or ischemia-induced dysrhythmias.

**Coronary arteriography *via* cardiac catheterization:**  Provides the ultimate diagnosis of CAD. Arterial lesions (plaque) are located, and the amount of occlusion is determined. At this time, feasibility for coronary artery bypass grafting (CABG) or angioplasty is determined. For details, see "Cardiac Surgery," p. 94, and "Collaborative Management," below.

**Serum enzymes:**  To rule out acute MI.

## COLLABORATIVE MANAGEMENT

**Management of risk factors:**  Eliminating tobacco, reducing BP, reducing serum lipid levels, controlling weight and stress, and initiating an exercise program.

**Oxygen by nasal cannula:**  During angina attacks.

**Pharmacotherapy**

*Sublingual NTG:*  During angina to increase microcirculation, perfusion to the myocardium, and venodilatation.

*Beta blockers:*  To decrease $O_2$ demand of the myocardium.

*Angiotensin-converting enzyme such as enalapril:*  To reduce $O_2$ demands by decreasing BP.

*Long-acting nitrates or topical NTG:*  For anginal prophylaxis.

*Calcium channel blockers such as nifedipine, diltiazem:*  To decrease coronary artery vasospasm and decrease $O_2$ demand.

**Diet:**  Low in cholesterol (Table 2-2), saturated fat (Table 2-3), Na (Table 3-2, p. 115), calories, and triglycerides, as appropriate.

**Percutaneous transluminal coronary angioplasty (PTCA):**  A procedure that improves coronary blood flow by using a balloon inflation catheter to compress plaque material into the vessel wall. Performed in the cardiac catheterization laboratory with a local anesthetic and mild sedation, it is a common alternative to bypass surgery for individuals with discrete lesions.

**Directional coronary atherectomy:**  A relatively new procedure for removal of atherosclerotic deposits in the coronary arteries. It involves use of a special catheter and contains a balloon (for stabilization of the catheter), a cutting device that "shaves" the lesion, and a nose cone in which the shaved lesions are placed. Usually it is performed in the catheterization laboratory.

## NURSING DIAGNOSES AND INTERVENTIONS

**Pain** (angina) related to decreased oxygen supply to the myocardium

*Desired outcomes:*  Within 30 min of onset of pain, patient's subjective perception of angina decreases, as documented by a pain scale. Objective indicators, such as grimacing and diaphoresis, are absent.

• Assess the location, character, and severity of pain. Record the severity on

### T A B L E  2 - 2   Guidelines for a Low-Cholesterol Diet

| Foods to avoid | Foods allowed |
|---|---|
| Egg yolks (no more than three per week) | Egg whites, cholesterol-free egg substitutes |
| Foods made with many egg yolks (e.g., sponge cakes) | Lean, well-trimmed meats; minimize servings of beef, lamb, and pork |
| Fatty cuts of meat, fat on meats | Fish (except shellfish), chicken, and turkey (without the skin) |
| Skin on chicken and turkey | |
| Luncheon meats or cold cuts | |
| Sausage, frankfurters | Dried peas and beans as meat substitutes |
| Shellfish (e.g., lobster, shrimp, crab) | Nonfat (skim) or lowfat (2%) milk |
| Whole milk, cream, whole milk cheese | Partially skim-milk cheeses |
| Ice cream | Ice milk and sherbet |
| Commercially prepared foods with hydrogenated shortening (saturated fat) | Polyunsaturated oils for cooking and food preparation: corn, safflower, cottonseed, sesame, and sunflower |
| Coconut and palm oils and products made with them (e.g., cream substitutes) | Margarines that list one of the above oils as their first ingredient |
| Butter, lard, hydrogenated shortening | Foods prepared "from scratch" with the above suggested oils |
| Meats and vegetables prepared by frying | |
| Seasonings containing large amounts of sugar and saturated fats | Meats (in acceptable quantity) and vegetables prepared by broiling, steaming, or baking (never frying) |
| Sauces and gravies | |
| Salad dressings containing cream, cheeses, or mayonnaise | Spices, herbs, lemon juice, wine, flavored wine vinegars |

From Steuble BT. In Swearingen PL, Keen JH: *Manual of critical care: applying nursing diagnoses to adult critical illness,* ed 2, St Louis, 1991, Mosby–Year Book, Inc.

### T A B L E  2 - 3   Guidelines for a Diet Low in Saturated Fat

| Foods to avoid | Foods to choose |
|---|---|
| Red meat, especially when highly "marbled;" salami, sausages, bacon | Lean cuts of meat, fresh fish, poultry with skin removed before cooking, grilled meats |
| Whole milk, whipping cream | Lowfat or skim milk |
| Tropical oils (coconut, palm oils; cocoa butter) | Monosaturated cooking oils, such as olive or canola oil |
| Candy | |
| Sweet rolls, donuts | Fresh fruit, vegetables |
| Ice cream | Whole grain breads, cereals |
| Salad dressings | Nonfat yogurt, sherbet |
| Peanut butter, peanuts, hot dogs, potato chips | Vinegar, lemon juice |
| | Unbuttered popcorn |
| Butter | Margarine (safflower oil listed as the first ingredient) |

From Steuble BT. In Swearingen PL, Keen JH: *Manual of critical care: applying nursing diagnoses to adult critical illness,* ed 2, St Louis, 1991, Mosby–Year Book, Inc.

a subjective 0 (no pain) to 10 (worst pain) scale. Also record the number of NTG tablets needed to relieve each episode, the factor or event that precipitated the pain, and alleviating factors. Document angina relief obtained, using the pain scale.

- Keep sublingual NTG within reach of patient, and explain that it is to be administered as soon as angina begins, repeating q5min × 3 if necessary.
- Stay with patient and provide reassurance during periods of angina. If indicated, request that visitors leave the room.
- Monitor HR and BP during episodes of chest pain. Be alert to and report irregularities in HR and changes in systolic BP >20 mm Hg from baseline.
- Monitor for presence of headache and hypotension after administering NTG. Keep patient recumbent during angina and NTG administration.
- Administer $O_2$ as prescribed to increase $O_2$ supply to the myocardium.
- Emphasize to patient the importance of immediately reporting angina to health-care team.
- Avoid activities and factors that are known to cause stress and may precipitate angina.
- Discuss the value of relaxation techniques, including tapes, soothing music, biofeedback, meditation, or yoga. See **Health-seeking behaviors,** which follows.
- Administer beta blockers and calcium channel blockers as prescribed to decrease cardiac work load and $O_2$ demand.
- Administer long-acting and/or topical nitrates to decrease $O_2$ demand and likelihood of angina.

**Activity intolerance** related to generalized weakness and imbalance between oxygen supply and demand secondary to tissue ischemia (MI)

*Desired outcome:* During activity, patient rates perceived exertion at ≤3 on a 0-10 scale and exhibits cardiac tolerance to activity as evidenced by RR ≤20 breaths/min, HR ≤120 bpm (or within 20 bpm of resting HR), systolic BP within 20 mm Hg of patient's resting systolic BP, and absence of chest pain and new dysrhythmias.

- Observe for and report increasing frequency of angina, angina that occurs at rest, angina that is unrelieved by NTG, or decreased exercise tolerance without angina.
- Assess patient's response to activity. Be alert to chest pain, increase in HR (>20 bpm), change in systolic BP (20 mm Hg over or under resting BP), excessive fatigue, and SOB. Ask patient to rate perceived exertion (see p. 711 for detail).
- Assist patient with recognizing and limiting activities that increase $O_2$ demands, such as exercise and anxiety.
- Maintain $O_2$ as prescribed for angina episodes.
- Have patient perform ROM exercises, depending on tolerance and prescribed activity limitations. Because cardiac intolerance to activity can be further aggravated by prolonged bed rest, consult with physician about in-bed exercises and activities that can be performed by the patient as the condition improves. Examples are found in Appendix One, "Caring for Patients on Prolonged Bed Rest," **High risk for activity intolerance,** p. 711, and **High risk for disuse syndrome,** p. 713.

**Altered nutrition:** More than body requirements of calories, sodium, or fats

*Desired outcome:* Within the 24-h period before hospital discharge, patient demonstrates knowledge of the dietary regimen by planning a 3-day menu that includes and excludes appropriate foods.

- If patient is over ideal body weight, explain that a low-calorie diet is necessary.
- Teach patient how to decrease dietary intake of saturated (animal) fats and increase intake of polyunsaturated (vegetable oil) fats. See Table 2-3.
- Teach patient to limit dietary intake of cholesterol to <300 mg/day (see Table 2-2).

- Teach patient to limit dietary intake of refined/processed sugar.
- Teach patient to limit dietary intake of sodium chloride (NaCl) to <4 g/day (mild restriction).
- Encourage intake of fresh fruits, natural carbohydrates, fish, poultry, legumes, fresh vegetables, and grains for a healthy, balanced diet.

**Health-seeking behaviors:**   Relaxation technique effective for stress reduction

*Desired outcome:*   Patient reports subjective relief of stress after using relaxation technique.

- Discuss with patient the importance of relaxation for decreasing nervous system tone (sympathetic), energy requirements, and $O_2$ consumption.
- Many techniques use breathing, concentration, or imagery to promote relaxation and decrease energy requirements. The following is an example of a technique that can be used easily by anyone. Speaking slowly and softly, give patient the following guidelines:
  - Find a comfortable position. Close your eyes.
  - Relax all your muscles. First, concentrate on your toes. Relax your toes. Now move to your feet. Relax the muscles of your feet. Continue with each muscle group, moving up your body, until finally you reach your facial muscles. Concentrate on your facial muscles and relax them.
  - Now breathe through your nose. Concentrate on feeling the air move in and out. As you exhale, say the word *one* silently to yourself. Again, continue feeling the air move in and out of your lungs. Continue for approximately 20 min.
  - Try to clear your mind of worries; be passive. Let relaxation occur. If distractions appear, gently push them away. Continue breathing through your nose, repeating *one* silently.
  - After approximately 20 min, slowly begin to allow yourself to become aware of your surroundings. Keep your eyes closed for a few moments.
  - Open your eyes.
- Encourage patient to practice this technique two to three times/day or whenever feeling stressed or tense. Acknowledge that this technique may feel strange at first but that it becomes easier and more effective with each practice.
- Explain that baroque music, played softly, helps many individuals achieve an even greater state of relaxation.

**Knowledge deficit:**   Precautions and side effects of nitrates

*Desired outcome:*   Within the 24-h period before hospital discharge, patient verbalizes understanding of the precautions and side effects of the prescribed medication.

- Instruct patient to report to physician or staff the presence of a headache associated with NTG, in which case the physician may alter the dose.
- Teach patient to assume a recumbent position if a headache occurs. Explain that the vasodilation effect of the drug causes a decrease in BP, which can result in orthostatic hypotension and transient headache.

**Knowledge deficit:**   Precautions and side effects of beta-blockers

*Desired outcome:*   Within the 24-h period before hospital discharge, patient verbalizes understanding of the precautions and side effects of beta-blockers.

- Instruct patient to be alert to depression, fatigue, dizziness, erythematous rash, respiratory distress, and sexual dysfunction, which can occur as side effects of beta-blockers. Explain the importance of notifying physician promptly if these side effects occur.
- Explain that weight gain and peripheral and sacral edema can occur as side effects of beta-blockers. Teach patient how to assess for edema and the importance of reporting signs and symptoms promptly if they occur.
- Explain that BP and HR are assessed before administration of beta blockers because the drug can cause hypotension and excessive slowing of the heart.

- Caution patient not to omit or abruptly stop taking β-blockers, because this can result in rebound angina or even MI.

**Knowledge deficit:** Disease process and life-style implications of CAD

*Desired outcome:* Within the 24-h period before hospital discharge, patient verbalizes knowledge about the disease process of CAD and the concomitant life-style implications.

- Teach patient about CAD, including the pathophysiologic processes of cardiac ischemia, angina, and infarction.
- Assist patient with identifying risk factors for CAD and risk factor modification as follows.
  - Diet low in cholesterol and saturated fat
  - Smoking cessation
  - Regular activity/exercise programs
- Discuss symptoms that necessitate medical attention, such as chest pain unrelieved by NTG.
- Discuss guidelines for sexual activity, such as resting before intercourse, finding a comfortable position, taking prophylactic NTG, and postponing intercourse for 1-1½ h after a heavy meal.
- Discuss medical procedures, such as cardiac catheterization, and surgical procedures, such as PTCA and CABG, if appropriate.

## PATIENT-FAMILY TEACHING AND DISCHARGE PLANNING

Give patient and significant others verbal and written information about the following:

- Medications, including drug name, dosage, purpose, schedule, precautions, and potential side effects. Discuss the potential for headache and dizziness after NTG administration. Caution patient about using NTG more frequently than prescribed and notifying physician if 3 tablets do not relieve angina.
- Importance of reducing intake of caffeine, which causes vasoconstriction and increases HR.
- Dietary changes: low saturated fat (Table 2-3), low Na (see Table 3-2, p. 115), low cholesterol (Table 2-2), and the need for weight loss if appropriate.
- Prescribed exercise program and importance of maintaining a regular exercise schedule. Remind patient of the need to measure pulse, stop if pain occurs, and stay within prescribed exercise limits. See Table 2-4 for a progressive at-home walking program.
- Indicators that necessitate medical attention: progression to unstable angina, loss of consciousness, decreased exercise tolerance, unrelieved pain, angina

## T A B L E  2 - 4   Guidelines for a Progressive At-Home Walking Program

| Week | Distance | Time |
| --- | --- | --- |
| 1 | 100-200 feet | 2 times a day |
| 2 | 200-400 feet | 2 times a day |
| 3 | ¼ mile | 8-10 min |
| 4 | ½ mile | 15 min |
| 5 | 1 mile | 30 min |
| 6 | 1¾ mile | 30 min |
| 7 | 2 miles | 40 min |

From Steuble BT. In Swearingen PL, Keen, JH: *Manual of critical care: applying nursing diagnoses to adult critical illness*, ed 2, St Louis, 1991, Mosby–Year Book, Inc.

that is unrelieved by NTG, increasing frequency of angina, and need to increase the number of NTG tablets to relieve angina.
- Elimination of smoking; refer patient to a "stop smoking" program, as ap-
propriate.
- Importance of involvement and support of significant others in patient's life-
style changes.
- Importance of getting BP checked at regular intervals (at least once a month
if the patient is hypertensive).
- Importance of avoiding strenuous activity for at least an hour after meals to
avoid excessive $O_2$ demands.
- Importance of reporting to health-care provider any change in the pattern or
frequency of angina.
- Sexual activity guidelines:
  - Rest is beneficial before sexual activity.
  - Medications such as NTG may be taken prophylactically if pain occurs
  with activity.
  - Postpone sexual activity for 1-1½ h after a meal.

# Myocardial infarction

Ischemic heart disease accounts for approximately one-third of all deaths in
the United States, and of patients with ischemic heart disease, half die because of myocardial infarction (MI). Most MIs are caused by critical narrowing of the coronary arteries due to atherosclerosis (see "Coronary Artery Disease"). Occlusion also can be caused by thrombus formation or coronary artery spasm. When ischemia is prolonged and unrelieved, irreversible damage
(infarction) occurs. MI can occur in various areas of the heart, depending on
the location of the coronary artery occlusion and distribution of blood supply.

## ASSESSMENT

**Signs and symptoms:**   Chest pain, substernal pressure and burning, pain that
radiates to the jaw and arm. Weakness, diaphoresis, nausea, vomiting, and
acute anxiety also can occur. The HR can be abnormally slow (bradycardia)
or rapid (tachycardia).

**Physical assessment:**   Possible minor hypotension, increasing RR, and crackles (rales) if ventricular failure occurs. Temperature elevations to 39.4 °C (104
°F) can occur secondary to the inflammatory process. Intensity of $S_1$ and $S_2$
heart sounds may be decreased, and pulmonary congestion will occur if papillary muscle rupture has occurred. $S_3$ and $S_4$ sounds may be present if heart
failure has occurred.

**History of:**   Sudden onset of intense chest pain that is unrelieved by stopping activity or taking nitroglycerine (NTG), positive family history, cigarette
smoking, hypercholesterolemia, obesity, diabetes mellitus, stressful or sedentary life-style.

## DIAGNOSTIC TESTS

**Serum enzymes:**   Will reveal myocardial muscle damage. The following enzyme levels will increase: creatinine phosphokinase (CPK), the MB isoen-
zyme, SGOT, and lactic dehydrogenase (LDH).

**Serial ECGs:**   For comparison to the baseline. Lead changes, including ST-
segment elevation, T-wave inversion, and formation of Q waves, identify the
area of infarct.

**Chest x-ray:**   Usually reveals cardiomegaly and signs of left ventricular failure.

**Radionuclide studies (using technetium pyrophosphate):**   May help localize area of infarct. The imaging agent concentrates in the infarcted zone, enabling visualization by scan.

**Echocardiography:**  Detects abnormalities of left ventricular wall motion, which usually correspond to the ECG site of infarction.

**Hemodynamic monitoring in the CCU:**  Measures cardiac output and pulmonary artery pressures, which may reflect significant myocardial injury and dysfunction.

**Coronary angiography:**  Determines areas of stenosis or occlusion and suitability for coronary artery bypass grafting (CABG) or percutaneous transluminal coronary angioplasty (PTCA). See discussion with "Cardiac Catheterization and Angioplasty," p. 91.

**ABG analysis:**  May reveal hypoxemia (decreased $Pao_2$) and hyperventilation (decreased $Paco_2$).

**Multiple-gated acquisition (MUGA) scan:**  Evaluates left ventricular function and detects aneurysms and wall motion abnormalities.

**CBC:**  May reveal leukocytosis secondary to the inflammatory process.

**Erythrocyte sedimentation rate (ESR) and WBC count:**  Increase in the presence of an inflammatory process.

**Indium-111 antimyosin antibody imaging:**  A diagnostic tool that is showing promise for detecting infarcted cells and tissue. The antibody is injected and taken up by damaged but not intact cells.

## COLLABORATIVE MANAGEMENT

**Relief of acute pain:**  NTG by IV drip until pain is relieved or IV morphine sulfate in small increments (2 mg).

**$O_2$:**  Usually 2-4 L/min by nasal cannula or mask for 2-3 days to increase the patient's $O_2$ supply. Hypoxia is common and adds stress to the compromised myocardium.

**Transfer to CCU:**  For close monitoring, if needed.

**Limiting infarct size by decreasing cardiac work load:**  beta blockade, controlled exercise program, risk-factor management, bed rest with commode privileges.

**Treatment and prevention of dysrhythmias:**  Antiarrhythmic agents (e.g., lidocaine) for premature ventricular beats; atropine for bradycardias.

**Management of fluid imbalance:**  Oral or IV fluids for dehydration; diuretics for fluid overload.

**Treatment of ventricular failure:**  See "Heart Failure."

**Dietary management:**  Low-cholesterol (Table 2-2), low-fat (Table 2-3), low-Na (Table 3-2, p. 115) diet as indicated.

**Medical reperfusion to limit infarct size**

*Thrombolytic therapy with streptokinase, tissue plasminogen activator (TPA), or the newest thrombolytic agent, anisoylated plasminogen streptokinase activator complex (APSAC), a streptokinase plasminogen complex that has been altered so that the plasminogen has a greater affinity for fibrin:*  To lyse (break down) the fibrin clot. Usually, it is done in the cardiac catheterization laboratory, ICU, or emergency room.

*PTCA:*  To compress plaque in the coronary artery. See discussion under "Cardiac Catheterization and Angioplasty," p. 91.

**Surgical reperfusion:**  CABG (see "Cardiac Surgery," p. 94).

## NURSING DIAGNOSES AND INTERVENTIONS

**Pain** related to ischemia and infarction of myocardial tissue

*Desired outcomes:*  Patient's subjective perception of pain decreases within 30 min of onset as documented by a pain scale. Objective indicators, such as grimacing and diaphoresis, are absent.

- Assess location, character, duration, and intensity of pain, using a pain scale of 0 (no pain) to 10 (worst pain). Assess associated symptoms, such as nausea and diaphoresis.
- Assess and document BP and HR with episodes of pain. BP and HR may

increase because of sympathetic stimulation or decrease because of ischemia and decreased cardiac function.

- Administer prescribed pain medications (usually morphine sulfate) and document quality of relief obtained, using the pain scale, and the time interval from administration to expressed relief.
- Provide reassurance during episodes of pain; stay with patient if possible.
- Observe for and report side effects of pain medications, such as hypotension, slowed RR, and difficulty with urination.
- Administer $O_2$ as prescribed, usually 2-4 L/min per nasal cannula.

**Decreased cardiac output** related to negative inotropic changes (decreased cardiac contractility) secondary to ischemia and infarction

*Desired outcome:*   Patient has adequate cardiac output within 1 h of treatment/intervention as evidenced by systolic BP ≥90 mm Hg, HR ≤100 bpm, urinary output ≥30 ml/h, RR 12-20 breaths/min with normal depth and pattern (eupnea), absence of crackles (rales), and edema ≤1+ on a 0-4+ scale.

- Assess for and document the following as indicators of decreased cardiac output: restlessness and/or change in LOC, extra heart sounds (e.g., $S_3$), systolic BP <90 mm Hg, and HR >100 bpm.
- Observe for and report any indicators of fluid accumulation in the lungs, such as dyspnea, crackles (rales), and SOB.
- Be alert to and report decreasing urine output (particularly <30 ml/h) and increasing specific gravity ( >1.030).
- Assess for peripheral (sacral, pedal) edema.
- Maintain IV infusion as prescribed. Usually fluids are monitored closely to prevent failure and circulatory overload.
- As prescribed, administer medications, such as beta blockers and vasodilators, to decrease cardiac work load and prevent a decrease in cardiac output.
- Prepare patient for possible transfer to CCU.

**Activity intolerance** related to imbalance between oxygen supply and demand secondary to decreased strength of cardiac contraction and decreased cardiac output

*Desired outcome:*   During exercise/activity, patient rates perceived exertion at ≤3 on a 0-10 scale and exhibits cardiac tolerance to activity as evidenced by systolic BP within 20 mm Hg of resting systolic BP, RR ≤20 breaths/min, and HR ≤120 bpm (or ≤20 bpm over resting HR).

- Monitor patient for signs of activity intolerance and ask patient to rate perceived exertion (see **High risk for activity intolerance** in Appendix One, "Caring for Patients on Prolonged Bed Rest," p. 711, for details).
- Observe for and report any symptoms of decreased cardiac output or cardiac failure, such as decreasing BP, cold extremities, oliguria, decreased peripheral pulses, and increased HR.
- Monitor I&O, and be alert to urinary output <30 ml/h. Auscultate lung fields q2h for presence of crackles (rales), which can occur with fluid retention and cardiac failure.
- Palpate peripheral pulses at frequent intervals. Be alert to irregularities and decreased amplitude, which can signal cardiac failure.
- Administer $O_2$ and medications as prescribed.
- During acute periods of decreased cardiac output and as prescribed, support patient in maintaining bed rest by keeping personal articles within reach, providing a calm and quiet atmosphere, and limiting visitors to ensure periods of undisturbed rest.
- Assist patient to commode when bathroom privileges are allowed.
- Assist patient with passive or assistive ROM exercises, as determined by activity tolerance and activity limitations. Consult with physician about the type and amount of in-bed exercises the patient can perform as the condition improves. Examples of in-bed exercises are found in Appendix One, "Caring for Patients on Prolonged Bed Rest," **High risk for activity intol-**

**erance,** p. 711, and **High risk for disuse syndrome,** p. 713. Also, discuss with physician patient's participation in an exercise program after hospital discharge.

- As appropriate, teach patient self-measurement of HR for gauging exercise tolerance.
- Ensure that patient has undisturbed rest periods of ≥90 min. Plan activities accordingly.

**Impaired gas exchange** related to alveolar-capillary membrane changes secondary to fluid accumulation in the lungs

***Desired outcome:*** Patient has adequate gas exchange within 30 min of treatment/intervention as evidenced by a state of eupnea. For a minimum of 24 h before hospital discharge, patient's $Pao_2$ is ≥80 mm Hg, $Paco_2$ is 35-45 mm Hg, and $O_2$ saturation is ≥95%.

- Assess ABG levels and be alert to evidence of hypoxemia (decreased $Pao_2$), decreased $O_2$ saturation, or hyperventilation (decreased $Paco_2$).
- Auscultate lung fields q2h for presence of crackles (rales), which occur with fluid accumulation.
- Monitor for sudden changes in respiratory pattern (increased dyspnea or decreased RR), which can occur with an extension of the infarction and decreased cardiac output; report immediately if they occur.
- Monitor BP. In the absence of marked hypotension, place patient in semi-Fowler's position to ease dyspnea.
- Administer $O_2$ as prescribed. Deliver $O_2$ with humidity to help prevent its drying effects on oral and nasal mucosa.
- Administer prescribed analgesics (usually morphine sulfate) to decrease cardiac work load by vasodilatation and ease respiratory effort.

---

**Note:** See "Coronary Artery Disease" for **Health-seeking behaviors:** Relaxation technique effective for stress reduction, p. 54, and **Knowledge deficit:** Disease process and life-style implications of CAD, p. 55. Also see Appendix One, "Caring for Preoperative and Postoperative Patients," p. 693, and psychosocial nursing diagnoses and interventions in "Caring for Patients with Cancer and Other Life-Disrupting Illnesses, p. 753.

---

## PATIENT-FAMILY TEACHING AND DISCHARGE PLANNING

Give patient and significant others verbal and written information about the following:

- Process of MI and extent of the patient's injury.
- Indicators that necessitate immediate medical attention: unrelieved pain, decreased activity tolerance, sudden onset of SOB, weight gain.
- Medications, including drug name, purpose, dosage, schedule, precautions, and potential side effects. Provide instructions for taking prophylactic NTG before activities, such as sexual activity.
- Exercise program specific to patient's condition. Guidelines for walking are provided in Table 2-4. Caution patient to start slowly, walk 3-5 times/week, warm up and cool down with stretching exercises, notify physician of any change in exercise tolerance, not overexert, and stop when tired.
- Importance of avoiding overexertion and getting rest when tired.
- Resumption of sexual activity as directed, usually after 2-4 weeks, but will vary with each patient.
- Diet regimen as prescribed. See Tables 2-2, 2-3, and 3-2, p. 115, for descriptions of low-cholesterol, low-fat, and low-Na diets.
- Cessation of smoking; refer patient to programs that specialize in this process.
- Phone number and address of local American Heart Association branch, local heart rehabilitation programs, family physician, and primary nurse.

- Referral to stress management programs, if appropriate. See "Coronary Artery Disease" for **Health seeking behaviors:** Relaxation technique effective for stress reduction, p. 54.

## Heart failure

Heart (cardiac) failure is the state in which the heart is unable to pump blood at a rate sufficient to meet metabolic requirements of the tissues. Heart failure can occur as a result of myocardial or cardiac muscle damage, such as after large infarcts, or when an adequate cardiac muscle is stressed or forced to work harder over a period of time. When the heart is unable to pump sufficient blood to meet metabolic demands, it relies on three main compensatory mechanisms:
**Increasing cardiac fluid** to increase fiber length and subsequent force of contraction (Frank-Starling law). The fluid that fills the ventricles before systole is termed *preload,* and it is a critical factor in patients with cardiac failure. It is important to have enough volume to stretch the fibers, but not so much of a stretch that decreased contractility and decreased cardiac output occur.
**Increasing catecholamine discharge** (epinephrine and norepinephrine) to increase contractility. This causes systemic vasoconstriction, which in turn increases work load of the heart by increasing resistance. This is called *afterload.*
**Myocardial hypertrophy** to increase the mass of working contractile tissue. The hypertrophy will be either right-sided, left-sided, or both, depending on the cause of failure. Conditions that can result in primary right-sided heart failure include right ventricular myocardial infarction (MI), chronic obstructive pulmonary disease, left-to-right shunts, and pulmonary valve stenosis. Primary left-sided heart failure is caused by conditions such as left ventricular MI, aortic valve stenosis, mitral regurgitation, and hypertension. Over time, left-sided failure can result in the involvement of both sides of the heart.

### ASSESSMENT

**Signs and symptoms:**   Orthopnea, fatigue, weakness, nocturia, cardiac cachexia (malnutrition/wasting), and confusion, which can occur late in the disease. In addition, decreased right ventricular output can cause increased CVP, distended neck veins, and peripheral edema; decreased left ventricular output can cause dyspnea and SOB, as well as other indicators of pulmonary edema.
**Physical assessment:**   Decreased BP, dysrhythmias, tachycardia, tachypnea, increased venous pulsations and pressure, crackles (rales), pitting edema, ascites, galloping heart sounds, and pulsus alternans (alternating strong and weak heart beats). Hepatomegaly may occur in the presence of right-sided or left-sided heart failure.
**History of:**   Noncompliance with medication or diet regimen, sleeping on extra pillows to enhance respirations, decreased exercise tolerance, increasing SOB, coronary artery disease (CAD), and risk factors for CAD (see p. 50).

### DIAGNOSTIC TESTS

**Chest x-ray:**   Will show the presence of cardiomegaly and engorged pulmonary vasculature.
**Serum electrolytes:**   May reveal hyponatremia (dilutional); hyperkalemia if glomerular filtration is decreased; or hypokalemia, which can result from some diuretics.
**Serum enzymes:**   May reveal an elevated SGOT level with hepatic congestion and decreased liver function.
**Serum bilirubin:**   May reveal hyperbilirubinemia in the presence of liver dysfunction.
**CBC:**   May reveal decreased Hgb and Hct levels in the presence of anemia.

## COLLABORATIVE MANAGEMENT

**Treatment of underlying cause:** Surgical repair of abnormalities such as valvular lesions or treatment of conditions such as hypertension or endocarditis.

**Treatment of precipitating factors:** Such as infection or dysrhythmias.

**Physical and emotional rest.**

**Low-Na diet:** In less severe disease states, this may mean elimination of table salt only. See Table 3-2, p. 115.

**Weight control:** If appropriate.

**Pharmacotherapy**

*Diuretics:* To control fluid accumulation and reduce blood volume.

*Vasodilators:* To decrease cardiac work load by decreasing sympathetic nervous system vasoconstriction. Although there is some controversy about when to initiate vasodilator therapy, it is believed that it is appropriate when patients develop symptoms with light activity or when they are being treated with digitalis. This provides a combination of increased contractility (digitalis) and decreased afterload (vasodilator). The administration of IV vasodilators such as sodium nitroprusside and nitroglycerine (NTG) necessitates the patient's transfer to the CCU.

*Inotropic drugs (usually digitalis):* Administered during acute exacerbation to increase the strength of contractions. Administration of inotropic drugs necessitates the patient's transfer to the CCU for close monitoring of vasoactive effects.

## NURSING DIAGNOSES AND INTERVENTIONS

**Activity intolerance** related to generalized weakness and imbalance between oxygen supply and demand secondary to decreased strength of cardiac contraction

*Desired outcome:* During activity/exercise, patient rates perceived exertion at ≤3 on a 0-10 scale and exhibits cardiac tolerance to activity as evidenced by RR ≤20 breaths/min with normal depth and pattern (eupnea), HR ≤120 bpm (or within 20 bpm of resting HR), systolic BP within 20 mm Hg of resting systolic BP, and absence of chest pain or new dysrhythmias.

- Monitor HR, BP, and RR during periods of patient activity. Note signs of activity intolerance, such as HR >120 bpm, RR >20 breaths/min, and systolic BP >20 mm Hg from resting range. Ask patient to rate perceived exertion (see Appendix One, p. 711, for a description).
- Monitor VS q2h or as necessary and report decreasing BP, increasing HR, or increasing RR, which can occur with worsening failure related to sympathetic nervous system discharge and fluid retention.
- Administer vasodilators and other cardiac drugs such as digitalis as prescribed.
- If symptoms worsen, discuss with patient the need for activity limitations. Assist patient with ADL to prevent SOB, and plan nursing care and limit visitors to allow for periods of undisturbed rest.
- Discuss ways to decrease activities at home, such as not climbing stairs.
- If appropriate, refer patient to an occupational therapist to learn how to conserve energy so that ADL can be performed with a minimum of exertion.
- Assist patient with passive or assistive ROM exercises, depending on activity tolerance and prescribed activity limitations. Because cardiac intolerance to activity can be further aggravated by prolonged bed rest, consult with physician about the type and amount of in-bed exercises that can be initiated as the patient's condition improves. For details, see Appendix One, "Caring for Patients on Prolonged Bed Rest," **High risk for activity intolerance,** p. 711, and **High risk for disuse syndrome,** p. 713.

**Fluid volume excess** related to compromised regulatory mechanisms secondary to decreased cardiac output

*Desired outcome:* For a minimum of 24 h before hospital discharge, patient is normovolemic as evidenced by urinary output ≥30 ml/h, balanced I&O, stable weight (or weight loss attributable to fluid loss), edema ≤1+ on a 0-4+ scale, HR ≤100 bpm, and absence of crackles (rales).

- Auscultate lung fields at least q8h; report presence of crackles (rales), which occur with fluid volume excess and heart failure.
- Monitor and document I&O at least q8h. Report imbalances, including urinary output <30 ml/h, which can occur with decreased renal blood flow.
- Monitor weight daily, and report unusual gains. Be alert to the presence of pitting edema. To assess for pitting edema, apply firm pressure to the edematous area with a finger. If the indentation remains after the finger has been removed, pitting edema is present.
- Auscultate heart sounds; be alert to $S_3$ gallop, an early sign of heart failure.
- Administer diuretics as prescribed. Observe for indicators of decreased effective circulating volume, such as hypotension, decreased CVP ( <5 cm $H_2O$), and tachycardia. Monitor potassium ($K^+$) levels, and notify physician of levels <3.5 mEq/L.
- If appropriate, teach patient the importance of decreasing intake of Na (or table salt). See Table 3-2, p. 115, for a list of foods high in Na.
- If fluids are limited, help relieve patient's thirst by offering ice chips or popsicles. Record the amount of intake on the I&O record.

**Knowledge deficit:**    Precautions and side effects of diuretic therapy
***Desired outcome:***    Within the 24-h period before hospital discharge, patient verbalizes knowledge of the precautions and side effects of diuretic therapy.

- Depending on type of diuretic used, teach patient to report signs and symptoms of the following:
  - *Hypokalemia:* Anorexia, irregular pulse, nausea, apathy, muscle cramps.
  - *Hyperkalemia:* Muscle weakness, hyporeflexia, and irregular HR, which can occur with K-sparing diuretics.
  - *Hyponatremia:* Fatigue, weakness, and edema (owing to fluid extravasation).
- For patients on long-term diuretic therapy, explain the importance of follow-up monitoring of blood levels of $Na^+$ and $K^+$.
- As appropriate, instruct patient to use care when rising from a sitting or recumbent position to prevent injury from orthostatic hypotension.

**Knowledge deficit:**    Precautions and side effects of digitalis therapy
***Desired outcome:***    Within the 24-h period before hospital discharge, patient verbalizes understanding of the precautions and side effects associated with digitalis therapy.

- Teach patient the technique and importance of assessing HR before taking digitalis. Explain that he or she should obtain HR parameters from the physician, but that digitalis is usually withheld when it is <60 bpm if the usual HR before digitalis administration is greater. Teach patient to notify physician if he or she has omitted a dose because of the low HR.
- Explain that serum $K^+$ levels are monitored routinely because low levels can potentiate digitalis toxicity.
- Explain that the apical HR and peripheral pulses are assessed for irregularity, which is a sign of digitalis toxicity.
- Teach patient to be alert to other indicators of digitalis toxicity, including nausea, vomiting, anorexia, diarrhea, blurred vision, yellow-haze vision, and mental confusion. Explain the importance of reporting signs and symptoms promptly to physician or staff if they occur.

**Knowledge deficit:**    Precautions and side effects of vasodilators
***Desired outcome:***    Within the 24-h period before hospital discharge, patient verbalizes knowledge of the precautions and side effects associated with vasodilators.

- Explain that a headache can occur after administration of a vasodilator and that lying down will help alleviate the pain.
- Teach the importance of assessment for weight gain and signs of peripheral

or sacral edema, any of which can occur as side effects of vasodilator therapy.
- Instruct patient to alert physician to side effects of this therapy.

---

**Note:** See "Coronary Artery Disease" for **Altered nutrition,** p. 53, and **Knowledge deficit:** Precautions and side effects of beta blockers, p. 54. See "Myocardial Infarction" for **Impaired gas exchange,** p. 59. Also see Appendix One, "Caring for Patients on Prolonged Bed Rest, p. 711, and psychosocial nursing diagnoses in "Caring for Patients with Cancer and Other Life-Disrupting Illnesses," p. 753.

---

### PATIENT-FAMILY TEACHING AND DISCHARGE PLANNING

Give patient and significant others verbal and written information about the following:
- Medications, including drug name, purpose, dosage, schedule, precautions, and potential side effects. Stress the importance of taking medications regularly and not stopping them without physician consultation. Teach patient and significant others how to measure HR for digitalis therapy.
- Diet: Advise patient that Na restriction may be lessened as cardiac function improves. Assist patient with diet planning or refer to a nutrition specialist if major dietary changes are necessary. Low-Na guidelines are found in Table 3-2, p. 115.
- Signs and symptoms that necessitate medical attention: irregular pulse, bradycardia, unusual SOB, increased orthopnea, decreased exercise tolerance, and unusual or steady weight gain.
- Importance of quitting smoking, which causes vasoconstriction and increases cardiac work load. As appropriate, refer patient to "stop smoking" programs.
- Importance of limiting exertional activities at home (e.g., minimize bending and lifting and avoid stair climbing). Stress, though, the importance of a progressive increase in activity.
- Emergency telephone numbers to call if needed.
- Importance of follow-up care; confirm date and time of next medical appointment.

# Section Two:   Inflammatory Heart Disorders

The disorders described in this section are inflammations or infections involving mainly the heart muscle and its linings, the pericardium and endocardium. The inflammation can be acute or chronic, and prognosis usually depends on extent of the involvement, structures involved, and secondary disorders that occur.

## Pericarditis

Pericarditis is an inflammation of the stiff, fibrous sac (pericardium) that surrounds, supports, and protects the heart. The pericardium is composed of a fibrous outer layer and a serous inner layer. The inflammatory condition produces friction between the layers during cardiac movement. Acute pericarditis causes exudate production and formation of chronic fibrinous adhesions. Pericarditis also may involve formation of pericardial effusions. Pericarditis occurs in a vast number of medical disorders. The most common causes are viral or bacterial infections, uremia, acute myocardial infarction (MI), neoplastic disease, and trauma.

## ASSESSMENT

**Chronic indicators:**   Elevated CVP and signs secondary to systemic venous congestion, including edema, ascites, and hepatic congestion. If fibrous constriction is severe, symptoms of left-sided heart failure may appear, such as dyspnea, cough, and orthopnea.

**Acute indicators:**   Chest pain localized to the retrosternal and left precordial regions, or pain that mimics acute abdominal pain or ischemic pain. Unlike ischemic pain, however, it is often increased with deep inspirations, movement, or lying down and eased by sitting up and leaning forward. Other indicators include dyspnea, if the increased pericardial fluid is severe enough to cause constriction of the bronchi, and fever.

**Physical assessment:**   Characteristic pericardial friction rub (a scratching, grating, high-pitched sound) heard on auscultation.

## DIAGNOSTIC TESTS

**Serial ECGs:**   Typically show widespread ST-segment elevation in most leads, unlike localized ischemic ST-segment elevation.

**CBC and other hematologic studies:**   Often show presence of increased WBCs (leukocytosis) and increased erythrocyte sedimentation rate (ESR) in the presence of inflammation.

**Cardiac enzymes:**   Probably will be normal, although the MB fraction of creatinine phosphokinase (CPK) may increase with epicardial inflammation.

**Echocardiogram:**   Reveals increase in pericardial fluid, which occurs with infection or irritation.

## COLLABORATIVE MANAGEMENT

**Treatment of underlying disorder.**

**Bed rest:**   Until pain and fever are relieved.

**Pharmacotherapy**

*Nonsteroidal antiinflammatory drugs (NSAIDs):*   See Table 8-1, p. 519.

*Corticosteroids*   (e.g., prednisone 60-80 mg qd in divided doses for 5-7 days and tapered thereafter): If symptoms are unrelieved by NSAIDs.

*Antibiotics:*   Given only in the presence of purulent pericarditis.

**Emergency pericardiocentesis:**   If cardiac tamponade (accumulation of fluid that restricts ventricular filling and reduces cardiac output) develops. This procedure involves needle aspiration of the fluid in the pericardial sac to relieve pressure and allow for normal cardiac muscle contraction. Usually it is done under local anesthetic in the ICU, operating room, or cardiac catheterization lab.

**Partial or total pericardectomy:**   To allow normal cardiac movement and function if pericarditis is recurrent and has produced scar tissue and constriction. This procedure involves the removal of part (a pericardial "window") or all of the pericardium to prevent constriction by scar tissue, exudate, or bleeding.

## NURSING DIAGNOSES AND INTERVENTIONS

**Activity intolerance** related to imbalance between oxygen supply and demand secondary to inflammation of the cardiac muscle and restriction of contraction

*Desired outcome:*   During activity, patient rates perceived exertion at ≤3 on a 0-10 scale and exhibits cardiac tolerance to activity as evidenced by systolic BP within 20 mm Hg of resting systolic BP, RR ≤20 breaths/min, HR ≤20 bpm above resting HR, and absence of chest pain or new dysrhythmia.

- Monitor patient for evidence of activity intolerance and ask patient to rate perceived exertion. For details, see Appendix One, p. 711.
- Ensure that patient maintains bed rest during febrile period and understands the rationale for doing so.
- Anticipate patient's needs by placing personal articles within easy reach.

- Advise patient about the importance of frequent periods of rest during convalescence.
- Monitor VS for changes indicative of cardiac or pulmonary decompensation, such as decreasing BP and increasing heart and respiratory rates.
- Assist patient with turning at least q2h, and provide passive ROM exercises at frequent intervals to help prevent complications of immobility. As the patient's condition improves, consult with physician about in-bed exercises that require more cardiac tolerance. Examples are found in **High risk for activity intolerance,** p. 711, and **High risk for disuse syndrome,** p. 713, in Appendix One.

**Altered peripheral, cardiopulmonary, cerebral, and renal tissue perfusion (or high risk for same)** related to interrupted blood flow secondary to dysfunctional cardiac muscle
*Desired outcome:* Within 24 h of admission, patient has adequate tissue perfusion as evidenced by distal pulses >2+ on a 0-4+ scale; HR ≤100 bpm; BP ≥90/60 mm Hg; RR ≤20 breaths/min with normal depth and pattern (eupnea); normal heart sounds; orientation to person, place, and time; and urinary output ≥30 ml/h.

- Observe for and report increasing restlessness or anxiety and changes in mentation, which can occur with decreased cerebral perfusion.
- Palpate distal pulses at least q2-4h to assess peripheral perfusion.
- Be alert to signs of cardiac tamponade, including narrowed pulse pressure, increased HR, hypotension, dyspnea, distended neck veins, and distant or decreased heart sounds. Report significant findings to physician, and prepare for emergency pericardiocentesis.
- Assess for pulsus paradoxus (decrease in pulse volume, and systolic BP >10 mm Hg during inhalation as compared to exhalation), which is produced by pericardial restriction and subsequent decreased ventricular filling. The assessment is performed as follows:
  - Apply BP cuff to the patient's arm; palpate the brachial pulse.
  - Place the stethoscope over the pulse point, and inflate the cuff to above the level of the patient's normal systolic BP.
  - Slowly deflate the cuff. Ask patient to exhale.
  - Listen for the first sound that occurs after the patient exhales. Note the manometer reading and tell patient to breathe normally.
  - Continue to deflate the BP cuff slowly until sounds are heard during inhalation and exhalation. Note the reading.
  - Calculate the difference in mm Hg between the two readings. This is the measurement of pulsus paradoxus.
- Instruct patient to perform foot and leg exercises (see description in Appendix One, p. 715) q4h to enhance venous circulation.
- If patient exhibits signs of decreased cerebral perfusion, reorient and institute safety precautions as necessary.
- Monitor urinary output to determine renal perfusion. Be alert to output <30 ml/h for 2 consecutive h.

**Pain** (friction rub) related to inflammatory process
*Desired outcomes:* Within 24 h of initiation of antiinflammatory medication, patient's subjective perception of pain decreases, as documented by a pain scale. Objective indicators, such as grimacing, are absent.

- Auscultate heart sounds for the presence of friction rub as an indicator of pericardial inflammation.
- Assess and document character, intensity, and duration of pain. Establish a pain scale with the patient, rating the pain from 0 (no pain) to 10 (worst pain). Administer pain medications as prescribed, and document their effectiveness using the pain scale. Advise patient to notify staff as soon as pain occurs so that the medication can be administered early.
- Use the following interventions to enhance the effectiveness of the medica-

tion: Support the patient in a side-lying position with pillows, or place the patient in Fowler's position; provide emotional support; and control environmental stimuli by limiting visitors, dimming lights, and maintaining quiet.
- Administer $O_2$ as prescribed, typically 2-3 L/min by nasal cannula.
- Administer NSAIDs, steroids, or antibiotics as prescribed to manage the pericardial inflammation.

**Ineffective breathing pattern** related to decreased lung expansion secondary to guarding due to pericardial pain

*Desired outcome:*   Within 1 h of the intervention(s), patient's RR is 12-20 breaths/min with normal depth and pattern (eupnea).
- Assess breath sounds and respirations at least q4h. Report the presence of crackles (rales) or areas of diminished breath sounds, which may occur due to atelectasis caused by decreased depth of respirations (guarding).
- Assess the breathing effort for adequate depth at least q2h, and teach the patient to breathe deeply. Teach the use of an incentive spirometer.
- Place the patient in semi-Fowler's or high-Fowler's position to ease pressure on the heart, which will help decrease the effort of breathing.

---

**Note:**   Also see Appendix One, "Caring for Patients on Prolonged Bed Rest," p. 711.

---

### PATIENT-FAMILY TEACHING AND DISCHARGE PLANNING

Give patient and significant others verbal and written information about the following:
- Importance of frequent rest periods during convalescence.
- Importance of prompt treatment if symptoms of pericarditis recur.
- Procedure for measuring temperature, which can be an indicator of recurring inflammation.
- Importance of avoiding individuals with upper respiratory infections (URIs) and promptly seeking medical attention if flu or cold symptoms occur.
- Medications, including drug name, purpose, dosage, schedule, precautions, and potential side effects.

*In addition*
- Explain that feelings of wellness do not necessarily mean that the inflammation has completely resolved.

# Infective endocarditis

Inflammation of the inner lining of the atria, ventricles, and covering of the heart valves is called infective endocarditis. This infection involves the left side of the heart more frequently than the right side and is characterized by vegetations (fibrous networks of platelets, blood cells, and pathogenic organisms) that are found most frequently on the mitral and aortic valves. Vegetations on the valves can prevent adequate closure and adherence of the valve flaps, resulting in regurgitation or stenosis. When the vegetations affect the chamber lining, muscle fibers eventually undergo degenerative changes, and the patient becomes at risk for emboli because parts of the vegetations can break off. In addition, there is a tendency for fibrin and platelets to deposit on the vegetations, and these may embolize as well. Endocarditis usually is classified as acute or subacute. Manifestations of infective endocarditis are the result of infection (systemic and local), the effects of emboli or valvular dysfunction, or antigen-antibody complexes causing injury to the microvasculature.

## ASSESSMENT

**Chronic indicators:** Murmurs (sign of valvular involvement); and dyspnea, distended neck veins, peripheral edema, pulmonary congestion, splenomegaly, and activity intolerance (signs of congestive heart failure [CHF]).

**Acute indicators:** Temperature elevation, malaise, anorexia, weight loss, tachycardia, pallor, diaphoresis, and joint pain.

**Physical assessment:** Presence of a murmur. If heart failure has developed as a result of valvular dysfunction, the following may be present: crackles, SOB, edema, neck vein distention, and hepatomegaly. **Note:** If embolization has occurred, signs may include evidence of decreased renal, cerebral, and peripheral perfusion.

**History of:** URI, flu, or other infectious process.

## DIAGNOSTIC TESTS

**Blood cultures:** To identify causative organism.

**Erythrocyte sedimentation rate (ESR):** Usually elevated owing to inflammatory process.

**WBC count:** May be normal in subacute forms and can range from 15,000-20,000-µl in acute disease.

**Two-dimensional echocardiography:** May be used to detect intracardiac complications such as valvular disorders or wall motion abnormalities. This test uses sound waves (or echoes), which allow visualization of the cardiac wall and valvular movement.

**Echo with Doppler:** May be performed to evaluate valvular involvement. Adding the Doppler to the echocardiogram provides more or different information than would be found using the echo alone.

## COLLABORATIVE MANAGEMENT

**Specific antibiotic therapy:** Will depend on the causative organism and its susceptibility or sensitivity to drugs. In the subacute form of the disorder, it is satisfactory to wait until the organism is identified, but with acute endocarditis, broad-spectrum antibiotic therapy is instituted immediately after blood cultures are drawn and then adjusted if necessary after organism identification. Intermittent IV antibiotics are given q4-6h. The duration of therapy usually is 4-6 weeks.

**Bed rest.**

**Well-balanced diet:** To maintain resistance to infection.

**Surgical repair or valve replacement:** Performed when CHF does not respond to medical management; when an infection does not respond to antimicrobial therapy within 1 week; when repeated episodes of embolization occur, especially when vascular occlusions are found in the eyes, brain, coronary arteries, and kidneys; when repeated infections occur (e.g., relapse after 3 months); and when fungal endocarditis is found. (See discussion of mitral valve replacement in "Mitral Stenosis," p. 70.)

**Treatment of heart failure, if present:** See "Heart Failure," p. 60.

## NURSING DIAGNOSES AND INTERVENTIONS

**High risk for infection** related to invasive procedures and inadequate secondary defenses (decreased immune response) secondary to prolonged antibiotic therapy

*Desired outcome:* Patient is free of infection as evidenced by normothermia, normal skin temperature and color at IV sites, HR ≤100 bpm, and straw-colored and clear urine.

- Use aseptic technique when working with IV lines, urinary catheters, and wounds.
- Monitor patient's body temperature and WBC count for increases from baseline assessment. Both already may be increased as a result of the primary ·

infection, but unexplained increases may occur after resolution of the acute phase as a result of a secondary infection.

- For patients with indwelling urinary catheters, monitor urine for signs of infection, including cloudiness and foul odor. Cleanse the urethral meatus and surrounding area daily, using soap and water.
- Rotate IV sites and change tubing and dressings q48-72h or per agency protocol.

**Knowledge deficit:** Disease process, therapeutic regimen, and assessment for infection

*Desired outcome:* Within the 24-h period before hospital discharge, patient verbalizes understanding of the disease process and measures that prevent bacteremia.

- Assess patient's level of knowledge about the disease and therapy.
- As indicated, explain the disease process and the need for prolonged antibiotic therapy.
- Because of the increased risk of bacteremia, discuss the need for antibiotic prophylaxis before dental procedures and all major and minor surgical procedures and of early treatment of common infections (e.g., urinary tract infections, URIs, and wound infection).
- Teach patient the early indicators of infection (see descriptions in "Care of the Renal Transplant Recipient," p. 141, and Table 5-4, p. 360) and the importance of reporting indicators to physician promptly. Teach patient how to measure body temperature and the importance of monitoring temperature weekly if asymptomatic and more frequently if weakness, fatigue, or symptoms of a cold or flu occur.

---

**Note:** See "Pulmonary Embolus" for **Altered protection** related to risk of prolonged bleeding or hemorrhage secondary to anticoagulant therapy, p. 17. See "Cardiomyopathy" for **Altered cardiopulmonary and peripheral tissue perfusion** (embolus formation), p. 48. See "Myocardial Infarction" for **Impaired gas exchange,** p. 59. See "Pericarditis" for **Activity intolerance,** p. 64. See "Mitral Stenosis" for **Decreased cardiac output,** p. 70. See "Osteomyelitis" for **Knowledge deficit:** Side effects from prolonged use of potent antibiotics, p. 544. Also see Appendix One, "Caring for Preoperative and Postoperative Patients," p. 693 and "Caring for Patients on Prolonged Bed Rest," p. 711.

---

## PATIENT-FAMILY TEACHING AND DISCHARGE PLANNING

Give patient and significant others verbal and written information about the following:

- Need for prolonged antibiotic therapy, including prophylaxis before dental procedures (including teeth cleaning) and surgery.
- Other medications to be taken at home, including drug name, purpose, dosage, schedule, precautions, and potential side effects. **Note:** The patient may be required to self-administer IV antibiotics at home to decrease the length of hospital stay; teach the technique if indicated.
- Importance of medical follow-up to check valve function; confirm date and time of next medical appointment.
- Signs and symptoms of URI and other infections (see pp. 141 and 360) that can precipitate recurrence of endocardial infection, and indicators of recurrence of endocarditis and the importance of getting prompt medical attention if they occur.
- Importance of reporting signs of increasing cardiac failure *stat*. These include steady weight gain, decreased exercise tolerance, fatigue, and dyspnea.

• Importance of regular temperature measurement (e.g., weekly if asymptomatic and more frequently if weakness, fatigue, or symptoms of a cold or flu occur).

# Section Three:    Valvular Heart Disorders

## Mitral stenosis

The most common cause of mitral valve stenosis is rheumatic heart disease, although it also can be caused by a virus or malignancy. In the diseased mitral valve, the orifice becomes narrowed either by calcification or thickening of the valve leaflets. Because the mitral valve is located between the left atrium and ventricle, stenosis results in decreased ventricular filling and increased left atrial and pulmonary pressures. As the severity of the stenosis increases, maintenance of cardiac output becomes more difficult. In addition, high pulmonary pressures cause fluid extravasation into the alveoli, which results in pulmonary edema.

Individuals with valvular disorders are predisposed to endocarditis (see "Infective Endocarditis," p. 66). Bacteria in the bloodstream have a tendency to lodge in the malfunctioning valves because of calcium deposits or turbulent blood flow, so special care should be taken whenever a systemic infection is present or the patient is undergoing major or minor surgical procedures, such as dental work.

### ASSESSMENT

**Chronic indicators:**  Decreased exercise tolerance secondary to decreased cardiac output; increased pulmonary artery pressures.

**Acute indicators:**  Dyspnea usually is the first symptom of worsening stenosis. Orthopnea, hemoptysis, thromboembolism, and chest pain with subsequent right ventricular failure may occur with elevated pulmonary pressure. In some patients, chest pain occurs secondary to decreased $O_2$ perfusion.

**Physical assessment:**  Decreased arterial pulse volume, as determined by palpation or Doppler ultrasonic probe; increased venous pulsations; low-pitched diastolic murmur; elevated CVP; and hepatomegaly. Left ventricular impulse (the point of maximal impulse [PMI]) may be displaced by an enlarged right ventricle. Normally, it is best heard over the mitral area, fifth intercostal space, midclavicular line.

### DIAGNOSTIC TESTS

**Chest x-ray:**  May reveal an enlarged left atrium and right ventricle.

**Echocardiography:**  Can readily diagnose mitral stenosis by poor valve leaflet separation and thickened leaflets; also may demonstrate pulmonary hypertension.

**ECG:**  Although not useful for a definitive diagnosis, it will demonstrate characteristic changes associated with left atrial and right ventricular enlargement, such as tall P waves and right axis deviation.

**Cardiac catheterization:**  To determine extent of the stenosis (see "Cardiac Catheterization and Angioplasty," p. 91).

### COLLABORATIVE MANAGEMENT

**Restriction of physically strenuous activities.**

**Antibiotic prophylaxis for endocarditis:**  Before and after invasive procedures, including dental work (see "Infective Endocarditis," p. 67).

**Pharmacotherapy**

*Oral diuretics:*   To reduce pulmonary artery pressures and relieve dyspnea.

*Positive inotropic drugs such as digitalis glycosides:*   To increase the strength of contraction for patients with ventricular failure.

*Oral anticoagulants (warfarin sodium):*   May be prescribed to prevent thromboemboli.

**Mitral commissurotomy:**   To relieve stenosis by incising the valve and removing calcifications. This procedure involves a heart-lung bypass. Usually the chest is entered through the left fifth intercostal space. The left atrial appendage is incised, and a dilator is inserted and guided through the mitral orifice.

**Percutaneous mitral valve balloon valvuloplasty:**   An alternative to surgery for some patients, this procedure is done in the cardiac catheterization laboratory, using local anesthetic. A balloon dilating catheter is inserted into the valve and inflated across the area of stenosis.

**Mitral valve replacement:**   For patients who continue to be symptomatic after a commissurotomy. Using a midline sternotomy incision, a prosthetic mitral valve is inserted while the patient is on a heart-lung bypass machine. Usually the patient remains in the ICU for 48 h after the procedure.

## NURSING DIAGNOSES AND INTERVENTIONS

**Decreased cardiac output** related to decreased preload secondary to decreased ventricular filling

*Desired outcome:*   By a minimum of the 24-h period before hospital discharge, patient has adequate cardiac output as evidenced by urine output ≥30 ml/h; systolic BP within 20 mm Hg of baseline systolic BP; HR 60-100 bpm with regular rhythm; pedal pulse amplitude >2+ on a 0-4+ scale; extremities warm and of normal color; and orientation to person, place, and time. By a minimum of the 48-h period before hospital discharge, patient is free of new dysrhythmias.

- Monitor BP and HR q4h unless patient is unstable. Report changes such as irregular heart rhythm, HR <60 bpm or >100 bpm, or systolic BP >20 mm Hg over or under baseline.
- Monitor urine output, noting amount that is <30 ml/h for 2 h.
- Assess pedal pulses and color and temperature of the extremities along with other assessment factors. Be alert to pulse amplitude ≤2+ and to extremities that are cool, pale, and mottled.
- Administer inotropic drugs as prescribed to increase cardiac contractility.
- Notify physician about significant findings.

**Activity intolerance** related to generalized weakness and imbalance between oxygen supply and demand secondary to decreased left ventricular filling

*Desired outcome:*   By a minimum of the 24-h period before hospital discharge, patient rates perceived exertion at ≤3 on a 0-10 scale and exhibits cardiac tolerance to activity as evidenced by HR ≤20 bpm over resting HR, systolic BP within 20 mm Hg of resting systolic BP, and RR ≤20 breaths/min with normal depth and pattern (eupnea).

- Monitor VS with patient activity, and report significant (20 mm Hg or greater) decrease or increase in BP. Be alert to indicators of activity intolerance, including SOB, dyspnea, and fatigue. Ask patients about perceived exertion (see description, p. 711).
- Assess for orthostatic changes in BP that occur when the patient moves from supine to standing position.
- Assess peripheral pulses, capillary refill, and temperature and color of the extremities as indicators of cardiac output.
- Provide rest periods at frequent intervals, especially between care activities.
- Confer with physician about in-bed exercises that can be incorporated as the patient's condition improves. Examples are found in Appendix One, **High risk for activity intolerance,** p. 711, and **High risk for disuse syn-**

**drome,** p. 713. Increase ambulation progressively and to the patient's tolerance.

**Fluid volume excess** related to compromised regulatory mechanisms secondary to right-sided heart failure

*Desired outcome:*  Within 24 h of treatment, patient is normovolemic as evidenced by CVP 5-12 cm $H_2O$, balanced I&O, stable weight, urine output $\geq 30$ ml/h, edema $\leq 1+$ on a 0-4+ scale, flattened neck veins, and lungs clear on auscultation.

- Observe for and report the following indicators of right-sided heart failure: increasing CVP ($\geq 12$ cm $H_2O$), peripheral edema, dyspnea, hepatic enlargement on palpation, and jugular vein distention.
- Monitor I&O and administer fluids only as prescribed to ensure that patient maintains adequate volume without overload. Weigh patient daily, and report significant I&O imbalance.
- If fluids are limited, offer ice chips and popsicles to help patient control thirst. Record the amount of intake.
- As prescribed, administer inotropic drugs, such as digitalis, to increase the strength of cardiac contraction.
- Administer diuretics as prescribed to decrease volume load.

**High risk for infection** (with concomitant endocarditis) related to tissue destruction and increased exposure secondary to lodging of bacteria in the malfunctioning valve

*Desired outcome:*  Patient is free of infection as evidenced by normothermia, WBC count $\leq 11,000$ /$\mu$l, and HR $\leq 100$ bpm.

- Maintain aseptic technique for all invasive procedures.
- Monitor temperature q4h, and report significant increases.
- Be alert to rising HR, which can signal presence of an infection.
- Administer prescribed antibiotics on time.
- Maintain hydration, as prescribed, through oral and prescribed IV fluids, making sure that patient has adequate volume without overload.

**Knowledge deficit:**  Disease process and treatments/management

*Desired outcome:*  Within the 24-h period before hospital discharge, patient verbalizes knowledge of valvular disorder, its treatment/management, and the potential for developing endocarditis.

- Discuss patient's valve disorder and associated physiologic effects and symptoms. Describe treatment options, including commissurotomy, percutaneous balloon valvuloplasty, and valve surgery.
- Assess patient's knowledge about the potential for endocarditis. As indicated, explain how endocarditis affects the heart and its valves and why individuals with valvular disorders are predisposed toward developing this disorder.
- Teach patient the following indicators of endocarditis: temperature increases, malaise, anorexia, tachycardia, and pallor. Explain the importance of reporting the symptoms early.
- Teach patient the indicators of frequently encountered infections (e.g., upper respiratory, urinary tract, and wound). For a description, see "Care of the Renal Transplant Recipient," p. 141, and Table 5-4, p. 360. Stress the importance of reporting symptoms promptly should they occur, since a systemic infection can lead to endocarditis.
- Discuss the importance of antibiotic prophylaxis before and after any major or minor surgical procedures.

---

**Note:**  See "Pulmonary Embolus" for **Altered protection** related to risk of prolonged bleeding or hemorrhage secondary to anticoagulant therapy, p. 17. See "Heart Failure" for **Knowledge deficit:** Precautions and side effects of diuretic therapy, p. 62, and **Knowledge deficit:** Precautions and side effects of digitalis therapy, p. 62. As appropriate, see nursing diagnoses and interventions in "Cardiac Catheterization and Angioplasty," p. 92, and "Cardiac Surgery," p. 95. Also see Appendix One, "Caring for Preoperative and Postoperative Patients," p. 693.

## PATIENT-FAMILY TEACHING AND DISCHARGE PLANNING

Give patient and significant others verbal and written information about the following:

- Medications, including drug name, purpose, dosage, schedule, precautions, and potential side effects.
- Gradually increasing exercise, avoiding heavy lifting (>10 lb), incorporating rest periods.
- Name and phone number of a resource person (e.g., physician, primary nurse) should questions arise after hospital discharge.
- Referral to cardiac rehabilitation program if appropriate.
- Resumption of sexual activity as directed by physician.
- Indicators that necessitate immediate medical attention: decreased exercise tolerance, signs of infection, SOB, bleeding.
- Importance of consulting physician before using over-the-counter (OTC) medications, especially aspirin products for individuals taking oral anticoagulants. Aspirin can affect coagulation times.
- Importance of follow-up care; confirm date and time of next medical appointment.

# Mitral regurgitation

Abnormalities of the mitral valve can cause mitral regurgitation (MR). MR can be caused by a number of conditions, including myocardial infarction (MI), coronary artery disease (CAD), papillary muscle dysfunction, cardiomyopathy, or inflammatory heart disorders. The significant effects of MR occur during ventricular systole. Normally, the mitral valve is closed during ventricular systole, but with MR the valve allows approximately half of the ventricular volume back into the left atrium rather than forcing it forward into the aorta. The heart may be able to compensate for a period of time, but eventually cardiac output decreases and heart failure occurs. Additionally, the increase in pulmonary vascular volume causes pulmonary hypertension (see p. 44).

## ASSESSMENT

**Chronic indicators:**  A majority of patients with MR remain asymptomatic, although weakness and low exercise tolerance secondary to low cardiac output may be present. Anxiety, intermittent palpitations, and chest discomfort can also occur.

**Acute indicators:**  Fatigue, exhaustion, dyspnea, palpitations, and signs of pulmonary edema (see p. 86) and heart failure (see p. 60).

**Physical assessment:**  Holosystolic murmur heard at the apex, radiating toward the axilla; possible presence of $S_3$ heart sounds; characteristic ejection click.

## DIAGNOSTIC TESTS

**ECG:**  Will show left atrial enlargement, possibly with atrial fibrillation.

**Chest x-ray:**  Will demonstrate cardiomegaly with left ventricular and left atrial enlargement.

**Echocardiography:**  Provides a definitive diagnosis and reveals severity of the disorder.

**Radionuclide imaging:**  Often useful in follow-up; progressive increases in end-systolic or end-diastolic volumes can indicate a worsening condition.

**Angiography and ventriculogram:** Will show decreased contraction and dilatation.

## COLLABORATIVE MANAGEMENT

**Endocarditis prophylaxis with antibiotics:** Initiated before major or minor surgical procedures, dental procedures, or any activity that may result in bacteremia.

**Pharmacotherapy**

*Beta-blockade:* To decrease cardiac work load and prevent chest pain and irregularities in rhythm.

*Digitalis:* To increase strength of contraction.

*Vasodilators:* To decrease afterload and increase cardiac output.

*Diuretics:* To control fluid accumulation and prevent pulmonary edema.

*Anticoagulants (heparin or warfarin):* To prevent embolization.

**Diet:** Low in Na (see Table 3-2, p. 115).

**Mitral valve replacement:** If necessary. (See "Mitral Stenosis," p. 70.)

**Medical treatment for heart failure:** As appropriate. See p. 61.

## NURSING DIAGNOSES AND INTERVENTIONS

**Activity intolerance** related to generalized weakness and imbalance between oxygen supply and demand secondary to decreased cardiac output with valvular regurgitation

*Desired outcome:* By a minimum of 24 h before hospital discharge, patient rates perceived exertion at ≤3 on a 0-10 scale and exhibits cardiac tolerance to activity as evidenced by HR ≤20 bpm over resting HR, systolic BP within 20 mm Hg of resting systolic BP, and RR ≤20 breaths/min with normal depth and pattern (eupnea).

- Assess patient's VS during activities, being alert to HR >20 bpm over resting HR, systolic BP >20 mm Hg over or under resting systolic BP, and RR >20 breaths/min. Ask patient to rate perceived exertion (see p. 711 for description).
- Provide frequent rest periods, especially between care activities.
- As necessary, assist patient with ADL to avoid SOB.
- Discuss ways to decrease energy output at home.
- Progressively increase ambulation to patient's tolerance. Be alert to dyspnea, fatigue, and SOB with activity. Modify or restrict activities as indicated. See **High risk for activity intolerance,** p. 711, and **High risk for disuse syndrome,** p. 713, in Appendix One.

---

**Note:** See "Pulmonary Embolus" for **Altered protection** related to risk of prolonged bleeding or hemorrhage secondary to anticoagulant therapy, p. 17. See "Coronary Artery Disease" for **Knowledge deficit:** Precautions and side effects of beta blockers, p. 54. See "Heart Failure" for **Fluid volume excess,** p. 61, **Knowledge deficit:** Precautions and side effects of diuretic therapy, p. 62, **Knowledge deficit:** Precautions and side effects of digitalis therapy, p. 62, and **Knowledge deficit:** Precautions and side effects of vasodilators, p. 62. See "Mitral Stenosis" for **High risk for infection** (with concomitant endocarditis), p. 71, **Decreased cardiac output,** p. 70, and **Knowledge deficit:** Disease process and treatments/management, p. 71. Also see "Cardiac Catheterization," p. 92, "Cardiac Surgery," p. 95, and Appendix One, "Caring for Preoperative and Postoperative Patients," p. 693.

---

## PATIENT-FAMILY TEACHING AND DISCHARGE PLANNING

See "Heart Failure," p. 63, and "Cardiac Surgery," p. 96, depending on patient's clinical course.

# Aortic stenosis

Aortic stenosis is a condition that obstructs outflow from the left ventricle. It is either congenital or acquired, and it results from adhesions and fusion of the valve cusps. Usually, normal left ventricular output can be maintained by compensatory left ventricular hypertrophy, but eventually progressive stenosis causes signs of low cardiac output, such as cool extremities, fluid accumulation, decreased urinary output, and cardiac failure.

## ASSESSMENT

**Signs and symptoms:**   Often patients are asymptomatic until approximately age 60 when angina, orthostatic hypotension, syncope with exertion, orthopnea, signs of pulmonary edema, and cardiac failure are seen. Signs of left ventricular failure may also be present, including dyspnea and SOB.

**Physical assessment:**   Decreased systolic BP, decreased pulse pressure (the difference between systolic and diastolic pressures), increased left ventricular impulse (point of maximal impulse [PMI] palpable at fifth intercostal space, midclavicular line as a "lift" of the chest wall during ventricular systole), and systolic ejection murmur (best heard at the apex of the heart, second intercostal space).

## DIAGNOSTIC TESTS

**ECG:**   Will show presence of left ventricular hypertrophy as evidenced by left axis deviation and increased amplitude of QRS complexes.

**Chest x-ray:**   May reveal aortic valve calcification.

**Cardiac catheterization with angiography:**   Demonstrates degree of thickness of the stenotic valve and the pressure gradient across the valve.

**Echocardiography:**   Allows visualization of the narrowed valve opening. Two-dimensional echocardiography can be helpful in determining severity of the stenosis.

## COLLABORATIVE MANAGEMENT

**Antibiotics:**   As a prophylaxis against endocarditis.

**Treatment of congestive heart failure (CHF):**   If present. See this section in "Heart Failure," p. 61.

**Aortic valve replacement:**   Appropriate for patients with left ventricular dysfunction and symptoms of decreased cardiac output and functional disability. Aortic valve replacement is performed using heart-lung bypass, and the patient is in ICU for 2-3 days postoperatively. **Note:** Artificial mechanical valves, as well as those obtained from animals, may be used. Patients with artificial valves are maintained on lifetime anticoagulant therapy.

**Percutaneous aortic valve valvuloplasty:**   An alternative to surgery for some patients. The procedure uses a balloon-dilating catheter, which is advanced to the stenotic valve and then inflated to dilate the valve. The procedure is performed under local anesthetic in the cardiac catheterization laboratory.

## NURSING DIAGNOSES AND INTERVENTIONS

See "Pulmonary Embolus" for **Altered protection** related to risk of prolonged bleeding or hemorrhage secondary to anticoagulant therapy, p. 17. See "Coronary Artery Disease" for **Knowledge deficit:** Precautions and side effects of beta blockers, p. 54. See "Heart Failure" for **Fluid volume excess,** p. 61, **Knowledge deficit:** Precautions and side effects of diuretic therapy, p. 62, **Knowledge deficit:** Precautions and side effects of digitalis therapy, p.62, and **Knowledge deficit:** Precautions and side effects of vasodilators, p. 62. See "Mitral Stenosis" for **Decreased cardiac output,** p. 70, **Activity intolerance,** p. 70, **High risk for infection** (with concomitant endocarditis), p. 71., and **Knowledge deficit:** Disease process and treatments/management, p. 71. As appropriate, see "Cardiac Catheterization and Angioplasty," p. 92, "Cardiac Surgery," p. 95, and Appendix One, "Caring for Preoperative and Postoperative Patients," p. 693.

# Aortic regurgitation

Many disorders can cause aortic valve regurgitation, but the most common is rheumatic fever. The cusps of the valve become fibrotic and retract, preventing valve closure during diastole. Incompetence of this valve allows backward flow, which results in a large ventricular volume. If the condition develops slowly, the patient remains asymptomatic longer because the left ventricle hypertrophies to accommodate a larger volume.

## ASSESSMENT

**Signs and symptoms:**  With slowly developing regurgitation, the patient can remain asymptomatic for years. When the heart begins to fail, signs associated with left ventricular failure develop, including dyspnea, orthopnea, decreasing BP, changes in mentation, peripheral vasoconstriction, and pulmonary edema.

**Physical assessment:**  Widened aortic pulse pressure (the difference between systolic and diastolic pressures), low diastolic BP, high systolic BP until heart failure develops, low-pitched diastolic murmur located in the second intercostal space to the right of the sternum, tachycardia, crackles (rales), and increased pulmonary arterial pressures.

## DIAGNOSTIC TESTS

**ECG:**  Will demonstrate left axis deviation and left ventricular conduction defects with chronic aortic regurgitation. With acute regurgitation, nonspecific ST-segment changes or left ventricular hypertrophy will be seen.

**Chest x-ray:**  Results depend on the severity and duration of the disorder, but it eventually demonstrates cardiac enlargement and left ventricular dilatation.

**Cardiac catheterization with angiography:**  Useful in determining severity of the regurgitation

**Echocardiography:**  May identify the cause of regurgitation by revealing damaged cusps or vegetations caused by endocarditis.

## COLLABORATIVE MANAGEMENT

**Pharmacotherapy**

*Positive inotropic agents, such as digitalis:*  To maintain ventricular function by increasing the strength of ventricular contractions.

*Vasodilators:*  To decrease afterload.

**Treatment of heart failure:**  See "Heart Failure," p. 61.

**Surgical interventions:**  Heart failure is not uncommon in patients with aortic regurgitation, even with aggressive medical treatment. Therefore, aortic valve replacement is usually recommended. Indications for this surgery include chronic aortic regurgitation that has become symptomatic, and ventricular dysfunction during exercise.

## NURSING DIAGNOSES AND INTERVENTIONS

See "Pulmonary Embolus" for **Altered protection** related to risk of prolonged bleeding or hemorrhage secondary to anticoagulant therapy, p. 17. See "Coronary Artery Disease" for **Knowledge deficit:** Precautions and side effects of beta blockers, p. 54. See "Heart Failure" for **Fluid volume excess,** p. 61, **Knowledge deficit:** Precautions and side effects of diuretic therapy, p. 62, **Knowledge deficit:** Precautions and side effects of digitalis therapy,

p. 62, and **Knowledge deficit:** Precautions and side effects of vasodilators, p. 62. See "Mitral Stenosis" for **High risk for infection** (with concomitant endocarditis), p. 71, and **Knowledge deficit:** Disease process and treatments/management, p. 71. As appropriate, see "Cardiac Catheterization and Angioplasty," p. 92, "Cardiac Surgery," p. 95, and Appendix One, "Caring for Preoperative and Postoperative Patients," p. 693.

### PATIENT-FAMILY TEACHING AND DISCHARGE PLANNING
See "Heart Failure," p. 63, and "Cardiac Surgery," p. 96, depending on patient's clinical course.

## Section Four:    Cardiovascular Conditions Secondary to Other Disease Processes

### Cardiac and noncardiac shock (circulatory failure)

A shock state exists when tissue perfusion decreases to the point of cellular metabolic dysfunction. Shock is classified according to the causative event.
**Hematogenic (hemorrhagic or hypovolemic) shock:**    Occurs when blood volume is insufficient to meet metabolic needs of the tissues, as with severe hemorrhage.
**Cardiogenic shock:**    Occurs when cardiac failure results in decreased tissue perfusion, as in myocardial infarction (MI).
**Distributive shocks:**    Characterized by displacement of a significant amount of vascular volume. Three types are:
*Neurogenic shock:*    Resulting from a neurologic event (e.g., head injury) that causes massive vasodilatation and decreased perfusion pressures.
*Anaphylactic shock:*    Caused by a severe systemic response to an allergen (foreign protein), resulting in massive vasodilatation, increased capillary permeability, decreased perfusion, decreased venous return, and subsequent decreased cardiac output.
*Septic shock:*    Occurs when bacterial toxins cause an overwhelming systemic infection.
    Regardless of the cause, shock results in cellular hypoxia secondary to decreased perfusion and ultimately in cellular, tissue, and organ dysfunction. A prolonged shock state can result in death, so early recognition and intervention are essential.

### ASSESSMENT
**Early signs and symptoms:**    Cool, pale, and clammy skin; decreased pulse strength; dry and pale mucous membranes; restlessness; hyperventilation; anxiety; nausea; thirst; weakness.
**Physical assessment:**    Rapid HR; decreased systolic BP and increased diastolic BP secondary to catecholamine (sympathetic nervous system [SNS]) response.
**Late signs and symptoms:**    Decreased urinary output, hypothermia, drowsiness, diaphoresis, confusion, and lethargy, all of which can progress to a comatose state.
**Physical assessment:**    Irregular HR; continually decreasing BP, usually with systolic pressure palpable at 60 mm Hg or less; rapid and possibly irregular RR.
    See Table 2-5 for a depiction of the clinical signs by shock type.

**T A B L E  2 - 5   Shock: Systemic Clinical Signs**

| | Cardiogenic | Septic | Hypovolemic | Neurogenic | Anaphylactic |
|---|---|---|---|---|---|
| *Cardiovascular* | ↓ BP, ↑ HR, ↓ pulses | *Early:* ↑ BP, ↑ pulses; *Late:* ↓ BP, ↓ pulses | ↓ BP, ↑ HR, Flat neck veins | Vasodilatation, ↑ BP (early) | ↓ BP, ↑ HR, ↓ pulses |
| *Respiratory* | Dyspnea, rales | *Early:* ↑ RR, *Late:* ↓ RR, Crackles | Lungs clear | Lungs clear | Dyspnea to air hunger; wheezes and complete obstruction |
| *Neurologic* | Confusion, lethargy, drowsiness | ↓ LOC | ↓ LOC | Normal or ↓ LOC | ↓ LOC |
| *Renal* | ↓ Urinary output | ↓ Urinary output | ↓ Urinary output | Normal or ↓ urinary output | ↓ Urinary output |
| *Cutaneous* | Cool skin | *Early:* warm *Late:* cool | Cool skin | Warm, secondary to vasodilatation | Urticaria, angioedema |

## DIAGNOSTIC TESTS

Diagnosis is usually based on the presenting symptoms and clinical signs.

**ABG values:** Will reveal metabolic acidosis ($HCO_3^-$ <22 mEq/L and pH <7.40) caused by anaerobic metabolism.

**Serial measurement of urinary output:** Less than 30 ml/h is indicative of decreased perfusion and decreased renal function.

**Blood urea nitrogen (BUN) and creatinine:** Increase with decreased renal perfusion.

**Blood glucose:** Hyperglycemia may be present owing to epinephrine-induced glycogenolysis.

*For septic shock*

**Serial creatinine and BUN levels:** To assess for potential renal complications and dysfunction.

**Serum electrolyte levels:** Identify renal complications and dysfunctions as evidenced by hyperkalemia and hypernatremia.

**Blood culture:** To identify the causative organism.

**WBC and erythrocyte sedimentation rate (ESR):** Elevated in the presence of infection.

*For hematogenic shock*

**CBC:** Hct and Hgb will be decreased because of decreased blood volume.

*For anaphylactic shock*

**WBC count:** Will reveal increased eosinophils, a type of granulocyte that appears in the presence of allergic reaction.

## COLLABORATIVE MANAGEMENT

Interventions are determined by clinical presentation and severity of the shock state. Patients are transferred to ICU to assess severity of the shock state and closely monitor status.

*For cardiogenic shock*

**Vascular support:** Intra-aortic balloon counterpulsation is used to augment perfusion pressures.

**Optimize blood volume:** Either with volume expanders such as dextran or with diuretics if fluid overload is the problem.

**Pharmacotherapy**

*Sympathomimetics:* For example, dopamine infusion at low doses (2-5 μg/kg/min) to increase renal perfusion and decrease systemic vasoconstriction. Moderate doses (5-8 μg/kg/min) help strengthen cardiac contraction.

*Vasopressors:* To stimulate vasoconstriction. Usually they are used in conjunction with vasodilators to achieve the desired effect without the negative effects of one drug alone. Levophed, for example, may be used in combination with regitine, which counteracts the severe end organ and peripheral damage caused by the severe vasoconstriction associated with Levophed.

*Vasodilators:* To increase peripheral perfusion and reduce afterload vasoconstriction caused by the vasopressors (see above).

*Osmotic diuretics:* To increase renal blood flow.

$O_2$ **support:** As needed, to increase $O_2$ availability to the tissues.

**Correction of acidosis and electrolyte imbalances.**

*For anaphylactic shock*

**Pharmacotherapy**

*Epinephrine* (0.5 ml, 1:1000 in 10 ml saline)*:* To promote vasoconstriction and decrease the allergic response by counteracting vasodilatation caused by histamine release.

*Bronchodilators:* To relieve bronchospasm.

*Antihistamines:* To prevent relapse and relieve urticaria.

*Hydrocortisone:* For its antiinflammatory effects.

*Vasopressors:* May be necessary for reversing shock state.

$O_2$ **and airway support:** As needed.

*For hemorrhagic shock*
**Control of hemorrhage:**   If possible, depending on the location and cause.
**Fresh whole blood:**   To increase $O_2$ delivery at the tissue level when >2 L of blood have been lost. Often a combination of packed RBCs and a crystalloid solution is administered.
**Albumin or dextran:**   Sometimes used to increase vascular volume.
**Ringer's solution:**   Often used as an isotonic solution to replace electrolytes and ions lost with bleeding.
*For septic shock*
**Antibiotic therapy:**   Specific to causative organism.
**Fluid administration:**   To maintain adequate vascular volume.
**Vasopressors:**   May be required to reverse vasodilatation and maintain perfusion.
**Positive inotropic drugs:**   To augment cardiac contractility.

## NURSING DIAGNOSES AND INTERVENTIONS

**Altered peripheral, cardiopulmonary, cerebral, and renal tissue perfusion** related to decreased circulating blood volume
*Desired outcome:*   Within 1 h of treatment, patient has adequate perfusion as evidenced by peripheral pulse amplitude >2+ on a 0-4+ scale; brisk capillary refill (<2 sec); BP within patient's normal range; CVP ≥5 cm $H_2O$; HR regular and ≤100 bpm; orientation to person, place, and time; and urine output ≥30 ml/h.

- Assess and document peripheral perfusion status. Report significant findings such as coolness and pallor of the extremities, decreased amplitude of pulses, and delayed capillary refill.
- Monitor BP at frequent intervals; be alert to readings >20 mm Hg below patient's normal range or to other indicators of hypotension such as dizziness, altered mentation, or decreased urinary output.
- If hypotension is present, place patient in a supine position to promote venous return. Remember that BP must be ≥80/60 mm Hg for adequate coronary and renal artery perfusion.
- Monitor CVP (if line is inserted) to determine adequacy of venous return and blood volume; 5-10 cm $H_2O$ usually is considered an adequate range. Values near zero can indicate hypovolemia, especially when associated with decreased urinary output, vasoconstriction, and increased HR, which are found with hypovolemia.
- Observe for indicators of decreased cerebral perfusion, such as restlessness, confusion, and decreased LOC. If positive indicators are present, protect patient from injury by raising side rails and placing bed in its lowest position. Reorient patient as indicated.
- Monitor for indicators of decreased coronary artery perfusion, such as chest pain and an irregular HR.
- Monitor urinary output hourly. Notify physician if it is <30 ml/h in the presence of adequate intake. Check weight daily for evidence of gain.
- Monitor lab results for elevated BUN (>20 mg/dl) and creatinine (>1.5 mg/dl) levels; report increases.
- Monitor serum electrolyte values for evidence of imbalances, particularly $Na^+$ (>147 mEq/L) and $K^+$ (>5.0 mEq/L). Be alert to signs of hyperkalemia such as muscle weakness, hyporeflexia, and irregular HR. Also monitor for signs of hypernatremia, such as fluid retention and edema.
- Administer fluids as prescribed to increase vascular volume. The type and amount of fluid depend on the type of shock and the patient's clinical situation.
  - *Cardiogenic shock:* Fluids are probably limited to prevent overload, yet dehydration must be avoided to ensure support of vascular space and cardiac muscle.

- *Hypovolemic shock:* The amount lost is replaced. As much as 1,000 ml/h of Ringer's solution may be administered if volume loss is severe. Most often this includes blood replacement.
- *Septic shock:* Ringer's solution, plasma, and blood are administered.
- Prepare for transfer of patient to ICU if appropriate.

**Impaired gas exchange** related to altered oxygen supply secondary to decreased respiratory muscle function occurring with altered metabolism

***Desired outcome:*** Within 1 h of intervention, patient has adequate gas exchange as evidenced by $O_2$ saturation $\geq$95%; $Pao_2$ $\geq$80 mm Hg; $Paco_2$ $\leq$45 mm Hg; pH $\geq$7.35; presence of eupnea; and orientation to person, place, and time.

- Monitor ABG results. Be alert to and report presence of hypoxemia (decreased $O_2$ saturation, decreased $Pao_2$), hypercapnia (increased $Paco_2$), and acidosis (decreased pH, increased $Paco_2$). Report significant findings.
- Monitor respirations q30 min; note and report presence of tachypnea or dyspnea. Be alert to restlessness, irritability, and confusion, which are indicators of hypoxia.
- Teach patient to breathe slowly and deeply to promote oxygenation.
- Ensure that the patient has a patent airway; suction secretions as needed to assist with gas exchange.
- Administer $O_2$ as prescribed.

---

**Note:** Also see psychosocial nursing diagnoses and interventions in Appendix One, "Caring for Patients with Cancer and Other Life-Disrupting Illnesses," p. 753.

---

## PATIENT-FAMILY TEACHING AND DISCHARGE PLANNING

For interventions, see discussion with patient's primary diagnosis.

# Dysrhythmias and conduction disturbances

Dysrhythmias are abnormal rhythms of the heart's electrical system. They can originate in any part of the conduction system, such as the sinus node, atrium, atrioventricular (A-V) node, His-Purkinje system, bundle branches, and ventricular tissue. Although a variety of diseases may cause dysrhythmias, the most common are coronary artery disease (CAD) and myocardial infarction (MI). Other causes include electrolyte imbalance, changes in oxygenation, and drug toxicity. Cardiac dysrhythmias may result from the following mechanisms.

**Disturbances in automaticity:** May involve an increase or decrease in automaticity in the sinus node (i.e., sinus tachycardia or sinus bradycardia). Premature beats may arise *via* this mechanism from the atria, junction, or ventricles. Abnormal rhythms, such as atrial or ventricular tachycardia, also may occur.

**Disturbances in conductivity:** Conduction may be too rapid, as in conditions caused by an accessory pathway (e.g., Wolff-Parkinson-White syndrome) or too slow (e.g., A-V block). *Reentry* is a situation in which a stimulus reexcites a conduction pathway through which it already has passed. Once started, this impulse may circulate repeatedly. For reentry to occur, there must be two different pathways for conduction: one with slowed conduction and one with unidirectional block.

**Combinations of altered automaticity and conductivity:** Observed when several dysrhythmias are noted (e.g., first-degree A-V block, or a disturbance in conductivity; and premature atrial contractions, or a disturbance in automaticity).

## ASSESSMENT

**Signs and symptoms:**  Can vary on a continuum from absence of symptoms to complete cardiopulmonary collapse. General indicators include alterations in LOC, vertigo, syncope, seizures, weakness, fatigue, activity intolerance, SOB, dyspnea on exertion, chest pain, palpitations, sensation of "skipped beats," anxiety, and restlessness.

**Physical assessment:**  Increases or decreases in HR, BP, and RR; dusky color or pallor; crackles (rales); cool skin; decreased urine output; and paradoxical pulse and abnormal heart sounds (e.g., paradoxical splitting of $S_1$ and $S_2$).

**ECG:**  Some findings seen with various dysrhythmias include abnormalities in rate such as sinus bradycardia or sinus tachycardia, irregular rhythm such as atrial fibrillation, extra beats such as premature atrial contractions (PACs) and premature junctional contractions (PJCs), wide and bizarre-looking beats such as premature ventricular contractions (PVCs) and ventricular tachycardia (VT), a fibrillating baseline such as ventricular fibrillation (VF), and a straight line as with asystole.

**History and risk factors:**  CAD, recent MI, electrolyte disturbances, drug toxicity.

## DIAGNOSTIC TESTS

**12-lead ECG:**  To detect dysrhythmias and identify possible cause.

**Serum electrolyte levels:**  To identify electrolyte abnormality, which can precipitate dysrhythmias. The most common are hyperkalemia and hypokalemia.

**Drug levels:**  To identify toxicities (e.g., of digoxin, quinidine, procainamide, aminophylline) that can precipitate dysrhythmias.

**Ambulatory monitoring (e.g., 24-h Holter monitor or cardiac event recorder):**  To identify subtle dysrhythmias and associate abnormal rhythms by means of the patient's symptoms.

**Electrophysiologic study:**  Invasive test in which two to three catheters are placed into the heart, giving the heart a pacing stimulus at varying sites and of varying voltages. The test determines origin of dysrhythmia, inducibility, and effectiveness of drug therapy in dysrhythmia suppression.

**Exercise stress testing:**  Used in conjunction with 24-h Holter monitoring to detect advanced grades of PVCs (those caused by ischemia) and to guide therapy. During the test, ECG and BP readings are taken while the patient walks on a treadmill or pedals a stationary bicycle; response to a constant or increasing work load is observed. The test continues until the patient reaches target heart rate, or symptoms such as chest pain, severe fatigue, dysrhythmias, or abnormal BP occur.

**ABG values:**  To document trend of hypoxemia.

## COLLABORATIVE MANAGEMENT

**Antiarrhythmic drugs:**  See Table 2-6.

**Automatic implantable cardioverter-defibrillator (AICD):**  To treat lethal cardiac dysrhythmias. It is recommended for patients who have had at least two episodes of sudden death dysrhythmias (cardiac arrest), for patients with CAD who have had a cardiac arrest, and for those in whom conventional antiarrhythmic therapy has failed. The pulse generator, which is powered by lithium batteries, is surgically inserted into a "pocket" formed in the umbilical region. The AICD is programmed to deliver the electrical stimulus at a predetermined rate and/or after assessing the morphology of the ECG.

Postoperative complications include atelectasis, pneumonia, seroma at the generator "pocket," pneumothorax, and thrombosis. Lead migration and lead fracture are the two most common structural problems. Interference from unipolar pacemakers and "myopotentials" (electrical interference) are common mechanical complications.

**Ablation:**  A procedure in which a catheter is placed in the heart *via* cardiac

# T A B L E  2 - 6   Antiarrhythmic Drugs

### Class I:

Local anesthetics and other drugs that decrease automaticity of ventricular conduction, delay ventricular repolarization, decrease conduction velocity, increase conduction *via* A-V node, and suppress ventricular automaticity. Class IA decreases depolarization moderately and prolongs repolarization. Class IB decreases depolarization and shortens repolarization. Class IC significantly decreases depolarization with minimal effect on repolarization.

| A | B | C |
|---|---|---|
| quinidine (PO, IV) | lidocaine (IV, IM) | encainide (PO) |
| procainamide (PO, IV, IM) | phenytoin (PO) | |
| disopyramide (PO) | mexiletine (PO) | |
| | tocainide (PO) | |

### Class II:

β-blockers that slow sinus automaticity, slow conduction *via* A-V node, control ventricular response to supraventricular tachycardias, and shorten the action potential of Purkinje fibers.

propranolol (PO, IV)
metoprolol (PO, IV)
atenolol (PO)
acebutolol (PO)

### Class III:

Increase the action potential and refractory period of Purkinje fibers, increase ventricular fibrillation threshold, restore injured myocardial cell electrophysiology toward normal, and suppress reentrant dysrhythmias.

bretylium (IV, IM)
amiodarone (PO, IV)

### Class IV:

Calcium channel blockers that depress automaticity in the sinoatrial (S-A) and A-V nodes, block the slow calcium current in the A-V junctional tissue, reduce conduction *via* the A-V node, and are useful in treating tachyarrhythmias due to A-V junction reentry.

verapamil (IV)
diltiazem (PO)
nifedipine (PO)

---

catheterization and an electrical heat stimulus is applied to the area in which the dysrhythmia originates. The heat stimulus causes controlled, localized necrosis of the area. This procedure is currently under investigation in several institutions and is used when the patient has not responded to antiarrhythmic drug therapy.

**Dietary guidelines:**   Usually patients with recurrent dysrhythmias are placed on a diet that restricts or reduces caffeine and is low in cholesterol (see Table 2-2).

**Surgical procedures**

*Left ventricular aneurysmectomy and infarctectomy:*   Excision of possible focal spots of ventricular dysrhythmias.

*Myocardial revascularization:*   Performed alone or in conjunction with electrophysiologic mapping, with excision or cryoablation of the dysrhythmia focus.

*Encircling ventriculotomy:*   Excises the diseased portion of the ventricle without compromising myocardial blood supply.

*Stellate ganglionectomy and block:*   Alters the electrical stability of the myocardium and the predisposition to ventricular dysrhythmias.

## NURSING DIAGNOSES AND INTERVENTIONS

**Decreased cardiac output** related to altered rate, rhythm, or conduction or negative inotropic changes secondary to cardiac disease

*Desired outcome:*   Within 1 h of treatment/intervention, patient has adequate cardiac output as evidenced by BP ≥90/60 mm Hg, HR 60-100 bpm, and normal sinus rhythm on ECG.

- Monitor patient's heart rhythm continuously; note BP and symptoms if dysrhythmias occur or increase in occurrence.
- If symptoms of decreased cardiac output occur, prepare to transfer patient to the CCU.
- Document dysrhythmias with rhythm strip. Use a 12-lead ECG as necessary to identify the dysrhythmia.
- Monitor patient's laboratory data, particularly electrolyte and digoxin levels. Serum $K^+$ levels <3.5 mEq/L or >5.0 mEq/L can cause dysrhythmias.
- Administer antiarrhythmic agents as prescribed; note patient's response to therapy.
- Provide $O_2$ as prescribed. $O_2$ may be beneficial if dysrhythmias are related to ischemia.
- Maintain a quiet environment, and administer pain medications promptly. Both stress and pain can increase sympathetic tone and cause dysrhythmias.
- If life-threatening dysrhythmias occur, initiate emergency procedures and cardiopulmonary resuscitation (as indicated).
- When dysrhythmias occur, stay with patient; provide support and reassurance while performing assessments and administering treatment.

**Knowledge deficit:**   Mechanism by which dysrhythmias occur and life-style implications

*Desired outcome:*   Within the 24-h period before hospital discharge, patient and significant others verbalize knowledge about causes of dysrhythmias and the implications for patient's life-style modifications.

- Discuss causal mechanisms for dysrhythmias, including resulting symptoms. Use a heart model or diagrams, as necessary.
- Teach the signs and symptoms of dysrhythmias that necessitate medical attention: unrelieved and prolonged palpitations, chest pain, SOB, rapid pulse (>150 bpm), dizziness, and syncope. Teach patient and significant others how to check pulse rate for a full minute.
- Teach patient and significant others about medications that will be taken after hospital discharge, including drug name, purpose, dosage, schedule, precautions, and potential side effects. Stress that patient will be maintained on long-term antiarrhythmic therapy and that it could be life-threatening to stop or skip these medications without physician approval because doing so may decrease blood levels effective for dysrhythmia suppression.
- Advise patient and significant others about the availability of support groups and counseling; provide appropriate community referrals. Patients who survive sudden cardiac arrest may experience nightmares or other sleep disturbances at home. Explain that anxiety and fear, along with periodic feelings of denial, depression, anger, and confusion, are normal following this experience.
- Stress the importance of leading a normal and productive life, even though patient may fear breakthrough of life-threatening dysrhythmias. If patient is going on vacation, advise him or her to take along sufficient medication and to investigate health-care facilities in the vacation area.
- Advise patient and significant others to take CPR classes; provide addresses of community programs.

- Teach the importance of follow-up care; confirm date and time of next appointment, if known. Explain that outpatient Holter monitoring is performed periodically.
- Explain that individuals with recurrent dysrhythmias should follow a general low-cholesterol diet (see Table 2-2) and reduce intake of products containing caffeine, including coffee, tea, chocolate, and colas.
- As indicated, teach patient relaxation techniques, which will reduce stress and enable patient to decrease sympathetic tone (see p. 54).

## PATIENT-FAMILY TEACHING AND DISCHARGE PLANNING
See patient's primary diagnosis.

# Cardiac arrest

**Note:** *This section is intended as an overview only. In the event of a cardiac arrest, the reader should refer to cardiac arrest procedures established by the institution.*

Cardiac arrest occurs when the heart stops beating, or when the contraction is ineffective in maintaining cardiac output (as in ventricular tachycardia [VT] or ventricular fibrillation [VF]). Many conditions can precipitate cardiac arrest, including myocardial infarction (MI), heart failure, shock state, severe electrolyte disturbances, drowning, electrocution, drug overdose, and hypoxia. Often the events that precipitate cardiac arrest occur in a vicious cycle. For example, a cardiac rhythm disturbance leads to decreased cardiac output, which leads to decreased tissue perfusion, which results in hypoxia, which leads to more rhythm disturbances, and the cycle goes on. Management of the prearrest stage is directed toward breaking this cycle and correcting the condition to prevent cardiac arrest. To help prevent an arrest from occurring, accurate and prompt nursing assessment is crucial. However, an arrest can occur without prior warning. This is an emergency situation, which requires *immediate* medical intervention.

## ASSESSMENT
**Signs and symptoms:**  Loss of consciousness—inability to arouse the patient by shaking and shouting.
**Physical assessment:**  Absence of carotid pulse, audible or palpable BP, and respirations.

## COLLABORATIVE MANAGEMENT
**Management of prearrest phase:**  Includes treatment for shock, $O_2$ therapy or airway support, transfer to ICU, antiarrhythmic drugs, and pain relief.
**Basic life support:**  Cardiopulmonary resuscitation (CPR) to maintain ventilation and circulation until normal cardiac rhythm is restored.
**Ventilation:**  To prevent hypoxia and subsequent anaerobic metabolism. The method depends on the patient's clinical presentation. Mouth-to-mask breathing, $O_2$ mask with 100% $O_2$ if the patient is breathing, oral or nasal airways, endotracheal intubation, and manual ventilation may be used. **Note:** Mouth-to-mask breathing is the preferred method of providing adjunct ventilation (rather than mouth-to-mouth). It is the nurse's responsibility to ensure availability of the mask before an emergency and know how to use it properly.
**Closed chest compressions:**  An adjunct to circulation. If done properly, cardiac compression can provide 25%-30% of the normal cardiac output.
**IV access line:**  In arrest situations, it is often difficult to establish a peripheral IV line because of vascular collapse or constriction. In addition, with decreased peripheral perfusion, absorption of drugs can be variable. The physi-

cian may instead insert a central venous catheter into the femoral, jugular, or subclavian vein.

**Treatment of cardiac rhythm abnormalities:** Lidocaine to suppress ventricular ectopic beats; atropine for bradycardias; defibrillation or epinephrine to combat ventricular fibrillation.

**Stimulation of effective cardiac contractions**

*Inotropic drugs:* To increase strength of cardiac contractions.

*Maintenance of acid-base and electrolyte balance:* Disorders such as acidosis, hyperkalemia, hypocalcemia, and hypomagnesemia are identified and corrected.

**Restoration of effective ventilation and circulation and stable cardiac rhythm before transfer to ICU.**

## NURSING DIAGNOSES AND INTERVENTIONS

**Decreased cardiac output** related to altered mechanical and electrical factors secondary to cardiac arrest

*Desired outcome:* Within 15 min of arrest, patient has adequate cardiac output as evidenced by systolic BP $\geq$90 mm Hg, HR 60-100 bpm with regular rhythm, peripheral pulse amplitude >2+ on a 0-4+ scale, equal radial/apical pulses, and RR 12-20 breaths/min with normal depth and pattern (eupnea).

- Ensure adequate oxygenation by maintaining a patent airway; provide $O_2$ support as prescribed.
- Maintain closed chest compressions until cardiac rhythm is restored.
- Maintain or establish an IV line. Typically, 5% dextrose in water ($D_5W$) is run at a rapid rate unless otherwise prescribed.
- Assess and document BP at frequent intervals (q5-15min), and report changes in pressure to physician immediately.
- Administer antiarrhythmic agents, such as lidocaine, bretylium, quinidine, and procainamide; and inotropic drugs, such as dopamine hydrochloride, as prescribed.
- Assess and document HR; report irregularities or apical/radial deficit (for example, apical rate 80 bpm/radial rate 50 bpm).
- Monitor ventilatory status, and be alert to indicators of hypoxia or inadequate ventilation, such as changes in breathing rhythm, adventitious breath sounds, or breath sounds that are not equal in both lungs. Be alert to ABG results that signal hypoxemia, hypercapnia, or acidosis, such as low pH (<7.35), low $Pao_2$ (<80 mm Hg), decreased $O_2$ saturation (<90%-95%), and high $Paco_2$ (>45 mm Hg). Report significant findings.
- Monitor femoral pulses for peripheral perfusion. Be alert to and report decreasing amplitude of pulse pressures.

Also see psychosocial nursing diagnoses in Appendix One, "Caring for Patients with Cancer and Other Life-Disrupting Illnesses," p. 753.

## PATIENT-FAMILY TEACHING AND DISCHARGE PLANNING

See discussion under patient's primary diagnosis.

## Pulmonary edema

Acute pulmonary edema is an emergency situation in which hydrostatic pressure in the pulmonary vessels is greater than the vascular colloid osmotic pressure that holds fluid in the vessels. As a result, fluid floods the alveoli. When the alveoli contain fluid, their ability to participate in gas exchange is reduced and hypoxia will occur. The most common cause or precipitating factor in acute pulmonary edema is acute left ventricular failure, or an acute exacerbation of congestive heart failure. Other causes include hypertension, volume overload, or nervous system disorders such as head trauma and grand mal seizures, which result in sympathetic nervous system hyperactivity and produce shifts in blood volume to the pulmonary system to increase pulmonary capillary pressure. Pulmonary edema can develop suddenly, or it can develop slowly over a period of hours or days. Prompt determination of cause and treatment are critical.

## ASSESSMENT

**Signs and symptoms:**  Anxiety, restlessness, frothy and blood-tinged sputum, orthopnea, extreme dyspnea. The patient exhibits "air hunger" and may thrash about and describe a sensation of drowning.

**Physical assessment:**  Crackles (rales), tachycardia, tachypnea, engorged neck veins, $S_3$ heart sound, and murmurs (with valve dysfunction, such as mitral regurgitation).

**History of:**  Recent myocardial infarction (MI) or "heart problems" in the past; hypertension; fluid overload, often from IV fluids.

## DIAGNOSTIC TESTS

**ABG values:**  Will reveal hypoxemia.

**Chest x-ray:**  Will delineate interstitial fluid and may reveal an increased heart size or pericardial tamponade (fluid accumulation in the pericardial space, resulting in compression of the heart muscle and interference with normal cardiac function).

**ECG:**  May reveal evidence of old or new MI.

## COLLABORATIVE MANAGEMENT

**Transfer to ICU**

$O_2$:  High flow either by nonrebreathing mask or endotracheal intubation and mechanical ventilation.

**High-Fowler's position:**  To decrease venous return.

**Morphine sulfate:**  In small increments (2-4 mg IV slowly) to decrease anxiety, WOB, and sympathetic vasoconstriction. **Note:** Morphine is avoided when pulmonary edema is associated with bronchial asthma, chronic obstructive pulmonary disease, or $CO_2$ retention.

**Diuretics:**  To reduce fluid volume and decrease venous return to the heart. Usually they are injected over a 2-min period.

**Other pharmacotherapy**

*Vasodilators such as nitroprusside:*  May be used to reduce systemic and venous pressures. Nitroglycerine (0.3-0.6 mg sublingual or transdermal) may also be given for venodilatation and to decrease preload.

*Digitalis:*  To decrease ventricular rate and strengthen contractions for patients who are not already using the drug.

*Theophylline:*  To reduce bronchodilatation if bronchospasm further complicates the pulmonary edema. The tachycardia caused by theophylline, however, may further decrease cardiac output, so the risk/benefit must be considered.

**Identification and treatment of precipitating factors.**

## NURSING DIAGNOSES AND INTERVENTIONS

**Impaired gas exchange** related to alveolar-capillary membrane changes secondary to fluid accumulation in the alveoli

*Desired outcome:*  Within 30 min of treatment/intervention, patient has adequate gas exchange as evidenced by normal breath sounds and skin color, presence of eupnea, HR ≤100 bpm, $Pao_2$ ≥80 mm Hg, and $Paco_2$ ≤45 mm Hg.

- Auscultate lung fields for breath sounds; be alert to the presence of crackles (rales), which signal alveolar fluid congestion.
- Assist patient into high-Fowler's position to decrease WOB and enhance gas exchange.
- Teach patient to take slow, deep breaths to increase oxygenation.
- Administer $O_2$ as prescribed. If ABGs are tested, monitor the results for the presence of hypoxemia (decreased $Pao_2$) and hypercapnia (increased $Paco_2$).

- Be alert to signs of increasing respiratory distress: increased RR, gasping for air, cyanosis, or rapid HR.
- Administer diuretics as prescribed. Monitor $K^+$ levels because of the potential for hypokalemia ($K^+$ <3.5 mEq/L) in patients taking certain diuretics.
- Administer vasodilators such as nitrates as prescribed to increase venous capacitance (venous dilatation) and decrease pulmonary congestion.
- As indicated, have emergency equipment (e.g., airway and manual resuscitator) available and functional.
- As indicated, prepare to transfer patient to ICU.

**Fluid volume excess** related to compromised regulatory mechanisms secondary to decreased cardiac output
*Desired outcome:*    Within 2 h of intervention/treatment, patient becomes normovolemic as evidenced by balanced I&O, normal breath sounds, and urine output ≥30 ml/h. Within 1 day of treatment/intervention, edema is ≤1+ on a 0-4+ scale, and weight becomes stable within 2-3 days.

- Closely monitor I&O, including insensible losses from diaphoresis and respirations.
- Record weight daily and report steady gains.
- Assess for edema (interstitial fluids), especially in dependent areas such as the ankles and sacrum.
- Assess the respiratory system for indicators of fluid extravasation such as crackles (rales) or pink-tinged, frothy sputum.
- Monitor IV rate of flow to prevent volume overload. Use a commercial infusion controller, if possible.
- Unless contraindicated, provide ice chips or popsicles to help patient control thirst. Record the amount on the I&O record.
- Administer diuretics as prescribed and record patient's response.
- Administer morphine sulfate if prescribed to induce vasodilatation and decrease venous return to the heart.

**Altered cardiopulmonary, peripheral, and cerebral tissue perfusion** related to interrupted blood flow secondary to decreased cardiac output
*Desired outcome:*    Within 2 h of intervention/treatment, patient has adequate tissue perfusion as evidenced by BP within 20 mm Hg of patient's baseline; HR ≤100 bpm with regular rhythm; RR ≤20 breaths/min with normal depth and pattern (eupnea); brisk capillary refill (<2 sec); and orientation to person, place, and time.

- Monitor BP q15min, or more frequently if unstable. Be alert to decreases >20 mm Hg over patient's baseline or associated changes, such as dizziness and altered mentation.
- Check pulse rate q15-30min. Monitor for irregularities, increased HR, or skipped beats, which can signal decompensation and decreased function.
- Monitor for indicators of peripheral vasoconstriction (from sympathetic nervous system compensation), such as cool extremities, pallor, and diaphoresis. Evaluate capillary refill. Optimally, pink color should return within 1-2 sec after applying pressure to nailbeds.
- Monitor for indicators of decreased cerebral perfusion, such as restlessness, anxiety, confusion, lethargy, stupor, and coma. Institute safety precautions accordingly.
- Administer inotropic drugs, such as digitalis, as prescribed.
- Administer vasodilators as prescribed, and monitor the effects closely. Be alert to problems such as hypotension and irregular heartbeats.
- Implement measures for decreasing venous return and increasing peripheral perfusion, such as placing patient in high-Fowler's position.

**Fear** related to potentially life-threatening situation
*Desired outcomes:*    Within 24 h of this diagnosis, patient communicates fears and concerns and relates the attainment of increasing physical and psychologic comfort.

- Provide the opportunity for patient and significant others to express feelings and fears. Be reassuring and supportive.
- Help make the patient as comfortable as possible with prompt pain relief and positioning, typically high-Fowler's.
- Keep the environment as calm and quiet as possible.
- Explain all treatment modalities, especially those that may be uncomfortable (e.g., $O_2$ face mask and rotating tourniquets).
- Remain with patient if at all possible, providing emotional support for both the patient and significant others.
- Also see this nursing diagnosis in Appendix One, "Caring for Patients with Cancer and Other Life-Disrupting Illness," p. 756.

---

**Note:** See "Coronary Artery Disease" for **Knowledge deficit:** Precautions and side effects of nitrates, p. 54. See "Heart Failure" for **Knowledge deficit:** Precautions and side effects of diuretic therapy, p. 62, **Knowledge deficit:** Precautions and side effects of digitalis therapy, p. 62, and **Knowledge deficit:** Precautions and side effects of vasodilators, p. 62. See psychosocial nursing diagnoses and interventions in Appendix One, "Caring for Patients with Cancer and Other Life-Disrupting Illnesses," p. 753.

---

PATIENT-FAMILY TEACHING AND DISCHARGE PLANNING
See the patient's primary diagnosis.

# Section Five:    Special Cardiac Procedures

## Pacemakers

A mechanical pacemaker delivers an electrical impulse to the heart to stimulate contraction when the heart's natural pacemakers fail to maintain normal rhythm. Patients for whom pacemakers are indicated have a history of syncopal episodes, dizziness, intolerance to exercise, blacking out, or an episode of cardiac arrest. When patients suffer from temporary or transient rhythm disturbances such as severe bradycardia or a conduction block, a temporary pacemaker can be inserted. Temporary pacemakers are seen most often in ICUs and on an emergency basis. The lead wire is inserted through a peripheral vein into the right side of the heart where it lodges in the tissue to deliver the electrical impulse. An alternative method is transcutaneous pacing, which employs two large skin electrodes connected to a pulse generator.

Some patients who have had temporary pacemakers inserted are observed for the possibility of permanent pacing. Permanent pacemakers are indicated for patients with a complete or incomplete conduction block that recurs or is not transient. Symptomatic bradycardia, Stokes-Adams syncope (an intermittent heart block), and uncontrollable tachydysrhythmias also are indications for permanent pacing. The pacemaker is implanted subcutaneously under local anesthesia, and it is completely internal.

## UNIVERSAL CODING

The increasing complexity of pacemakers has led to the development of a five-letter code for universal language by the Intersociety Commission on Heart Disease. However, the first three letters remain the basis for classification.
**First letter:**   Chamber that is paced.
*V:*   Ventricle.
*A:*   Atrium.
*D:*   Dual (both).

**Second letter:**   Chamber that is sensed.
*V:*   Ventricle.
*A:*   Atrium.
*D:*   Dual (both).
*O:*   None.
**Third letter:**   Mode of response.
*T:*   Triggered by ventricular activity.
*I:*   Inhibited by ventricular activity.
*D:*   Dual (both)—atrial triggered, ventricular inhibited.
*O:*   Neither (works continuously).
*R:*   Reverse (pacing occurs when tachycardia is sensed).
**Fourth letter:**   Programmable functions.
*P:*   Programmable.
*M:*   Multiprogrammable.
*O:*   None.
**Fifth letter:**   Special antitachycardia functions.
*B:*   Burst ventricular pacing to break ventricular tachycardia.
*N:*   Silent during normal rates.
*S:*   Scans and delivers progressive stimuli.
*E:*   Externally activated.

## PACEMAKER TYPES

**Asynchronous or fixed rate:**   Discharges an impulse to the ventricle at a pre-scribed rate, without a sensing mechanism. Asynchronous or fixed-rate pace-makers can be VOO, AOO, or DOO.
**Ventricular demand:**   Senses intrinsic cardiac function and discharges only when the ventricle fails to do so (at the prescribed rate). This type of pace-maker is coded VVI or VVT.
**Synchronous:**   Senses the activity in the atrium and stimulates the ventricle. This type of pacemaker is coded VAT.
**Sequential:**   Senses the activity in the atrium and ventricle and stimulates both sequentially if no intrinsic activity occurs. This type of pacemaker is coded DVI, VDD, or DDD.
**Rate-responsive:**   Increasing numbers of patients have this type of pace-maker, which is designed to increase rate in response to activity. For exam-ple, it "senses" changes in right ventricular blood temperature, cardiac output, $O_2$ saturation, and stroke volume and responds accordingly.

   Temporary pacemakers often are inserted in the ICU where the patient can be monitored continuously. Permanent pacemakers are implanted in the oper-ating room, after which the patient is transferred to the telemetry unit for 24-48 h of close monitoring. After implantation, a sling or other immobilizer may be applied for 24 h if a brachial approach was used. Exercise is encouraged the day following insertion to prevent "frozen joints."

## NURSING DIAGNOSES AND INTERVENTIONS

**Knowledge deficit:**   Pacemaker insertion procedure, pacemaker function, and precautions to take after hospital discharge
*Desired outcomes:*   Before the procedure, patient verbalizes knowledge about the insertion procedure and the function of the pacemaker. Before hospital dis-charge, patient describes precautions to take after hospital discharge.
*Before pacemaker insertion*
- Assess patient's knowledge about the insertion procedure and function of the pacemaker. As appropriate, describe the procedure and explain that the pacemaker stimulates the patient's own heart to beat when the heart becomes lazy or slows down.
- Begin a teaching program specific to the patient's rhythm disorder and type of pacemaker inserted, including normal function of the heart, patient's dis-

order of rhythm that requires a pacemaker, and how the patient's pacemaker works.

- Reinforce explanation by physician about the length of time of the procedure, use of local anesthetic, and postprocedure care.
- Explain that after the procedure patient can expect the following: continuous ECG monitoring, stiffness and soreness at the insertion site, and no vigorous activity. Explain that patient should request pain medication as soon as pain is felt.

### After pacemaker insertion

- Explain activity restrictions as directed by physician, such as no heavy lifting, and give instructions about the amount and type of exercise allowed. Resumption of sexual activity probably will not be affected, but this will depend on patient's underlying condition.
- Teach patient the signs and symptoms that necessitate medical attention, such as decreasing pulse rate, irregular pulse, dizziness, shortness of breath, ankle swelling, passing out, and signs of infection. Teach patient the technique for measuring radial pulse.
- Stress the necessity of follow-up care, usually at pacemaker clinic; confirm date of next appointment. Telephonic monitoring of pacemakers is used frequently as a method of assessing patients between visits. If this method is to be used, inform patient about this type of monitoring.
- Teach patient the expected life of the pacemaker battery, which is approximate and can vary from 5-10 years, depending on the type of battery. It is important to know the manufacturer of the specific pacemaker because some start to show signs of battery failure 2 years before absolute failure.

**Altered cardiopulmonary and peripheral tissue perfusion (or risk of same)** related to interrupted blood flow secondary to pacemaker malfunction

*Desired outcome:* On an ongoing basis, patient has adequate perfusion as evidenced by BP within 20 mm Hg of baseline BP, peripheral pulse amplitude >2+ on a 0-4+ scale, and apical/radial pulses regular, equal, and at rate ≥ that established for pacemaker.

- Monitor perfusion by assessing BP at frequent intervals.
- Assess rate and regularity of apical and radial pulses. At minimum, it should be the rate established for the pacemaker.
- Assess for apical/radial deficit, which if present indicates that the heart is mechanically contracting but that there is no peripheral perfusion (e.g., the apical pulse rate is 80 bpm with auscultation, but the palpable radial pulse is 42 bpm).
- Be alert to pulse irregularity, which can signal pacemaker malfunction or decreasing patient response.
- Ensure that patient maintains strict bed rest for the prescribed amount of time postoperatively to prevent pacemaker dislodgment.
- Maintain patient's arm in a sling or other immobilizer to prevent pacemaker dislodgment caused by arm movement.
- Alert physician to significant findings.

**Pain** related to pacemaker insertion

*Desired outcomes:* Within 1 h of intervention, patient's subjective perception of pain decreases, as documented by a pain scale. Objective indicators, such as grimacing, are absent.

- Assess for pain, using a pain scale of 0 (no pain) to 10 (worst pain), and medicate as prescribed. Evaluate relief obtained, using the pain scale.
- Assist patient with positioning for comfort, using pillows for support as needed.
- Adjust the sling or shoulder support to avoid incisional pressure and other pressure areas.
- For additional information about pain, see this nursing diagnosis in Appendix One, p. 694.

**Note:**   Also see Appendix One, "Caring for Preoperative and Postoperative Patients," p. 693.

## PATIENT-FAMILY TEACHING AND DISCHARGE PLANNING

Give patient and significant others verbal and written information about the following:

- Activity restrictions as directed by physician, such as no heavy lifting, and instructions about the amount and type of exercise allowed. Resumption of sexual activity probably will not be affected, but this will depend on patient's underlying condition.
- Technique for measuring radial pulse.
- Signs and symptoms that necessitate medical attention, such as decreasing pulse rate, irregular pulse, dizziness, passing out, and signs of infection.
- Necessity of follow-up care, usually at pacemaker clinic; confirm date of next appointment. Telephonic monitoring of pacemakers is used frequently as a method of assessing patients between visits. If this method is to be used, inform patient about this type of monitoring.
- Medications, including drug name, purpose, dosage, schedule, precautions, and potential side effects.
- Importance of using caution around strong magnetic fields, which can alter the function of the pacemaker (this is not a problem for newer pacemakers). **Note:** Strong magnetic fields such as microwave ovens can convert some pacemakers to a "fixed-rate" mode. Once the patient moves away from the magnetic field, the pacemaker will return to the normal programmed function.
- Expected life of the pacemaker battery, which is approximate and can vary from 5-10 years, depending on the type of battery. It is important to know the manufacturer of the specific pacemaker because some start to show signs of battery failure 2 years before absolute failure.

# Cardiac catheterization and angioplasty

**Cardiac catheterization** is an invasive diagnostic procedure used to assess the extent of coronary artery disease or valvular heart disease. It involves insertion of a radiopaque catheter through a peripheral vessel into the heart. With *left heart catheterization*, the catheter is advanced retrogradely, usually through the femoral artery, into the left ventricle and the coronary arteries. Subsequently, pressure measurements are made and the amount of cardiac output is determined to diagnose valvular stenosis and resistance to blood flow. Then dye is injected so that the heart structures, including ventricular chambers, coronary arteries, great vessels, and valves, can be visualized with fluoroscopy. *Right heart catheterization* involves advancement of a catheter from a peripheral vein into the right side of the heart to the pulmonary artery. This catheter measures pulmonary vascular pressures.

Associated procedures may include *electrophysiologic studies* (EPS) to assess conduction system abnormalities and ectopic (irregular) beats. If indicated, *transvenous intracardiac pacing wires* also may be inserted to assess conduction defects and determine the exact location of the disorder. Another procedure performed in the cardiac catheterization laboratory is the *intracoronary injection of streptokinase*, a therapeutic measure used to dissolve a clot or thrombus that is occluding a coronary artery. This procedure restores circulation to the myocardial muscle distal to the occlusion.

Patients are sedated before cardiac catheterization and given a local anesthetic so that they can be awake to alert the physician to any chest pain and cooperate with position changes. Usually cardiac catheterization is an elective, scheduled procedure, but it also might be performed in emergency situations.

**Percutaneous transluminal coronary angioplasty (PTCA)** is an invasive procedure for improving blood flow through stenotic coronary arteries. A balloon-tipped catheter is inserted into the coronary arterial lesion, and the balloon is inflated to compress the plaque material against the vessel wall, thereby opening the narrowed lumen. PTCA is indicated for the surgical candidate whose angina is refractory to medical treatment. It also is being performed in individuals with postinfarction angina, postbypass angina, and chronic stable angina. The ideal candidate has single vessel disease with a discrete, proximal, noncalcified lesion.

During the procedure the patient is sedated lightly; given a local anesthetic at the insertion site, usually the femoral artery; and ECG electrodes are placed on the chest. A pulmonary artery catheter is passed through the vena cava and right atrium into the heart to measure heart pressure. A pacing wire may be inserted as well. An introducer sheath is inserted into the femoral artery, a guide wire is passed into the aorta and coronary artery, and the balloon catheter is passed over the guide wire to the stenotic site. The patient may be asked to take deep breaths and cough to facilitate passage of the catheter. Heparin is given to prevent clot formation, and intracoronary nitroglycerine (NTG) and sublingual nifedipine are administered to dilate coronary vessels and prevent spasm. The balloon is inflated repeatedly for 60-90 sec at a pressure of 4-11 atm. Subsequently, radiopaque dye is injected to determine whether the stenosis has been reduced to less than 50% of the vessel diameter, which is the goal of the procedure. The introducer sheath is left in the femoral artery for up to 12 h after PTCA for heparin infusion or in case of need for repeat angiography, and the patient usually is in a special care unit.

Complications after PTCA include acute coronary artery occlusion, myocardial infarction (MI), coronary artery spasm, bleeding, circulatory insufficiency, renal hypersensitivity to contrast material, hypokalemia, vasovagal reaction, dysrhythmias, and hypotension. Restenosis can occur 6 weeks to 6 months after PTCA, although the patient may not experience angina.

**Laser angioplasty** is a newer treatment for some patients with coronary artery occlusions. It is similar to cardiac catheterization and involves application of a laser beam to the occlusion or lesion in the coronary artery to ablate the lesion and allow reperfusion.

## NURSING DIAGNOSES AND INTERVENTIONS

**Knowledge deficit:** Catheterization procedure and postcatheterization regimen

***Desired outcome:*** Before the procedure, patient verbalizes knowledge about cardiac catheterization and the postcatheterization regimen.

- Assess patient's knowledge about the catheterization procedure. As appropriate, reinforce physician's explanation of the procedure, and answer any questions or concerns of the patient and significant others. If possible, arrange for an orientation visit to the catheterization laboratory before the procedure.
- Before the cardiac catheterization, have the patient practice techniques (e.g., Valsalva's maneuver, coughing, and deep breathing) that will be used during the catheterization.
- Explain that after the procedure bed rest will be required, and that VS, circulation, and the insertion site will be checked at frequent intervals to ensure integrity. In addition, explain that sandbags may be used over the insertion site, and that flexing of the insertion site (arm or groin) is contraindicated to prevent bleeding.
- Stress the importance of promptly reporting signs and symptoms of hemorrhage, hematoma formation, or embolization.

**Altered cardiopulmonary, peripheral, and cerebral tissue perfusion** related to interrupted arterial flow secondary to the catheterization procedure

*Desired outcome:* Within 1 h after the procedure, patient has adequate perfusion as evidenced by HR regular and within 20 bpm of baseline HR; apical/radial pulse equality; BP within 20 mm Hg of baseline BP; peripheral pulse amplitude >2+ on a 0-4+ scale; warmth and normal color in the extremities; and orientation to person, place, and time.

- Monitor BP q15min until stable on 3 successive checks, q2h for the next 12 h, and q4h thereafter. If the systolic pressure drops 20 mm Hg below previous recordings, lower HOB and notify physician. **Note:** If the insertion site was the antecubital space, measure BP in the unaffected arm.
- Be alert to and report indicators of decreased perfusion, including cool extremities, decreased amplitude of peripheral pulses, cyanosis, decreased LOC, and SOB.
- Monitor patient's HR, and notify physician if dysrhythmias occur. If the patient is not on a cardiac monitor, auscultate apical and radial pulses with every BP check, and report irregularities or apical/radial discrepancies.
- If the femoral artery was the insertion site, maintain HOB at a 30-degree elevation to prevent acute hip joint flexion.

**High risk for fluid volume deficit** related to hemorrhage or hematoma formation due to arterial puncture and/or osmotic diuresis owing to the dye

*Desired outcomes:* Patient remains normovolemic as evidenced by HR ≤100 bpm; BP ≥90/60 mm Hg (or within 20 mm Hg of baseline range); and orientation to person, place, and time. The patient's dressing is dry, and there is no swelling at the puncture site.

- Be alert to indicators of shock or hemorrhage, such as a decrease in BP, increase in HR, and decreasing LOC.
- Inspect dressing on the groin or antecubital space for presence of frank bleeding or hematoma formation (fluctuating swelling).
- Monitor peripheral perfusion, and be alert to decreased amplitude or absence of distal pulses, delayed capillary refill, coolness of the extremities, and pallor, which can signal embolization or hemorrhagic shock.
- To minimize the risk of bleeding, caution patient about flexing the elbow or hip for 6-8 h, or as prescribed.
- If bleeding occurs, maintain pressure at the insertion site as prescribed. Typically this is done with a pressure dressing or a 2½-5 lb sandbag.

**Altered peripheral (involved limb) tissue perfusion (or risk of same)** related to interrupted arterial flow secondary to embolization

*Desired outcome:* Patient has adequate perfusion in the involved limb as evidenced by peripheral pulse amplitude >2+ on a 0-4+ scale; normal color, sensation, and temperature; and brisk capillary refill (<2 sec).

- Assess peripheral perfusion by palpating peripheral pulses q15min for 30 min, then q30min for 1h, then hourly for 2h, or per protocol.
- Monitor for and report any indicators of embolization in the involved limb, such as faintness or absence of pulse, coolness of extremity, mottling, decreased capillary refill, cyanosis, and complaints of numbness, tingling, and pain at the insertion site. Instruct patient to report any of these indicators promptly.
- If there is *no* evidence of an embolus or thrombus formation, instruct patient to move fingers or toes and rotate wrist or ankle to promote circulation.
- Ensure that patient maintains bed rest for 4-6 h, or as prescribed.

**Altered renal tissue perfusion (or risk of same)** related to interrupted blood flow secondary to decreased cardiac output or reaction to contrast dye

*Desired outcome:* Patient has adequate renal perfusion as evidenced by urinary output ≥30 ml/h, good skin turgor, and moist mucous membranes.

- Because contrast dye for cardiac catheterization may cause osmotic diure-

sis, monitor for indicators of dehydration, such as poor skin turgor, dry mucous membranes, and high urine specific gravity.
- Monitor I&O. Notify physician if urinary output is <30 ml/h in the presence of an adequate intake.
- If urinary output is insufficient despite adequate intake, restrict fluids. Be alert to and report indicators of fluid overload, such as crackles (rales) on auscultation of lung fields, distended neck veins, and SOB. Notify physician about significant findings.
- If patient does not exhibit signs of cardiac or renal failure, encourage daily intake of 2-3 L of fluids, or as prescribed, to flush the contrast dye out of the system.

---

**Note:** See "Coronary Artery Disease" for **Pain,** p. 52, **Knowledge deficit:** Precautions and side effects of nitrates, p. 54, and **Knowledge deficit:** Precautions and side effects of beta blockers, p. 54.

---

## PATIENT-FAMILY TEACHING AND DISCHARGE PLANNING

Give patient and significant others verbal and written information about the following:
- Use of NTG, including purpose, dosage, schedule, precautions, and potential side effects, such as headache and dizziness. Caution patient to avoid using NTG more frequently than prescribed and to notify physician if 3 tablets do not relieve pain.
- Use of calcium antagonists, beta blockers, antiarrhythmic agents, and antihypertensive agents, including the drug name, purpose, dosage, schedule, precautions, and potential side effects. Advise patient about the importance of taking the medications regularly and not discontinuing them without physician approval.
- Signs and symptoms necessitating immediate medical attention, including chest pain unrelieved by NTG, decreased exercise tolerance, increasing SOB, and loss of consciousness.
- Activity and dietary limitations as prescribed.
- Importance of follow-up with physician; confirm date and time of next appointment.

## Cardiac surgery

Cardiac surgery is performed to correct a variety of heart disorders. For example, *coronary artery bypass grafting* (CABG) is a technique used to treat blocked coronary arteries; a portion of the saphenous vein or internal mammary artery is used to shunt blood around the blocked portions of arteries to maintain flow to the heart muscle. *Valve replacement,* another type of cardiac surgery, is performed for patients with valvular stenosis or valvular incompetence of the mitral, tricuspid, pulmonary, or aortic valve. Cardiac surgery is also performed to correct heart defects that are either acquired or congenital, such as ventricular aneurysm, ventricular or atrial septal defects, transposition of the great vessels, and tetralogy of Fallot.

Unless an emergency occurs, patients usually are admitted to the hospital the day before surgery. Most institutions that perform cardiac surgery have special units called transitional care, special care, or "step-down" units where preoperative cardiac patients are admitted. After surgery, most patients are in an ICU for 24-72 h and then transferred to a medical-surgical unit. However, this is highly variable and depends on the patient's postoperative course and need for close cardiac monitoring.

## NURSING DIAGNOSES AND INTERVENTIONS

**Knowledge deficit:**    Diagnosis, surgical procedure, preoperative routine, and postoperative course
*Desired outcome:*    Before surgery, patient verbalizes knowledge about the diagnosis, surgical procedure, and preoperative and postoperative regimens.

- Assess patient's level of knowledge about the diagnosis and surgical procedure, and provide information where necessary. Encourage questions, and allow time for verbalization of concerns and fears.
- If appropriate for the patient, provide orientation to the ICU and equipment that will be used postoperatively.
- Provide instructions for deep breathing and coughing in the preoperative teaching.
- Reassure patient that postoperative discomfort will be relieved with medication. **Note:** Pain following a midline sternotomy (the usual incision with cardiac surgery) usually is less than that with conventional thoracotomy because the somatic nerves are not divided by the surgical incision.
- Advise patient that in the immediate postoperative period, speaking will be impossible because of the presence of an endotracheal tube, which will assist with breathing. Also explain that a chest tube will be present. Teach patient how he or she will move, deep breathe, and cough with a chest tube in place. (See Chapter 1 for care considerations for patients with chest tubes.)

**Activity intolerance** related to generalized weakness and bed rest secondary to cardiac surgery
*Desired outcome:*    By a minimum of 24 h before hospital discharge, patient rates perceived exertion at ≤3 on a 0-10 scale and exhibits cardiac tolerance to activity after cardiac surgery as evidenced by HR ≤120 bpm, systolic BP within 20 mm Hg of resting systolic BP, and RR ≤20 breaths/min with normal depth and pattern (eupnea).

- Ask patient to rate perceived exertion during activity, and monitor for evidence of activity intolerance. For details, see **High risk for activity intolerance** in Appendix One, "Caring for Patients on Prolonged Bed Rest," p. 711. Notify physician of significant findings.
- Monitor VS at frequent intervals, and be alert to indicators of cardiac failure, including hypotension, tachycardia, crackles (rales), tachypnea, and decreased amplitude of peripheral pulses. Notify physician of significant findings.
- Monitor BP and note a decrease >20 mm Hg of resting systolic BP. **Note:** A mean BP of 50 mm Hg is required for adequate brain perfusion.
- To help minimize myocardial oxygen consumption, ensure that the patient has frequent rest periods.
- As prescribed, administer medications that decrease myocardial $O_2$ consumption, such as beta-blockers or calcium antagonists.
- Assist patient with ROM and other exercises, depending on tolerance and prescribed activity limitations. Consult with physician about patient's readiness to participate in exercises that require increased cardiac tolerance. For a discussion of in-bed exercises that may be used, see **High risk for activity intolerance,** p. 711, and **High risk for disuse syndrome,** p. 713, in Appendix One.

---

**Note:**    See "Pulmonary Embolus" for **Altered protection** related to risk of prolonged bleeding or hemorrhage secondary to anticoagulant therapy, p. 17. See "Coronary Artery Disease" for **Altered nutrition:** More than body requirements of salt, calories, and fat, p. 53, and **Health-seeking behaviors:** Relaxation technique effective for stress reduction, p. 54. See "Atherosclerotic Arterial Occlusive Disease" for **Altered renal tissue perfusion,** p. 100. See Appendix One, "Caring for Preoperative and Postoperative Patients," in particular **Ineffective breathing pattern,** p. 703, and **High risk for infection,** p.

705. See Appendix One, "Caring for Patients on Prolonged Bed Rest," in particular **Altered peripheral tissue perfusion,** p. 715.

## PATIENT-FAMILY TEACHING AND DISCHARGE PLANNING

Give patient and significant others verbal and written information about the following:

- Medications, including drug name, dosage, schedule, purpose, precautions, and potential side effects.
- Untoward symptoms requiring medical attention for patients taking warfarin, such as bleeding from the nose, hemoptysis, hematuria, melena, and excessive bruising. In addition, stress the following: Take warfarin at the same time every day; notify physician if *any* signs of bleeding occur; keep appointments for physical therapy (PT) checks; avoid OTC medications unless approved by physician; carry a Medic-Alert bracelet or card; avoid constrictive or restrictive clothing; and use soft-bristled toothbrushes and electric razors.
- Maintenance of low-Na (see Table 3-2, p. 115), low-fat (see Table 2-3), and low-cholesterol (see Table 2-2) diet.
- Importance of pacing activities at home and allowing frequent rest periods.
- Technique for assessing radial pulse, temperature, and weight, if these indicators require monitoring at home, and reporting significant changes to physician.
- Introduction to local American Heart Association activities.
- Telephone number of nurse available to discuss concerns and questions or clarify instructions that are unclear.
- Importance of follow-up visits with physician; confirm date and time of next appointment.
- Signs and symptoms that necessitate immediate medical attention: chest pain, dyspnea, SOB, weight gain, and decrease in exercise tolerance.
- Activity restrictions (e.g., no heavy lifting [≥10-20 lb], pushing, or pulling for at least 6 weeks); prescribed exercise program; and resumption of sexual activity, work, and driving a car, as directed.
- Care of the incision site; importance of assessing for signs of infection, such as drainage, fever, persistent redness, and local warmth and tenderness.
- Referral to a cardiac rehabilitation program.
- Discussion of the patient's home environment and the potential need for changes or adaptations (e.g., too many steps to climb, ADL that are too strenuous).

# Section Six:   Disorders of the Peripheral Vascular System

## Atherosclerotic arterial occlusive disease

*Arteriosclerosis* is a normal aging process of changes occurring in the arteries, including thickening of the walls, loss of elasticity, increase in calcium deposits, and usually, an increase in external diameter and a decrease in internal diameter. In contrast, *atherosclerosis* refers to a pathologic process of focal changes in the arteries, usually involving the accumulation of lipids, carbohydrates, calcium, blood components, and fibrous tissue. Although the two processes differ, they usually occur simultaneously.

The process of atherosclerotic disease results in narrowing of the arterial lumen, which limits blood flow. Thrombosis or aneurysm can occur, depending on the reaction of the tissue that is supplied by the atherosclerotic vessels. Arterial occlusion and insufficiency are usually found in the lower extremities in patients over age 50. *Raynaud's disease* is a type of impairment that tends to affect younger individuals and women. It is characterized by vasospasm of small arteries and arterioles in the extremities, particularly associated with an oversensitivity to the sympathetic nervous system (SNS) effects of cold and possibly stress. The cause of Raynaud's disease is unknown.

## ASSESSMENT

**Signs and symptoms:**    Severe, cramping pain (called intermittent claudication) that follows exercise and is relieved by rest. It is indicative of ischemia secondary to decreased blood flow. The patient also may have delayed healing, collapsed veins, decreased sensory or motor function, leg ulcers, or gangrene.

**Physical assessment:**    Decreased pulse amplitude, decreased hair distribution, and bluish discoloration of the extremities and areas of decreased circulation. The skin may appear shiny and the nails thickened. Audible bruits may be assessed with a stethoscope over partially occluded vessels. Capillary filling will be ≥2 sec (with normal circulation, capillary filling occurs in <2 sec), and amplitude of peripheral pulses will be decreased.

**Risk factors:**    Hypertension, cigarette smoking, diabetes mellitus, family history of atherosclerotic disease, and hyperlipoproteinemia. Use of beta blocker drugs can exacerbate patient's symptoms because of their peripheral vasoconstricting effect.

## DIAGNOSTIC TESTS

**Angiography of peripheral vasculature:**    Will locate obstruction and reveal extent of vascular lesions. This invasive study usually is done only if surgery is planned.

**Duplex imaging:**    Uses ultrasound to assess arteries for plaque formation and measurement of flow and pressure.

**Doppler flow studies:**    Uses a transducer that emits sound waves through a probe to determine the amount of blood flow in arteries in which palpable pulses are difficult to obtain.

**Digital subtraction angiography:**    Uses computerized tomography (CT) to visualize arteries radiologically and determine presence and extent of occlusion.

**Exercise testing:**    To determine the amount of exercise that precipitates ischemia and claudication.

**Oscillometry:**    Uses a BP cuff connected to a manometer to locate occlusive sites, as evidenced by decreased pressure readings.

## COLLABORATIVE MANAGEMENT

**Regular lower extremity exercise program:**    To increase circulation. This can include a walking program or Buerger-Allen exercises. Activity may be contraindicated for some patients with severe disease, who may instead require bed rest to decrease $O_2$ demands to the tissues.

**Cessation of cigarette smoking:**    To prevent increased vasoconstriction and severity of the circulation deficit.

**Control of hyperlipidemia and cholesterol levels:**    To help prevent progression of atherosclerosis. This is accomplished through a low-fat (Table 2-3), low-cholesterol (Table 2-2) diet or the controversial antilipemic drugs, which may be used if diet control is ineffective. Examples of these drugs include clofibrate and cholestyramine.

**Control of hypertension:**    Administration of agents such as thiazide diuretics.

**Provision of warmth:**    To promote arterial flow. **Caution:** Care must be taken not to apply extreme heat, because the patient's sensitivity to temperature is often decreased, and burns can result.

**Pharmacotherapy**

*Mild analgesics:*  For relief of pain.

*Antiplatelet agents such as aspirin:*  May be used to help prevent platelet adherence and thromboembolism. The use of anticoagulants such as warfarin to prevent thrombus formation is controversial.

*Thrombolytics:*  For example, streptokinase, to lyse the clot.

*Pentoxyphylline:*  To increase flexibility of erythrocytes, which enhances their movement through the microcirculation, prevent aggregation of RBCs and platelets, and decrease viscosity. This has the potential to increase circulation at the capillary level.

*Calcium channel blockers:*  For example, diltiazem, to reduce vasospasm.

*Lovastatin (Mevacor):*  To reduce serum cholesterol level.

**Surgical management:**  For patients who are severely limited by the occlusion and for whom the occlusion is fairly localized.

*Endarterectomy:*  Removal of the atheromatous obstruction *via* an arterial incision.

*Bypass vascular grafting:*  Removal or bypass of the obstructed segment by suturing a graft proximally and distally to the obstruction. The most common procedures are aortofemoral, aortoiliac, and femoropopliteal bypasses. Graft material may be the patient's saphenous vein or prosthetic materials such as Gortex or Dacron.

*Percutaneous transluminal angioplasty* (PTA):  May be used to treat focal arterial obstruction. A balloon-tipped catheter is inserted through the vein or artery to the area of the occlusion. The balloon is gradually inflated to ablate the obstruction.

*Laser angioplasty:*  Technique similar to PTA. A fiberoptic catheter is inserted and threaded to the area of occlusion. Energy from a laser is applied, and the occlusion is oliterated.

*Amputation:*  See discussion in Chapter 8.

## NURSING DIAGNOSES AND INTERVENTIONS

**Impaired extremity tissue integrity** related to altered arterial circulation secondary to atherosclerotic process

*Desired outcome:*  Patient's extremity tissue remains intact.

- Assess leg(s) for ulcerations that can occur with decreased arterial circulation.
- Teach patient to elevate HOB to increase circulation to the lower extremities. Explain that this can be accomplished at home by raising the HOB on 6-inch blocks.
- Teach patient that walking and ROM exercises for the hip, knee, and ankle promote collateral circulation.
- Discuss an exercise program with physician, and describe the routine to the patient. Often this includes walking to the patient's tolerance (without pain).
- If prescribed, teach the patient Buerger-Allen exercises. **Note:** Bed rest without exercise may be prescribed to decrease $O_2$ demand in acute, severe cases.
  - Teach patient to lie flat in bed with the legs elevated above the level of the heart for 2-3 min.
  - Have the patient sit on the edge of the bed for 2-3 min with the legs relaxed and dependent.
  - Have the patient in the same position, flex, extend, invert, and evert the feet, holding each position for 30 sec.
  - Finally, have the patient lie flat with the legs at heart level and covered with a warm blanket for approximately 5 min.
- Teach patient to assess peripheral pulses, warmth, color, hair distribution, and capillary filling. To check for capillary filling, teach the patient to press

on a nailbed until blanching occurs and release the pressure. Explain that with normal capillary filling, color (pink) returns in 1-2 sec.

- As appropriate, teach patient that smoking results in a decrease in both blood flow to the extremities and extremity temperature, particularly to the fingers and toes.
- Discuss the importance of keeping warm by wearing socks when walking or in bed. Caution patient about using heating pads, which increase metabolism and may promote ischemia if circulation is limited.
- Caution patient to cover all exposed areas when going outside in cooler weather.
- Teach patient to maintain moderate room temperatures and avoid extremes.
- Administer antiplatelet agents as prescribed to help prevent platelet adherence.

**Chronic pain** related to atherosclerotic obstructions

*Desired outcomes:* By hospital discharge, patient's subjective perception of chronic pain decreases as documented by a pain scale. Objective indicators, such as grimacing, are absent.

- Assess for the presence of pain, using a pain scale from 0 (no pain) to 10 (worst pain). Administer pain medications as prescribed; document effectiveness using the pain scale.
- Teach patient to rest and stop exercising before claudication (severe, cramping pain) occurs.
- Because the pain may be chronic and continuous, explore alternate methods of pain relief such as visualization, guided imagery, biofeedback, meditation, and relaxation exercises or tapes. For an example of a relaxation exercise, see "Coronary Heart Disease," **Health-seeking behaviors,** on p. 54.
- Institute measures to increase circulation to ischemic extremities, such as Buerger-Allen exercises and walking.
- Administer calcium channel blockers such as diltiazem hydrochloride as prescribed to reduce vasospasm.
- Advise patient about the possibility of "rest" pain, which occurs at night when recumbent and decreases when the legs are in a dependent position.

**Knowledge deficit:** Potential for infection and impaired tissue integrity due to decreased arterial circulation

*Desired outcome:* By hospital discharge, patient verbalizes knowledge about the potential for infection and impaired tissue integrity, as well as measures to prevent these problem⁻

- Teach patient how to assess for signs of infection or problems with skin integrity and to report significant findings to physician.
- Caution patient about the increased potential for easily traumatizing the skin (e.g., from bumping the lower extremities).
- Stress the importance of wearing shoes or slippers that fit properly.
- Instruct patient to cut toenails straight across to prevent ingrown toenails.
- Advise patient to cover corns or calluses with pads to prevent further injury.
- Encourage patient to keep the feet clean and dry, using mild soap and warm water for cleansing, and applying a mild lotion to prevent dryness.
- Advise patient not to scratch or rub the skin on the feet because this can result in abrasions that easily can become infected.
- Suggest that patient keep the feet warm with loose-fitting socks and warm soaks. Caution patient to check the temperature of warm soaks and bath water carefully to protect the skin from burns.
- Discuss potential surgical interventions, such as endarterectomy, bypass vascular grafting, and angioplasty.

**Altered peripheral tissue perfusion (or risk of same)** related to interrupted arterial flow with postsurgical graft occlusion

***Desired outcome:***   Patient has adequate peripheral perfusion as evidenced by peripheral pulse amplitude >2+ on a 0-4+ scale, BP within 20 mm Hg of baseline BP, and absence of the six *P*s in the involved extremities.

- Assess peripheral pulses and the involved extremity for the six *P*s: pain, pallor, pulselessness, paresthesia, polar (coolness), and paralysis. Report significant findings.
- Monitor BP, another indicator of peripheral perfusion pressure. Report to physician any significant increase or decrease (>15-20 mm Hg, or as directed).
- If necessary, use the Doppler ultrasonic probe to check pulses, holding the probe to the skin at a 45-degree angle to the blood vessel. In the presence of blood flow, wavelike "whooshing" sounds will be heard. Record the presence or absence of pulsations, as well as the rate, character, frequency, and intensity of the sounds.
- To prevent pressure on the tissue, use foam protectors to keep sheets and blankets off the legs and feet.
- For the first 48-72 h after surgery (or as directed), prevent acute joint flexion in the presence of a graft, which can occlude blood flow.

**Altered renal tissue perfusion** related to interrupted blood flow during surgery and potential embolization

***Desired outcome:***   Within 1 h after surgery, patient has adequate renal perfusion as evidenced by urinary output ≥30 ml/h.

---

**Note:**   During many vascular surgical procedures, the aorta is clamped temporarily to facilitate endarterectomy and grafting. Although all body systems are affected to a degree, the renal system is especially sensitive to the lack of blood flow.

---

- Monitor I&O. Report output <30 ml/h.
- Monitor results of renal function tests. Be alert to increases in serum creatinine (>1.5 mg/dl) and BUN (>20 mg/dl), which occur with decreasing renal function.
- Monitor for signs of fluid retention (e.g., distended neck veins, crackles [rales], and peripheral edema).
- In the absence of acute cardiac or renal failure, encourage adequate fluid intake (2-3 L/day) to help maintain adequate renal blood flow and promote fluid balance.

---

**Note:**   As appropriate, also see Appendix One, "Caring for Preoperative and Postoperative Patients," p. 693.

---

## PATIENT-FAMILY TEACHING AND DISCHARGE PLANNING

Give patient and significant others verbal and written information about the following:

- "Stop smoking" programs, if appropriate.
- Importance of avoiding factors and activities that cause vasoconstriction (e.g., tight clothing and crossing the legs at the knee).
- Exercise program as prescribed by physician; importance of rest periods if claudication occurs.
- Skin and foot care.
- Measures that optimize arterial blood flow such as keeping warm and raising HOB on blocks to promote circulation to the lower extremities.
- Medications, including drug name, purpose, dosage, schedule, precautions, and potential side effects.

# Aneurysms: abdominal, thoracic, and femoral

An aneurysm is a localized, outpouching sac that is formed at a weak point in an arterial wall. The most likely cause of aneurysm is hereditary lack of elastin, although vessel wall trauma, congenital defect, infection, and atherosclerosis may be other causes. Loss of vessel wall elasticity and atherosclerotic deposits cause the vessel to weaken, resulting in gradual dilation. Unless this condition is recognized and surgically treated, rupture and exsanguination can occur. Although aneurysms can develop in any vessel, peripheral vessel aneurysms are most commonly found in the abdominal aorta, thoracic aorta, and femoral arteries. *Dissecting aneurysms* occur in aortic vessels that have atherosclerotic lesions and develop intimal tears, allowing bleeding into the layers of the vessel, which causes weakening and hematoma formation.

Until the aneurysm reaches sufficient size to press on adjacent organs, the individual may be asymptomatic. Complications include rupture and bleeding, exsanguination, and embolization. Most individuals with aneurysms are hypertensive.

## ASSESSMENT

**Chronic indicators**
*Abdominal aneurysm:* Patient describes sensation of heartbeat in the abdomen. Chronic abdominal pain in the middle or lower abdomen also may be present.
*Thoracic aneurysm:* Patient may be asymptomatic for years. Pressure from the aneurysm on adjacent structures can result in dull pain in the upper back, dyspnea, cough, dysphagia, and hoarseness.
*Femoral aneurysm:* Signs of decreased distal arterial blood flow. See the indicators discussed with "Atherosclerotic Arterial Occlusive Disease."
**Acute indicators (rupture or dissection):** Sudden onset of severe pain, often described as tearing or ripping; pallor; diaphoresis; and sudden loss of consciousness.
*Pain with aneurysm at ascending aorta:* Nonradiating, central chest pain.
*Pain with aneurysm at distal aorta:* Radiation to back, abdomen, and legs.
**Physical assessment:** Decreased BP and peripheral pulses, tachycardia, cyanosis, and cool and clammy skin. Patient may have pulsating abdominal mass or systolic bruit over the abdomen (abdominal aneurysm) or a diastolic murmur (thoracic aneurysm).

## DIAGNOSTIC TESTS

**Chest x-ray:** May reveal the outline of an aneurysm, especially if there is calcification.
**Aortography:** Uses contrast dye to locate the lesion and identify its size as well as the condition of the proximal and distal vessels.
**Ultrasound:** May assist in diagnosis when x-ray and physical examination are inconclusive. The sound waves may help determine the size, shape, and location of the aneurysm.
**Digital subtraction angiography:** To confirm diagnosis *via* CT which visualizes the arteries radiographically.
**ECG:** May help differentiate the pain of thoracic aneurysm from that of myocardial infarction (MI).
**CT scan:** To determine the site of the intimal tear and size of the aneurysm.
**Arteriography:** Important before surgery to identify proximal and distal blood vessels.

## COLLABORATIVE MANAGEMENT

**Decrease BP:** Using antihypertensive agents such as atenolol or hydralazine.
**Decrease aortic pulsatile flow:** Using medications that decrease myocardial contractility, such as propranolol.

**Analgesics:**   For pain relief.
**Surgical interventions:**   Indicated if the aneurysm is larger than 4 cm in diameter, peripheral embolization has occurred, there is rupture (a surgical emergency), or a stable aneurysm suddenly becomes tender or causes severe pain. The most common procedure is reconstructive and involves resection of the aneurysm and restoration of vascular flow with an autogenous graft, such as the patient's saphenous vein or a synthetic graft.

## NURSING DIAGNOSES AND INTERVENTIONS

**High risk for fluid volume deficit** related to postsurgical bleeding/hemorrhage
*Desired outcome:*   Patient is normovolemic as evidenced by systolic BP ≥90 mm Hg (or within 20 mm Hg of patient's baseline) and <180 mm Hg, HR ≤100 bpm, peripheral pulse amplitude >2+ on a 0-4+ scale, balanced I&O, and urine output ≥30 ml/h.

- After the patient has been transferred from the ICU, monitor BP and peripheral pulses q30min during the first hour; then q2h or as necessary.
- Check the operative site for the presence of frank bleeding.
- Assess apical and peripheral pulses, and report the presence of tachycardias or a decreased amplitude of peripheral pulses, which can occur with bleeding.
- Monitor abdomen for increasing girth.
- Be alert to patient complaints of low back pain, which, in addition to signs of hypovolemic shock, may signal retroperitoneal hemorrhage.
- Monitor urine output hourly and report volume <30 ml/h.
- Instruct patient to alert staff members promptly to signs and symptoms such as dizziness, lightheadedness, or palpitations (tachycardia), which may occur with hemorrhage due to sympathetic nervous system compensation.

**Altered peripheral tissue perfusion (or risk of same)** related to interrupted arterial flow secondary to postoperative embolization
*Desired outcome:*   Patient has adequate peripheral perfusion as evidenced by peripheral pulse amplitude >2+ on a 0-4+ scale, brisk capillary refill (<2 sec), and baseline extremity sensation, motor function, color, and temperature.

- Assess peripheral pulses at least hourly, and report decreases in amplitude or absence of a pulse.
- Report to physician any changes in color, capillary refill, temperature, sensation, and motor function of the extremities.
- Maintain patient on bed rest until otherwise directed.
- Keep patient flat to maintain graft patency and ensure healing with decreased risk of embolization.
- Instruct patient to report impaired sensation promptly to staff members.

---

**Note:**   Also see Appendix One, "Caring for Preoperative and Postoperative Patients," p. 693.

---

## PATIENT-FAMILY TEACHING AND DISCHARGE PLANNING

Give patient and significant others verbal and written information about the following:

- Importance of regular medical follow-up to ensure graft patency and prompt identification of the development of a new aneurysm.
- Prevention of recurrence of aneurysm by avoiding factors that accelerate atherosclerosis, such as cigarette smoking, obesity, and hypertension.
- Necessity of a regularly scheduled exercise program that alternates exercise with rest.
- Indicators of wound infection and thrombus or embolus formation, and the need to report them promptly to physician should they occur.

- Medications, including drug name, purpose, dosage, schedule, precautions, and potential side effects.
- Telephone number of nurse available to discuss concerns and questions or clarify instructions that are unclear.
- Importance of follow-up visits with physician; confirm date and time of next appointment.
- Potential for aneurysm rupture if surgery is not immediately planned.
  - Teach patient and significant others the symptoms of rupture, including sudden onset of severe pain, often described as tearing or ripping; pallor; diaphoresis; and sudden loss of consciousness.
  - Emphasize the importance of seeking immediate medical attention should any signs and symptoms of rupture occur. Provide numbers of emergency services in the area.
- Potential need for ultrasound for other family members to rule out aneurysm.

# Arterial embolism

An embolus is a fragment of a thrombus, globule of fat, clump of tissue, fragment of an atherosclerotic lesion, bacteria, or a bubble of air that moves in the circulation, lodges in a vessel, and ultimately obstructs flow.

Emboli can be venous (see "Venous Thrombosis/Thrombophlebitis") or arterial. An arterial embolism most commonly arises from thrombi that develop in the chambers of the heart secondary to valvular heart disease, atrial fibrillation (a dysrhythmia with ineffective atrial contraction), myocardial infarction, congestive or chronic cardiac failure, or vascular injury or disease. Emboli also can arise from atherosclerotic plaque lesions in any vessel. The clinical course following embolism depends on the size of the embolus, the vessel(s) affected, the degree of obstruction, and whether distal tissue is involved. Also see "Pulmonary Embolus."

## ASSESSMENT

**Signs and symptoms:**   Sudden onset of severe pain and a gradual decrease in sensory and motor functioning (i.e., presence of the six $P$s of arterial occlusion: pain, pulselessness, pallor, polar [coolness], paresthesia, and paralysis) as early as 12-18 h after occlusion.

**Physical assessment:**   Possible presence of a darkened or mottled extremity; diminished or absent pulse(s). Necrosis or gangrene can occur if there is total occlusion and absence of collateral flow.

**History of:**   Vascular injury or surgery, infection such as cellulitis, valvular heart disease, cardiac dysrhythmias.

## DIAGNOSTIC TESTS

**Ultrasonic Doppler flow studies:**   Will reveal decreased or absent arterial blood flow distal to the embolus.

**Angiography:**   Provides visualization of the embolus in the arterial tree and collateral circulation.

## COLLABORATIVE MANAGEMENT

**Bed rest:**   To prevent further embolization.

**Anticoagulation with oral anticoagulant or heparin *via* continuous IV drip:**   To prevent proximal and distal embolization.

**Thrombolytic drugs such as urokinase or streptokinase:**   To speed up the process of clot lysis; used in individuals who are poor surgical risks or as an alternative to surgical procedures.

**Analgesics:**   To relieve pain caused by distal vasospasm and ischemia.

**Embolectomy:**   Surgical removal of the embolus.

## NURSING DIAGNOSES AND INTERVENTIONS

**Altered peripheral tissue perfusion** related to interrupted arterial flow secondary to embolization (preoperative period)

*Desired outcome:*   Optimally, patient's peripheral perfusion is adequate as evidenced by peripheral pulse amplitude >2+ on a 0-4+ scale and normal extremity color, temperature, sensation, and motor function.

- Maintain patient on bed rest to prevent further embolization.
- Monitor peripheral circulation. Keep extremities warm (room temperature). Advise patient to avoid chilling by wearing socks or slippers.
- Protect extremities from trauma. Provide foam protectors to keep sheets and blankets off tissue that has decreased circulation.
- If prescribed, keep the lower extremities slightly dependent (but not >45 degrees) to promote circulation.
- Teach patient and significant others signs and symptoms of embolization, which necessitate immediate medical attention: sudden onset of severe pain and a gradual decrease in sensory and motor functioning; presence of tingling, numbness, coolness, and cyanosis.

---

**Note:**   See "Pulmonary Embolus" for **Altered protection** related to risk of prolonged bleeding or hemorrhage secondary to anticoagulant therapy, p. 17. Also see Appendix One, "Caring for Preoperative and Postoperative Patients," p. 693, as appropriate.

---

## PATIENT-FAMILY TEACHING AND DISCHARGE PLANNING

Give patient and significant others verbal and written information about the following:

- Prescribed exercise plan to prevent stasis of the blood.
- Signs and symptoms that necessitate immediate medical attention: extremity pain, coolness, pallor, and cyanosis.
- Indicators of wound infection, if surgery was performed.
- Oral anticoagulant therapy: need for regular medical checkups and immediate reporting of epistaxis, ecchymosis, hemoptysis, melena, or hematuria; administration at the same time every day; not changing regular dietary habits (e.g., becoming a vegetarian without first consulting physician or nurse; many green, leafy vegetables are high in vitamin K, which reverses the effect of warfarin; vegetarian diets may necessitate an increase in warfarin dosage to achieve therapeutic anticoagulation); importance of consulting with physician before taking any over-the-counter medications, especially aspirin products, which affect platelet aggregation and potentiate the anticoagulant effect of warfarin.
- Other medications, including drug name, purpose, dosage, schedule, precautions, and potential side effects.
- Risk factor modification, such as smoking cessation, control of hypertension, and dietary modifications to decrease the potential for atherosclerosis and acute arterial occlusion.

# Venous thrombosis/Thrombophlebitis

Although venous thrombosis and thrombophlebitis are different disorders, clinically they are referred to as a single entity, and the terms are used interchangeably to refer to the development of a venous thrombus or thrombi, with associated inflammation. Disturbances in the venous system can have a variety of causes and precipitating factors, including stasis of blood, hemoconcentration, venous trauma, inflammation, or altered coagulation. Venous stasis can occur with heart failure, shock states, immobility from prolonged bed rest, structural disorders of the veins, or as a side effect of anesthesia. Vessel trauma can result from chemical irritation caused by IV solutions or direct trauma. Altered coagulation states usually are related to liver disease or withdrawal from anticoagulants. Venous thrombosis and thrombophlebitis most often occur in the lower extremities, and the most serious complication is embolization.

## ASSESSMENT

**Signs and symptoms:** Unilateral leg swelling (edema), pain, tenderness, erythema, local warmth, and prominence of superficial veins. Sometimes the first sign is a pulmonary embolus (PE) (see "Pulmonary Embolus," p. 13).
**Physical assessment:** A knot or bump occasionally can be felt on palpation.

---

**Caution:** Because of the risk of embolization, never test for a positive Homan's sign in the presence of clinical indicators of venous thrombosis or thrombophlebitis.

---

**Risk factors:** Prolonged bed rest and immobility, leg trauma, recent surgery, use of oral contraceptives, obesity, varicose veins.

## DIAGNOSTIC TESTS

**Contrast phlebography (venography):** A contrast dye is injected into the venous system that is to be studied, allowing visualization of the veins by showing filling or absence of filling.
**Doppler ultrasound:** Identifies changes in blood flow secondary to presence of a thrombus.
**Duplex imaging:** Use of ultrasound to assess veins for flow and pressure.
**I-fibrinogen injection test:** Useful screening device for early detection of thrombosis because the isotope identifies clots that are forming.
**Impedence plethysmography:** Estimates blood flow using measures of resistance and normal changes that occur during pulsatile blood flow.

## COLLABORATIVE MANAGEMENT

**Prevention:** Involves identifying patients at risk, increasing fluid intake to at least 2-3 L/day, promoting leg exercises to prevent stasis, prescribing elastic stockings and early ambulation, administering minidoses of heparin to prevent clot formation, and use of alternating compression devices.
**Therapeutic anticoagulation:** Prevents development of a PE. Heparin is used during the acute phase, and long-term warfarin therapy is used after the acute phase.
**Thrombolytic therapy:** Instituted to lyse and digest the clot. Streptokinase or urokinase may be used.
**Bed rest:** During the acute phase, with support hose and leg elevation to decrease venous stasis.
**Analgesics for pain:** Usually acetaminophen.
**Exercise regimen:** Walking or leg exercises after the acute phase.
**Warm moist packs:** To reduce discomfort and pain.
**Thrombectomy:** Necessary when the danger of PE is extreme, the patient cannot tolerate anticoagulation, or extremity damage from the absence of venous drainage is imminent.

## NURSING DIAGNOSES AND INTERVENTIONS

**Altered peripheral and cardiopulmonary tissue perfusion (or risk of same)** related to interrupted blood flow secondary to embolization from thrombus formation
*Desired outcome:* Patient has adequate peripheral and cardiopulmonary perfusion as evidenced by normal extremity color, temperature, and sensation; RR 12-20 breaths/min with normal depth and pattern (eupnea); HR ≤100 bpm; BP within 20 mm Hg of baseline BP; and normal breath sounds.

- Be alert to and promptly report early indicators of peripheral thrombus formation: pain, edema, erythema, and impaired sensation. If indicators appear, maintain patient on bed rest and notify physician promptly.
- Monitor for and immediately report signs of PE: sudden onset of chest pain, dyspnea, tachypnea, tachycardia, hypotension, hemoptysis, shallow respirations, crackles (rales), decreased breath sounds, and diaphoresis. Should they occur, prompt medical attention is crucial.
- Administer anticoagulants as prescribed. Double-check drip rates and doses with a colleague.
- Minimize the risk of PE by keeping patient on bed rest, providing ROM exercises, and applying support hose as prescribed.

**Pain** related to inflammatory process caused by thrombus formation

***Desired outcomes:***  Within 1 h of intervention, patient's subjective perception of pain decreases, as documented by a pain scale. Objective indicators, such as grimacing, are absent.

- Monitor patient for the presence of pain. Document the degree of pain, using a pain scale from 0 (no pain) to 10 (worst pain). Administer analgesics as prescribed, and document relief obtained using the pain scale.
- Ensure that the patient maintains bed rest during the acute phase to minimize painful engorgement and the potential for embolization.
- If prescribed, apply warm, moist packs. Be sure that the packs are warm (but not extremely so) and not allowed to cool. If appropriate, use a Kock-Mason dressing (warm towel covered by plastic wrap and a K-pad to provide continuous moist heat).
- To promote venous drainage and reduce engorgement, keep the legs elevated above heart level (but not >45 degrees).

**Altered peripheral tissue perfusion (or risk of same)** related to interrupted venous flow secondary to venous engorgement or edema

***Desired outcome:***  Patient has adequate peripheral perfusion as evidenced by absence of discomfort and normal extremity temperature, color, sensation, and motor function.

- Assess for signs of inadequate peripheral perfusion, such as pain and changes in skin temperature, color, and motor or sensory function. Be alert to venous engorgement (prominence) in the lower extremities.
- Elevate patient's legs above heart level (but not >45 degrees) to promote venous drainage.
- As prescribed for patients without evidence of thrombus formation, apply antiembolic hose, which compress superficial veins to increase blood flow to the deeper veins. Remove the stockings for approximately 15 min q8h. Inspect the skin for evidence of irritation.
- Encourage patient to perform ankle circling and active or assisted ROM exercises of the lower extremities to prevent venous stasis. Perform passive ROM if patient cannot.

---

**Caution:**  If there are any signs of acute thrombus formation, such as calf hardness or tenderness, the exercises are contraindicated because of the risk of embolization. Notify physician.

---

- Encourage deep breathing, which creates increased negative pressure in the lungs and thorax to assist in the emptying of large veins.
- Arterial circulation usually will not be impaired unless there is arterial disease or severe edema compressing arterial flow. Assess pulses regularly, however, to confirm the presence of good arterial flow.

**Knowledge deficit:**  Disease process with venous thrombosis/thrombophlebitis and treatment/management measures after hospital discharge

***Desired outcome:***  Before hospital discharge, patient verbalizes knowledge of the disease process and treatment/management measures that are to occur after hospital discharge.

- Discuss the process of venous thrombosis/thrombophlebitis and ways to prevent thrombosis and discomfort, such as avoiding restrictive clothing, avoiding prolonged periods of standing, and elevating legs above heart level when sitting.

- Teach patient the signs of venous stasis ulcers, such as redness and skin breakdown. Stress the importance of avoiding trauma to the extremities and keeping the skin clean and dry.
- Discuss the prescribed exercise program. Walking usually is considered the best exercise.
- Teach patient how to wear antiembolic hose if prescribed. The hose must fit properly without wrinkling and should be snug over the feet and progressively less snug as they reach the knee or thigh.
- Describe indicators that necessitate medical attention: persistent redness, swelling, tenderness, weak or absent pulses, and ulcerations in the extremities.

---

**Note:** See "Pulmonary Embolus" for **Altered protection** related to prolonged bleeding or hemorrhage secondary to anticoagulant therapy, p. 17. See "Varicose Veins" for **Impaired tissue integrity** related to altered circulation secondary to venous engorgement, p. 108.

---

## PATIENT-FAMILY TEACHING AND DISCHARGE PLANNING

See **Knowledge deficit**, p. 106, for topics to discuss (both verbally and through written information) with the patient and significant others.
*In addition:*

- If the patient is discharged from the hospital on warfarin therapy, provide information about the following:
  - As directed, see physician for scheduled prothrombin time (PT) checks.
  - Take warfarin at same time each day; do not skip days unless directed to by the physician.
  - Wear a Medic-Alert bracelet.
  - Avoid alcohol consumption and changes in diet (e.g., changing to a vegetarian diet), both of which can alter the body's response to warfarin.
  - When making appointments with other physicians and dentists, inform them that warfarin is being taken.
  - Be alert to indicators that necessitate immediate medical attention: hematuria, melena, epistaxis, ecchymosis, hemoptysis, dizziness, and weakness.
  - Avoid taking over-the-counter medications (e.g., aspirin, which potentiates the anticoagulant effect of warfarin) without consulting physician or nurse.

# Varicose veins

Varicose veins are enlarged, tortuous, and dilated, and they occur as a result of incompetent valves or increased venous pressure. As the vessels dilate, they lose their elasticity and become less functional. This can result in venous stasis and subsequent thrombus formation. Varicose veins are most often found in the lower extremities.

## ASSESSMENT

**Signs and symptoms:** If only the superficial veins are involved, the patient can be asymptomatic except for the appearance of dilated veins. Increases in venous pressure can cause swelling, pain, leg fatigue, and muscle aches and cramps. As the condition progresses, discomfort increases and ulcerations can develop.

**Physical assessment:** Increased firmness of calf muscles, redness, and swelling; tenderness elicited at the affected site; leg ulcer(s).

**Risk factors:**   Pregnancy, prolonged periods of standing, familial history, obesity, lack of exercise.

## DIAGNOSTIC TESTS

**Brodie-Trendelenburg test:**   Demonstrates the presence of backward flow through incompetent venous valves. While the patient is supine, the leg is elevated to empty the venous system. A tourniquet is then applied to occlude the superficial veins, and the patient is asked to stand. If the communicating valves are incompetent, blood will flow superficially and engorge the superficial veins. This test determines the appropriate treatment.

**Doppler flow studies:**   Detect backward blood flow through incompetent valves.

**Phlebography:**   Allows visualization of veins *via* injection of contrast medium to reveal dilatations, incompetent valves, and thrombi.

## COLLABORATIVE MANAGEMENT

**Prevention through health teaching**

**Support hose or antiembolic hose:**   To compress the superficial veins, decrease engorgement, and shunt venous flow to the deeper, stronger veins.

**Weight reduction program:**   If obesity is a contributing factor.

**Walking or leg-exercise program:**   To prevent venous stasis.

**Vein ligation and stripping:**   When pain from the varicose veins is severe or the risk of thrombus formation increases. Usually this involves ligation of the saphenous vein at the groin, where the saphenous and femoral veins meet. Another small incision is made at the ankle, and a wire is passed into the vein, "stripping" it as it passes. For tortuous veins, multiple incisions may be required.

**Injection sclerotherapy:**   Injection of a sclerosing agent into the vein to obliterate and cause permanent fibrosis.

## NURSING DIAGNOSES AND INTERVENTIONS

**Pain** related to preoperative venous engorgement or surgical procedure

*Desired outcomes:*   Within 1 h of intervention, patient's subjective perception of pain decreases, as documented by a pain scale. Objective indicators, such as grimacing, are absent.

- Monitor patient for the presence of pain using a pain scale from 0 (no pain) to 10 (worst pain). Administer analgesics as prescribed, and document their effectiveness using the pain scale.
- To prevent increased venous pressure and promote venous drainage, encourage patient to keep legs elevated above level of the heart.
- Maintain elastic wraps and antiembolic hose for support and venous drainage.
- To promote circulation and prevent venous stasis, initiate postoperative leg exercises and ambulation as soon as possible after surgery (as directed by physician). To minimize discomfort, advise patient not to sit with the legs dependent or stand still for prolonged periods.
- Suggest to patient that for long periods of sitting when the legs cannot be elevated above heart level, elevating the feet 5-10 inches off the floor (for example, by resting the feet on several books) may help decrease venous stasis.

**Impaired tissue integrity** related to altered circulation secondary to venous engorgement

*Desired outcome:*   Patient's tissue remains intact.

- Apply elastic stockings when the veins are most likely to be empty (e.g., after patient has been recumbent or legs have been elevated for 20 min). This will help minimize distention.
- Remove the stockings at prescribed intervals to minimize swelling proximal to the hose. Assess the skin during the period when the hose are removed,

and be alert to signs of stasis dermatitis (i.e., skin that is thin, shiny, and bluish in color) and for ulcerations. Be sure that the patient's skin is cleansed and dried thoroughly before reapplying the stockings.
- Ensure that the tops of the stockings do not roll, because this would cause a tourniquet effect and further compromise circulation. Also be sure that there are no creases or wrinkles in the hose, which would cause pressure areas.
- Protect the extremities from trauma. If indicated, use foam protectors to keep bedding off the compromised tissues.
- Teach patient not to cross legs, which worsens venous stasis.

---

**Note:** See "Venous Thrombosis/Thrombophlebitis" for **Altered peripheral tissue perfusion (or risk of same),** related to interrupted venous flow secondary to venous engorgement or edema, p. 106, and **Knowledge deficit:** Disease process with venous thrombosis/thrombophlebitis and treatment/management measures following hospital discharge, p. 106. As appropriate, also see Appendix One, "Caring for Preoperative and Postoperative Patients," p. 693.

---

## PATIENT-FAMILY TEACHING AND DISCHARGE PLANNING
Give patient and significant others verbal and written information about the following:
- Medications, including drug name, purpose, dosage, schedule, precautions, and potential side effects.
- Importance of preventive measures, including the following: Wear support hose, elevate legs when possible, avoid prolonged periods of sitting and standing still, initiate a walking or exercise program, change positions at frequent intervals, and start a weight reduction program, if appropriate.
- Necessity of frequent rest periods for at least the first 6 weeks after surgery.
- Importance of regular medical follow-up.
- Avoiding constricting clothing or knee-high stockings, which can obstruct venous flow.

### Selected Bibliography

Acute Pain Management Guideline Panel: *Acute pain management: operative or medical procedures and trauma,* Clinical practices guideline, Agency for Health Care Policy and Research Pub No 92-0032, Rockville, MD, 1992, Public Health Service, US Department of Health and Human Services.

Allen JL: Physical and psychosocial outcomes after coronary artery bypass graft surgery, *Heart Lung* 19(1):49-54, 1990.

Baas LS: Cardiovascular dysfunctions. In Swearingen PL, Keen JH: *Manual of critical care: applying nursing diagnoses to adult critical illness,* ed 2, St Louis, 1991, Mosby–Year Book.

Beekman RH et al: Therapeutic cardiac catheterization for pulmonary valve and pulmonary artery stenosis, *Cardiol Clin* 7(2):331-340, 1989.

Bilodeau ML, Capasso, VC: Peripheral arterial thrombolytic therapy, *Crit Care Nurs Clin North Am* 2(4):673-680, 1990.

Blake GJ: Metoprolol for myocardial infarction, *Nursing 91* 21(1):91, 1991.

Brooks-Brunn J: Thrombolytic intervention and its effect on mortality in acute myocardial infarction: review of clinical trials, *Heart Lung* 17(6):756-760, 1988.

Cimini DM: Indium-111 antimyosin antibody imaging: a promising new technique in the diagnosis of MI, *Crit Care Nurs* 12(6):44-51, 1992.

Daily EK: Percutaneous balloon valvuloplasty in adult patients with valvular heart disease, *Crit Care Nurs Clin North Am* 1(2):339-389, 1989.

Ford KA: Carotid artery aneurysm: a case study, *J Vasc Nurs* 9(1):2-6, 1991.

Ford KA: Laser-assisted angioplasty in the patient with peripheral arterial disease, *J Vasc Nurs* 8(3):6-8, 1990.

Frohlich ED: Calcium antagonists for initial therapy of hypertension, *Heart Lung* 18(4):370-376, 1989.

Guyton AC: *Textbook of medical physiology,* ed 8, Philadelphia, 1991, WB Saunders Co.

Henderson E: Thrombolytic therapy in acute myocardial infarction: an overview, *J Emerg Nurs* 15(2) part 2: 145-149, 1989.

Henneman EA, Henneman PL: Intracacies of blood pressure measurement: reexamining the rituals, *Heart Lung* 18(3):263, 1989.

Interqual: The ISD-A review system with adult ISD criteria, August 1992, Northhampton, NH, and Marlboro, MA, Interqual, Inc.

Johnson SM, Anderson B: Carotid endarterectomy: a review, *Crit Care Clin North Am* 3(3):499-506, 1991.

Kim MJ, McFarland GK, McLane AM: *Pocket guide to nursing diagnoses,* ed 5, St Louis, 1993, Mosby–Year Book.

McHugh M, Collier M, Morris G: Alternatives to mouth-to-mouth rescue breathing, *Nurs Management* 21(12):37-39, 1990.

Mercer M: Providing electrical support for the heart: rate-responsive pacers, *RN* 55(5):34-37, 1992.

Merva JA: Providing electrical support for the heart: Temporary pacemakers, *RN* 55(5):28-33, 1992.

Misinski M: Pathophysiology of acute myocardial infarction: a rationale for thrombolytic therapy, *Heart Lung* 17(6):743-740, 1988.

Moore HS: Preventing coronary artery reocclusion following t-PA, *Crit Care Nurs* 10(10):52-58, 1990.

Morton PG: Latest advances in thrombolytic therapy, *J Intravenous Nurs* 14(3):181-189, 1991.

Ohler L et al: Aortic valvuloplasty: medical and critical care nursing perspectives, *Focus Crit Care* 16(4):275-291, 1989.

Porth CM: *Pathophysiology: concepts of altered health states,* ed 3, Philadelphia, 1990, JB Lippincott Co.

Pratt CM, O'Rourke R: Application and interpretation of submaximal exercise testing and ambulatory ECG recordings in patients with acute myocardial infarction, *Chest* 93(1):29s-32s, 1988.

Prevost DB: Diagnostic arteriography and percutaneous transluminal angioplasty of the lower extremities, *J Vasc Nurs* 8(4):6-12, 1990.

Rice V: Shock, a clinical syndrome: an update, *Crit Care Nurs* 11(4):20-27, 1991.

Senerchia C: Methods to limit reinfarction and ischemia after thrombolytic therapy, *Crit Care Clin North Am* 2(4):635-642, 1990.

Sipperly MD: Expanding the role of coronary angioplasty: current implications, limitations, and nursing considerations, *Heart Lung* 18(5):507-513, 1989.

Sirles AT, Selleck CS: Cardiac disease and the family: impact, assessment, and implications, *J Cardiovasc Nurs* 3(2):23-32, 1989.

Sommers MS: Potential for injury: trauma after cardiopulmonary resuscitation, *Heart Lung* 20(3):287-293, 1991.

Steuble BT: Cardiovascular dysfunctions. In Swearingen PL, Keen JH: *Manual of critical care: applying nursing diagnoses to adult critical illness,* ed 2, St Louis, 1991, Mosby–Year Book.

Steuble BT: Multi-system stressors. In Swearingen PL, Keen JH: *Manual of critical care: applying nursing diagnoses to adult critical illness,* ed 2, St Louis, 1991, Mosby–Year Book.

Stewart JV, Sheehan AM: Permanent pacemakers: the nurse's role in patient education and follow-up care, *J Cardiovasc Nurs* 5(3):32-43, 1991.

Sulzbach LM: Measurement of pulsus paradoxus, *Focus Crit Care* 16(2):142-145, 1989.

Teplitz L: Transcutaneous pacemakers, *J Cardiovasc Nurs* 5(3):44-57, 1991.

Tognoni G et al: Thrombolysis in acute MI, *Chest* 99(4):121S-127S, 1991.

Trausch PA: Infective endocarditis: nursing care and prevention, *Prog Cardiovasc Nurs* 3(2):45-53, 1988.

Underhill S et al: *Cardiac nursing,* ed 2, Philadelphia, 1989, JB Lippincott Co.

Witherell CL: Questions nurses ask about pacemakers, *Am J Nurs* 90(12):20-28, 1990.

Section One   Renal Disorders   113
    Glomerulonephritis   113
    Nephrotic syndrome   118
    Acute pyelonephritis   120
    Renal calculi   123
    Hydronephrosis   125
    Renal artery stenosis   127
Section Two   Renal Failure   129
    Acute renal failure   129
    Chronic renal failure   135
Section Three   Care of the Renal Transplant Recipient   140
Section Four   Renal Dialysis   142
    Care of the patient undergoing peritoneal dialysis   143
    Care of the patient undergoing hemodialysis   145
Section Five   Disorders of the Urinary Tract   147
    Ureteral calculi   147
    Urinary tract obstruction   152
    Cancer of the bladder   154
Section Six   Urinary Disorders Secondary to Other Disease Processes   158
    Urinary incontinence   158
    Urinary retention   165
    Neurogenic bladder   167
Section Seven   Urinary Diversions   172
Selected Bibliography   178

## Section One:   Renal Disorders

### Glomerulonephritis

Glomerulonephritis (GN) is the name of a group of diseases that damage the renal glomeruli. When the glomerulus is injured, protein and RBCs are allowed to enter the renal tubule and be excreted in the urine. GN can be acute or chronic. Most individuals with acute GN improve dramatically within weeks and recover completely within 1-2 years, but renal damage continues to progress for those with chronic GN. Chronic GN is the most common cause of chronic renal failure. Most forms of GN are the result of immunologic processes (e.g., poststreptococcal infection, systemic lupus erythematosus).

See "Acute Renal Failure" and "Chronic Renal Failure" as appropriate.

## ASSESSMENT

Indicators can range from subtle to blatant, depending on the patient's level of renal function.

**Acute indicators:**  Hematuria, proteinuria, oliguria, dull bilateral flank pain, headache, low-grade fever.

**Chronic indicators:**  Fatigue, lethargy, anorexia, nausea, nocturia, headache, weakness.

**Physical assessment:**  Presence of edema (peripheral, periorbital, sacral), crackles (rales), elevated BP, pallor.

**History of:**  Recent upper respiratory infection (URI) or other infection; systemic lupus erythematosus or other autoimmune disease; bloody urine.

## DIAGNOSTIC TESTS

**Urinalysis and 24-hour urinary protein excretion:**  Hematuria with red cell casts and proteinuria are the cardinal findings.

**Blood urea nitrogen (BUN) and serum creatinine:**  If elevated, may indicate decreased renal function.

**Plasma complement, antinuclear antibody titer, antistreptolysin O titer, throat and blood cultures, hepatitis B antigen, and immunoelectrophoresis of the serum and urine:**  Optional tests to determine cause of GN.

**Renal biopsy:**  Indicated when tissue diagnosis is needed to direct therapy or provide prognostic data. Usually a percutaneous (closed) renal biopsy is performed. Postbiopsy care includes keeping the patient supine with a rolled towel under the biopsy site for 12 h and frequent monitoring of VS (q15min initially). Two possible complications of renal biopsy are bleeding and infection. Severe pain, hypotension, persistent gross hematuria, or fever should be reported to the physician immediately. Samples of urine from the first several voidings may be saved to assess for hematuria.

## COLLABORATIVE MANAGEMENT

**Bed rest:**  For patients with acute GN. Limited activity may be necessary for weeks to months.

**Pharmacotherapy**

*Corticosteroids and cytotoxic agents:*  To suppress the immune system and reduce antibody formation.

*Anticoagulants:*  To reduce nonimmunologic mediators of glomerular damage.

*Antibiotics:*  If causative factor is bacterial.

*Diuretics:*  To remove excess fluid (Table 3-1).

*Antihypertensives:*  To control BP.

**Plasmapheresis:**  To remove immune complexes or antiglomerular basement antibodies. It is used only in patients with Goodpasture's syndrome and rapidly progressing GN.

**Diet:**  Restriction of sodium (Na) (Table 3-2) and fluids if edema or hypertension is present. A high-carbohydrate diet is encouraged to maintain nutrition and prevent tissue catabolism. If renal function is markedly decreased, protein and phosphorus may be limited to prevent retention of excess nitrogenous wastes and hyperphosphatemia.

**Peritoneal dialysis or hemodialysis:**  To maintain homeostasis or prevent uremic complications if renal function is markedly decreased (see "Renal Dialysis," p. 142).

## NURSING DIAGNOSES AND INTERVENTIONS

**Activity intolerance** related to generalized weakness and prolonged bed rest

*Desired outcomes:*  Patient maintains bed rest until BP and protein excretion are normal or near normal. After resumption of activity, patient exhibits car-

**T A B L E 3 - 1    Diuretics**

| Generic name | Common brand names | Usual dosage/24 h (mg) |
|---|---|---|
| acetazolamide | Diamox | 250-375    (qod) |
| amiloride HCl* | Midamor | 5-10 |
| chlorothiazide sodium | Diuril | 250-1,000 |
| chlorthalidone | Hygroton | 25-100 |
| ethacrynic acid | Edecrin | 25-200 |
| furosemide | Lasix | 20-160 |
| hydrochlorothiazide | Esidrix | 25-100 |
| metolazone | Zaroxolyn, Diulo | 2.5-10 |
| spironolactone* | Aldactone | 25-200 |
| triamterene* | Dyrenium | 50-300 |

*Although most diuretics can cause hypokalemia, these diuretics might cause hyperkalemia. For this reason they are often used in combination with thiazide diuretics.

**T A B L E 3 - 2    Foods High in Sodium Content**

Bouillon
Celery
Cheeses
Dried fruits
Frozen, canned, or packaged foods
Monosodium glutamate (MSG)
Mustard
Olives
Pickles
Preserved meat
Salad dressings and prepared sauces
Sauerkraut
Snack foods (e.g., crackers, chips, pretzels)
Soy sauce

diac tolerance as evidenced by systolic BP and HR within 20 mm Hg or bpm of resting levels and RR ≤20 breaths/min with normal depth and pattern (eupnea).
- During period of enforced bed rest, assist patient with ADL as necessary. For patients with acute GN, bed rest usually lasts 10 days-2 weeks.
- Provide bed exercises within the prescribed activity limitations. Establish a progressive activity regimen that will allow patient to return to normal activities without complications. For more information, see Appendix One, "Caring for Patients on Prolonged Bed Rest," for **High risk for activity intolerance,** p. 711, and **High risk for disuse syndrome,** p. 713.
- Before patient resumes activities, ensure that BP is within patient's normal range and urine protein excretion is near normal. Normal ranges for protein excretion are 2-8 mg/dl (random) and 40-150 mg/24 h. Notify physician if elevations occur after patient resumes activities.

**Fluid volume excess** related to compromised regulatory mechanisms secondary to decreased renal function
***Desired outcomes:***  With successful therapy, patient is normovolemic as ev-

idenced by urine output of at least 30-60 ml/h (or patient's normal range), stable weight, edema $\leq 1+$ on a 0-4+ scale, and subjective statement that thirst is controlled. BP and HR are within patient's normal range, CVP is 5-12 cm $H_2O$, and RR is 12-20 breaths/min with normal depth and pattern (eupnea). Within the 24-h period before hospital discharge, patient lists foods that are high in Na and plans a 3-day menu that excludes foods high in Na.

- Monitor I&O closely. Notify physician about sudden changes in output.
- Monitor weight daily. Report unusual or steady gains or losses (e.g., 0.5-1 kg/day).
- Observe for indicators of fluid overload: edema, hypertension, crackles (rales), tachycardia, lethargy, distended neck veins, SOB, and increased CVP. **Note:** Not all patients with edema are fluid-overloaded. Edema also can occur because of decreased serum albumin secondary to urinary losses.
- Offer ice chips or popsicles to minimize thirst in the fluid-restricted patient; be sure to record the amount on the intake record. Frequent mouth care also may help minimize thirst.
- Provide patient with data about foods high in Na content (Table 3-2), which should be avoided. Mustard and soy sauce, which traditionally are high in Na content, are available in low-salt versions. Many over-the-counter preparations are high in Na (e.g., mouthwashes and antacids). Advise patient and significant others to read all labels carefully.

**Knowledge deficit:**   Signs and symptoms of fluid and electrolyte imbalance (caused by decreased renal function or diuretic therapy)

***Desired outcomes:***   Within 36 h of admission, patient verbalizes knowledge about the signs and symptoms of fluid and electrolyte imbalance and the importance of reporting them promptly to physician or staff if they occur.

- Alert patient and significant others to signs and symptoms of the following:
  - *Hypokalemia:* Muscle weakness, lethargy, dysrhythmias, nausea, and vomiting.
  - *Hyperkalemia:* Abdominal cramping, diarrhea, irritability, and muscle weakness (if severe).
  - *Hypocalcemia:* Twitching, numbness and tingling of fingers and circumoral region, and muscle cramps.
  - *Hyperphosphatemia:* Precipitation of calcium phosphate in the soft tissue (e.g., cornea, lungs, kidneys, gastric mucosa, heart, blood vessels) and periarticular region of the large joints (e.g., hips, shoulders, and elbows).
  - *Uremia:* Anorexia, nausea, metallic taste in the mouth, irritability, confusion, lethargy, restlessness, and pruritus (itching).
- Instruct patient to report the above signs and symptoms to physician or staff promptly should they occur.

**Knowledge deficit:**   Side effects of corticosteroids and cytotoxic agents

***Desired outcome:***   Within the 24-h period before hospital discharge, patient verbalizes knowledge of the side effects of corticosteroids and cytotoxic agents and the importance of reporting them promptly to staff or physician should they occur.

- Corticosteroids and cytotoxic agents are potent medications with potentially serious side effects that are used in GN to suppress the immune system and reduce antibody formation. Alert patient on corticosteroids to the potential for the following, depending on dose and duration of therapy: poor resistance to infection, increasing BP, mental changes, hyperglycemia, capillary fragility, and gastrointestinal (GI) bleeding. Stress the importance of avoiding individuals known to have infections. If the patient has been on corticosteroid therapy over a prolonged period, Na and water retention, hypokalemia, and indicators similar to Cushing's syndrome can occur, as manifested by edema, buffalo hump, hirsutism, moon face, skin striae and thinning, weight gain, peptic ulcer, headache, nervousness, insomnia, and metabolic acidosis, in addition to the initial indicators described previously.

- If patient has been on corticosteroids for 1 week or longer, caution against abrupt withdrawal, which can result in adrenal insufficiency. Therapy must be withdrawn with gradual reductions in dosage. Signs and symptoms that can occur with abrupt withdrawal include fever, malaise, fatigue, anorexia, orthostatic hypotension, dyspnea, muscle and joint pain, and hypoglycemia.
- Alert patient on cytotoxic agents about the potential for the following: infection, cystitis with hematuria, and abnormal hair loss. See Appendix One, "Caring for Patients with Cancer and other Life-Disrupting Illnesses," p. 719, for additional information about cytotoxic agents.
- Stress the importance of notifying physician or staff promptly if any of these symptoms occur.

**High risk for infection** related to immunosuppression with corticosteroid therapy, immobility, invasive techniques, and impaired skin integrity

*Desired outcome:* Patient is free of infection as evidenced by normothermia and absence of adventitious breath sounds. Respiratory secretions are of normal color, consistency, and quantity.

- Because the respiratory system is a common site for infection in the immunocompromised patient, be alert to indications of infection, such as increased body temperature, adventitious breath sounds, and increased, thickened, or colored airway secretions. If secretions are noted, encourage coughing or provide suctioning at frequent intervals. **Note:** Individuals who are uremic and older adults tend to run subnormal temperatures, so even slight fevers can be significant. Remember that steroids may mask the signs and symptoms of infection.
- Use meticulous sterile technique when performing invasive procedures or manipulating urinary catheters, IV lines, or venous catheters.
- Provide oral hygiene and skin care at frequent intervals. Edema, bed rest, and uremia all increase the potential for skin breakdown, which further increases the risk of infection.
- Teach patient the necessity of avoiding infections and seeking treatment promptly if infections occur after hospital discharge. Teach the signs and symptoms of URI, otitis media, urinary tract infection (UTI), and impetigo. (See **High risk for infection** in "Care of the Renal Transplant Recipient," p. 141.)

---

**Note:** See "Pulmonary Embolus" for **Altered protection** related to risk of prolonged bleeding or hemorrhage secondary to anticoagulation therapy, p. 17. See nursing diagnoses and interventions in Appendix One, "Caring for Patients on Prolonged Bed Rest," p. 711.

---

## PATIENT-FAMILY TEACHING AND DISCHARGE PLANNING

Give patient and significant others verbal and written information about the following:

- Medications, including drug name, purpose, dosage, schedule, precautions, and potential side effects.
- Diet, including fact sheet listing foods that should be avoided or limited. Inform patient that diet and fluid restrictions may be altered as renal function changes.
- Indicators that require medical attention: irregular pulse, fever, unusual SOB or edema, sudden change in urine output, or unusual weakness.
- Technique for measuring temperature and pulse and recording I&O.
- Necessity for continued medical evaluation; confirm date and time of next physician appointment, if known.
- Importance of adjusting and gradually increasing activities to avoid fatigue.
- Necessity of avoiding infections and seeking treatment promptly should they occur. Teach the signs and symptoms of URI, otitis media, UTI, and im-

petigo (see **High risk for infection,** p. 141, in "Care of the Renal Transplant Recipient").

*In addition*
- Coordinate family and social service support for the patient who must continue bed rest or restrict activity at home. Consider such factors as meals, loss of income, housework, child care, and transportation.

## Nephrotic syndrome

Nephrotic syndrome (NS) is a complex of symptoms that can occur with any disease that causes glomerular damage and consequent increased glomerular permeability to protein. The hallmarks of NS are increased urinary excretion of protein, decreased serum albumin, increased serum lipids, hypercoagulability, and edema. The two main causes of NS are glomerulonephritis and diabetic nephropathy, and its course and prognosis depend on the status of the disease that caused it. In adults, NS often progresses to chronic renal failure.

See "Glomerulonephritis" and "Chronic Renal Failure" as appropriate.

### ASSESSMENT

**Signs and symptoms:**   Anorexia, nausea, diarrhea, lethargy, fatigue. Patient may also have ascites, pleural effusion, decreased urinary output, and weight gain.

**Physical assessment:**   Pallor; edema (periorbital, abdominal, sacral, dependent); and either hypertension or hypotension, depending on the primary renal disease and effective circulating volume.

**History of:**   Glomerulonephritis, diabetes mellitus, lupus erythematosus, or infectious disease.

### DIAGNOSTIC TESTS

**24-h protein excretion:**   To diagnose the syndrome. NS is defined as urinary excretion of >3.5 g/day of protein. Protein loss can be >10 g/day.

**Urinalysis:**   Will show sediment-containing casts, oval fat bodies, and RBCs.

---

**Note:**   All urine samples should be sent to the lab immediately after they are obtained, or refrigerated if this is not possible. Urine left at room temperature has greater potential for bacterial growth, turbidity, and alkalinity, any of which can distort the results. Specimens for urine culture should *not* be refrigerated.

---

**Serum tests:**   Will show low albumin, elevated cholesterol and triglycerides, and low total calcium. BUN and creatinine may be elevated. Additional lab tests might be performed, depending on the suspected cause of NS.

**Renal biopsy:**   Often necessary to determine the cause, direct the therapy, and indicate the prognosis of NS. See "Glomerulonephritis," p. 114, for further discussion.

### COLLABORATIVE MANAGEMENT

**Bed rest:**   During periods of severe edema.

**Diet:**   Low in Na (see Table 3-2), low in saturated fat (Table 2-3, p. 52), rich in high-biologic value protein (1.5 g/kg body weight/day), with adequate caloric intake. Liberal protein intake is required to provide necessary amino acids for albumin synthesis. In chronic nephrotic syndrome, protein intake may be restricted in order to limit urinary excretion of protein.

**Pharmacotherapy** may include the following:

*Diuretics:*   Used cautiously to reduce edema and control hypertension if present (see Table 3-1).

*Antibiotics:*   To treat infection.

*Corticosteroids, anticoagulants, or cytotoxic agents:*   To treat glomerulone-phritis (GN). See "Glomerulonephritis," p. 114. Anticoagulants may also be used in patients with thromboembolic complications.
*Antihypertensive agents:*   To treat hypertension.

## NURSING DIAGNOSES AND INTERVENTIONS

**High risk for fluid volume deficit** related to loss secondary to pharmacother-apy or related to failure of regulatory mechanisms secondary to disease pro-cess; *or*
**Fluid volume excess** related to compromised regulatory mechanisms resulting in renal retention of Na and water
*Desired outcomes:*   With successful treatment, patient is normovolemic as ev-idenced by balanced I&O, urine output of at least 30-60 ml/h (or patient's normal range), stable weight, normal breath sounds, edema ≤1+ on a 0-4+ scale, CVP 5-12 cm $H_2O$, and BP and HR within patient's normal range. Within the 24-h period before hospital discharge, patient verbalizes knowl-edge of foods high in Na and the rationale for avoiding them.

- Monitor I&O closely; document every shift.
- Monitor patient's weight daily. Report unusual or steady gains or losses.
- Observe for and document changes in hydration and VS after administration of diuretics, antihypertensives, or osmotic agents.
- Limit Na intake as prescribed. Teach patient about foods that are high in Na (Table 3-2).
- Measure abdominal girth every shift in patients with ascites.
- Auscultate lung fields every shift for evidence of pleural effusion (i.e., bron-chial or decreased breath sounds), and be alert to signs of respiratory dis-tress, such as increased RR and SOB. Notify physician about significant changes.
- Observe for indicators of decreased effective circulating volume (e.g., hy-potension, hypotension with position changes, tachycardia, and decreased CVP), which can occur as a result of ascites formation, Na restriction, and administration of diuretics or certain antihypertensives.

**Altered nutrition:**   Less than body requirements, related to anorexia and uri-nary losses of protein
*Desired outcomes:*   Following treatment, patient has adequate nutrition as ev-idenced by stable weight, normal or near normal values of serum albumin (3.5-5.5 g/dl), and a positive nitrogen (N) state. Patient maintains a diet rich in high-biologic-value protein and relates knowledge about high-protein foods within 24 h of admission.

- Provide prescribed diet in small, frequent feedings.
- Teach patient about foods rich in high-biologic-value protein (e.g., meat, poultry, fish, lentils, and eggs).
- Develop a diet plan with dietitian, patient, and significant others, adjusting it to patient's preference.
- Encourage significant others to bring in patient's favorite high-protein foods as allowed.
- Record calorie intake and weigh patient daily.

**High risk for infection** related to treatment with immunosuppressive agents, prolonged immobility, invasive procedures, and disease process
*Desired outcomes:*   Patient is free of infection as evidenced by normother-mia, normal breath sounds, and respiratory secretions of normal consistency, color, and odor. Within the 24-h period before hospital discharge, patient ver-balizes knowledge of the indicators of infection and the importance of seeking medical attention promptly if they occur.

---

**Note:**   Nephrotic syndrome causes an increased susceptibility to infection, which is believed to occur because of the loss of serum-immune globulins in the urine. The risk of infection is further increased if the patient is being treated with immunosuppressive agents.

---

- Minimize the risk of exposing patient to individuals with infections by providing a private room, if possible. Alert significant others about this concern.
- For other interventions, see this nursing diagnosis in "Glomerulonephritis," p. 117.

---

**Note:**   Because these patients are at increased risk for thrombus formation, see "Pulmonary Embolus" for **Altered protection** related to risk of prolonged bleeding or hemorrhage secondary to anticoagulant therapy, p. 17. See "Glomerulonephritis" for **Activity intolerance,** p. 114, **Knowledge deficit:** Signs and symptoms of fluid and electrolyte imbalance, p. 116, and **Knowledge deficit:** Side effects of corticosteroids and cytotoxic agents, p. 116. See nursing diagnoses and interventions in Appendix One, "Caring for Patients on Prolonged Bed Rest, p. 711.

---

## PATIENT-FAMILY TEACHING AND DISCHARGE PLANNING

Give patient and significant others verbal and written information about the following:

- Medications, including drug name, purpose, dosage, schedule, precautions, and potential side effects.
- Diet: Advise patient and significant others that diet and fluid restrictions may be altered as renal function changes. Provide lists of advocated and restricted foods.
- Signs and symptoms that require medical attention: irregular pulse, fever, unusual SOB or edema, sudden change in urinary output, unusual weakness, and increase in weight of >1 kg/week.
- Need for continued medical evaluation; confirm time and date of next physician appointment, if known.
- Importance of avoiding infections and seeking treatment promptly should signs and symptoms appear. Teach the indicators of upper respiratory infection, otitis media, impetigo, and urinary tract infection. For details, see **High risk for infection,** p. 141, in "Care of the Renal Transplant Recipient."
- Importance of skin care, especially over edematous areas.
*In addition*
- Coordinate family and social service support for the patient who must continue bed rest or limited activity at home. Consider such factors as meals, loss of income, housework, child care, and transportation.

# Acute pyelonephritis

Acute pyelonephritis is an infection of the renal parenchyma and pelvis, which usually occurs secondary to an ascending urinary tract infection (UTI). UTIs typically result from anatomic or functional obstruction to urine flow (e.g., from prostatic hypertrophy or renal calculi, or instrumentation, such as catheterization or cystoscopy). Hematogenous infection also can occur in acute pyelonephritis when bacteria reach the kidney *via* the bloodstream.

The incidence of acute pyelonephritis increases with advancing age. In the absence of anatomic obstruction or instrumentation, acute pyelonephritis is almost exclusively a disease of females. The infecting organism may be a type of fecal flora, such as *Escherichia* or *Klebsiella*, or normal flora from the periurethral skin (e.g., *Staphylococcus saprophyticus*). Recurrent infections are common; chronic renal failure is a rare complication.

## ASSESSMENT

**Signs and symptoms:**   Fever, chills, flank pain, nausea, vomiting, malaise, frequency and urgency of urination, dysuria, cloudy and foul-smelling urine, and nocturia. **Note:** These indicators can be nonspecific, especially in the elderly.

**Physical assessment:**   Tender, enlarged kidneys; abdominal rigidity; and costovertebral tenderness.

**History of:**   UTI or obstruction; recent urologic procedure; pregnancy.

## DIAGNOSTIC TESTS

Unless an anatomic or preexisting renal disease is present, renal function should remain normal.

**Urine culture:**   Should be positive for the causative organism. **Note:** Asymptomatic bacteriuria is common in elders.

**Urinalysis:**   Will reveal presence of WBCs, WBC casts, RBCs, and bacteria.

---

**Note:**   All urine samples should be sent to the lab immediately after they are obtained, or refrigerated if this is not possible. Urine left at room temperature has greater potential for bacterial growth, turbidity, and alkalinity, any of which can distort the test results. Urine cultures should *not* be refrigerated.

---

**Blood culture:**   Positive for the causative organism in hematogenous infection. It is obtained from patients who appear septic or are hypotensive.

**Intravenous pyelogram (IVP) or retrograde pyelogram:**   May be performed if there are recurrent episodes or if obstruction is suspected.

## COLLABORATIVE MANAGEMENT

**Bed rest.**

**Pharmacotherapy**

*Antibiotics:*   For the infection; initially parenteral, then oral. Low-dose antimicrobial prophylaxis may be indicated for women with recurrent UTI.

*ASA or acetaminophen:*   To control the fever and treat the discomfort.

**Surgical intervention:**   May be necessary if an obstruction is present.

## NURSING DIAGNOSES AND INTERVENTIONS

**Pain** related to dysuria secondary to infection

*Desired outcomes:*   Within 1 h of intervention, patient's subjective perception of discomfort decreases, as documented by a pain scale. Objective indicators, such as grimacing, are absent or diminished.

- Monitor patient for the presence of costovertebral angle (CVA) pain and tenderness, abdominal pain, and dysuria. Devise a pain scale with patient, rating pain from 0 (absent) to 10 (worst pain). As appropriate, administer the prescribed analgesics, and document their effectiveness, using the pain scale.
- If it is not contraindicated, increase the patient's fluid intake to help relieve dysuria.
- Notify physician about unrelieved or increasing flank pain.
- As appropriate, assist patient with repositioning if it is effective in relieving discomfort.
- Use nonpharmacologic interventions when possible (e.g., relaxation techniques, guided imagery, and distraction).

**High risk for infection** (or its recurrence) related to chronic disease process

*Desired outcomes:*   Patient is free of infection as evidenced by normothermia; urine that is clear and of normal odor; HR ≤100 bpm; BP ≥90/60 mm Hg (or within patient's normal range); absence of flank, CVA, and labial pain;

and absence of dysuria, urgency, and frequency. Within the 24-h period before hospital discharge, patient verbalizes knowledge about the signs and symptoms of infection and the importance of reporting them promptly if they occur.

- Monitor patient's temperature at least q4h. Report temperature >38° C (100° F) to physician. Monitor for the presence of flank, CVA, and labial pain; foul-smelling or cloudy urine; malaise; headache; and frequency and urgency of urination. Teach these indicators to the patient and stress the importance of reporting them promptly to physician or staff if they occur.
- Monitor BP and pulse at least q4h. The presence of hypotension and tachycardia can be indicative of sepsis and bacteremic shock.
- Administer prescribed antibiotics as scheduled. Draw prescribed antibiotic serum levels at correct times to ensure reliable results. **Note:** Most antibiotics are measured at peak (30-60 min after infusion) and trough (30-60 min before the next dose) levels.
- Use urinary catheters only when mandatory. Use meticulous sterile technique when inserting, irrigating, or obtaining specimens. Provide perineal care daily. For indwelling catheters, maintain unobstructed flow, and always keep the urinary collection container below the level of the patient's bladder to prevent reflux of urine. Tape the catheter to the thigh or abdomen to decrease meatal irritation. **Note:** Intermittent catheterization carries less of a risk of UTI than indwelling catheterization.
- Offer cranberry, plum, or prune juices, which leave an acid ash in the urine and inhibit bacteriuria.
- Treat fever with prescribed antipyretics and tepid baths as needed.
- Teach female patients the importance of wiping the perianal area from front to back, wearing undergarments with cotton crotch, and voiding before and immediately after sexual intercourse to minimize the risk of introducing bacteria into the urinary tract.
- Stress the importance of emptying the bladder at least q3-4h and once during the night to help prevent UTI caused by residual urine.

**Altered nutrition:**   Less than body requirements, related to nausea and anorexia

*Desired outcome:*   Patient maintains an adequate diet within 24 h of admission.

- Provide patient who is nauseated or anorexic with frequent small meals and carbonated beverages.
- Treat nausea and vomiting with prescribed medications.
- Record accurate calorie intake and weigh patient daily.
- Alert physician about inadequate nutritional intake.
- For additional information see "Providing Nutritional Support," p. 665.

**Fluid volume deficit** related to decreased intake secondary to anorexia or active loss secondary to vomiting and diaphoresis

*Desired outcomes:*   Following treatment patient becomes normovolemic as evidenced by balanced I&O, stable weight, urinary output ≥30-60 ml/h, and BP and HR within patient's normal range. Within 24 h of admission, patient verbalizes knowledge about the importance of a fluid intake of at least 2-3 L/day.

- Maintain adequate fluid intake to avoid fluid volume deficit. An intake of at least 2-3 L/day is usually indicated; however, the appropriate amount depends on the patient's output, which includes gastric, fecal, urinary, sensible, and insensible losses. Obtain guidelines for the desired amount of fluid intake/restriction from physician. Teach nonrestricted patients the importance of maintaining a fluid intake of at least 2-3 L/day.
- Monitor I&O and daily weight as indicators of hydration status.
- Report indicators of volume deficit: poor skin turgor, thirst, dry mucous membranes, tachycardia, or orthostatic hypotension.

## PATIENT-FAMILY TEACHING AND DISCHARGE PLANNING

Give patient and significant others verbal and written information about the following:

- Medications, including drug name, purpose, dosage, schedule, precautions, and potential side effects.
- Importance of taking medications for prescribed length of time, even if feeling "well."
- Necessity of reporting the following indicators of UTI to physician: urgency, frequency, dysuria, flank pain, cloudy or foul-smelling urine, and fever.
- Importance of perineal hygiene for female patients and the necessity of wiping from front to back, wearing undergarments with cotton crotch, and voiding before and after intercourse.
- Importance of emptying the bladder at least q3-4h and once during the night to help prevent UTI caused by residual urine.
- Necessity of maintaining a fluid intake of at least 2-3 L/day and drinking fruit juices (cranberry, plum, prune) that leave an acid ash in the urine.
- Importance of continued medical follow-up because of the high incidence of recurrence.

# Renal calculi

The kidneys excrete several substances that singly or in combination are highly insoluble. Normally these substances are excreted with minimal crystal formation; but diet, medications, metabolic abnormalities, systemic disease, or infection can increase the tendency for crystals to form and stones to develop. Altered urine pH and concentration also can be important factors in stone formation.

Stones can lodge and cause obstruction or be passed in the urine. Giant staghorn calculi occasionally develop and fill the entire renal pelvis. The most common types of stones are made of calcium, struvite, uric acid, and cystine. Renal calculi are often recurrent and a common medical problem. Complications include infection and hydronephrosis.

## ASSESSMENT

**Signs and symptoms:**   The primary symptom is pain, with the location and severity depending on the area in which the stone has lodged. Vague back pain occurs when the stone lodges in the calyces or pelvis. Renal colic (severe flank pain radiating to the groin) is typical when the stone has lodged at the junction of the pelvis and ureter. Other indicators are hematuria, nausea, vomiting, syncope, and fever.

**Physical assessment:**   Diaphoresis, pallor, and obvious distress.

**History of:**   Previous stone formation, urinary tract infection (UTI), or urinary tract obstruction; diet high in calcium, purine, or oxalate; gout or administration of uricosuric agents; or treatment of neoplastic disease (due to increased production of uric acid).

## DIAGNOSTIC TESTS

See "Ureteral Calculi," p. 148.

## COLLABORATIVE MANAGEMENT

See "Ureteral Calculi," p. 149, for a discussion of management, including extracorporeal shock wave lithotripsy.

**Surgical interventions:**   Indications for surgery include complete obstruction; persistent infection; severe, uncontrollable pain; renal pelvic calculus that is too large to pass spontaneously.

*Pyelolithotomy:* (incision into the renal pelvis).

*Nephrolithotomy:* (incision into the renal parenchyma).
*Nephrectomy:* (removal of the kidney if it is severely damaged).

## NURSING DIAGNOSES AND INTERVENTIONS FOR THE SURGICAL PATIENT

**High risk for fluid volume deficit** related to postoperative bleeding after pyelolithotomy or nephrolithotomy
*Desired outcome:* Patient remains normovolemic as evidenced by balanced I&O, stable weight, good skin turgor, and BP and HR within patient's normal range.
- Monitor I&O, daily weight, VS, and skin turgor as indicators of volume status. **Note:** Skin turgor is not a reliable indicator of volume deficit in older adults because of the decreased elasticity of their skin.
- Observe for signs of hemorrhage. Urine usually is dark red or pink for approximately 48 h postoperatively in the patient who has had a pyelolithotomy or nephrolithotomy. Urine should not be bright red or contain clots.
- For additional information, see this nursing diagnosis in Appendix One, "Caring for Preoperative and Postoperative Patients," p. 703.

**High risk for impaired skin integrity** related to wound drainage
*Desired outcome:* Patient's skin remains clear and intact.
- After a pyelolithotomy, there can be drainage of urine from the incision for several days. Apply an ostomy pouch with a skin barrier to collect drainage and protect the skin.
- Closely monitor skin integrity, especially in older adults, who are at increased risk for skin breakdown.
- Ensure that the wound drainage tube remains in its proper position; notify physician immediately if it dislodges because it can be difficult to reinsert after 30 min.

**Knowledge deficit:** Potential for recurrence of calculi and interventions that can be taken to prevent it
*Desired outcome:* Within the 24-h period before hospital discharge, patient verbalizes knowledge about the potential for recurrence of calculi and the steps that can be taken to prevent it.
- When appropriate, teach patient a diet that prevents recurrence of stones. Provide lists of foods that should be limited or avoided, including those that are high in calcium (e.g., dairy products), purine (e.g., meats, fish, poultry), and oxalate (e.g., beets, figs, nuts, spinach, black tea, chocolate, instant and decaffeinated coffee, carbonated beverages).
- Encourage a daily fluid intake of at least 3 L/day in nonrestricted patients. A high fluid intake is especially important in preventing recurrent stones in patients with cystinuria.
- Teach patient about the need for continued use of medications and medical follow-up because of the high rate of recurrence.
- Teach patient about the importance of maintaining the prescribed urinary pH to prohibit stone precipitation and the necessity of urine pH testing. Demonstrate urine pH testing as appropriate.
- Caution patient about the importance of seeking prompt medical treatment for signs and symptoms of UTI (e.g., fever, flank or labial pain, cloudy or foul-smelling urine), obstruction (e.g., anuria, oliguria, and pain that is dull and aching or sharp and sudden), and recurrence of stones (e.g., renal colic, hematuria, nausea, vomiting).

---

**Note:** See "Ureteral Calculi," p. 147, for more information about stone formation. Also see nursing diagnoses and interventions in Appendix One, "Caring for Preoperative and Postoperative Patients," p. 693.

---

## PATIENT-FAMILY TEACHING AND DISCHARGE PLANNING

Give patient and significant others verbal and written information about the following:

- Medications, including drug name, purpose, dosage, schedule, precautions, and potential side effects.
- When appropriate, a diet that prevents recurrence of stones. Provide lists of foods that should be limited or avoided, including those that are high in calcium (e.g., dairy products), purine (e.g., meats, fish, poultry), and oxalate (e.g., beets, figs, nuts, spinach, black tea, chocolate, instant and decaffeinated coffee, and carbonated beverages). Encourage a daily fluid intake of at least 3 L/day in nonrestricted patients. A high fluid intake is especially important in preventing recurrent stones in patients with cystinuria.
- Need for continued use of medications and medical follow-up because of the high rate of recurrence.
- Requirements for maintaining alterations in urinary pH to prohibit stone precipitation and the necessity of urine pH testing.
- Importance of seeking prompt medical treatment for signs and symptoms of UTI (e.g., fever, flank or labial pain, cloudy or foul-smelling urine) or obstruction (e.g., anuria, oliguria, and pain that is dull and aching or sharp and sudden).
- Care of drains or catheters if patient is discharged with them.
- Care of the surgical incision and indicators of wound infection, which necessitate medical attention: persistent erythema, swelling, pain, local warmth, and purulent drainage.
- Postoperative activity precautions: avoiding heavy lifting (>10 lb) for the first 6 weeks, being alert to fatigue, getting maximum amounts of rest, and gradually increasing activities to tolerance.

# Hydronephrosis

Hydronephrosis is the dilatation of the renal pelvis and calyces secondary to the obstruction of urinary flow. It results from any condition or abnormality that causes urinary tract obstruction. If the obstruction is not corrected, the affected kidney eventually atrophies and fails. Obstruction in the urethra or bladder will affect both kidneys, while obstruction in a single ureter or kidney will affect only the involved kidney.

Dramatic postobstructive diuresis can occur after the release of the obstruction. Inappropriate loss of $Na^+$ and $H_2O$ can in turn lead to volume depletion.

## ASSESSMENT

Indicators are determined by the level, severity, and duration of obstruction.

**Kidney/ureteral obstruction:** Flank pain and abdominal tenderness, renal colic, gross hematuria.

**Bladder neck/urethral obstruction:** Frequency, hesitancy, dribbling, incontinence, nocturia, signs and symptoms of renal insufficiency, suprapubic pain, anuria.

**Physical assessment:** Enlarged kidney(s), distended bladder (if bladder neck obstruction is present), crackles (rales), and possibly hypertension and edema if patient is fluid-overloaded.

**History of:** Urinary tract infection (UTI), nephrolithiasis, benign prostatic hypertrophy, neurogenic bladder, or other obstruction.

## DIAGNOSTIC TESTS

**BUN and serum creatinine:** To determine level of renal function.

**Urinalysis:** To determine the presence of stone formation or infection.

**Renal ultrasound:** Noninvasive technique that uses high-frequency sound

waves to assess renal size, contour, and structural changes. Because it does not rely on dye uptake, it can be used to evaluate poorly functioning kidneys.
**Abdominal x-ray, intravenous pyelogram, and retrograde pyelogram:**   To identify cause and location of obstruction.

## COLLABORATIVE MANAGEMENT

Management of hydronephrosis depends on the cause and duration of the urinary tract obstruction. Major causes of obstruction in the pelvis and ureter are calculi (see "Renal Calculi") and neoplasms. Major causes of obstruction in the bladder and urethra are neoplasms (see "Cancer of the Bladder"), neurogenic bladder (see "Neurogenic Bladder)," and prostatic hypertrophy (see "Benign Prostatic Hypertrophy"). Also see "Urinary Tract Obstruction" for a general discussion of urinary tract obstruction. See "Acute Renal Failure" and "Chronic Renal Failure" as appropriate.

Management of hydronephrosis might include the insertion of a nephrostomy tube into the renal pelvis to drain urine and relieve pressure. It is inserted percutaneously under local anesthesia or in an open surgical procedure. The tube may be permanent or temporary.

## NURSING DIAGNOSES AND INTERVENTIONS

**High risk for infection** related to invasive procedure (insertion/presence of nephrostomy tube)
**Desired outcome:**   Patient is free of infection as evidenced by normothermia, BP and HR within patient's normal range, urine that is clear and normal in odor and color, and absence of dysuria.

- Maintain sterile technique when providing dressing changes and nephrostomy tube care.
- Observe for and report indicators of infection, such as fever, pain, purulent drainage, and tachycardia. Document changes in color, odor, or clarity of urine. Infection is common with hydronephrosis.
- Do not change, clamp, or irrigate the nephrostomy tube unless specifically prescribed by physician.

---

**Caution:**   Because of the tiny renal pelvis, never insert more than 5 ml at one time into the tube unless a larger amount has been specifically prescribed by the physician.

---

- Keep the urine collection container and tubing in a dependent position. Avoid kinks in the tubing.

**High risk for injury** related to insertion/presence of nephrostomy tube
**Desired outcome:**   Patient remains free of signs of nephrostomy tube complications as evidenced by urine that is clear and of normal color after the first 24-48 h, a urine output of 30-60 ml/h, and absence of discomfort/pain.

- Report gross hematuria (urine that is bright red, possibly with clots). Transient hematuria can be expected for 24-48 h after tube insertion.
- Notify physician of leakage around the catheter, which can occur with blockage, as well as a sudden decrease in urine output, which can signal a dislodged catheter.
- Report a sudden onset of or increase in pain, which can indicate perforation of a body organ by the catheter.
- Keep the tube securely taped to the patient's flank with elastic tape. If the tube becomes accidently dislodged, cover the site with a sterile dressing; notify physician immediately.
- **Note:** Before removing the nephrostomy tube, the physician may request that it be clamped for several hours at a time to evaluate patient tolerance. While the tube is clamped, monitor the patient for the following indications of ureteral obstruction: flank pain, diminished urinary output, and fever.

**Fluid volume deficit** related to active loss secondary to postobstructive diuresis

*Desired outcome:* With intervention/treatment patient becomes normovolemic as evidenced by stable weight, good skin turgor, BP ≥90/60 mm Hg, HR ≤100 bpm, and CVP ≥5 cm $H_2O$ (or VS within patient's normal range).

- Monitor I&O hourly. Initially, output should exceed intake.
- Monitor weight daily. Alert physician to steady weight loss.
- Observe for and report indicators of volume depletion, including postural hypotension, tachycardia, poor skin turgor, elevated hematocrit (Hct), and decreased CVP. Monitor VS q30min for the first few hours after release of obstruction.
- As prescribed, encourage fluids in nonrestricted patients who are hypovolemic.

---

**Note:** See "Glomerulonephritis" for **Knowledge deficit:** Signs and symptoms of fluid and electrolyte imbalance, p. 116.

---

## PATIENT-FAMILY TEACHING AND DISCHARGE PLANNING

Give patient and significant others verbal and written information about the following:

- Medications, including drug name, purpose, dosage, schedule, precautions, and potential side effects.
- Care of the nephrostomy catheter, if discharged with one; procedure to follow should the catheter become dislodged.
- Frequency of and procedure for dressing changes. Patient or significant others should demonstrate safe dressing-change technique before hospital discharge.
- Need for continued medical follow-up; confirm date and time of next physician appointment, if known.
- Signs and symptoms that necessitate medical attention: fever, cloudy or foul-smelling urine, flank or labial pain, increased catheter drainage, and drainage around the catheter site.

# Renal artery stenosis

Stenosis of the renal artery or one of its main branches usually is the result of fibromuscular dysplasia or arteriosclerotic changes. A reduction in the lumen of the renal artery causes a decrease in blood flow to the affected kidney, which in turn stimulates the renin-angiotensin system, causing systemic hypertension. The elevation in blood pressure usually is proportional to the degree of ischemia in the affected kidney. If the hypertension is left untreated, the nonischemic kidney will develop arteriolar hyperplasia. When both kidneys are involved, renal failure can occur.

## ASSESSMENT

**Signs and symptoms:**   Headache, nose bleeds, tinnitus.
**Physical assessment:**   Auscultation of a bruit in the mid-epigastric area. BP can be severely elevated.
**History of:**   Accelerated hypertension with abrupt onset; hypertensive retinopathy.

## DIAGNOSTIC TESTS

**Intravenous pyelogram:**   Visualizes kidneys *via* excretion of iodine-containing contrast medium; will demonstrate an ischemic kidney.
**Renal arteriography:**   Injection of contrast medium into the renal arteries to visualize renal vasculature. The arteriogram can be false-positive in the older

adult. Complications include allergic reaction to the contrast medium, contrast medium–induced acute renal failure, hemorrhage, embolus, and infection.

**Radioisotope renogram:**   Will demonstrate a delayed transit time of the radioisotope through the affected kidney; may be performed in combination with the captopril test (see *Captopril test,* below).

**Renal vein renin levels:**   Will show a difference between the two kidneys in unilateral disease. The renin level from the ischemic kidney should be 1.5 times that of the nonischemic kidney.

**Plasma renin level:**   Will be increased owing to stimulation of the renin-angiotensin system.

**Captopril test:**   A significant increase in plasma renin levels after a dose of captopril suggests renovascular hypertension. Captopril inhibits the enzyme that converts angiotensin I to angiotensin II. Individuals with hypertension caused by increased renin levels will respond to captopril by producing more renin.

**BUN and serum creatinine:**   To determine the level of renal function.

**Serum $K^+$ levels:**   Often decreased secondary to increased secretion of aldosterone.

## COLLABORATIVE MANAGEMENT

Renovascular hypertension can be treated medically, invasively *via* percutaneous transluminal angioplasty, or surgically. Patients with diffuse arteriosclerotic vascular disease or bilateral renal artery lesions may be considered poor surgical risks. Type and duration of the disease are additional factors that can contribute to the decision to treat patients medically.

*Invasive procedure*

**Percutaneous transluminal angioplasty:**   Performed if the patient is a suitable candidate and the necessary equipment and personnel are available. Angioplasty involves the insertion of a balloon-tipped catheter to dilate the narrowed vessel. It can be performed under local anesthetic and requires minimal hospitalization.

*Surgical interventions*

**Arterial endarterectomy with follow-up anticoagulant therapy.**

**Resection or bypass of the lesion (aortorenal bypass graft):**   Performed for those patients who are unsuitable candidates for endarterectomy or angioplasty, or when angioplasty has been unsuccessful or is unavailable. Revascularization may be achieved using the patient's saphenous vein or internal iliac artery or a synthetic graft.

## NURSING DIAGNOSES AND INTERVENTIONS

**Knowledge deficit:**   Rationale for frequent assessments after aortorenal bypass graft, angioplasty, or endarterectomy and the technique for measuring BP

*Desired outcome:*   Before the procedure, patient verbalizes knowledge about the renal procedure he or she will undergo and the rationale for frequent VS checks and demonstrates BP measurement technique before hospital discharge.

- Monitor BP frequently during the first 48 h after aortorenal bypass graft. Explain to patient and significant others that hypertension during this period usually is temporary but may require treatment. When angioplasty is successful, hypertension should decrease within 4-6 h postprocedure.
- Explain the rationale for measuring VS q15min immediately after angioplasty. Monitor the integrity of the pulses distal to the angioplasty site.
- Alert patient and significant others to the potential for bleeding and hematoma formation at the angioplasty site, as well as symptoms of hidden bleeding, including hypotension and tachycardia. Explain that if a hematoma is noted, it will be circled with ink and the time will be noted to detect further bleeding.
- Explain the rationale for measuring BP under the same conditions each day:

sitting, standing, lying down. Teach the technique for measuring BP to the patient and significant others before hospital discharge.
- Explain that BP may remain elevated after the renal procedure and that antihypertensive medications still may be required. Review the purpose, action, dose, and potential side effects of all medications with patient and significant others before hospital discharge.
- Stress the need for continued medical evaluation of BP and renal function.

---

**Note:** See nursing diagnoses and interventions in Appendix One, "Caring for Preoperative and Postoperative Patients," p. 693.

---

### PATIENT-FAMILY TEACHING AND DISCHARGE PLANNING
Give patient and significant others verbal and written information about the following:
- Medications, including drug name, purpose, dosage, schedule, precautions, and potential side effects.
- Diet: low in Na (see Table 3-2). Include lists of foods high in K (see Table 3-4) if patient is taking diuretics that cause hypokalemia. Provide sample menus, and have the patient demonstrate understanding of the diet by planning meals for 3 days.
- Technique for measuring BP. Patient or significant others should demonstrate proficiency before discharge.
- Care of incision or angioplasty site. Teach patient the indicators of wound infection (e.g., erythema, purulent discharge, local warmth, fever) and the importance of reporting them promptly to the physician.
- Need for continued medical follow-up to evaluate effectiveness of the treatment.
- Importance of avoiding other risk factors for hypertension: obesity, smoking, stress.

# Section Two:   Renal Failure

## Acute renal failure

Acute renal failure (ARF) is a sudden loss of renal function, which may or may not be accompanied by oliguria. The kidneys lose the ability to maintain biochemical homeostasis, causing retention of metabolic wastes and dramatic alterations in fluid, electrolyte, and acid-base balance. Although the alteration in renal function usually is reversible, ARF is associated with an overall mortality rate of 40%-60%. However, mortality rate varies greatly with the cause of ARF, the patient's age, and preexisting medical problems.

The causes of ARF are classified according to development as prerenal, intrarenal, and postrenal. A decrease in renal function secondary to decreased renal perfusion but without renal parenchymal damage is called *prerenal failure*. Causes of prerenal failure include fluid volume deficit, shock, and decreased cardiac function. If hypoperfusion has not been prolonged, restoration of renal perfusion will restore normal renal function. A reduction in urine output because of obstruction to urine flow is called *postrenal failure*. Conditions causing postrenal failure can include neurogenic bladder, tumors, and urethral strictures. Early detection of prerenal and postrenal failure is essential since, if prolonged, they can lead to parenchymal damage.

The most common cause of *intrarenal failure,* or renal failure that develops secondary to renal parenchymal damage, is acute tubular necrosis (ATN). Although typically associated with prolonged ischemia (prerenal failure) or exposure to nephrotoxins (antibiotics, heavy metals, or radiographic contrast media), ATN also can occur after transfusion reactions, septic abortions, or crushing injuries. The clinical course of ATN can be divided into the following three phases: oliguric (lasting approximately 7-21 days), diuretic (7-14 days), and recovery (3-12 months). Causes of intrarenal failure other than ATN include acute glomerulonephritis (GN), malignant hypertension, and hepatorenal syndrome.

## ASSESSMENT

**Electrolyte disturbance:**   Muscle weakness, dysrhythmias, pruritus.
**Fluid volume excess:**   Oliguria, pitting edema, hypertension, pulmonary edema.
**Metabolic acidosis:**   Kussmaul respirations (hyperventilation), lethargy, headache.
**Uremia (retention of metabolic wastes):**   Altered mental state, anorexia, nausea, diarrhea, pale and sallow skin, purpura, decreased resistance to infection, anemia, fatigue. **Note:** Uremia adversely affects all body systems.
**Physical assessment:**   Pallor; edema (peripheral, periorbital, sacral); crackles (rales); and elevated BP in patient who has fluid overload.
**History of:**   Exposure to nephrotoxic substances, recent blood transfusion, prolonged hypotensive episodes or decreased renal perfusion, abortion, or a recent urinary tract infection (URI).

## DIAGNOSTIC TESTS

**BUN and serum creatinine:**   Assess the progression and management of ARF. Although both BUN and creatinine will increase as renal function decreases, creatinine is a better indicator of renal function because it is not affected by diet, hydration, or tissue catabolism.
**Creatinine clearance:**   Measures the kidney's ability to clear the blood of creatinine and approximates the glomerular filtration rate. It will decrease as renal function decreases. Creatinine clearance is normally decreased in the elderly. **Note:** Failure to collect all urine during the period of study can invalidate the test.
**Urinalysis:**   Can provide information about the cause and location of renal disease as reflected by abnormal urinary sediment (casts and cellular debris).
**Urinary osmolality and urinary Na$^+$ levels:**   To rule out renal perfusion problems (prerenal). In ATN the kidney loses the ability to adjust urine concentration and conserve Na$^+$.

---

**Note:**   All urine samples should be sent to the lab immediately after collection, or refrigerated if this is not possible. Urine left at room temperature has greater potential for bacterial growth, turbidity, and alkalinity, any of which can distort the reading.

---

**Renal ultrasound:**   Provides information about renal anatomy and pelvic structures, evaluates renal masses, and detects obstruction and hydronephrosis
**Renal scan:**   Provides information about the perfusion and function of the kidneys.

## COLLABORATIVE MANAGEMENT

The goal is to remove the precipitating cause, maintain homeostatic balance, and prevent complications until the kidneys are able to resume function. Initially, prerenal or postrenal causes are ruled out or treated. A trial of fluid and diuretics may be used to rule out prerenal problems.
**Restrict fluids:**   Replace losses plus 400 ml/24 h. **Note:** Insensible fluid

losses are only partially replaced to offset the water formed during the metabolism of protein, carbohydrates, and fats.

**Pharmacotherapy**

---

**Note:** Medications that are handled primarily by the kidney (Table 3-3) will require modification of dosage or frequency to prevent medication toxicity. Renal failure also may decrease hepatic metabolism and protein binding of certain medications, resulting in increased medication effect.

---

*Diuretics:* In nonoliguric ARF for fluid removal (see Table 3-1).
*Furosemide (Lasix) or mannitol:* May be given early in ARF to limit or prevent the development of oliguria.
*Antihypertensives:* To control BP.
*Aluminum hydroxide antacids, calcium carbonate, or calcium acetate:* To control hyperphosphatemia.

---

**T A B L E  3 - 3  Drug Usage in Renal Failure**

---

Drugs that are handled primarily by the kidney have an increased effect in patients with renal failure. Usually they require modification of dosage or frequency. Some of these medications are:

| **Antibiotics** | **Antiarrhythmics** |
|---|---|
| *carbenicillin | digoxin |
| *cefazolin | *procainamide |
| *gentamicin | **Hypoglycemic agents** |
| *kanamycin | insulin |
| *tobramycin | **Sedatives** |
| vancomycin | *phenobarbital |

Drugs that usually do not require dosage modification include:

| **Antibiotics** | **Antihypertensive agents** | **Sedatives** |
|---|---|---|
| *chloramphenicol | hydralazine | diazepam |
| clindamycin | clonidine HCl | chlordiazepoxide HCl |
| dicloxacillin | prazosin HCl | |
| erythromycin | minoxidil | |
| nafcillin sodium | *methyldopa | |

| **Diuretics** | **Hypoglycemic agent** | **Antiinflammatory** |
|---|---|---|
| furosemide | tolbutamide | indomethacin |
| metolazone | | |

| **Narcotics** | **Antiarrhythmics** |
|---|---|
| codeine | propranolol |
| morphine | *quinidine gluconate |

---

*Dialyzable drugs, which might require extra dosage after dialysis.

**T A B L E  3 - 4    Foods High in Potassium Content**

| | |
|---|---|
| Apricots | Nuts |
| Artichokes | Oranges, orange juice |
| Avocado | Peanuts |
| Banana | Potatoes |
| Cantaloupe | Prune juice |
| Carrots | Pumpkin |
| Cauliflower | Spinach |
| Chocolate | Swiss chard |
| Dried beans, peas | Sweet potatoes |
| Dried fruit | Tomatoes, tomato juice, tomato sauce |
| Mushrooms | Watermelon |

*Cation exchange resins (Kayexalate):*   To control hyperkalemia. Severe hyperkalemia also may be treated with *IV sodium bicarbonate,* which shifts $K^+$ into the cells temporarily, or *glucose and insulin.* Insulin also helps move $K^+$ into the cells, and glucose helps prevent dangerous hypoglycemia, which could result from the insulin. *IV calcium* is given to reverse the cardiac effects of life-threatening hyperkalemia.

*Calcium or vitamin D supplements:*   For hypocalcemic patients.

*Sodium bicarbonate:*   To treat acidosis. It is used cautiously in hypocalcemic or fluid-overloaded patients.

*Vitamins B and C:*   To replace losses if patient is on dialysis.

*Packed cells:*   For active bleeding or if anemia is poorly tolerated.

**Diet:**   High carbohydrate, low protein (high biologic value), low K (Table 3-4), and low Na (see Table 3-2). Carbohydrates are increased to provide adequate calories and limit protein catabolism. Na is limited to prevent thirst and fluid retention. K is limited because of the kidney's inability to excrete excess $K^+$. Protein is limited to minimize retention of nitrogenous wastes. **Note:** Because of the loss of $K^+$ during the diuretic phase, K might need to be increased during that time.

**Total parenteral nutrition (TPN):**   May be necessary for patients unable to maintain adequate oral/enteral intake.

**Peritoneal dialysis or hemodialysis:**   Administered if the above therapy is inadequate for maintaining homeostasis or preventing complications (see "Renal Dialysis," p. 142.

## NURSING DIAGNOSES AND INTERVENTIONS

**Fluid volume excess** related to compromised regulatory mechanisms secondary to renal dysfunction: *Oliguric phase*

*Desired outcome:*   Patient adheres to prescribed fluid restrictions and becomes normovolemic as evidenced by decreasing or stable weight, normal breath sounds, edema ≤1+ on a 0-4+ scale, CVP ≤12 cm $H_2O$, and BP and HR within patient's normal range.

- Closely monitor and document I&O.
- Monitor weight daily. The patient should lose 0.5 kg/day if not eating; a sudden weight gain suggests excessive fluid volume.
- Observe for indicators of fluid volume excess, including edema, hypertension, crackles (rales), tachycardia, distended neck veins, SOB, and increased CVP.
- Carefully adhere to prescribed fluid restriction. Provide oral hygiene at frequent intervals, and offer fluids in the form of ice chips or popsicles to minimize thirst. Hard candies also may be given to decrease thirst. Spread al-

lotted fluids evenly over a 24-h period, and record the amount given. Instruct patient and significant others about the need for fluid restriction. **Note:** Patients nourished *via* TPN are at increased risk for fluid overload because of the necessary fluid volume involved.

**High risk for fluid volume deficit** related to active loss secondary to excessive urinary output: *Diuretic phase*

**Desired outcome:** Patient remains normovolemic as evidenced by stable weight, balanced I&O, good skin turgor, CVP ≥5 cm $H_2O$, and BP and HR within patient's normal range.

- Closely monitor and document I&O.
- Monitor weight daily. A weight loss ≥0.5 kg/day may reflect excessive volume loss.
- Observe for indicators of volume depletion, including poor skin turgor, hypotension, tachycardia, and decreased CVP.
- As prescribed, encourage fluids in the dehydrated patient.
- Report significant findings to physician.

**Altered nutrition:** Less than body requirements related to nausea, vomiting, anorexia, and dietary restrictions

**Desired outcome:** Within 2 days of admission, patient has stable weight and demonstrates normal intake of food within restrictions, as indicated.

- The presence of nausea, vomiting, and anorexia may signal increased uremia. Alert physicians to symptoms, and monitor BUN levels. BUN levels >80-100 mg/dl usually require dialytic therapy.
- Provide frequent small meals.
- Administer prescribed antiemetics as necessary.
- Coordinate meal planning and dietary teaching with patient, significant others, and renal dietitian. Dietary restriction may include reduced protein, Na, K, and fluid intake.

**Activity intolerance** related to generalized weakness secondary to uremia and anemia

**Desired outcome:** Following interventions/treatment, patient rates perceived exertion at ≤3 on a 0-10 scale and exhibits improving endurance during activity as evidenced by HR ≤20 bpm over resting HR, systolic BP ≤20 mm Hg over or under resting systolic BP, and RR ≤20 breaths/min with normal depth and pattern (eupnea).

- Monitor patient during activity for signs of activity intolerance, and ask patient to rate perceived exertion. For detail, see **High risk for activity intolerance,** p. 711, in Appendix One, "Caring for Patients on Prolonged Bed Rest."
- Hct will decrease and stabilize at around 20%-25%. Usually patients are not transfused unless their Hct drops below 20%-25% or their anemia is poorly tolerated. Notify physician of increased weakness, fatigue, dyspnea, chest pain, or a further decrease in Hct.

---

**Caution:** Muscle weakness can be an indicator of dangerous hyperkalemia and should be reported immediately.

---

- Assist with ADL as necessary; encourage independence to patient's tolerance.
- Establish a progressive activity regimen within patient's activity limitations that will help patient return to normal activities without complications. For more information, see Appendix One, "Caring for Patients on Prolonged Bed Rest," **High risk for activity intolerance,** p. 711, and **High risk for disuse syndrome,** p. 713.

**Altered protection** related to neurosensory, musculoskeletal, and cardiac changes secondary to uremia, electrolyte imbalance, and metabolic acidosis

**Desired outcomes:** Following treatment, patient verbalizes orientation to person, place, and time and is free of injury caused by neurosensory, musculo-skeletal, or cardiac disturbances. Within the 24-h period before hospital discharge, patient verbalizes the signs and symptoms of electrolyte imbalance and metabolic acidosis and the importance of reporting them promptly should they occur.

- Assess for and alert patient to indicators of the following:
  - *Hypokalemia* (may occur during the diuretic phase): Muscle weakness, lethargy, dysrhythmias, and nausea and vomiting (secondary to ileus).
  - *Hyperkalemia:* Muscle cramps, dysrhythmias, muscle weakness, peaked T waves on ECG.

---

**Note:**  A normal serum $K^+$ level is necessary for normal cardiac function. Hyperkalemia is a common and potentially fatal complication of ARF during the oliguric phase.

---

  - *Hypocalcemia:* Neuromuscular irritability and paresthesias.
  - *Hyperphosphatemia:* Soft tissue calcifications.
  - *Uremia:* Anorexia, nausea, metallic taste in the mouth, irritability, confusion, lethargy, restlessness, and itching.
  - *Metabolic acidosis:* Rapid, deep respirations; confusion.
- Avoid giving patient foods high in K (see Table 3-4). Many salt substitutes also contain K and should be avoided.
- Minimize tissue catabolism by controlling fevers, maintaining adequate nutritional intake (especially calories), and preventing infections. If caloric intake is inadequate, body protein will be used for energy. A high-carbohydrate diet helps to minimize tissue catabolism and production of nitrogenous wastes.
- Prepare patient for the possibility of altered taste and smell.
- Patients with renal failure are at risk for increased magnesium levels because of decreased urinary excretion of dietary magnesium, and thus magnesium-containing medications should be avoided (e.g., patients using magnesium-containing antacids such as Maalox typically are switched to aluminum hydroxide preparations such as AlternaGel or Amphojel).
- Administer aluminum hydroxide antacids as prescribed to control hyperphosphatemia. Experiment with different brands or try capsules for patients who refuse certain liquid antacids. Phosphate binders vary in their aluminum or calcium content, however, and one may not be exchanged for another without first ensuring that the patient is receiving the same amount of elemental aluminum or calcium.
- Assure patient and his or her significant others that irritability, restlessness, and altered thinking are temporary. Facilitate orientation through calendars, radios, familiar objects, and frequent reorientation.
- Ensure safety measures (e.g., padded side rails, airway) for patients who are confused or severely hypocalcemic. For patients who exhibit signs of hyperkalemia, have emergency supplies (e.g., manual resuscitator bag, crash cart, and emergency drug tray) available.

**High risk for infection** related to uremia
***Desired outcome:***  Patient is free of infection as evidenced by normothermia, WBC count $\leq 11,000$ µl, urine that is clear and of normal odor, normal breath sounds, and absence of erythema, swelling, and drainage at the catheter sites.

---

**Note:**  One of the primary causes of death in ARF is sepsis.

---

- Monitor temperature and secretions for indicators of infection. Even minor increases in temperature can be significant because uremia masks the febrile response and inhibits the body's ability to fight infection.

- Use meticulous aseptic technique when changing dressings or manipulating venous catheters, IV lines, or indwelling catheters.
- Avoid use of indwelling urinary catheters because they are a common source of infection. When it is indicated, use intermittent catheterization instead.
- Provide oral hygiene and skin care at frequent intervals. Use emollients and gentle soap to avoid drying and cracking of skin, which can lead to breakdown and infection. Take care to rinse off all soap when bathing patient because soap residue may further irritate skin.

**Constipation** related to restrictions of fresh fruit and fluids, prolonged bed rest, and side effects of medications (e.g., phosphate-binding antacids)

***Desired outcomes:*** Within 1-3 days of intervention, patient states that bowel movements are within normal pattern. Before hospital discharge, patient verbalizes the foods and activities that promote bowel movements.

- Monitor and record the quality and number of bowel movements.
- Provide prescribed stool softeners and bulk-building supplements (e.g., Metamucil) as necessary.
- Suggest alternate dietary sources of fiber, such as unsalted popcorn or unprocessed bran.
- Encourage exercise and activity as appropriate.
- Provide Fleet, oil retention, or tap water enemas as prescribed, *only* if the previous measures fail. Avoid use of large-volume water enemas because excess fluid can be absorbed from the GI tract.

---

**Note:** Also see nursing diagnoses and interventions in "Care of the Patient Undergoing Peritoneal Dialysis," p. 143, and "Care of the Patient Undergoing Hemodialysis," p. 145, as appropriate.

---

### PATIENT-FAMILY TEACHING AND DISCHARGE PLANNING

Give patient and significant others verbal and written information about the following:

- Medications, including drug name, purpose, dosage, schedule, precautions, and potential side effects.
- Diet: Include fact sheet that lists foods to restrict.
- Care and observation of the dialysis access if the patient is being discharged with one (see "Renal Dialysis," p. 142).
- Importance of continued medical follow-up of renal function.
- Signs and symptoms of potential complications. These should include indicators of infection (see **High risk for infection,** p. 134), electrolyte imbalance (see **Altered protection,** p. 133), **fluid volume excess** (see p. 132), and bleeding (especially from the GI tract for patients who are uremic).

*In addition*

- If the patient requires dialysis after discharge, coordinate discharge planning with dialysis unit staff. Arrange visit to dialysis unit if possible.

## Chronic renal failure

Chronic renal failure (CRF) is a progressive, irreversible loss of kidney function that develops over days to years. Eventually it can progress to end-stage renal disease (ESRD), at which time renal replacement therapy (dialysis or transplantation) is required to sustain life. Prior to ESRD the individual with CRF can lead a relatively normal life managed by diet and medications. The length of this period is variable, depending on the cause of renal disease and the patient's level of renal function at the time of diagnosis.

There are many causes of CRF, some of the most common being glomerulonephritis (GN), diabetes mellitus, hypertension, and polycystic kidney disease. Regardless of the cause, the clinical presentation of CRF, particularly as the individual approaches ESRD, is similar. Retention of nitrogenous wastes and accompanying fluid and electrolyte imbalances adversely affect all body systems. Alterations in neuromuscular, cardiovascular, and gastrointestinal function are common. Renal osteodystrophy is an early and frequent complication. The collective manifestations of CRF are termed *uremia*.

## ASSESSMENT

**Fluid volume abnormalities:**   Crackles (rales), hypertension, edema, oliguria, or anuria.

**Electrolyte disturbances:**   Muscle weakness, dysrhythmias, pruritus, tetany.

**Uremia—retention of metabolic wastes:**   Weakness, malaise, anorexia, dry and discolored skin, peripheral neuropathy, irritability, clouded thinking, ammonia odor to breath. **Note:** Uremia adversely affects all body systems.

**Metabolic acidosis:**   Deep respirations, lethargy, headache.

**Potential acute complications**

*Congestive heart failure:*   Crackles, dyspnea, orthopnea.

*Pericarditis:*   Chest pain, SOB.

*Cardiac tamponade:*   Hypotension, distant heart sounds, pulsus paradoxus (exaggerated inspiratory drop in systolic BP).

**Physical assessment:**   Pallor, dry and discolored skin, edema (peripheral, periorbital, sacral). With fluid overload, crackles and elevated BP may be present.

**History of:**   GN, diabetes mellitus, polycystic kidney disease, hypertension, systemic lupus erythematosus, chronic pyelonephritis, and analgesic abuse, especially the combination of phenacetin and aspirin.

## DIAGNOSTIC TESTS

**BUN and serum creatinine:**   Both will be elevated. **Note:** Nonrenal problems, such as dehydration or GI bleeding, also can cause the BUN to increase, but there will not be a corresponding increase in creatinine.

**Creatinine clearance:**   Measures the kidney's ability to clear the blood of creatinine and approximates the glomerular filtration rate. Creatinine clearance will decrease as renal function decreases. Dialysis is usually begun when the creatinine clearance is less than 10 ml/min. Creatinine clearance normally is decreased in the elderly. **Note:** Failure to collect all urine specimens during the period of study will invalidate the test.

**X-ray of the kidneys, ureters, and bladder (KUB):**   Documents the presence of two kidneys, changes in size or shape, and some forms of obstruction.

**Intravenous pyelogram (IVP), renal ultrasound, renal biopsy, renal scan (using radionuclides), and computerized axial tomography (CT) scan:** Additional tests for determining the cause of renal insufficiency. Once the patient has reached ESRD, these tests are not performed.

**Serum chemistries, chest and hand x-rays, and nerve conduction velocity test:**   To assess for development and progression of uremia and its complications.

## COLLABORATIVE MANAGEMENT

Prior to ESRD, medical management is aimed at slowing the progression of CRF and avoiding complications. Once the patient reaches ESRD, management is aimed at alleviating uremic symptoms and providing dialysis or renal transplantation.

**Diet:**   Carbohydrates are increased in protein-restricted patients to ensure adequate caloric intake and prevent catabolism. Depending on existing renal function, Na is limited to prevent thirst and fluid retention (see Table 3-2), K is limited because of the kidney's inability to excrete excess $K^+$ (see Table 3-4), and protein is limited to minimize retention of nitrogenous wastes. Protein restriction may slow the progression of CRF in some patients. Protein intake should be that of high biologic value only.

**Fluid restriction:** For patients at risk for developing fluid volume excess. Fluid weight gain should be limited to 3%-4% of an individual's "dry" weight (i.e., weight with stable fluid balance).

**Pharmacotherapy**

*Aluminum hydroxide, calcium carbonate, or calcium acetate:* To control hyperphosphatemia.

*Antihypertensives:* To control BP.

*Multivitamins and folic acid:* For patients with dietary restrictions or who are on dialysis (water-soluble vitamins are lost during dialysis).

*Anabolic steroids, parenteral iron, ferrous sulfate, recombinant human erythropoietin (Epogen):* To treat anemia.

*Diphenhydramine:* To treat pruritus.

*Sodium bicarbonate:* To treat acidosis.

*Vitamin D preparations and calcium supplements:* To treat hypocalcemia and prevent bone disease.

*Deferoxamine:* To treat iron or aluminum toxicity.

---

**Note:** Medications that are excreted primarily by the kidney require modification of dosage or frequency. Dialyzable medications may need to be increased or held and given postdialysis (Table 3-3).

---

**Packed cells:** To treat severe or symptomatic anemia.

**Maintenance of homeostasis and prevention of complications** by avoiding the following: Volume depletion, hypotension, use of radiopaque contrast medium, and nephrotoxic substances. Pregnancy is contraindicated.

**Renal transplantation or dialysis:** If the above therapies are inadequate.

## NURSING DIAGNOSES AND INTERVENTIONS

**Activity intolerance** related to generalized weakness secondary to anemia and uremia

*Desired outcome:* Following treatment, patient rates perceived exertion at ≤3 on a 0-10 scale and exhibits improving endurance to activity as evidenced by HR ≤20 bpm over resting HR, systolic BP ≤20 mm Hg over or under resting systolic pressure, and RR ≤20 breaths/min with normal depth and pattern (eupnea).

---

**Note:** Anemia is better tolerated in the uremic than in the nonuremic patient.

---

- Anemia is usually proportional to the degree of azotemia. Hct can be as low as 20% or less, but usually stabilizes at around 20%-25%. Typically these patients are not transfused unless the Hct drops below 20% or anemia is poorly tolerated. Monitor patient during activity, and ask patient to rate perceived exertion (see **High risk for activity intolerance,** p. 711, in Appendix One, "Caring for Patients on Prolonged Bed Rest," for details). Notify physician of increased weakness, fatigue, dyspnea, chest pain, or further decreases in Hct. In addition:
  - Provide and encourage optimal nutrition.
  - Administer epoetin alfa (Epogen) if prescribed.
  - Administer anabolic steroids (e.g., nandrolone) if prescribed. Prepare female patients for side effects, including increasing facial hair, deepening voice, and menstrual irregularities.
  - Coordinate lab studies to minimize blood drawing.
  - Observe for and report evidence of occult blood and blood loss.
  - Report symptomatic anemia: weakness, SOB, chest pain.
  - Do not administer ferrous sulfate at the same time as antacids. The two

medications should be given at least 1 h apart to maximize absorption of the ferrous sulfate.
- Administer parenteral iron if prescribed. Anaphylaxis is a possible complication.
- Assist patient with identifying activities that cause increased fatigue and adjusting those activities accordingly.
- Assist the patient with ADL while encouraging maximum independence to the patient's tolerance.
- Establish with the patient realistic, progressive exercises and activity goals that are designed to increase endurance. Ensure that they are within the patient's prescribed limitations. Examples are found in **High risk for activity intolerance,** p. 711, and **High risk for disuse syndrome,** p. 713, in Appendix One, "Caring for Patients on Prolonged Bed Rest."

**Impaired skin integrity** related to pruritus and dry skin secondary to uremia and edema

*Desired outcome:*   Patient's skin remains intact and free of erythema and abrasions.

- Pruritus is common in uremic patients, causing frequent and intense scratching. Pruritus often decreases with a reduction in BUN and improved phosphorus control. Encourage use of phosphate binders and the reduction of dietary phosphorus if elevated phosphorus level is a problem. Foods high in phosphorus content include meats (especially organ meats—brain, kidney, liver), fish, poultry, milk and milk products (e.g., cheese, ice cream, cottage cheese), whole grains (e.g., oatmeal, bran, barley), seeds (e.g., pumpkin, sesame, sunflower), nuts (e.g., Brazil nuts, peanuts), eggs and egg products (e.g., eggnog, soufflés), and dried peas and beans. Give phosphate binders with meals for maximum effects. If necessary, administer antihistamines as prescribed. Keep patient's fingernails short.
- Because uremia retards wound healing, instruct the patient to monitor scratches for evidence of infection and seek early medical attention should signs and symptoms of infection appear.
- Uremic skin is often dry and scaly because of reduction in oil gland activity. Encourage use of skin emollients. Patients should avoid hard soaps and excessive bathing. Advise patient to bathe every other day and use bath oils as needed if dry skin is a problem.
- Clotting abnormalities and capillary fragility place the uremic patient at increased risk for bruising. Advise patient and significant others that this can occur.
- Provide scheduled skin care and position changes for individuals with edema.

**Knowledge deficit:**   Need for frequent BP checks and adherence to antihypertensive therapy and the potential for change in insulin requirements for individuals who are diabetic

*Desired outcomes:*   Within the 24-h period before hospital discharge, patient verbalizes knowledge about the importance of frequent BP checks and adherence to antihypertensive therapy. The patient with diabetes mellitus (DM) verbalizes knowledge about the potential for change in insulin requirements.

---

**Note:**   Patients with CRF may experience hypertension because of fluid overload, excess renin secretion, or arteriosclerotic disease.

---

- Teach patient about the importance of getting BP checked at frequent intervals and adhering to the prescribed antihypertensive therapy. Control of hypertension may slow the progression of chronic renal insufficiency.
- Teach patients with DM that insulin requirements often decrease as renal function decreases. Instruct these patients to be alert to indicators of hypoglycemia, including confusion, blurred vision, diaphoresis, and hypotension.

**Altered protection** related to neurosensory, musculoskeletal, and cardiac changes secondary to electrolyte and acid-base imbalances
*Desired outcomes:* Following successful treatment, patient verbalizes orientation to person, place, and time and remains free of injury caused by neurosensory, musculoskeletal, and cardiac disturbances. Within the 24-h period before hospital discharge, patient verbalizes the importance of avoiding foods and products that are high in K in particular, and, if indicated, Na, phosphorus, and protein content.

---

**Note:** K is limited because of the kidneys' inability to excrete excessive $K^+$. (For foods high in K content, see Table 3-4.) Depending on existing renal function, Na is limited to prevent thirst and fluid retention. (For foods high in Na content, see Table 3-2.) Dietary restriction of protein and phosphorus early in the course of the disease may slow the progression of chronic renal insufficiency. (For foods high in phosphorus content, see **Impaired skin integrity,** above.) Protein intake often is limited to that of high biologic value only. Carbohydrates are increased in patients on protein restriction to ensure adequate caloric intake and prevent catabolism.

---

- Hyperkalemia is a common complication of ESRD. Avoid salt substitutes (potassium chloride [KCl]), "light" salts (which contain KCl), and K-containing medications such as potassium penicillin G. Teach patient and significant others to read all over-the-counter labels.
- If the patient requires multiple blood transfusions, observe for indicators of hyperkalemia because old banked blood may contain as much as 30 mEq/L of K. Use fresh-packed cells when possible.
- Compliance with the prescribed dietary restrictions of K, Na, protein, and phosphorus should decrease symptoms and limit complications. To promote dietary compliance, encourage use of spices such as garlic, onions, and oregano to enhance the flavor of the foods patient is allowed. Provide fact sheets that list foods that are to be restricted or limited. Inform patient that diet and fluid restrictions may be altered as renal function decreases. Provide sample menus and have the patient demonstrate understanding by preparing 3-day menus that incorporate dietary restrictions.
- For other interventions, see this nursing diagnosis in "Acute Renal Failure," p. 133.

---

**Note:** See "Acute Renal Failure" for **Fluid volume excess** (oliguric phase), p. 132, **Altered nutrition,** p. 133, **High risk for infection,** p. 134, and **Constipation,** p. 135. See psychosocial nursing diagnoses and interventions in Appendix One, "Caring for Patients with Cancer and Other Life-Disrupting Illnesses, p. 753.

---

## PATIENT-FAMILY TEACHING AND DISCHARGE PLANNING
Give patient and significant others verbal and written information about the following:
- Medications, including drug name, purpose, dosage, schedule, precautions, and potential side effects.
- Diet, including fact sheet listing foods that are to be restricted or limited. Inform patient that diet and fluid restrictions may be altered as renal function decreases. Provide sample menus and have the patient demonstrate understanding by preparing 3-day menus that incorporate dietary restrictions.
- Care and observation of dialysis access if the patient has one (see "Renal Dialysis," p. 142).
- Signs and symptoms that necessitate medical attention: irregular pulse, fe-

ver, unusual SOB or edema, sudden change in urine output, and unusual muscle weakness.

- Need for continued medical follow-up; confirm date and time of next physician appointment.
- Importance of avoiding infections and seeking treatment promptly should one develop. Instruct the patient in the indicators of frequently encountered infections, including upper respiratory infection (URI), urinary tract infection (UTI), impetigo, and otitis media. For details, see **High risk for infection,** p. 141, in "Care of the Renal Transplant Recipient."

*In addition*

- For the patient with or approaching ESRD, provide data concerning the various treatment options and support groups. The local chapter of the National Kidney Foundation can be helpful in identifying support groups and organizations in the area. Patient and significant others should meet with the renal dietitian and social worker before discharge.
- Coordinate discharge planning and teaching with the dialysis unit or facility. If possible, have patient visit dialysis unit before discharge.
- For the individual with ESRD, the importance of coordinating all medical care through the nephrologist and the importance of alerting all medical and dental personnel to ESRD status, owing to the increased risk of infection and the need to adjust medication dosages. In addition, dentists may want to premedicate ESRD patients with antibiotics prior to dental work and avoid scheduling dental work on the day of dialysis owing to the heparinization that is used with dialytic therapy.

# Section Three:    Care of the Renal Transplant Recipient

Annually, approximately 10,000 patients with end-stage renal disease (ESRD) receive renal transplants. A small but increasing number of patients with ESRD and diabetes are receiving a combined kidney/pancreas transplant. Although patients receive transplants at major medical centers and are cared for postoperatively in specialized units, they may be admitted to any hospital for treatment of a rejection episode, medication complication, or unrelated illness. The majority of the transplanted kidneys come from cadavers, although living family members or friends also might donate. The organs for combined kidney/pancreas transplants come from a single cadaveric donor. Unless the graft is donated from an identical twin, transplant success depends on the suppression of graft rejection. This is accomplished by carefully matching donors to recipients through tissue typing before transplantation and immunosuppression after transplantation. Rejection is the major complication of renal transplant. Other long-term complications include infection, hypertension, cardiovascular disease, chronic liver disease (secondary to infection or medications), bone demineralization, cataracts, and GI hemorrhage.

## IMMUNOSUPPRESSION

**Necessary for the life of the graft.**

**Puts patient at increased risk for infection and development of malignancy in the long term.**

**Usual immunosuppressive medications**

*Azathioprine (Imuran):*   Side effects include decreased WBC and platelet count.

*Prednisone:*   Side effects include muscle wasting, aseptic necrosis of bone, cataracts, bleeding, Na retention, altered carbohydrate metabolism, mood and behavior changes, and cushingoid changes.

*Cyclosporine (Sandimmune):* Side effects include nephrotoxicity, hepato-toxicity, hirsutism, tremors, gum hyperplasia, hypertension, infection, malig-nancy. Route is either PO or IV. If IV, administer slowly over a period of 2-4 h and monitor for anaphylaxis. If route is PO, use a glass container; mix with orange juice or chocolate milk to make it more palatable. Do not allow solu-tion to stand.

*Antilymphocyte sera (ATGAM):* Given IV. Side effects include increased risk of infection and malignancy. In addition, immediate side effects include chills, fever, rash, joint pain, and anaphylaxis.

*Monoclonal antibody (Orthoclone, OKT-3):* Given IV. Side effects include increased risk of infection and malignancy. In addition, immediate side ef-fects include fever, chills, headache, nausea, and bronchospasm. Patients re-ceiving initial doses require close monitoring owing to the high incidence of side effects.

## REJECTION

**Acute:** 1 week-4 months after surgery; potentially reversible; treated with increased immunosuppression.

**Chronic:** Months to years after transplant; irreversible; managed conserva-tively with diet and antihypertensives until dialysis is required.

**Indicators of rejection:** Oliguria, tenderness over graft site (located in iliac fossa), sudden weight gain (2-3 lb/day), fever, malaise, hypertension, and in-creased BUN and serum creatinine. In addition, hyperglycemia will develop with combined kidney/pancreas transplants.

## NURSING DIAGNOSES AND INTERVENTIONS

**High risk for infection** related to invasive procedures, exposure to infected individuals, and immunosuppression

*Desired outcomes:* Patient is free of infection as evidenced by normother-mia, HR ≤100 bpm (or within patient's normal range), and absence of ery-thema or purulent drainage at wounds or catheter exit sites. Patient verbalizes the indicators of infection and the importance of reporting them promptly to physician or staff.

- Observe for indicators of infection, such as fever and unexplained tachycar-dia. Instruct the patient to be alert to signs and symptoms of commonly en-countered infections and the importance of reporting them promptly. These include *urinary tract infection* (UTI)—cloudy and malodorous urine; uri-nary burning, frequency, and urgency; *upper respiratory tract infection (URI)*—malodorous, purulent, colored, and copious secretions; productive cough; *otitis media*—malaise, earache; *impetigo*—inflamed or draining ar-eas on the skin.
- Teach patient to avoid exposure to individuals known to have infections.
- Use aseptic technique with all invasive procedures and dressing changes.

**Knowledge deficit:** Signs and symptoms of rejection, side effects of immu-nosuppressive agents, transplantation complications, and importance of pro-tecting the existing hemodialysis vascular access

*Desired outcome:* Within the 24-h period before hospital discharge, patient verbalizes knowledge of the signs and symptoms of rejection, the side effects of immunosuppressive therapy, complications of transplantation, and the im-portance of protecting the hemodialysis vascular access.

- Explain the importance of renal function monitoring: I&O, daily weight, and BUN and serum creatinine values. As renal function decreases, BUN and creatinine values will increase.
- Alert patient to the following signs and symptoms of rejection: oliguria, ten-derness over the kidney (located in the iliac fossa), sudden weight gain, fe-ver, malaise, hypertension, and increased BUN (>20 mg/dl) and serum cre-atinine (>1.5 mg/dl). Provide patient with a notebook in which to record

daily VS and weight measurements. Remind patient to bring the notebook to all out-patient visits and to report abnormal values promptly should they occur.

- Explain that significant decreases in WBC and platelet counts can be a side effect of immunosuppressive agents, and therefore serial monitoring is essential.
- Explain that GI bleeding is a potential side effect of immunosuppressive agents. Alert patient to the signs and symptoms of GI bleeding (e.g., tarry stools, "coffee-ground" emesis, increasing fatigue and weakness) and the importance of reporting them promptly should they occur.
- In the patient who has undergone renal transplantation, hypertension may develop for a variety of reasons, including cyclosporine or steroid use, rejection, or renal artery stenosis. Teach patient and/or significant others how to measure BP, and provide guidelines for values that necessitate notification of physician or staff member.
- If the patient has a patent fistula or graft (hemodialysis vascular access), explain that it must be handled with care because the patient will need it if a return to dialysis is indicated. Explain that taking BPs, drawing blood, and starting IVs are contraindicated in the fistula arm, and therefore patient should warn others about these contraindications.
- Stress the need for continued medical evaluation of the transplantation.

# Section Four:    Renal Dialysis

**Note:**    This section does not include care of the patient during dialysis but rather provides essential background data, including nursing care of patients who undergo dialysis.

Peritoneal dialysis and hemodialysis are lifesaving procedures used to treat severely decreased or absent renal function. Dialysis can be either temporary, until the kidneys are able to resume adequate function, or permanent. Dialysis is defined as the selective movement of water and solutes from one fluid compartment to another across a semipermeable membrane. The two fluid compartments are the patient's blood and the dialysate (electrolyte and glucose solution). With hemodialysis, the semipermeable membrane is an artificial one; while with peritoneal dialysis, the peritoneum serves as a natural dialysis membrane.

**Indications for dialysis:**    Acute renal failure or acute episodes of renal insufficiency that cannot be managed by diet, medications, and fluid restriction; end-stage renal disease (ESRD); drug overdose; hyperkalemia; fluid overload; or metabolic acidosis.

**Functions of dialysis:**    Correction of electrolyte abnormalities; removal of excess fluid and metabolic wastes; correction of acid-base abnormalities. **Note:** Dialysis does not compensate completely for the lack of functioning kidneys. Medications and dietary and fluid restrictions are necessary to supplement dialysis.

**Peritoneal dialysis:**    Slower; does not require heparinization; can be performed by trained medical-surgical nurses; requires a minimum of equipment.

**Hemodialysis:**    Faster; requires heparinization, specially trained staff, expensive and complex equipment; patient must have adequate vasculature for access.

**Continuous arteriovenous hemofiltration (CAVH):**    One of the newest forms of renal replacement therapy, its use is currently limited to patients in critical-care settings because it requires continuous monitoring and canulation of a high-flow vessel, usually the femoral artery. Blood flows from an arterial line through the hemofilter and returns to the patient's circulation *via* a venous access. Ultrafiltrate (fluid, metabolic wastes, and electrolytes) drains from the hemofilter into a collection device.

# Care of the patient undergoing peritoneal dialysis

Peritoneal dialysis uses the peritoneum as the dialysis membrane. Dialysate is instilled into the peritoneal cavity *via* a special catheter, and movement of solutes and fluid occurs between the patient's capillary blood and the dialysate. At set intervals the peritoneal cavity is drained and new dialysate is instilled.

## COMPONENTS OF PERITONEAL DIALYSIS

**Catheter:**   Silastic tube that is either implanted as a surgical procedure for chronic patients or inserted at the bedside for acute dialysis.

**Dialysate:**   Sterile electrolyte solution similar in composition to normal plasma. The electrolyte composition of the dialysate can be adjusted according to individual need. The most commonly adjusted electrolyte is $K^+$. Glucose is added to the dialysate in varying concentrations to remove excess body fluid *via* osmosis. **Note:** Some glucose crosses the peritoneal membrane and enters the patient's blood. Patients with diabetes mellitus may require additional insulin. Observe for and report indicators of hyperglycemia (e.g., complaints of thirst or changes in sensorium).

## TYPES OF PERITONEAL DIALYSIS

**Intermittent peritoneal dialysis (IPD):**   The patient is dialyzed for periods of 8-10 h, 4-5 times per week. A predetermined amount of dialysate (usually 2 L) is instilled for a set length of time (usually 20-30 min). It is then allowed to drain by gravity, and the process is repeated. IPD can be performed manually with individual bottles and bags, or mechanically using a proportioning machine or cycler. The patient is restricted to a chair or bed. Peritoneal dialysis also can be performed as an acute, temporary procedure. Continuous hourly exchanges are performed for 48-72 h. The patient is restricted to bed.

**Continuous ambulatory peritoneal dialysis (CAPD):**   The patient attaches a specialized bag of dialysate to the peritoneal catheter; allows the dialysate to drain in; clamps the catheter, leaving the bag attached; and goes about his or her daily routine. After 4 h (8 h at night) the clamp is opened and the dialysate is allowed to drain out. Using aseptic technique, the patient attaches a new bag of dialysate, and the process is repeated. Dialysis exchanges are done continuously, 7 days a week. CAPD is used primarily for ESRD.

**Continuous cycling peritoneal dialysis (CCPD):**   This is a combination of IPD and CAPD. A cycler performs three dialysate exchanges at night. In the morning a fourth exchange is instilled and left in the peritoneal cavity for the entire day. At the end of the day, the fourth exchange is allowed to drain out, and the process is repeated. The patient is ambulatory by day and restricted to bed at night.

## NURSING DIAGNOSES AND INTERVENTIONS

**High risk for infection** related to invasive procedure (direct access of the catheter to the peritoneum)

***Desired outcomes:***   Patient is free of infection as evidenced by normothermia and absence of the following: abdominal pain, cloudy outflow, nausea, malaise, and erythema, drainage, and tenderness at the exit site. Before hospital discharge, patient verbalizes the signs and symptoms of infection and demonstrates sterile technique for bag, tubing, and dressing changes.

- The most common complication of peritoneal dialysis is peritonitis. Monitor for and report indications of peritonitis, including fever, abdominal pain, cloudy outflow, nausea, and malaise.

---

**Caution:** To minimize the risk of peritonitis, it is essential that sterile technique be used when connecting and disconnecting the catheter from the dialysis system.

---

- The dialysate must remain sterile because it is instilled directly into the body. Maintain sterile technique when adding medications to the dialysate.
- Follow agency policy for dressing the catheter exit site.
- Observe for and report redness, drainage, or tenderness at exit site. Culture any exudate and report the results to the physician.
- Report to physician if dialysate leaks around the catheter exit site. This can indicate an obstruction or the need for another purse-string suture around the catheter site. Continued leakage at the site can lead to peritonitis.
- Instruct the patient in the preceding interventions and observations if peritoneal dialysis will be performed after discharge.

**High risk for fluid volume deficit** related to hypertonicity of the dialysate; *or* **Fluid volume excess** related to inadequate exchange

*Desired outcomes:*  Postdialysis the patient is normovolemic as evidenced by balanced I&O, stable weight, good skin turgor, CVP 5-12 cm $H_2O$, RR 12-20 breaths/min with normal depth and pattern (eupnea), and BP and HR within patient's normal range. The volume of dialysate outflow is $\geq$ inflow.

- Fluid retention can occur because of catheter complications that prevent adequate outflow, or a severely scarred peritoneum that prevents adequate exchange. Observe for and report indicators of fluid overload, such as hypertension, tachycardia, distended neck veins, or increased CVP. Also be alert to incomplete dialysate returns. Accurate measurement and recording of outflow are critical.
- Outflow problems can occur because of the following:
  - *Full colon:* Use stool softeners, high-fiber diet, or enemas if necessary.
  - *Catheter occlusion by fibrin* (usually occurs soon after insertion): Obtain order to irrigate with heparinized saline.
  - *Catheter obstruction by omentum:* Turn patient from side to side, elevate HOB, or apply firm pressure to the abdomen. **Note:** Notify physician for unresolved outflow problems.
- Monitor I&O and weight daily. A steady weight gain indicates fluid retention.
- Respiratory distress can occur because of compression of the diaphragm by the dialysate. If this occurs, elevate the HOB, drain the dialysate, and notify physician.
- Bloody outflow may appear with initial exchanges. Report gross bloody outflow.
- Coordinate laboratory studies to limit blood drawing because patients with renal failure are anemic owing to altered RBC production and longevity.
- Volume depletion can occur with excessive use of hypertonic dialysate. Observe for and report indicators of volume depletion, including poor skin turgor, hypotension, tachycardia, and decreased CVP.

**Altered nutrition:**  Less than body requirements, related to protein loss in the dialysate

*Desired outcomes:*  At a minimum of 24 h before hospital discharge patient exhibits adequate nutrition as evidenced by stable weight and serum albumin 3.5-5.5 g/dl. Patient's protein intake is 1.2-1.5 g/kg body weight/day.

- Protein crosses the peritoneum and a significant amount is lost in the dialysate. An increased intake of protein is necessary to prevent excessive tissue catabolism. Protein loss increases with peritonitis. Ensure adequate dietary intake of protein: 1.2-1.5 g/kg body weight daily.
- Peritoneal dialysis patients typically have fewer dietary restrictions than those on hemodialysis. Ensure that a dietary evaluation and teaching pro-

gram are performed when the patient changes from one type of dialysis to the other.

- Provide a list of restricted and encouraged foods with menus that illustrate their integration into the daily diet. Ensure patient's understanding by having him or her plan a 3-day menu that incorporates the appropriate foods and restrictions.

**Altered protection** related to neurosensory, musculoskeletal, or cardiac changes secondary to uremia and serum electrolyte imbalance

***Desired outcome:*** Patient verbalizes orientation to person, place, and time and remains free of injury caused by neurosensory, musculoskeletal, or cardiac changes.

- Instruct patient and staff to observe for and report indications of the following:
  - *Increased uremia:* Confusion, lethargy, and restlessness. Monitor BUN and serum creatinine values. Increases in value can signal the need for increased dialysis. BUN should be <80-100 mg/dl. Serum creatinine values will vary, depending on the individual's muscle mass.
  - *Hyperkalemia:* Muscle cramps and muscle weakness. Monitor serum $K^+$ values. Normal range is 3.5-5.0 mEq/L.
  - *Hypokalemia* (secondary to dialysis): Abdominal pain, lethargy, and dysrhythmias. Monitor serum $K^+$ values. Normal range is 3.5-5.0 mEq/L.

---

**Note:** Alert physician to the development of an irregular pulse because it can be indicative of dangerous hypokalemia. This is especially important for patients on digitalis because hypokalemia potentiates digitalis toxicity.

---

- Promptly report abnormal laboratory values to the physician. The dialysate or length of dialysis time may require adjustment to compensate for the abnormal values.
- For other interventions, see this nursing diagnosis in "Acute Renal Failure," p. 133.

## Care of the patient undergoing hemodialysis

During hemodialysis, blood is removed *via* a special vascular access, heparinized, pumped through an artificial kidney (dialyzer), and then returned to the patient's circulation. Hemodialysis is either a temporary, acute procedure performed as needed, or it is performed chronically 2-4 times a week for 2-5 h each treatment.

### COMPONENTS OF HEMODIALYSIS

**Artificial kidney** (dialyzer): Composed of a blood compartment and dialysate compartment, separated by a semipermeable membrane that allows the diffusion of solutes and the filtration of water. Protein and bacteria do not cross the artificial membrane.

**Dialysate:** An electrolyte solution similar in composition to normal plasma. Each of the constituents may be varied according to patient need. The most commonly altered component is K. Glucose may be added to prevent sudden drops in serum osmolality and serum glucose during dialysis.

**Vascular access:** Necessary to provide a blood flow rate of 200-500 ml/min for an effective dialysis.

### NURSING DIAGNOSES AND INTERVENTIONS

**High risk for fluid volume deficit** related to excessive fluid removal or bleeding resulting from dialysis; *or*

**Fluid volume excess** related to compromised regulatory mechanism resulting in fluid retention secondary to renal failure

*Desired outcomes:*  Postdialysis patient is normovolemic as evidenced by balanced I&O, stable weight, RR 12-20 breaths/min with normal depth and pattern (eupnea), CVP 5-12 cm $H_2O$, HR and BP within patient's normal range, and absence of abnormal breath sounds and abnormal bleeding. Following instruction, patient relates the signs and symptoms of fluid volume excess and deficit.

- Monitor I&O and daily weight as indicators of fluid status. A steady weight gain indicates retained fluid. The patient's weight is an important guideline for determining the quantity of fluid that needs to be removed during dialysis. Weigh patient at the same time each day, using the same scale, and wearing the same amount of clothing (or with same items on the bed if using a bed scale).
- Instruct patient and staff to observe for and report indications of fluid volume excess: edema, hypertension, crackles (rales), tachycardia, distended neck veins, SOB, and increased CVP.
- After dialysis observe for and report indicators of fluid volume deficit, including hypotension, decreased CVP, and tachycardia. Describe the signs and symptoms to the patient and explain the importance of reporting them promptly should they occur. Be aware that because of autonomic neuropathy, the patient with uremia may not develop a compensatory tachycardia when hypovolemic. **Note:** Antihypertensive medications usually are held before and during dialysis to help prevent hypotension during dialysis. Clarify medication prescriptions with the physician.
- Monitor for postdialysis bleeding (gums, needle sites, incisions), which can occur because of use of heparin during dialysis. Alert patient to the potential for bleeding from these areas.
- To prevent hematoma formation, do not give IM injection for at least 1 h after dialysis.
- GI bleeding is common in patients with renal failure, especially after heparinization. Test all stools for the presence of blood. Report significant findings.

**High risk for fluid volume deficit** related to bleeding/hemorrhage that can occur with vascular access puncture or disconnection

**Altered peripheral tissue perfusion (or risk of same)** related to interrupted blood flow that can occur with clotting in the vascular access; *and*

**High risk for infection** related to invasive procedure (creation of the vascular access for hemodialysis)

*Desired outcomes:*  Patient's vascular access remains intact and connected, and patient is normovolemic (see description in preceding nursing diagnosis). Patient has adequate tissue perfusion as evidenced by normal skin temperature and color and brisk capillary refill (<2 seconds) distal to the vascular access. Patient's access is patent as evidenced by presence of bright red blood within shunt tubing or presence of thrill with palpation and bruit with auscultation of fistula or graft. Patient is free of infection as evidenced by normothermia and absence of erythema, local warmth, exudate, swelling, and tenderness at the exit site.

- After the surgical creation of the vascular access, assess for patency, auscultate for bruit, and palpate for thrill. Report severe or unrelieved pain, and observe for and report numbness, tingling, and swelling of the extremity distal to the access, any of which can signal impaired tissue perfusion. Expect postoperative swelling along the fistula; elevate the extremity accordingly.
- Notify physician if the extremity distal to vascular access becomes cool, has decreased capillary refill, or is discolored, because these problems can occur with vascular insufficiency.
- Follow the three principles of nursing care common to all types of vascular

access: prevent bleeding, prevent clotting, and prevent infection. Explain the monitoring and care procedures to the patient. Remember that the vascular access is the patient's lifeline. Monitor it closely and handle it with care. Vascular accesses include the following:

- **Subclavian or femoral lines:** External, temporary catheters inserted into a large vein.
  - *Prevent bleeding*: Anchor catheter securely because it might not be sutured in. Tape all connections. Keep clamps at bedside in case line becomes disconnected. If the line is removed or accidentally pulled out, apply firm pressure to site for at least 10 min.

---

**Caution:** An air embolus can occur if a subclavian line accidentally becomes disconnected. If this occurs, immediately clamp the line. Turn the patient onto a left-side-lying position to help prevent the air from blocking the pulmonary artery, and lower the HOB into Trendelenburg's position to increase intrathoracic pressure. This will decrease the flow of inspiratory air into the vein. Administer 100% oxygen by mask and obtain VS. Notify physician *stat!*

---

  - *Prevent clotting:* Keep line patent by priming with heparin or by constant infusion with a heparinized solution. Follow protocol or obtain specific order from physician. Attach a label to all lines that are primed with heparin to alert other personnel.
  - *Prevent infection:* Perform aseptic dressing changes according to agency protocol. Observe for and report indications of infection, including presence of erythema, local warmth, exudate, swelling, and tenderness at exit site. Report and culture any drainage.
- **Fistula or graft:** Internal, permanent connection between an artery and a vein, or the insertion of an internal graft that is joined to an artery and vein. Grafts can be straight or U-shaped. They are located in the arm or thigh.
  - *Prevent bleeding:* Inspect needle puncture sites for postdialysis bleeding. If bleeding occurs, apply just enough pressure over the site to stop it. Release the pressure and check for bleeding q5-10min.
  - *Prevent clotting:* Do not take BP, start IV, or draw blood in the arm with the graft or fistula. Have patient avoid tight clothing, jewelry, name bands, or restraint on affected extremity. Palpate for thrill and auscultate for bruit at least every shift and after hypotensive episodes. Notify physician *stat* if bruit or thrill is absent.
  - *Prevent infection:* Observe for and report indications of infection: presence of erythema, local warmth, swelling, exudate, and unusual tenderness at the fistula site. Culture and report any drainage.

---

**Note:** See "Care of the Patient Undergoing Peritoneal Dialysis" for **Altered protection,** p. 145.

---

# Section Five:    Disorders of the Urinary Tract

## Ureteral calculi

Ureteral calculi (stones) are a common urologic condition. Although the cause of stones is unknown in 50% of reported cases, it is believed that they originate in the kidney and are passed through the kidney to the ureter. About 90% of all stones pass from the ureter into the bladder and out of the urinary system spontaneously. See "Renal Calculi," for related information.

## ASSESSMENT

**Signs and symptoms:**  Pain that is sharp, sudden, and intense or dull and aching; located in the flank area; and frequently radiating toward the groin. Pain can be intermittent as the stone moves along the ureter and subside when it enters the bladder. Nausea, vomiting, diarrhea, abdominal pain, and paralytic ileus can occur. Patient may experience frequency, void in small amounts, and have hematuria.

**Physical assessment:**  Hypertension, pallor, diaphoresis, tachycardia, and tachypnea may be noted; chills and fever may be present in the acute stage. There can be absence of bowel sounds secondary to ileus, and the abdomen may be distended and tympanic. The patient will be restless and unable to find a position of comfort.

**History of:**   Sedentary life-style; residence in geographic area in which water supply is high in stone-forming minerals; vitamin A deficiency; vitamin D excess; hereditary cystinuria; treatment with acetazolamide, which is given for glaucoma; inflammatory bowel disease; recurrent urinary tract infections (UTI); prolonged periods of immobilization; gout; decreased fluid intake; and familial history of calculi or renal disease such as renal tubular acidosis.

## DIAGNOSTIC TESTS

**Serum tests:**   To assess calcium levels >5.3 mEq/L, phosphorus levels >2.6 mEq/L, and uric acid levels >7.5 mg/dl, which have been implicated in the formation of stones.

**BUN and creatinine tests:**   To evaluate renal-urinary function. Abnormalities are reflected by high BUN and serum creatinine and low urine creatinine. **Note:** Be aware that BUN results are affected by fluid volume excess and deficit. Volume excess will reduce BUN levels, while volume deficit will increase levels. For the older adult, serum creatinine level may not be a reliable measure of renal function because of reduced muscle mass and a decreased glomerular filtration rate. These tests must be evaluated based on an adjustment for the patient's age, hydration status, and in comparison to other renal-urinary tests.

**Urinalysis:**   To provide baseline data on the functioning of the urinary system, detect metabolic disease, and assess for the presence of UTI. A cloudy or hazy appearance, foul odor, pH >8.0, and the presence of WBCs and WBC casts signal UTI. A pH <5 is associated with uric acid calculi.

**Urine culture:**   To determine the type of bacteria present in the genitourinary tract. To avoid contamination, a midstream specimen should be collected.

**24-h urine collection:**   To test for high levels of uric acid, cystine, oxalate, calcium, phosphorus, or creatinine.

---

**Note:**   All urine samples should be sent to the lab immediately after they are obtained, or refrigerated if this is not possible (specimens for culture are *not* refrigerated). Urine left at room temperature has greater potential for bacterial growth, turbidity, and alkaline pH, any of which can distort the reading.

---

**Kidney, ureter, bladder (KUB) x-ray:**   To outline gross structural changes in the kidneys and urinary system. Typically, calcification is seen. Serial radiography monitors progressive movement of the stone.

**Intravenous pyelogram (IVP)/excretory urogram:**   Used to visualize the kidneys, renal pelvis, ureters, and bladder, this test also outlines radiopaque stones within the ureters.

**Renal ultrasound:**   To identify ureteral dilatation and presence of stones in the ureters.

**CT scan with or without injection of contrast medium:**   To distinguish cysts, tumors, calculi, and other masses; and determine presence of ureteral dilatation and bladder distention.

## COLLABORATIVE MANAGEMENT

**Pharmacotherapy during the acute stage**
*Narcotic and antispasmodic agents:* To relieve pain and ureteral spasms. **Note:** Both morphine and meperidine increase ureteral peristalsis, which aids in passage of the stone, but also can increase pain in the process.
*Antiemetics:* For nausea and vomiting.
*Antibiotics:* For infection.
**Prophylactic pharmacotherapy**
*For uric acid stones:* Allopurinol or sodium bicarbonate is given to reduce uric acid production or alkalinize the urine, keeping the pH at ≥6.5.
*For calcium stones:* Sodium cellulose phosphate, when used with a calcium-restricted diet, reduces risk of stone formation. Orthophosphates (potassium acid phosphate and disodium and dipotassium phosphates) are given to decrease urinary excretion of citrate and pyrophosphate, and thus inhibit stone formation. Thiazides also reduce excretion of citrate and reduce urinary calcium.
*For cystine stones:* Sodium bicarbonate or sodium-potassium citrate solution is given to increase urinary pH (≥7.5). Penicillamine can be given to lower cystine levels in the urine. Alpha-mercaptopripionylglycine produces similar action to penicillamine but produces fewer side effects.
**IV therapy:** For patients who are dehydrated.
**Increase fluid intake:** To help flush stone from the ureter to the bladder and out through the system.
**Diet:** Specific to patient's stone type. (See **Health-seeking behaviors,** p. 151, for detail.)
**Endoscopic removal of calculi** *via* **cystoscope:** A basketing catheter is placed beyond the stone and rotated in a downward movement to capture and remove the stone.
**Ureteral catheters (stents):** Positioned above the stone to promote ureteral dilatation, allowing the calculus to pass. These catheters also can be used for intermittent or continuous irrigation with an acidic solution to combat alkalinity. They may be placed temporarily after removal of the stone to allow for healing and promote patency of the ureter in the presence of edema.
**Ureterolithotomy:** Removal of calculi that are unable to pass through the ureter. The ureter is surgically incised, and the stone is manually removed.
**Percutaneous ultrasonic lithotripsy (PUL):** Used when the stone is easily accessible, such as in the renal pelvis, calyx, or upper ureter. A small tube is placed through a nephrostomy tract against the stone. An ultrasonic probe is passed through this tube, allowing ultrasound waves to shatter the stone. Fragments are removed by suction or irrigation.
**Extracorporeal shock wave lithotripsy (ESWL):** The patient is anesthetized (epidural or general) and placed in a water bath. The affected area is positioned under an electric shock generator, which shatters the calculi. Usually, 1,000-2,000 shock waves over a period of 30-45 min are adequate to break the calculi into fine particles. The fragments pass naturally in the patient's urine within a few days.
**Chemolysis:** Installation of solutions (acids, alkalines, chelate, and thiol) *via* nephrostomy and ureteral catheters to dissolve stones or stone fragments left by other treatments.

## NURSING DIAGNOSES AND INTERVENTIONS

**Pain** related to presence of the calculus or the surgical procedure to remove it
*Desired outcomes:* Patient's subjective perception of pain decreases within 1 h of intervention, as documented by a pain scale. Objective indicators, such as grimacing, are absent or diminished.
- Assess and document quality, location, intensity, and duration of pain. Devise a pain scale with the patient that ranges from 0 (no pain) to 10 (worst pain). Notify physician of sudden and/or severe pain.

- Notify physician of a sudden cessation of pain, which can signal the passage of the stone. (Strain all urine for solid matter, and send it to the laboratory for analysis.)
- Medicate patient with prescribed analgesics, narcotics, and antispasmodics; evaluate and document the response based on the pain scale.
- Provide warm blankets, heating pad to affected area, or warm baths to increase regional circulation and relax tense muscles.
- Provide back rubs. These are especially helpful for postoperative patients who were in the lithotomy position during surgery.

**Altered urinary elimination** (dysuria, urgency, or frequency) related to obstruction caused by ureteral calculus
*Desired outcomes:*  Patient relates the return of a normal voiding pattern within 2 days. Patient demonstrates the ability to record I&O and strain urine for stones.

- Determine and document patient's normal voiding pattern.
- Monitor quality and color of the urine. Optimally it is straw-colored and clear and has a characteristic urine odor. Dark urine is often indicative of dehydration, and blood-tinged urine can result from the rupture of ureteral capillaries as the calculus passes through the ureter.
- In patients for whom fluids are not restricted, encourage a fluid intake of at least 2 L/day to help flush calculus through ureter into the bladder and out through the system.
- Record accurate I&O; teach patient how to record I&O.
- Strain all urine for evidence of solid matter; teach patient the procedure.
- Send any solid matter to the laboratory for analysis.

**Altered urinary elimination** related to obstruction or positional problems of the ureteral catheter
*Desired outcome:*  Following intervention, patient has output from the ureteral catheter and is free of spasms or flank pain, which could signal obstruction or dislodgment.

- Occasionally patients return from surgery with a ureteral catheter. If patient has more than one catheter, label one *right* and the other *left;* keep all drainage records separate.
- Monitor output from ureteral catheter. Amount will vary with each patient and depend on catheter dimension. If drainage is scanty or absent, milk the catheter and tubing gently to try to dislodge the obstruction. If this fails, notify physician.
- **Caution:** Never irrigate the catheter without specific physician instructions to do so. If irrigation is prescribed, use gentle pressure and aseptic technique. Always aspirate with sterile syringe before instillation to prevent ureteral damage from overdistention. Use another sterile syringe to insert amounts no greater than 3 ml per instillation.
- Typically patient will require bed rest if ureteral catheter is indwelling. Explain to patient that semi-Fowler's and side-lying positions are acceptable. Fowler's position should be avoided, however, because sutures are seldom used and gravity can cause catheter to move into the bladder.
- Ureteral catheters are often attached to the urethral catheter after placement in the ureters. Carefully monitor the urethral catheter for movement, and ensure that it is securely attached to the patient. **Note:** After the ureteral catheters have been removed (usually simultaneously with the urethral catheter), monitor for indicators of ureteral obstruction, including flank pain, nausea, and vomiting.

**High risk for impaired skin integrity** related to wound drainage
*Desired outcome:*  Patient's skin surrounding the wound site remains intact.

- Monitor incisional dressings frequently during the first 24 h, and change or reinforce as needed. Excoriation can result from prolonged contact of urine with the skin.

- Note and document odor, consistency, and color of drainage. Immediately after surgery, drainage may be red.
- To facilitate frequent dressing changes, use Montgomery straps rather than tape to secure dressing.
- If drainage is copious after drain removal, apply wound drainage or ostomy pouch with a skin barrier over the incision. Use a pouch with an antireflux valve to prevent contamination from reflux.

**Health-seeking behaviors:** Dietary regimen and its relationship to stone formation

*Desired outcome:* Within the 24-h period before hospital discharge, patient verbalizes knowledge about foods and liquids to limit to prevent stone formation and demonstrates this knowledge by planning a 3-day menu that excludes or limits these foods.

- Assess patient's knowledge about diet and its relationship to stone formation.
- Advise patient to maintain a urine output of >2 L/day. Increasing the urine output reduces saturation of stone-forming solutes.
- Teach patient to maintain adequate hydration of 2-3 L/day. Good hydration after meals and exercise is important because the patient's solute load is highest at these times. **Caution:** Persons with cardiac or renal disease require special fluid intake instructions from their physician.
- Teach patient the technique for measuring urine specific gravity *via* a hydrometer. Explain that to minimize stone formation, specific gravity should remain <1.010.
- As appropriate, provide the following information:
  - *For uric acid stones:* Limit intake of foods high in purines, such as lean meat, legumes, whole grains. Limit protein intake to 90 g/day.
  - *For calcium stones:* Limit intake of foods high in calcium, such as milk, cheese, green leafy vegetables, yogurt. Limit Na intake (see Table 3-2). Explain to patient that a low-Na diet helps reduce intestinal absorption of calcium. Limit intake of refined carbohydrates and animal proteins, which cause hypercalciuria. Encourage patient to eat foods high in natural fiber content (e.g., bran, prunes, apples). Foods high in natural fiber content provide phytic acid, which binds dietary calcium. Explain that sodium cellulose phosphate, 5 g tid, may be given to bind with intestinal calcium and thus increase the excretion of calcium.
  - *For oxalate stones:* Limit intake of foods high in oxalate, such as chocolate, caffeine-containing drinks (including instant and decaffeinated coffees), beets, spinach, and peanuts. Large doses of pyridoxine may help with certain types of oxalate stones, and cholestyramine, 4 g qid, may be prescribed to bind with oxalate enterally. Explain that vitamin C supplements should be avoided because as much as half is converted to oxalic acid.

---

**Note:** Also see nursing diagnoses and interventions in Appendix One, "Caring for Preoperative and Postoperative Patients," p. 693.

---

## PATIENT-FAMILY TEACHING AND DISCHARGE PLANNING

Give patient and significant others verbal and written information about the following:

- Medications, including drug name, purpose, dosage, schedule, precautions, and potential side effects.
- Indicators of UTI or recurrent calculi, which necessitate medical attention: chills, fever, hematuria, flank pain, cloudy and foul-smelling urine, frequency, and urgency.
- Care of incision, including cleansing and dressing. Teach patient signs and

symptoms of local infection, including redness, swelling, local warmth, tenderness, and purulent drainage.
- Care of drains or catheters if patient is discharged with them.
- Importance of daily fluid intake of at least 3 L/day in nonrestricted patients.
- Dietary changes as specified by physician.
- Activity restrictions as directed for patient who has had surgery: avoid lifting heavy objects (>10 lb) for the first 6 weeks, be alert to fatigue, get maximum rest, increase activities gradually to tolerance.
- Use of nitrazine paper to assess pH of urine. Desired pH will be determined by type of stone formation to which the patient is prone. Instructions for use are on nitrazine container.
- Importance of walking or other exercise to decrease risk of stone formation.

# Urinary tract obstruction

Urinary tract obstruction usually is the result of blockage from pelvic tumors, calculi, and urethral strictures. Additional causes include neoplasms, benign prostatic hypertrophy, ureteral or urethral trauma, inflammation of the urinary tract, pregnancy, and pelvic or colonic surgery in which ureteral damage has occurred. Obstructions can occur suddenly or occur slowly, over weeks to months. They can occur anywhere along the urinary tract, but the most common sites are the ureteropelvic and ureterovesical junctions, bladder neck, and urethral meatus. The obstruction acts like a dam, blocking the passage of urine. Muscles in the area contract to push urine around the obstruction, and dilatation of the structures behind the obstruction begins to occur. The smaller the site of obstruction, the greater the damage. Hydrostatic pressure increases, and filtration and concentration processes in the tubules and glomerulus are compromised. Obstructions in the upper urinary tract can lead to bilateral involvement of the ureters and kidneys, leading to hydronephrosis, renal insufficiency, and kidney destruction. Obstructions in the lower urinary structures, such as the bladder neck or urethra, can lead to urinary retention and urinary tract infection.

## ASSESSMENT

**Signs and symptoms:**　Anuria, pain that is sharp and intense or dull and aching, nausea, vomiting, local abdominal tenderness, hesitancy, straining to start a stream, dribbling, oliguria, and nocturia.

**Physical assessment:**　Bladder distention (absent if obstruction is above the bladder), mass in flank area, and "kettle drum" sound over bladder with percussion.

**History of:**　Recent fever (possibly caused by the obstruction); hypertensive episodes (caused by increased hormone production from the body's attempt to increase renal blood flow).

## DIAGNOSTIC TESTS

**Serum $K^+$ and $Na^+$ levels:**　To determine renal function. Normal range for $K^+$ is 3.5-5.0 mEq/L; normal range for $Na^+$ is 137-147 mEq/L.

**BUN and creatinine:**　To evaluate renal-urinary status. Normally, their values will be elevated with decreased renal-urinary function. **Note:** These values must be considered based on the patient's age and hydration status. For the older adult, serum creatinine level may not be a reliable indicator, owing to decreased muscle mass and a decreased glomerular filtration rate. Hydration status can affect BUN: fluid volume excess can result in reduced values, while volume deficit can cause higher values.

**Urinalysis:**　To provide baseline data on the functioning of the urinary system, detect metabolic disease, and assess for the presence of urinary tract infection (UTI). A cloudy, hazy appearance; foul odor; pH >8.0; and presence of WBCs and WBC casts are signals of a UTI.

**Urine culture:** To determine type of bacteria present in the genitourinary tract. To minimize contamination, a sample should be obtained from a midstream collection.

**Hgb and Hct:** To assess for systemic bleeding and anemia, which may be related to decreased renal secretion or erythropoietin.

**Kidney, ureter, bladder (KUB) radiography:** This x-ray identifies the size, shape, and position of the kidneys, ureters, and bladder and abnormalities such as tumors, calculi, or malformations.

**Intravenous pyelogram:** To evaluate the cause of urinary dysfunction by visualizing the kidneys, renal pelvis, ureters, and bladder.

**Cystoscopy:** To determine degree of bladder outlet obstruction and facilitate visualization of any tumors or masses.

**Cystogram:** Radiopaque dye is instilled *via* cystoscope or catheter. This allows visualization of the bladder and evaluation of the vesiculoureteral reflex.

## COLLABORATIVE MANAGEMENT

**Catheterization:** To establish drainage of urine.

**Pharmacotherapy**

*Narcotics:* For pain relief.

*Antispasmodics:* For relief of spasms.

*Antibiotics:* For bacterial infection.

*Corticosteroids:* For reduction of local swelling.

**IV therapy:** For acutely ill, dehydrated patients.

**Surgically establish drainage:** *Via* catheters or drains (ureteral, urethral, or suprapubic) above point of obstruction.

**Surgical removal of obstruction or dilatation of strictures.**

## NURSING DIAGNOSES AND INTERVENTIONS

**High risk for fluid volume deficit** related to postobstructive diuresis

*Desired outcomes:* Patient is normovolemic as evidenced by HR ≤100 bpm (or within patient's normal range), BP ≥90/60 mm Hg (or within patient's normal range), RR ≤20 breaths/min, and orientation to person, place, and time (within patient's normal range). Within 2 days after bladder decompression, output approximates input, patient's urinary output is normal for patient (or ≥30-60 ml/h), and weight becomes stable.

- Using sterile technique, insert a urinary catheter to drain the patient's bladder. Monitor the patient carefully during catheterization; clamp the catheter if the patient complains of abdominal pain or has a symptomatic drop in systolic BP of ≥20 mm Hg. Current research (Bristoll et al, 1989; Dodds and Hans, 1990) suggests that rapid bladder decompression of >750-1,000 ml does not result in shock syndrome as previously believed.
- Monitor I&O hourly for 4 h and then q2h for 4 h after bladder decompression. Notify physician if output exceeds 200 ml/h or 2 L over an 8-h period. This can signal postobstructive diuresis, which can lead to major electrolyte imbalance. If this occurs, anticipate initiation of IV infusion.
- Monitor VS for signs of shock: decreasing BP, changes in LOC or mentation, tachycardia, tachypnea, thready pulse.
- Anticipate the need for urine specimens for analysis of electrolytes and osmolality and blood specimens for analysis of electrolytes.
- Observe for and report indicators of the following:
  - *Hypokalemia:* Abdominal cramps, lethargy, dysrhythmias.
  - *Hyperkalemia:* Diarrhea, colic, irritability, nausea, muscle cramps, weakness, irregular apical or radial pulses.
  - *Hypocalcemia:* Muscle weakness and cramps, complaints of tingling in fingers, positive Trousseau's and Chvostek's signs.

- *Hyperphosphatemia:* Excessive itching.
- Monitor mentation, noting signs of disorientation, which can occur with electrolyte disturbance.
- Weigh patient daily using the same scale and at the same time of day (e.g., before breakfast). Weight fluctuations of 2-4 lb (0.9-1.8 kg) normally occur in a patient who is undergoing diuresis.

**Pain** related to bladder spasms

***Desired outcomes:*** Within 1 h of intervention, patient's subjective perception of discomfort decreases, as documented by a pain scale. Objective indicators, such as grimacing, are absent or diminished.

- Assess for and document patient complaints of pain in the suprapubic or urethral area. Devise a pain scale with the patient, rating the pain from 0 (no pain) to 10 (worst pain). Reassure patient that spasms are normal with obstruction.
- Medicate with antispasmodics or analgesics as prescribed. Document the pain relief obtained, using the pain scale.
- Teach patient the procedure for slow diaphragmatic breathing.
- If the patient is losing urine around the catheter and has a distended bladder (with or without bladder spasms), check the catheter and drainage tubing for evidence of obstruction. Inspect for kinks and obstructions in drainage tubing, compress and roll catheter gently between fingers to assess for gritty matter within catheter, milk drainage tubing to release obstructions, or instruct patient to turn from side to side. Obtain prescription for catheter irrigation if these measures fail to relieve the obstruction.
- In nonrestricted patients, encourage intake of fluids to at least 2-3 L/day to help reduce frequency of spasms.
- Instruct patient in the use of nonpharmacologic methods of pain relief, such as guided imagery, relaxation techniques, and distraction. See relaxation technique described under "Coronary Artery Disease," **Health-seeking behaviors,** p. 54.

---

**Note:** See " Hydronephrosis" for **High risk for injury** related to insertion/presence of nephrostomy tube, p. 126. See "Ureteral Calculi" for **High risk for impaired skin integrity** related to wound drainage, p. 150. See nursing diagnoses and interventions in Appendix One, "Caring for Preoperative and Postoperative Patients," p. 693.

---

## PATIENT-FAMILY TEACHING AND DISCHARGE PLANNING

Give patient and significant others verbal and written information about the following:

- Medications, including drug name, dosage, purpose, schedule, precautions, and potential side effects.
- Indicators that signal recurrent obstruction and require prompt medical attention: pain, fever, decreased urinary output.
- Necessity of limiting activities during postoperative period.
- Care of drains or catheters if patient is discharged with them; care of the surgical incision if present.
- Indicators of *wound infection:* persistent redness, local warmth and tenderness, drainage, swelling; and *UTI:* dysuria, flank or suprapubic pain, cloudy or foul-smelling urine, chills, and fever.

# Cancer of the bladder

Cancer of the bladder is the most common form of urinary system cancer, and it occurs most often in persons 50-70 years of age. Causes are not clearly understood, but individuals with a history of industrial exposure to such chemicals as β-naphthylamine or benzidine or occupational exposure to dyes, rubber, leather and leather products, and paint are at a higher risk to develop this disease. Additional environmental factors affecting the development of bladder cancer are cigarette smoking, diets high in fat and protein, and deficiency in vitamin A. Other factors, including coffee drinking, chronic bladder infection, vesical calculus disease, phenacetin and cyclophosphamide use, and pelvic radiation therapy, are under investigation.

Bladder cancer often begins in the bladder lumen, but the bladder neck wall and ureteral orifices also can be involved. Cancers from nearby sites, particularly the prostate and uterine cervix, as well as the sigmoid colon, rectum, or uterus, also can invade the bladder. Cellular proliferation can occur throughout the transitional epithelium, which lines the kidneys, ureters, and mucosa of the bladder. Metastasis most commonly occurs in the bones, liver, and lungs and spreads throughout the lymph nodes.

## ASSESSMENT

**Signs and symptoms:**   Painless and intermittent hematuria, dysuria, urgency, burning with urination, increased frequency, small volumes of urine, and nocturia. Depending on tumor size, the patient may experience suprapubic pain. If the tumor causes urinary obstruction, see "Urinary Tract Obstruction," for further data. In later stages, low back pain, pelvic pain, and leg edema can occur.

**Physical assessment:**   Usually normal. A tumor can be palpated only after the disease has become deeply invasive.

## DIAGNOSTIC TESTS

**Urinalysis, urine culture:**   To check for pus, RBCs, WBCs, WBC casts, and a pH >8.0, which occur with infection.

**Urine cytology:**   To assess for cells that have been sloughed off from tumors/ neoplasms. The urine sample is taken from a voided specimen.

**CBC:**   To check for presence of infection (WBC >11,000 μl) and anemia (RBCs, Hct, and Hgb less than normal).

**Serum or urine carcinoembryonic antigen (CEA):**   To determine the amount of the tumor marker for bladder cancer. This antigen is produced by the tumor, and therefore the greater the amount, the higher the tumor grade.

**Intravenous pyelogram (IVP):**   Can reveal filling defects within the urinary tract and presence of tumor obstruction.

**Ultrasonography/magnetic resonance imaging (MRI):**   These tests are used to diagnose the cancer. Ultrasonography helps determine degree of tumor invasion in the bladder wall, and MRI can facilitate recognition of early bladder cancer and assist in staging of the bladder neoplasm.

**Biopsy in conjunction with cystoscopy:**   A cystoscope is inserted through the urethra and into the bladder to visualize the structures. If abnormalities are seen, a section of the tissue is removed for biopsy. Because the procedure is very uncomfortable under a local anesthetic, general anesthesia is usually used.

**Cystogram (cystography):**   To outline tumors that are present in the bladder. A radiopaque medium is introduced into the bladder *via* a urethral catheter. X-rays are taken both before and after urination.

## COLLABORATIVE MANAGEMENT

**Grading and staging the disease:**   To formulate a prognosis and guide treatment. The degree of grading and staging is determined by the extent of metastasis and tissue involvement: the greater the metastasis, the higher the grade and stage.

**Transurethral resection of the bladder and tumor (TURBT):**   Removal of the tumor with electrocautery *via* cystoscope and rectoscope. Water is used during this procedure because it causes the tumor cells released by the procedure to swell and lyse. TURBT is used to treat superficial bladder tumors.

**Photodynamic (laser) or electrical fulguration:**   Laser or electrical cauterization of small, well-delineated lesions. Usually it is followed by intravesical infusion of chemotherapy directly into the the bladder. **Note:** Patients undergoing photodynamic therapy become photosensitive and should avoid any exposure to sunlight for 4-6 weeks. Skin gradually can be exposed to sunlight after this period.

**Chemotherapy:**   With superficial bladder tumors, the patient may receive a bladder instillation of thiotepa *via* catheter 24-48 h postoperatively or as a treatment without surgery. Mitomycin, doxorubicin, or bacille Calmette-Guérin (BCG) can be used. These drugs reduce the recurrence rate of tumor growth. For invasive tumors, cisplatin and methotrexate are the most commonly used single agents for treatment and palliation of symptoms. Doxorubicin and vinblastine also are used. In addition, all four drugs are used in combination chemotherapy regimens to improve tumor response.

**Palliative radiation therapy:**   Used primarily in the late stages for pain relief, but it can also be used early in treatment.

**Radon seeds:**   May be implanted around the base of the tumor in an attempt to eradicate the bladder tumor and prevent regrowth. Typically, this is done after a transurethral resection (TUR) and fulguration of the bladder tumor. Severe cystitis is likely to occur from the irradiation.

**Supervoltage radiation therapy:**   Often used in conjunction with surgery or chemotherapy to shrink very large tumors or for pain relief if the cancer has metastasized widely.

**Pharmacotherapy**
- *Analgesics and narcotics:* For pain relief.
- *Antibiotics:* For therapy-induced infections.

**Segmental resection:**   Performed if the dome of the bladder is involved. The top half of the bladder is removed *via* an abdominal incision.

**Cystectomy:**   Removal of the entire bladder. Radical cystectomy involves removal of the entire bladder, portions or all of the urethra, and the distal ends of both ureters. In addition, seminal vesicles and the prostate gland are removed in males and the ovaries, uterus, fallopian tubes, and anterior vaginal wall are removed in females.

**Urinary diversion:**   See "Urinary Diversions," p. 172, for discussion.

## NURSING DIAGNOSES AND INTERVENTIONS

**High risk for fluid volume deficit** related to postsurgical hemorrhage after TURBT or segmental resection; *or*

**Fluid volume excess (or risk of same)** related to excessive fluid intake secondary to irrigation

***Desired outcome:***   Patient is normovolemic as evidenced by BP ≥90/60 mm Hg (or within patient's normal range), HR ≤100 bpm (or within patient's normal range), and orientation to person, place, and time (within patient's normal range).

- Monitor and record VS and I&O; record color and consistency of catheter drainage at least q8h. Drainage may be dark red after surgery, but it should lighten to pink or blood-tinged within 24 h. **Note:** Patients who have undergone TURBT may have clots passing through the drainage tubing. Continuous bladder irrigation (CBI) is often used to flush bloody drainage from the bladder to prevent clot formation, which can occlude the urethral catheter. For more information about patient care after a transurethral resection, see "Benign Prostatic Hypertrophy," p. 615.
- Be alert to hypotension and rapid HR, and watch for bright red, thick drainage or drainage that does not lighten after irrigation, any of which can signal arterial bleeding within the operative area and necessitate immediate surgical intervention.
- Monitor TURBT patient's postoperative mental status, being alert to changes

in mentation, such as confusion, which can denote a change in electrolyte balance and necessitate medical intervention. Water intoxication and hyponatremia (as evidenced by headache, lassitude, apathy, confusion, weakness, hypertension, muscle spasms, convulsions, coma) can occur because of the high volumes of irrigation fluid that are used with a transurethral resection.

**High risk for infection** related to invasive procedure (presence of suprapubic catheter), increased environmental exposure (opening of a closed drainage system), or use of intravesical chemotherapy
*Desired outcome:* Patient is free of infection as evidenced by WBC ≤11,000 µl, normothermia, and orientation to person, place, and time (within patient's normal range).

- Using aseptic technique, cleanse the area surrounding the suprapubic catheter with an antimicrobial solution, such as povidone-iodine. Apply sterile 4x4 gauze pad(s) over the catheter exit site and tape securely. Change the dressing as soon as it becomes wet, and use a pectin wafer skin barrier to protect the insertion site if indicated. **Note:** If a trocar system is used, clean around the plastic cover and keep the area dry. Tape the plastic edges securely to the skin to prevent accidental removal.
- Wash hands *before* and *after* manipulating the catheter, and use aseptic technique when opening the closed drainage system, changing dressings, and irrigating the catheter.
- Irrigate catheter *only* if there is an obstruction and by physician prescription.
- Protect the catheter by keeping it securely taped to the patient's lateral abdomen.
- If the catheter is accidentally pulled out of the insertion site, immediately cover the site with a sterile 4x4 gauze pad and notify physician.
- To keep urine dilute to help prevent urinary tract infection (UTI), encourage a fluid intake of at least 2-3 L/day in nonrestricted patients.
- Keep the drainage collection container below the level of the patient's bladder to prevent infection from reflux of urine.

**Altered urinary elimination** related to obstruction of suprapubic catheter or anuria/dysuria secondary to removal of catheter
*Desired outcome:* Patient's urinary output is appropriate for the amount of intake within 3 days after surgery.

- Keep drainage records from suprapubic catheter separate from those of other catheters and drains.
- Prevent external obstruction of the catheter, assessing frequently for patency. Irrigate *only* if internally obstructed and with physician order.
- Before removal of suprapubic catheter, physician may request a 3-4-h clamping routine to assess patient's ability to void normally. After patient has voided, unclamp the catheter and measure the residual urine that flows into the drainage collection container. Once the residual urine is <100 ml after each of two successive voidings, notify physician. Usually the catheter can be removed at that time.
- After removal of the catheter, evaluate patient's ability to void by recording the time and amount during the first 24 h. Patients with segmental resections will void frequently and in small amounts at first because the bladder capacity is approximately 60 ml. Explain to the patient that the bladder will expand to 200-400 ml within a few months.
- If patient cannot void 8-12 h after catheter removal and experiences abdominal pain or has a distended bladder, notify physician for intervention.
- If patient experiences burning with urination, encourage an increased intake of fluids and apply heat over the bladder area with a warm blanket, heating pad, or sitz bath, any of which will increase circulation to the area and relax the muscles.

- Obtain specimen for urine culture as prescribed if patient complains of burning, urgency, or frequency. The culture will differentiate between sterile pyuria and bacterial cystitis.

---

**Note:** See "Urinary Tract Obstruction" for **Pain** related to bladder spasms, p. 154. See Appendix One, "Caring for Preoperative and Postoperative Patients," p. 693, and "Caring for Patients with Cancer and Other Life-Disrupting Illnesses," p. 719 (in particular **Altered urinary elimination** related to hemorrhagic cystitis secondary to cyclophosphamide treatment; oliguria or renal toxicity secondary to cisplatinum or high-dose methotrexate administration; or dysuria secondary to cystitis, p. 752).

---

## PATIENT-FAMILY TEACHING AND DISCHARGE PLANNING

Give patient and significant others verbal and written information about the following:

- Medications, including drug name, purpose, dosage, route, schedule, precautions, and potential side effects.
- Indicators of complications from photodynamic therapy, such as redness or swelling over areas exposed to sun, the importance of reporting them to health-care provider, and the necessity of avoiding sun exposure for 4-6 weeks after the last treatment.
- Expectations of severe urinary frequency and urgency, blood-tinged urine, and dysuria during the first week after cauterization.

# Section Six:    Urinary Disorders Secondary to Other Disease Processes

## Urinary incontinence

Urinary incontinence occurs when an individual experiences involuntary loss of urine. The ability to urinate requires complex interactions between nerve pathways, the detrusor muscle, the internal sphincter, the external sphincter, and a higher urethral pressure than bladder pressure. Since incontinence occurs when bladder pressure exceeds urethral resistance, structural or musculature weakness or damage places an individual at increased risk. A spinal cord lesion above S–2 through S–4 may result in loss of sensation or awareness of bladder filling because of interruption of the nerve pathways. Thus, the bladder acts in response to bladder pressure, which becomes higher than that in the urethra. Urinary incontinence can be short term, caused by an acute illness, or it can be chronic. General causes can be classified as interference with neural control (e.g., cerebrovascular accident [CVA], spinal cord injury [SCI]); interference with bladder function (e.g., inflammatory states, loss of or increased contractility, constipation or impaction); interference with urethral sphincter mechanism (e.g., "stress" incontinence in women, posttransurethral resection of the prostate [TURP] incontinence in males); and environmental interferences (e.g., radiation therapy, medications such as diuretics or anticholinergics). These conditions manifest as stress, urge, overflow, or functional incontinence or as combinations of two factors.

## ASSESSMENT

**Signs and symptoms:**   Polyuria; dysuria; low back or flank pain; loss of urine with increased intraabdominal pressure, such as during laughing, sneezing, coughing, lifting; involuntary urination occurring soon after the urge to void is sensed; involuntary passage of urine occurring at predictable intervals; inability to reach the commode on time when environmental barriers exist or disorientation occurs; nocturia.

**History of:** Neurologic dysfunctions, such as Parkinson's disease, CVA, brain injury, normal pressure hydrocephalus, SCI or spinal cord lesions, multiple sclerosis (MS); acute or chronic diminishing of cerebral functioning; abdominal or bladder surgery; use of such medications as loop diuretics, anticholinergics, and adrenergic agents; radiation therapy for bladder cancer; meningitis; impaired mobility; diabetes mellitus (due to autonomic neuropathy and decreased detrusor contractility); multiparity; and low back syndrome.

Voiding problems may be verified *via* use of a diary in which the patient documents and describes duration, frequency, volume, and type of incontinence as well as fluid intake. An evaluation is made of environmental and social factors that may affect continence, such as access to toilets, living arrangements, and caregiver availability.

## DIAGNOSTIC TESTS

**Urinalysis:** To provide baseline data on the functioning of the urinary system, detect metabolic disease, and assess for the presence of urinary tract infection (UTI). A cloudy or hazy appearance, foul odor, pH $>8.0$, and presence of WBCs and WBC casts are indicative of UTI. **Note:** Obtain urine sample before rectal or genital examination. Urine collected after either examination may be contaminated by vaginal or prostatic secretions.

**Urine culture:** To determine the type of bacteria present in the genitourinary tract. To minimize the risk of contamination, a specimen should be obtained from a midstream collection.

**Urodynamic studies:** To evaluate cause and extent of the incontinence.

*Uroflowmetry:* Provides information about bladder strength and the opening ability of the urethral sphincter. The force of the urine stream is tested, using a specially designed commode.

*Cystometry:* Measures the pressure-volume relationship of the bladder. The bladder is filled at a rate of 50 ml/min to the maximum capacity of the bladder, and the bladder's ability to accommodate pressure changes is evaluated. In a normal individual, the bladder will fill smoothly without contractions and empty when the individual desires. The ability of the patient to detect bladder fullness also is noted.

*Urethral pressure profile:* Most helpful in detecting stress incontinence, this test identifies the amount of closing pressure the urethra can produce, *via* a dual-tip, microtip, pressure-sensitive catheter, which enables simultaneous measurement of the intraurethral and intravesical pressures.

*Sphincter electromyography:* Evaluates the function of the striated urinary sphincter. Results of this test are compared to the results from cystometry to identify abnormalities in coordination between the bladder and sphincter function.

**Postvoid residual:** Measures amount of urine in the bladder after a normal voiding. Amounts $>100$ ml imply retention problems.

**BUN and creatinine:** Serum values increase as renal-urinary function declines. **Note:** These values can be affected by hydration status and age. Fluid volume deficit can falsely increase the values, while volume excess can decrease the values. Creatinine values may be misleading in the older adult because of the loss of muscle mass and decreased glomerular filtration rate.

## COLLABORATIVE MANAGEMENT

### Behavioral interventions

*Bladder training:* Incorporation of a progressively increased time interval between voidings. The patient is taught to resist the urge to void and thus delay voiding until a set time. Intervals are set close together intitially and then further apart. Fluid intake also is adjusted. The goal with bladder training is reduction of small voidings and thus more normal bladder function.

*Habit training:*   The patient voids according to a set schedule on a planned basis. The schedule is set according to the patient's voiding habits. The goal is for the patient to remain dry. Habit training differs from bladder training in that there is no attempt to encourage the patient to resist or delay voiding, and the caregiver takes the initiative in maintaining the schedule and toileting the patient.

*Prompted voidings:*   An addition to habit training, the caregiver checks the patient regularly, asks whether he or she is wet or dry, and then requests that the patient use the toilet. If successful, positive feedback about maintaining continence is given; if unsuccessful, the caregiver gives no feedback. This technique is used with cognitively impaired or dependent individuals. The goal is to have the patient recognize incontinent status and learn to ask for assistance when needed.

**Catheter drainage of urine:**   Either intermittent or continuous.

**Vaginal cones:**   Cone-shaped devices of varying weights may be used to improve pelvic muscle tone and strength in females. The cones are inserted intravaginally (light ones first) and the patient must retain the device for 15 min bid. The cone's weight may provide heightened proprioceptive information to achieve the desired pelvic muscle contraction as well as increase pelvic muscle strength.

**Pelvic muscle (Kegel) exercise program:**   To increase strength of voluntary periurethral and pelvic muscles *via* exercise of the pubococcygeus muscle. These exercises, which must be performed frequently during a day (i.e., 100 times), are done by tightening the periovaginal muscles and anal sphincter as though controlling urination or defecation.

**Fluid intake:**   At least 2-3 L/day in nonrestricted patients.

**External (condom) catheter:**   For male patients, if appropriate.

**Surgical procedures to restore bladder-urethral structure:**   There are many surgical procedures that may be employed to reestablish normal vesicourethral structure. Examples of the most common include the following:

*Urethral suspension (Marshall-Marchetti-Krantz; Stamey) procedure:*   For stress incontinence. The bladder is elevated in the abdominal cavity *via* suprapubic transverse incision to lengthen the urethra, thereby creating resistance in the urethral lumen. The *Pereya* procedure uses both vaginal and suprapubic approaches.

*Pubovaginal sling urethropexy:*   After harvesting a small strip of rectus fascia through a small suprapubic incision, a transvaginal approach is used. The area lateral to the urethra is joined to the junction of the pelvic floor and overlying symphysis pubis.

*Artificial urinary sphincter.*

**Medications used for urge incontinence:**   Anticholinergics or smooth muscle relaxants, such as imipramine or oxybutynin, may be prescribed to inhibit uncontrolled bladder contractions and enhance functional bladder capacity. Calcium channel blockers such as verapamil and nifedapine, which are used for cardiovascular problems, also can depress the bladder, thereby relieving urge incontinence. However, they also can cause urinary retention. **Note:** Anticholinergics must be used cautiously in the older adult because they can increase the occurrence of acute confusion.

**Medications used for stress incontinence:**   Alpha-adrenergic drugs, such as pseudoephedrine, ephedrine, or phenylpropanolamine, assist smooth muscle contraction of the bladder neck. Estrogen therapy, which decreases muscle atrophy, is given to improve urgency and frequency.

## NURSING DIAGNOSES AND INTERVENTIONS

---

**Note:** Patients with urinary incontinence may have overlapping conditions. For example, they may experience functional incontinence, which is made more severe by UTI superimposed on urge incontinence.

---

**Stress incontinence** related to degenerative changes or weakness in pelvic muscles and structural supports secondary to menopause, childbirth, obesity, or surgical procedure interfering with normal vesicourethral structure

***Desired outcome:*** After implementation of bladder training program, patient becomes continent.

### Bladder training program

- Assess and document the patient's voiding pattern: time, amount voided, amount of fluid intake, timing of fluid intake followed by voiding, and related information such as the degree of wetness experienced (e.g., number of incontinence pads used in a day, degree of underwear dampness) and the exertion factor causing the wetness (e.g., laughing, sneezing, bending, lifting). Teach patient to keep a voiding diary that incorporates this information.

- Determine the amount of time between voidings to estimate how long the patient can hold urine. Establish a voiding schedule that does not exceed this time period.

- Assist patient with scheduling times for emptying the bladder, such as (initially) q1-2h when awake and q4h at night. If successful, attempt to lengthen the time intervals between voiding. Provide patient and significant others with a written copy of the schedule. **Note:** Patients need to empty their bladders at least q4h to reduce the risk of UTI caused by urinary stasis.

- Estimate and document urinary output when patient is incontinent in clothes or bed linens. For example, a wet spot of approximately 2 inches in diameter is equal to approximately 5 ml urine.

- Teach patient techniques that strengthen the sphincter and structural supports of the bladder, such as the Kegel exercises (see **Knowledge deficit,** p. 163).

- In nonrestricted patients, encourage a fluid intake of at least 2-3 L/day. Be aware that patients with urinary incontinence often will reduce their fluid intake to avoid incontinence at the risk of dehydration and UTI.

- Educate patient about dietary irritants (e.g., caffeine, alcoholic beverages) that may increase stress incontinence.

**Urge incontinence** related to bladder irritation or reduced bladder capacity secondary to radiation treatment for bladder cancer, UTI, increased urine concentration, use of caffeine or alcohol, or enlarged prostate

***Desired outcome:*** After implementation of the toileting program, patient becomes continent.

- Assess and document patient's usual pattern of voiding, including frequency and timing of incontinent episodes.

- Adhere to the toileting program (see interventions with **Stress incontinence,** earlier).

- Teach nonrestricted patient to increase fluid intake to $\geq 3$ L/day but to avoid caffeinated drinks or alcohol, which are natural diuretics and bladder irritants.

- Explain the types of fluids patient should drink that are not irritating to the bladder, such as water, fruit juices, herbal drinks, and decaffeinated sodas, teas, and coffees.

- Encourage the intake of cranberry juice, prunes, and plums, which leave an acid ash in the urine to minimize the occurrence of UTI.

- Teach patient to keep a voiding record for at-home use, documenting accurate information about frequency and timing of incontinent episodes.

- Encourage patient to decrease fluid intake a few hours before bedtime and to void before sleep.

- Keep a urinal or bedpan at the bedside and instruct patient in its use.
- Teach patient deep, slow breathing technique, which can be used when the urge to void occurs prematurely.
- If the patient is ambulatory but has a cognitive impairment, label the bathroom door with signs that denote *toilet* to the patient, such as a picture of a commode. Adhere closely to the toileting program, reminding patient to void at the scheduled intervals.
- Administer prescribed anticholinergics or smooth muscle relaxants, which inhibit detrusor contractions or decrease detrusor instability.

**Functional incontinence** related to sensory, cognitive, or mobility deficits or related to environmental changes

***Desired outcome:***   After implementation of habit training program, the patient becomes continent.

- Assess and document patient's pattern of voiding: time, amount voided, amount of fluid intake, timing of fluid intake followed by voiding, and other related factors.
- Determine environmental obstacles that would prevent patient from toileting appropriately, and intervene accordingly. For example, remove obstacles between the bed and bathroom, leave a light on in the bathroom, attach the call light to the bed sheet.
- Assess patient's bowel status for the potential for constipation, which causes straining and weakens sphincter tone.
- Monitor patient for the increased need to void after taking medications such as diuretics, which increase urine production or the sensation of urgency.

*Habit training*

- Based on the assessed pattern of incontinence, establish a planned schedule for voiding.
- Offer bedpan, urinal, or assistance to the bathroom at least q2h.
- Maintain the planned schedule for voiding and note the time of any incontinent episode that occurs between the scheduled voidings. If the patient's incontinence pattern consistently does not match the voiding schedule, change the voiding schedule.

*In addition*

- Administer diuretics in the morning or early afternoon to reduce the risk of nighttime incontinence.
- If the patient has an intravenous infusion, consult with physician about advisability of reducing the infusion rate at nighttime.
- For bedridden patients, keep call light within patient's reach and answer call quickly.
- For confused patients, keep a clock and calendar in the room and remind patient of the time and date as appropriate. Toilet patient as described above. If the patient is acutely confused, calmly let the patient know that you do not see or hear what he or she does, but do not argue (e.g., if the patient cries, "Help, I'm in jail," you might say, "It must feel like jail being tied to all these tubes"). This approach, rather than constantly trying to reorient the patient, will minimize her or his agitation until the underlying cause of the disorientation has been resolved. When the patient is calm, you can reorient to the environment, but if he or she becomes agitated, stop the attempt to reorient.
- If the patient has permanent or severe cognitive impairment, reorient to his or her baseline and toilet the patient as described previously.

**High risk for impaired skin integrity** related to incontinence of urine

***Desired outcome:***   Patient's perineal skin remains intact.

- Assess the patient for wetness of the perineal area at frequent intervals. Inform the patient that prolonged exposure to urine can cause maceration and to alert staff as soon as wetness occurs.
- Keep bed linen dry. As necessary, use and change absorbent materials, such as protective underwear or underpads.

- Keep the perineum clean with mild soap and water; dry it well.
- Expose the perineum to air whenever possible by using a sheet draped over a bed cradle; ensure the patient's privacy.
- Use sealants and moisture-barrier ointments to protect the patient's skin.
- Make sure that plastic pads or sheet protectors do not contact the patient's skin directly because maceration can result from the increased perspiration they cause. Cover these pads with pillow cases or place them under the sheets.
- Educate patient in the use of containment devices, such as briefs with pads, adult absorptive briefs, and external catheters.
- Initiate habit or bladder training to reduce episodes of incontinence.

**Body image disturbance** related to odor, discomfort, and embarrassment secondary to incontinence
**Desired outcomes:** After intervention(s), patient verbalizes feelings and frustrations without self-deprecating statements. Within the 24-h period before hospital discharge, patient verbalizes knowledge about actions that will control either incontinence or odor and discomfort.

- Encourage patient to discuss feelings and frustrations.
- Offer reassurance and encouragement, and provide information about treatment, especially about those activities that are within the patient's own control.
- Be realistic with the patient; if incontinence cannot be controlled, reassure patient that odor and discomfort *can* be controlled.
- Explore with patient the methods for relief of discomfort and odor control: maintenance of good hygiene, frequent changes of undergarments, use and frequent changes of incontinence pads.
- Although fluid intake of at least 2-3 L/day is essential for minimizing the risk of UTI, suggest that the patient limit fluids when away from the home environment and increase them on return. A decrease also should be incorporated into the evening hours to prevent nighttime incontinence.
- Refer patient to support groups, such as HIP (Help for Incontinent People): Box 544, Union, SC 29379, (803)-579-7900; and The Simon Foundation: Box 835, Wilmette, IL, 60091, (800)-23-SIMON.
- For additional information, see this nursing diagnosis in Appendix One, "Caring for Patients with Cancer and Other Life-Disrupting Illnesses," p. 760.

**Knowledge deficit:** Pelvic muscle (Kegel) exercise program to strengthen perineal muscles (effective for individuals with mild-moderate stress incontinence or for those with functional incontinence who are able to participate)
**Desired outcome:** Within the 24-h period before hospital discharge, patient verbalizes and demonstrates knowledge about the pelvic muscle (Kegel) exercise program.

- Explain that Kegel exercises will strengthen the pelvic area muscles, which will help regain bladder control.
- Assist patient with identifying the correct muscle group:
  - To strengthen the proximal muscle, instruct patient to attempt to shut off urinary flow after beginning urination, hold for a few seconds, and then start the stream again. Explain to patient that if this can be accomplished, the correct muscle is being exercised.
  - To strengthen the distal muscle, teach patient to contract the muscle around the anus as though to stop a bowel movement.

---

**Note:** A common error when attempting to identify the correct muscle group is contraction of the buttocks, quadriceps, and abdominal muscles.

---

- Teach patient to repeat these exercises 10-20 times, four times per day. Advise patient that these exercises may require 2-9 months before any benefit is obtained.

**Knowledge deficit:**   Use of external (condom) catheter
*Desired outcomes:*   Within the 24-h period before hospital discharge, patient or significant other successfully returns demonstration of condom catheter application and verbalizes knowledge about the rationale for its use.

- Instruct male patients or significant other in the procedure for application of a condom catheter.
- Teach the importance of keeping pubic hair trimmed or moved away from the penis to avoid contact with the adhesive used with the catheter.
- Instruct patient to cleanse and dry the penis thoroughly before and after every condom application. With uncircumcised patients, the foreskin should be retracted to cleanse the area under the prepuce and then returned to its original position.
- Teach patient or significant other to monitor skin under the external device daily for redness, rashes, or open areas.
- For ambulatory patients, demonstrate connecting the condom catheter to a leg drainage bag; for patients on bed rest, demonstrate connecting the catheter to a bedside urinary collection container, such as that used with an indwelling catheter.
- Advise patient to remove and replace the catheter as directed. Most manufacturers recommend that external catheters be changed and replaced daily.
- If appropriate for the patient, suggest that the condom catheter be used only during the night.

---

**Note:**   Both internal and external catheters should be used only if other methods for urinary continence fail, because both lead to increased incidence of UTI.

---

See "Neurogenic Bladder" for **Reflex incontinence,** p. 168. For surgical patients, see nursing diagnoses and interventions in Appendix One, "Caring for Preoperative and Postoperative Patients," p. 693. In particular, see **High risk for infection** related to presence of indwelling urinary catheter, p. 705.

## PATIENT-FAMILY TEACHING AND DISCHARGE PLANNING

Give patient and significant others verbal and written information about the following:

- Medications, including drug name, dosage, purpose, schedule, precautions, and potential side effects.
- Diet: importance of increasing dietary fiber to help prevent constipation and keep stools soft.
- Indicators of UTI, which necessitate medical attention: fever, chills, cloudy or foul-smelling urine, frequency, urgency, burning with urination, hematuria, increasing or recurring incontinence.
- Care of catheters and drains if the patient is discharged with them.
- Importance of maintaining fluid intake of at least 3 L/day and avoiding caffeine and alcohol, which act as bladder irritants and increase the risk of urgency.
- Maintenance of schedule for bladder training program.
- Use of perineal muscles to improve bladder tone.
- Care of perineal skin.
- Support groups (see **Body image disturbance,** p. 163).

*For surgical patients*

- Care of the incision, including cleansing and dressing; and indicators of infection: purulent drainage, persistent redness, swelling, warmth along incision line.
- Activity restrictions: no heavy lifting (>10 lb) and resting when fatigued. Explain that prolonged periods of sitting can cause relaxation of the muscu-

lature of the bladder and sphincter, leading to incontinence. Encourage mild activity, such as walking, to improve muscle tone.

# Urinary retention

When urine is produced and accumulates in the bladder but is not released, the condition is called urinary retention. In the acute care setting, urinary retention is most commonly seen as a postoperative complication following surgical procedures using general or spinal anesthesia. Another major cause is obstruction (e.g., from benign prostatic hypertrophy, tumor, calculi, urethral stricture, fibrosis, meatal stenosis, or fecal impaction). Other causes include decreased sensory stimulation to the bladder, anxiety, or muscular tension. Medications such as opiates, sedatives, antihistamines, antispasmodics, major tranquilizers and antidepressants, and antidyskinetics also can interfere with the normal micturition reflex.

## ASSESSMENT

**Signs and symptoms:**   Sudden inability to void, intense suprapubic pain, restlessness, diaphoresis, voiding small amounts (20-50 ml) at frequent intervals.

**Physical assessment:**   "Kettle drum" sound with bladder percussion, bladder distention, bladder displacement to one side of the abdomen.

## DIAGNOSTIC TESTS

**Urinalysis:**   Provides baseline data regarding urinary system function, detects metabolic disease, and evaluates for the presence of urinary tract infection (UTI). A cloudy or hazy appearance, foul odor, pH >8.0, and the presence of WBCs and WBC casts are all signals of UTI.

**Urine culture:**   To determine the type of bacteria present in the genitourinary tract. To minimize contamination, a midstream specimen should be collected.

**BUN and creatinine:**   To evaluate renal-urinary function. Generally, serum values increase in the presence of dysfunction. **Note:** BUN values are affected by the patient's hydration status: fluid volume excess can result in decreased values, while volume deficit can result in increased values. Creatinine may not be a reliable indicator of renal function in the older adult owing to decreased muscle mass and decreased glomerular filtration rate.

**Urinary function tests:**   To evaluate cause of the urinary retention.

*Cystoscopy:*   A lighted, tubular scope is inserted into the bladder to allow visualization of tumors or masses.

*Cystogram:*   Radiopaque dye is instilled into the bladder *via* cystoscope or catheter to enable visualization of the bladder and evaluation of the vesiculoureteral reflex.

*Cystometrogram:*   Water or saline is instilled into the bladder *via* a catheter to create pressure against the bladder wall to evaluate bladder tone.

**Kidney, ureter, bladder (KUB) radiography:**   Used diagnostically, this x-ray identifies the size, shape, and position of the kidneys, ureters, and bladder and abnormalities such as tumors, calculi, or malformations.

**Intravenous pyelogram:**   Visualizes the kidney, renal pelvis, ureters, and bladder to evaluate for the cause of urinary dysfunction.

## COLLABORATIVE MANAGEMENT

**Catheterization:**   For drainage of urine.

**Pharmacotherapy**

*Cholinergics:*   To stimulate bladder contractions.

*Analgesia:*   For pain relief.

*Antibiotics:*  If infection is present.
**IV therapy:**  For hydration of the acutely ill patient.
**Surgery:**  Performed if obstruction is the cause of the retention. (See "Urinary Tract Obstruction," p. 152.)

## NURSING DIAGNOSES AND INTERVENTIONS

**Urinary retention** related to weak detrusor muscle, blockage, inhibition of reflex arc, or strong sphincter
*Desired outcome:*  Patient reports a normal voiding pattern within 2 days; or, if appropriate, the patient demonstrates self-catheterization before hospital discharge.

- Assess the bladder for distention by inspection, percussion, and palpation; measure and document I&O.
- If appropriate, try noninvasive measures for release of urine: position patient in a normal position for voiding; have patient listen to the sound of running water or place hands in a basin of warm water. If these measures are ineffective, try pouring warm water over the perineum. Unless contraindicated, Credé's method (pressure applied from the umbilicus to the pubis) may be used to stimulate a weak micturitional reflex.
- Maintain privacy for patient who is trying to use the commode, bedpan, or urinal. Remember that cold bedpans can cause muscle tension, so use a plastic bedpan or warm a metal bedpan before giving it to the patient. Encourage relaxation technique, such as deep breathing or visualization, to relax the body.
- Provide an adequate amount of time for the patient's urge to void to occur. Do not rush the patient.
- Notify physician if patient is unable to void, has bladder distention, or has suprapubic or urethral pain.
- If catheterization is prescribed, monitor patient's BP and HR during the procedure. If the patient complains of abdominal pain or has a symptomatic drop of >20 mm Hg systolic BP, clamp the catheter until patient's BP returns to within normal limits. For additional information see **High risk for fluid volume deficit** related to post-obstructive diuresis in "Urinary Tract Obstruction," p. 153.
- Catheterization may be difficult beyond the prostatic gland in men with benign prostatic hypertrophy (BPH) or in those over age 65, a large percentage of whom have undiagnosed BPH. For these patients, use a coudé (bent tip) catheter instead of a straight catheter. The tip on this catheter is stiff and does not bend against an obstacle. Lubricate the catheter tip generously with a minimum of 5 ml of lubricating jelly before insertion.
- Teach patient the technique for intermittent self-catheterization, if appropriate. Catheterization should be accomplished on a set q4h schedule to prevent bladder distention, which can injure the bladder mucosa and increase the risk of infection. Teach the patient clean technique for use at home.

---

**Note:**  See "Urinary Tract Obstruction" for **High risk for fluid volume deficit** related to post-obstructive diuresis, p. 153, and **Pain** related to bladder spasms, p. 154. Also see "Neurogenic Bladder" for **Dysreflexia** related to distended bladder, p. 170.

---

## PATIENT-FAMILY TEACHING AND DISCHARGE PLANNING

Give patient and significant others verbal and written information about the following:

- Medications, including drug name, purpose, dosage, schedule, precautions, and potential side effects.

- Indicators of UTI and recurrent retention, which necessitate medical attention: suprapubic or urethral pain, fever, recurring or increasing difficulty with voiding.
- Self-catheterization technique, if appropriate.

# Neurogenic bladder

Neurogenic bladder, also known as neuromuscular bladder dysfunction, neurologic bladder dysfunction, or neuropathic bladder disorder, is a complex phenomenon resulting from disruption of the signals from the bladder to the brain. Caused by a myriad of diseases, injuries, or lesions, the interruption of the signal can be found in either the central nervous system or at the level of the spinal cord. Certain conditions leave the sacral reflex intact while affecting the brain's ability to receive or interpret the signal.

Conditions such as multiple sclerosis (MS), cerebrovascular accident (CVA), dementia, tumors, and lesions above level T–12 lead to reflex or uninhibited bladder control. Interruption of the signal at the spinal level leads to autonomous neurogenic bladder, from which the patient has no sensation of needing to void and no micturition reflex. Voiding occurs irregularly and is uncontrolled. Lack of muscle control results in loss of bladder contraction, leading to overflow incontinence. Conditions leading to overflow incontinence include sacral cord trauma, tumors, transection of the pelvic parasympathetic nerves during abdominal surgery, and herniated disk. Loss of the sensation to void results in atonic bladder. Displayed by dribbling, voiding in small amounts, or complaints of loss of sensation of bladder fullness, this condition occurs with damage to the posterior nerve roots or in the presence of diabetes mellitus.

## ASSESSMENT

**Upper motor neuron disturbance (spastic bladder):**   Urinary frequency, residual urine, urinary retention, recurrent urinary tract infections (UTIs), spontaneous loss of urine, urge incontinence, and lack of urinary control.
**Lower motor neuron disturbance (flaccid bladder):**   Urinary retention, recurrent UTIs, inability to perceive the need to void.
**History of:**   Spinal cord injury (SCI), spinal tumor, MS, diabetes mellitus, CVA, Parkinson's disease, Alzheimer's disease, herpes zoster.

## DIAGNOSTIC TESTS

**Urinalysis:**   To provide baseline data on the functioning of the urinary system, detect metabolic disease, and assess for the presence of UTI. A cloudy or hazy appearance, foul odor, pH >8.0, and presence of WBCs and WBC casts are indicative of UTI.
**Urine culture:**   To determine the type of bacteria present in the genitourinary tract. To minimize the risk of contamination, a specimen should be obtained from a midstream collection.
**Urodynamic studies:**   To evaluate cause and extent of the incontinence.
*Uroflowmetry:*   Provides information about bladder strength and the opening ability of the urethral sphincter. The force of the urine stream is tested, using a specially designed commode.
*Cystometry:*   Measures the pressure-volume relationship of the bladder. The bladder is filled at a rate of 50 ml/min to its maximum capacity, and the bladder's ability to accommodate pressure changes is evaluated. In a normal individual, the bladder will fill smoothly without contractions and empty when the individual desires. The ability of the patient to detect bladder fullness also is noted.
*Urethral pressure profile:*   Most helpful in detecting stress incontinence, this

test identifies the amount of closing pressure the urethra can produce. For a description of this test, see "Urinary Incontinence," p. 159.

*Sphincter electromyography:*  Evaluates the function of the striated urinary sphincter. Results of this test are compared to the results from cystometry to identify abnormalities in coordination between the bladder and sphincter function.

**BUN and creatinine:**  Serum values increase as renal-urinary function declines. **Note:** These values can be affected by hydration status and age. Fluid volume deficit can falsely increase the values, while volume excess can decrease the values. Creatinine values may be misleading in the older adult because of the loss of muscle mass and decreased glomerular filtration rate.

**Intravenous pyelogram (IVP):**  Enables visualization of the kidneys, renal pelvis, ureters, and bladder to determine cause of the dysfunction.

**Postvoid residual:**  The patient is catheterized 15-20 min after voiding to assess for residual urine >100 ml.

**Cystoscopy:**  To determine loss of muscle fibers and elastic tissue.

## COLLABORATIVE MANAGEMENT

**Pharmacotherapy**

*Parasympatholytics or anticholinergics (e.g., propantheline bromide and oxybutynin chloride):*  To treat hyperreflexive neurologic conditions.

*Parasympathomimetics (e.g., bethanechol chloride):*  To treat hypotonic bladders by increasing bladder tone.

*Antibiotics:*  For infection, if indicated.

**Catheterization:**  Either intermittent or continuous.

**Increase fluid intake:**  To prevent infection, minimize calcium concentration in urine, and prevent formation of urinary calculi.

**Increase patient mobility:**  To augment renal blood flow and minimize urinary stasis.

**Low-calcium diet:**  To prevent calculus formation.

**Neuroprosthetics (bladder pacemaker):**  Electrodes are implanted on the ventral (motor) nerve roots of the sacral nerves that will produce detrusor contraction when stimulated. These electrodes are then connected to a subcutaneous receiver that can be controlled from outside the body. The bladder can be controlled selectively by the external transmitter.

**Continent vesicostomy:**  Surgical closure of urethral neck of the bladder to form an internal reservoir for urine and create an opening or valve in the bladder wall so that the patient can insert a catheter intermittently to remove urine.

**Artificial urinary sphincter implantation:**  Surgical placement of a hydraulically activated sphincter mechanism around the bladder neck or urethra. To empty the bladder, patient activates the device by squeezing the bulbs, which are implanted under the labia or scrotum.

## NURSING DIAGNOSES AND INTERVENTIONS

**Reflex incontinence** related to neurologic impairment secondary to injury or disease that affects the transmission of signals from the reflex arc to the cerebral cortex

*Desired outcomes:*  The patient or significant other participates in a habit training program. Patient experiences a decrease in or absence of incontinent episodes.

*Habit training program*

- Assess patient's voiding pattern: time, amount voided, amount of fluid intake, timing of fluid intake followed by voiding, and other related factors.
- Determine the amount of time between voidings to estimate the amount of time patient can hold urine. Establish a voiding schedule that does not exceed this period.
- Regulate fluids to achieve adequate hydration and a desirable voiding

pattern. For example, teach patient to drink measured amounts of fluids (e.g., 8 oz q2h) and attempt to void 30 min later, based on voiding schedule.

- Assist patient with scheduling times for emptying the bladder, such as q1-2h when awake and q4h at night. If successful, attempt to lengthen the time intervals between voidings. Provide patient and significant others with a written copy of the schedule.

*In addition*

- Monitor for bladder retention by assessing I&O, inspecting the suprapubic area, and percussing and palpating the bladder. Be alert to the presence of swelling proximal to the symphysis pubis, a "kettle drum" sound with percussion, and dribbling of urine.
- As appropriate, teach patient techniques that stimulate the voiding reflex. Examples include tapping the suprapubic area with the fingers, pulling the pubic hair, or digitally stretching the anal sphincter. The latter is effective because the rectal nerves follow basically the same path as the urethral nerves; however, this maneuver is contraindicated in patients with an SCI at or above T–6 because it can cause autonomic dysreflexia (AD, see next nursing diagnosis). Valsalva's maneuver also can be used to stimulate voiding: The patient bears down as though having a bowel movement to increase intrathoracic and intraabdominal pressure.
- If an artificial inflatable sphincter is used, instruct the patient to deflate the valve q4h, which allows the bladder to empty. Remind the patient to wear a Medic-Alert tag or bracelet to alert emergency personnel to the presence and use of the device.
- If a condom catheter is used, see **Knowledge deficit:** Use of external (condom) catheter in "Urinary Incontinence," p. 164, for appropriate nursing interventions.
- For males with extensive sphincter damage, a penile clamp might be prescribed. Before and after use, instruct patient (or significant other) to cleanse the penis with soap and water, dry it thoroughly, and sprinkle powder along the shaft. Explain that the clamp is placed horizontally behind the glans after voiding, and removed q3h. Stress the importance of inspecting the skin for redness along the area in which the clamp presses. If breakdown occurs (i.e., redness does not disappear after massage), the clamp must be discontinued. If swelling appears along the glans, advise patient to set the clamp at a looser setting. **Caution:** Minimize the potential for injury by alternating the penile clamp with a condom catheter.
- If intermittent catheterization is prescribed, teach the procedure to the patient or significant other. Emphasize the need to follow a routine (e.g., q4h) to minimize the potential for UTI caused by stasis and bladder distention.
- If Credé's method is prescribed, patients with arm and hand strength should be taught the procedure as an alternative to self-catheterization: Place the ulnar surface of the hand horizontally along the umbilicus; while bearing down with the abdominal muscles, press the hand downward and toward the bladder in a kneading motion until urination is initiated; continue q30sec until urination ceases.
- In nonrestricted individuals, encourage a fluid intake of at least 3 L/day, which dilutes the urine and increases output, thereby minimizing the risk of developing an infection and calculi.
- To help prevent urinary stasis, which can lead to UTI, and to increase cardiac output, which nourishes the kidneys, encourage as much mobility as the patient can tolerate.
- If diuretics are prescribed, administer them in the morning or early afternoon to reduce the risk of nighttime incontinence.
- If the patient has an intravenous infusion, consult with physician about advisability of reducing infusion rate at night to minimize the risk of nighttime incontinence.

- If the patient has a permanent cognitive impairment, use visual clues, such as a sign on the bathroom door that says *toilet* or a picture of a toilet.

**Dysreflexia (or risk for same)** related to distended bladder

*Desired outcomes:*   Patient is free of the indicators of AD as evidenced by HR $\geq$60 bpm, BP within patient's normal limits, skin dry and of normal color above the level of SCI (if appropriate), normal vision, and absence of headache, nausea, piloerection (goose bumps) below the level of injury (if appropriate), and nasal congestion. Patient/significant others verbalize understanding of the indicators, prevention, and treatment of AD.

---

**Note:**   Autonomic dysreflexia is a life-threatening condition that can occur in patients with neurogenic bladder, especially those with SCI at or above level T–8.

---

- Be alert to the following indicators of AD: headache, bradycardia, excessively high BP, blurred vision, flushing and sweating above the level of injury, piloerection and pallor below the level of injury, and nausea.
- If signs of AD occur, raise the HOB immediately to help lower the BP, and assess for bladder distention. Have the patient empty the bladder in the accustomed manner, or check for patency of the indwelling catheter. **Caution:** Irrigation of the urinary catheter can increase bladder pressure and intensify the AD. If the catheter is obstructed, either recatheterize the patient using liberal amounts of anesthetic jelly or irrigate the catheter gently, using $\leq$30 ml normal saline. Follow agency policy.
- Monitor patient's BP for trends. Be aware that continuing increases in BP can be life-threatening, leading to CVA, status epilepticus, and death.
- Administer appropriate medications as prescribed, such as phenoxybenzamine hydrochloride, a long-acting vasodilator that increases blood flow to the skin, mucosa, and abdominal viscera and lowers both supine and standing BP. Notify physician if symptoms do not disappear after the bladder is emptied, if the bladder is full and cannot be emptied, or if the medication does not relieve symptoms.
- Encourge a fluid intake of at least 3 L/day, which dilutes the urine and increases output, thereby minimizing the risk of developing an infection, calculi, and ultimately AD.
- To help prevent urinary stasis, which can lead to UTI and consequently to AD, encourage as much mobility as the patient can tolerate.
- Teach patient and significant others the indicators, prevention, and treatment of AD and the importance of seeking help immediately if indicators occur.
- For additional information about AD, see **Dysreflexia (or risk of same)** in "Spinal Cord Injury," p. 237.

**Total incontinence** related to neuropathy preventing transmission of reflex indicating bladder fullness or related to lower motor neuron disturbance secondary to SCI below S–3–S–4

*Desired outcomes:*   Patient or significant other follows habit training program; incontinent episodes decrease to less than 3 per week.

*Habit training program*

- Assess and document patient's voiding pattern: time, amount voided, amount of fluid intake, timing of fluid intake followed by voiding, and other related factors.
- Determine the amount of time between voidings to estimate how long the patient can hold urine. Establish a voiding schedule that does not exceed this time period.
- Assist patient with scheduling times for emptying the bladder, such as q1-2h when awake and q4h at night. If successful, attempt to lengthen the time intervals between voiding. Provide patient and significant other with a written copy of the schedule.

- If the patient takes fluids orally, provide the necessary amounts for optimal hydration (3 L/day) during the day and decrease the amount given during the evening and nighttime hours.
- Provide information about incontinence aids, such as incontinence pads and easy-to-remove clothing.
- For male patients, demonstrate use of external (condom) catheters for nighttime use (see p. 164).

*In addition*

- Administer diuretics in the morning or early afternoon to reduce the risk of nighttime incontinence.
- If the patient has an intravenous infusion, consult with physician about advisability of reducing the infusion rate at nighttime.

**Knowledge deficit:**   Function and care of long-term indwelling catheters after continent vesicostomy (continent urinary reservoir)

***Desired outcomes:***   Before continent vesicostomy, patient verbalizes rationale for the use of a suprapubic catheter and vesicostomy tube, including the approximate amount of time they will be indwelling. Within the 24-h period before hospital discharge, patient or significant other demonstrates proficiency with intermittent catheterization, tube irrigation, and dressing changes.

- Preoperatively, explain that the patient will return from surgery with a suprapubic catheter and vesicostomy tube in place.
- Explain that the patient will be discharged with the catheter and readmitted for catheter removal in approximately 6 weeks. After removal of the indwelling catheter, intermittent catheterization will be performed hourly, progressing to 2-4 h and ultimately to 4-6 h. Continuous drainage will be used overnight. After removing the indwelling catheter, ensure that the patient or significant other demonstrates proficiency with the following:
  - Washing hands with soap and water before catheterization.
  - Selecting a clean catheter and placing it on a clear paper towel.
  - Cleaning the stoma site with povidone-iodine solution and removing mucus that has drained from the stoma.
  - Inserting the catheter carefully into the stoma and draining the bladder of urine. Lubricants usually are not necessary. If lubrication is needed, however, teach patient to use one that is water soluble, *never* products made from petroleum jelly, which can damage the catheter.
  - If mucus clogs the catheter, removing the catheter from the stoma, rinsing it with hot water, and reinserting the catheter to continue the drainage.
- Encourage patient's participation in care, including tube irrigation, which removes mucus from the pouch, and dressing changes. Demonstrate the procedure for irrigation once it has been prescribed. Typically, sterile normal saline (30-50 ml) is used for irrigation. Instruct the patient to wash hands before handling the catheters to help prevent contamination and to cleanse around the catheter site daily with an antimicrobial solution, such as povidone-iodine.

---

**Note:**   As appropriate, see "Urinary Incontinence" for **High risk for impaired skin integrity,** p. 162, and **Body image disturbance,** p. 163.

---

## PATIENT-FAMILY TEACHING AND DISCHARGE PLANNING

Give patient and significant others verbal and written information about the following:

- For patients with artificial sphincters, the indicators of UTI and erosion: pain, fever, swelling, urinary retention, or incontinence.
- For more information, see this discussion in "Urinary Incontinence," p. 164.

# Section Seven:    Urinary Diversions

When the bladder must be bypassed or is removed, a urinary diversion is created. Urinary diversions most commonly are created for individuals with bladder cancer. However, malignancies of the prostate, urethra, vagina, uterus, or cervix may require the creation of a urinary diversion if anterior, posterior, or total pelvic exenteration must be done. Individuals with severe, nonmalignant urinary problems, such as radiation damage to the bladder, vesicovaginal fistula, urethrovaginal fistula, neurogenic bladder, radiation or interstitial cystitis, or urinary incontinence that cannot be managed conservatively, also are candidates for urinary diversion. A radical cystectomy may or may not accompany the placement of a urinary diversion. While most urinary diversions are permanent, some act as a temporary bypass of urine, and undiversion (reversal) can be performed if there is a change in the patient's condition.

The urinary stream may be diverted at multiple points: the renal pelvis (pyelostomy or nephrostomy); the ureter (ureterostomy); the bladder (vesicostomy); or *via* an intestinal "conduit." Cutaneous ureterostomy was the diversion most commonly performed in the past. Vesicostomies are most commonly performed in children as a temporary diversion. Construction of an intestinal (ileal) conduit is now the most common type of urinary diversion. Newer techniques allow reconstruction of a new bladder from intestinal segments, resulting in a more normal urinary pattern. In addition, because males have an external urinary sphincter that can be left in place when the bladder is removed, men may undergo attachment of a reconstructed bladder to the urethra, which will enable urination without the use of catheterization.

**Intestinal (ileal) conduit:**   Any segment of bowel may be used to create a passageway for urine, but the ileal conduit is the usual procedure. A 15-20 cm section of the ileum is resected from the intestine to form a passageway for the urine. The proximal end is closed, and the distal end is brought out through the abdomen, forming a stoma. The ureters are resected from the bladder and anastomosed to the ileal segment. The intestine is reanastomosed, and therefore bowel function is unaffected.

**Cutaneous ureterostomy:**   The ureters are resected from the bladder and brought out through the surface of the abdomen, either separately or with one attached to the other inside the body, resulting in only one abdominal stoma. Typically, the stoma is flush with the abdomen rather than protruding. Stenosis and ascending urinary tract infections (UTIs) are a common problem with this diversion.

**Continent urinary diversion:**   There are several different continent procedures, but the two that are most commonly performed are the Indiana reservoir and the Kock continent urostomy. All continent urinary diversions are constructed with the following three components: a reservoir or reconstructed bladder, a continence mechanism, and an antireflux mechanism. For example, the Indiana reservoir uses 15-18 cm of the distal ileum and 20-24 cm of the cecum sutured together to create the pouch, which stores eventually up to 800 ml of urine. The antireflux mechanism is established *via* use of the ileocecal valve, which acts as a one-way valve keeping urine in the reservoir until a catheter is passed through the skin-level stoma. The presence of a tapered ileal segment further strengthens the continence mechanism by creating increased resistance to urine outflow pressures. The ureters are attached at an angle to the wall of the cecum, preventing reflux of urine to the kidneys.

## NURSING DIAGNOSES AND INTERVENTIONS

**Anxiety** related to threat to self-concept, interaction patterns, or health status secondary to urinary diversion surgery

*Desired outcome:*   Before surgery, patient communicates fears and concerns, relates the attainment of increased psychologic and physical comfort, and exhibits effective coping mechanisms.

• Assess patient's perceptions of his or her impending surgery and resulting body function changes. Provide opportunities for patient to express fears and concerns (e.g., "You seem very concerned about next week's surgery"). Listen actively to the patient. Recognize that anger, denial, withdrawal, and demanding behaviors may be coping responses.

- Acknowledge patient's fears and concerns.
- Provide brief, basic information regarding physiology of the procedure and the equipment that will be used after surgery, including tubes and drains.
- Show patient pouches that will be used after surgery. Assure patient that the pouch usually cannot be seen through clothing and that it is odor-resistant.
- For patient about to undergo a continent urostomy, explain that a pouching system may be needed for a short time after surgery. Reassure patient that teaching about accessing the continent urostomy will be done before hospital discharge.
- Discuss ADL with patient. Inform patient that showers, baths, and swimming can continue and that diet is not affected after the early postoperative period.
- As appropriate, ask patient what information has been relayed by the surgeon about the sexual implications of the surgery. This will help establish an open relationship between the patient and primary nurse and inform the nurse if the patient has understood the information given by the surgeon. Some males undergoing radical cystectomy with urinary diversion may become impotent, but recent surgical advances have enabled preservation of potency for others. The pelvic plexus, which innervates the corpora cavernosa, will be damaged permanently. Autonomic nerve damage results in loss of erection and ejaculation; however, because sensation and orgasm are mediated by the pudendal nerve (sensorimotor), they are not affected.
- Arrange for a visit by the enterostomal therapy (ET) nurse during the preoperative period. Collaborate with the surgeon, ET nurse, and patient to identify and mark the most appropriate site for the stoma. Showing the patient the actual spot for placement may help alleviate anxiety by reinforcing that the impact on life-style and body image will be minimal.

**Altered protection** related to neurosensory, musculoskeletal, and cardiac changes secondary to hyperchloremic metabolic acidosis with hypokalemia (can occur secondary to reabsorption of $Na^+$ and $Cl^-$ from the urine in the ileal segment, which results in compensatory loss of $K^+$ and $HCO_3^-$)

***Desired outcome:*** Patient verbalizes orientation to person, place, and time (within patient's normal range) and remains free of injury caused by neurosensory, musculoskeletal, and cardiac changes.

- For patients with ileal conduits, assess for indicators of hypokalemia and metabolic acidosis, including nausea and changes in LOC (from sleepy to combative), muscle tone (convulsions to flaccidity), and irregular HR.
- If patient is confused or exhibits signs of motor dysfunction, keep the bed in the lowest position and raise the side rails. Notify physician of significant findings.
- Encourage oral intake as directed, and assess for the need for IV management. The physician may prescribe IV fluids with K supplements.
- If patient is hypokalemic and allowed to eat, encourage foods high in K, such as bananas, cantaloupes, and apricots. See Table 3-4 for other foods that are high in K.
- Encourage patient to ambulate by the second or third day after surgery. Mobility will help prevent urinary stasis, which increases the risk of electrolyte problems.

**High risk for impaired skin integrity** related to presence of urine or sensitivity to the appliance material

***Desired outcome:*** Patient's peristomal skin remains nonerythematous and intact.

- For patient with significant allergy history, patch-test the skin for a 24-h period, at least 24 h before ostomy surgery, to assess for allergies to the different tapes that might be used on the postoperative appliance. If erythema, swelling, itching, weeping, or other indicators of tape allergy occur, document the type of tape that caused the reaction and note on the cover of the chart "Allergic to _____tape."

• Inspect the integrity of the peristomal skin with each pouch change and question the patient about the presence of itching or burning, which can signal leakage. Change the pouch routinely (per agency or surgeon preference) or immediately if leakage is suspected.

• Assess for inflamed hair follicles (folliculitis) or a reaction to the tape. Report the presence of a rash to the physician since this often occurs with a yeast infection and will require topical medication.

• Assess the stoma, pouch, or skin for crystalline deposits, which are signals of alkaline urine.
   • Teach patient to monitor urine pH every week and to maintain pH below 6.0.
   • Teach patient to decrease urine pH by drinking acetic fluids such as cranberry or orange juice or taking ascorbic acid in a dose consistent with patient's size.
   • Teach patient signs of ascorbic acid toxicity: nausea, vomiting, heartburn, diarrhea, flushing, and insomnia.

• When changing the pouch, measure the stoma with a measuring guide and ensure that the opening of the skin barrier is cut to the exact size of the stoma to protect the peristomal skin. Protect the skin from maceration caused by pooling of urine on the skin:
   • *For a patient using a two-piece system or pouch with a barrier:* Size the barrier to fit snugly around the stoma. If using a barrier and attaching an adhesive pouch, size the barrier to fit snugly around the stoma and size the pouch to clear the stoma by at least ⅛ inch.
   • *For a patient using a one-piece "adhesive-only" pouch:* If the pouch has an antireflux valve, size the pouch to clear the stoma and any peristomal creases so that the pouch adheres to a flat, dry surface. An antireflux valve prevents pooling of urine on the skin. If the pouch does not have an antireflux valve, size the pouch so that it clears the stoma by ⅛ inch in order to prevent stomal trauma while minimizing the amount of exposed skin. Use a copolymer film sealant wipe on peristomal skin before applying adhesive-only pouch. This will provide a moisture barrier and reduce epidermal trauma when the pouch is removed.

• Wash the peristomal skin with water or a special cleansing solution marketed by ostomy supply companies. Dry the skin thoroughly before applying the skin barrier and pouch.

• When changing the pouch, instruct the patient to hold a gauze pad on (but not in) the stoma to absorb the urine and keep the skin dry.

• After applying the pouch, connect it to the bedside drainage system if the patient is on bed rest. When the patient is no longer on bed rest, empty the pouch when it is ⅓-½ full by opening the spigot at the bottom of the pouch and draining the urine into the patient's measuring container. Do not allow the pouch to become too full, because this could break the seal of the appliance with the patient's skin. Instruct the patient accordingly.

• Change the incisional dressing as often as it becomes wet, using sterile technique.

• Teach patient to treat peristomal skin irritation in the following ways after hospital discharge:
   • Dry the skin with a hair dryer on a cool setting.
   • Dust the peristomal skin with an absorptive powder (e.g., Karaya or Stomahesive).
   • If desired, blot the skin with water or a sealant wipe to "seal" in the powder.
   • Use a porous tape to prevent moisture trapping.

- Notify physician or ET nurse of any severe or nonresponsive skin problems.

**Impaired stomal tissue integrity (or risk of same)** related to altered circulation

*Desired outcomes:* Patient's stoma is pink or bright red and shiny. The stoma of a cutaneous urostomy is raised, moist, and red.

- Inspect the stoma at least q8h and as indicated. The stoma of an ileal conduit will be edematous and should be pink or red in color with a shiny appearance. A stoma that is dusky or cyanotic in color is indicative of insufficient blood supply and impending necrosis and must be reported to the physician immediately.
- Also assess the degree of swelling, and inform the patient that the stoma will shrink considerably over the first 6-8 weeks and less significantly over the next year. For patients with ileal conduit, evaluate stomal height and plan care accordingly (see **High risk for impaired skin integrity,** p. 173). The stoma formed by a cutaneous ureterostomy is usually raised during the first few weeks after surgery, red in color, and moist.

**Altered urinary elimination** related to postoperative use of ureteral stents, catheters, or drains and to urinary diversion surgery

*Desired outcome:* Patient's urinary output is ≥30 ml/h and the urine is clear, straw-colored, and with normal, characteristic odor.

- Monitor color, clarity, and volume of urine output *via* stoma, stents, and/or catheter.
  - *Ureterostomy:* Urine drainage *via* stoma and/or ureteral stents.
  - *Intestinal conduit:* Urine drainage *via* stoma. The patient also may have ureteral stents and/or conduit catheter/stent in the early postoperative period to stabilize the ureterointestinal anastomoses and maintain drainage from the conduit during early postoperative edema.
  - *Continent urinary diversions or reservoirs:* The Kock urostomy usually has a reservoir catheter and also may have ureteral stents. The Indiana (ileocecal) reservoir usually has ureteral stents exiting from the stoma through which most of the urine drains, and may have a reservoir catheter exiting from a stab wound, which serves as an overflow catheter. The continent urinary diversion with urethral anastomosis will have a urethral catheter in place that will drain urine, which initially will be light red to pink in color with mucus, but should clear in 24-48 h. This catheter will remain in place for 21 days to ensure adequate healing of the anastomosis.
- Monitor for evidence of anastomotic breakdown/intraabdominal urine leakage, which may occur in an individual with intestinal conduit or continent diversion: decreasing urinary output from stoma or stents, flank pain, increasing abdominal girth, and increasing drainage from Penrose drains.
- Monitor functioning of the ureteral stents, which protrude from the stoma under the pouch. These stents maintain the patency of the ureters and assist in the healing of the anastomosis. Right stents usually are cut at a 90-degree angle, while left stents are cut at a 45-degree angle. Each usually produces approximately the same amount of urine, although the amount produced by each is not important as long as each drains adequately and total drainage from all sources is ≥30 ml/h. Urine should be pink for the first 24-48 h and become straw-colored by the third postoperative day. Absent or lessening amounts of urine may indicate a blocked stent or problems with the ureter. **Note:** Stents may become blocked with mucus. As long as urine is draining adequately around the stent and the volume of output is adequate, this is not a problem.
- Monitor functioning of the stoma catheters. In continent urinary diversions, a catheter is placed in the reservoir to prevent distention and promote healing of the suture lines. This new reservoir exudes large amounts of mucus, necessitating irrigation of the catheter with 30-50 ml of normal saline, which is instilled gently and allowed to empty *via* gravity. Expect the output to

include pink or light red urine with mucus and small red clots for the first 24 h. Urine should become amber-colored with occasional clots in 3 post-operative days. Mucus production will continue but should decrease in volume.

- Monitor functioning of the drains. Any urinary diversion may have Penrose drains in place to maintain integrity of the ureterointestinal anastomosis. Excessive lymph fluid and urine can be removed *via* these drains without putting pressure on the suture lines. Drainage from the Penrose drain may be light red to pink in color for the first 24 h and then lighten to amber color and decrease in amount. In a continent urinary diversion, an increase in drainage after amounts have been low might signal reservoir leakage. Notify physician if this occurs.
- Monitor I&O, and record the total amount of urine output from the urinary diversion for the first 24 h postoperatively. Differentiate and record separately amounts from all drains, stents, and catheters. Notify physician of an output <60 ml during a 2-h period, because in the presence of adequate intake this can indicate a ureteral obstruction, a leak in the urinary diversion, or impending renal failure. Assess for other indicators of ureteral obstruction: flank pain, nausea, vomiting, and anuria.
- Monitor drainage from Foley catheter or urethral drain (if present). Patients who have had a cystectomy may have a urethral drain, while those with a cystectomy will have a Foley catheter in place. Note color, consistency, and volume of drainage, which may be red or pink with mucus. Report sudden increase (which would occur with hemorrhage) or decrease (which can signal blockage that can lead to infection). Report signficant findings to physician.
- Advise patient that after removal of urethral catheter or drain, mucus drainage will continue from the urethral meatus for several months.
- To keep the urinary tract well irrigated, encourage an intake of at least 2-3 L/day in the nonrestricted patient.

**High risk for infection** related to invasive surgical procedure and risk of ascending bacteriuria with urinary diversion

*Desired outcome:*   Patient is free of infection as evidenced by normothermia, WBC count ≤11,000 μl, and absence of purulent drainage, erythema, puffiness, warmth, and tenderness along the incision.

- Monitor the patient's temperature q4h during the first 24-48 h after surgery. Notify physician of fever spikes.
- Inspect the dressing frequently following surgery. Infection is most likely to become evident after the first 72 h. Assess for the presence of purulent drainage on the dressing, and notify physician accordingly. Change the dressing when it becomes wet, using sterile technique. Use extra care to prevent disruption of the drains.
- Note the condition of the incision. Be alert to indicators of infection, including erythema, tenderness, local warmth, puffiness, and purulent drainage.
- Monitor and record the character of the urine at least q8h. Mucus particles are normal in the urine of patients with ileal conduits and continent urinary diversions because of the nature of the bowel segment used. Cloudy urine, however, is abnormal and can signal an infection. The urine should be yellow or pink-tinged during the first 24-48 h after surgery. Assess for other indicators of UTI, including flank pain, chills, and fever.
- Note the position of the stoma relative to the incision. If they are close together, apply the pouch first to avoid the overlap of the pouch with the suture line, which can increase the risk of infection. If necessary, cut the pouch down on one side, or place it at an angle to avoid contact with drainage, which may loosen the adhesive. To help prevent contamination and cross-contamination, wash your hands before and after caring for the patient.

- Patients with cystectomies without anastomosis to the urethra may have an indwelling urethral catheter to drain serosanguineous fluid from the peritoneal cavity. **Caution:** Do not irrigate this catheter, because irrigation can result in peritonitis.
- Encourage a fluid intake of at least 2-3 L/day as this helps flush urine through the urinary tract, preventing stasis.

**High risk for fluid volume deficit** related to postsurgical bleeding/hemorrhage
***Desired outcomes:*** Patient is normovolemic as evidenced by balanced I&O; urinary output ≥30 ml/h; and BP, HR, and RR within patient's baseline range. Urine becomes amber- to straw-colored after 2-3 postoperative days.

- Monitor I&O, and note the amount and character of the urine output at least q4h. Initially the urinary output will be blood-tinged, but it should become clear within 2-3 days. The amount of urinary output should be normal (≥30 ml/h for 2 consecutive h).
- Be alert to the presence of gross hematuria, along with decreasing BP, tachycardia, and tachypnea, which can signal hemorrhage.
- Report significant findings to the physician.

**Knowledge deficit:**   Self-care regarding urinary diversion
***Desired outcome:***   Patient or significant other demonstrates proper care of stoma and urinary diversion before hospital discharge.

- Assess patient's or significant other's readiness to participate in care.
- Involve ET nurse in patient teaching if available.
- Assist patient with organizing the equipment and materials that are needed to accomplish home care. Usually the patient is discharged with disposable pouching systems. The majority of these patients remain in disposable systems for the long term. Those who will use reusable systems usually are not fitted for 6-8 weeks following surgery.
- Teach patient how to remove and reapply pouch, how to empty it, and how to use gravity drainage system at night, including procedures for rinsing and cleansing the drainage system.
- Teach patient the signs and symptoms of UTI, peristomal skin breakdown, and the appropriate therapeutic responses, including maintenance of an acidic urine (if not contraindicated), the importance of adequate fluid intake, and techniques for checking urine pH, which should be assessed weekly. Explain that urine pH should remain ≤6.0. Persons with urinary diversions have a higher incidence of UTIs than the general public, so it is important to keep their urinary pH acidic. If it is >6.0, advise patient to increase fluid intake and, with physician approval, to increase vitamin C intake to 500-1,000 mg/day, which will increase urine acidity.
- Teach patient with continent diversion the technique for reservoir catheter irrigation.
- Teach patient with continent urinary diversion with urethral anastomosis the signals of the urge to void: (1) feeling of vague abdominal discomfort and (2) feeling of abdominal pressure or cramping.
- Instruct patient with continent urinary diversion with urethral anastomosis about the procedure to void: relax the perineal muscles and employ Valsalva's maneuver.
- Emphasize the importance of follow-up visits, particularly for those patients with continent urinary diversions, who will be taught how to catheterize the reservoir and use a small dressing over the stoma rather than an appliance.
- Provide patient with a list of ostomy groups and ET nurses in the area for referral and assistance.
- Provide patient with enough equipment and materials for the first week following hospital discharge. Remind patient that proper cleansing of ostomy appliances will reduce the risk of bacterial growth and decrease the risk of UTI.

**Note:**  See "Fecal Diversions" for **Body image disturbance,** p. 437. See nursing diagnoses and interventions in Appendix One, "Caring for Preoperative and Postoperative Patients," p. 693, and "Caring for Patients with Cancer and Other Life-Disrupting Illnesses," p. 719.

## PATIENT-FAMILY TEACHING AND DISCHARGE PLANNING

Give patient and significant others verbal and written information about the following:

- Medications, including drug name, dosage, schedule, precautions, and potential side effects.
- Indicators that necessitate medical intervention: fever, chills, nausea, vomiting, abdominal pain and distention, cloudy urine, incisional pain or redness, peristomal skin irritation, or abnormal changes in stoma shape or color from the normal bright and shiny red.
- Community resources, including local United Ostomy Association, the American Cancer Society, and an ET nurse in the area, if appropriate.
- Maintenance of fluid intake at least 2-3 L/day to maintain adequate kidney function.
- Monitoring of urine pH, which should be checked weekly. Urine pH should remain at 6.0 or less. Individuals with urinary diversions have a higher incidence of UTIs than the general public, so it is important to keep their urinary pH acidic. If it is above 6.0, advise patient to increase fluid intake and, with physician approval, to increase vitamin C intake to 500-1,000 mg/day, which will increase urine acidity
- Care of stoma and application of urostomy appliances. The patient should be proficient in the application technique before hospital discharge.
- Care of urostomy appliances. Remind patient that proper cleansing will reduce the risk of bacterial growth, which would contaminate the urine and increase the risk of UTI.
- Importance of follow-up care with physician and ET. Confirm date and time of next appointment.

### Selected Bibliography

Aaberg RA, Flaherty R, Smith RB: Renal artery occlusive disease, *Crit Care Nurs Clin North Am* 3(3): 507-514, 1991.

Anderson J, Wilson J: Urolithiasis, *Topics in Emergency Medicine* 13(1): 47-54, 1991.

Baer CL: Acute renal failure: recognizing and reversing its deadly course, *Nursing 90* 20(6): 34-39, 1990.

Brenner BM, Rector FC, editors: *The kidney,* Philadelphia, 1991, WB Saunders Co.

Brettschneider N, Orihuela E: Carcinoma of the bladder, *Urol Nurs* 10(1): 14-21, 1990.

Bristol SL, et al: The mythical danger of rapid urinary drainage, *Am J Nurs* 89(3): 344-345,1989.

Carpenter CB, Lazarus JM: *Dialysis and transplantation in the treatment of renal failure.* In Wilson JD et al, editors: *Harrison's principles of internal medicine,* ed 12, New York, 1991, McGraw-Hill.

Cotton SL, Holechek MJ: Management of anemia using recombinant human erythropoietin in patients with chronic hemodialysis, *ANNA Journal* 16(7): 463-468, 1989.

Davidson M, et al: Continent Indiana reservoir: nursing management, *Ostomy/Wound Management* 31: 50-57, 1990.

Dodds P, Hans A: Distended urinary bladder drainage practices among hospital nurses, *Appl Nurs Res* 3(2): 66-72, 1990.

Eschbach JW, Adamson JW: Recombinant human erythropoietin: implications for nephrology, *Am J Kidney Dis* 11 (3): 203-209, 1988.

Feikles R: Long-term complications of renal transplantation, *J Urol Nurs* 10(1): 1086-1098, 1991.

Finn WF: Diagnosis and management of acute tubular necrosis, *Med Clin North Am* 74(4): 873-890, 1990.

Glenn J, editor: *Urologic surgery,* ed 4, Philadelphia, 1991, JB Lippincott Co.

Goodship TH, Mitch WE: Nutritional approaches to preserving renal function, *Adv Intern Med* 33: 337-356, 1988.

Harasyko C: Kidney transplantation, *Nurs Clin North Am* 24(4): 851-863, 1989.

Horne MM, Swearingen PL: *Pocket guide to fluid, electrolyte, and acid-base balance,* ed 2, St Louis, 1993, Mosby–Year Book.

Interqual: The ISD—A review system with adult ISD criteria, August 1992, Northhamptom, NH and Marlboro, MA, Interqual, Inc.

Jacobson HR, Striker GE, Klahr S: *The principles and practice of nephrology,* Philadelphia, 1991, BC Decker, Inc.

Kaschak-Newman D, et el: Restoring urinary continence, *Am J Nurs* 91(1): 28-36, 1991.

Kim MJ, McFarland GF, McLane AM: *Pocket guide to nursing diagnoses,* ed 5, St Louis, 1993, Mosby–Year Book.

Klein E: Option in surgical treatment of bladder cancer, *J Enterostomal Ther Nurs* 19(4): 122-125, 1992.

LaPorte J, Baum N: Kidney stones: how to identify the cause and prevent recurrence, *Postgrad Med* 87(5): 219-226, 1990.

Lederer JR et al: *Care planning pocket guide: a nursing diagnosis approach,* ed 5, Redwood City, Calif, 1993, Addison-Wesley.

Lewis DJ, Robinson JA, Robinson K: Spice of life: a strategy to enhance dietary compliance, *ANNA Journal* 17(5): 387-389, 401, 1990.

Lingaas L: Transplants: trials and triumphs, *UCSF Magazine* 13(3): 1-23, 1992.

Lonergan E: Aging and the kidney: adjusting treatment to physiologic change, *Geriatrics* 43(3): 27-33, 1988.

McNally J et al, editors: *Guidelines for oncology nursing practice,* Philadelphia, 1991, WB Saunders Co.

Pagana K, Pagana T: *Mosby's diagnostic and laboratory test reference,* St Louis, 1992, Mosby–Year Book.

Price CA: Continuous renal replacement therapy: the treatment of choice for acute renal failure, *ANNA J* 18(3): 263-267, 1991.

Rauscher J, Farber R, Parra R: Carney procedure: a continent urinary diversion technique, *AORN J* 54(1): 34-44, 1991.

Rose BD: *Pathophysiology of renal disease,* ed 3, New York, 1989, McGraw-Hill Book Co.

Rousseau P, Fuentevilla-Clifton A: Urinary incontinence in the aged, *Geriatrics* 47(6): 22-48, 1992.

Schlueter W, Battle DC: Chronic obstructive nephropathy, *Semin Nephrol* 8(1):17-28, 1988.

Smith-Young A, Whitehead E: Types, etiologies, diagnostics, and evaluation of urinary incontinence, *J Urol Nurs* 9(1): 781-791, 1990.

Swearingen PL: *Addison-Wesley photo-atlas of nursing procedures,* ed 2, Redwood City, Calif, 1991, Addison-Wesley.

Thielen JB: Air emboli: a potentially lethal complication of central venous lines, *Focus Crit Care* 17(5): 374-383, 1990.

Tootla J, Easterling A: Current options in bladder cancer management, *RN* 55(4):42-48, 1992.

Trusler LA: Simultaneous kidney-pancreas transplantation, *ANNA J* 18(5):487-491, 1991.

Ulrich BT, editor: *Nephrology nursing—concepts and strategies,* Norwalk Conn, 1989, Appleton & Lange.

US Department of Health and Human Services: *Urinary incontinence in adults: clinical practice guideline,* Public Health Service, Agency for Health Care Policy and Research, Rockville, Md, March 1992.

Voith A: Alterations in urinary elimination: concepts, research, and practice, *Rehabilitation Nurs* 13(3):122-131, 1988.

Walsh B: Urostomy and urinary pH, *J Enterostomal Ther Nurs* 19(4): 110-113, 1992.

Warkentin R: Implentation of a urinary continence program, *J Gerontol Nurs* 18(1): 31-37, 1992.

Weiskittel PD: *Renal-urinary dysfunctions.* In Swearingen PL, Keen JH, editors: *Manual of critical care: applying nursing diagnoses to adult critical illness,* ed 2, St Louis, 1991, Mosby–Year Book.

# 4 NEUROLOGIC DISORDERS

Section One   Inflammatory Disorders of the Nervous System   181
   Multiple sclerosis   182
   Guillain-Barré syndrome   188
   Bacterial meningitis   194
   Encephalitis   199
Section Two   Degenerative Disorders of the Nervous System   202
   Parkinsonism   203
   Alzheimer's disease   213
Section Three   Traumatic Disorders of the Nervous System   224
   Intervertebral disk disease   224
   Spinal cord injury   232
   Head injury   247
Section Four   Nervous System Tumors   258
   Brain tumors   258
   Spinal cord tumors   266
Section Five   Vascular Disorders of the Nervous System   269
   Cerebral aneurysm   269
   Cerebrovascular accident   276
Section Six   Seizure Disorders   288
Section Seven   General Care of Patients with Neurologic Disorders   298
Selected Bibliography   316

# Section One:   Inflammatory Disorders of the Nervous System

Inflammation of nervous system tissue results from a wide variety of causes, including bacterial or viral infections, autoimmune processes, or chemical toxins. The inflammatory response may cause increased vascular permeability with exudation of fluids from the vessels, resulting in swelling. Inflammation involving the myelin nerve sheath can cause the destruction or stripping away of the myelin. The resulting demyelinization interferes with the conduction of electric nerve impulses. Inflammation of other brain tissue, such as may occur in acute infectious processes, usually results in swelling, which in turn can cause increased intracranial pressure (IICP) and the potential for brain herniation.

# Multiple sclerosis

Multiple sclerosis (MS) is an inflammatory disorder causing scattered and sporadic demyelinization of the central nervous system (CNS). Myelin permits nerve impulses to travel quickly through the nerve pathways of the CNS. In response to the inflammation the myelin nerve sheaths peel off the axon cylinders. This demyelinization interrupts electrical nerve transmission and causes the wide variety of symptoms associated with MS. If the myelin regenerates, electric nerve impulse transmission may be restored. If the inflammation is severe and causes irreversible destruction of myelin, the involved areas are replaced by dense glial scar tissue that forms areas of sclerotic plaque, which may permanently damage the conductive pathways of the CNS. Nerve fibers also may degenerate. Deficits present after 3 months usually are permanent.

The MS disease course is highly variable, with several general categories of progression. Motor or coordination symptoms from onset and/or frequent attacks during the first 2 years of the disease usually indicate a poorer outlook. In the *benign* form of MS (20% of patients), attacks are few and mild. Complete or nearly complete clearing of symptoms occurs with little or no disability. In the *exacerbating-remitting* form (25%), attacks (exacerbations) occur early on in the illness and become increasingly frequent. Less complete clearing of symptoms occurs, and there may be relatively long periods of stability (remission). The *chronic-relapsing* form (40%) has fewer remissions, and symptom resolution is less complete after an exacerbation. An increasing number of symptoms occurs with each exacerbation, and they become cumulative. In the *chronic-progressive* form (15%), onset usually is insidious and without remissions. A slow, progressive accumulation of symptoms and deficits occurs.

Although the cause of MS is unknown, autoimmune processes, slow-acting viral infections, and allergic reactions to infectious agents, such as viruses, are suspected causes. MS is more common among people living in cool, temperate climates. It is 12-15 times more common among siblings of individuals who have the disease, suggesting a possible inheritance mechanism. Infection and trauma are common precipitating factors, as are episodes of fatigue and physical or emotional stress. Exacerbations may be fewer during pregnancy but increase immediately postpartum. Heat and fever tend to aggravate symptoms.

## ASSESSMENT

Onset of MS can be extremely rapid, causing disability within days, or it can be insidious, with exacerbations and remissions. Signs and symptoms vary widely, depending on the site and extent of demyelinization, and they can change from day to day. Usually, early symptoms are mild.

**Damage to motor nerve tracts:**   Weakness, paralysis, and spasticity. Fatigue is common. Diplopia may occur secondary to ocular muscle involvement.

**Damage to cerebellar or brain stem regions:**   Intention tremor, nystagmus, or other tremors; incoordination, ataxia; weakness of facial and throat muscles resulting in difficulty chewing, dysphagia, and dysarthria. Slurred speech often occurs early, while "scanning speech" (slow speech with pauses between syllables) is usually seen in later stages.

**Damage to sensory nerve tracts:**   Decreased perception of pain, touch, and temperature; paresthesias, such as numbness and tingling; decrease or loss of proprioception; and decrease or loss of vibratory sense. Optic neuritis is an early common symptom, which may cause partial or total loss of vision, visual clouding, and pain with eye movement.

**Damage to cerebral cortex (especially frontal lobes):**   Mood swings, inappropriate affect, euphoria, apathy, irritability, depression, and hyperexcitability.

**Damage to motor and sensory control centers:**  Urinary frequency, urgency, or retention; urinary and fecal incontinence; constipation.

**Sacral cord lesions:**  Impotence; diminished sensations that result in inhibited sexual response.

**Physical assessment:**  Ophthalmoscopic inspection may reveal temporal pallor of optic disks. Reflex assessment may show increased deep tendon reflexes (DTRs) and diminished abdominal skin and cremasteric reflexes.

## DIAGNOSTIC TESTS

**Note:** MS is sometimes called the "great masquerader." Diagnostic testing is often done to exclude disorders with similar symptoms. The diagnosis of MS usually will be made after other neurologic disorders have been ruled out, when the patient has experienced two or more exacerbations of neurologic symptoms, and when the patient has two or more areas of demyelinization or plaque formation throughout the CNS, as demonstrated by diagnostic tests, such as the MRI and evoked potential studies, or by the patient's clinical symptoms.

**Magnetic resonance imaging (MRI):**  To reveal presence of plaques and demyelinization in the CNS. This is the test of choice when MS is suspected.

**Evoked potential studies:**  May be slow or absent due to interference of nerve transmission from demyelinization or plaque formation. Stimulation of a sensory organ, such as the eye or ear, or of a peripheral nerve triggers a measurable electrical response (evoked potential) along the visual, auditory, and somatosensory nerve pathways. Measuring these evoked potentials enables evaluation of the integrity of these nerve pathways.

**Lumber puncture (LP) and cerebrospinal fluid (CSF) analysis:**  To evaluate CSF levels of oligoclonal bands of immunoglobulin G (IgG), protein, gamma globulin, myelin basic protein, and lymphocytes, any of which may be elevated in the presence of MS. Increased gamma globulin levels indicate hyperactivity of the immune system due to chronic demyelinization. Oligoclonal bands of IgG are seen in 85%-95% of patients with MS. Although these bands can be elevated in some other inflammatory diseases, they help confirm the diagnosis of MS. Detecting oligoclonal bands of IgG requires examination of the CSF gamma globulin by electrophoresis. During acute MS attacks, destruction of the myelin sheath will release myelin basic protein into the CSF. Lymphocytes also increase during acute demyelinization.

**Computerized axial tomography (CT) scan:**  To demonstrate presence of plaques and rule out mass lesions. This scan is less effective than MRI in detecting areas of plaque and demyelinization.

**EEG:**  Shows abnormal slowing in one-third of patients with MS due to altered nerve conduction.

**Positron emission tomography (PET):**  May show altered locations and patterns of cerebral glucose metabolism.

---

**Note:**  See **Knowledge deficit:** Neurologic diagnostic tests, p. 311, in "General Care of Patients with Neurologic Disorders" for care considerations for patients undergoing MRI, evoked potential studies, LP, CT scan, EEG, and PET.

---

## COLLABORATIVE MANAGEMENT

Generally, treatment is symptomatic and supportive. Various treatments are under investigation, but no treatment currently is available that has demonstrated an ability to alter the overall disease course. Adrenocorticotropic hormone (ACTH) is the only drug that has been shown to hasten recovery from acute exacerbations, but there is no evidence that it improves the degree of recovery.

**Bed rest:**  During acute exacerbation.

**Pharmacotherapy**

*Steroidal antiinflammatory agents (e.g., ACTH, prednisone, and dexamethazone):*   May be prescribed during an exacerbation in an attempt to reduce symptoms by decreasing inflammation and associated edema of the myelin, thereby hastening onset of remission. Dosage regimens usually include initial high-dose therapy with tapering over a month's time. Antacids, histamine $H_2$-receptor blockers, potassium (K) supplements, diuretics, blood pressure medications, and psychotropic agents may be given to counter the steroidal side effects.

*Antispasmodics and muscle relaxants (e.g., baclofen or dantrolene sodium):*   May be given to decrease spasticity.

*Smooth muscle relaxants (e.g., propantheline bromide):*   To decrease urinary frequency and urgency.

*Smooth muscle stimulants (e.g., bethanechol chloride):*   May be given to help prevent urinary retention.

*Stool softeners (e.g., docusate), laxatives (e.g., bisacodyl), and suppositories:*   To maintain a bowel program that prevents fecal impaction and minimizes incontinence.

*Antidepressants (e.g., amitriptyline):*   May benefit depression related to cerebral lesions.

*Tranquilizers (e.g., diazepam):*   May be given for both its anxiety-reducing and muscle relaxant effects, which may help spasms and tremors.

*Amantadine:*   Has been effective in relieving fatigue associated with MS (see "Parkinsonism," p. 206, for side effects/patient teaching).

*Propranolol:*   To decrease tremors, but is not always effective. *Isoniazid* is under investigation for treatment of tremors, but it may cause liver toxicity at levels necessary for control.

*Carbamazepine:*   Used to help control some types of neuritic pain (see "Seizure Disorders," p. 297, for side effects and patient teaching).

**Physical medicine:**   Physical therapy (PT), occupational therapy (OT), and assistive devices or braces may be prescribed so that patient can maintain mobility and independence with ADL. Muscle-strengthening and conditioning exercises and gait training (to develop alternative muscle groups not yet weakened by demyelination) as well as stretching exercises are also frequently indicated. Weighting the affected limbs may help with mild tremors.

**ROM exercises:**   To maintain or increase joint function and prevent contractures.

**Bowel and bladder program:**   To prevent incontinence, constipation, and urinary retention. This program may include bowel and bladder training, intermittent catheterization, and external drainage appliances.

**Speech therapy:**   To improve speech deficits using accessory respiratory muscles and tongue and facial muscles.

**Counseling or psychotherapy:**   To help patient and significant others adapt to the disability and deal with emotions and feelings that are either a direct or indirect result of the disease process. Sexual counseling also should be included.

**Treatment of complications:**   Complications, such as respiratory or urinary tract infection (UTI), may require treatment with antibiotics or other measures.

**Surgical interventions:**   To treat complications, such as contractures, spasticity, decreased mobility, and pain. Intrathecal phenol may give 3-12 months of relief from spasms refractory to drug treatment, but it produces a flaccid paralysis with sensory loss and possibly bladder and bowel dysfunction. Other interventions may include peripheral nerve block with phenol, tendotomy, myotomy, peripheral neurectomy, rhizotomy, or stereotaxic thalamotomy. A penile prosthesis may be performed for men whose impotence occurs secondary to MS.

**Controversial therapies**

*Immunosuppressive drug therapy:* Agents such as cyclophosphamide (Cytoxan, see p. 723) and azathioprine (Imuran, see p. 140) may slow and stabilize chronic progressive MS.

*Total lymphoid irradiation:* To suppress the body's immune system and slow down chronic progressive MS by reducing the immunoinflammatory response that leads to demyelinization of the nerve sheaths. For more information about radiation therapy, see Appendix One, "Caring for Patients with Cancer and Other Life-Disrupting Illnesses," p. 735.

*Interferon drug therapy:* Appears to reduce the exacerbation rate and stabilize the patient's overall clinical status. The mechanism of beneficial effect is unknown but probably related to the drug's ability to enhance the body's immune system rather than its antiviral action (see p. 731 for more information).

*Copolymer I (a random polymer-stimulating myelin basic protein):* Appears to decrease the number of exacerbations in patients with exacerbating-remitting MS.

*Plasmapheresis:* To reduce the patient's antibodies to CNS tissue by removing the plasma portion of the blood, which contains circulating antibodies. This therapy usually involves several exchanges that provide short-term improvement only.

## NURSING DIAGNOSES AND INTERVENTIONS

**Knowledge deficit:** Factors that aggravate and exacerbate MS symptoms

*Desired outcome:* By day 3 (or before hospital discharge), patient and significant others verbalize knowledge about factors that exacerbate, prevent, or ameliorate symptoms of MS.

- Inform patient and significant others that heat, both external (hot weather, bath) and internal (fever), tends to aggravate weakness and other symptoms of MS.
- Teach preventive measures, such as avoiding hot baths and using acetaminophen or aspirin to reduce fever, if present.
- Because infection often precedes exacerbations, caution patient to avoid exposure to persons known to have infections of any kind.
- Teach the indicators of common infections (see "Care of the Renal Transplant Recipient," p. 141, and Table 5-4, p. 360) and the importance of seeking prompt medical treatment should they occur. For example, the MS patient is susceptible to UTI because of urinary retention. Because of the disease process, the patient may not feel any pain with urination. Teach the patient to monitor for increased frequency, urgency, or incontinence and to check the urine for changes in odor or the presence of cloudiness or blood. Instruct patients to check body temperature periodically for fever. Signals that a UTI has reached the kidneys include chills and flank pain.
- Teach patient the relationship between stress and fatigue to the exacerbations. Encourage patients to get sufficient rest, stop activity short of fatigue, schedule activity and rest periods, and reduce factors that cause stress in their lives. See "Coronary Artery Disease" for **Health-seeking behaviors:** Relaxation technique effective for stress reduction, p. 54.
- As appropriate, explain to the patient that there may be an increase in exacerbations postpartum. Provide information about birth control measures to female patients who desire counseling.
- As appropriate, reassure patient and significant others that most persons with MS do not become severely disabled. Encourage continued activity and normal life-style even when limitations are necessary.

**Knowledge deficit:** Precautions and potential side effects of prescribed medications

*Desired outcome:* By day 3 (or before hospital discharge), patient verbalizes accurate information about the prescribed medications.

- Provide patient with verbal instructions and written handouts that describe the name, purpose, dose, and schedule of the prescribed medications.
- For patients taking ACTH, prednisone, or dexamethasone, provide additional instructions for the following:
  - Common side effects: sodium (Na) and fluid retention, hypertension, gastric ulcers, stomach upset, weakness, hypokalemia, mood changes, impaired wound healing, and masking of infections.
  - Importance of monitoring weight and BP for evidence of fluid retention; taking the medication with food, milk, or buffering agents to help prevent gastric irritation; avoiding aspirin, indomethacin, caffeine, or other gastrointestinal (GI) irritants while taking this medication; and tapering rather than abruptly stopping the drug when it is discontinued. Advise patient to report symptoms of K deficiency, such as anorexia, nausea, and muscle weakness, and to eat foods high in K (see Table 3-4). Encourage a diet low in Na content (see Table 3-2) to minimize the potential for fluid retention. Monitor for and report black, tarry stools, which may signal occult blood. Physician follow-up is important while the patient is taking these drugs.
- If the patient is taking baclofen or dantrolene, provide instructions for the following:
  - Common side effects: drowsiness, dizziness, fatigue, and nausea. In addition, dantrolene can cause diarrhea, muscle weakness, hepatitis, and photosensitivity.
  - Importance of taking the medication with food, milk, or a buffering agent to reduce gastric upset or nausea. Explain that although drowsiness is usually transient, patient should avoid activities that require alertness until their effect on the CNS is known. The patient also should avoid alcohol intake because of its additive CNS depression effects. Baclofen can lower a person's seizure threshold and should be used cautiously in susceptible patients. Baclofen also may raise blood glucose levels, and individuals with diabetes mellitus may need an insulin dose adjustment. Monitor patients during transfers/ambulation initially because some weak patients cannot tolerate the loss in spasticity that may be permitting them to bear weight. Patients on dantrolene should monitor for and report occurrence of fever, jaundice, dark urine, clay-colored stools, and itching (all of which signal hepatitis) or severe diarrhea; avoid exposure to the sun; and use sunscreens if exposure is unavoidable.
- If bethanechol chloride has been prescribed, provide instructions for the following:
  - Common side effects: hypotension, diarrhea, abdominal cramps, urinary urgency, and bronchoconstriction.
  - Importance of taking the drug on an empty stomach to avoid nausea and vomiting; notifying physician if lightheadedness occurs because this can signal hypotension; and seeking medical attention if an asthmatic attack occurs. Caution patient to make position changes slowly and in stages to prevent fainting caused by orthostatic hypotension.
- If the patient is taking propantheline bromide, provide instructions for the following:
  - Common side effects: dryness of the mouth, blurred vision, constipation, palpitations, tachycardia, decreased sweating, and urinary retention or overflow incontinence.
  - Measures that relieve constipation; measures for remaining cool in hot or humid weather because heat stroke is more likely to develop while on the medication; importance of notifying physician immediately if urinary retention or overflow incontinence occurs. In addition, if the patient can chew and swallow effectively, explain that sugarless gum, hard candy, or

artificial saliva products may reduce mouth dryness. Encourage slow position changes and monitoring for dizziness because postural hypotension may occur when the drug is first started.

**Chronic pain** and spasms related to motor and sensory nerve tract damage

*Desired outcomes:* Within 1-2 h of intervention, patient's subjective evaluation of pain and spasms improves, as documented by a pain scale. Objective indicators, such as grimacing, are absent or reduced.

- Because heat tends to aggravate MS symptoms, maintain a comfortable room temperature. Advise patient to keep environment cool in warm weather and avoid hot baths.
- To reduce muscle tightness and spasms, provide passive, assisted, or active ROM q2h and periodic stretching exercises. Teach these exercises to patient and significant others and encourage their performance several times daily. Explain that sleeping in a prone position may help decrease flexor-spasms of the hips and knees.
- Administer antispasmodics as prescribed.
- For other interventions, see **Pain,** p. 308, in "General Care of Patients with Neurologic Disorders."

---

**Note:** For patients undergoing plasmapheresis see "Guillain-Barré Syndrome" for **Knowledge deficit:** Therapeutic plasma exchange procedure, p. 192. See "Spinal Cord Injury" for **Constipation,** p. 238, **High risk for disuse syndrome,** p. 240, **Urinary retention** *or* **Reflex incontinence,** p. 242, and **Sexual dysfunction,** p. 245. See "General Care of Patients with Neurologic Disorders" for **High risk for trauma** related to unsteady gait, p. 298, **High risk for injury** related to impaired pain, touch, and temperature sensations, p. 299, **Impaired corneal tissue integrity,** p. 300, **Altered nutrition:** Less than body requirements, p. 300, **High risk for fluid volume deficit** related to decreased intake, p. 301, **High risk for aspiration,** p. 302, **Self-care deficit,** p. 302, **Impaired verbal communication,** p. 304, **Constipation,** p. 305., **Sensory/perceptual alterations** (visual), p. 307, **Impaired swallowing,** p. 308, and **Knowledge deficit:** Neurologic diagnostic tests (for discussions of EEG, MRI, CT scan, evoked potential studies, PET, and LP), p. 311. For patients with impaired nutrition, see "Providing Nutritional Support," p. 665. For patients who are immobile, see related nursing diagnoses in "Pressure Ulcers," p. 687, and Appendix One, "Caring for Patients on Prolonged Bed Rest," p. 711. Also see Appendix One, "Caring for Patients with Cancer and Other Life-Disrupting Illnesses" for patients undergoing immunosuppressive drug or radiation therapy, p. 719, and for related psychosocial nursing diagnoses, p. 753, as appropriate.

---

## PATIENT-FAMILY TEACHING AND DISCHARGE PLANNING

The patient with MS may have a wide variety of symptoms that cause disability, ranging from mild to severe. Give patient and significant others verbal and written information about the following, as appropriate:

- Remission/exacerbation aspects of the disease process. Explain the effects of demyelinization on sensory and motor function and factors that aggravate symptoms.
- Referrals to community resources, such as local and national MS society chapters, public health nurse, visiting nurse association, community support groups, social workers, psychological therapists, vocational rehabilitation agencies, home health agencies, extended and skilled care facilities, and financial counseling. The National Multiple Sclerosis Society can be reached at 205 East 42nd Street, New York, NY 10017, (800)-624-8236.
- Safety measures relative to decreased sensation, visual disturbances, and motor deficits.

- Medications, including drug name, purpose, dosage, frequency, precautions, and potential side effects.
- Exercises that promote muscle strength and mobility; measures for preventing contractures and skin breakdown; transfer techniques and proper body mechanics; use of assistive devices and other measures to minimize neurologic deficits.
- Measures for relieving pain, muscle spasms, or other discomfort.
- Indications of constipation, urinary retention, or UTI; implementation of bowel and bladder training programs; self-catheterization technique or care of indwelling urinary catheters.
- Indications of upper respiratory infection; implementation of measures that help prevent regurgitation, aspiration, and respiratory infection.
- Dietary adjustments that may be appropriate for neurologic deficit (e.g., soft, semisolid foods for patients with chewing difficulties or a high-fiber diet for patients experiencing constipation).
- Importance of follow-up care, including visits to physician, PT, and OT, as well as speech, sexual, or psychological counseling.

# Guillain-Barré syndrome

Guillain-Barré syndrome (G-BS) is a rapidly progressing polyneuritis of unknown cause. An inflammatory process causes lymphocytes to enter the perivascular spaces and destroy the myelin sheath covering the peripheral or cranial nerves. Posterior (sensory) and anterior (motor) nerve roots can be affected because of this segmental demyelinization, and the individual may experience both sensory and motor losses. Respiratory insufficiency may occur in as many as half the individuals affected. Life-threatening respiratory muscle weakness can develop as rapidly as 24-72 h after onset of initial symptoms. In about 25% of cases, motor weakness progresses to total paralysis.

Peak severity of symptoms usually occurs within 1-3 weeks after onset of symptoms. There follows a plateau stage that usually lasts 1-2 weeks. Remyelinization with return of function then occurs, but it may take months to years for a full recovery. Full neurologic recovery occurs in about 50% of patients. Residual neurologic deficits tend to be mild motor or reflex alterations in the feet or legs and are the result of axonal nerve degeneration.

G-BS may follow a recent viral illness, such as upper respiratory infection or gastroenteritis, a rabies or flu vaccination, lupus erythematosus, or Hodgkin's disease or other malignant process. While the exact cause of G-BS is unknown, it is believed to be an autoimmune response to a viral infection.

## ASSESSMENT

Weakness is the most common indicator. Typically, numbness and weakness begin in the legs and ascend symmetrically upward, progressing to the arms and facial nerves. Peak severity usually occurs within 10-14 days of onset. G-BS does not affect LOC, cognitive function, or pupillary function.

**Anterior (motor) nerve root involvement:**   Weakness or flaccid paralysis. Weakness or paralysis of respiratory muscles can be life-threatening. There is a loss of reflexes, muscle tension, and tone, but muscle atrophy usually does not occur.

**Autonomic nervous system involvement:**   Sinus tachycardia, bradycardia, hypertension, hypotension, cardiac dysrhythmias, facial flushing, diaphoresis, inability to perspire, loss of sphincter control, urinary retention, adynamic ileus, and increased pulmonary secretions may occur. Autonomic nervous system involvement may occur unexpectedly and can be life-threatening. Autonomic disturbances usually do not persist for longer than 2 weeks.

**Cranial nerve involvement:**   Inability to chew, swallow, speak, or close the eyes.

**Posterior (sensory) nerve root involvement:** Paresthesias, such as numbness and tingling, which usually are minor compared to the degree of motor loss. Ascending sensory loss often precedes motor loss. The patient may experience muscle cramping, tenderness, or pain that may become severe.

**Physical assessment:** Symmetrical motor weakness, impaired position and vibration sense, hypoactive or absent deep tendon reflexes, hypotonia in affected muscles, and decreased ventilatory capacity.

## DIAGNOSTIC TESTS

Diagnostic tests are performed to rule out other diseases, such as acute poliomyelitis. The diagnosis of G-BS is based on clinical presentation, history of recent viral illness, and CSF findings.

**Lumbar puncture (LP) and CSF analysis:** Usually show an elevated protein (especially IgG) without an increase in cell count. Although CSF pressure usually is normal, in severe disease it may be elevated.

**EMG (electromyography):** Reveals slowed nerve conduction velocities soon after paralysis appears. Findings occur due to segmental demyelinization. Denervation potentials appear later.

**Serum CBC:** Will show presence of leukocytosis early in illness, possibly due to the inflammatory process associated with demyelinization.

**Evoked potentials (auditory, visual, and brain stem):** May be used to distinguish G-BS from other neuropathologies.

---

**Note:** See "General Care of Patients with Neurologic Disorders" for **Knowledge deficit:** Neurologic diagnostic tests, p. 311, for care considerations for patients undergoing LP, EMG, and evoked potential studies.

---

## COLLABORATIVE MANAGEMENT

The patient is likely to be in ICU when the neurologic deficit is progressing and is at risk for respiratory failure and autonomic dysfunction.

**Respiratory support:** Serial vital capacity measurements and ABG analysis to monitor for respiratory muscle weakness or paralysis. Endotracheal tube, tracheostomy, or mechanical ventilation are used as necessary, generally when vital capacity falls below a preset level.

**Pharmacotherapy**

*Glucocorticosteroids (e.g., prednisone, adrenocorticotropic hormone [ACTH]):* May include a 1-week trial to determine whether symptoms decrease. In the absence of marked improvement, it is discontinued.

*Analgesia (e.g., acetaminophen, codeine, morphine):* For muscle pain. Other medications that may be tried to relieve uncomfortable paresthesias include perphenazine, phenytoin, carbamazepine, or amitriptyline.

*Stool softeners (e.g., docusate), laxatives (e.g., bisacodyl), and suppositories:* To maintain a bowel program that prevents fecal impaction and minimizes incontinence.

**Exercise and activity:** Activity other than bed rest and passive ROM is restricted during the acute phase. After the patient stabilizes, active ROM or active assistive ROM is implemented, and a physical therapy (PT) and rehabilitation program is initiated. Occupational therapy (OT) and assistive devices or braces are employed so that patient can maintain mobility and independence with ADL. Muscle-strengthening exercises, conditioning exercises, and gait training also are frequently prescribed.

**Antiembolism hose:** To prevent thrombophlebitis in the legs.

**Nutritional support:** A high-fiber diet may be prescribed to help prevent constipation. If the patient cannot chew or swallow effectively because of cranial nerve involvement, gastric, gastrostomy, or parenteral feedings may be initiated. The patient is advanced to a solid diet upon return of the gag reflex and swallowing ability.

**Management of bowel and bladder dysfunction:**   A regular bowel program should be started to prevent fecal impaction. Indwelling urinary catheters, intermittent catheterizations, or external urinary collection devices may be needed until strength and mobility return.

**Management of acute autonomic dysfunction:**   Short-acting antihypertensive agents for hypertension; intravascular volume expanders or vasopressors for hypotension; cardiac monitoring of dysrhythmias; gastric suction, nutrition, and parenteral fluids for adynamic ileus; and catheterization and medications for urinary retention. Phenoxybenzamine may be used to help with paroxysmal hypertension, headache, sweating, anxiety, and fever. Diabetes insipidus (see p. 343) and syndrome of inappropriate antidiuretic hormone (SIADH, see p. 351) have been reported, so urine output, state of hydration, and serum and urine electrolytes should be monitored.

**Plasmapheresis:**   To reduce the patient's antibodies to peripheral and cranial nerve tissue by removing the plasma portion of the blood, which contains the circulating antibodies. If performed within 7-14 days of the onset of symptoms, removal of these autoantibodies appears to lessen the duration and severity of the disease.

**Treatment of complications:**   For example, antibiotic therapy for aspiration pneumonia or anticoagulant therapy for deep vein thrombosis (DVT) or emboli.

**Controversial therapies:**   Immunosuppressive drug therapy with agents such as cyclophosphamide (Cytoxan) (see p. 723) and azathioprine (Imuran) (see p. 140) may slow and stabilize disease progression, probably by suppressing the immunoinflammatory response that leads to demyelinization of the peripheral nerve sheath. High IV-dose gamma globulin also is being tried in severe cases to affect antibody response.

## NURSING DIAGNOSES AND INTERVENTIONS

**Ineffective breathing pattern** related to neuromuscular weakness or paralysis of the facial, throat, and respiratory muscles (severity of symptoms peaks around week 1-3)

*Desired outcome:*   Deterioration in patient's breathing pattern (e.g., $Pao_2$ <80 mm Hg, vital capacity <1 L [or <12-15 ml/kg], and tidal volume <75% of predicted value) is detected and reported promptly, resulting in immediate and effective medical treatment.

- Test for ascending loss of sensation by touching patient lightly with a pin or fingers at frequent intervals (hourly or more frequently initially). Assess from the level of the iliac crest upward toward the shoulders. Measure the highest level at which decreased sensation occurs. Decreased sensation frequently precedes motor weakness, so if it ascends to the level of the T-8 dermatome, anticipate that intercostal muscles (used with respirations) soon will be impaired. Also monitor for upper arm and shoulder weakness, which precedes respiratory failure, by checking patient for the presence of arm drift and the ability to shrug the shoulders. Arm drift is detected in the following way: Have the patient hold both arms out in front of the body, level with the shoulders and with the palms up. Instruct patient to close the eyes while holding this position. Weakness is present if one arm pronates or drifts down or out from its original position. Alert physician to significant findings.

- Assist patient with oral intake to detect changes or difficulties that may indicate ascending paralysis. Assess patient q8h and before oral intake for cough reflexes, gag reflexes, and difficulty swallowing.

- Observe patient for changes in LOC and orientation, which may signal reduced oxygenation to the brain. Monitor patient's respiratory rate, rhythm, and depth. Watch for accessory muscle use, nasal flaring, dyspnea, shallow respirations, apnea, and loss of abdominal breathing. Auscultate for diminished breath sounds. Monitor patient for breathlessness while speaking. To observe for breathlessness, ask patient to take a deep breath and slowly count as high as possible. A reduced ability to count to a higher number before breathlessness occurs may signal grossly reduced ventilatory function. Alert physician to significant findings.

- Monitor effectiveness of breathing by checking serial vital capacity results on pulmonary function tests. If the vital capacity is <1L or is rapidly trending downward, or if the patient exhibits signs of hypoxia such as tachycardia, increasing restlessness, mental dullness, or cyanosis, report findings immediately to physician.
- Monitor ABG levels and pulse oximetry to detect hypoxia or hypercapnia.
- Raise HOB to promote optimal chest excursion.
- The patient may require tracheostomy, endotracheal intubation, or mechanical ventilation to support respiratory function. Prepare patient emotionally for such procedures or for the eventual transfer to ICU or transition care unit for closer monitoring.
- For other interventions, see **High risk for aspiration** in "General Care of Patients with Neurologic Disorders," p. 302.

**High risk for disuse syndrome** related to paralysis/immobilization secondary to neuromuscular impairment and prolonged bed rest
***Desired outcome:*** Patient exhibits complete (or baseline) ROM in all joints without subjective or objective indicators of pain.

- Assess functional ability on a regular basis and at least daily; compare to baseline. Notify physician of significant findings.
- Perform passive ROM and avoid active exercise during acute phase of G-BS. Vigorous exercise may exacerbate symptoms and prolong recovery by increasing the time needed for remyelinization.
- Coordinate care to ensure a balance between activity and rest.
- Elevate extremities above heart level if possible to prevent or reduce edema.
- For other interventions see this nursing diagnosis in Appendix One, "Caring for Patients on Prolonged Bed Rest," p. 713.

**Pain** related to muscle tenderness; hypersensitivity to touch; or discomfort in shoulders, thighs, and back
***Desired outcomes:*** Within 1-2 h of intervention, patient's subjective perception of discomfort decreases, as documented by a pain scale. Objective indicators, such as grimacing, are absent or diminished.

- For patients with muscle tenderness, consider use of massage, moist heat packs, cold application, or warm baths, which may be very soothing for the muscles.
- For patients with hypersensitivity, assess the amount of touch that can be tolerated, and incorporate this information into the patient's plan of care.
- Reposition patient at frequent intervals to decrease muscle tension and fatigue. Some individuals find that a supine "frog-leg" position is particularly comfortable.
- Provide passive ROM to reduce joint stiffness.
- For other interventions, see this nursing diagnosis in "General Care of Patients with Neurologic Disorders," p. 308.

**Altered cardiopulmonary and cerebral tissue perfusion (or high risk of same)** related to interrupted sympathetic outflow with concomitant BP fluctuations secondary to autonomic dysfunction
***Desired outcomes:*** When underlying autonomic dysfunction ceases (usually in about 2 weeks), patient has optimal cardiopulmonary and cerebral tissue perfusion as evidenced by systolic BP ≥90 mm Hg and ≤160 mm Hg and orientation to person, place, and time. BP fluctuations, if they occur, are detected and reported promptly.

- Monitor BP, noting wide fluctuations; report significant findings to physician. Changes in BP that result in severe hypotension or hypertension may occur because of unopposed sympathetic outflow or loss of outflow to the peripheral nervous system, causing changes in vascular tone. Short-acting hypertensive agents may be required for persistent hypertension.

- Monitor carefully for changes during activities such as coughing, suctioning, position changes, or straining at stool.
- For patients with hypotension or postural hypotension, see this nursing diagnosis in "Spinal Cord Injury," p. 244.

**Altered nutrition:**   Less than body requirements, related to adynamic ileus
*Desired outcome:*   Patient has adequate nutrition as evidenced by maintenance of baseline body weight.

- Auscultate abdominal sounds, noting presence, absence, or changes that may signal onset of ileus. Be alert to abdominal distention or tenderness, nausea and vomiting, and absence of stool output. Notify physician of significant findings.
- Patients with adynamic ileus generally require gastric suctioning to decompress the stomach. Because these patients are unable to take foods orally, parenteral nutrition may be required (see "Providing Nutritional Support," p. 665).
- For general interventions, see **Altered nutrition,** p. 300, in "General Care of Patients with Neurologic Disorders."

**Fear** related to threat to biologic integrity
*Desired outcome:*   Within 24 h of this diagnosis, patient verbalizes known sources of fear and the attainment of increased psychologic and physical comfort.

- For the patient in whom the neurologic deficit is still progressing, arrange for a transfer to a room close to the nurses' station to help alleviate the fear of being suddenly incapacitated and helpless.
- Be sure that patient's call light is within easy reach. Frequently assess patient's ability to use it.
- Provide continuity of patient care through assignment of staff and use of care plan.
- Perform assessments at frequent intervals, letting patient know you are there. Provide care in a calm and reassuring manner.
- For other interventions, see **Fear** in Appendix One, "Caring for Patients with Cancer and Other Life-Disrupting Illnesses," p. 756.

**Knowledge deficit:**   Therapeutic plasma exchange procedure
*Desired outcome:*   Before scheduled date of each procedure, patient verbalizes accurate information about the plasma exchange procedure.

- Before the plasma exchange procedure, the patient's physician explains the reason for the procedure, its risks, and anticipated benefits or outcome. Determine patient's level of understanding of the physician's explanation, and clarify or reinforce information accordingly.
- Determine patient's past experience with plasmapheresis, the positive or negative effects, and the nature of any fears or concerns. Document and communicate this information to others involved in the patient's care.
- Explain in words the patient can understand that the goal of plasma exchange is to remove autoimmune factors from the blood to decrease or eliminate the patient's symptoms. These antibodies to the patient's peripheral and cranial nerve tissue are reduced by the removal of the plasma portion of the blood, which contains the circulating antibodies. The procedure is similar to hemodialysis. Blood is removed from the patient and separated into its components. The patient's plasma is discarded; the other blood components (e.g., RBCs, WBCs, platelets) are saved and returned to the patient with donor plasma or replacement fluid. If started within 1-2 weeks of G-BS symptoms, the exchange process seems to decrease the duration and severity of the disease. Multiple exchanges over a period of weeks can be expected.
- The patient is at risk for the following complications during this procedure: fluid volume deficit, hypotension, hypokalemia, hypocalcemia, cardiac dysrhythmias, clotting disorders, anemia, phlebitis, infection, hypothermia, and air embolism. Explain these complications accordingly.

- This procedure requires good blood flow. Inform patient that the antecubital vein most often is used as the access site, but if the patient has poor peripheral veins, the physician may need to insert a central intravenous line or a femoral catheter. If the antecubital site is used, place a sign alerting others to avoid using this site for routine laboratory sticks.
- Explain that the patient can expect the procedure to take 2-4 h, although it may take considerably longer, depending on condition of the patient's veins, blood flow, and hematocrit (Hct) level.
- Explain that the patient can expect pre- and postprocedure blood work for clotting factors and electrolyte levels. The patient may be placed on cardiac monitoring to assess for electrolyte imbalance, particularly if taking prednisone or digitalis. Weight and VS will be taken pre- and postprocedure, with frequent VS checks during the procedure. Calcium gluconate or potassium chloride (KCl) may be administered to correct electrolyte imbalances.
- Instruct patient to report chills, fever, hives, sweating, or lightheadedness, which may signal reaction to donor plasma.
- Teach patient to report thirst, faintness, or dizziness, which can occur with hypotension or hypovolemia. The patient should take oral fluids during the procedure, if possible.
- Instruct patient to report numbness or tingling around the lips or in the hands, arms, and legs; muscle twitching; cramping; or tetany, which can occur with hypocalcemia. Fatigue, nausea, weakness, or cramping may signal hypokalemia.
- Inform patient that medications may be held until after the procedure to prevent their removal from the blood.
- If the patient does not have a urinary catheter, remind him or her to void before and during the procedure, if necessary, to avoid any mild hypotension caused by a full bladder. I&O will be monitored closely because decreased urine output may signal hypovolemia.
- Explain that the patient's temperature will be checked during the procedure, and warm blankets will be provided to prevent hypothermia.
- Explain that the patient probably will feel fatigued 1-2 days after the procedure because of decreased plasma protein levels. Encourage extra rest and a high-protein diet during this time.
- Teach patient to monitor IV access site for signs of infection such as warmth, redness, swelling, or drainage and to report significant findings.
- Teach patient to monitor for signs of bruising or bleeding. The anticoagulant citrate dextrose is used in the extracorporeal machine circuitry to prevent clotting. This may cause excessive bleeding at the access site. A pressure dressing may be kept in place over the access site for 2-4 h postprocedure. Caution patient about avoiding cutting self or bumping into objects and to sustain pressure over cuts. Inform patient that black, tarry stools usually signal the presence of blood and should be reported.

---

**Note:** For patients with urinary incontinence, retention, neurogenic bladder, or urinary tract infection (UTI), see related discussions in Chapter Three, "Renal-Urinary Disorders." For patients with autonomic dysfunction see "Spinal Cord Injury" for **Altered peripheral and cardiopulmonary tissue perfusion,** p. 244. See "General Care of Patients with Neurologic Disorders" for **High risk for trauma** related to unsteady gait, p. 298; **High risk for injury** related to impaired pain, touch, and temperature sensations, p. 299; **Impaired corneal tissue integrity,** p. 300; **High risk for fluid volume deficit,** p. 301; **Self-care deficit,** p. 302; **Impaired verbal communication,** p. 304; **Constipation,** p. 305; **Sensory/perceptual alterations,** p. 307; **Impaired swallowing,** p. 308, **Altered body temperature,** p. 310, and **Knowledge deficit:** Neurologic diagnostic tests, p. 311. For patients who are immobile, see related nursing diagnoses in "Pressure Ulcers," p. 687, and Appendix One, "Caring for Patients on Prolonged Bed Rest," p. 711. Also see Appendix One,

"Caring for Patients with Cancer and Other Life-Disrupting Illnesses" for care of patients undergoing immunosuppressive drug therapy, p. 719, and patient and family psychosocial nursing diagnoses, p. 753, as appropriate.

## PATIENT-FAMILY TEACHING AND DISCHARGE PLANNING

Most patients with G-BS eventually recover fully, but because the recovery period can be prolonged, the patient often goes home with some degree of neurologic deficit. Discharge planning and teaching will vary according to the degree of disability. Give patient and significant others verbal and written information about the following, as appropriate:

- The disease process, expected improvement, and importance of continuing in the rehabilitation or PT program to promote as full a recovery as possible.
- Referrals to community resources, such as public health nurse, visiting nurse association, community support groups, social workers, psychologic therapy, home health agencies, and extended and skilled care facilities. The Guillain-Barré Syndrome Foundation International can be contacted at Box 262, Wynnewood, PA 19096, (215)-667-0131.
- Safety measures relative to the decreased sensorimotor deficit.
- Exercises that promote muscle strength and mobility; measures for preventing contractures and skin breakdown; transfer techniques and proper body mechanics; and use of assistive devices.
- Indications of constipation, urinary retention, or UTI; implementation of bowel and bladder training programs; and, if appropriate, care of indwelling catheters or self-catheterization technique.
- Indications of URI; measures for preventing regurgitation, aspiration, and respiratory infection.
- Medications, including drug name, purpose, dosage, schedule, precautions, and potential side effects.
- Importance of follow-up care, including visits to physician, PT, and OT.

# Bacterial meningitis

Bacterial meningitis is an infection that results in inflammation of the meningeal membranes covering the brain and spinal cord. Bacteria in the subarachnoid space multiply and cause an inflammatory reaction of the pia and arachnoid meninges. Purulent exudate is produced, and the inflammation and infection spread quickly through the CSF that circulates around the brain and spinal cord. Bacteria and exudate can create vascular congestion, plugging the arachnoid villa. This obstruction of CSF flow and decreased reabsorption of CSF can lead to increased intracranial pressure (IICP), brain herniation, and death.

Meningitis generally is transmitted in one of four ways: *via* airborne droplets or contact with oral secretions from infected individuals; from direct contamination (e.g., from a penetrating skull wound; a skull fracture, often basilar, causing a tear in the dura; lumbar puncture [LP]; ventricular shunt; or surgical procedure); *via* the bloodstream (e.g., pneumonia, endocarditis); or from direct contact with an infectious process that invades the meningeal membranes, as can occur with osteomyelitis, sinusitis, otitis media, mastoiditis, or brain abscess. *Hemophilus influenzae* is the leading infecting agent of bacterial meningitis. Meningococcal meningitis, caused by *Neisseria meningitidis*, is the next leading cause, followed by pneumococcal meningitis, caused by *Streptococcus pneumoniae*. Any bacteria can cause a meningitis, and some, such as that caused by *Staphylococcus aureus*, can be difficult to treat because of their resistance to antibiotic therapy. Adhesions and fibrotic changes in the arachnoid layer and subspace may cause obstruction or reabsorption problems with CSF, resulting in hydrocephalus. The prognosis, however, is good, and complete neurologic recovery is possible if the disorder is recognized early and antibiotic treatment is initiated promptly. However, if left untreated, the mortality rate is 70%-100%.

## ASSESSMENT

**Infection:** Fever, chills, malaise.

**IICP and herniation:** Severe headache, decreased LOC (irritability, drowsiness, stupor, coma), nausea and vomiting, a decreasing Glasgow Coma Score (see p. 248), VS changes (increased BP, decreased HR, widening pulse pressure), changes in respiratory pattern, decreased pupillary reaction to light, pupillary dilatation or inequality.

**Meningeal irritation:** Back stiffness and pain, nuchal rigidity.

**Other:** Generalized seizures and photophobia. In the presence of *H. influenzae,* there may be deafness or joint pain.

**Physical assessment**

- A positive Brudzinski's sign may be elicited due to meningeal irritation: When the neck is passively flexed forward, both legs flex involuntarily at the hip and knee.
- A positive Kernig's sign also may be found: When the thigh is flexed 90 degrees at the hip, the individual is unable to extend the leg completely without pain.
- In the presence of meningococcal meningitis, a pink macular rash, petechiae, ecchymoses, purpura, and increased deep tendon reflexes (DTRs) may occur.

## DIAGNOSTIC TESTS

**LP, CSF analysis, and Gram stain and culture:** To identify causative organism. Glucose is generally decreased, and protein is usually increased. Typically, the CSF will be cloudy or milky because of increased WBCs, and CSF pressure will be increased because of the inflammation and exudate, causing an obstruction in outflow of CSF from the arachnoid villa. This test, in the presence of IICP, can cause brain herniation. If CSF pressure is elevated, check neurologic status and VS at frequent intervals for signs of brain herniation (decreased LOC; pupillary changes such as dilatation, inequality, or decreased reaction; irregular respirations; and hemiparesis).

**Culture and sensitivity testing of blood, sputum, urine, and other body secretions:** To identify infective organism and/or its source and determine appropriate antibiotic.

**Counterimmunoelectrophoresis (CIE):** For detection of bacterial antigens of pneumococci, meningococci, and *H. influenzae* in the CSF, blood, and urine.

**Sinus, skull, and chest x-rays:** Taken after treatment is started to rule out sinusitis, pneumonia, and cranial osteomyelitis.

**Radioimmunoassay (RIA), latex particle agglutination (LPA), or enzyme-linked immunosorbent assay (ELISA):** To detect microbial antigens in the CSF to identify the causative organism.

**CT scan with contrast:** To rule out hydrocephalus or mass lesions such as brain abscess and detect exudate in the CSF spaces.

---

**Note:** See **Knowledge deficit:** Neurologic tests, p. 311, in "General Care of Patient with Neurologic Disorders" for care considerations for patients undergoing LP, CT scan, and MRI.

---

## COLLABORATIVE MANAGEMENT

**Respiratory precautions:**  Patients with *N. meningitidis, H. influenzae,* or in whom the causative organism is in doubt require observation with special respiratory isolation precautions for 24 h after initiation of the appropriate antibiotic therapy. The patient should be placed in a private room. Infection may be spread by contact with airborne droplets or oral secretions. Masks should be used, along with adherence to body substance isolation (BSI, see p. 777).

**Parenteral antibiotics:**  Because treatment cannot be delayed until the results of the culture are returned, high doses are started immediately, based on Gram stain results. The antibiotic must penetrate the blood-brain barrier into the CSF. Adjustments in therapy can be made after CIE and culture and sensitivity test results are in. Antibiotics may include the following: penicillin G, ampicillin, nafcillin, oxacillin, chloramphenicol, gentamicin, kanamycin, or vancomycin.

**Prophylactic antibiotic treatment of significant others and close contacts:**  Rifampin is generally administered. Other antibiotics, such as sulfadiazine or minocycline, also may be used.

**Other pharmacotherapy**

*Glucocorticosteroids (e.g., dexamethasone, prednisone):*  High-dose therapy to stabilize the cell membrane and reduce inflammation and cerebral edema. Use is somewhat controversial.

*Osmotic diuretics (e.g., mannitol) and loop diuretics (e.g., furosemide):*  To decrease cerebral edema.

*Antiepilepsy drugs (e.g., diazepam and phenytoin):*  To control seizures.

*Analgesics (e.g., acetaminophen and codeine):*  For headache and other pain.

*Antipyretics (e.g., acetaminophen):*  For control of fever to reduce cerebral metabolism.

*Mild sedatives (e.g., diphenhydramine):*  To promote rest.

*Antacids and histamine $H_2$-receptor blockers (e.g., ranitidine):*  To reduce gastric acidity and prevent hemorrhage or ulcer formation.

*Stool softeners and laxatives (e.g., docusate sodium):*  To prevent constipation and straining at stool, which would increase intracranial pressure (ICP).

*Tranquilizers (e.g., chlorpromazine):*  To control shivering, which can increase ICP.

**Support respirations:**  *Via* $O_2$, suctioning, airway maintenance, or intubation as necessary.

**Bed rest with elevation of HOB and seizure precautions:**  To promote venous drainage, help reduce cerebral congestion and edema, and prevent injury from possible seizure activity.

**Fluid management:**  Limitation of fluids to ⅔ maintenance (about 1,500 ml) to keep patient underhydrated and reduce cerebral edema and effects of inappropriate antidiuretic hormone (ADH) secretion. I&O is measured, and the patient usually has an indwelling urinary catheter. Hypotonic IV solutions, such as 5% dextrose in water ($D_5W$), are avoided because they increase cerebral edema.

**Nutritional support:**  Parenteral or enteral feedings or modified diet, depending on patient's LOC and ability to swallow.

**Measures to reduce hyperthermia:**  Tepid sponges or cooling blankets to reduce fever.

**Antiembolism hose:**  To prevent thrombophlebitis in the legs from venous stasis.

**Treatment of complications:**  Examples include disseminated intravascular coagulation, syndrome of inappropriate antidiuretic hormone (SIADH), respiratory or heart failure, and septic shock. A shunt may be needed if hydrocephalus from arachnoid adhesions and fibrotic changes persists.

**Intrathecal antibiotics:**  Sometimes used if it is believed that systemic antibiotics alone will not be curative in the presence of particular bacteria (e.g., *Pseudomonas, Enterobacter, Staphylococcus).*

**Physical medicine:**   Physical therapy (PT) and rehabilitation program may be needed, depending on neurologic deficits.

## NURSING DIAGNOSES AND INTERVENTIONS

**Knowledge deficit:**   Side effects and precautions for the prescribed antibiotics

*Desired outcome:*   Before beginning the medication regimen, patient and significant others verbalize knowledge about the potential side effects and precautions for the prescribed antibiotics.

- For significant others and contacts placed on prophylactic rifampin, explain the prescribed dose and schedule. Rifampin should be taken 1 h before meals for maximum absorption. Emphasize the importance of taking this drug as a preventive measure against meningitis, and describe potential side effects, such as nausea, vomiting, diarrhea, orange urine, headache, and dizziness. Caution against wearing contact lenses, as the drug will permanently color them orange. In addition, rifampin reduces the effectiveness of oral contraceptives and is contraindicated during pregnancy.
- Instruct significant others and patient's other contacts who are taking rifampin to report the onset of jaundice (yellow skin or sclera), allergic reactions, and persistence of GI side effects.
- For other interventions, see **Knowledge deficit:** Adverse side effects from prolonged use of potent antibiotics, p. 544, in "Osteomyelitis."

**Knowledge deficit:**   Rationale and procedure for BSI
*Desired outcome:*   Before visitation, patient and significant others verbalize knowledge about the rationale for BSI and comply with the prescribed restrictions and precautionary measures.

---

**Note:**   Patients with *N. meningitidis, H. influenzae,* or meningitis caused by an unidentified organism will be placed in a private room and will require special respiratory isolation precautions for 24 h after initiation of appropriate antibiotic therapy. Masks should be worn, and other BSI procedures observed.

---

- For patients with meningitis caused by *H. influenzae* or *N. meningitidis,* explain the method of disease transmission *via* airborne droplets and oral secretions and the rationale for private room and special precautions.
- Provide instructions for covering the mouth before coughing/sneezing and properly disposing of tissue.
- Instruct patients with specific respiratory precautions to stay in their rooms. If they must leave the room for a procedure or test, explain that a mask must be worn to protect others from contact with airborne droplets.
- For individuals in contact with the patient, explain the importance of wearing a surgical mask and using good handwashing technique. Gloves should be worn when handling any body fluid, especially oral secretions. For more information, see Appendix Two, p. 777.
- Reassure patient that special respiratory precautions are temporary and will be discontinued once patient has been on the appropriate antibiotic for 24 to 48 h.

**Pain** related to headache, photophobia, and neck stiffness secondary to meningitis

*Desired outcomes:*   Within 1-2 h of intervention, patient's subjective perception of discomfort decreases, as documented by a pain scale. Objective indicators, such as grimacing, are absent or diminished.

- Provide a quiet environment and a darkened room. Restrict visitors as necessary to reduce noise. Sunglasses may promote comfort from photophobia.

- Promote bed rest and assist with ADL as needed to decrease movement that may cause pain.
- Apply an ice bag to the head or cool cloth to the eyes to help diminish the headache.
- Support patient in a position of comfort. Many persons with meningitis are comforted in a position with the head in extension and the body slightly curled. The HOB elevated to 30 degrees also may help. Keep the neck in alignment during position changes.
- Provide gentle passive ROM and massage to the neck and shoulder joints and muscles to help relieve stiffness. If the patient is afebrile, apply moist heat to the neck and back to promote muscle relaxation and decrease pain.
- Patients tend to be hyperirritable, with hyperalgesia. Sounds are loud. Keep communication simple and direct, in a soft and calm tone of voice. Touching startles the patient. Avoid needless stimulation. Consolidate activities. Loosen constricting bed clothing. Avoid restraining patient. Reduce stimulation to the minimal amount needed to accomplish required activity.
- For other interventions see this nursing diagnosis in "General Care of Patients with Neurologic Disorders," p. 308.

**High risk for trauma** related to oral, musculoskeletal, and airway vulnerability secondary to seizure activity
*Desired outcomes:* Patient exhibits no signs of oral or musculoskeletal injury or airway compromise after seizure. Significant others verbalize knowledge of actions that are necessary during seizure activity.
- Monitor for twitching of the hands, feet, or mouth. Twitching signals generalized central nervous system (CNS) irritability and may herald the onset of seizures. This sign requires further evaluation and possible interventions to prevent complications.
- For other interventions, see this nursing diagnosis in "Seizure Disorders," p. 292.

---

**Note:** See "Head injury" for **High risk for disuse syndrome,** p. 256, and **Fluid volume excess** related to SIADH, p. 256. See "Seizure Disorders" for **Impaired tissue integrity** related to IV administration of phenytoin, p. 293. See "General Care of Patients with Neurologic Disorders" for **High risk for trauma** related to unsteady gait, p. 298; **High risk for injury** related to impaired pain, touch, and temperature sensations, p. 299; **Impaired corneal tissue integrity,** p. 300; **Altered nutrition:** Less than body requirements, p. 300; **High risk for fluid volume deficit,** p. 301; **High risk for aspiration,** p. 302; **Self-care deficit,** p. 302; **Constipation,** p. 305; **Altered cerebral tissue perfusion,** p. 305; **Impaired swallowing,** p. 308; **Altered body temperature,** p. 310; and **Knowledge deficit:** Neurologic diagnostic tests, p. 311. For patients needing nutritional support, see nursing diagnoses in "Providing Nutritional Support," p. 673. For patients who are immobile, see related nursing diagnoses in "Pressure Ulcers," p. 687, and Appendix One, "Caring for Patients on Prolonged Bed Rest," p 711. In addition, see Appendix One, "Caring for Patients with Cancer and Other Life-Disrupting Illnesses," p. 753, for appropriate patient and family psychosocial nursing diagnoses and interventions.

---

## PATIENT-FAMILY TEACHING AND DISCHARGE PLANNING

The extent of teaching and discharge planning will depend on whether or not patient has any residual damage. As appropriate, give patient and significant others verbal and written information about the following:
- Referrals to community resources, such as public health nurse, visiting nurse association, community support groups, social workers, psychologic therapy, vocational rehabilitation agency, home health agencies, and extended and skilled care facilities.

- Medications, including purpose, dosage, schedule, precautions, and potential side effects for patient's medications, as well as those for the prophylactic antibiotics taken by family and significant others.

*In addition*

- For patients with residual neurologic deficits, teach the following as appropriate: exercises that promote muscle strength and mobility; measures for preventing contractures and skin breakdown; transfer techniques and proper body mechanics; safety measures if the patient has decreased pain and sensation or visual disturbances; use of assistive devices; indications of constipation, urinary retention, or urinary tract infection (UTI); bowel and bladder training programs; self-catheterization technique or care of indwelling catheters; and seizure precautions if indicated.

# Encephalitis

Encephalitis is an inflammation of the brain that can cause severe neuronal dysfunction. In response to infection the brain tissue becomes inflamed, leading to cerebral edema. The brain's ganglion cells may degenerate, leaving diffuse nerve cell destruction and necrotic areas. The cerebral edema can be severe, leading to increased intracranial pressure (IICP), herniation, and death.

Encephalitis usually is caused by a viral infection. Other infecting agents, such as bacteria, fungi, or amebas, occur but are quite rare. Viral encephalitis may be the result of an arbovirus infection that is transmitted by an infected mosquito or tick bite. Postinfectious encephalitis occurs after a vaccination or as a complication of other infections, such as measles, chicken pox, and herpes simplex type I virus. The prognosis varies according to the type of infection. Some cases of encephalitis leave few or no residual side effects, and the neurologic symptoms often subside in several weeks. Other types of encephalitis, such as eastern equine encephalitis (an arbovirus infection), can have a high mortality rate (up to 66%), and survivors frequently have severe residual damage. Herpes simplex encephalitis has a mortality rate ranging from 30%-70%, depending on when the antiviral drug therapy is started, and survivors are often left with seizures, aphasia, or severe mental deterioration, such as dementia.

## ASSESSMENT

**Infection:** Fever, chills, malaise.
**IICP and brain herniation:** Headache; changes in LOC such as irritability, confusion, and drowsiness, symptoms that can progress to stupor and coma; a falling Glasgow Coma Scale score (see p. 248); nausea and vomiting; VS changes (hypertension, bradycardia, widening pulse pressure); changes in respiratory pattern; and pupillary changes, such as inequality and decreased reaction to light.
**Meningeal irritation:** Neck stiffness/rigidity; pain.
**Focal:** Symptoms vary. Patient may have seizures or photophobia, ataxia, and sensorimotor deficits. Eastern equine encephalitis, for example, can destroy major portions of a lobe or hemisphere and leave the individual with hemiplegia, aphasia, blindness, deafness, and/or seizures. Herpes simplex encephalitis has a special affinity for the frontal and temporal lobes of the brain, resulting in alterations in the senses of smell and taste, seizures, aphasia, organic psychosis, and dementia.

## DIAGNOSTIC TESTS

**Lumbar puncture (LP) and CSF analysis:** May reveal increased CSF pressure, increased WBC and protein levels, and normal glucose. CSF analysis helps differentiate between viral encephalitis and bacterial encephalitis.

**CT scan:**   To rule out other neurologic problems. A scan showing frontal/ temporal lobe edema is suggestive of herpes simplex encephalitis.
**EEG:**   May show generalized or focal slowing of electrical activity.
**Brain biopsy:**   May be done to identify the infecting agent. This requires the drilling of burr holes into the skull to obtain a specimen. The specimen then undergoes an immunofluorescent exam and culture to identify the virus present. Usually the test is done only to determine if the encephalitis is caused by a treatable virus infection, such as herpes simplex. If the diagnosis of herpes simplex is fairly certain based on other clinical evidence, the physician may decide to initiate drug therapy and forego this test.
**MRI:**   To rule out other neurologic problems. A scan showing frontal/temporal lobe edema is suggestive of herpes simplex encephalitis.

---

**Note:**   See "General Care of Patients with Neurologic Disorders" for **Knowledge deficit:** Neurologic diagnostic tests, p. 311, for care considerations for patients undergoing LP, CT scan, or MRI.

---

## COLLABORATIVE MANAGEMENT

Except for herpes simplex encephalitis, the treatment is supportive only.
**Antiviral agent (e.g., acyclovir):**   For herpes simplex encephalitis. Acyclovir is less toxic and more effective than the previously used antiviral agent vidarabine. To be most effective, therapy with acyclovir should be initiated before the patient becomes comatose.
**Supportive pharmacotherapy**
*Antiepilepsy drugs (e.g., phenytoin, diazepam):*   To treat or prevent seizures.
*Glucocorticosteroids (e.g., dexamethasone):*   To reduce cerebral edema and inflammation. For herpes simplex encephalitis, steroids may potentiate the spread of herpes in nervous tissue, so generally they are not used until definite indications of IICP appear.
*Osmotic diuretics (e.g., mannitol) and loop diuretics (e.g., furosemide):*   To decrease cerebral edema.
*Mild sedatives (e.g., diphenhydramine):*   For restlessness.
*Analgesics (e.g., acetaminophen):*   For headache and other pain.
*Antipyretics (e.g., acetaminophen):*   For control of fever to reduce cerebral metabolism.
*Antacids and histamine $H_2$-receptor blockers (e.g., ranitidine):*   To reduce gastric acidity and prevent hemorrhage or ulcer formation.
*Stool softeners and laxatives (e.g., docusate sodium):*   To prevent constipation and straining at stool, which would increase ICP.
*Tranquilizers (e.g., chlorpromazine):*   To control shivering, which can increase ICP.
*Antiinfective agents:*   Amphotericin B and other antibiotics are being tried with amebic meningoencephalitis, but they generally are ineffective.
**Bed rest with HOB elevated and seizure precautions:**   To promote venous drainage, help reduce cerebral congestion and edema, and prevent injury from possible seizure activity.
**Fluid and electrolyte management:**   IV fluids are given to maintain a balanced electrolyte status. Generally, fluids are limited to two-thirds maintenance (about 1,500 ml) to maintain a state of underhydration, which helps reduce cerebral edema. I&O are measured, and the patient usually has an indwelling urinary catheter. Hypotonic IV solutions, such as $D_5W$, are avoided because they increase cerebral edema.
**Support of respirations:**   Via $O_2$, suctioning, airway maintenance, or intubation.
**Nutritional support:**   Enteral or parenteral feedings for stuporous or comatose patients, as needed. A soft or semisolid diet may be prescribed for some patients, depending on their neurologic deficit.

**Measures to reduce hyperthermia:**  Tepid sponge baths or cooling blankets to reduce fever.

**Antiembolism hose:**  To prevent thromboembolism in the legs from venous stasis.

**Physical medicine:**  Physical therapy, occupational therapy, and assistive devices or braces may be prescribed so that the patient can maintain mobility and independence with ADL. Muscle-strengthening and conditioning exercises and gait training also may be prescribed.

**ROM exercises:**  To maintain or increase joint function and prevent contractures.

**Speech therapy:**  To assist the aphasic or dysarthric patient.

## NURSING DIAGNOSES AND INTERVENTIONS

**Knowledge deficit:**  Disease process of encephalitis and precautions that must be taken

*Desired outcome:*  Within 24 h before hospital discharge, patient and significant others verbalize knowledge about encephalitis and the precautions that must be taken.

- Determine patient's and significant others' level of understanding of encephalitis, and intervene accordingly.
- Explain that encephalitis usually is caused by a viral infection, such as an arbovirus infection, which is transmitted by an infected mosquito or tick. Postinfectious encephalitis may occur after a vaccination or as a complication of other infections, such as measles, chicken pox, or herpes simplex type I virus. Exposure to a virus, however, does not guarantee the development of encephalitis. Encephalitis is relatively rare because the virus must first cross the blood-brain barrier.
- Reassure patient and significant others that the patient usually is not contagious. Others can touch and be close to the patient. If the patient has herpes simplex lesions, however, contact with the lesions should be avoided. Teach good handwashing technique and BSI. Emphasize that these techniques also should be used in everyday life.
- For encephalitis caused by mosquito or tick, reassure patient that the virus is not transmitted from person-to-person. Emphasize the importance of mosquito control. In the home environment, the patient should eliminate breeding places by screening the doors and windows. In addition, patient should use mosquito repellent on exposed skin, and insecticides and aerosols according to directions. Repellents should be used when in areas contaminated with ticks.
- For more information about BSI, see Appendix Two, p. 777.

**Fluid volume excess (or risk of same)** related to decreased urine output secondary to kidney damage from treatment with acyclovir for herpes simplex encephalitis

*Desired outcome:*  Throughout drug therapy with acyclovir, patient is normovolemic as evidenced by balanced I&O, stable weight, eupnea, HR ≤100 bpm, nondistended neck veins, stable neurologic status, CVP ≤2 mm Hg (≤5 cm $H_2O$), edema ≤1 on a 0-4+ scale, and absence of crackles (rales).

- Monitor I&O, weight, breath sounds, and renal function tests (serum creatinine, blood urea nitrogen [BUN], and electrolytes). Also assess for edema, SOB, tachycardia, distended neck veins, and increased CVP. Notify physician of significant findings.
- To decrease risk of kidney damage from precipitation of drug in renal tubules, ensure adequate hydration during administration, and avoid rapid or bolus injection by giving the drug *via* infusion pump over at least 1 h.
- Although acyclovir is generally well tolerated, be alert to other side effects of IV therapy, including dizziness, hypotension, occasional headache, sweating, or nausea. Rare side effects include lethargy, delirium tremens, and seizures. Hepatic and bone marrow dysfunction also may occur, but usually

in the immunocompromised patient only. Oral acyclovir also may cause nausea, vomiting, diarrhea, and stomach pain.
- Rotate IV sites to prevent phlebitis. Wrap the extremity in a warm towel if discomfort occurs during infusion.

---

**Note:** For patients with urinary incontinence, retention, or neurogenic bladder, see related nursing diagnoses in "Renal-Urinary Disorders." See "Alzheimer's Disease" for **Sensory/perceptual alterations** related to impaired sensory reception, transmission, integration, and evaluation, p. 219, and **High risk for trauma** related to lack of awareness of environmental hazards, p. 216. See "Head Injury" for **High risk for disuse syndrome,** p. 256, and **Fluid volume excess** (secondary to SIADH), p. 256. See "Cerebrovascular Accident" for **Impaired physical mobility,** p. 282, **Sensory/perceptual alterations** related to neurologic deficit, p. 283, and **Impaired verbal communication,** p. 284. See "Seizure Disorders" for **High risk for trauma** related to oral, musculoskeletal, and airway vulnerability secondary to seizure activity, p. 292, and **Impaired tissue integrity** related to IV administration of phenytoin, p. 293. See "General Care of Patients with Neurologic Disorders" for **High risk for trauma** related to gait unsteadiness, p. 298; **High risk for injury** related to decreased pain, touch, and temperature sensations, p. 299; **Impaired corneal tissue integrity,** p. 300; **Altered nutrition,** p. 300; **High risk for fluid volume deficit,** p. 301; **High risk for aspiration,** p. 302; **Self-care deficit,** p. 302; **Constipation,** p. 305; **Altered cerebral tissue perfusion,** p. 305; **Pain,** p. 308; **Impaired swallowing,** p. 308; **Altered body temperature,** p. 310; and **Knowledge deficit:** Neurologic diagnostic tests, p. 311. For patients who have varying degrees of immobility, see related nursing diagnoses and interventions in "Pressure Ulcers," p. 687, and Appendix One, "Caring for Patients on Prolonged Bed Rest," p. 711. Also see Appendix One, "Caring for Patients with Cancer and Other Life-Disrupting Illnesses," p. 753, for patient and family psychosocial nursing diagnoses and interventions as appropriate.

---

## PATIENT-FAMILY TEACHING AND DISCHARGE PLANNING

The amount of teaching and discharge planning will depend on the degree of neurologic deficit. See Patient-Family Teaching and Discharge Planning (second through tenth entries only) in "Multiple Sclerosis," as appropriate.
*In addition*
- Teach interventions that increase effective communication in the presence of aphasia or dysarthria. See "Cerebrovascular Accident" for **Impaired verbal communication,** p. 284.
- Provide instructions regarding seizure precautions, factors that may precipitate seizures, and actions to be taken should they occur. See "Seizure Disorders," p. 288.

# Section Two:    Degenerative Disorders of the Nervous System

The central nervous system (CNS), peripheral nervous system, and autonomic nervous system are responsible for controlling and coordinating the functions of all body systems. With degenerative nerve disorders, the function of the nerve cells, dendrites, or axons is progressively altered or decreased. A variety of mechanisms, including outright destruction of the neurons and decreases in neurotransmitter synthesis uptake or release, account for this change in neuronal function.

# Parkinsonism

Parkinson's disease is a slowly progressive degenerative disorder of the CNS affecting the brain centers that regulate movement. For unknown reasons, cell death occurs in the substantia nigra of the midbrain. When healthy, the substantia nigra projects dopaminergic neurons into the corpus striatum and releases the neurotransmitter dopamine in that area. Degeneration of these neurons leads to an abnormally low concentration of dopamine in the basal ganglia. The basal ganglia control muscle tone and voluntary motor movement *via* a balance between two main neurotransmitters, dopamine and acetylcholine. The deficit of dopamine, which has an inhibitory effect, allows the relative excess of acetylcholine. The excitatory effect of acetylcholine causes overactivity of the basal ganglia, which interferes with normal muscle tone and the control of smooth, purposeful movement, causing the characteristic symptoms of Parkinson's disease: muscle rigidity, tremors, and slowness of movement.

Possible causes include viral encephalitis, neurotoxins, cerebrovascular disease, head injury, phenothiazide use, and exposure to carbon monoxide. Improper synthesis of a heroinlike substance results in the product n-methyl 4-phenyl 1236 tetrahydropyridine (MPTP), which causes a severe form of Parkinson's disease in those who have taken this illegal recreational drug. The vast majority of Parkinson's disease occurs without an apparent or known cause, however. Approximately 1% of all individuals over age 50 have this disease. Parkinsonism is usually progressive, and death can result from aspiration pneumonia or choking. *Parkinsonian crisis,* a medical emergency, is usually precipitated by emotional trauma or failure to take the prescribed medications.

## ASSESSMENT

Initially, symptoms are mild and include stiffness or slight hand tremors. They gradually increase and can become disabling. Cardinal features are tremors, rigidity, and bradykinesia. Assessment findings vary in degree and are highly individualized.

**Bradykinesia:**   Slowness, stiffness, and difficulty initiating movement. The patient may have a masklike, blank facial expression; "unblinking" stare; difficulty chewing and swallowing; drooling due to decreased frequency of swallowing; and a high-pitched, monotonal, weak voice. Speech may be slow and slurred. The patient also has loss of automatic associated movements, such as the ability to swing the arms when walking.

**Loss of postural reflexes:**   Causes the typical stooped, forward-leaning, shuffling, propulsive gait with short, rapidly accelerating steps; stumbling; and difficulty maintaining or regaining balance, which makes the individual prone to stumbling and falling.

**Increased muscle rigidity:**   Limb muscles become rigid on passive motion. Typically, this rigidity results in jerky ("cogwheel") motions.

**Tremors:**   Increase when the limb is at rest and stop with voluntary movement and during sleep (nonintentional tremor). "Pill-rolling" tremor of the hands and "to-and-fro" tremor of the head are typical.

**Autonomic:**   Excessive diaphoresis, seborrhea, postural hypotension, decreased libido, hypomotility of the GI tract, and urinary hesitancy. Vision may blur as a result of lost accommodation.

**Other:**   Dementia (e.g., forgetfulness, irritability, paranoia, hallucination) commonly is associated with Parkinson's disease. However, not all patients develop impaired intellectual and mental functioning. Some patients may experience akathisia, a condition of motor restlessness in which the individual has a compelling need to walk about constantly. Handwriting becomes progressively smaller, cramped, and tremulous.

**Physical assessment:**   Usually a positive blink reflex is elicited by tapping a finger between the patient's eyebrows. Blinking may occur 5-10 times/min instead of the normal 20 times/min. A positive palmomental (palm-chin) reflex can be elicited (muscles of the chin and corner of mouth contract when the patient's palm is stroked). Diminished postural reflexes are present on neurologic exam; however, there is risk of injury with this test because the patient may quickly lose balance and fall.

**Parkinsonian crisis:**   This sudden and severe increase in bradykinesia, muscle rigidity, and tremors can lead to tachycardia, hyperpnea, hyperprexia, and muscle paralysis, causing an inability to swallow or maintain a patent airway.

**Oculogyric crisis:**   Fixation of the eyes in one position, generally upward, sometimes for several hours. This is relatively rare.

## DIAGNOSTIC TESTS

Diagnosis usually is made on the basis of physical assessment and characteristic symptoms, and after other neurologic problems have been ruled out.

**Urinalysis:**   May reveal decreased dopamine level, which supports the diagnosis.

**Medication withdrawal:**   Long-term therapy with large doses of medications, such as haloperidol or phenothiazines, can produce Parkinsonlike symptoms. If caused by these medications, symptoms will disappear when the drug is discontinued.

**EEG:**   Often shows abnormalities, such as diffuse, nonspecific slowing of theta waves.

**Lumbar puncture (LP) with CSF analysis:**   May show decreased levels of dopamine or its metabolite in the CSF.

**Tremor studies:**   Serial measurements of functional activity will show decreased performance.

**Cineradiographic study of swallowing:**   May show abnormal pattern and delayed relaxation of cricopharyngeal muscles.

---

**Note:**   See "General Care of Patients with Neurologic Disorders," **Knowledge deficit:** Neurologic diagnostic tests, p. 311, for care considerations for patients undergoing EEG and LP.

---

## COLLABORATIVE MANAGEMENT

**Pharmacotherapy:**   See Table 4-1 for a description of the mechanisms, action, and side effects of anti-Parkinson drugs.

*Dopamine replacement (e.g., levodopa or levodopa-carbidopa combination):*   Given in increasing amounts until symptoms are reduced or patient's tolerance to side effects is reached. It may be used as initial therapy or later when other medications can no longer control Parkinson's symptoms.

*Antiviral agents (e.g., amantadine):*   Less effective than levodopa but has less severe side effects. May be used as the initial therapy or as an adjunct to anticholinergics or levodopa. Effects diminish in a few months, so this drug may be used intermittently.

*Dopamine agonist (e.g., bromocriptine):*   Administered with a concomitant reduction of dopamine replacement dosage. It may be used to reduce levodopa-induced dyskinesia, such as involuntary movements and the frequency of "on-off" responses.

*Monoamine oxidase (MAO) type B inhibitor (e.g., selegiline):*   Used as an adjunct with levodopa to inhibit the breakdown of levodopa, resulting in less fluctuation in blood levels.

*Anticholinergics (e.g., ethopropazine, trihexyphenidyl, cycrimine, procyclidine, biperiden, or benztropine mesylate):*   Often used in conjunction with dopamine replacement therapy but may be used alone if the patient's symptoms are mild or if the patient cannot tolerate levodopa. Anticholinergics may improve tremor and rigidity but often do little for bradykinesis or balance problems.

*Antihistamines (e.g., diphenhydramine, orphenadrine hydrochloride):* Usually given in conjunction with anticholinergic drugs but may be used alone if the patient's symptoms are mild.

*Phenothiazine derivative (e.g., ethopropazine):* Generally used in combination with other anti-Parkinson drugs to reduce rigidity, tremors, and spasms.

*Laxatives and stool softeners (e.g., docusate sodium):* To prevent constipation.

*Antitremor (e.g., propranolol):* May be used to decrease tremors.

*Antidepressants (e.g., nortriptyline, imipramine, amitriptyline):* Treat depression as well as some Parkinsonism symptoms; help to block reuptake of dopamine and have some anticholinergic properties.

*Antiemetics (e.g., trimethobenzamide, domperidone).*

**Physical medicine and exercise program:** Massage; muscle stretching; active/passive ROM, especially on hands and feet; walking and gait training exercises; suggestions for maintaining mobility; occupational therapy (OT) evaluation for assistive devices to help in self-care with ADL.

**Treatment of complications of dopamine replacement therapy**

*Choreiform or involuntary movements (e.g., facial grimacing, tongue protrusion, or restlessness).*

—Dose reduction or redistribution throughout the day.

—Drug "holiday": Treatment is somewhat controversial. After temporary withdrawal, levodopa is resumed at a much lower dose. Generally the patient can be maintained for several months to years at this much lower dose, with fewer drug-related adverse side effects and good mobility. This treatment requires hospitalization, because during withdrawal the patient may become completely immobile and dependent. Medications are tapered gradually. These individuals often need psychologic support because, without the drug's mitigating effects, this may be the first time they experience the full impact and immobility of their disease.

*Severe mental status changes (e.g., agitation, confusion, psychosis).*

—Dose reduction.

—Drug holiday.

*"End of dose" wearing-off phenomenon:* Return of signs and symptoms before next dose is due.

—Administer smaller, more frequent doses.

—Use slow-release medication preparations.

—Encourage low-protein diet.

*Vivid dreaming.*

—Reduce the last dose of levodopa given at night.

*On-off response:* This is a rapid fluctuation or change in the patient's condition. The individual is "on" one moment, in a state of relative mobility, and "off" the next, in a state of complete or nearly complete immobility. Attacks can occur over a 2-3 min period of time or may last several h. Initially the attacks may occur 3-4 h after anti-Parkinson medication is given. Later in the disease they may occur at any time. Cause is uncertain but appears to be related to fluctuating drug levels in the brain as loss of striatal ability to store dopamine progresses. Usually this response occurs after the patient has been on medication for several years.

—Smaller, more frequent doses to titrate and space the levodopa doses during the 24-h day.

—Combining levodopa with anticholinergic medications, dopamine agonists, or amantadine may be helpful.

—Use of substained-release forms of levodopa.

—Drug holiday. Not used too often since on-off response usually is very short-lived.

**Treatment for Parkinsonian crisis:** This crisis necessitates respiratory and

# T A B L E  4 - 1   Anti-Parkinson Drugs

| Medication | Mechanism of action | Side effects |
|---|---|---|
| **Dopamine replacements** | | |
| levodopa | Levodopa is the metabolic precursor of dopamine. Levodopa crosses the blood-brain barrier and restores dopamine levels in the extrapyramidal centers in the brain. Before levodopa crosses the blood-brain barrier, much of it is converted into dopamine by the peripheral metabolism (GI tract and liver). This causes many of the drug's side effects | Choreiform and involuntary movements (e.g., facial grimacing, tongue protusion); on-off response; severe depression with possible suicidal overtones; GI bleeding; orthostatic hypotension; anorexia; nausea and vomiting; dry mouth; constipation; urinary retention; confusion; agitation; hallucination |
| carbidopa-levodopa, benserazide-levodopa | Carbidopa prevents peripheral metabolism of levodopa, thereby increasing the amount of levodopa available for transport to the brain. Carbidopa does not cross the blood-brain barrier and therefore does not affect the metabolism of levodopa in the brain. Carbidopa reduces the amount of levodopa needed | No reactions to carbidopa alone. Adverse reactions are to levodopa |
| **Antivirals** | | |
| amantadine | Mechanism of action not understood. This medication appears to increase the release of dopamine from neuronal storage sites. It has an anticholinergic effect as well | Most side effects are like those of levodopa but are milder and dose-related. They include insomnia, peripheral edema, CHF, depression, nervousness, slurred speech, ataxia, orthostatic hypotension, blurred vision, anorexia, nausea, vomiting, dry mouth, constipation, urinary retention, confusion, irritability, hallucination |

| Drug | Action | Side effects |
|---|---|---|
| *Dopamine agonists* bromocriptine, lisuride, pergoline | Have a direct stimulating effect on dopamine receptors, thereby enhancing their activity | Produce less nausea and vomiting than levodopa, but otherwise have similar side effects, including orthostatic hypotension, blurred vision, nausea, vomiting, dry mouth, constipation, urinary retention, confusion, paranoia, insomnia, ataxia, digital vasospasm |
| *Anticholinergics* ethopropazine, trihexyphenidyl, cycrimine, procyclidine, biperiden, benztropine mesylate | Reduce the excitatory action of acetylcholine on cholinergic neuron receptors. In Parkinson's disease, there is an imbalance between the dopamine deficit, with its inhibitory action, and acetylcholine, with its excitatory action. Anticholinergics reduce acetylcholine action and work to reestablish this balance | Side effects are dose-related and include decreased sweating, orthostatic hypotension, tachycardia, dry mouth, blurred vision, photophobia, nausea, drowsiness, constipation, urinary retention or overflow incontinence, confusion, mental slowness, insomnia, nervousness, headache |
| *Antihistamines* diphenhydramine, orphenadrine HCl | Have a central cholinergic blocking action, prolonging dopamine action by inhibiting its uptake and storage. Used in conjunction with anticholinergics | GI effects are fairly minimal. Other side effects include drowsiness, mild hypotension, dry mouth, anorexia, constipation, urinary retention |
| *Phenothiazine derivative* ethopropazine | Has a central cholinergic blocking action. Differs from other phenothiazines in that it is used to control extrapyramidal symptoms. Used in conjunction with other anti-Parkinson drugs | Depression, drowsiness, hypotension, dizziness, ataxia, blurred vision, nausea, vomiting, dry mouth, constipation |
| *MAO B inhibitor* selegiline | Inhibits breakdown of levodopa | Nausea, lightheadedness, dizziness, abdominal pain, insomnia, confusion, dry mouth |

cardiac support. The patient is placed in a quiet, calm environment with subdued lighting. Sodium phenobarbital or sodium amobarbital is given IM or IV.

**Speech therapy:**    Speech evaluation for patient with verbal deficits.

**Antiembolism hose:**    To help prevent postural hypotension.

**Counseling or psychotherapy:**    To help patient and significant others adapt to the disability and deal with emotions and feelings, such as depression, that are either a direct or indirect result of the disease process or drug therapy. Occasionally, electroconvulsive therapy is used for persistent and serious depression.

**Diet:**    A controlled, low-protein diet may be prescribed if the patient is on dopamine replacement therapy because high protein intake reduces the medication's effectiveness. A high-fiber diet may be given to prevent constipation.

**Adrenal transplant:**    Involves grafting one of the patient's own adrenal medullary glands to the caudate nucleus of the brain. The medullary portion of the adrenal gland produces dopamine for the peripheral nervous system. When grafted, the adrenal medullary may continue to produce dopamine in the CNS, reducing or eliminating Parkinson's disease symptoms and the need for medication. Postural problems causing falls often improve, but other benefits often are variable and minimal. This procedure involves three major surgeries: (1) stereotactic localization of the caudate nucleus, (2) craniotomy (see "Brain Tumors," p. 260), and (3) laparotomy for adrenalectomy. Prepare the patient for transfer to the ICU following surgery.

**Stereotaxic surgery:**    Rarely performed now because of the effectiveness of drug therapy. It involves the use of electrical coagulation, freezing, radioactivity, or ultrasound to destroy portions of the globus pallidus of the ventrolateral nucleus of the thalamus to prevent involuntary movement and help relieve tremors and rigidity of the extremities.

**Controversial therapies:**    Fetal neuronal tissue transplants eventually may be found to produce dopamine in the CNS and reduce or alleviate symptoms.

## NURSING DIAGNOSES AND INTERVENTIONS

**High risk for trauma** related to unsteady gait secondary to bradykinesis, tremors, and rigidity

*Desired outcome:*    Following instruction, patient demonstrates effective ambulatory techniques and preventive measures and remains free of trauma.

- During ambulation, encourage patient to deliberately swing the arms to assist the gait and raise the feet to help prevent falls. Advise patients to step over an imaginery object or line, which will help them raise their feet higher and increase their stride.
- Have patient practice movements that are especially difficult (e.g., turning). Teach patient to walk in a wide arc rather than pivot when turning.
- Teach head and neck exercises to help improve patient's posture. Remind patient repeatedly to maintain an upright posture, especially when walking.
- Advise patient to stop occasionally to slow down the walking speed. Teach patients to concentrate on listening to their feet as they touch the floor and count the cadence to prevent too fast a gait. Encourage patient to lift toes and to walk with the heel touching the floor first.
- Remind patient to maintain a wide-based gait.
- Provide a clear pathway while the patient is walking. Teach patient to avoid crowds, scatter rugs, uneven surfaces, fast turns, narrow doorways, and obstructions.
- Encourage patient to perform ROM exercises daily and to exercise for flexibility, strength, gait, and balance. Emphasize that routine exercises, along with prescribed medications, may prevent or delay disability.
- Encourage patient not to hurry or rush because this may precipitate falls. Slowness of gait and inability to get to the bathroom fast enough may cause

incontinence. Encourage males to keep urinal at the bedside. A commode at the bedside may be helpful for females.

- For other interventions, see **High risk for trauma** in "General Care of Patients with Neurologic Disorders," p. 298.

**Health-seeking behaviors:** Methods for overcoming difficulty initiating movement

*Desired outcome:* Following instruction, patient demonstrates measures that enhance the ability to initiate desired movement.

- Teach patient that rocking from side to side may help initiate leg movement. Marching in place a few steps before resuming forward motion also may be helpful. If the patient's feet remain "glued" to the floor despite these measures, suggest that he or she think of something else for a few moments and then try again.
- Teach patients to get out of a chair by getting to the edge of the seat, placing their hands on the arm supports, bending forward slightly, moving their feet back, and then rhythmically rocking in the chair a few times before trying to get up. Advise patients to sit in chairs with backs and arms and to purchase elevated toilet seats or sidebars in the bathroom to assist with rising and prevent falls.
- "Freezing" is variable and can fluctuate with stress or the patient's emotional state. Teach patients and significant others to recognize situations that can cause freezing episodes so that they can anticipate and plan to avoid them. Attempting two movements simultaneously, such as trying to change direction quickly while walking, can cause freezing. Distracting environmental, visual, or auditory stimuli also can precipitate a freezing episode. Doorways; narrow passages; or a change in floor color, texture, or slope pose problems for many patients.

**Knowledge deficit:** Side effects of and precautionary measures for taking anti-Parkinson medications

*Desired outcome:* Following instruction and before hospital discharge, patient and significant others verbalize knowledge about the side effects of and necessary precautionary measures for taking anti-Parkinson medications.

---

**Note:** Teach patient and significant others to report adverse side effects promptly because many side effects are dose-related and can be controlled by an adjustment in the dosage.

---

### Side effects common to most anti-Parkinson medications

- Stress the importance of taking medication on schedule and not forgetting a dose. Missing a dose may adversely affect mobility. Patient and physician can adjust the dose schedule so that the medication peaks at mealtime or times when patient needs mobility most.
- Teach patient to take medications with meals to decrease the potential for nausea and stomach upset. Encourage the patient with anorexia to eat frequent, small nutritious snacks and meals.
- Advise patients to counteract orthostatic hypotension by making position changes slowly and in stages. Teach patient to dangle legs a few minutes before standing. Antiembolism hose may help some patients. Encourage male patients to urinate from a sitting rather than standing position if possible. Report dizziness to physician.
- To lessen dry mouth and maintain the integrity of the oral mucous membrane, teach patient to use sugarless chewing gum or hard candy, frequent mouth rinses with water, or artificial saliva products.
- Advise patient to report any urinary hesistancy or incontinence because this may signal urinary retention. Individuals taking anticholinergics may find that voiding before taking the medication relieves this problem. See "Urinary Retention," p. 165, for additional measures.

- Constipation is a common problem with these medications. For interventions, see **Constipation,** p. 716, in Appendix One, "Caring for Patients on Prolonged Bed Rest."
- Many of these drugs can cause or aggravate mental status changes such as confusion, mental slowness or dullness, and even agitation, paranoia, and hallucinations. Teach patient to report these signs to the physician promptly for possible dose adjustment.
- For patient with blurred vision, orient to surroundings, identify self when entering the room, keep walkways unobstructed, and encourage patient to ask for assistance when ambulating.

### Side effects specific to levodopa

- Teach patient to avoid vitamin preparations or fortified cereals that contain pyridoxine (vitamin $B_6$), which reduces the effectiveness of levodopa. The physician may limit the patient's intake of foods high in pyridoxine, such as wheat germ, whole grain cereals, legumes, and liver.
- Teach patient that a dietary intake high in protein may interfere with the effectiveness of levodopa. While the diet should meet the Recommended Daily Allowance of protein, the patient should avoid excessive amounts of meat, eggs, dairy products, and legumes.
- Instruct patient to report muscle twitching or spasmodic winking because these are early signs of overdose.
- Abnormal involuntary movements, such as facial grimacing and tongue protusion, signal that an adjustment in dose may be needed. The physician may prescribe a reduced dose, redistribution throughout the day, or a medically supervised drug holiday.
- Explain signs and symptoms of Parkinsonian crisis. Emphasize the need for immediate medical intervention with this crisis because respiratory and cardiac support may be necessary. Teach patient that to avoid this crisis, it is necessary to take levodopa as scheduled and not to stop the medication abruptly. Teach significant others to place patient in a quiet, calm environment with subdued lighting until medical help arrives if Parkinsonian crisis occurs.
- Explain the signs of the on-off response and the importance of seeking medical intervention should they occur. Titrating the dose, spacing the doses differently, using sustained-release forms of levodopa, and combining levodopa with other anti-Parkinson medications may be prescribed to counter the on-off effect. If these interventions are ineffective, a medically supervised drug holiday may be prescribed.
- Monitor for behavioral changes. Severe depression with suicidal overtones can be caused by this drug and should be reported immediately. The physician may prescribe a dose reduction or, if this is ineffective, a medically supervised drug holiday.
- Explain that the patient's medication may cause dark-colored urine and sweat.
- Caution patient to avoid alcohol because it impairs levodopa's effectiveness.
- Explain the importance of medical follow-up while taking this drug to monitor for such problems as increased intraocular pressure and changes in glucose control.

### Side effects specific to amantadine

- Teach patient that taking this drug earlier in the day may prevent insomnia.
- Teach patient and significant others to monitor for and report any SOB, peripheral edema, significant weight gain, or change in mental status because these signs often signal congestive heart failure.
- Instruct patient not to stop taking this medication abruptly because doing so may precipitate Parkinsonian crisis.
- A diffuse, rose-colored mottling of the skin, usually confined to the lower extremities, may develop. The condition may subside with continued therapy and will disappear in a few weeks to months after the drug is discon-

tinued. Exposure to cold or standing may make the color more prominent. Teach patient to report this condition if it occurs, but reassure him or her that the condition is more cosmetic than serious.

- Patients with a history of seizures may have an increase in the number of seizures. Instruct patient to monitor and promptly report to physician a loss of seizure control.
- Caution patient to avoid alcohol and CNS depressants because these agents potentiate the effects of amantadine.
- Explain that most side effects of amantadine are dose-related.

*Side effects specific to dopamine agonists*

- Caution patient to avoid alcohol when taking this medication because he or she will experience less tolerance.
- Bromocriptine can cause digital vasospasm. Teach patient to avoid exposure to cold and to report the onset of finger or toe pallor.

*Side effects specific to anticholinergic medications*

- Teach patient that this medication may decrease perspiration. Explain that patient should avoid strenuous exercise and keep cool during the summer to avoid heat stroke.
- Teach patient not to stop taking this medication abruptly because doing so can result in Parkinsonian crisis.
- Teach patient to monitor for tachycardia or palpitation and to report either condition.

*Side effects specific to selegiline hydrochloride (Eldepryl)*

- Stress the importance of taking this medication only in the prescribed dose. Selegiline is a selective MAO type B inhibitor and in the recommended dose of ≤10 mg/day does not cause the hypertensive crisis that can occur when tyramine-containing foods (e.g., cheese, red wine, beer, and yogurt) are eaten. Dosages >10 mg/day may result in hypertension if these foods are eaten. Usually, dietary modifications to reduce intake of tyramine-containing foods are recommended, but they are not imperative.
- Avoidance of meperidine and other opioids is suggested. At recommended doses, no drug interactions have been noted. However, fatal drug interactions have occurred with patients taking other nonselective MAO inhibitors and could conceivably occur if higher-than-recommended doses were taken.
- Teach patient that taking the drug earlier in the day may prevent insomnia.

**Health-seeking behaviors:** Facial and tongue exercises that enhance verbal communication and help prevent choking

*Desired outcome:* Following the demonstration and within the 24-h period before hospital discharge, patient demonstrates facial and tongue exercises and states the rationale for their use.

- Explain to patient that special exercises can help strengthen and control facial and tongue muscles, which in turn will improve verbal communication and help prevent choking. Emphasize that routine exercises of the facial and tongue muscles, along with the prescribed medications, may prevent or delay disability.
- Teach the following exercises, and have patient return the demonstration: Hold a sound for 5 seconds, sing the scale, read aloud, and extend the tongue and try to touch the chin, nose, and cheek. Encourage patient to practice increasing voice volume.
- Provide a written handout that lists and describes the preceding exercises. Encourage patient to perform them hourly while awake.
- Teach patient the importance of stating feelings verbally because monotone speech and lack of facial expression impede nonverbal communication.

**Knowledge deficit:** Adrenal brain graft surgery

*Desired outcome:* Before the procedure, patient verbalizes accurate information about adrenal brain graft surgery.

- Determine patient's level of understanding of the procedure. As indicated, explain that the surgery involves grafting of one of the patient's own adrenal medullary glands to the caudate nucleus of the brain. The medullary portion of the adrenal gland produces dopamine for the peripheral nervous system. When grafted, the adrenal medullary gland may continue to produce dopamine in the CNS, thereby reducing or eliminating Parkinson's disease symptoms or the need for medication. The graft involves three surgeries: (1) stereotaxic localization of the caudate nucleus, (2) craniotomy, and (3) laparotomy to obtain the adrenal gland, which is positioned atop the kidney.

- Explain that the patient may have to undergo laboratory tests and CT scan to determine if both adrenal glands are normal, because the unharvested gland will have to compensate for both.
- Also explain that the patient may undergo cerebral blood flow tests (see discussions of "Digital Subtractive Angiography," and "Cerebral Angiography," p. 314) to evaluate perfusion of brain tissue and thus ensure adequate oxygenation and nutrients for healing. In addition, the patient may require several LPs to obtain CSF for testing levels of monoamine, a metabolite of dopamine. The comparison of serial postoperative levels to baseline levels will give an indication of graft viability.
- Teach patient how to splint the laparotomy site to reduce pain. Inform the patient that the wound will be monitored at scheduled intervals for signs of bleeding. Purplish coloration of the flank may signal retroperitoneal hematoma.
- The patient will be monitored after surgery for endocrine effects that signal nonfunctioning of the remaining adrenal gland, including hypoglycemia (see p. 373), hyperkalemia (see p. 134), and hypervolemia (see p. 132). Teach patient to report headache, irritability, weakness, thirst, nausea, anorexia, or intractable abdominal pain (also see "Addison's Disease," p. 338, for related nursing diagnoses).
- For additional interventions see "Brain Tumors" for **Knowledge deficit:** Craniotomy procedure, p. 263.

---

**Note:**   See "General Care of Patients with Neurologic Disorders" for **Impaired corneal tissue integrity,** p. 300; **Altered nutrition,** p. 300; **High risk for fluid volume deficit,** p. 301; **High risk for aspiration,** p. 302; **Self-care deficit,** p. 302; **Impaired verbal communication,** p. 304; **Constipation,** p. 305; **Impaired swallowing,** p. 308; and **Knowledge deficit:** Neurologic diagnostic tests, p. 311. For patients with varying degrees of immobility, refer to p. 687, related nursing diagnoses in "Pressure Ulcers," and Appendix One, "Caring for Patients on Prolonged Bed Rest," p. 711. For patients undergoing surgery see Appendix One, "Caring for Preoperative and Postoperative Patients," p. 693. Also see Appendix One, "Caring for Patients with Cancer and Other Life-Disrupting Illnesses," p. 753, for psychosocial nursing diagnoses and interventions for patients and significant others as appropriate.

---

## PATIENT-FAMILY TEACHING AND DISCHARGE PLANNING

Give patient and significant others verbal and written information about the following:

- Referrals to community resources, such as local and national Parkinson's Society chapters, public health nurse, visiting nurses association, community support groups, social workers, psychologic therapy, vocational rehabilitation agency, home health agencies, and extended and skilled care facilities. Provide the following addresses: American Parkinson Disease Association, 116 John Street, New York, NY 10038, (212)-732-9550 or (800)-223-APDA; United Parkinson's Foundation, 360 West Superior Street, Chicago, IL 60610, (312)-664-2344; Parkinson's Disease Foundation, Inc, 640 West 168th Street, New York, NY 10032, (212)-923-4700 or (800)-457-6676; Parkinson's Education Program, 3900 Birch Street, #105, Newport Beach, CA 92660, (800)-344-7872; and National Parkinson Foundation, Inc, 1501 NW 9th Avenue, Miami, FL 33136, in Florida call (800)-433-7022, all other states call (800)-327-4545.

- Related safety measures for patients with bradykinesis, muscle rigidity, and tremors.
- Emphasis that disability may be prevented or delayed through exercises and medications.
- Techniques for unlocking a position (see p. 209).
- Evaluation of home environment and tips for home accident prevention.
- Measures to prevent or lessen postural hypotension.
- Signs and symptoms of Parkinsonian crisis (see p. 204) and the need for immediate medical attention.
- For other interventions, see Patient-Family Teaching and Discharge Planning (third through tenth entries only) in "Multiple Sclerosis," p. 187.

# Alzheimer's disease

Alzheimer's disease is a progressive disorder of the brain characterized by changes and degeneration of the cerebral cortical nerve cells and nerve endings, resulting in abnormal neurofibrillary tangles and neuritic plaques that affect nerve conduction between cells. This process causes irreversible impairment of memory and deterioration of intellectual functions. Although the cause is unknown, aluminum poisoning, viruses, autoimmune disease, genetics, and neurotransmitter deficiency are possible causes, of which the last two are considered the most probable. Genetics as a factor seems to be more strongly linked if there is a younger age at the time of onset. The primary neurotransmitter that appears to be deficient is acetylcholine. Neurotransmitters such as somatostatin, norepinephrine, serotonin, and dopamine also may be reduced, but to a lesser degree. The primary risk factor for Alzheimer's disease is age. Onset is insidious, and it can strike individuals as young as 40 years of age. The disease progresses to total disability and eventually results in death from problems such as infection or aspiration, usually within 3-15 years.

## ASSESSMENT

The appearance and severity of signs and symptoms vary from individual to individual. Alzheimer's disease is characterized by progressive memory failure, intellectual deterioration, and personality change. It is classified into four stages: early, middle, late, and terminal, depending on the patient's degree of impairment. Initial indicators are mild, but short-term memory loss is a cardinal early sign. It may take several years before a definite diagnosis can be made. Often a diagnosis is not made until the middle stage, when the patient is having trouble recognizing objects or things, carrying out previously performed skills or activities, and/or communicating. By the late stage, memory and intellectual ability are absent. The terminal stage finds the individual in both a mental and physical vegetative condition.

**Memory:**   Initially, memory loss is slight, usually consisting of inability to retain recently acquired information. The individual may lose things and forget dates. The individual also may forget how to use common objects and tools, while retaining the power and coordination necessary for performing these activities. Long-term memory eventually is lost. The individual becomes lost in the home or other familiar surroundings. Gradually he or she loses the ability to recognize or name common objects and familiar people, including members of the immediate family.

**Cognitive process:**   The individual demonstrates increasing inability to think through problems, poor decision-making ability, shortened attention span, lack of insight, inability to perform arithmetic calculations, and loss of reading and writing capabilities. Gradually the ability to manage familiar activities, such as shopping or cooking, fails. The individual will become hesitant and reluctant to carry out minor and familiar tasks. As the ability to reason and abstract declines, the individual fails to recognize unsafe behaviors, resulting in a potential for injury. Hallucinations often occur due to misperception of the environment. There is increasing difficulty following even simple two- or three-step instructions. Eventually there is a total loss of intellectual ability and comprehension and an inability to participate in any activities. In the last stages, there may be instinctual and emotional awareness of family voices, touching, or presence, but there is no intellectual or conscious awareness or conscious interaction with the environment.

**Personality changes:**   The realization that memory and intellect are deteriorating may result in depression, frustration, bitterness, anxiety, and apathy. Difficulty with tasks that are beyond the individual's capacity leads to easy frustration. As insight declines, depression becomes less of a problem. There is often emotional lability, panic, fear, bewilderment, and perplexity. As awareness of the environment declines, apathy may become more prominent. Symptoms of paranoia, delusion, agitation, and hallucination may appear, resulting in suspiciousness and accusing others of stealing things that have been misplaced. Previous psychotic traits are exaggerated. As the ability to communicate lessens and the world becomes more frightening, the potential for violence and agitation increases. The patient may have catastrophic reactions and emotional outbursts when faced with a complex task.

**Social behavior:**   Decreased ability to handle social interaction, loss of social graces, loss of inhibitions, helplessness, dependency.

**Communication patterns:**   Difficulty finding words, loss of spontaneity in speech, inability to express thoughts, incoherent speech. The individual gradually loses all language ability and becomes unable to communicate other than with such behaviors as yelling, noisiness, or striking out. Eventually, this limited ability may be lost and he or she may be able only to grunt or express pain by grimacing.

**Sleep pattern:**   Restlessness, pacing, and wandering occur. Sleep/wake cycles are maintained, but generally there is decreased need for sleep. Nocturnal awakenings and reversals of normal sleep patterns are common. Toward the final stages, the individual often sleeps excessively.

**Self-care:**   Progressive neglect of routine tasks and personal hygiene; weight loss owing to refusal to eat and lack of awareness of the importance of nutrition; increasing inability to dress, bathe, toilet, and feed self or recognize where to urinate or defecate. Eventually the individual becomes totally dependent on others for all self-care activities.

**Mobility/posture:**   Stooped and shuffling gait; progressive balance and coordination problems; falling; inability to walk and use arms, hands, and legs for purposeful movement. The individual becomes bedridden. Joint contractures and muscle rigidity are common in the final stages.

**Other:**   In the last stages of the disease, myoclonus and seizures can occur. Spontaneous involuntary movement occurs, but the ability to open the eyes and track is maintained. Brain stem reflexes are present, and grasping, snout (evidenced by tapping the nose, which results in a marked facial grimace), and sucking reflexes can be elicited. Control of sphincter muscles is gone, and the individual may be incontinent of stool and urine. Chewing and swallowing incoordination develop, and death usually occurs as a result of aspiration pneumonia.

## DIAGNOSTIC TESTS

Many disorders that can cause a progressive dementia syndrome (e.g., head injuries, brain tumors, depression, arteriosclerosis, drug toxicity, metabolic disorders, and alcoholism) need to be ruled out. This is especially important because some dementias are reversible. The only definitive test for Alzheimer's is the brain biopsy, but usually this is done only post mortem. The diagnosis usually is made on the basis of the neurologic and mental status examination and after other causes have been ruled out.

**Mental status examination:** To test orientation, memory, calculation, abstraction, judgment, and mood.

**Neurologic examination:** Indicators that may signal Alzheimer's disease include release signs, such as snout, grasp, and sucking reflexes; olfactory deficits; impaired stereognosis (inability to recognize the touch or smell of a familiar object when placed in the hand); short-stepped, bradykinetic gait; tremor; and abnormalities on cerebellar testing.

**Positron emission tomography (PET):** May show lower cerebral cortex metabolic rates for glucose, even in the early stages of the disease.

**CT scan:** May reveal brain atrophy and symmetrical bilateral ventricular enlargement, which help support the diagnosis. It also helps rule out other neurologic problems, particularly mass lesions.

**MRI:** May reveal brain atrophy and symmetrical bilateral ventricular enlargement, which help support the diagnosis. Because of its ability to detect both biochemical and anatomic changes, this test may identify Alzheimer's disease at a very early stage.

**EEG:** May reveal generalized slowed brainwave activity and reduced voltage, which support the diagnosis.

**Brain biopsy:** Will demonstrate the presence of neurofibrillary tangles and neuritic plaques.

**In addition:** The following tests may be performed to rule out other causes of dementia: skull and chest x-rays, lumbar puncture (LP), serum tests (e.g., liver, thyroid, syphillis), urinalysis, arteriograms, drug screen, and brain scan.

---

**Note:** See "General Care of Patients with Neurological Disorders," **Knowledge deficit,** p. 311, for care considerations for patients undergoing PET, MRI, CT scan, and EEG.

---

## COLLABORATIVE MANAGEMENT

Generally, treatment is supportive only. No recognized treatment or cure exists at this time.

**Pharmacotherapy:** Medications, if prescribed, are used to treat symptoms or behavioral manifestations. These include:

*Early stage*

*Ergoloid mesylate:* Sometimes shown to be effective in improving cognitive performance in early stages of dementia. However, its effect is only temporary and declines as the disease advances. Side effects include postural hypotension, transient nausea, and GI disturbances.

*Tricyclic or other antidepressants (e.g., desipramine, trazodone, nortriptyline, amitriptyline):* To relieve depression and elevate mood. Side effects include drowsiness, dizziness, orthostatic hypotension, urinary retention, and lowered seizure threshold.

*Stimulants (e.g., methylphenidate, dextroamphetamine):* May be given for loss of spontaneity or inattention.

*Experimental drugs:* May be used in an attempt to improve cognitive function on a temporary basis. Cholinergic therapy aims to correct the acetylcholine deficiency in the brain. Various drugs include choline derivative (e.g., choline chloride, lecithin), anticholinesterase inhibitor (e.g., physostigmine and tetrahydroaminoacridine), and cholinergic receptor stimulants (e.g., bethanechol). Intrathecal infusion of medication directly into the CSF *via* continuous infusion pumps also is being tried. Other experimental drug therapy includes dopamine precursors, opioid antagonists (e.g., naloxone), serotonin precursors, neuropeptides, and transcerebral vasodilators (e.g., papaverine, cyclandelate, isoxsuprine, and dihydroergotoxine).

*Middle stage*
***Antipsychotic agents (e.g., haloperidol):***   Used for combative or extremely agitated patients.
***Tranquilizers or sedatives (e.g., chloral hydrate, dipenhydramine, triazolam, and oxazepam):***   Used to control hyperactivity, restlessness, and sleep disturbances. Lorazepam and alpraxolam may be used for agitation.
*Late stage*
***Antiepilepsy drugs (e.g., phenytoin):***   To control seizures.
***Laxatives and stool softeners (e.g., psyllium, docusate):***   For constipation.
*Terminal stage*
***Oral morphine:***   Small doses may be given for patients who have developed hypersensitivity to touch or restlessness.
***Atropine or scopolomine:***   May be given to decrease respiratory secretions and the need for frequent, uncomfortable suctioning.
**Diet:**   A high-fiber diet may be given to prevent constipation. For restless, hyperactive patients, a high-calorie diet or supplements may be prescribed. Caffeine is avoided because of its stimulating effect. In later stages, tube feedings may be an option for some patients. Although vitamin (e.g., niacin, $B_{12}$) folate, zinc and lecithin treatments have not been proven effective in treating Alzheimer's disease, they are relatively harmless and the family may find some consolation in their use.
**Counseling or psychotherapy:**   Counseling focus generally is on the significant others to help them deal with the depression, grief, guilt, and emotions caused by the patient's progressive disability and behavior. In all but the early stages, Alzheimer patients quickly lose the insight and intellectual ability that would make counseling beneficial to them.

## NURSING DIAGNOSES AND INTERVENTIONS

**High risk for trauma** related to lack of awareness of environmental hazards secondary to cognitive deficit
***Desired outcomes:***   Patient is free of symptoms of physical trauma. At least 24 h before patient's hospital discharge, significant others identify and plan to eliminate or control potentially dangerous factors in the patient's home environment.

- Orient patient to new surroundings. Reorient as needed. Keep necessary items, including water, telephone, and call light, within easy reach. Assess patient's ability to use these items. Keep bed in its lowest position. Side rail position (up or down) will vary with the patient. The patient may be at risk of falling from climbing over side rails.
- Maintain an uncluttered environment to minimize the risk of environmental confusion and tripping. Ensure adequate lighting to help prevent falls in the dark.
- Prevent exposure to hot food or equipment that can burn the skin. Discourage use of heating pads. Check temperature of heating device and bath water before patient is exposed to them.
- Encourage patient to use low-heeled, nonskid shoes for walking. Teach the use of wide-based gait to give unsteady patients a broader base of support. Assess patient for the presence of ataxia, and assist with walking as necessary. Use gestures or turn patient's body in the direction he or she is to go. Canes and walkers may be too complicated for patients with Alzheimer's disease.
- Request that significant others assist with watching restless patients. Provide attendant care if necessary. Avoid restraining patient because this usually increases agitation. If restraints must be used, reassure patient that he or she is not being punished, that you are trying to help him or her regain control, and the restraints will be removed when the staff is certain the patient will not cause self-injury. **Note:** For many persons with Alzheimer's disease, walking will reduce agitation.

- Check patient at frequent intervals. If necessary, move patient closer to the nursing station, away from stairways or unit exits, or seat patient in a chair at the nursing station. Consider obtaining a picture of the patient to assist in a search if necessary.
- Watch for nonverbal clues of pain or distress, such as restlessness, wincing, wrinkled brow, cautious breathing, rapid or shallow breathing, poor appetite, or crying. Report significant findings.
- Try to make tubes as unobtrusive as possible to prevent their removal. Place IV tubing high on the dominant arm. Dress patient in a long-sleeved gown with a cuff, with IV tubing going up the arm and out the neck. Place binders over the dressing to help prevent picking. Position hand splints to eliminate pincer grasp.

## Suggestions for home safety

- Encourage significant others to evaluate the home environment carefully for potential safety hazards. Caution them to remove harmful objects (e.g., matches and scissors) from the bedside, and store medications and chemicals (e.g., insect spray, cleaning supplies, lighter fluid) in locked cabinets to prevent accidental ingestion, because these patients tend to put objects in their mouths. Remove plants that are toxic, plastic fruit, and toiletries because patient may attempt to eat them. The temperature of the home hot water heater should be turned down to prevent accidental scalding. Lock up hazardous power tools, lawn mowers, or kitchen appliances. Place gates or guard rails on porches as needed. Safety plugs should be placed in electrical outlets. Hand rails and grab bars also may be helpful. Remind significant others to check the house carefully before leaving because the patient may leave the stove on or water running. It may be necessary to remove knobs from stove burners and the oven.
- Advise significant others to dress these individuals according to the physical environment and individual need. These patients may not know or be able to communicate if they are too cold or too warm.
- Advise significant others to keep the patient's home environment simple and familiar. Rearranging furniture can increase the patient's confusion and potential for falls. Encourage use of nightlights in patient's home.
- If the patient tends to wander, encourage significant others to have an identification bracelet made with patient's name, phone number, and diagnosis. An identifying label can be sewn into clothes. Alert neighbors and local police to call if they notice the patient wandering. Keep a good current picture of patient available to help in searching in case he or she becomes lost. Covering door handles with cloth hangings or pictures may be sufficient to prevent patient from exiting. Locks on doors to keep patient inside may be necessary but should not require a key, because this may hamper escape in the case of a fire. Door or exit alarms can be installed on home doors. Daily walks or exercise tend to decrease the amount of wandering.
- Caution significant others that patients who are disoriented should be allowed to smoke only while being observed. Advise them to get a smoke detector and take control of matches.
- Advise significant others that patient should be restricted from driving. Document advisement. Significant others can inform the state automobile licensing bureau about the need for retesting to take the burden of restriction off the family. Suggest that significant others hide car keys or disable the car if necessary to prevent patient from driving.

**Altered nutrition:**   Less than body requirements, related to decreased intake secondary to cognitive and motor deficit; and to increased nutritional needs secondary to constant pacing and restlessness
*Desired outcome:*   Patient maintains baseline body weight.

- Because patient may not eat food that does not look familiar or is on hospital plates, request that significant others assist with menu planning or bring in meals and dishes the patient recognizes. These persons often are over-

whelmed with choices and need help with menu selection.
- When patient is no longer able to handle a fork, knife, and spoon, cut up food for patient and/or provide finger foods.
- For the patient who is in constant motion, provide small snacks around the clock and a high-calorie diet unless contraindicated.
- Try to limit the number of foods on the plate or serve foods in courses because too many foods can be overwhelming for patient.
- If patient clenches teeth and refuses to eat, stimulate the oral suck reflex by stroking the cheeks or stimulating the mouth with a spoon. Use patient's forgetfulness to advantage by taking a short break from feeding and returning in a few moments when patient may be more receptive.
- Provide privacy. Accept eating with hands and whimsical food mixtures. Tolerate spills without scolding, and obtain nonspill cups when needed. Be creative. A punch card or ticket so that the patient can "pay for the meal" may persuade some to eat.
- For other interventions, see **Altered nutrition** in "General Care of Patients with Neurologic Disorders," p. 300.

**Altered urinary elimination** related to urinating in inappropriate places or incontinence secondary to cognitive deficit
*Desired outcome:* Patient urinates in the toilet stool (commode) on an ongoing basis.
- Make sure patient knows location of the bathroom. If possible, locate patient within sight of the bathroom, ensure a clear path, and provide adequate light at night. Take patient to the bathroom q1-2h; avoid a sense of hurry. Restrict fluids in the evenings to minimize the risk of enuresis.
- Identify bathroom door with a picture of a toilet to help patient locate the bathroom.
- Assess for nonverbal clues such as restlessness or holding self, which can signal the need to void.
- As appropriate, provide disposable underpants. Indwelling and external catheters may increase confusion. Male patients may be able to accept condom catheters to help manage incontinence.
- Incontinence may signal a urinary tract infection (UTI). Investigate the cause of the incontinence to see whether it is treatable.
- After patient has voided, assess him or her for cleanliness and dryness of the perianal area; intervene accordingly to help ensure skin integrity.

**Bowel incontinence** or defecating in inappropriate places, related to inability to find bathroom or decreased awareness or loss of sphincter control secondary to cognitive deficit
*Desired outcome:* Following intervention(s), patient has no or fewer episodes of bowel incontinence.
- Show patient location of the bathroom. Identify the bathroom door with a picture of a toilet to help patient locate the bathroom.
- Assess patient's normal bowel habits. Take patient to the bathroom at the time of day patient normally has a bowel movement (for example, after meals).
- Evaluate patient for nonverbal indications of the need to eliminate wastes, such as restlessness, picking at clothes, facial expressions or grunting sounds indicative of bearing down, or the passing of flatus.
- As appropriate, provide disposable underpants.
- After bowel elimination, assess patient for cleanliness of perianal area to maintain skin integrity. The patient may forget to wipe the perianal area or clean the area only partially.
- For other suggestions, see **Constipation,** p. 716, in Appendix One, "Caring for Patients on Prolonged Bed Rest."

**Self-care deficit** related to memory loss and coordination problems secondary to cognitive and motor deficits

*Desired outcome:* On an ongoing basis, patient's physical needs are met by self, staff, or significant others.

- Provide care for the totally dependent patient, and assist those who are not totally dependent. Allow ample time to perform activities, encouraging patient's independence. Ask patient to perform only one task at a time; go through each step separately. Do not hurry patient. Involve significant others with care activities if they wish to be involved. Ask them when patient normally bathes at home, and establish this as part of a daily routine. Provide a consistent caregiver. Use simple visual and verbal cues and gestures for self-care.
- Place a stool in the shower if sitting will enhance self-care. Use a hand-held shower head to prevent water from hitting patient's head, which can be frightening.
- To facilitate dressing and undressing, encourage significant others or patient to buy shoes without laces and clothing that is loose-fitting or has snaps, Velcro closures, or elastic waistbands. Offer clothing items one at a time, sequentially. Allow agitated patients for whom hygiene is not a problem to sleep in their shoes and clothing, and attempt a clothes change later.
- Provide a commode chair or elevated toilet seat as needed.
- If the patient becomes combative or agitated, postpone ADL and try again a short time later. The patient may forget the reason for the resistance.

**Sensory/perceptual alterations** related to impaired sensory reception, transmission, integration, and evaluation secondary to degeneration of neuronal functioning

*Desired outcome:* Following the intervention(s) and on an ongoing basis, patient interacts appropriately with the environment.

- Monitor for and record short-term memory deficit. Once a level of comprehension has been determined, avoid repeatedly asking if patient knows who and where he/she is and what time it is, because this may cause frustration and agitation. At frequent intervals, orient patient to reality, time, and place in the following ways: Call patient by name; keep clocks and calendars in the room; inform patient of the day and time; correct patient gently; minimize disturbing noise; ensure adequate lighting to prevent shadow formation; request that significant others bring in familiar objects and family pictures; speak with patient about his or her interests, both present and past; allow patient to reminisce; ensure that staff members show name tags and identify themselves; explain upcoming events; and set up regular schedules for hygiene, eating, and waste elimination.
- Approach patient in a calm, slow, relaxed, nonthreatening, friendly manner. Treat patient with dignity and respect. Remain calm and patient when repeating questions. Be nonjudgmental and objective, even when confronted with inappropriate behaviors.
- Keep patient's personal belongings where they can be used and seen.
- Evaluate patient's cognitive impairment for any relation to medication use, such as sedatives or tranquilizers. If found, inform physician.
- Provide a quiet, calm, pleasant environment. Simple, minimally decorated rooms are best. The patient may not recognize self in a mirror. Cover or remove artwork and mirrors if patient misinterprets images (e.g., wallpaper patterns may be disturbing to some patients). Turning off the public address system in the patient's room may prevent patient stimulation and misinterpretation of sound.
- Provide stimulation that the patient can handle. Soft music may be appropriate, but television might be too overwhelming because the images change quickly and may be misperceived.
- Limit visitors as appropriate because crowds and complex social interaction often are beyond the patient's ability to tolerate.
- Check to ensure that persons who need eyeglasses or hearing aids wear them

as appropriate. Eyeglasses should be clean and with a current prescription; hearing aids should be functioning with working batteries.
- If patient becomes agitated, reduce environmental stimuli. Use a soft, reassuring voice and gentle touch. Avoid quick, unexpected movements.

**Impaired verbal communication** related to aphasia and altered sensory reception, transmission, and integration secondary to cognitive deficits

***Desired outcome:*** Following the intervention(s), patient communicates needs to staff, follows instructions, and answers questions.

- Provide a supportive and relaxed environment for patients who are unable to form words or sentences or who are unable to speak clearly or appropriately. Acknowledge patient's frustration about the inability to communicate. Maintain a calm, positive attitude; eliminate distracting noises, such as radio or television. Observe for nonverbal communication cues, such as gestures. Consider pain as a possible cause of restlessness, moaning, guarding, and yelling; provide analgesia as needed. Avoid meperidine, if possible, because of its common side effect of restlessness. Anticipate patient's needs.
- Explain activities in short, easily understood sentences. Use simple gestures, point to objects, or use demonstration if possible. When giving directions, be sure to break tasks into small, understandable units, using simple terms. Ask patient to do only one task at a time. Give patient time to accomplish one task before progressing to the next.
- Be sure that you have the patient's attention. Repeat patient's name or gently touch patient to get his or her attention. Use touch to communicate if the patient is receptive to it. Speak slowly and calmly, using a clear, low-pitched voice. Use short, simple words and sentences, but speak as though patient understands you. Ask only one question at a time, and formulate questions that can be answered by "yes" or "no." Wait for a response. If patient does not respond (i.e., after 15 sec), repeat the question again, exactly as before, to help patient mentally process the question.
- Listen to and include patient in conversation.

**Anxiety** related to actual or perceived threats or changes (e.g., from bewildering hospital environment and multiple tests and procedures)

***Desired outcome:*** Within 1 h of intervention, patient's anxiety is absent or reduced as evidenced by HR ≤100 bpm, RR ≤20 breaths/min with normal depth and pattern, and an absence of or decrease in irritability and restlessness.

- Remain calm with patient. Use slow, deliberate gestures. Patients with Alzheimer's disease frequently mirror the emotions of others. Use a low, soothing voice and a gentle touch. The tone of voice is often more important than the actual words used.
- Provide time for patient to verbalize feelings of fear, concern, and anxiety. Listen with regard. Patients with Alzheimer's disease often have trouble finding the correct words and may not be capable of stringing more than a few words together. Provide calm and realistic assurance, and stay with patient during periods of acute anxiety.
- To help reduce anxiety and establish ongoing rapport, provide patient with a consistent caregiver. Avoid changing patient's room.
- Patients who still have reading capability may find reassurance with notes, orienting signs, or lists of names, phone numbers, or activities (e.g., the phone numbers of significant others or a note reminder of the reason they are in the hospital), which may reassure them that they are not lost or abandoned.
- Encourage significant others to bring in familiar items.
- Permit patient to hoard inanimate objects because this may provide the individual with a sense of security. Enable patients to keep personal belongings, such as purses or wallets, in bed with them.
- Assist with finding misplaced items. Label drawers and belongings.
- Refrain from forcing activities or giving patient too many choices.

- Encourage ambulation. Often, walking helps reduce anxiety and agitation.
- Encourage unlimited visiting hours for familiar significant others.
- Encourage patient to avoid caffeine, which has a stimulating effect.

**High risk for violence** related to irritability, frustration, and disorientation secondary to degeneration of cognitive thinking

***Desired outcome:*** Patient demonstrates control of his or her behavior with absence of violence.

- Ask caregiver how patient usually acts when tired or overwhelmed, and ask what caregiver does to calm patient. Document this information.
- Monitor patient for signs of increasing anxiety, fright, or panic (e.g., inability to verbalize feelings, suspiciousness of others, fear of others or self, irritability, and agitation), which can precede a violent act.
- Encourage verbalization of feelings rather than suppression because frustration can lead to violence. Praise efforts at self-control.
- Try to identify what is immediately distressing to patient (e.g., full bladder, catheter, pain), and attempt to remedy it. Respond to the emotion. Respond to the patient's questions in simple, concrete replies that relate directly to the patient's questions, frustrations, or anger. Avoid making promises that cannot reasonably be kept. Do not confront or argue with patient and become authoritarian. If the situation cannot be remedied by calming the patient, use distraction and try to defuse the situation by redirecting attention away from the source of irritation. Talk about other topics, and vary the topics periodically. Provide diversional activities, offer juice, or walk with patient until the agitation has lessened. A request for patient's help (e.g., with folding and unfolding towels, making a bed) may promote calm behavior by returning a sense of mastery or control.
- Remain calm and keep gestures slow and deliberate. Keep your hands open and below your waist where they can be seen. Approach patient slowly in a confident, relaxed, and open manner. Avoid sudden changes or surprises. Keep your voice low and soft, and smile. Humor and gentle laughter may help change the patient's mood. Some patients may respond positively to gentle touch.
- Reduce environmental stimuli, including people entering the room. Provide a private room if possible. Reduce noise level by turning the television volume down or off.
- Do not give routine care when patient is upset or agitated. Leave the room briefly, and return when the patient is calmer and more approachable. If the patient cannot be left alone, sit quietly with no talking except gentle reassurance. Use the patient's forgetfulness to your advantage.
- If patient is not combative unless approached, simply supervise from a safe distance. If you must approach patient, do so from the side rather than face-to-face. Stand off to one side and maintain distance of at least one arm's length from the patient.
- If patient is upset or agitated, avoid turning your back on patient. Avoid cornering patient or being cornered. Think of escape routes for yourself, and be alert to potential weapons patient may use. Get help; protect yourself.
- Never attempt to deal with a physically aggressive patient by yourself. If other interventions fail, use physical or chemical restraints as necessary for your own or patient's safety.
- Document the signs and symptoms, precipitating factor, time of onset, duration, and successful interventions. Prevent further episodes by controlling precipitating stressors (e.g., controlling pain, simplifying schedule, limiting visitors).

**Sleep pattern disturbance** related to restlessness and disorientation secondary to cognitive deficits

***Desired outcome:*** Following the intervention(s), patient sleeps at least 6 h per night, or an amount of time appropriate for the patient.

- Space activities with quiet periods so that patient does not become excessively tired and require a daytime nap.
- Prevent patients from falling asleep during the day through such measures as periodic short walks, planned activities, and keeping them upright as much as possible. **Note:** If patient does nap during the day but also sleeps well at night, there is no need to impose a specific sleep schedule.
- Patients who nap should do so in an easy chair, if possible, rather than in bed. The easy chair may serve as a cue that their sleep is just a nap.
- Avoid continuous use of restraints because restraints often increase agitation and limit the patient's ability to rest.
- Adhere to regular bedtime schedules and rituals such as a bedtime snack. Keep the room lighted until the patient is ready for sleep. Provide soft music, and tell patient that it is time for sleep.
- Administer tranquilizers and sedatives as prescribed to facilitate sleeping.
- Avoid turning on overhead light at night, which may cue patient to think it is time to get up.

**Altered family processes** related to situational crisis (illness of family member)

*Desired outcome:*   Within the 24-h period before patient's hospital discharge, significant others verbalize knowledge of measures that will assist with coping for the care of the patient after hospital discharge.

- Encourage significant others to interpret patient's behavior as a reflection of the disease process rather than a willful act. Advise them that generally another illness, surgery, or disease process will exaggerate the patient's disorientation. Once these problems are corrected, the patient usually returns to his or her previous cognitive level.
- Encourage patient's major caregiver to have other significant others or hired help take care of patient regularly so that he or she can have scheduled respites. A neighbor looking in or a home-health aide on a part-time, overnight, or live-in basis is another option. Local day-care programs also are useful. If the patient is a veteran, he or she may be eligible for some respite programs offered by the Veterans Administration. Advise caregiver that some home health agencies or day-care programs have sliding payment scales for their services. Refer to community sources that supply equipment for home use. Encourage use of other support services, such as homemakers, choreworkers, home-delivered food, and volunteer drivers. Support significant others in asking for help.
- If significant other is unaccustomed to handling finances, refer him or her to a place where help with financial management is available. Often, patients with Alzheimer's disease lose the ability to manage finances and balance checkbooks and may give away money inappropriately. Eventually the patient's checkbook and credit cards will have to be taken away. Phone use may require monitoring because these patients cannot differentiate between local and long-distance calls. As appropriate, suggest that significant others post important phone numbers and secure long-distance numbers to help prevent excessively high phone bills.
- Encourage early financial planning, and suggest professional financial counseling. Families should locate and identify the patient's various assets, sources of income, and liabilities and make arrangements for their security and daily management.
- Encourage early family legal planning and consultation. This is especially important because an individual must have mental capacity and competence to sign documents. Legal planning may involve wills, intervivos trusts, subpayee assignment for social security, traditional and durable power of attorney, guardianship, and conservatorship. Advise family that some free legal services are available to the elderly in most areas.
- Explain to significant others that if patient refuses medication or is unable

to swallow pills, obtaining a liquid form of the drug or crushing the pills and mixing them with soft food may help.

- Some individuals with this disease go through a phase in which, because of increased motor activity and lessening social inhibitions, they have increased sexual demands. This may result in increased sexual encounters. Be sure the family is aware that this is a symptom of the disease process. Furthermore, the patient eventually will lose the ability to be intimate and tender. Sex will become a mindless act. Mates may feel rejected, frustrated, humiliated, or repulsed. Suggest that professional counseling be obtained to assist the patient's spouse or loved one in dealing with these feelings. Suggest that the use of gentle dissuasion or distraction may be effective with these patients. Remind patient that certain public behavior is unacceptable.
- Encourage caregivers to maintain their own friendships and attend social functions. The patient's embarrassing behaviors and the demands of giving care can lead to withdrawal from society.
- Encourage significant others to focus on specific problems as they occur and establish priorities. Help them develop a plan of care and schedule of daily activities.
- Encourage professional counseling and support so that significant others can work through such feelings as anger, guilt, embarrassment, and depression and develop effective coping strategies and mechanisms. Each new and subtle loss of patient function brings another round of grieving. Decisions about institutionalization and the extent of health-care measures also are emotionally difficult. Behaviors such as hoarding, unjust accusations, angry outbursts, and clinging can precipitate burnout in the caregiver. Caregivers and significant others must be reassessed continually for their ability to care for the patient at home.
- Encourage participation in local or national support groups, such as Alzheimer's Disease and Related Disorders Association (ADRDA).
- For other interventions, see **Altered family processes** in Appendix One, "Caring for Patients with Cancer and other Life-Disrupting Illnesses," p. 763.

---

**Note:** For patients experiencing seizures, see "Seizure Disorders," p. 288. See "General Care of Patients with Neurologic Disorders" for **High risk for fluid volume deficit,** p. 301, **High risk for aspiration** p. 302, **Impaired swallowing,** p. 308, and **Knowledge deficit:** Neurologic diagnostic tests, p. 311. For patients experiencing varying degrees of immobility, see related nursing diagnoses in "Pressure Ulcers," p. 687, and Appendix One, "Caring for Patients on Prolonged Bed Rest," p. 711. Also see Appendix One, "Caring for Patients with Cancer and Other Life-Disrupting Illnesses," p. 753, for psychosocial nursing diagnoses for patients and significant others, as appropriate.

---

## PATIENT-FAMILY TEACHING AND DISCHARGE PLANNING

The degree and scope of discharge teaching and planning will depend on the severity of the patient's condition. Give patient and significant others verbal and written information about the following, as appropriate:

- Referrals to community resources, local and national Alzheimer's disease chapters, public health nurse, visiting nurses association, community support groups, social workers, psychologic therapy, home health agencies, and extended and skilled care facilities. Provide the address and phone numbers of the ADRDA, 919 North Michigan Avenue, Suite 1000, Chicago, IL 60611, (800)-272-3900 or (312)-335-8700, and "Help Line" (708)-933-1000.
- Safety measures for preventing injury relative to cognitive deficits.

- Measures that assist in reorienting and communicating with patient in view of cognitive deficits.
- Importance of scheduled respites and involvement in support groups for significant others.
- Medications, including drug name, purpose, dosage, frequency, precautions, and potential side effects.
- Exercises that promote muscle strength and mobility; measures for preventing contractures and skin breakdown; transfer techniques and proper body mechanics; and use of assistive devices, if appropriate.
- Techniques for dealing with incontinence; indications of constipation or infection; implementation of bowel and bladder training programs; and indwelling catheter care, if appropriate.
- Indications of upper respiratory infection (URI) and measures that prevent regurgitation, aspiration, and infection.
- Techniques for encouraging adequate food and fluid intake and performance of ADL.
- Importance of seeking financial and legal counseling.

# Section Three:    Traumatic Disorders of the Nervous System

## Intervertebral disk disease

The intervertebral disk is a semifluid-filled fibrous capsule that facilitates movement of the spine and acts as a shock absorber. The ability of the disk to withstand stressors is not unlimited and diminishes with aging. Pressure on the disk eventually may force elastic material from the center of the disk, called the nucleus pulposus, to break or herniate through the fibrous rim of the disk. The rupture or bulging of an interverterbral disk causes its typical symptoms by pressing on and irritating the spinal nerve roots or spinal cord itself. Herniated nucleus pulposus usually is the result of injury or a series of insults to the vertebral column from lifting or twisting. When the disk ruptures without a known discrete injury, it is believed to be caused by degenerative changes. Deterioration can occur suddenly, or it may happen gradually, with symptoms appearing months or years after the initial injury. Almost all herniated disks occur in the lumbar spine, with 90% of the problems occurring at L–4-L–5 and L–5-S–1. Cervical disk problems most frequently occur at C–5-C–6 and C–6-C–7 and generally are caused by degenerative changes or trauma, such as whiplash or hyperextension. Thoracic disk problems are rare.

### ASSESSMENT
**General indicators:**    Onset can be sudden, with intense unilateral pain, or with pain that is dull, diffuse, deep, and aching. Symptoms vary according to the level of injury and nerves involved. Usually, pain is increased with movement or activities that increase intraabdominal or intrathoracic pressure, such as sneezing, coughing, and straining. Often pain is improved by lying down. Immediate medical attention is essential if there is any paralysis, extreme sensory loss, or altered bowel or bladder function.

**Cervical disk disease:**    Pain or numbness in the upper extremities, shoulders, thorax, occipital area, or back of the head or neck. Pain can radiate down the forearms and into the hands and fingers. Usually the neck has restricted mobility, and there can be cervical muscle spasm and loss of the normal cervical lordosis. The patient may have upper extremity muscle weakness with diminished biceps or triceps reflex.

**Lumbar disk disease:**   Pain in the lumbosacral area with possible radiculopathy (sciatica) to the buttock, down the posterior surface of the thigh and calf, and to the lateral border of the foot. Frequently there is altered mobility, as evidenced by decreased ability to stand upright, listing to one side, asymmetrical gait, limited ability to flex forward, and restricted side movement caused by pain and muscle spasms. The individual walks cautiously, bearing little weight on the affected side, and often finds sitting or climbing stairs particularly painful. Reflex muscle spasms can cause bulging of the back with concomitant flattening of the lumbar curve and possible scoliosis at the level of the affected disk. Usually, there is depression of the patellar and Achilles tendon reflexes.

**Physical assessment:**   Possible findings include depressed reflexes, muscle atrophy, paresthesias (described as "pins and needles"), or anesthesia (numbness) in the dermatome of the involved nerves. The following tests are two of several that are performed to confirm the presence of lumbar disk disease:

*Straight leg raise test:*   Examiner extends and raises patient's leg. The test is positive if patient has pain on the posterior aspect of the leg. People without injury usually can have a leg raised to 90 degrees without significant discomfort.

*Sciatic nerve test:*   Examiner extends and raises patient's leg until pain is elicited and then lowers the leg to a comfortable level. The examiner then dorsiflexes the foot to stretch the sciatic nerve. If this causes pain, the test is positive for sciatic nerve involvement.

**Risk factors:**   Repetitive bending or lifting involving a twisting motion, continuous vibration, smoking, poor physical condition, obesity, above average height, osteoporosis, prolonged sitting, depression, severe scoliosis, spondylolisthesis, or genetic predisposition.

## DIAGNOSTIC TESTS

**MRI:**   May reveal that the disk is impinging on the spinal cord or nerve root or related pathology, such as tumors or spondylosis.

**CT scan of the spine:**   May reveal disk protrusion/prolapse or related pathology, such as tumors, spondylosis, or spinal stenosis.

**Myelogram:**   May show characteristic deformity and filling defect or related pathology, such as tumors, spondylolisthesis, spondylosis, spinal stenosis, or Paget's disease. Generally this test is performed only if surgery is considered.

**X-ray of the spine:**   May show narrowing of the vertebral interspaces in affected areas, loss of curvature of the spine, and spondylosis (formation of bone spurs around vertebral joints).

**Diskography:**   Using fluoroscopy, contrast medium is injected into the disk space to identify degenerated or extruded disks.

**Electromyography (EMG):**   May show denervation patterns of specific nerve roots to indicate the level and site of injury.

---

**Note:**   See "General Care of Patients with Neurologic Disorders," **Knowledge deficit,** Neurologic diagnostic tests, p. 311, for care considerations for patients undergoing the following tests: MRI, CT scan, and myelography.

---

## COLLABORATIVE MANAGEMENT

**Bed rest:**   To limit motion of vertebral column, relieve nerve root compression, and enhance shrinkage of the disk.

**Bedboards under the mattress:**   To support normal spine curvature and minimize spinal flexion.

**Orthotics (e.g., splints, braces, girdles, and cervical collars):**   To limit motion of the vertebral column. Generally, long-term use of braces is discouraged because it prohibits development of necessary musculature.

**Pelvic/cervical skin traction:**   To reduce muscle spasm and distract vertebral bodies to reduce bulging or rupture of the disk. **Note:** There is some controversy regarding whether traction actually provides any therapeutic benefit. However, some individuals find that it increases comfort.

**Pelvic traction girdle:**   Device used in an attempt to widen the intervertebral space. The patient pulls the side handles in an axial direction to flex the pelvis. Alternatively, the handles can be attached to weights. There is also a gravity lumbar traction in which the patient in a chest harness is elevated slightly so that traction is applied *via* the patient's own weight.

**Other therapeutic modalities:**   Include thermotherapy, hydrotherapy, massage, diathermy/ultrasound electrotherapy, transcutaneous electrical nerve stimulation (TENS), dorsal column stimulation, and stress reduction techniques.

**Physical therapy and a graded exercise program:**   To strengthen the legs, back, and abdominal muscles and teach correct body mechanics. It is initiated once acute symptoms subside.

**Local injection of anesthetic or cortisone into paraspinal or paravertebral regions and epidural or subarachnoid spaces:**   To reduce pain and muscle spasms and increase function.

**Antiembolism hose:**   To prevent thrombophlebitis while the patient is on bed rest. Hose should be worn until the amount of time out of bed ambulating is equal to the amount of time spent in bed.

**Pharmacotherapy**

*Analgesics (e.g., aspirin, acetaminophen, and narcotics):*   Administer sufficient medication to achieve pain relief or adequate pain reduction. Narcotics generally are used for acute pain episodes. Because of the potential for narcotics abuse, individuals with chronic back pain are discharged with nonnarcotic analgesia.

*Muscle relaxants (e.g., carisoprodol, chlorzoxazone, cyclobenzaprine, metaxalone, methocarbamol, and diazepam):*   To reduce muscle spasm. Common side effects are drowsiness, fatigue, dizziness, dry mouth, and GI upset.

*Corticosteroids (e.g., dexamethasone):*   May be given for a short period of time to reduce cord edema, if present.

*Nonsteroidal antiinflammatory drugs:*   See Table 8-1, p. 519, for names and usual dosage.

*Stool softeners or laxatives (e.g., docusate):*   To prevent constipation or straining that would be painful.

---

**Note:**   Surgery is done without delay if signs of spinal cord compression are present, such as motor or sensory loss or loss of sphincter control. Otherwise, surgery is considered only after symptoms fail to respond to conservative therapy.

---

**Chemonucleolysis:**   Injection of enzymes (chymopapain, collagenase) directly into the disk has been used to dissolve fibrocartilage or collagen materials of the nucleus pulposus in an attempt to relieve pressure on the spinal cord or nerve roots. Chemonucleolysis provides pain relief in 50%-80% of patients but may take up to 3 months to do so. Fluoroscopy is used to confirm proper position of the needle. Because of the 1% incidence of allergic reaction and potential for severe anaphylaxis, chymopapain is injected in the operating room with an anesthesiologist or nurse anesthetist in attendance. Allergic reactions quickly can progress to laryngeal edema, laryngospasm, bronchospasm, and cardiac arrest if the patient is not treated promptly. Additional complications include nerve root injury, bowel or bladder dysfunction, and transverse myelitis. Chemonucleolysis is done less often now because of its fairly frequent side effects.

**Diskectomy with laminectomy:**   An incision is made, allowing removal of part of the vertebra (laminectomy) so that the herniated portion of the disk can be removed (diskectomy). If multiple intervertebral disk spaces are explored, a drain may be present when the patient returns to the room. Complications include paralytic ileus, urinary retention, CSF leakage with possible fistula formation, meningitis, hematoma at the operative site, nerve root injury causing wrist or foot drop, arachnoiditis, and postural deformity.

**Microdiskectomy:**   The herniated portion of the disk and small parts of the lamina are removed, using microsurgical techniques. This surgery results in less tissue damage, less pain, fewer spasms, and increased postoperative spinal stability. Patients often are out of bed the first day and may be discharged in 2-3 days.

**Percutaneous lumbar disk removal:**   Degenerated disk material is aspirated through a cannula that has been placed into the intervertebral disk *via* fluoroscopy. This procedure cannot be used on patients with L–5-S–1 disk disease or if the disk has extruded into the spinal cord. This is a relatively less invasive method of relieving pain from herniated disks. The procedure is done under local anesthetic and may be performed on an outpatient basis. Complications include back spasm or transient syncope.

**Spinal fusion:**   May be indicated for patients with recurrent low back pain, spondylolisthesis, or subluxation of the vertebra. Bone chips are taken from the iliac crest or tibia and placed between the vertebrae in the prepared area of the unstable spine to fuse and stabilize the area. Internal fixation may be necessary to provide added stability until the fusion has healed fully.

Patients undergoing anterior cervical fusion may have difficulty swallowing or managing secretions because of postoperative edema and hematoma formation secondary to retraction of the trachea and esophagus during surgery. Hoarseness also can occur secondary to nerve irritation. Complaints of excessive pressure in the neck or severe, uncontrolled incisional pain may signal excessive bleeding.

## NURSING DIAGNOSES AND INTERVENTIONS

**Health-seeking behaviors:**   Proper body mechanics and other measures that prevent back injury
*Desired outcome:*   Within the 24-h period before hospital discharge, patient verbalizes knowledge of measures that prevent back injury and demonstrates proper body mechanics.

- Teach patient proper body mechanics: Stand and sit straight with the chin and head up and the pelvis and back straight; bend at the knees and hips rather than at the waist, keeping the back straight; when carrying objects, hold them close to the body, avoiding twisting when lifting. Turn using the entire body. Do not strain to reach things. If an object is overhead, raise yourself to its level, or move things out of the way if they are obstructing the object. Avoid lifting anything heavier than 20 lb. Have patient demonstrate proper body mechanics, if possible, before hospital discharge.
- Teach patient about the following measures for keeping the body in alignment: Sit close to the pedals when driving a car, and use a seat belt and firm backrest to support the back; support the feet on a footstool when sitting so that the knees are elevated to hip level or higher; obtain a firm mattress or bedboard; use a flat pillow when sleeping to avoid strain on the neck, arms, and shoulders; sleep in a side-lying position with the knees bent or in a supine position with the knees and legs supported on pillows; avoid sleeping in a prone position; avoid reaching or stretching to pick up objects. Avoid sitting on furniture that does not support the back.
- Encourage patient to perform the following measures to relieve pressure on the back: Reduce to a proper weight for age, height, and sex; continue the exercise program prescribed by physician for strengthening abdominal, thoracic, and back muscles; use the thoracic and abdominal muscles when lifting to keep a significant portion of the weight off the vertebral disks.

- Teach patient the rationale and procedure for Williams flexion exercises, which are performed while lying on the floor with the knees flexed.
  - *Pelvic tilt:* To strengthen the abdominal muscles. Stomach and buttock muscles are tightened and the pelvis is tilted with the lower spine kept flat against the floor.
  - *Knee-to-chest raise:* To help make a stiff back limber. Each knee is individually raised to the chest, returned to the starting position, and then both knees are raised simultaneously to the chest.
  - *Nose-to-knee touch:* To stretch hip muscles and strengthen abdominal muscles. Raise the knee to the chest, and then pull the knee to the chest with the hands. Raise the head and try to touch the nose to the knee. Keep the lower back flat on the floor.
  - *Half sit-ups:* To strengthen abdomen and back. Slowly raise the head and neck to the top of the chest. Reach both hands forward to knees and hold for a count of five. Repeat, keeping lower back flat on the floor.
- Instruct patient to wear supportive shoes with a moderate heel height for walking.
- Teach patient the following technique for sitting up at the bedside from a supine position: Log-roll (described, p. 225) to the side, and then raise to a sitting position by pushing against the mattress with the hands while swinging the legs over the side of the bed. Instruct patient to maintain alignment of the back during the procedure.
- Caution patient that pain is the signal to stop or change an activity or position.
- Teach patient that the following indicators necessitate medical attention: increased sensory loss, increased motor loss/weakness, and loss of bowel and bladder function.

**Health-seeking behaviors:**   Pain control measures
*Desired outcome:*  Following instruction and within the 24-h period before hospital discharge, patient verbalizes knowledge about pain control measures and demonstrates ability to initiate these measures when appropriate.

- Teach patient about the physiologic mechanisms of pain.
- Instruct patient about methods of controlling pain and their individual applications. Methods include distraction, use of counterirritants, massage, hydrotherapy, dorsal column stimulation, use of TENS, behavior modification, relaxation techniques, hypnosis, music therapy, imagery, biofeedback, and diathermy. In addition, suggest the application of local heat or cold massage to painful areas. The latter can be achieved by freezing water in a paper cup, tearing off the top of the cup to expose the ice, and massaging in a circular motion, using the remaining portion of the cup as a handle.
- Suggest that patient use a stool to rest the affected leg when standing.
- Advise patient to sit in a straight-back chair that is high enough to get out of easily. Raised toilet seats also may be useful. Straddling a straight-back chair and resting the arms on the chair back is comfortable for many individuals.
- Encourage use of a firm mattress, to support normal spinal curvature, and extra pillows as needed for positioning. Some patients find the normal bed height too low and use blocks to raise it to a more comfortable height.
- Instruct patient on bed rest to roll rather than lift off the bedpan. The patient may find a fracture bedpan more comfortable than a regular bedpan.
- Caution patient to avoid sudden twisting or turning movements. Explain the importance of log-rolling when moving from side to side.
- Advise patient to avoid factors that enhance spasms, such as staying in one position too long, fatigue, chilling, and anxiety.
- Suggest positions of comfort, such as lying on the side with the knees bent or lying supine with the knees supported on pillows. A small pillow supporting the nape of the neck may be helpful with cervical pain. Usually the patient is on bed rest or limited activity during the period of acute pain.

Once increased activity is allowed, teach patient to avoid prolonged periods of sitting, which stress the back.

- Inform patient that applying a heating pad to the back for 15-30 min before getting out of bed in the morning will help allay stiffness and discomfort. Heating pads should be used only for short intervals and only if patient's temperature sensations are intact. Remind patient to place a towel or cloth between heating pad and skin to prevent burns.

**Knowledge deficit:** Diskectomy with laminectomy or fusion procedure

*Desired outcomes:* Before surgery, patient verbalizes knowledge about the surgical procedure, preoperative routine, and postoperative regimen. Patient demonstrates activities and exercises correctly.

- Assess patient's knowledge about the surgical procedure, preoperative routine, and postoperative regimen. Provide ample time for instruction and clarification.
- Teach patient the technique for deep breathing, which will be performed immediately after surgery (coughing may be contraindicated in the immediate postoperative period to prevent disruption of the fusion or surgical repair). Also teach patient use of incentive spirometry.
- Document baseline neurovascular checks, including color, capillary refill, pulse, warmth, muscle strength, movement, and sensation. Explain that VS and neurologic status will be evaluated at frequent intervals after the surgery and compared to baseline. Reassure patient that this is normal and does not indicate that anything is wrong. Teach patient the following indicators of impairment, which necessitate immediate attention by the health-care staff: paresthesias, weakness, paralysis, radiculopathy, and changes in bowel or bladder function. Patients undergoing fusion lose more blood during surgery than those undergoing laminectomy. Signs of hypovolemia, such as decreased BP, increased HR, and thirst, may be present. Teach patient to report faintness or dizziness.
- Explain that the surgical dressing will be inspected for excess drainage or oozing at frequent intervals. Bleeding with a laminectomy usually is minimal. Patients with fusions may have slight bloody oozing postoperatively. Serous drainage usually is checked with a glucose reagent strip. The presence of glucose is a signal of CSF leakage. Lumbar dressings will be checked after each bed pan use. Wet or contaminated dressings require changing. Inform patients undergoing fusions that they will have a second dressing at the donor site.
- Instruct patient to report any nausea or vomiting, which is not uncommon, so that antiemetics can be given. Explain that the patient will be monitored for bowel and bladder dysfunction postprocedure. The abdomen will be checked for bowel sounds and distention. The patient may be asked to void within 8 h of the procedure to check for urinary retention. Caution patient to avoid straining at stool.
- Explain that fever may occur during the first few days postoperatively but that this does not necessarily signal an infection. The patient will be assessed for other indicators of infection, such as heat, redness, irritation, swelling, or drainage at the wound site. Instruct patient to report headache, neck stiffness, or photophobia.
- Inform patient that postoperative pain often is caused by nerve root irritation and edema. Spasms are common on the third or fourth postoperative day and should not discourage patient. Pain may take days or weeks to resolve. The patient should request medication for pain as needed and not let the pain get out of control. Muscle relaxants may be prescribed to supplement pain control. Patient-controlled analgesia (PCA) and nonsteroidal antiinflammatory drugs (NSAIDs) also may be used for postoperative pain control.
- Inform patient that in the immediate postoperative period he or she will probably be required to lie supine for several hours to minimize the possibility

of wound hematoma formation. After this period, HOB of the laminectomy patient usually can be raised to 20 degrees to facilitate eating and bed pan use. The patient undergoing spinal fusion may be kept flat and on bed rest considerably longer than the patient with laminectomy.

- Only the log-roll method is used for turning. Teach patient the following technique: Position a pillow between the legs, cross the arms across the chest while turning, and contract the long back muscles to maintain the shoulders and pelvis in straight alignment. Explain that initially, patient will be assisted in this procedure. Use a turning sheet and sufficient help when log-rolling patient.

- Teach patient the following technique for getting out of bed: Log-roll to the side, splint the back, and rise to a sitting position by pushing against the mattress while swinging the legs over the side of the bed. While in the hospital with an electric bed, the HOB may be raised to facilitate a sitting position. Initially the patient will be helped to a sitting position and should not push against the mattress. Patients with a cervical laminectomy should not pull themselves up with their arms. When assisting patients with a cervical laminectomy to a sitting position, caution them not to put their arms on the nurse's shoulder.

- Explain that antiembolism hose and possibly sequential compression sleeves will be applied after surgery to prevent thrombus formation. Teach techniques for ankle circling and calf pumping to promote venous circulation in the legs. Teach patient to report calf pain, tenderness, or warmth.

- Advise patient that physician will prescribe certain postoperative activity restrictions. Sitting for limited, prescribed periods of time will be permitted in a straight-back chair. Teach patient not to sit for long periods of time on the edge of the mattress because it does not provide enough support. Explain that weakness, dizziness, and lightheadedness may occur on a first walk.

- Instruct patient to avoid stretching, twisting, flexing, or jarring the spine to prevent vertebral collapse, shifting of the bone graft, or a bleeding episode. Explain that the spine should be kept aligned and in a neutral position.

- If patient is scheduled for a cervical laminectomy, explain that a cervical collar will be worn postoperatively. Review use and application of cervical collar. Teach these patients not to pull with their arms on objects such as side rails.

- Instruct patient in use of braces or corsets, if prescribed. Braces should be applied while in bed. Wearing underwear under the brace will help protect the skin from irritation. The person undergoing a fusion procedure often wears a supportive brace or corset for ≤3 months to keep the operative site immobile so that the graft will heal and not dislodge.

- Explain that the physician will give patient instructions for at-home activity restrictions, including driving or riding in the car, sexual activity, lifting and carrying objects, tub bathing (generally, soaking the incision is avoided until about 1 week after the sutures are out), going up and down stairs, the amount of time to be spent in and out of bed, and back exercises.

- Teach patient the following symptoms of postoperative wound infection, which require medical attention: swelling, discharge, persistent redness, local warmth, fever, and pain.

- For additional interventions, see this nursing diagnosis in Appendix One, "Caring for Preoperative and Postoperative Patients," p. 693.

**Impaired swallowing (or risk of same)** related to postoperative edema or hematoma formation secondary to anterior cervical fusion

*Desired outcome:*  Patient regains uncompromised swallowing ability (usually by the third postoperative day) as evidenced by presence of normal breath sounds and absence of food in the oral cavity or choking/coughing.

- As part of the preoperative teaching, instruct patient in the potential for difficulty with swallowing following anterior cervical fusion. Caution patient of the need to report promptly any significant postoperative difficulty with swallowing.

- Monitor for edema of the face or neck or tracheal compression or deviation that could compromise respiratory function. Listen for hoarseness, which can indicate laryngeal nerve irritation and signal an ineffective cough or swallowing difficulty in a particular patient.
- Monitor patient for complaints of excessive pressure in the neck or severe uncontrolled incisional pain, which can signal excessive bleeding.
- Check for gag and swallowing reflexes before oral intake. Begin the postoperative diet with clear fluids, and progress to more solid foods only after patient demonstrates ability to ingest fluids safely.
- To minimize the risk of aspiration, position patient in Fowler's position, or semi-Fowler's position at minimum, when initiating fluid intake.
- Also see **High risk for aspiration,** p. 302, in "General Care of Patients with Neurologic Disorders."

**Knowledge deficit:**   Chemonucleolysis procedure
*Desired outcome:*   Before the procedure, patient verbalizes information about chemonucleolysis, including risks and anticipated outcome.

- During the preoperative period, reinforce physician's explanation of the chemonucleolysis procedure, including its purpose, risks, and anticipated benefits and outcome.
- As indicated, explain that chemonucleolysis involves injection of an enzyme directly into the disk to dissolve parts of the nucleus pulposus to relieve pressure on the spinal cord or nerve roots.
- Evaluate patient for allergies to iodine, papaya, or products that may contain papaya derivatives, such as meat tenderizer, beer, dental powder, digestive aids, and contact lens cleansers. Report allergies to physician.
- A delayed allergic reaction following the procedure is possible. Instruct patient to report immediately any urticaria, itching, dizziness (hypotension), nasal or chest congestion, wheezing, or respiratory distress.
- Document baseline distal neurologic status carefully, especially motor or sensory deficits of the legs and feet. Explain that VS and neurologic status will be monitored frequently after the procedure. IM injections (both pre- and postprocedure) are given in a site other than the patient's affected area to avoid confusing the patient's disk pathology with injection site pain. Instruct patient to report any numbness or weakness, especially if this is a change from baseline neurologic status, because this may signal nerve root injury.
- Explain that patient will be monitored for bowel and bladder dysfunction postprocedure. The abdomen will be checked for bowel sounds and distention. Patients should report any nausea or vomiting and may be asked to void within 8 h of the procedure to check for urinary retention.
- Inform patient that he or she will be on bed rest for 2-24 h after the procedure, depending on surgeon's preference.
- Explain that back stiffness, soreness, pain, or spasm may occur after the procedure and that patient should alert staff member so that analgesia can be given. Chemonucleolysis provides pain relief in 50%-80% of patients, but it may take up to 3 months to do so. Pain actually may be worse after the procedure.
- Instruct patient to report immediately any numbness, weakness, paraplegia, paraparesis, or change in bowel or bladder function after hospital discharge. These symptoms may signal an acute transverse myelitis, which can develop several days after the procedure.
- For additional interventions, see this nursing diagnosis in Appendix One, "Caring for Preoperative and Postoperative Patients," p. 693.

**Impaired tissue integrity (or risk of same)** related to altered circulation or shearing forces secondary to cervical or pelvic traction
*Desired outcome:*   Patient's skin remains unbroken; the tissue blanches.

- Pelvic traction: Ensure that patient is positioned correctly with the HOB elevated 30 degrees and the knees flexed 10-20 degrees. Be especially alert to the condition of the tissue at the iliac crests, coccyx, and intergluteal fold. Wearing an undershirt or a pajama top may help protect the skin from the pelvic belt. Inspect for erythemic areas at least q2h. If the area is reddened and does not blanch or erythema does not resolve after removing pressure or padding, notify physician promptly about your findings.
- Cervical traction: Maintain bed in low-Fowler's position, and keep a small rolled towel under patient's shoulders to enhance hyperextension. Apply cornstarch to skin that is in contact with the halter. Check the chin, ears, and occipital areas for the presence of erythema or irritation at least q2h. Adjust or pad the halter as needed.
- Pad any areas of increased pressure beneath the traction.
- Maintain alignment between the patient's body and the weights to keep the traction forces even.

---

**Note:**  See "General Care of Patients with Neurologic Disorders" for **High risk for injury** related to impaired pain, touch, and temperature sensation, p. 299, and **Knowledge deficit:** Neurologic diagnostic tests, p. 311. For surgical patients, see Appendix One, "Caring for Preoperative and Postoperative Patients," p. 693, for related nursing diagnoses and interventions. For patients experiencing varying degrees of immobility, see "Pressure Ulcers," p. 687, and Appendix One, "Caring for Patients on Prolonged Bed Rest," p. 711.

---

## PATIENT-FAMILY TEACHING AND DISCHARGE PLANNING

Give patient and significant others verbal and written information about the following:

- Prescribed exercise regimen, including rationale for each exercise, technique for performing the exercise, number of repetitions of each, and frequency of the exercise periods. If possible, ensure that patient demonstrates understanding of the exercise regimen and proper body mechanics before hospital discharge.
- Wound incision care. Indicators of postoperative wound infection, which necessitate medical attention, include swelling, discharge, persistent redness, local warmth, fever, and pain.
- Use and care of a brace or immobilizer, if appropriate.
- Medications, including name, rationale, dosage, schedule, precautions, and potential side effects.
- Anticonstipation routine, which should be initiated during hospitalization.
- Pain control measures.
- Telephone number of a resource person, should questions arise after hospital discharge.
- Postsurgical activity restrictions as directed by physician. These may affect the following: driving and riding in a car, returning to work, sexual activity, lifting and carrying, tub bathing, going up and down steps, and the amount of time spent in or out of bed.
- Signs and symptoms of worsening neurologic function and the importance of notifying physician immediately if they develop. These include numbness, weakness, paralysis, or bowel and bladder dysfunction.

## Spinal cord injury

The spinal cord injuries (SCIs) discussed in this section are caused by vertebral fractures or dislocations that sever, lacerate, stretch, or compress the spinal cord and interrupt neuronal function and transmission of nerve impulses.

Blood supply to the spinal cord also may be interrupted. The spinal cord swells in response to injury, and this, along with hemorrhage, can cause additional compression, ischemia, and compromised function. Neurologic deficits resulting from compression may be reversible if the resulting edema and ischemia do not lead to spinal cord degeneration and necrosis. Common causes of injury include motor vehicle accident, diving or other sporting accidents, falls, and gunshot wounds. SCIs are classified in a number of different ways according to type (open, closed), cause, site (level of spinal cord involved), mechanism of injury (compression, hyperflexion, hyperextension, rotational, penetrating), stability, and degree of spinal cord function loss (complete, incomplete). A *spinal cord concussion* is a transient loss of cord function due to a traumatic event and resulting in immediate flaccid paralysis that resolves completely in a matter of minutes or hours.

**Prognosis:**   Any evidence of voluntary motor function, sensory function, or sacral sensation below the level of injury is indicative of an incomplete SCI, with the potential for partial or complete recovery. After an acute injury, the spinal cord usually goes into a condition called spinal shock, in which there can be total loss of spinal cord function below the level of injury. During spinal shock there is no reflex activity. Resolution of spinal shock with return of reflexes usually occurs within 1-6 weeks but may take 6 months or more. If there is no evidence of returning motor function after local reflexes have returned, the spinal cord is considered irreversibly damaged. Generally, SCI does not cause immediate death unless it is at C-1 through C-3, which results in respiratory muscle paralysis. Individuals who survive these injuries require a ventilator for the rest of their lives. If the injury occurs at C-4, respiratory difficulties may result in death, although some individuals who have survived the initial injury have been successfully weaned from the ventilator. Injuries below C-4 also can be life-threatening because of ascending cord edema, which can cause respiratory muscle paralysis. Immediately after injury, common complications that require treatment include hypotension (systolic BP <80 mm Hg), bradycardia, paralytic ileus, urinary retention, pneumonia, and stress ulcers. Other long-term, life-threatening, potential complications of SCI include autonomic dysreflexia, decubitus ulcers, pneumonia, sepsis, urinary calculi, and urinary tract infection (UTI).

## ASSESSMENT

**Acute indicators:**   Loss of sensation, weakness, or paralysis below the level of the injury; localized pain or tenderness over the site of injury; headache; hypothermia or hyperthermia; and alterations in bowel and bladder function.

*Cervical injury:*   Possible alterations in LOC, weakness or paralysis in all four extremities (quadriparesis or quadriplegia), paralysis of respiratory muscles or signs of respiratory problems, such as flaring nostrils and use of accessory muscles for respirations. Any cervical injury can result in a low body temperature (to 96° F), slowed pulse rate (<60 bpm) caused by vagal stimulation of the heart, hypotension (systolic BP <80 mm Hg) caused by vasodilation, and decreased peristalsis.

*Thoracic and lumbar injuries:*   Paraparesis/paraplegia or altered sensation in the legs; hand and arm involvement in upper thoracic injuries.

*Acute spinal shock:*   Can last from 2 days to 6 months but usually resolves in 1-6 weeks. Indicators depend on the severity of the injury and include total loss of spinal cord function, loss of skin sensation, flaccid paralysis or absence of reflexes below the level of injury, paralytic ileus and constipation secondary to atonic bowel, bladder distention secondary to atonic bladder, low/falling BP secondary to loss of vasomotor tone and decreased venous return, and anhidrosis (absence of sweating) below level of injury. Autonomic instability is more dramatic in higher (e.g., cervical) lesions. Resolution of spinal shock is indicated by the return of the bulbocavernosus reflex (slight muscle contraction when the glans penis is squeezed or the urinary catheter is pulled) and the anal reflex (puckering of the anus on digital exam or gentle scratching around the anus). The remaining reflexes may take weeks to return.

**Chronic indicators:**  As spinal shock resolves, muscle tone, reflexes, and some function may return, depending on severity and level of injury. The return of reflexes usually results in muscle spasticity. Chronic autonomic dysfunction may be manifested as fever; mild hypotension; anhidrosis; and alterations in bowel, bladder, and sexual function. Injuries at or below L–1 may result in permanent flaccid paralysis.

*Upper motor neuron (UMN) involvement:*  UMNs are nerve cell bodies that originate in high levels of the central nervous system (CNS) and transmit impulses from the brain down the spinal cord. Injury will interrupt this impulse transmission, causing muscle or organ dysfunction below the level of injury. However, since the injury does not interrupt reflex arcs coming from those muscles or organs to the spinal cord, hypertonic reflexes, clonus paralysis, and spastic paralysis are seen. The patient will have a positive Babinski reflex.

*Lower motor neuron (LMN) involvement:*  LMNs are anterior horn cell bodies that originate in the spinal cord. LMNs transmit nerve impulses to muscles and organs and are involved in reflex arcs that control involuntary responses. Damage to LMNs will abolish voluntary and reflex responses of muscles and organs, resulting in flaccid paralysis, hypotonia, atrophy, and muscle fibrillations and fasciculations. The patient will have an absent Babinski reflex. The spinal cord ends at the T–12-L–1 level. Below that level, a bundle of nerve roots from the spinal cord fill the spinal canal and are called the cauda equina. Injuries at or below L–1 that damage the nerve fiber after it leaves the spinal cord result in flaccid paralysis because of interrupted reflex arc activity.

*Bowel and bladder dysfunction:*  Usually there is loss of conscious sensation of the need to void or defecate. UMN bowel and bladder involvement results in reflex incontinence. Flaccid LMN bladder involvement causes urinary retention with overflow incontinence. Flaccid LMN bowel involvement causes fecal retention/impaction.

**Autonomic dysreflexia (AD):**  For patients with injuries at or above T–6, the uninhibited autonomic reflex response to stimuli can be life-threatening as reflex activity returns. Signs and symptoms include gross hypertension (up to 240-300/150 mm Hg), pounding headache, blurred vision, bradycardia, nausea, and nasal congestion. Above the level of the injury, flushing and sweating may occur. Below the level of injury there are often piloerection (goose bumps) and skin pallor, which signal vasoconstriction. Seizures, subarachnoid hemorrhage, cerebrovascular accident (CVA), or retinal hemorrhage may occur.

**Physical assessment**

*Acute (spinal shock):*  Absence of deep tendon reflexes (DTRs) below level of injury; absence of cremasteric reflex (scratching or light stroking of the inner thigh for male patients causes the testicle on that side to elevate) for T–12 and L–1 injuries; absence of penile or anal sphincter reflex.

*Chronic:*  Generally, increased DTRs occur if the spinal cord lesion is of the UMN type.

## DIAGNOSTIC TESTS

**X-ray of spine:**  To delineate fracture, deformity, or displacement of vertebrae, as well as soft tissue masses, such as hematomas.

**CT scan:**  To reveal changes in the spinal cord, vertebrae, and soft tissue surrounding the spine.

**Myelography:**  Shows blockage or disruption of the spinal canal and is used if other diagnostic exams are inconclusive. Radiopaque dye is injected into the subarachnoid space of the spine, using a lumbar or cervical puncture.

**MRI:** Reveals changes in the spinal cord and surrounding soft tissue.

**ABG/pulmonary function tests:** To assess effectiveness of respirations and detect the need for $O_2$ or mechanical ventilation.

**Cystometry:** To assess capacity and function of the bladder after resolution of spinal shock for the best type of bladder training program.

**Pulmonary fluoroscopy:** To evaluate the degree of diaphragm movement and effectiveness in individuals with high cervical injuries.

**Evoked potential studies:** To help locate the level of spinal cord lesion by evaluating the integrity of the nervous system's anatomic pathways and connections. Stimulation of a peripheral nerve triggers a discrete electrical response along a neurologic pathway to the brain. This response or lack of response to stimulation is measured in this test.

---

**Note:** See "General Care of Patients with Neurologic Disorders," **Knowledge deficit:** Neurologic diagnostic tests, p. 311, for care considerations for patients undergoing CT scan, myelography, MRI, and evoked potentials.

---

## COLLABORATIVE MANAGEMENT

### Acute care

**Immobilization of injury site:** Essential for preventing further damage. See "Surgery/immobilization" in this list below.

**Bed rest on a firm surface:** For example, Roto Rest Kinetic Treatment Table.

**Pharmacotherapy**

*Corticosteroids (methylprednisolone):* Mega IV dose given within 8 h of injury reduces damage and improves functional recovery by protecting the neuromembrane from further destruction. Dosage is IV bolus of 30 mg/kg followed by continuous IV infusion of 5.4 mg/kg/h for a 23-h period.

*Osmotic diuretics (e.g., mannitol):* Sometimes used for 10 days to reduce cord edema after the initial injury and minimize ascending cord edema.

*Analgesics (e.g., acetaminophen, codeine) and sedatives:* To decrease pain and anxiety.

*Antacids; histamine $H_2$-receptor blockers (e.g., ranitidine):* To prevent gastric ulceration, which may occur owing to increased production of gastric secretions with SCI and steroid use.

*Anticoagulants (e.g., heparin or warfarin):* To prevent thrombophlebitis and reduce the potential for pulmonary emboli.

*Stool softeners (e.g., docusate sodium):* To keep stool soft and prevent fecal impaction while the bowel is atonic.

*Vasopressors:* To treat hypotension in the immediate postinjury stage caused by loss of vasomotor tone. *Fluid therapy* also may be given for hypotension. *Atropine* may be given for bradycardia. Typically, patient will be on a cardiac monitor and in ICU during this stage.

**Aggressive respiratory therapy:** For all patients with SCIs. Patients with injuries above C–5 are intubated and put on a ventilator. Nasal intubation or tracheostomies may be used to prevent neck extension (and thus further damage) during intubation. Intermittent positive pressure breathing (IPPB) and chest physiotherapy are used to prevent and treat atelectasis. Respiratory therapy is ongoing past the acute stage.

**Nasogastric decompression during spinal shock phase:** To prevent aspiration of gastric contents and treat paralytic ileus.

**Bladder decompression during spinal shock phase:** Either intermittent catheterization or continuous drainage.

**Surgery/immobilization:** May include traction, fusion, laminectomy, and closed or open reduction of fractures. The surgical goal is to immobilize the spine and, if indicated, decompress the spinal cord to help prevent additional neurologic deficit. If indicated, bone fragments are removed and the spine is surgically fused within 5-10 days of the injury. Complete healing may take 3-4 months.

*Cervical spine:*    Immobilized with devices such as Crutchfield tongs, Vinke Gardner Wells tongs, or halo traction. Halo traction does not need to be removed for surgery; it enables early mobilization, and some types can be used in an MRI.

*Thoracic spine:*    May be immobilized with a surgical corset, plaster Minerva jacket, plastic body jacket, Harrington rods, or spinal fusion.

*Lumbar spine injuries:*    Usually treated with closed reduction and hyperextension or extension with traction techniques, followed by immobilization in a plastic jacket or spica cast. If these interventions are unsuccessful or if neurologic symptoms occur, a laminectomy is usually performed. A new halo-type device that provides femoral distraction has been developed for lumbar injuries.

*Sacral (cauda equina) fracture:*    Usually treated with a laminectomy and spinal fusion.

**Tracheostomy:**    If patient needs long-term ventilation.

**Physical and occupational therapy:**    Passive ROM is started on all joints. After the injury is stabilized, an aggressive rehabilitation program is initiated, including muscle-strengthening and conditioning exercises to develop alternative muscle groups needed for independence; a sitting program; massage; and instruction in adaptive devices, equipment, and transfer techniques as appropriate. Patients with sacral injuries have the potential to walk and should be instructed in the use of braces, crutches, or a cane as appropriate. Functional electrical stimulation of paralyzed muscles assists some paraplegic patients with walking. A therapy program is ongoing throughout the patient's rehabilitation.

**Antiembolism hose or sequential alternating compression sleeves:**    To prevent thrombophlebitis and reduce the effects of orthostatic hypotension.

**Nutrition:**    Parenteral nutrition and fluids until the GI tract starts functioning and oral intake is possible. A diet high in calories, protein, and fiber usually is prescribed.

**Bowel program during spinal shock:**    Usually consists of manual disimpaction and small-volume enemas while the bowel is atonic.

**Counseling and psychotherapy:**    To help patient and significant others adjust to the disability. This is ongoing and should address sexual functioning and vocational rehabilitation.

**Experimental treatments**

*Endorphin blocking agents:*    Used immediately postinjury to prevent the hypotensive action of endorphins that may contribute to cord ischemia.

*Hyperbaric oxygen therapy:*    Used immediately postinjury to attempt to prevent ischemic cord destruction.

*Spinal cord cooling:*    Used immediately postinjury to reduce edema, thus improving cord circulation. A small pad through which cool saline solution circulates is placed on the epidural layer of the cord for several hours postinjury. A major complication is infection caused by exposure of the cord during cooling.

*Immunosuppressive therapy (e.g., cyclophosphamide):*    To try to reduce cellular or immune responses after injury.

*Chronic care*

**Pharmacotherapy**

*Muscle relaxants (e.g., diazepam).*

*Antispasmodics (e.g., baclofen and dantrolene):*    To decrease spasms.

*Antibiotics (e.g., methenamine mandelate):*    To prevent bladder infection.

*Stool softeners (e.g., docusate sodium), laxatives (e.g., bisacodyl), and suppositories:*    To maintain a bowel program that prevents fecal impaction and minimizes incontinence. **Note:** Suppositories are avoided or used with caution in individuals at risk for AD.

*Anticholinergics (e.g., oxybutynin, propantheline):* To reduce bladder spasms causing reflex incontinence.

**Dietary management:** Limiting milk and other dairy products to minimize the risk of renal calculi, and promoting juices (e.g., cranberry, plum, and prune) that leave an acid ash in the urine and decrease urinary pH, thus reducing the potential for infection. Vitamin C also may be used to acidify the urine. An adequate diet also should include high roughage and fiber to promote soft stools. If not contraindicated, fluids are encouraged to promote adequate hydration.

**Management of AD:** AD is a medical emergency that can occur for patients with SCIs at or above level T−6. The noxious stimulus (e.g., a distended bladder) must be found and alleviated as quickly as possible. The following may be administered during crisis to control hypertension: vasodilators, such as hydralazine, nitroprusside, or amyl nitrate; hypotensive nondiuretic thiazides, such as diazoxide; adrenergic blockers, such as IV phentolamine; ganglionic blocking agents, such as reserpine, guanethidine, or mecamylamine; and fast-acting calcium channel blockers, such as nifedipine. Tetracaine or lidocaine may be instilled into the bladder to reduce bladder excitability. (For nursing interventions, see **Dysreflexia,** below.)

**Surgical interventions**

*Diaphragm pacer insertion:* This is a phrenic nerve stimulator that may allow selected ventilatory patients to be off the respirator for short periods of time. Electrodes are implanted over the phrenic nerve and, when activated, cause the diaphragm to contract, generating a breath.

*Intrathecal baclofen:* A programmable pump is implanted to deliver a continuous dose of baclofen into the sheath of the spinal canal to control spasticity.

*Tenotomies, myotomies, muscle transplants, peripheral neurectomies, and rhizotomy:* These are some of the surgical approaches that may be used to treat spasticity that cannot be managed by medications or more conservative measures such as stretching or ROM.

*Intrathecal injection of phenol:* To relieve muscle spasm for up to 3-6 months.

## NURSING DIAGNOSES AND INTERVENTIONS

**Dysreflexia (or risk of same)** related to exaggerated unopposed autonomic response to noxious stimuli for individuals with SCI at or above T−8.

---

**Note:** AD is seen most commonly in patients with injuries at or above T−6, but cases have been reported in patients with injuries as low as T−8.

---

*Desired outcomes:* On an ongoing basis, patient is free of symptoms of AD as evidenced by BP within patient's baseline range, HR 60-100 bpm, and absence of headache and other clinical indicators of AD. Following instruction, patient and significant others verbalize factors that cause AD, treatment and prevention, and when immediate emergency treatment is indicated.

- Monitor for indicators of AD, including hypertension (>20 mm Hg above baseline but may go as high as 240-300/150 mm Hg), pounding headache, bradycardia, blurred vision, nausea, nasal congestion, flushing and sweating above the level of injury, and piloerection (goose bumps) or pallor below the level of injury.
- If AD is suspected, raise HOB immediately to 90 degrees, or assist patient into a sitting position to lower the BP.
- Call for someone to notify physician; stay with patient and try to find and ameliorate the noxious stimulus. Speed is essential. Monitor BP q3-5min

during the hypertensive episode. Remain calm and supportive of patient and significant others.

- Assess the following sites for causes, and implement measures for removing the noxious stimulus:

**Bladder (most likely cause):**   Distention, UTI, calculus and other obstructions, bladder spasms, catheterization, and bladder irrigations performed too quickly or with too cold a liquid.

- Do not use Credé's method for a distended bladder.
- Catheterize patient (ideally using anesthetic jelly) if there is a possibility or question of bladder distention. Notify physician *stat*.
- If a catheter is already in place, check the tubing for kinks and lower the drainage bag. For obstruction, such as sediment in the tubing, irrigate the catheter as indicated, using no more than 30 ml of normal saline. If catheter patency is uncertain, recatheterize patient using anesthetic jelly.
- If the bladder is not distended, check for signs of UTI and/or urinary calculi, including cloudy urine, hematuria, and positive lab or x-ray results. Obtain urine specimen for culture and sensitivity studies as indicated.

**Bowel (second most likely cause):**   Constipation, impaction, insertion of suppository or enema, and rectal examination.

- Do not attempt rectal examination without first anesthetizing the rectal sphincter with anesthetic jelly.
- Use large amounts of anesthetic jelly in the anus and rectum before disimpacting bowel to remove the potential stimulus. Allow 5 min for the anesthetic jelly to work, as manifested by a falling BP, before disimpacting.

**Skin:**   Pressure, infection, injury, heat, pain, or cold.

- Loosen clothing and remove antiembolism hose, leg bandages, ABD binder, or constrictive sheets as appropriate.
- For male patients, check for a pressure source on the penis or testicles, and remove the pressure, if present.
- Check the skin surface below level of injury. Monitor for the presence of a pressure area or sore, infection, laceration, rash, sunburn, ingrown toenail, or infected area. If indicated, apply a topical anesthetic.
- Observe for and remove the source of heat or cold (e.g., ice pack or heating pad).

**Additional causes:**   Surgical manipulation, sexual activity, menstruation, and labor.

- Administer antihypertensive agents such as hydralazine, diazoxide, or nifedipine, as prescribed.
- On resolution of the crisis, answer patient's and significant others' questions about AD. Discuss signs and symptoms, treatment, and methods of prevention. Encourage patient to wear a medical-alert type bracelet or tag.

---

**Note:**   Prevention is the best way to deal with AD. A good bowel regimen and skin integrity program are key factors in preventing the noxious stimuli that constipation or pressure areas may cause. Loosen clothing, bedsheets, and contricting bands; turn patient off side to relieve other possible sources of pressure. Keep the bed free of sharp objects and wrinkles. Adhere to turning schedules. Measures should be instituted to reduce the potential for UTI and urinary calculi, and the patient should be taught self-inspection of skin and urinary catheter and the importance of using anesthetic jelly for catheterization and disimpaction.

---

**Constipation** or fecal impaction related to immobility and decreased peristalsis, atonic bowel, and loss of sensation and voluntary sphincter control secondary to sensorimotor deficit

***Desired outcome:***   Patient has bowel movements that are soft and formed every 2-3 days or within patient's preinjury pattern.

- During acute phase of spinal shock, assess patient's bowel function by auscultating for bowel sounds, inspecting for the presence of abdominal distention, and monitoring for nausea and vomiting and fecal impaction. Notify physician of significant findings. In the presence of fecal impaction, gentle manual removal or a small cleansing enema may be prescribed. Because the atonic intestine distends easily, administer small-volume enemas only. Avoid long-term use of enemas.
- Lesions above the conus medullaris (located at the lower two levels of the thoracic region where the cord begins to taper) generally leave the S-3, S-4, and S-5 spinal cord nerve segments intact. If this spinal reflex arc is intact, the patient will have a UMN bowel and be capable of stimulating (training) the reflex evacuation of the bowel. Lesions below the conus medullaris (T-12) may injure the S-3, S-4, and S-5 nerve segments, resulting in disruption of the reflex arc and causing an LMN flaccid bowel. A flaccid bowel usually is managed with increased intraabdominal pressure techniques, manual disimpaction, and small-volume enemas.
- For the UMN reflex bowel, once bowel activity returns, teach patient to attempt bowel movement 30 min after a meal or warm drink. This regimen will allow patient's gastrocolic and duodenalcolic mass peristalsis reflexes to assist with evacuation. Increasing intraabdominal pressure by bearing down, bending forward, or applying manual pressure to the abdomen also will help promote bowel evacuation. Abdominal belts may be used if the patient is unable to strain at stool. A prescribed, medicated suppository also may be used if necessary. If allowed, provide a bedside commode rather than a bedpan. Check patient's ability to maintain balance on a commode.
- **Caution:** For patients with injuries at T-8 or above, promote use of stool softeners and high-fiber diet. Use suppositories and enemas only when essential and with extreme caution because they can precipitate AD. Use anesthetic jelly liberally when performing a rectal examination or inserting a suppository or enema.
- For patients with hand mobility (who are not at risk for AD), teach the technique for suppository insertion and digital stimulation of the anus to promote reflex bowel evacuation. For digital stimulation, insert finger and gently rotate in a circular motion for about 30 seconds (or longer) until the internal sphincter relaxes. Stop if sphincter spasms are felt or if signs of AD occur. Repeat q10min several times until adequate evacuation occurs. Suppository inserters and rectal stimulation devices are available for patients with limited hand mobility.
- For other interventions, see **Constipation** in Appendix One, "Caring for Patients on Prolonged Bed Rest," p. 716.

**Ineffective airway clearance** related to neuromuscular paralysis/weakness or restriction of chest expansion secondary to halo vest obstruction

*Desired outcome:* Following intervention, patient has a clear airway as evidenced by RR 12-20 breaths/min with normal depth and pattern (eupnea) and absence of adventitious breath sounds.

- Monitor ventilation capability by checking vital capacity, tidal volume, and pulmonary function tests. Monitor serial ABG values and/or pulse oximetry readings. If vital capacity is less than 1 L or if patient exhibits signs of hypoxia ($Pao_2$ <80 mm Hg, tachycardia, increased restlessness, mental dullness, cyanosis), notify physician immediately.
- Monitor for ascending cord edema, which may be signalled by increasing difficulty with secretions, coughing, respiratory difficulties, bradycardia, fluctuating BP, and increased motor and sensory losses at a higher level than baseline findings. Notify physician immediately.
- Maintain patent airway. Keep patient's head in neutral position and suction as necessary. Be aware that suctioning may cause severe bradycardia in the patient with AD. If indicated, prepare patient for a tracheostomy, endotracheal intubation, and/or mechanical ventilation to support respiratory func-

tion. If appropriate, arrange for a transfer to ICU for continuous monitoring.

- If patient is wearing halo vest traction, assess respiratory status at least q4h. Ensure that the vest is not restricting chest expansion. Teach the use of incentive spirometry. Be alert to the following indicators of pulmonary embolus: SOB, hemoptysis, tachycardia, and diminished breath sounds. Pain may or may not be present with pulmonary emboli, depending on the level of SCI.
- If the patient's cough is ineffective, implement the following technique, known as "assisted coughing": Place the palm of the hand under the patient's diaphragm (below the xiphoid process and above the naval). As the patient exhales forcibly, push up into diaphragm to assist in producing a more forceful cough. Assisted cough may be contraindicated in patients with spinal instability.
- Feed patients in Stryker frames or Foster beds in the prone position to minimize the potential for aspiration. Raise stable patients in halo traction to high-Fowler's position if it is not contraindicated.
- For additional interventions, see **High risk for aspiration,** p. 302, in "General Care of Patients with Neurologic Disorders."

**High risk for disuse syndrome** related to paralysis, immobilization, or spasticity secondary to SCI
*Desired outcomes:*   After stabilization of the injury, patient exhibits complete ROM of all joints. By time of discharge, patient demonstrates measures that enhance mobility, reduce spasms, and prevent complications.

- Once the injury is stabilized, assist patient with position changes. For example, a prone position, if not contraindicated, helps prevent sacral decubiti and hip contractures. Assist patient into this position on a regular schedule.
- For patients with spasticity, use hand splints or cones to assist with maintaining a functional grasp.
- To help prevent foot contractures for patients with spasticity, it may be helpful to fit patient with splints or high-top tennis shoes that are cut off at the toes so that each shoe ends just proximal to the metatarsal head. These shoes help keep the feet dorsiflexed but prevent contact of the balls of the feet with a hard surface, which can cause spasticity. Avoid footboards for these patients because the hard surface may trigger spasticity and promote plantarflexion.
- Teach patient that some of the factors that trigger spasms include cold, anxiety, fatigue, emotional distress, infections, bowel or bladder distention, ulcers, pain, tight clothing, and lying too long in one position. Controlling these factors may reduce the number of spasms experienced.
- Teach patients with spasticity proper positioning, ROM, and daily sustained stretching exercises. Steady, continuous, directional stretching once or twice a day is especially important because it may decrease the amount of spasticity for several hours. Cooling and icing techniques, heat, vibration therapy, and transcutaneous electrical nerve stimulation (TENS) of the spastic muscles also may be helpful.
- Because tactile stimulation may trigger spasms, touch by caregivers should be limited. When touch is necessary, do it in a firm, gentle, and steady manner.
- For additional interventions, see **High risk for disuse syndrome** in Appendix One, "Caring for Patients on Prolonged Bed Rest," p. 713.

**High risk for injury** related to incorrect neck position, irritation of cranial nerves, impaired lateral vision secondary to presence of halo vest traction, and lack of access for external cardiac compression
*Desired outcome:*   At time of discharge (and ongoing during use of halo traction), patient exhibits no adverse changes in motor, sensory, or cranial nerve function and is free of symptoms of injury caused by impaired vision.

- Assess position of the patient's neck to the body. Alert physician to the presence of flexion or hyperextension. Assess any difficulty with swallowing, as this may signal improper position of the neck and chin. Keep a torque screwdriver in a secure place so that physician can readily adjust tension on bars to return the patient's neck position to neutral.
- Evaluate degree of sensation and movement of the upper extremities, and assess cranial nerve function. Changes in cranial nerve function can occur if the cranial pins compress or irritate a nerve. Notify physician of sudden changes in motor, sensory, or cranial nerve function (e.g., weakness, paresthesias, ptosis, and difficulty chewing or swallowing). Jaw pain may occur when chewing is attempted, and this needs to be differentiated from cranial nerve problems. A soft diet, cut into small pieces, will help jaw pain.
- Assess pins, bolts, and vest structure for looseness. Clicking sounds may signal a loose pin. Never use the superstructure of the halo traction in turning or moving patient. Notify physician if pins or vest becomes loose or dislodged. Stabilize patient's head as necessary.
- Instruct patient to avoid pulling clothes over the top of the halo apparatus because this may loosen pins. Patient should instead step into and pull clothes up over feet and legs. Advise patient to buy strapless bras, tube tops, clothes that are several sizes larger, or to modify neck openings (e.g., with Velcro closures, ties).
- Avoid loosening a buckle without physician's directive. Buckle holes should be marked so that they are always cinched correctly to the appropriate snugness.
- If patient is ambulatory, teach him or her how to survey the environment while walking, either by using a mirror or by turning the eyes to their extreme lateral positions. A cane may help determine the height of curbs and detect unseen objects or uneven walking surfaces. Explain that trunk flexibility is limited, and achieving balance can be difficult because of the top-heavy weight of the vest. Ambulating with a walker initially may help the patient learn to adjust. Abdominal- and back-strengthening exercises may aid balance and walking. Advise patient to walk only in low-heeled shoes. Extra space allowance may be needed when passing through doorways and to avoid bumping into objects.
- Teach patient that bending over can be hazardous because of top-heaviness. A shower chair that rolls usually can fit over a toilet seat, providing an extra 3-6 in. in height. Slip-on shoes should be worn and assistive devices used to reach or pick up objects.
- To get out of bed, teach patients to roll onto their side at the edge of bed and then drop their legs over the side of the bed while pushing up their trunk sideways.
- Recommend backing into the car seat with the body bent forward for getting into a car. Caution patient against driving, because of the limited field of vision.
- Teach patient that a high table will help bring objects into view and that a swivel chair at home will permit easier visualization of the environment.
- Explain that the patient will need the assistance of another person to shampoo hair safely. Shampooing a short haircut is easiest, and hair should be blown dry because toweling the hair may loosen pins.
- Ensure that an open-end wrench is taped to the halo vest so that the bolts can be released and the vest removed promptly if external cardiac compression is needed. One type of halo vest permits the anterior vest to be lifted up after release of two side belts. Teach significant others how to release the vest in an emergency.

**High risk for impaired skin integrity** and/or **impaired tissue integrity (or risk of same)** related to altered circulation and mechanical factors secondary to presence of halo vest traction or tongs
***Desired outcome:*** At time of discharge (and ongoing), patient's skin is clear

and unbroken; tissue underlying and surrounding the halo vest blanches appropriately.
- Inspect the skin around the vest edges for erythema and other signs of irritation. Massage these nonerythematous areas routinely to promote circulation and help prevent breakdown. Teach skin inspection, which may require use of a mirror, flashlight, or another person. Teach patient to alert medical personnel if breakdown, sensitive spots, odor, dirty vest liner, or loose pins are present.
- Investigate complaints of discomfort or uncomfortable fit. A finger should be able to fit between the vest and patient's skin. Weight loss or gain can affect the fit. Pad the vest as needed until it can be properly adjusted or trimmed by physician. Protect the vest from moisture and soiling. Be alert to foul odor from the cast openings, which can signal pressure necrosis beneath the vest.
- Instruct/assist patient with changing body position q2h. Support the vest while patient is in bed. Use pads to prevent pressure on prominent body areas such as the forehead or shoulder. Use a small pillow under the head for comfort at sleep time.
- Skin care should include cleansing with soap and warm water. Usually, releasing one vest belt at a time is allowed for washing. Avoid use of lotion and powder, which can cake under the vest. Rub unbroken skin with alcohol to toughen the skin. Replace soiled linens promptly. Patient's perspiration may be dried with a hair blower on a cool setting.
- If a rash appears, the patient may be allergic to the vest's lining. A synthetic liner, knitted body stockinette, or T-shirt may correct this problem.
- Provide oral care. A flexible disposable straw can be used both to sip clear water for rinsing teeth and to expel the rinse water into a sink or basin.
- In the event of skin breakdown, keep patient's skin cleansed, dried, and covered with a transparent dressing. Notify physician and orthotist accordingly because skin breakdown requires a brace adjustment.
- Place rubber corks over the tips of the halo device to diminish annoying sound vibrations if the apparatus is bumped and to prevent lacerations from possible sharp edges.
- Check tong placement. If slippage has occurred, immobilize patient's head with a sandbag and notify physician. Pain may signal erosion of bone and displacement into muscle. Check drainage for the presence of CSF (see p. 255). Ensure that traction weights are hanging freely.
- Provide analgesia, as needed, for mild headache and discomfort.
- For a discussion of pin care, see "Fractures," p. 552, for **Knowledge deficit:** Function of external fixation, pin care, and signs and symptoms of pin site infection.

**Urinary retention or reflex incontinence** related to neurologic impairment (spasticity or flaccidity occurring with SCI)
*Desired outcomes:*  Patient has urinary output without incontinence. Patient empties bladder with residual volumes of <50 ml by time of discharge. Following instruction, patient demonstrates triggering mechanism and gains some control over voiding.

---

**Note:**  Bladder dysfunction is complicated and should be assessed by cystometric testing to determine the best type of bladder program. Lesions above the conus medullaris (located at the lower two levels of the thoracic region where the cord begins to taper) generally leave the S−2, S−3, and S−4 spinal cord nerve segments intact. If this spinal reflex arc is intact the patient will have a UMN-involved bladder, resulting in a spastic bladder. This bladder has tone, occasional bladder contractions, and periodically will empty on its own, resulting in reflex incontinence. The UMN-involved bladder is "trainable" with techniques that stimulate reflex voiding. Lesions below the conus medullaris (T–12) may injure the S–2, S–3, and S–4 nerve segments, which will disrupt the reflex arc, causing an LMN-involved flaccid bladder. This bladder has no tone and will distend until it overflows, resulting in overflow incontinence.

---

*General guidelines for individuals with bladder dysfunction*
- Initially patient will have an indwelling urinary catheter or scheduled intermittent catheterizations. If intermittent catheterization is used and episodes of incontinence occur or more than 500 ml urine is obtained, catheterize the patient more often.
- Teach patient and significant others the procedure for intermittent catheterization, care of indwelling catheters, and indicators of UTI (e.g., fever, cloudy and/or foul-smelling urine, malaise, anorexia, restlessness, incontinence).
- Habit/bladder scheduling program consists of gradually increasing the time between catheterizations or periodically clamping indwelling catheters. The goal is a gradual increase in bladder tone. When the bladder can hold 300-400 ml of urine, measures to stimulate voiding are attempted.
- Make sure patient takes fluids at even intervals throughout the day. Restrict fluids before bedtime to prevent nighttime incontinence. Alcohol and caffeine-containing foods and beverages (e.g., cola, chocolate, coffee, tea) have a diuretic effect and may cause incontinence. In addition, caffeine-containing products may increase bladder spasms and reflex incontinence.
- Patients using bladder-emptying techniques should void at least q3h. To obtain the postvoid residual urine, catheterize the patient after an attempt to empty the bladder. Residual amounts >100 ml usually indicate the need for a return to a scheduled intermittent catheterization program.

*Guidelines for patients with UMN-involved spastic reflex bladder*
- Explain to these patients that eventually they may be able to empty the bladder automatically and so may not require catheterization.
- Teach patient techniques that stimulate the voiding reflex, such as tapping the suprapubic area with the fingers, gently pulling the pubic hair, digitally stretching the anal sphincter, stroking the glans penis, stroking the inner thigh, or lightly punching the abdominal area just proximal to the inguinal ligaments. Perform the selected technique for 2-3 min or until a good urine stream has started. Wait 1 min before trying another stimulation technique.
  - *Bladder tapping:* Position self in a half-sitting position. Tapping is performed over the suprapubic area, and the patient may shift the site of stimulation within that area to find the most effective site. Tapping is performed rapidly (7-8 times/sec) with one hand for approximately 50 single taps. Continue tapping until a good stream starts. When the stream stops, wait about 1 min and repeat tapping until the bladder is empty. One or two tapping attempts without response indicates that no more urine will be expelled.
  - *Anal stretch technique (contraindicated in individuals with lesions at T–8 or above because of the potential for AD):* Position self on commode or toilet. Lean forward on the thighs and insert 1 or 2 lubricated fingers into the anus to the anal sphincter. Spread the anal sphincter gently by spreading the fingers apart or pulling in a posterior direction. Maintain the stretching position, take a deep breath, and hold breath while bearing down to void. Relax and repeat until the bladder is empty.
- Teach patients with abdominal muscle control to bear down using Valsalva's maneuver when attempting to trigger voiding.

*Guidelines for patients with LMN-involved flaccid bladders*
- Increasing intraabdominal pressure can overcome sphincter pressure, which may empty the bladder. This may be contraindicated, however, depending on the risk of ureteral reflux.

- Explain that occasionally these patients may be able to empty their bladders manually well enough to avoid catheterization. Need for catheterization can be determined by checking residual urine volume.
- Teach patient bladder-emptying techniques, such as straining or Valsalva's maneuver, to increase intraabdominal pressure. If Credé's method is prescribed, teach patient the following technique: Place the ulnar surface of the hand horizontally along the umbilicus; while bearing down with the abdominal muscles, press the hand downward and toward the bladder in a kneading motion until urination is initiated; continue 30 sec or until urination ceases. For both of these techniques, wait a few minutes and repeat the procedure to ensure complete emptying of the bladder.
- If the patient's bladder cannot be trained to empty completely, intermittent catheterization or external collection devices usually are indicated, and the patient may be a candidate for an artificial inflatable sphincter device or urinary diversion.

---

**Note:** See related discussions in "Urinary Incontinence," p. 158, "Urinary Retention," p. 165, and "Neurogenic Bladder," p. 167.

---

**Altered cardiopulmonary and cerebral tissue perfusion** related to relative hypovolemia secondary to decreased vasomotor tone with SCI
*Desired outcomes:* By a minimum of the 24-h period before hospital discharge (or as soon as vasomotor tone improves), patient has adequate cardiopulmonary and cerebral tissue perfusion as evidenced by systolic BP ≥90 mm Hg and orientation to person, place, and time. For a minimum of 48 h before hospital discharge, patient is free of dysrhythmias.

- Monitor patient for hypotension (drop in systolic BP >20 mm Hg, systolic BP <90 mm Hg), lightheadedness, dizziness, fainting, and confusion.
- Monitor HR and rhythm. Sinus tachycardia/bradycardia may develop because of impaired sympathetic innervation or unopposed vagal stimulation. Document dysrhythmias.
- Monitor I&O. Give prescribed IV fluids cautiously because impaired vascular tone can make the patient sensitive to small increases in circulating volume. Intravascular volume expanders or vasopressors may be required for hypotension.
- Implement measures that prevent episodes of decreased cardiac output due to postural hypotension:
  - Change position slowly.
  - Perform ROM exercises q2h to prevent venous pooling.
  - Prevent patient's legs from crossing, especially when in a dependent position.
  - Patients with SCI at higher levels, especially above T–6, may require abdominal binders in addition to antiembolic hose because these individuals are prone to more severe hypotensive reactions, even with minor changes, such as raising the HOB.
  - Work with the physical therapist (PT) to implement a gradual sitting program that will help patient progress from a supine to upright position. The goal is to increase the patient's ability to sit upright while avoiding adverse effects, such as hypertension, dizziness, and fainting. This may include a bed that can rotate gradually from a horizontal position to a vertical position or a chair that has multiple positions progressing from flat to sitting.
  - For additional information, see **Altered cerebral tissue perfusion** in Appendix One, "Caring for Patients on Prolonged Bed Rest," p. 715.

**Altered peripheral and cardiopulmonary tissue perfusion** related to interrupted blood flow (venous stasis) with corresponding risk of thrombophlebitis and pulmonary emboli secondary to immobility and decreased vasomotor tone
*Desired outcome:* For a minimum of the 24-h period before hospital dis-

charge and ongoing, patient has adequate peripheral and cardiopulmonary tissue perfusion as evidenced by absence of heat, erythema, and swelling in calves and thighs; HR ≤100 bpm, RR ≤20 breaths/min with normal depth and pattern (eupnea), and $Pao_2$ ≥80 mm Hg.

- Monitor for indicators of thrombophlebitis: erythema, warmth, decreased pulses, and swelling in the calves or thighs. Measure calves and thighs daily while the patient is supine or before activity, and monitor for increased circumference. An increase of ≥2 cm in one day is significant. The presence of pain or tenderness depends on the level of SCI. Notify physician about significant findings.
- Protect patient's legs from injury during transfers and turning. Avoid IM injections in the legs, and do not massage them.
- Provide ROM to legs qid. If not contraindicated, place patient in Trendelenburg position for 15 min q2h to promote venous drainage.
- Monitor for indicators of pulmonary emboli: tachycardia, SOB, hemoptysis, decrease in $Pao_2$, and decreased or adventitious breath sounds. Presence of pain depends on the level of injury. Notify physician about significant findings.
- For other interventions, see this nursing diagnosis in Appendix One, "Caring for Patients on Prolonged Bed Rest," p. 715.

**Sexual dysfunction** related to altered body function secondary to SCI

***Desired outcome:*** Within the 24-h period before hospital discharge, patient discusses concerns about sexuality and verbalizes knowledge of alternative methods of sexual expression, and over time expresses acceptance of changes in sexual functioning.

- Evaluate your own feelings about sexuality. Refer patient to someone (e.g., knowledgeable staff member, professional sexual therapy counselor) who can address patient's sexual concerns if you are uncomfortable discussing these issues with the patient.
- Provide a supportive environment that gives the patient permission to have and express sexual concerns. Sexuality can be discussed as it relates to an erection that occurs during a bath or to objective findings noted during a physical assessment. Elicit patient's knowledge, concerns, and questions. Expect acting out behavior related to the patient's sexuality. This is a normal response to the patient's anxiety about his or her sexual response and prognosis.
- Provide limited information about normal sexual response and changes caused by SCI. Sexual functioning may be different but still possible with SCI. The general rule for men is the higher the lesion, the greater the chance of retaining the ability to have an erection but with less chance to ejaculate. For example, 25% of male SCI patients can attain erections permitting coitus, but less than 10% of paraplegics (SCIs resulting in paralysis of the lower limbs) are able to ejaculate. Women may have problems with lubrication and transient loss of ovulation. Ovulation usually returns, and women can become pregnant and deliver vaginally. Uterine contractions of labor in women with an SCI lesion T–8 or above, however, may cause AD. Provide information about birth control and oral contraception for women who desire it. Oral contraceptives may be contraindicated because of the risk of thrombophlebitis.
- Sexual activity may seem impossible to the SCI patient. Specific suggestions that may provide gratification include oral-genital sex, digital stimulation, cuddling, mutual masturbation, anal eroticism, and massage. Specific suggestions for managing common problems include decreasing fluid intake 2-3 h before sexual encounter, emptying the bladder and bowels (if necessary) before a sexual encounter, (for men) folding back indwelling catheter along the penis and holding it in place with a condom, (for women) taping the catheter to the abdomen and leaving it in place, taking a warm bath before sexual activity to reduce spasticity, planning sexual activity for a time

of day in which both partners are rested, experimenting with a variety of positions, and applying topical anesthetics to areas that are hypersensitive to touch. Explain that water-soluble lubricants are useful, if needed, but that petroleum-based lubricants can cause UTI and should be avoided. Adductor spasms in women may pose a barrier but can be overcome if a rear entry is acceptable. Penile implants may be an option for some men.

- Nurses may not be able to answer all the patient's concerns and questions. When this occurs, acknowledge patient's concerns and refer to someone with more expertise.
- Suggest that patient's partner be included in discussion about sexual concerns. Explaining the physical condition caused by the SCI and preparing the partner for scars, lack of muscle tone, atrophy, and the presence of a catheter are important and will provide the partner with an opportunity to discuss sexual concerns as well.
- For additional interventions, see **Altered sexuality pattern** in Appendix One, "Caring for Patients on Prolonged Bed Rest," p. 718.

---

**Note:** See "Renal Calculi," p. 124, and "Ureteral Calculi," p. 149, for nursing diagnoses for the prevention and treatment of renal or ureteral calculi. See "Multiple Sclerosis" for **Knowledge deficit:** Precautions and potential side effects of prescribed medications, p. 185. For patients undergoing diskectomy with laminectomy or spinal fusion, see **Knowledge deficit:** Diskectomy with laminectomy or fusion procedure, p. 229, and **Impaired swallowing,** p. 230. See "General Care of Patients with Neurologic Disorders" for **High risk for trauma** related to unsteady gait, p. 298; **High risk for injury** related to impaired pain, touch, and temperature sensations, p. 299; **Altered nutrition:** Less than body requirements, p. 300; **High risk for fluid volume deficit,** p. 300; **Self-care deficit,** p. 301; **Pain** and spasms, p. 308; **Altered body temperature,** p. 310; and **Knowledge deficit:** Neurologic diagnostic tests, p. 311. Also see "Peptic Ulcers," p. 392, for related nursing diagnoses and interventions. For patients with varying degrees of immobility, see related nursing diagnoses and interventions in "Pressure Ulcers," p. 687, and Appendix One, "Caring for Patients on Prolonged Bed Rest," p. 711. For individuals undergoing surgery, see Appendix One, "Caring for Preoperative and Postoperative Patients," p. 693. For psychosocial nursing diagnoses, see Appendix One, "Caring for Patients with Cancer and Other Life-Disrupting Illnesses," p. 753, as appropriate.

---

## PATIENT-FAMILY TEACHING AND DISCHARGE PLANNING

Give patient and significant others verbal and written information about the following:

- Spinal cord functioning and the effects trauma has on how the body works.
- Referrals to community resources, such as public health nurse, visiting nurses association, community support groups, social workers, psychologic therapy, vocational rehabilitation agency, home health agencies, and extended and skilled care facilities. As appropriate, provide the following addresses: Information Center for Individuals with Disabilities, Fort Point Place, 1st Floor, 27-43 Wormwood Street, Boston, MA 02110-1606, (617)-727-5540; National Spinal Cord Injury Association, 600 West Cummings Park, Suite 2000, Woburn, MA 01801, (617)-935-2722; and American Paralysis Association, 500 Morris Avenue, Springfield, NJ 07081, (800)-225-0292 or in New Jersey (201)-379-2690. Spinal Cord Injury Hotline: (800)-526-3456.
- Safety measures relative to decreased sensation, motor deficits, and orthostatic hypotension, and the symptoms, preventive measures, and interventions for AD.
- Use and care of a brace or immobilizer as appropriate.

- What patient can expect if transferred to a rehabilitation center.
- Techniques and devices for performing ADL, including bathing, grooming, turning, feeding, and other self-care activities to patient's maximum potential. The patient may need a home accessibility evaluation and a driving evaluation and training.
- Indicators of urinary calculi and dietary measures to prevent their formation (see p. 147).
- Indicators of deep vein thrombosis and measures to prevent it (see p. 104).
- For additional information, see teaching and discharge planning interventions (the fourth through tenth entries only) in "Multiple Sclerosis," p. 187, as appropriate.

# Head injury

Head injuries (HIs) can cause varying degrees of damage to the skull and brain tissue. Primary injuries occur at the time of impact and include skull fracture, concussion, contusion, scalp laceration, brain tissue laceration, and tear or rupture of cerebral vessels. Problems that arise soon after the primary injury and are the result of that injury include hemorrhage and hematoma formation from the tear or rupture of vessels, ischemia from interrupted blood flow, cerebral swelling and edema, infection, and IICP or herniation, any of which can interrupt neuronal function. These secondary injuries or events increase the extent of initial injury and result in poorer recovery and higher risk of death. Cervical neck injuries are commonly associated with HIs. Because of the potential for spinal cord injury, all HI patients should be assumed to have cervical neck injury until it is conclusively ruled out by cervical spine x-ray.

Most HIs result from a direct impact to the head. Depending on the force and angle of impact, the brain may suffer injury directly under the point of impact or in the region opposite the point of impact owing to brain rebound action within the skull, or tissue tearing or shearing may occur elsewhere because of the rotational action of the brain within the cranial vault. HIs may be classified by location, severity, extent, or mechanism. Common causes include motor vehicle accidents, falls, and sports-related injuries, such as those occurring in football or boxing. Acts of violence often result in missile or implement HIs, such as gunshot or stab wounds.

## ASSESSMENT

The Glasgow Coma Scale (Table 4-2) standardizes observations for objective assessment of a patient's LOC. This or some other objective scale should be used to prevent confusion with terminology and to detect changes or trends quickly in the patient's LOC.

**Concussion:**  Mild diffuse HI in which there is temporary, reversible neurologic impairment typically involving loss of consciousness and possible amnesia of the event. There is no visible damage to brain structure on CT or MRI examination. After the concussion, the patient may have headache, dizziness, nausea, lethargy, and irritability. Although full recovery usually occurs in a few days, a postconcussion syndrome with headaches, dizziness, irritability, emotional lability, lethargy, and decreased judgment, concentration, and memory abilities may continue for several weeks or months.

**Diffuse axonal injury (DAI):**  A diffuse brain injury caused by stretching and tearing of the neuronal projections owing to a shearing-type injury. No distinct focal lesion, such as infarction, ischemia, contusion, or intracerebral bleeding, is noted, but the patient has an immediate and prolonged unconsciousness of at least 6 h in duration. CT scan may show small hemorrhagic areas in the corpus collosum, cerebral edema, and small midline ventricles. Brain stem injury may be associated with DAI, resulting in autonomic dysfunction. The injury may be quite mild with full recovery, or in severe cases

## T A B L E  4 - 2   Glasgow Coma Scale

| Response | Rating | |
|---|---|---|
| Best eye-opening response (Record *C* if eyes closed because of swelling.) | Spontaneously | 4 |
| | To speech | 3 |
| | To pain | 2 |
| | No response | 1 |
| Best motor response (Record best upper limb response to painful stimuli.) | Obeys verbal command | 6 |
| | Localizes pain | 5 |
| | Flexion—withdrawal | 4 |
| | Flexion—abnormal | 3 |
| | Extension—abnormal | 2 |
| | No response | 1 |
| Best verbal response (Record *E* if endotracheal tube in place or *T* if tracheostomy tube in place.) | Conversation—oriented × 3 | 5 |
| | Conversation—confused | 4 |
| | Speech—inappropriate | 3 |
| | Sounds—incomprehensible | 2 |
| | No response | 1 |
| **Total score:** | 15 = normal | |
| | 13-15 = minor head injury | |
| | 9-12 = moderate head injury | |
| | 3-8 = severe head injury | |
| | ≤7 = coma | |
| | 3 = deep coma or brain death | |

the individual may be comatose for months, die, or be left in a vegetative state.

**Contusion:**  Bruising of the brain tissue, which produces a longer-lasting neurologic deficit than concussion. The size and severity of bruising varies widely, and the bruise or small diffuse venous hemorrhage usually is visible on CT scan. Traumatic amnesia often occurs, causing loss of memory not only of the trauma, but also of events occurring before the incident. Loss of consciousness is common, and it is generally more prolonged than that with concussion. Changes in behavior, such as agitation or confusion, can last for several hours to days. Headache, nausea, lethargy, motor paralysis, paresis, and possibly seizures can occur as well. Depending on the extent of damage, there is potential for either full recovery or permanent neurologic deficit, such as seizures, paralysis, paresis, or even coma and death.

**Brain laceration:**  Actual tearing of the cortical surface of the brain results in direct mechanical disruption of neural function, causing focal deficits. Blood vessel tearing causes hemorrhage, resulting in contusion, edema, or hematoma formation. Seizures often occur as well. Brain lacerations usually result from depressed skull fractures, penetrating injuries, missile or implement injuries, or rotational shearing injury within the skull. Shock waves from a bullet's high energy produces additional damage. A knife or other impalement object should be supported and left in the wound to control bleeding until it can be removed during surgery. Contusions and lacerations often are found together. The consequences of a laceration usually are more serious than those with a contusion because of the increased severity of trauma. Assessment findings are similar to those with contusion but generally are more pronounced.

**Skull fracture:**  Can be *closed* (simple) or *open* (compound), depending on whether the scalp is torn, thereby exposing the skull to the outside environment. Skull fractures are further classified as *linear* (hairline), *comminuted* (fragmented, splintered), or *depressed* (pushed inward toward the brain tissue). A blow forceful enough to break the skull is capable of causing significant brain tissue damage, and therefore close observation is essential. With a penetrating wound or basilar fracture (see below), there is potential for CSF leakage, meningitis, encephalitis, brain abscess, cellulitis, or osteomyelitis.

- *Basilar fractures:* Fractures of the base of the skull do not show up easily on skull/cervical x-rays. Indicators include blood from the nose, throat, ears; serous or serosanguinous drainage from the nose (rhinorrhea), throat, ears (otorrhea), eyes; Battle's sign (bruising noted behind the ear); "Racoon's eyes" (bruising around the eyes in the absence of eye injury); and bleeding behind the tympanum (eardrum) noted on otoscopic exam. Glucose in serous drainage signals the presence of CSF. CSF leakage indicates a tear in the dura, making the patient particularly susceptible to meningitis. Basilar fractures may damage the internal carotid artery and the cranial nerves. Hearing loss also may occur.
- *Temporal fractures:* May result in deafness or facial paralysis.
- *Occipital fractures:* May cause visual field and gait disturbances.
- *Sphenoidal fractures:* May disrupt the optic nerve, possibly causing blindness.

**Rupture of cerebral blood vessels**
- *Epidural (extradural) hematoma or hemorrhage:* Usually, bleeding between the dura mater (outer meninges) and skull causes hematoma formation. This creates pressure on the underlying brain and produces a local mass effect, causing IICP and shifting of tissue, which leads to brain stem compression and herniation. Indicators are primarily those of IICP: altered LOC, headache, vomiting, unilateral pupil dilation (on same side as the lesion), and possibly hemiparesis. Although some individuals never regain consciousness, most patients lose consciousness for a short period of time immediately after injury, regain consciousness, and have a lucid period lasting a few hours or 1-2 days. However, because arterial bleeding causes a rapid rise in ICP, a rapid decrease in LOC often ensues. The bleeding site often is the middle meningeal artery or vein, owing to temporal bone fracture. These patients are at high risk for brain stem herniation. A unilateral dilated fixed pupil is a sign of impending herniation and is a neurosurgical emergency. The patient should not be left alone, because respiratory arrest may occur at any time.
- *Subdural hematoma or hemorrhage:* Accumulation of venous blood between the dura mater (outer meninges) and arachnoid membrane (middle meninges) that is not reabsorbed. Hematoma formation creates pressure on the underlying brain and produces a local mass effect, causing IICP and shifting of tissue, leading to brain stem compression and herniation. This type of hematoma is classified as acute, subacute, or chronic depending on how quickly indicators arise. In acute subdural hematomas, indicators appear within 24-48 h, resulting from focal neurologic deficit (hemiparesis, pupillary dilation) and IICP (headache, decreased LOC). When indicators occur 2-14 days later, the hematoma is considered subacute. When indicators occur ≥2 weeks later, it is considered chronic. Early indicators can include headache, progressive personality changes, decreased intellectual functioning, and drowsiness. Later indicators may include unilateral weakness or paralysis and loss of consciousness and occasionally seizures. Patients with cerebral atrophy (e.g., elders and chronic alcohol users) are more prone to subdural hematoma formation.
- *Intracerebral hemorrhage:* Arterial or venous bleeding into the white matter of the brain. Signs of IICP may develop early if the bleeding causes a rapidly expanding space-occupying lesion. If the bleeding is slower, signs of IICP can take 36-72 h to develop. Indicators depend on location of the hematoma and can include altered LOC, headache, aphasia, hemiparesis,

hemiplegia, hemisensory deficits, pupillary changes, and loss of consciousness.

- *Subarachnoid hemorrhage:* Bleeding into the subarachnoid space below the arachnoid membrane (middle meninges) and above the pia mater (inner meninges next to brain). The patient often has a severe headache. Other general indicators include vomiting, restlessness, seizures, and loss of consciousness. Signs of meningeal irritation include nuchal rigidity and positive Kernig's (see p. 195) and Brudzinski's (see p. 195) signs. This patient may be a candidate for a shunt because of hemorrhagic interference with CSF circulation and reabsorption.

**Indicators of IICP**

- *Early indicators:* Alteration in LOC ranging from irritability, restlessness, and confusion to lethargy; possible onset or worsening of headache; beginning pupillary dysfunction, such as sluggishness; visual disturbances, such as diplopia or blurred vision; onset or increase in sensorimotor changes or deficits, such as weakness; onset or worsening of nausea.
- *Late indicators:* Continued deterioration of LOC leading to stupor and coma; projectile vomiting; hemiplegia; posturing; alterations in VS (typically increased systolic BP, widening pulse pressure, decreased pulse rate); respiratory irregularities, such as Cheyne-Stokes breathing; pupillary changes, such as inequality, dilatation, and nonreactivity to light; papilledema; and impaired brain stem reflexes (corneal, gag, swallowing).

---

**Note:**   The single most important early indicator of IICP is a change in LOC. Late indicators of IICP usually signal impending or occurring brain stem herniation. Signs generally are related to brain stem compression and disruption of cranial nerves and vital centers. Hypotension and tachycardia in the absence of explainable causes, such as hypovolemia, usually are seen as a terminal event in HI.

---

**Brain herniation:**   Brain herniation occurs when IICP causes displacement of brain tissue from one cranial compartment to another. See late indicators of IICP, above, for signs of impending or initial herniation. In the presence of actual brain herniation, the patient is in a deep coma, pupils become fixed and dilated bilaterally, posturing may progress to bilateral flaccidity, brain stem reflexes generally are lost, and respirations and VS deteriorate and may cease.

**Brain death:**   Criteria for determining brain death are not universally agreed upon. Check state and institutional guidelines. General criteria include absent brain stem reflexes (e.g., apnea, pupils nonreactive to light, no corneal reflex, no oculovestibular reflex to ice water calorics), absent cortical activity (e.g., several flat EEG tracings spaced over time), and coma irreversibility continued over a prescribed period of time, such as 24 h. Brain stem auditory evoked responses and cerebral blood flow studies also may be used to help establish brain death.

## DIAGNOSTIC TESTS

**Cervical spine and skull x-rays:**   To locate neck and skull fractures. Because of the close association between head injuries and spinal or vertebral injuries, cervical immobilization is essential until cervical x-rays rule out fracture and potential spinal cord injury (SCI).

**CT scan:**   To identify type, location, and extent of injury, such as accumulation of blood or a shift of midline structure caused by IICP.

**MRI:**   To identify the type, location, and extent of injury. Although not usually performed in acute, unstable patients, this test is the study of choice for subacute or chronic HI. It is superior to CT scan for detecting isodense chronic subdural hematomas or evaluating contusions and shearing injuries, especially in the brain stem area.

**EEG:**   May reveal abnormal electrical activity indicating neuronal damage due to ischemia or hemorrhage. EEG may be used to establish brain death in conjunction with other tests and may be done serially to assess development of pathologic wave.

**Evoked response potentials:**   Used to evaluate the integrity of the brain's anatomic pathways and connections. Stimulation of a sense organ, such as an ear, triggers a discrete electrical response (i.e., evoked potential) along a neurologic pathway to the brain. Measurement of the brain's response to auditory, visual, and/or somatosensory stimulation also aids in predicting neurologic outcome.

**Cerebral angiography:**   To reveal presence of a hematoma and status of blood vessels secondary to rupture or compression. Angiography usually is performed only if CT scan or MRI is unavailable or to evaluate possible carotid or vertebral artery dissection.

**Brain scan:**   To identify hematoma with chronic subdural hematoma. It is not done for acute disorders because of the lengthy uptake time of the radioactive isotope. For the most part, brain scan has been replaced by CT scan and MRI.

---

**Note:**   See "General Care of Patients with Neurologic Disorders," **Knowledge deficit:** Neurologic diagnostic tests, p. 311, for care considerations for patients undergoing CT scan, MRI, EEG, evoked potentials, cerebral angiography, and brain scan.

---

## COLLABORATIVE MANAGEMENT

**Maintenance of airway, respirations, and therapeutic O$_2$ levels:**   O$_2$ delivery, airway maintenance, intubation, and ventilation to prevent hypoxia. Hyperventilation may be necessary to reduce Paco$_2$ levels and promote cerebral vasoconstriction, which will reduce ICP. Nasal intubation or cricothyroidotomy may be performed to prevent neck hyperextension on patients in whom cervical neck injury has not yet been ruled out.

**Monitoring of VS/neurologic status:**   Baseline assessment is established, and patient is monitored frequently for changes

**Positioning:**   Bed rest with HOB elevated (or as prescribed) to promote venous drainage and help reduce cerebral congestion and edema. If a subdural drain is placed, the HOB may be flat while the drain is in place and for 24 h after removal to prevent air being pulled into the subdural space.

**Fluids and electrolytes:**   NPO status for 8-24 h (or longer if patient is unresponsive). Fluids are restricted usually to ⅔ maintenance (<1500 ml) to decrease cerebral edema. I&O are measured carefully, and the patient usually has an indwelling catheter. Supplementation of electrolytes is done in response to laboratory results. Hypotonic IV solutions, such as D$_5$W, are contraindicated because they increase cerebral edema.

**Gastrointestinal decompression:**   Initially the patient may have a gastric tube for gastric decompression to prevent vomiting and aspiration. With basilar skull fractures the tube may be inserted through the mouth to avoid passing the tube *via* the nose through the fracture area and into the brain.

**Nutritional support:**   Total parenteral nutrition (TPN), intralipids, tube feedings, or progressive diet, depending on patient's LOC, ability to swallow, and GI tract functioning.

**Treatment of secondary complications:**   E.g., cerebral edema, IICP, syndrome of inappropriate antidiuretic hormone (SIADH), disseminated intravascular coagulation (DIC), adult respiratory distress syndrome (ARDS), diabetes insipidus, infection, and seizures.

**Pharmacotherapy:**   Narcotics and other medications that alter mentation are generally avoided.

*Antiepilepsy drugs (e.g., phenytoin, phenobarbital, IV diazepam):*   Prophylaxis for seizures with or following penetrating wounds.

*Glucocorticosteroids (e.g., dexamethasone):*   To decrease cerebral edema. There is some controversy regarding effectiveness of glucocorticoids in reducing cerebral edema.

*Osmotic diuretics (e.g., mannitol) and loop diuretics (e.g., furosemide):*   To decrease cerebral edema.

*Antibiotics and tetanus prophylaxis:*   In the presence of penetrating wounds and basilar fractures.

*Antipyretics (e.g., acetaminophen):*   For fever, so that patient's metabolic needs are not increased.

*Analgesics (e.g., acetaminophen, codeine):*   For pain.

*Mild sedatives (e.g., diphenhydramine):*   For restlessness.

*Blood pressure medications:*   To control hypertension and hypotension so that optimal cerebral blood flow is maintained and cerebral edema is reduced.

*Antacids and histamine H$_2$-receptor blockers (e.g., ranitidine):*   To reduce gastric acidity and prevent gastric ulcer formation.

*Stool softeners and laxatives (e.g., docusate sodium):*   To prevent constipation and straining at stool, which would increase ICP.

*Tranquilizers (e.g., chlorpromazine):*   To control shivering, which can increase ICP.

*Tricyclic antidepressants (e.g., amitriptyline, doxepin):*   To increase neurotransmitters in the CSF.

*Skeletal muscle relaxants (e.g., pancuronium):*   To decrease the skeletal muscle tension that is seen with abnormal flexion and extension posturing, which can increase ICP. This therapy requires transfer of patient to ICU for intubation and ventilation.

*Barbiturate coma therapy:*   To reduce cerebral metabolic rate during uncontrolled intracranial hypertension. This therapy requires transfer of patient to ICU for intubation and ventilation.

*Exogenous antidiuretic hormone (e.g., vasopressin or desmopressin):*   To treat diabetes insipidus.

**Hypothermia:**   Hypothalamic dysfunction from swelling or injury may cause hyperthermia. Induced hypothermia *via* a cooling blanket is a controversial treatment used to obtain a subnormal body temperature and thereby minimize metabolic needs.

**Antiembolism hose:**   To prevent thrombophlebitis and pulmonary emboli.

**Bowel and bladder program:**   A bowel program is initiated to prevent straining at stool. Initially the patient usually has an indwelling urinary catheter. A bladder training program may be necessary, depending on the presence and type of neurologic deficit.

**Physical medicine:**   Physical therapy, occupational therapy, and assistive devices or braces may be prescribed to promote mobility and independence with ADL, depending on presence and type of neurologic deficit.

**Speech therapy:**   To evaluate and aid communication of aphasic or dysarthric patients.

**Seizure precautions:**   To prevent injury in the event of seizure activity.

**Cognitive rehabilitation:**   To promote the highest level of cognitive functioning (Table 4-3). Start coma stimulation techniques on appropriate patients to increase the quantity, quality, and duration of responses. Most cognitive recovery occurs in the first 6 months. Provide referrals, as appropriate, to cognitive retraining specialist.

**Surgical procedures**

*Suturing:*   To repair superficial laceration or dural tears.

*Craniotomy, craniectomy:*   To evacuate hematomas, control hemorrhage, remove bone fragment or foreign objects, debride necrotic tissue, or elevate depressed fractures. (See "Brain Tumors," p. 260, for patient care.)

*Trephination ("burr" holes):*   To evacuate hematomas or insert intracranial monitoring devices.

*Cranioplasty:*   To repair traumatic or surgical defects in the skull.

**T A B L E   4 - 3    Cognitive Rehabilitation Goals***

| Level | Response | Goal/Intervention |
|-------|----------|-------------------|
| I | None | *Goal:* Provide sensory input to elicit responses |
| II | Generalized | of increased quality, frequency, duration, |
| III | Localized | and variety. |
| | | *Intervention:* Give brief but frequent stimulation sessions, and present stimuli in an organized manner, focusing on one sensory channel at a time; e.g.: |
| | | *Visual:* Intermittent television, family pictures, bright objects |
| | | *Auditory:* Tape recordings of family or favorite song, talking to patient, intermittent TV or radio |
| | | *Olfactory:* Favorite perfume, shaving lotion, coffee, lemon, orange |
| | | *Cutaneous:* Touch or rub skin with different textures such as velvet, ice bag, warm cloth |
| | | *Movement:* Turn, ROM exercises, up in chair |
| | | *Oral:* Oral care, lemon swabs, ice, sugar on tongue, peppermint, chocolate |
| IV | Confused, agitated | *Goal:* Decrease agitation and increase awareness of environment. This stage usually lasts 2-4 weeks. |
| | | *Interventions:* Remove offending devices (e.g., nasogastric [NG] tube, restraints), if possible. |
| | | Do not demand patient follow-through with task. |
| | | Provide human contact unless this increases agitation. |
| | | Provide a quiet, controlled environment. |
| | | Use a calm, soft voice and manner around patient. |
| V | Confused, inappropriate | *Goal:* Decrease confusion and incorporate improved cognitive abilities into functional activity. |
| VI | Confused, appropriate | |
| | | *Interventions:* Begin each interaction with introduction, orientation, and interaction purpose. |
| | | List and number daily activity in the sequence in which it will be done throughout the day. |
| | | Maintain a consistent environment. |
| | | Provide memory aids (e.g., calendar, clock). |

*Adapted from Rancho Los Amigos Hospital, Inc, Levels of Cognitive Functioning (scale based on behavioral descriptions or responses to stimuli).

*Continued.*

## T A B L E  4 - 3  Cognitive Rehabilitation Goals—cont'd

| Level | Response | Goal/Intervention |
|-------|----------|-------------------|
| VI | Confused, appropriate—cont'd | Use gentle repetition, which aids learning. Provide supervision and structure. Reorient as needed. |
| VII<br>VIII | Automatic, appropriate<br>Purposeful | *Goal:* Integrate increased cognitive function into functional community activities with minimal structuring.<br>*Interventions:* Enable practicing of activities. Reduce supervision and environmental structure.<br>Help patient plan adaptation of ADL and home living skills to home environment. |

***Ventricular puncture, ventriculostomy:***　To remove excess CSF.
***Ventricular shunt:***　To provide drainage of CSF and reduce ICP. See "Brain Tumors," p. 261, for patient care.
***Placement of ICP monitoring device:***　To provide accurate and continual monitoring of patient's ICP. This necessitates transfer of patient to ICU for monitoring.
***Repair of CSF leak:***　Most CSF leaks from dural tears heal themselves in 5-10 days. If they do not, serial lumbar punctures or a lumbar subarachnoid drain may be needed to drain CSF, reduce CSF pressure, and promote healing. Acetazolamide or dexamethasone may be given to decrease CSF production. Radionuclide-labeled materials may be placed in the CSF to find the site of the leak. Basilar fractures are a common site of CSF leaks and make surgical repair difficult because of location inaccessibility.
　—With a lumbar drain the patient is on bed rest with HOB elevated up to 15-20 degrees and instructed not to cough, sneeze, or strain. Maintain HOB and collection container securely at prescribed levels. Maintain a sterile occlusive dressing. Possible complications include meningitis (see p. 194) or a tension pneumothorax (see p. 19) resulting from too rapid drainage of CSF, which causes air to siphon in through the dural tear, creating an intracranial mass effect. If neurologic signs deteriorate, clamp the lumbar drain tubing, place patient flat or in a slight Trendelenburg position, and provide supplemental $O_2$, which will promote absorption of intracranial air and relieve IICP.

## NURSING DIAGNOSES AND INTERVENTIONS

**Knowledge deficit:**　Caretaker's responsibilities for observing the patient who is sent home with a concussion
**Desired outcomes:**　Following instruction, caretaker verbalizes knowledge about the observation regimen. Caretaker returns patient to the hospital if neurologic deficits are noted.
*If patient goes home for observation, provide caretaker with verbal and written instructions for the following:*
• Avoid giving patient anything stronger than acetaminophen to relieve headache. Aspirin is usually contraindicated because it can prolong bleeding, if it occurs.
• Assess patient at least hourly for the first 24 h as follows: Awaken patient; ask patient's name, location, and caretaker's name; monitor for twitching or seizure activity. Return patient to the hospital immediately if he or she be-

comes increasingly difficult to awaken; cannot answer questions appropriately; cannot answer at all; becomes confused, restless, or agitated; develops slurred speech; develops twitching or seizures; develops or reports worsening headache or nausea/vomiting; has visual disturbances, such as blurred or double vision; develops weakness, numbness, clumsiness, or has difficulty walking; has clear or bloody drainage from the nose or ear; or develops a stiff neck.

- Ensure that patient rests and eats lightly for the first day or so after the concussion or until he or she feels well. Over the next 2-3 days, patient should avoid alcohol, driving, contact sports, swimming, using power tools, and taking medication for headache or nausea without calling the physician.
- Inform patient and significant others that some individuals may have a postconcussion syndrome in which they continue to have headaches, dizziness, or lethargy for several weeks or months after a concussion. Patient also may experience sleep disturbance, difficulty concentrating, poor memory, irritability, emotional lability, and difficulty with judgment or abstract thinking. Explain the importance of reporting these problems to the physician.

**High risk for infection** related to inadequate primary defenses secondary to basilar skull fractures, penetrating or open head injuries, or surgical wounds
***Desired outcomes:*** Patient is free of symptoms of infection as evidenced by normothermia, stable or improving LOC, and absence of headache, photophobia, or neck stiffness. Patient verbalizes knowledge about the signs and symptoms of infection and the importance of reporting them promptly.

- Monitor injury site or surgical wounds for indicators of infection, such as persistent erythema, warmth, pain, hardness, and purulent drainage. Notify physician of significant findings.
- Be alert to indicators of meningitis or encephalitis (fever, chills, malaise, back stiffness and pain, nuchal rigidity, photophobia, seizures, ataxia, sensorimotor deficits), which can occur after a penetrating, open head injury or cerebral surgical wound.
- When examining scalp lacerations and assessing for foreign bodies or palpable fractures, wear sterile gloves and follow aseptic technique. Cleanse the area gently, and cover scalp wounds with sterile dressings.
- Document drainage and its amount, color, and odor. If the patient has clear or bloody drainage from the nose, throat, or ears, notify physician of findings and assume that the patient has a dural tear with CSF leakage until proven otherwise. Complaints of a salty taste or swallowing frequently may signal CSF dripping down the back of the throat. Bending forward may produce nasal drainage that can be tested for CSF. Inspect the dressing and pillowcases for the presence of a halo ring, which may indicate CSF drainage. Clear drainage may be tested with a glucose reagent strip. Drainage may also be sent to the laboratory to test for Cl. The presence of glucose and Cl (CSF Cl is > serum Cl) in nonsanguineous drainage indicates that the drainage is CSF rather than mucus or saliva.
- If CSF leakage occurs, do not clean the ears or nose unless prescribed by physician. Place a sterile pad over the affected ear or under the nose to catch drainage, but do not pack them. Position patient so that fluids can drain. Change dressings when they become damp, using aseptic technique.
- To prevent introduction of bacteria into the nervous system in the presence of CSF leakage or possible basilar fracture, avoid nasal suction. Instruct patient to avoid Valsalva's maneuver and vigorous coughing to prevent tearing of the dura and increased CSF flow and to avoid nose-blowing, sneezing, or sniffing in of nasal drainage.
- If the patient is intubated, the tube for gastric decompression may be placed orally rather than nasally. If the nasogastric tube is placed nasally, the physician usually performs the intubation. Check placement of the tube, preferably by x-ray, before applying suction. NG tubes have been known to en-

ter the fracture site and curl up into the patient's cranial vault during insertion attempts. Visually check the back of the patient's throat for the NG tube to help confirm placement.

- Individuals with basilar skull fractures generally are placed flat in bed on complete bed rest. This position helps decrease pressure and the amount of CSF draining from a dural tear. Patients are placed on antibiotics to prevent infection and observed for healing and sealing of the dural tear within 7-10 days.
- Teach patient to report any indicators of infection promptly.

**High risk for disuse syndrome** related to prescribed immobility and/or decreased LOC

*Desired outcome:*   Patient exhibits full ROM of all joints.

- For patients at risk of IICP, perform passive ROM exercises rather than allow active or assisted ROM exercises, which can increase intraabdominal or intrathoracic pressure and hence ICP. For the same reason, avoid using the prone position.
- Once the risk of IICP is no longer significant, additional measures to enhance mobility and strength may be implemented. For discussion, see **High risk for activity intolerance,** p. 711, and **High risk for disuse syndrome,** p. 713, in Appendix One, "Caring for Patients on Prolonged Bed Rest."

**Pain** related to headaches secondary to head injury

*Desired outcome:*   Within 1 h of intervention, patient's subjective perception of pain decreases, as documented by a pain scale.

- Monitor and document the duration and character of the patient's pain, rating it on a scale of 0 (no pain) to 10 (worst pain).
- Administer analgesics as prescribed. Patients with head injuries generally do not have much pain, and the pain is usually relieved by analgesics, such as acetaminophen. Sometimes codeine is prescribed, but as a rule, other narcotics are contraindicated because they can mask neurologic indicators of IICP and cause respiratory depression.
- For additional interventions, see **Pain,** p. 308, in "General Care of Patients with Neurologic Disorders."

**Fluid volume excess** related to compromised regulatory mechanisms with increased ADH and increased renal resorption secondary to SIADH

*Desired outcome:*   By hospital discharge (or within 3 days of injury), patient is normovolemic as evidenced by stable weight, balanced I&O, urinary output ≥30 ml/h, urine specific gravity 1.010-1.030, BP within patient's baseline limits, absence of fingerprint edema over the sternum, and orientation to person, place, and time.

- Monitor I&O, daily weight, VS, urine specific gravity, and electrolyte and serum osmolarity studies. Sudden and significant weight gain, urine output <500 ml/24 h, urine specific gravity >1.030, and hypertension occur with SIADH. SIADH creates a dilutional hyponatremia; therefore, also be alert to serum Na levels <137 mEq/L, serum osmolality <280 mOsm/kg, low BUN, and increased urine Na and osmolality. Notify physician of significant changes.
- Monitor patient for changes in orientation and LOC (e.g., apprehension, irritability, confusion), incoordination, headache, anorexia, muscle cramps, and fatigue. These are mild symptoms of SIADH. As SIADH progresses, expect nausea, vomiting, and abdominal cramps. Symptoms of severe SIADH include weakness, lethargy, confusion, muscle twitching, and seizures. Expect seizure activity when serum Na level drops below 118 mEq/L. Serum Na level ≤115 mEq/L may result in loss of reflexes, coma, and death. Notify physician of significant findings. See "Syndrome of Inappropriate Antidiuretic Hormone," p. 351, for more information.
- Monitor patient for symptoms of IICP, and institute measures for its prevention (see **Altered cerebral tissue perfusion,** p. 305).

- Assess for fingerprint edema over the sternum, which reflects cellular edema. Because fluid is not retained in the interstitium with SIADH, peripheral edema will not necessarily occur.
- Maintain fluid restriction as prescribed. Depending on the serum Na value, fluids may be restricted to an amount as low as 500 ml/24 h. Remove water or ice chips from the bedside. Hypotonic solutions such as $D_5W$ usually are contraindicated because of their conversion to free $H_2O$.
- As appropriate, provide measured ice chips and frequent mouth care for thirst.
- Administer hypertonic saline (3%) as prescribed.
- As prescribed, give furosemide (Lasix) to promote diuresis; demeclocycline (Declomycin), which acts as an ADH inhibitor; and lithium, which interferes with the action of aldosterone.
- Ensure that HOB is elevated $\leq$10-20 degrees to promote venous return and left atrial filling pressure, thereby reducing release of ADH.
- Institute seizure precautions (see "Seizure Disorders," p. 288).

---

**Note:**    If the patient has urinary incontinence, retention, or neurogenic bladder, see Chapter Three, "Renal-Urinary Disorders" for related discussions. **Caution:** Credé's method and other measures that can increase intraabdominal and intrathoracic pressure are contraindicated for patients who are at risk of IICP. See "Alzheimer's Disease" for **Sensory/perceptual alterations,** p. 219, and **High risk for violence,** p. 221. See "Brain Tumors" for **Knowledge deficit:** Ventricular shunt procedure, p. 262, and **Knowledge deficit:** Craniotomy procedure, p. 263. See "Cerebrovascular Accident" for **Impaired verbal communication,** p. 284, **Impaired physical mobility,** p. 282, and **Sensory/perceptual alterations,** p. 283. See "Seizure Disorders," p. 292, for seizure-related nursing diagnoses. See "General Care of Patients with Neurologic Disorders" for **High risk for trauma,** p. 298, **High risk for injury** related to impaired pain, touch, and temperature sensation, p. 299, **Impaired corneal tissue integrity,** p. 300, **Altered nutrition,** p. 300, **High risk for fluid volume deficit,** p. 301, **High risk for aspiration,** p. 302, **Self-care deficit,** p. 302, **Constipation,** p. 305, **Altered cerebral tissue perfusion,** p. 305, **Sensory/perceptual alterations,** p. 307, **Impaired swallowing,** p. 308, **Altered body temperature,** p. 310, and **Knowledge deficit:** Neurologic diagnostic tests, p. 311. For patients with diabetes insipidus, see nursing diagnoses in "Diabetes Insipidus," p. 346. For patients with SIADH, see "Syndrome of Antidiuretic Hormone," p. 352." For patients undergoing surgical procedures, see Appendix One, "Caring for Preoperative and Postoperative Patients," p. 693. For patients with varying degrees of immobility, see related nursing diagnoses in "Pressure Ulcers," p. 687, and Appendix One, "Caring for Patients on Prolonged Bed Rest," p. 711. Also see Appendix One, "Caring for Patients with Cancer and Other Life-Disrupting Illnesses," p. 753, for appropriate psychosocial nursing diagnoses and interventions.

---

## PATIENT-FAMILY TEACHING AND DISCHARGE PLANNING

The head-injured patient can have varying degrees of neurologic deficit, ranging from mild to severe. As indicated by the patient's condition and prognosis, give patient and significant others verbal and written information about the following:

- Referrals to community resources, such as cognitive retraining specialist, head injury rehabilitation centers, visiting nurses association, community support groups, social workers, psychologic therapy, vocational rehabilitation agency, home health agencies, and extended and skilled care facilities. In addition, provide the following address: National Head Injury Foundation, 1140 Connecticut Avenue NW, Suite 812, Washington, DC 20036, (202)-296-6443 or (800)-444-6443.

- Safety measures related to decreased sensation, visual disturbances, motor deficits, and seizure activity.
- Measures that promote communication in the presence of aphasia.
- Wound care and indicators of infection.
- Measures that deal with cognitive or behavioral problems. As appropriate, include home evaluation for safety. Caution significant others that personality can change drastically after HI. The patient may demonstrate inappropriate social behavior, inappropriate affect, hallucination, delusion, and altered sleep pattern.
- If patient had a concussion, a description of problems that may occur at home and necessitate prompt medical attention (see **Knowledge deficit,** p. 254).
- For other information, see teaching and discharge planning interventions (the fourth through tenth entries only) in "Multiple Sclerosis," p. 187, as appropriate.

# Section Four:   Nervous System Tumors

## Brain tumors

The abnormal and uncontrolled cell growth of neoplastic or benign tumors can have a wide variety of effects on the brain. Most significant is the disruption of neuronal function caused by infiltration of the tissue, compression of brain tissue and blood vessels, or obstruction of normal flow of CSF. The increase in ICP from tumor growth and other factors, such as cerebral edema, will cause brain structures to shift, eventually leading to brain herniation and death. *Primary brain tumors,* composed of nervous system tissue, rarely metastasize outside the central nervous system (CNS). It is not uncommon, however, for primary brain tumors to metastasize to other parts of the CNS. *Secondary brain tumors* arise from cells that have metastasized from other parts of the body, such as the lung, breast, and skin. Although benign tumors tend to be more treatable than neoplastic tumors, they are considered serious because they are equally capable of destroying adjacent nerves through compression and increasing ICP, which in turn compromises vital centers.

**Tumor classification:**   Generally, brain tumors are classified according to their cell of origin. They may be further classified by cell differentiation (e.g., benign, malignant, grade I-IV) and by their location.

- *Gliomas:* Comprise 45% of all brain tumors and arise from brain connective tissue. Generally, they are infiltrative and often cannot be removed totally by surgery. As a group, gliomas usually are considered neoplastic.

  —Astrocytomas: The most common glioma, astrocytomas are graded from I to IV, with grade I cytologically (but not necessarily biologically) benign and grade IV the most malignant. Glioblastoma multiforme is a grade III-IV astrocytoma and is the most common (20% of all brain tumors), and a highly malignant glioma. It is usually found in the cerebral hemisphere and may metastasize to other parts of the CNS.

  —Oligodendrogliomas: The next most common glioma, arising out of cells involved in the process of myelination. Generally, they are slow-growing, often encapsulated, tumors, which often are cytologically (but not necessarily biologically) benign.

  —Medulloblastomas: This relatively rare glioma is highly malignant, often obstructs CSF flow, and metastasizes to the spinal cord. It is found primarily in children.

  —Ependymomas: This glioma arises out of the cells that line the cavities of the CNS, such as the ventricles, and usually obstructs CSF flow. These rare tumors are quite invasive and primarily are found in children and young adults.

- *Meningiomas:* Originate from pia or arachnoid membranes and make up around 15% of all brain tumors. They are slow-growing and, while technically benign, can invade the skull and cause brain tissue compression.
- *Schwannomas (e.g., acoustic neuroma):* Account for about 10% of brain tumors, affect the craniospinal nerve sheath, and are slow-growing. Although these tumors are cytologically benign, they may not be diagnosed until they are large in size and compressing sensitive brain stem centers.
- *Pituitary tumors:* See "Pituitary and Hypothalamic Tumors," p. 347.
- *Secondary (metastatic) tumors:* Most often occur in the cerebrum, may be multiple because of the "seeding" effect, and resemble the primary neoplasm histologically. Lung and breast carcinomas are the lesions that most frequently result in metastases to the brain.

## ASSESSMENT

Onset of signs and symptoms usually is insidious and progressive, although seizure activity may be the first sign in 15% of cases.

**General indicators:** Headache (especially in the morning), nausea, projectile vomiting, lethargy, forgetfulness, disorientation, personality changes, and seizure activity.

**Focal symptoms**

- *Frontal lobe:* Personality/mood changes, impaired judgment, weakness or paralysis (usually unilateral), apraxia, aphasia.
- *Parietal lobe:* Visual field deficit, sensory disturbance, impaired position sense, perceptual problems, such as altered stereognosis and dyslexia.
- *Temporal lobe:* Auditory changes, tinnitus, visual field deficit, sensory aphasia, impaired memory, personality changes, psychomotor seizures.
- *Occipital lobe:* Seizures, visual agnosia, visual field deficit.
- *Cerebellar:* Tremors, nystagmus, incoordination, loss of balance, gait disturbances, nuchal headache.
- *Ventricular or hypothalamic:* Diabetes insipidus, weight gain, somnolence, headache, disturbance of temperature regulation.
- *Cranial nerve:* Sense of smell alterations, ptosis, diplopia, alterations in ocular movement, drooping of facial muscles on the same side as the tumor, difficulty swallowing, loss of cough/gag reflex, loss of corneal reflex, protrusion of the tongue toward the side of the tumor.
- *Schwannoma:* Unilateral hearing loss with or without tinnitus, stiff neck. Other symptoms may include decreased facial sensation, facial muscle weakness or paralysis on same side as the hearing loss, and diplopia. Late symptoms include ataxia and arm coordination problems secondary to brain stem and cerebellar compression.

**Indicators of IICP:** See discussion in "Head Injury," p. 250.

**Indicators of brain stem herniation:** See discussion in "Head Injury," p. 250.

**Physical assessment:** Ophthalmoscopic examination may reveal papilledema if ICP is increased; visual field exam may reveal impairment such as hemianopia (blindness in part of the field of vision); and audiometry or vestibular function studies may show abnormalities such as hearing loss, especially with acoustic neuromas.

## DIAGNOSTIC TESTS

Diagnostic tests are done to rule out vascular causes, such as hemorrhage, abscess, and trauma, as well as to diagnose brain tumor. Any one or a combination of the following tests may be performed.

**MRI:** May reveal presence of tumor, tissue shift, and hydrocephalus. This diagnostic tool, because of its ability to detect biochemical changes, can help diagnose tumors at an early stage. It is also very good for visualizing brain stem and posterior fossa structures.

**CT scan:**  May detect tumor mass, tissue shift, and hydrocephalus. Serial screens may be done to track the tumor's response to therapy.

**X-rays of the skull and spinal cord:**  May reveal tumors that contain calcium or cause bony erosion.

**Positron emission tomography (PET):**  May distinguish tumor tissue from normal brain tissue by identifying abnormal metabolic activity of the tumor tissue.

**EEG:**  May localize abnormal brain wave activity, which may suggest tumor growth.

**Brain scan:**  May demonstrate presence of a space-occupying lesion *via* uptake of radioisotope. This test is helpful in localizing certain tumors such as meningiomas.

**Cerebral angiography:**  May show abnormal perfusion patterns, which suggest tumor location; also may reveal alterations in the position of vessels caused by the tumor, and may even outline the tumor *via* its circulation. The test may be performed preoperatively in order to plan surgical strategy.

**Lumbar puncture (LP) and CSF analysis:**  May be performed in the absence of any indicators of IICP. CSF may be clear to bloody; protein values and WBC count may be increased; glucose values may be decreased; and cytology may reveal the presence of cancer cells. This test usually is done when there is concern about the possibility of an infectious process.

**Lesion biopsy:**  Identifies pathologic cells and confirms diagnosis.

**Endocrine studies:**  May show abnormal hormonal levels that may signal a pituitary tumor. See "Pituitary and Hypothalamic Tumors," p. 348.

**Evoked potentials:**  Brain stem auditory evoked response may be reduced with acoustic neuromas.

**Stapedius reflex study:**  Measures the contraction of the stapedius muscle with high-intensity sound. The muscle should stay contracted as long as sound is present. With acoustic neuroma, the muscle initially may contract but then relax.

**Electronystagmography:**  Acoustic neuroma may cause a reduced caloric response.

**Tumor markers:**  To measure presence of substances that are unique or very specific to a class of tumor. This test will aid in the diagnosis of the tumor type and measure response to therapy.

**Other studies such as chest x-rays:**  To determine primary site(s) of metastatic brain tumors.

---

**Note:**  See "General Care of Patients with Neurologic Disorders," **Knowledge deficit:** Neurologic diagnostic tests, p. 311, for care considerations for patients undergoing MRI, CT scan, PET, EEG, brain scan, cerebral angiography, LP, and evoked potentials.

---

## COLLABORATIVE MANAGEMENT

The mode of treatment depends on the tumor's histologic type, anatomic location, and sensitivity to radiation. Treatment usually includes surgery, often in combination with radiation or chemotherapy. Immunotherapy also is being evaluated as a treatment modality. The location and accessibility of the tumor determines whether or not surgery can be performed. Tumors of the brain stem, medulla, pons, and corpus callosum tend to be inaccessible. Partial surgical resection may be done to debulk the tumor, decompress the brain, and relieve symptoms temporarily.

**Craniotomy/craniectomy:**  Surgical opening into the skull. The bone flap may be left open postoperatively to accommodate cerebral edema and prevent compression.

**Surgical techniques:**    Laser neurosurgery has proven useful in certain types of tumor removal, such as meningiomas. *Laser neurosurgery* tends to be more precise than conventional dissection, resulting in less tissue damage and less postoperative swelling. Drugs such as hematoporphyrin may be given to photosensitize tumor cells selectively in order to increase their precise destruction. *Stereotaxic neurosurgery* techniques using the CT scan and computer processing of stereoactive data allow the precise guidance of a surgical probe to the tumor for biopsy, ablative procedures, or radiation implants. Some deep tumors now can be removed or debulked without extensive damage to surrounding brain tissue. Sometimes ultrasound can be used during surgery to locate the tumor diagnostically and then remove the tumor layer by layer by fragmenting the tissue with an ultrasonic vibrating tip.

**Transsphenoidal hypophysectomy:**    For pituitary tumors (see "Pituitary and Hypothalamic Tumors," p. 349).

**Ventricular shunt for ventricular drainage:**    May be done to allow drainage of CSF. This procedure is usually performed if the brain tumor is inoperable and obstructs the flow of CSF, causing IICP. The shunt mechanically may carry CSF from the ventricles to another body part, such as the left atrium of the heart or peritoneal cavity. A surgical procedure called a third ventriculostomy produces an exit for ventricular fluid without tubes or synthetic materials by using a probe to create another drainage canal in the brain.

**Supportive pharmacotherapy**

*Antiepilepsy agents (e.g., phenytoin):*    Prophylaxis for seizures.

*Osmotic diuretics (e.g., mannitol) and loop diuretics (e.g., furosemide):*    To decrease cerebral edema and ICP.

*Glucocorticosteroids (e.g., dexamethasone):*    To reduce cerebral edema. May be used after radiotherapy to decrease radiation-induced edema.

*Antacids and histamine $H_2$-receptor blockers (e.g., ranitidine):*    To prevent/ treat stress ulcers by reducing gastric acidity.

*Analgesics (e.g., acetaminophen, codeine):*    For headaches.

*Antipyretics (e.g., acetaminophen):*    To reduce fever so that cerebral metabolic needs are not increased.

*Stool softeners and laxatives (e.g., docusate):*    To prevent constipation and straining at stool, which would increase ICP.

**Radiation therapy:**    To destroy remaining tumor cells or treat inaccessible tumors. External beam radiation is frequently begun as soon as the surgical incision has healed. It can be localized or include the entire brain and part of the spinal cord, depending on the type, location, and extent of the tumor.

Radiation can cause inflammation of the brain, which in turn increases ICP and neurologic symptoms. A cerebral radiation necrosis with symptoms similar to tumor recurrence may occur 6-36 months after treatment. An MRI, CT scan, or PET will distinguish radiation necrosis from tumor recurrence. Treatment is surgical removal of the necrotic mass and high-dose steroids.

With inoperable tumors, radiation therapy often becomes the primary modality. Proton beam irradiation seems effective against certain tumor types. Stereotaxic radiotherapy with a "gamma knife" is believed to be capable of destroying deep and inaccessible lesions in a single treatment. Multiple beams are focused at the tumor with such precision that surrounding tissue is spared. This irradiation is very useful with acoustic neuromas. Maximal shrinkage of tumors may take 1-4 years. Other techniques include the placement of radionuclide seeds into the tumors of patients with recurrent malignant gliomas. Placement of the seeds requires either a stereotaxic procedure or a craniotomy. Techniques being used to increase tumor cell sensitivity to radiation include localized tumor tissue heating (with an implanted microwave probe or electrode) and hyperbaric $O_2$ therapy. For more information about radiation therapy, see Appendix One, "Caring for Patients with Cancer and Other Life-Disrupting Illnesses," p. 735.

**Chemotherapy:**    Nitrosourea agents, such as carmustine (BCNU), lomustine

(CCNU), and methyl-CCNU, cross the blood-brain barrier and because of this are useful for patients with brain tumors. Other drugs used include cisplatin, methotrexate, 5-fluorouracil, procarbazine, and etoposide. Generally, chemotherapy is used only as an adjunct to surgery and radiation therapy. Chemotherapy on some tumors is used only after tumor regrowth or when the tumor is not sensitive to radiation therapy. Intraarterial (carotid), intrathecal, and intraventricular (Ommaya reservoir) delivery of chemotherapeutic agents such as methotrexate to the brain is being investigated in the hopes of getting higher drug doses to the tumor while limiting the degree of systemic side effects. Bone marrow sometimes is harvested and then returned to the patient to protect against bone marrow suppression. Immunotherapy using biologic response modifiers (BRM) such as interferons, interleukins, *Cornebacterium parvum*, tumor necrosis factor, and ImuVert strives to act on the host immune system to improve antitumor response or increase antitumor defenses. See Appendix One, "Caring for Patients with Cancer and Other Life-Disrupting Illnesses," p. 719, for more information about chemotherapy and immunotherapy.

**Conductive hyperthermia:**   This investigational technique to destroy brain tumors is based on the fact that the cancer cell is heat-sensitive and may be damaged by temperatures that do not harm normal cells. Hyperthermia catheters are inserted into the entire tumor mass using a stereotactic CT-guided technique. The tumor is then heated for a period of 3-4 days. Activity is restricted during this time, and the patient may have a headache. The catheters are removed before hospital discharge. The patient usually has 3 hyperthermia cycles at 6-8 week intervals.

*Depending on the presence and severity of neurologic deficits, the patient also may need the following:*

**Respiratory support and intubation:**   To maintain the airway and supply $O_2$ as needed.

**Fluid and nutritional support:**   The patient may require high-calorie, high-protein supplements and enteral feedings or parenteral nutrition because of swallowing/chewing deficits or side effects of radiation and chemotherapy, and IV fluids to prevent dehydration. See "Providing Nutritional Therapy," p. 665, for more information.

**Physical medicine:**   E.g., physical therapy (PT), occupational therapy (OT), and assistive devices or braces so that the patient can maintain mobility and independence with ADL. Muscle-strengthening exercises, conditioning exercises, and gait training are also frequently prescribed.

**ROM exercises:**   To maintain or increase joint function and prevent contractures. While the patient is at risk of IICP, the exercises are passive only. Once the risk of IICP is minimized, active or active-assistive ROM is employed.

**Bowel and bladder program:**   To prevent incontinence and constipation.

**Treatment of secondary complications:**   E.g., cerebral edema, IICP, SIADH, and diabetes insipidus.

## NURSING DIAGNOSES AND INTERVENTIONS

**Knowledge deficit:**   Ventricular shunt procedure

*Desired outcome:*  Following the explanation, patient verbalizes accurate information about the ventricular shunt procedure, including presurgical and postsurgical care.

• Determine patient's understanding of the procedure after physician's explanation, including purpose, risks, and anticipated benefits or outcome. Intervene accordingly.

• Explain that the procedure is performed to enable drainage of CSF when flow is obstructed (e.g., because of the presence of a tumor or blood). Shunt types vary but can extend from the lateral ventricle of the brain to one of the following: subarachnoid space of the spinal canal, right atrium of the heart, a large vein, or the peritoneal cavity.

- Explain that it is important to avoid lying on the insertion site after the procedure to prevent putting pressure on the shunt mechanism. The head and neck are kept in alignment to prevent kinking and compression of the shunt catheter. Explain that the shunt site will be monitored for redness, tenderness, bulging, or fluid collection, and swelling will be assessed along the shunt's course.
- If the shunt has a valve for controlling CSF drainage or reflux, explain that the valve will be pumped or compressed a certain number of times at prescribed intervals to flush the system of exudate and prevent plugging. Explain that the valve, which is usually located behind or above the ear and is the approximate diameter of a fingertip, can be felt to empty and then refill.
- Reassure patient and significant others that before hospital discharge specific instructions will be given about shunt care, recognition of shunt site infection and malfunction, and steps to take should they occur. Teach signs and symptoms of IICP (i.e., headache, change in LOC such as drowsiness, lethargy, irritability, personality changes), which can signal shunt malfunction.
- For additional interventions, see **High risk for infection,** p. 255, in "Head Injury" and this nursing diagnosis in Appendix One, "Caring for Preoperative and Postoperative Patients," p. 693.

**Knowledge deficit:**    Craniotomy procedure

*Desired outcome:*    Following the explanation, patient verbalizes accurate understanding of the craniotomy procedure, including presurgical and postsurgical care.

- After physician's explanation of the procedure, determine patient's level of understanding of the purpose, risks, and anticipated benefits or outcome. Intervene accordingly or reinforce physician's explanation as appropriate.
- Explain that a craniotomy is a surgical opening into the skull to remove a hematoma or tumor, repair a ruptured aneurysm, or apply arterial clips or wrap the involved vessel to prevent future rupture. As appropriate, explain that the bone flap may be left open postoperatively to accommodate cerebral edema and prevent compression. When the bone is removed, the procedure is called a craniectomy.
- Explain that before surgery, antiseptic shampoos may be given and the patient may be started on corticosteroids such as dexamethasone and antiepilepsy drugs. Explain that a baseline neurologic assessment will provide a basis for comparison with postoperative neurologic checks.
- During the immediate postoperative period, the patient is in the ICU. Explain the following considerations and interventions that are likely to occur.
  - Assessment of VS and neurologic status at least hourly. Patient will be asked to perform a variety of assessment measures, including squeezing tester's hand, moving extremities, extending the tongue, and answering questions. Emphasize the importance of performing these tasks to the best of the patient's ability.
  - Changes in body image that can occur because of loss of hair, presence of a head dressing, and the potential for and expected duration of facial edema.
  - Possible need for respiratory and airway support, including $O_2$, intubation, or ventilation. Typically patients are on a cardiac monitor for 24-48 h because dysrhythmias are not unusual after posterior fossa surgery or when blood is in the CSF.
  - Presence of large head dressing and drains, which will be inspected periodically for bleeding or CSF leakage. Stress the importance of not pulling or tugging on the dressing or drains.
  - NPO status for the first 36-48 h because of the risk of vomiting and choking. Explain that once fluids are allowed, they usually are limited to minimize cerebral edema.

- Periorbital swelling, which usually occurs within 24-48 h of supratentorial surgery. Explain that relief is obtained with applications of cold or warm compresses around the eyes.
- Insertion of indwelling urinary catheter to enable accurate measurement of I&O and monitor for problems such as diabetes insipidus.
- Measurement of core temperature (e.g., rectal, tympanic, bladder) at frequent intervals. A rectal probe or bladder catheter temperature probe may be used for continuous monitoring. Oral temperatures are avoided during the period while cognitive function is decreased.
- Teach patient that postsurgical positioning is a key factor during recovery.
  - *Supratentorial craniotomy:* Patient maintained with HOB elevated to 30 degrees or as prescribed. The patient will be assisted with turning and usually will be kept off the operative site, especially if the lesion was large. The head and neck will be kept in good alignment.
  - *Infratentorial craniotomy* (for cerebellar or brain stem surgery): HOB is kept flat or as prescribed. Pressure usually is kept off the operative site, especially with a craniectomy, so these patients are kept off their backs for 48 h. In posterior fossa surgery the supporting neck muscles are altered. Log-roll patient to alternate sides, keeping the head in good alignment. A soft cervical collar may be used to prevent anterior or lateral angulation of the neck. A small pillow may be used for comfort.
- Explain that bed rest will be enforced immediately after surgery.
- Teach patients undergoing infratentorial surgery that they are likely to experience the following:
  - Dizziness and hypotension, necessitating a longer period of bed rest.
  - Nausea, which should be reported so that antiemetics such as metochlorpramide or trimethobenzamide can be given.
  - Cranial nerve edema, which might result in swallowing difficulties, extraocular movements, or nystagmus, any of which should be reported promptly.
- Teach patient the following precautions that are taken to prevent increased intraabdominal and intrathoracic pressure, which can cause IICP:
  - Exhaling when being turned.
  - Not straining at stool.
  - Not moving self in bed, but rather letting staff members do all moving.
  - Importance of deep breathing and avoiding coughing and sneezing. If coughing and sneezing are unavoidable, they must be done with an opened mouth to minimize pressure buildup.
  - Avoiding hip flexion and lying prone.
  - For additional precautions against IICP, see **Altered cerebral tissue perfusion,** p. 305.
- Teach patient that precautions are taken for seizures (see **High risk for trauma** related to oral, musculoskeletal and airway vulnerability secondary to seizure activity, p. 292).
- Teach patient wound care and indicators of infection. Generally, a surgical cap is worn after removal of the head dressing. The patient must avoid scratching the wound or sutures and keep the incision dry. When the sutures are removed, the hair can be shampooed, being careful not to scrub around the suture line. Hair dryers are avoided until the hair is regrown. For more information, see **High risk for infection,** p. 255, in "Head Injury."
- Explain that patients undergoing acoustic neuroma excision may have hearing loss, facial weakness or paralysis, diminished or absent blinking, eye dryness, tinnitus, vertigo, headache, and occasionally swallowing, throat, and voice problems. Contralateral routing of signal hearing aids may improve hearing by directing the sound from the deaf ear to the hearing ear *via* a tiny microphone and transmitter. Background music or other "white noise" may mask tinnitus. Awareness of tinnitus eventually should lessen.

Balance exercises and walking with assistance will start the process of compensation by the functioning vestibular system.
- For additional interventions, see this nursing diagnosis in Appendix One, "Caring for Preoperative and Postoperative Patients," p. 693.

---

**Note:** If patient has urinary incontinence, retention, or neurogenic bladder, see related discussions in "Renal-Urinary Disorders." See "Alzheimer's Disease" for **Sensory/perceptual alterations,** p. 219. See "Head Injury" for **High risk for disuse syndrome,** p. 256, and, if the patient has SIADH, **Fluid volume excess,** p. 256. See "Cerebrovascular Accident" for **Impaired verbal communication,** p. 284; **Impaired physical mobility,** p. 282; and **Sensory/perceptual alterations,** p. 283. See "Seizure Disorders," p. 292, for nursing diagnoses related to seizures. See "General Care of Patients with Neurologic Disorders," pp. 298–316, for related diagnoses. If patient has diabetes insipidus, see related nursing diagnoses in "Diabetes Insipidus," p. 346. If patient has SIADH, see related nursing diagnoses in "Syndrome of Antidiuretic Hormone," p. 352. If patient has a pituitary tumor, see related nursing diagnoses in "Pituitary and Hypothalamic Tumors," p. 349. For patients with varying degrees of immobility, see related nursing diagnoses in "Pressure Ulcer," p. 687, and Appendix One, "Caring for Patients on Prolonged Bed Rest," p. 711. Also see Appendix One, "Caring for Preoperative and Postoperative Patients," p. 693, and "Caring for Patients with Cancer and Other Life-Disrupting Illnesses," p. 719, as appropriate.

---

## PATIENT-FAMILY TEACHING AND DISCHARGE PLANNING

Give patient and significant others verbal and written information about the following as appropriate:
- Safety measures specific to sensory deficits, motor deficits, incoordination, cognitive deficits, and seizures.
- Measures to promote communication in the presence of aphasia.
- Appropriate referrals to community resources, such as public health nurse, visiting nurses association, community support groups, social workers, psychologic therapy, vocational rehabilitation agency, home health agencies, and extended and skilled care facilities. In addition, provide the address for the American Cancer Society: 1599 Clifton Road NE, Atlanta, GA 30329, (404)-320-3333 or (800)-ACS-2345. The American Brain Tumor Association, 3725 North Talman, Chicago, IL, 60618, (312)-286-5571 or (800)-886-2282, also has set up local support groups and will try to assist brain tumor patients and their families. Provide the following address for patients with acoustic neuroma: Acoustic Neuroma Association, P.O. Box 12402, Atlanta, GA 30355, (404)-237-8023.
- Care of postoperative or postprocedure wounds and indicators of infection.
- Potential side effects and precautions for patients undergoing radiation therapy.
- Medications, including drug name, purpose, dosage, frequency, precautions, and potential side effects, especially for chemotherapeutic agents.
- Exercises that promote muscle strength and mobility, measures for preventing contractures and skin breakdown, transfer techniques and proper body mechanics, use of assistive devices, and other measures that promote independence with ADL.
- Measures for relieving pain, nausea, or other discomfort.
- Indications of constipation, urinary retention, or urinary tract infection; implementation of bowel and bladder training programs; and if appropriate, care of indwelling catheters.
- Indications of upper respiratory infections and measures to prevent regurgitation, aspiration, and respiratory infection.
- Importance of follow-up care, including visits to physician, PT, OT, speech

therapy, pyschologic counseling, and laboratory monitoring for side effects of radiation/chemotherapy.

- First aid measures for seizures.
- Causes of IICP and measures to prevent it.
- Care of ventricular shunt, if present. Include specific instructions for shunt care and information about how to identify shunt infection or malfunction and steps to take should they occur.
- Measures that assist with reorientating, dealing with behavioral or cognitive problems, and communicating with patient in view of cognitive deficits.

## Spinal cord tumors

The majority of spinal cord tumors interrupt neuronal function and nerve impulse transmission by compressing the spinal cord, its roots, or its blood supply, and eventually cause cord degeneration. Spinal cord tumors can occur anywhere along the length of the spinal cord, may obstruct or block CSF flow, and, if untreated, lead to paralysis and sensory deficits. Cervical tumors may cause respiratory muscle weakness or paralysis. *Intramedullary tumors* occur within the cord itself and are fairly rare. Symptoms of cord dysfunction may occur from onset as cord function is interrupted by direct invasion and compression. *Extramedullary tumors* occur outside the spinal cord and are further classified as intradural or extradural. *Intradural tumors,* such as meningiomas and schwannomas, arise from the membrane covering the spinal cord and nerve roots and account for the majority of all primary spinal cord tumors. Intradural tumors occur in the space between the cord and the dura. Intradural and intramedullary tumors usually are slow-growing and cytologically benign but still can be extremely disabling. *Extradural tumors* usually are secondary (metastatic) tumors that have been "seeded" from other sites in the body, such as the prostate, bone marrow, lymph tissue, breast, or lungs. They occur in the epidural space or in the vertebrae that surround the spinal cord and related tissue. Tumors may be classified according to their anatomic locations, cellular origin, location in relation to the vertebral column, and whether they are primary or secondary.

### ASSESSMENT

Indicators vary according to tumor site. Severity of symptoms generally depends on the rate of growth and degree of compression. Typically pain or radiculopathy in the back precedes compression signs of motor, sensory, and bowel or bladder dysfunction by weeks or months. Compression signs initially may be quite subtle but may rapidly progress to complete paralysis in a few days.

**Motor involvement:**   Weakness or paralysis of one or more body parts with the potential for spasticity below the level of the tumor. If the tumor interrupts the spinal cord reflex arc (e.g., a tumor at the level of the cauda equina), decreased or lost reflexes, flaccidity, muscle atrophy, and fasciculations can occur.

**Sensory involvement:**   Decreased sensation to pain, touch, and temperature with potential loss of position and vibration sense.

**Pain:**   Neck or back pain that persists despite bed rest is most severe over the tumor site and potentially radiates around the trunk or down the affected side because of nerve root irritation. The spinal processes can be quite tender to the touch. Pain often is aggravated by moving, straining, coughing, and sneezing. Pain may increase when the individual is recumbent.

**Bladder and bowel dysfunction:**   Initially, the patient may have difficulty starting a stream or may empty the bladder incompletely. The patient may have a spastic bladder, causing urinary retention; a flaccid bladder, causing incontinence; and bowel incontinence from loss of control. The patient also may be constipated.

**Physical assessment:**   Depending on location of the tumor, patient may exhibit increased, decreased, or absent deep tendon reflexes (DTRs).

## DIAGNOSTIC TESTS

**X-ray:**   May show changes in vertebrae such as destruction and collapse of bony matrix.

**MRI:**   To show tumor location and the presence of cord compression and rule out spinal abscess or syringomyelia. Because it can detect biochemical abnormalities, it may detect the tumor at a very early stage. MRI is of particular value in evaluating high cervical lesions, where the presence of bone makes the CT scan less effective.

**Spinal CT scan:**   To reveal tumor location and presence of cord compression.

**Bone scan:**   Shows increased radioactive tracer uptake where there is metastatic invasion of the vertebrae causing increased osteoblastic activity. **Note:** Check for pregnancy in appropriate patients, and notify physician accordingly. After procedure, patient should drink several glasses of water to facilitate clearance of free-circulating isotope.

**Lumbar puncture (LP) and CSF analysis:**   May show malignant cells in CSF. With partial blockage, there may be slightly increased levels of protein and a yellow tinge to the fluid; with complete blockage, there are definite increases in protein and the fluid is yellow below the blockage.

*Queckenstedt's test:*   Performed by compressing the jugular vein for 10 seconds during the LP. Normally, a rise in CSF pressure occurs. For patients in whom a tumor is partially blocking the spinal cord above the level of the LP, the test may cause a sluggish rise in CSF. With complete blockage, there will be no rise in CSF pressure.

**Myelography (sometimes with CT scan):**   Shows boundaries and level at which the tumor is located if the spinal canal is not totally obstructed. This procedure can be dangerous because withdrawal of CSF may cause increased compression of the cord by the tumor.

**Tissue biopsy:**   Confirms presence of a tumor.

**Positron emission tomography (PET):**   Will identify tumor location by showing abnormal metabolic activity.

---

**Note:**   See "General Care of Patients with Neurologic Disorders," **Knowledge deficit:** Neurologic diagnostic tests, p. 311, for care considerations for patients undergoing MRI, CT scan, LP, myelography, and PET.

---

## COLLABORATIVE MANAGEMENT

**Bed rest:**   For patients with cancer that has invaded the bony vertebral body. Body weight alone can cause vertebral collapse, resulting in possible cord laceration or compression.

**Pharmacotherapy**

*Glucocorticoids (e.g., dexamethasone):*   Often given in very high doses to decrease compression caused by cord edema. They are also given to reduce radiation-induced cord edema.

*Hormone therapy:*   For hormone-mediated metastatic tumor.

*Analgesics (e.g., acetaminophen, codeine, morphine):*   For pain, which can be quite severe.

*Stool softeners and laxatives (e.g., docusate):*   To prevent constipation and straining at stool.

*Antacids and histamine H$_2$-receptor blockers (e.g., ranitidine):*   To reduce gastric acidity and prevent ulcer formation during steroid use.

**Transcutaneous electrical nerve stimulation (TENS):**   Battery-operated device that delivers electrical impulses to the body to relieve pain.

**Surgery:**   Is the treatment of choice and may include a laminectomy or decompression or excision of primary tumors. Microsurgery techniques and the use of spinal cord evoked potentials during surgery has helped surgeons protect cord function. New surgical techniques permitting an anterior approach to the cord may enable better cord decompression and tumor excision. Generally, surgery is not indicated for metastatic tumors. Emergency surgical decompression of the spinal cord may save function in instances of sudden onset of partial paralysis or bowel or bladder dysfunction. Best surgical results occur when surgery is performed before neurologic deficits occur. (See "Intervertebral Disk Disease," p. 224, for care of patient with a laminectomy.) A cordotomy or palliative section of the sensory roots is sometimes done for intractable pain.

**Radiation therapy:**   May be performed preoperatively and postoperatively to reduce tumor mass and symptoms and help prevent recurrence. Radiation therapy is the primary treatment modality for secondary metastatic tumors and those tumors that cannot be removed totally. Cord inflammation and edema caused by radiation therapy can result in an increase in the neurologic deficit. The patient also is at risk of developing radiation necrosis 6-36 months (average 14 months) posttherapy. Onset usually is insidious and may progress to complete motor and sensory loss. MRI will rule out tumor recurrence and may show a swollen cord. There is no effective treatment, although high-dose corticosteroids may be used.

**Chemotherapy:**   May be used for some lymphomas and myelomas. Usually it is not used with other types of tumors.

**Physical medicine:**   May include physical therapy (PT), occupational therapy (OT), and assistive devices or braces so that patient can maintain mobility and independence with ADL. Muscle-strengthening exercises, conditioning exercises, and gait training are also frequently prescribed.

**ROM exercises:**   To maintain or increase joint function and prevent contractures.

**Bowel and bladder program:**   To prevent incontinence and constipation and to retrain the bowel and bladder, depending on the neurologic deficit.

## NURSING DIAGNOSES AND INTERVENTIONS

**Pain** (acute or chronic) related to tissue compression secondary to tumor growth

*Desired outcomes:*   Within 1 h of intervention, patient's subjective perception of pain decreases, as documented by a pain scale. Objective indicators, such as grimacing, are absent or diminished.

---

**Note:**   Symptoms of primary tumors usually develop slowly, while with metastatic tumors they develop rapidly. Intense localized pain generally is the first symptom, with localized tenderness over the spine.

---

- Assess patient's character and degree of pain, using a pain scale. Rate pain from 0 (no pain) to 10 (worst pain). Pain may signal the need for immediate medical treatment (e.g., corticosteroids, radiation therapy, decompressive laminectomy) to help prevent or minimize neurologic deficits that may be permanently disabling. Have patient alert staff members or physician to the following: backache; sensations of heaviness or weakness in the arms or legs; any incoordination; loss of sensations of light touch, pain, and temperature; incontinence or difficulty urinating or defecating; and sexual impotence.
- Advise patient that moving slowly with good body alignment may help minimize pain. A soft cervical collar may help neck alignment.
- Suggest that keeping knees and hips slightly flexed when in bed will help

reduce pain by preventing traction on nerve roots caused by full extension of the spinal cord.
- Inform patient that sneezing and straining can cause pain.
- For other interventions, see **Pain** in "General Care of Patients with Neurologic Disorders," p. 308.

---

**Note:** If patient has urinary incontinence, retention, or neurogenic bladder, see related discussions in "Renal-Urinary Disorders." See "Intervertebral Disk Disease" for **Knowledge deficit:** Diskectomy with laminectomy or fusion procedure, p. 229. See "Spinal Cord Injury," p. 237, for nursing diagnoses and interventions related to the care of patients with disorders of the spinal cord. See "General Care of Patients with Neurologic Disorders" for **Knowledge deficit:** Neurologic diagnostic tests, p. 311. See "Pressure Ulcers," p. 687, and Appendix One, "Caring for Patients on Prolonged Bed Rest," p 711, for nursing diagnoses and interventions for patients who are immobile. Also see Appendix One, "Caring for Preoperative and Postoperative Patients," p. 693, and "Caring for Patients with Cancer and Other Life-Disrupting Illnesses," p 719.

---

### PATIENT-FAMILY TEACHING AND DISCHARGE PLANNING

Give patient and significant others verbal and written information about the following:
- Safety measures relative to sensorimotor deficits.
- For more information, see third through eleventh entries in "Brain Tumor," p. 265.

# Section Five: Vascular Disorders of the Nervous System

## Cerebral aneurysm

An aneurysm is a localized weakness and dilation of an artery. With cerebral aneurysms, this dilation generally takes one of two forms: *fusiform,* in which the entire circumference of a vessel section is dilated; or *saccular,* in which there is dilation of the side of a vessel. Saccular aneurysms, also called "berry" aneurysms, are the most common. Depending on their size and location, unruptured aneurysms can produce neurologic symptoms by compressing brain tissue or cranial nerves. Usually, however, the aneurysm causes no symptoms until it ruptures. When this occurs, the hemorrhage usually bleeds into the subarachnoid space, although occasionally it may bleed directly into the intracranial tissue, causing direct neuronal damage. Rupture causes a sudden increase in ICP and a loss of cerebral perfusion pressure. Brain tissue may be compressed by the expanding mass effect of the bleeding. Cranial nerves and brain tissue are irritated by the presence of blood, and the brain begins to swell. Blood in the subarachnoid space prevents adequate circulation and reabsorption of CSF, which increases ICP further. In addition, interruption of blood flow to the areas supplied by the ruptured artery can cause brain ischemia and possibly infarction. The patient may experience permanent neurologic deficits, depending on the size and site of the bleed and the development of complications.

Aneurysms can be caused by a congenital defect in the arterial wall, degenerative processes, such as hypertension or atherosclerosis, or vessel trauma. Prognosis depends on the site and size of the ruptured aneurysm, but 45%-50% of affected individuals die immediately.

Common causes of death for individuals who survive the initial rupture include IICP, rebleeding, and vasospasm of the blood vessels. The patient is at greatest risk of rebleeding within the first 24-48 h following the initial rupture. Rebleeding, however, is a significant risk for the first 2 weeks because of the body's normal process of clot lysis at the rupture site. Approximately 20% of patients will rebleed within 2 weeks. Nearly two-thirds of patients experiencing rebleeding will die. Rebleeding may occur up to 6 months after the initial rupture.

The patient also is at risk of experiencing cerebral vasospasm, which decreases cerebral blood flow, leading to cerebral ischemia. The cerebral ischemia can increase the patient's neurologic deficits and may cause cerebral infarct and death. Vasospasm seems to be directly related to the amount of blood present in the subarachnoid space after rupture. Vasospasm usually starts within 3-4 days after the subarachnoid hemorrhage, peaks in 7-10 days, and usually resolves in about 3 weeks.

Following rupture, 20%-25% of patients may develop acute or chronic hydrocephalus. The presence of blood in the subarachnoid space appears to damage the arachnoid villa and decrease or prevent CSF reabsorption. This will increase ICP, leading to possible brain herniation. Other complications the patient may be at risk for are diabetes insipidus, syndrome of inappropriate antidiuretic hormone (SIADH) owing to pituitary gland or hypothalamus compression or damage, and cerebral salt wasting syndrome.

## ASSESSMENT

Indicators vary, depending on the site and amount of bleeding. Rupture often occurs with exertion, excitement, or a sudden rise in BP.

**Signs and symptoms**

- *Prodromal (as the aneurysm enlarges but before it ruptures):* Periodic headaches, transitory weakness, numbness, tingling on one side, transitory diplopia, blurred vision, ptosis, and transitory speech disturbances.
- *Acute (with leakage and rupture):* Sudden and severe headache, nausea and/or vomiting, and neck stiffness are among the most common symptoms.

**IICP and herniation:** Sudden, severe headache; nausea and vomiting; changes or alteration in LOC ranging from confusion, irritability, and restlessness to coma; a falling score on the Glasgow Coma Scale (see Table 4-2); pupillary dilatation and changes in their size and reaction to light; VS changes, such as increasing BP with widening pulse pressure and decreased pulse rate; irregular respiratory pattern.

**Meningeal irritation** (caused by blood in the subarachnoid space): Neck stiffness; neck, back, and leg pain; fever; photophobia; seizures.

**Cranial nerve irritation/compression:** Blurred vision and other visual disturbances, ptosis, inability to rotate the eyes, difficulty with swallowing or speaking, tinnitus.

**Focal symptoms:** Sensory loss, motor weakness, or paralysis on one side of the body.

**Autonomic disturbance** (from increased catecholamines immediately following rupture): ECG changes, flushing, sweating, dilated pupils, hypertension, tachycardia, increased blood sugar, increased temperature, ileus.

**Physical assessment:** Positive Kernig's and Brudzinski's signs confirm presence of meningeal irritation. (See description with "Bacterial Meningitis," p. 195.)

**Grading:** Individuals with ruptured aneurysms are often graded according to the severity of the bleeding or injury:

- *Grade 1:* Patient alert with no neurologic deficit; slight neck stiffness; minimal headache, if present.
- *Grade 2:* Patient alert with mild to severe headache; presence of stiff neck; may have minimal neurologic deficit, such as third cranial nerve palsies.

- *Grade 3:* Patient drowsy or confused; presence of stiff neck; may have mild focal neurologic deficits.
- *Grade 4:* Patient stuporous, semicomatose; presence of stiff neck; may have neurologic deficits, such as hemiparesis.
- *Grade 5:* Patient comatose and posturing.

## DIAGNOSTIC TESTS

**CT scan:**   To reveal presence of aneurysm(s) and the site, size, and amount of bleeding from the subarachnoid or intracerebral hemorrhage. The scan also may reveal the presence of hydrocephalus. The scan may not identify small aneurysms or those in vasospasm. CT scan may be used 1-2 days postrupture to assess the amount of bleeding in order to predict risk of vasospasm.

**Cerebral angiography:**   To pinpoint site, structure, and size of aneurysm(s) and presence of vasospasm. This test provides the definitive diagnosis of aneurysm, and it usually is performed before surgery to exclude the presence of vasospasm and review accessibility. Small aneurysms may be missed.

**MRI:**   Can reveal presence of even small amounts of blood or small aneurysms that are not visualized with the CT scan or angiography. Magnetic resonance angiography is being used in some areas to highlight cerebral vascularity.

**Lumbar puncture (LP) and CSF analysis:**   May reveal presence of bloody CSF, increased CSF pressure, and increased protein. Blood in the CSF indicates that a subarachnoid hemorrhage has occurred. This procedure is contraindicated for patients with IICP. The LP usually is done only when CT scan is nondiagnostic or unavailable.

**Skull x-ray:**   May reveal calcification in the wall of a large aneurysm.

**Cerebral blood flow studies (e.g., transcranial doppler sonography):**   To monitor for cerebral vasospasms, changes in blood flow states, loss of autoregulation, IICP, and brain death.

---

**Note:**   See "General Care of Patients with Neurologic Disorders," **Knowledge deficit:** Neurologic diagnostic tests, p. 311, for care considerations for patients undergoing CT scan, angiography, MRI, and LP.

---

## COLLABORATIVE MANAGEMENT

**Respiratory support:**   Airway maintenance, intubation, and ventilation as necessary. ABG values are often monitored for evidence of hypoxia. If indicated, $O_2$ is administered to prevent hypoxia and carbon dioxide retention, which can cause vasodilation of the cerebral arteries and cerebral edema.

**Activity restrictions:**   Strict bed rest in a quiet, dark room; limitation of visitors; restriction of ADL. Although active ROM is occasionally permitted, even the alert patient is usually limited to passive ROM. Restraints are avoided because they can result in IICP if the patient struggles against them.

**Elevation of HOB:**   To 30 degrees or as prescribed to reduce cerebral congestion.

**Pharmacotherapy**

*Antifibrinolytic agent (e.g., aminocaproic acid):*   To decrease the risk of rebleeding at the site of aneurysm by delaying the body's lysis of the blood clot. Use of this drug is controversial because although it reduces the risk of rebleeding, it appears to increase the risk of vasospasm. Use of antifibrinolytic agents has decreased in favor of early surgery to clip the aneurysm before development of vasospasm. If used, an IV loading dose of 5 g is generally given over 1 h followed by a continuous infusion of ≥30 g/day for 3 weeks or until the patient goes for surgical repair. Rapid IV infusion may cause hypotension, bradycardia, or dysrhythmias. The IV drug route is preferred over the oral route. The drug should be diluted 1 g/50 ml $D_5W$ or other compatible solution. Side effects include phlebitis at the insertion site (IV route) and nausea and diarrhea (oral route). Other side effects include headache, tinnitus, dizziness, fatigue, and generalized thrombosis.

***Corticosteroids (e.g., dexamethasone):***  To help decrease cerebral edema and ICP. Antacids and histamine $H_2$-receptor blockers, such as ranitidine, may be given concurrently to inhibit gastric secretions and reduce GI irritation.

***Antihypertensives (e.g., hydralazine):***  If indicated, to treat underlying hypertension.

***Laxatives and stool softeners (e.g., docusate sodium):***  To prevent straining with bowel movements.

***Sedatives/tranquilizers (e.g., phenobarbital):***  To reduce stress and restlessness and promote rest.

***Osmotic diuretics (e.g., mannitol):***  To reduce severe cerebral edema.

***Loop diuretics (e.g., furosemide):***  Being used by some physicians because it appears to decrease cerebral edema without causing the increase in intracranial blood volume that occurs with mannitol.

***Antiepilepsy drugs (e.g., phenytoin or phenobarbital):***  To control or prevent seizures.

***Antipyretics (e.g., acetaminophen):***  To control fever, which increases the brain's metabolic activity. Aspirin is avoided because it prevents platelet adhesion.

***Analgesics (e.g., acetaminophen and codeine):***  To manage pain. Aspirin is contraindicated because it prevents platelet adhesion.

**Fluid limitation:**  Generally, fluids are limited to 1,500-1,800 ml/day to keep patient slightly underhydrated and reduce cerebral congestion and ICP.

**Nutrition:**  Coffee and other stimulants are restricted. Very hot and very cold liquids also may be restricted. A high-fiber diet may be prescribed to prevent constipation. For patients with dysphagia, enteral or parenteral feedings may be necessary. A low-Na (see Table 3-2, p. 115) low-cholesterol (see Table 2-2, p. 51) diet is often prescribed to control hypertension and atherosclerosis.

**Antiembolism hose or sequential compression sleeves:**  To help prevent thrombophlebitis and deep-vein thrombosis.

**Avoiding rectal stimulation:**  Rectal suppositories, thermometers, enemas, and digital examinations are contraindicated because they can stimulate a type of Valsalva's maneuver in the patient, causing increased intrathoracic pressure and IICP, resulting in rupture or rebleeding.

**Seizure precautions:**  To prevent patient injury in the event of seizure.

**Cardiac monitoring:**  May be done to assess for and treat cardiac dysrhythmias, which are common immediately following subarachnoid hemorrhage.

**ICU monitoring:**  May be necessary, particularly if the patient develops cerebral vasospasm or IICP.

**Surgical management/interventional neuroradiology:**  The patient's surgical candidacy depends on LOC, extent of neurologic deficit, nature and location of the aneurysm, and presence of vasospasm. The timing of the surgery is based on the patient's status and surgeon's preference. Usually, it is performed within 2-14 days of the initial bleed. Surgery is not performed in the presence of vasospasm. Patients graded 1-2 are the best surgical candidates, and the trend is for them to have surgery within 1-3 days of the initial bleed. Computerized EEG may be used in the OR during the procedure for continuous monitoring of neuronal integrity. Brain activity as recorded on an EEG correlates with cerebral blood flow and can be used to identify ischemia in the anesthetized patient and thereby signal for interventions to prevent brain damage.

***Surgical repair with craniotomy:***  To isolate the aneurysm and prevent rebleeding, a craniotomy is performed and the aneurysm is repaired by clipping, ligating, coagulating, wrapping the aneurysm neck with muscle, or encasing the aneurysmal sac in plastic or surgical gauze. (For information on craniotomy patient care considerations, see "Brain Tumors," p. 263.)

*Carotid artery clamping:*   For internal carotid artery aneurysms, and sometimes for other inaccessible aneurysms, a carotid artery clamp may be used to reduce blood flow and blood pressure. After surgery, the carotid artery clamp is tightened slowly over several days, which allows time for collateral circulation to take over in the brain.

*Endovascular balloon occlusion of aneurysm or parent vessel:*   A small and extremely flexible catheter is threaded through the femoral artery at the groin and advanced up to the aneurysm or parent vessel. The balloon can be inflated with a liquid that solidifies within 45 min. Balloon occlusion within the aneurysm is ideal, but sometimes the parent vessel (usually the carotid) must be occluded. A test occlusion is done to see if the patient can tolerate the parent vessel occlusion. If signs of ischemia occur, the balloon procedure is stopped. A bypass is done, if possible, and the balloon occlusion usually is performed a few days later. See "Cerebrovascular Accident," p. 280, for cerebral artery bypass patient care considerations.

*Ventriculostomy:*   To permit temporary ventricular drainage for acute hydrocephalus.

*Daily LPs or lumbar drain:*   To provide temporary CSF drainage and restore the reabsorptive ability of the arachnoid villi by removing blood from the CSF.

*Ventricular shunt for ventricular drainage:*   Performed to allow long-term drainage of CSF in patients who develop chronic hydrocephalus after a subarachnoid hemorrhage. (See discussion of ventricular shunt in "Brain Tumors," p. 262.)

**Management of SIADH vs. cerebral salt wasting syndrome:**   Hyponatremia and decreased fluid volume increase the risk of vasospasm. It is critical to distinguish correctly between these two types of hyponatremia and fluid imbalance because their treatment is so different. SIADH (characterized by dilutional hyponatremia with increased plasma volume, weight gain, low BUN, and serum hypoosmolality) is treated with fluid restriction (see "Syndrome of Inappropriate Antidiuretic Hormone," p. 351, for more information). Cerebral salt wasting syndrome (characterized by hyponatremia with decreased plasma volume, weight loss, high BUN, serum hypoosmolality, and hypernatriuria) is treated with fluid replacement, volume expanders, and occasionally fludrocortisone to inhibit Na excretion and induce Na retention to counteract hyponatremia and volume depletion.

**Treatments for cerebral vasospasm:**   There is no completely effective treatment for cerebral vasospasm, but some techniques seem to reduce its incidence or severity. Some treatments necessitate ICU monitoring:

*Craniotomy:*   Done within 48 h to remove any blood clot that may aggravate vasospasm.

*Hemodilution (e.g., albumin, crystalloid fluid):*   The patient is kept well hydrated with IV fluids or volume expanders to decrease blood viscosity in order to improve cerebral blood flow through narrowed arteries.

*Hypervolemic (e.g., plasma protein fraction, whole blood, saline, albumin, hetastarch) or hypertensive (e.g., dopamine, phenylephrine) therapy:*   Usually only performed following aneurysm repair to increase cerebral perfusion pressure *via* increased blood volume and arterial pressure in order to reduce the ischemia and resulting neurologic deficits during vasospasm.

*Calcium channel blockers (e.g., nicardipine):*   Cause vasodilatation *via* smooth muscle relaxation and promote collateral circulation *via* dilatation of small pia arteries.

*Experimental treatments under investigation:*
—Balloon angioplasty: To dilate arteries that are in vasospasm.
—Theophylline, isoproterenol, nitroprusside: To increase cerebral perfusion through smooth muscle dilatation.

—Barbiturate coma: To decrease cerebral metabolic needs so that injury will be minimized until vasospasm subsides and cerebral blood flow improves.

## NURSING DIAGNOSES AND INTERVENTIONS

The following nursing diagnoses relate primarily to the patient whose aneurysm is graded 1-3. If the patient's aneurysm is graded 4-5, see nursing diagnoses in "Cerebrovascular Accident," p. 281, for patient care.

**Knowledge deficit:**   Aneurysms and the potential for rebleeding, rupture, or vasospasm

*Desired outcome:*   Following instruction and ongoing, patient verbalizes knowledge about the potential for rebleeding or vasospasm, measures to prevent their occurrence, and symptoms to report to the health-care staff.

- Assess patient for sensorimotor deficits, such as decreased or absent vision, impaired temperature and pain sensation, unsteady gait, weakness, or paralysis. Document baseline neurologic and physical assessments so that changes in patient status are detected promptly. Teach patient and significant others these indicators, and explain the importance of reporting them to the staff promptly.
- Teach these patients the importance of reducing activity level to avoid rebleeding or rupture. Strict bed rest may be prescribed. Emphasize the necessity of allowing others to help them with moving, ADL, and passive ROM, even though they may feel capable of self-care. Explain that the number and frequency of visitors will be limited and that individuals whose presence is stressful to the patient should not be allowed to visit. The telephone will be removed from the room, and television, radio, and reading may be restricted or limited to programs and books that are not overstimulating. The room will be darkened to promote rest, and sedatives and tranquilizers may be offered. Caffeine and other stimulants may be restricted, as well as nicotine, which can increase the risk of vasospasm.
- Teach patient measures that will prevent a sudden increase in ICP.
  - Avoid coughing and sneezing; if they are unavoidable, do so with an opened mouth.
  - Exhale when being turned.
  - Avoid straining with bowel movements.
  - Avoid extreme hip flexion or lying prone.
  - Avoid moving self up in bed because this requires a pushing movement. Do not grip, push, or pull on side rails or push feet against the mattress or foot of bed. Request help from staff member for all moving and turning movements.
- Explain that the HOB may be maintained at 30 degrees, and the patient may be asked to keep head and neck in good alignment to promote venous return to the heart and reduce cerebral congestion and ICP.
- Explain that the patient may be given a high-fiber diet and stool softeners to promote bowel elimination without straining.
- Describe, as appropriate, the following preventive measures: corticosteroids to prevent or reduce cerebral edema, antiepilepsy medications to prevent seizures, antihypertensive medications to keep BP within defined parameters, and a low-Na and low-cholesterol diet to help control BP.
- Teach patient to avoid taking aspirin or aspirin-containing products, which increase the risk of hemorrhage.
- Teach patient and significant others the indicators of cerebral vasospasm (p. 270), which can lead to ischemia and infarction. As appropriate, explain any prescribed treatment.

**Knowledge deficit:**   Effects of aminocaproic acid drug therapy

*Desired outcome:*   Following instruction and ongoing, patient verbalizes knowledge about the side effects of aminocaproic therapy, the measures to prevent complications from the drug therapy, and signs and symptoms that should be reported immediately to health-care staff if they occur.

- Teach patients on aminocaproic acid therapy the indicators of pulmonary embolus, including SOB, chest pain (especially that which increases with inspiration), and blood-tinged sputum, as well as indicators of deep-vein thrombosis, such as calf pain or tenderness and increased heat, swelling, or redness of the leg. Stress the importance of notifying staff immediately if they occur. Encourage patient to wear antiembolism hose.
- Monitor patient's IV site for signs of phlebitis. Instruct patient to report any tenderness or swelling at the site.
- Alert patient to the potential for loose stools, frequent stools (more than 3/day), cramps, and weakness with aminocaproic therapy. Instruct patient to report these problems promptly because, if the diarrhea is a side effect of oral aminocaproic therapy, the physician may switch patient to IV medication.
- Inform patients that because the drug may cause postural hypotension, they should make position changes very slowly and in stages. Faintness or dizziness should be reported promptly.
- Instruct patient to report any muscle weakness, muscle pain, sweating, fever, or myeloglobinuria (reddish-brown urine) because these may be signs of myopathy caused by this drug therapy.
- Teach patient to report nausea, tinnitus, nasal stuffiness, or fatigue, which are other side effects of aminocaproic drug therapy.

**Ineffective airway clearance (or risk of same)** related to imposed inactivity secondary to the risk of aneurysm rupture or rebleeding
***Desired outcomes:*** Following intervention and ongoing, patient's lungs are clear to auscultation. Secretions are thin and clear, and the patient remains normothermic.

- Assess patient for increased WOB or a change in the rate or depth of respirations. Auscultate lung fields for breath sounds, noting presence of crackles (rales), rhonchi, and diminished sounds. Assess for fever, purulent sputum, and cyanosis, and monitor patient's ABG values for hypoxemia ($Pao_2$ <80 mm Hg) or hypercapnia ($Paco_2$ >45 mm Hg). Notify physician of significant findings.
- Encourage patient to breath deeply and change positions q2h to help expand the lungs. Instruct patient to avoid coughing or sneezing because these activities increase intraabdominal and intrathoracic pressure, which in turn increase ICP and the risk of aneurysm rupture. Explain that if sneezing is unavoidable, it should be done with an open mouth.
- Maintain patient on oxygen as prescribed.
- Assist patient with using incentive spirometry, if prescribed.

**High risk for disuse syndrome** related to prescribed immobilization secondary to risk of aneurysm rupture or rebleeding
***Desired outcome:*** Patient exhibits complete ROM.

- To maintain joint mobility, perform passive ROM exercises during the period of activity restriction. Even if the patient feels well enough to perform assisted or active ROM, these activities are contraindicated because they increase ICP and the risk of rupture or rebleeding. Explain to patient the rationale for activity limitation.
- Maintain joint alignment and provide support to the joints and extremities with pillows, trochanter rolls, sandbags, and other positioning devices.
- When the patient is no longer on bed rest and activity restrictions, additional strengthening and conditioning exercises may be necessary to counteract the effects of prolonged bed rest. In addition, the patient may have residual neurologic deficits that necessitate gait training or the use of assistive devices to promote mobility. Obtain a physical therapy or occupational therapy referral as appropriate. For additional interventions, see **High risk for disuse syndrome** in Appendix One, "Caring for Patients on Prolonged Bed Rest," p. 713.

**Self-care deficit** related to imposed activity restrictions secondary to risk of aneurysm rupture or rebleeding
*Desired outcome:*    Patient's care activities are completed for him or her during the period of strict bed rest.
- During the period of strict bed rest and activity restrictions, perform care activities, even for patients who do not exhibit signs of neurologic deficit. Explain the reason for patient's activity restrictions.
- If patient has bathroom privileges, provide a commode as appropriate, and assist patient with transferring as necessary.

---

**Note:**    As appropriate, see "Head Injury" for **Fluid volume excess** related to SIADH, p. 256. For surgical patients, see "Brain Tumors" for **Knowledge deficit:** Ventricular shunt procedure, p. 262; and **Knowledge deficit:** Craniotomy procedure, p. 263. See "Cerebrovascular Accident" for **Knowledge deficit:** Cerebral artery bypass surgery, p. 285. As appropriate, see "Seizure Disorders," p. 292, for related nursing diagnoses. See "General Care of Patients with Neurologic Disorders" for **High risk for fluid volume deficit,** p. 301; **Constipation,** p 305; **Altered cerebral tissue perfusion,** p. 305; **Pain,** p. 308; and **Knowledge deficit:** Neurologic diagnostic tests, p. 311. As appropriate, see "Diabetes Insipidus" for **Altered protection** related to side effects of vasopressin, p. 347. For patients with varying degrees of immobility, see "Pressure Ulcers," p. 687, and Appendix One, "Caring for Patients on Prolonged Bed Rest," p. 711. Also see Appendix One, "Caring for Patients with Cancer and Other Life-Disrupting Illnesses," p. 753, as appropriate, for psychosocial interventions.

---

## PATIENT-FAMILY TEACHING AND DISCHARGE PLANNING
Give patient and significant others verbal and written information about the following:
- Wound care and indicators of wound infection for patients who have undergone surgery.
- Importance of avoiding strenuous physical activity. Check with physician regarding activity restrictions and limitations; instruct patient accordingly.
- Low-Na (see Table 3-2, p. 115), low-cholesterol (see Table 2-2, p. 51) diet if prescribed to control hypertension and artherosclerosis.
- Medications, including drug name, rationale, schedule, dosage, precautions, and potential side effects.
- Signs and symptoms of rupture and rebleeding, for which the patient is at risk for 6 months after the initial bleed.
- Care of the ventricular shunt, if present. Instructions should include indicators of shunt infection and steps to take in the event of shunt infection or malfunction.

*In addition:*
- See the teaching and discharge planning section in "Cerebrovascular Accident," p. 288, for additional interventions for patients who have residual neurologic deficits.

# Cerebrovascular accident

A cerebrovascular accident (CVA) is the sudden disruption of $O_2$ supply to the nerve cells, generally caused by obstruction or rupture in one or more of the blood vessels that supply the brain. *Ischemic CVA* has three main mechanisms: thrombosis, embolism, and systemic hypoperfusion. Thrombosis or embolism results in a blockage of blood supply to the brain tissue. The resulting ischemia, if prolonged, causes brain tissue necrosis (infarction), cerebral edema, and IICP. Most thrombotic strokes are caused by blockage due to atherosclerosis. Most embolic strokes are the result of emboli produced during atrial fibrillation of the heart. Ischemic stroke due to systemic hypoperfusion usually is the result of decreased cerebral blood flow owing to circulatory failure. Circulatory failure results from too little blood, too low a BP, or failure of the heart to pump blood adequately. Hypoxia from any cause also can produce this syndrome.

A transient ischemic attack (TIA), which is a temporary (less than 24-h) neurologic deficit that resolves completely without permanent damage, occurs when the artery cannot deliver enough blood to meet the brain's $O_2$ requirement. TIAs usually are associated with thrombosis but may be caused by any of the ischemic mechanisms just mentioned. TIAs may precede a permanent ischemic CVA by hours, days, months, or years. TIAs are a warning sign, and treatment may prevent a stroke. Most TIAs last an average of 5-10 min. A reversible ischemic neurologic deficit (or RIND) lasts longer than 24 h but otherwise is similar to a TIA.

*Hemorrhagic CVA* causes neural tissue destruction because of the infiltration and accumulation of blood. Ischemia and infarction may occur distal to the hemorrhage because of interrupted blood supply. Although a cerebral hemorrhage usually results from hypertension or an aneurysm, trauma also can cause hemorrhagic CVA. Bleeding may spread into the brain tissue itself, causing an intracerebral hemorrhage, or into the subarachnoid space. Usually there is a large rise in ICP with a hemorrhagic stroke due to cerebral edema and the mass effect of blood (see "Cerebral Aneurysm," p. 269, for discussion of subarachnoid hemorrhage).

A CVA may be classified as a "progressive stroke in evolution," in which deficits continue to worsen over time, or as a "completed stroke," in which maximum deficit has been acquired. Progressive strokes usually are the result of a thrombus formation and often take 1-3 or more days to become "completed." CVA is the third most common cause of death and the most common cause of neurologic disability. Half the survivors are left permanently disabled or experience another CVA. Improvement may continue for 1-2 years, but deficits at 6 months usually are considered permanent.

## ASSESSMENT

**General findings:** Classically, symptoms appear on the side of the body opposite the damaged site. For example, a CVA in the left hemisphere of the brain will produce symptoms in the right arm and leg. However, when the CVA affects the cranial nerves, the symptoms of cranial nerve deficit will appear on the same side as the site of injury. Similarly, an obstruction of an anterior cerebral artery can produce bilateral symptoms, as will severe bleeding or multiple emboli. Hemiplegia is fairly common. Initially, the patient usually has flaccid paralysis. As spinal cord depression resolves, more normal tone is seen and hyperactive reflexes occur.

**Signs and symptoms:** Vary with the size and site of injury and may improve in 2-3 days as the cerebral edema decreases. Changes in mentation including apathy, irritability, disorientation, memory loss, withdrawal, drowsiness, stupor, or coma; bowel and bladder incontinence; numbness or loss of sensation; weakness or paralysis on part or one side of the body; aphasia; headache; neck stiffness and rigidity; vomiting; seizures; dizziness or syncope; and fever may occur. A brain stem infarct leaving the patient completely paralyzed with intact cortical function is called "locked-in syndrome."

• *Cranial nerve involvement:* Visual disturbances including diplopia, blindness, hemianopia; inequality or fixation of the pupils; nystagmus; tinnitus; difficulty chewing and swallowing.

**Physical assessment:** Papilledema, arteriosclerotic retinal changes, or hemorrhagic retinal areas on ophthalmic exam. Hyperactive deep tendon reflexes (DTRs), decreased superficial reflexes, and positive Babinski's sign also may be present. To check for Babinski's response, stroke the lateral aspect of the sole of the foot (from the heel to the ball of the foot) with a hard object. Dorsiflexion of the great toe with fanning of the other toes is a positive sign. A positive Kernig's or Brudzinski's sign (see "Bacterial Meningitis," p. 195) is indicative of meningeal irritation.

**TIAs:** Typical symptoms include temporal episodes of slurred speech, weakness, numbness or tingling, blindness in an eye, blurred or double vision, dizziness or ataxia, and confusion.

**History of:** TIAs; hypertension; atherosclerosis; high serum cholesterol or triglycerides; diabetes mellitus; gout; smoking; cardiac valve diseases, such as those that may result from rheumatic fever, valve prosthesis, and atrial fibrillation; cardiac surgery; blood dyscrasias; anticoagulant therapy; neck vessel trauma; oral contraceptive use; family predisposition for arteriovenous malformation (AVM); aneurysm; or previous CVA.

## DIAGNOSTIC TESTS

The CT scan or MRI is the test most likely to be obtained for every patient with a suspected stroke. However, technologic advances have provided numerous diagnostic tests for CVA. The selection, sequence, and urgency of these tests will be determined by the patient's history and symptoms. For example, the patient who has a TIA will have a different set or sequence of tests than the patient who is in coma.

**CT scan:** To reveal site of infarction, hematoma, and shift of brain structures. CT scan is of particular value in identifying blood released early on during hemorrhagic strokes. CT scan is the test of choice for unstable patients. Generally there is difficulty identifying ischemic areas until they start to necrose at around 48-72 h.

**MRI:** To reveal site of infarction, hematoma, shift of brain structure, and cerebral edema. MRI is of particular value in identifying ischemic strokes early on.

**Phonoangiography/Doppler ultrasonography:** May identify presence of bruits if there is a partial occlusion of the carotid blood vessels.

**Oculoplethysmography:** To obtain indirect measurement of carotid blood flow by determining intraocular ophthalmic systolic pressure. Reduced pressure may signal carotid stenosis.

**Transcranial Doppler ultrasound:** A noninvasive test that provides information about pressure and flow in the intracranial arteries.

**Positron emission tomography (PET):** To provide information on cerebral metabolism and blood flow characteristics. This test is useful in identifying ischemic stroke by showing areas of reduced glucose metabolism.

**EEG:** Shows abnormal nerve impulse transmission, such as focal slowing, which will help locate the lesion and/or indicate the amount of brain wave activity present.

**Lumbar puncture (LP) and CSF analysis:** Not done routinely, especially in the presence of IICP, but may reveal increase in CSF pressure; clear to bloody CSF, depending on the type of stroke; and presence of infection or other nonvascular cause for bleeding. CSF glutamic oxalacetic transaminase (GOT) will be increased for 10 days postinjury. Blood in the CSF signals that a subarachnoid hemorrhage has occurred.

**Cerebral angiography:** To pinpoint site of rupture or occlusion and identify collateral blood circulation, aneurysms, or AVM.

**Digital subtractive angiography (DSA):** To visualize cerebral blood flow and detect vascular abnormalities, such as stenosis, aneurysm, and hematomas.

---

**Note:** See **Knowledge deficit:** Neurologic diagnostic tests, p. 311, for care considerations for patients undergoing CT scan, MRI, oculoplethysmography, PET, EEG, LP, cerebral angiography, and DSA.

## COLLABORATIVE MANAGEMENT

**Respiratory support:**   Maintenance of airway and delivery of $O_2$, as needed. IPPB and chest physiotherapy also may be prescribed. Mechanical ventilation occasionally may be used.

**IV fluids:**   To maintain fluid and electrolyte balance. Fluids may be limited while IICP is a risk.

**Positioning:**   Bed rest during acute stage. Activity level is increased as patient's condition improves. Maintain HOB as prescribed. HOB may be down or flat with thrombotic or embolic strokes to increase cerebral perfusion. HOB may be kept up with hemorrhagic strokes or patients at risk of IICP to decrease cerebral perfusion and improve venous outflow.

**Diet:**   NPO status and possible gastric tube if swallow and gag reflexes are diminished or if patient has decreased LOC. A low-Na (see Table 3-2, p. 115) and/or low-fat (see Table 3-3, p. 53), low-cholesterol (see Table 3-2, p. 52) diet may be prescribed to minimize other risk factors. Diet may consist of fluids and pureed, soft, or chopped foods, or tube feedings, depending on patient's LOC and ability to chew and swallow.

**Pharmacotherapy**

*Anticoagulants:*   May be used for patients with thrombotic CVAs or TIAs. Medications include heparin sodium and warfarin sodium to help prevent further thrombosis. If the stroke or neurologic deficit is in evolution (still progressing), anticoagulants may be useful for 24-72 h. Once the stroke is completed and neurologic status is stable, anticoagulants are no longer useful. Anticoagulants are contraindicated with hemorrhagic CVA. Anticoagulants may be continued if the stroke was caused by emboli.

*Antihypertensive agents (e.g., nifedipine):*   To control very high BP, which may cause cerebral edema and IICP. Mild to moderate hypertension may be needed to maintain cerebral perfusion and prevent further ischemia.

*Antiplatelet medications (e.g., aspirin in conjunction with dipyridamole or sulfinpyrazone):*   To prevent platelet aggregation that may lead to thrombus formation. Patients with TIAs or those at risk for additional thrombotic strokes may be started on this therapy to prevent future ischemic strokes from thrombosis. **Caution:** These medications should not be used in the presence of hemorrhagic CVA.

*Vasopressors (e.g., dopamine):*   To treat low BP, which may increase ischemia.

*Glucocorticosteroids (e.g., dexamethasone) and osmotic diuretics (e.g., mannitol):*   To prevent or reduce cerebral edema. Use is controversial.

*Antacids and histamine $H_2$-receptor blockers (e.g., ranitidine):*   To reduce the risk of GI hemorrhage from gastric ulcer caused by stress or corticosteroid therapy.

*Antiepilepsy drugs (e.g., phenytoin or phenobarbital):*   To control and prevent seizures.

*Sedatives/tranquilizers (e.g., diphenhydramine):*   To promote rest. These are used cautiously to avoid further impairment of neurologic function.

*Analgesics (e.g., acetaminophen):*   To control headache. If CVA is hemorrhagic, aspirin is avoided because it can cause an increase in bleeding.

*Stool softeners (e.g., docusate):*   To prevent straining, which can result in IICP.

*Antipyretics (e.g., acetaminophen):*   To reduce fever, which increases cerebral metabolic needs.

*Hemodilution (e.g., albumin, crystalloid fluids):*   Hydration is promoted *via* IV fluids and volume expanders to decrease blood viscosity in order to improve cerebral blood flow through narrowed arteries.

*Hypervolemic (e.g., plasma protein fraction, whole blood, saline, albumin, hetastarch):*   To increase cerebral perfusion pressure *via* increased blood volume.

*Medications under investigation*
—Calcium channel blockers (e.g., nimodipine): May reduce deficit by promoting collateral circulation *via* vasodilatation and thereby decrease cerebral ischemia.
—Pentoxifylline: Used to decrease blood viscosity and improve capillary microcirculation, thus improving perfusion and oxygenation to ischemic brain tissue. It is used primarily with TIAs.
—Thrombolytic enzymes (e.g., tissue plasminogen activator): To cause lysis of thrombus or embolus obstructing cerebral arteries in an acute nonhemorrhagic CVA.
—Ancord: A purified protein fraction of venom from the Malayan pit viper, which rapidly decreases circulating fibrinogen. The reduction in blood viscosity from this defibrinogenation produces a hemodilutional state, which increases cerebral blood flow to the ischemic brain. Impending infarction may be reversed with early intervention (e.g., ideally within 1-2 h but no more than 6 h from onset).
—Barbiturate coma: To decrease cerebral metabolic needs so that injury will be minimized until cerebral blood flow improves.
**Physical medicine and rehabilitation:**   May include physical therapy (PT), occupational therapy (OT), and assistive devices or braces so that patient can maintain mobility and independence with ADL. Muscle-strengthening exercises, conditioning exercises, swallowing facilitation exercises, and gait training are also frequently prescribed. Reinforce special mobilization techniques such as Bobath (focuses on restoring bilateral function and incoorporating affected side into weight bearing) or proprioceptive neuromuscular facilitation (PNF), which focuses on using reflex and patterning techniques.
**ROM:**   To maintain or increase joint function and prevent contractures. Exercises may include passive ROM, active ROM, or active-assistive ROM. Passive ROM is started immediately for all joints.
**Speech therapy:**   For aphasic and dysarthric patients.
**Antiembolism hose or sequential compression sleeves:**   To help prevent thrombophlebitis and deep-vein thrombosis.
**Bowel and bladder programs:**   A bowel program should be initiated to prevent constipation and incontinence. The patient initially may have an indwelling catheter but should soon start on a bladder program to prevent incontinence or retention.
*Typically, patients are placed in ICU in the immediate postoperative period for the following surgeries:*
**Carotid endarterectomy:**   Surgical removal of plaque in the obstructed artery to increase blood supply to the brain. The carotid is clamped while the artery is opened, the plaque removed, and the artery sutured or patched. Cerebral blood flow studies and EEG monitoring may be done during the procedure. A shunt is sometimes done while the carotid is occluded. This is treatment of choice for patients with TIAs or RINDSs when a lesion lies at or near the carotid bifurcation. This procedure is not generally done for patients who have experienced a CVA unless it is performed to correct a stenosis to the unaffected hemisphere.
**Cerebral artery bypass surgery:**   Anastomosis of an extracranial vessel to an intracranial vessel in order to increase blood flow to the brain. The patient typically has an occlusion in the internal carotid artery, which is not accessible through the neck. Most commonly, the superficial temporal artery is anastomosed to the middle cerebral artery to provide collateral circulation to the area distal to the stenosis. Another frequent bypass is the subclavian artery to the external carotid artery (ECA). Difficult posterior circulation bypasses also are being attempted and include anastomosis of the occipital branch of the ECA to the posterior inferior cerebellar artery. These procedures usually are limited to patients with TIAs and RINDs. The recipient artery also must be clamped 20-30 min in order to obtain a satisfactory anastomosis.

**Craniotomy:** May be performed for evacuation of a hematoma, repair of a ruptured aneurysm, or application of arterial clips or plastic spray to the involved vessel to prevent further rupture. Craniotomy also may be performed in order to do an embolectomy. This is a controversial procedure. If done, it must be performed within 6-12 h of the occlusion. (See "Brain Tumors," p. 263, for patient care.)

## NURSING DIAGNOSES AND INTERVENTIONS

**Unilateral neglect** related to disturbed perceptual ability secondary to neurologic insult

***Desired outcome:*** Following intervention and ongoing, patient scans the environment and responds to stimuli on the affected side.

- Assess patient's ability to recognize objects to the right or left of his or her visual midline; perceive body parts as his or her own; perceive pain, touch, and temperature sensations; judge distances; orient self to changes in the environment; differentiate left from right; maintain posture sense; and identify objects by sight, hearing, or touch. Document specific deficits.
- Neglect of and inattention to stimuli on the affected side occur more often with right hemisphere injury. Neglect cannot be totally explained on the basis of loss of physical senses (e.g., both ears are used in hearing, but with auditory neglect, patient may ignore conversation or noises that occur on the affected side). Assess patient for neglect of the affected side as follows:
  - *Visual neglect:* Patient does not turn his or her head to see all parts of an object (e.g., may read only half of a page or eat from only one side of the plate). When the patient exhibits signs of visual neglect, continue to place objects necessary for ADL and call bells on the unaffected side and approach patient from that side, but gradually increase stimuli on the affected side (e.g., while communicating with patient, physically move across her or his visual boundary and stand on that side to shift the patient's attention to the neglected side; encourage patient to turn his or her head past the midline and scan the entire environment. Place patient's food on the neglected side, and encourage patient to look to the neglected side and name the food before eating. Place a bright red tape or ribbon on the affected side, and encourage patient to scan and find it). Continuously clue patient to the environment. Initially place patient's unaffected side toward the most active part of the room, but as compensation occurs, reverse this. As the patient begins to compensate, place additional items out of his or her visual field.
  - *Self-neglect:* Patient does not perceive his or her arm or leg as being a part of the body. For example, when combing or brushing the hair, patient attends to only one (the unaffected) side of the head. Inadequate self-care and injury may occur. Encourage patients to touch or massage and look at their affected sides and make a conscious effort to care for neglected body parts; also, check them for proper position to ensure against contractures and skin breakdown. To enhance patient's self-recognition, periodically refer to the patient's body parts on the neglected side. When patient is in bed or up in a chair, provide safety measures, such as siderails and restraints, to prevent patient from attempting to get up, which can occur because of unawareness of the affected side. Teach patient to use unaffected arm to perform ROM exercises on the affected side. Integrate patient's neglected arm into activities. Position arm on the bedside table or wheelchair lapboard with the hand or arm past the midline, where patient can see it. Teach patient to attend to the affected side first when performing ADL, consciously look for the affected side, monitor its position, and check for exposure to sharp objects and irritants. Provide a mirror so that patients can watch themselves shave or brush their teeth and hair. Instruct patient to take precautions with hot or cold items or when around moving machinery. Teach the use of an arm sling to support the

affected arm when patient is out of bed and when in bed to elevate the affected arm. Stand on patient's affected side when ambulating with patient.

- *Auditory neglect:* Patient ignores individuals who approach and speak from his or her affected side, but communicates with those who approach or speak from the unaffected side. To stimulate patient's attention to the affected side, move across the auditory boundary while speaking, and continue speaking from the patient's neglected side to bring patient's attention to that area.
- Arrange the environment to maximize performance of ADL by keeping necessary objects, such as the call light, on patient's unaffected side. If possible, move the bed so that the patient's unaffected side faces the largest section of the room. Approach and speak to the patient from the unaffected side. If you must approach the affected side, announce yourself, to avoid startling the patient. Perform activities on the unaffected side unless you are specifically attempting to stimulate the neglected side. After attempting to stimulate the neglected side, return to patient's unaffected side for activities and communication. Inform significant others about patient's deficit and compensatory interventions.

**Impaired physical mobility** related to neuromuscular impairment with limited use of the upper and/or lower limbs secondary to CVA

*Desired outcome:* By a minimum of the 24-h period before hospital discharge, patient and significant others demonstrate techniques that promote ambulating and transferring.

- Teach patient methods for turning and moving, using the stronger extremity to move the weaker extremity. For example, to move the affected leg in bed or when changing from a lying to a sitting position, slide the unaffected foot under the affected ankle to lift, support, and bring the affected leg along in the desired movement.
- Encourage patient to make a conscious attempt to look at the extremities and check position before moving. Remind patient to make a conscious effort to lift and then extend the foot when ambulating.
- Instruct patient with impaired sense of balance to compensate by leaning toward the stronger side. (The tendency is to lean toward the weaker or paralyzed side.) As necessary, remind patient to keep body weight forward over the feet when standing.
- Protect impaired arms with a sling to support the arm and shoulder when the patient is up to help maintain anatomic position.
- General principles when transferring include:
  - Encourage weight-bearing on patient's stronger side.
  - Instruct patient to pivot on the stronger side and use the stronger arm for support.
  - Teach patient that transferring toward the unaffected side is generally easiest and safest.
  - Instruct patient to place the unaffected side closest to the bed or chair he or she wishes to transfer to.
  - Explain that when transferring, the affected leg should be under the patient with the foot flat on the ground.
  - Position a braced chair or locked wheelchair close to patient's stronger side. If patient requires assistance from staff member, teach patient not to support self by pulling on or placing hands around assistant's neck. Staff members should use their own knees and feet to brace the feet and knees of patients who are very weak.
- Obtain PT and OT referrals as appropriate. Reinforce special mobilization techniques (e.g., Bobath, PNF) per patient's individualized rehabilitation program. These techniques may vary from the above general principles (e.g., Bobath focuses on the use of the affected side in mobility training).

**Sensory/perceptual alterations** related to altered sensory reception, transmission, and/or integration secondary to neurologic damage

***Desired outcome:*** Following intervention and ongoing, patient interacts appropriately with his/her environment and does not exhibit evidence of injury caused by sensory/perceptual deficit.

- Patients who have a dominant (left) hemisphere injury usually have normal awareness of their body and spatial orientation despite possible lack of or decreased pain sensation, position sense, and visual field deficit on the right side of the body. These patients may need reminders to scan their environment but usually do not exhibit unilateral neglect. They tend to be slow, cautious, and disorganized when approaching an unfamiliar problem and benefit from frequent, accurate, and immediate feedback on their performance. Because of a short attention span and impaired logical reasoning the patient is easily distracted, so give short, simple messages or questions and step-by-step directions. Since the patient may have poor abstract thinking, keep conversation on a concrete level (e.g., say "water," not "fluid," "leg," not "limb"). These patients may have difficulty recognizing items by touch and benefit from touching them (e.g., washcloth, comb) and having caretaker name them.
- Patients with nondominant (right) hemisphere injury also may have decreased pain sensation, pain sense, and visual field deficit, but typically are unaware of or deny their deficits or lost abilities. They tend to be impulsive and too quick with movements. Typically, they have impaired judgment about what they can or cannot do and often overestimate their abilities. Encourage these patients to slow down and check each step or task as it is completed. These individuals are at risk for burns, bruises, cuts, and falls and may need to be restrained from attempting unsafe activities. They also are more likely to have unilateral neglect (see **Unilateral neglect,** p. 281). The patient generally retains the ability to think logically but sees specifics rather than the global picture (i.e., can see the trees but not the forest). Be careful what you say because it may be taken literally (e.g., if you say "ate the lion's share," the patient may think that someone literally ate the lion's portion of the meal). Impaired ability to recognize subtle distinctions may occur (e.g., the difference between a fork and spoon may become too subtle to detect).
- Patients with apraxia have an inability to carry out previously learned motor tasks, although they may be able to describe them in detail. Have these patients return your demonstration of the task. They may be able to be talked through a task or may be able to talk themselves through a task step-by-step.
- Patients may have visual field deficits in which they can only physically see a portion of the normal visual field. Encourage making a conscious effort to scan the rest of the environment by turning the head from side to side.
- Patients with nondominant (right) hemisphere injury also may have the following sensory/perceptual alterations:
  - Impaired ability to recognize, associate, or interpret sounds (e.g., voice quality, animal noises, musical pieces, types of instruments): Direct patient's attention to a particular sound (e.g., if a cat meows on the television, state that it is the sound a cat makes and point to the cat on the screen).
  - Visual-spatial misperception: E.g., patient may underestimate distances and bump into doors or confuse the inside and outside of an object, such as an article of clothing. These patients may lose their place when reading or adding up numbers and therefore never complete the task. These patients will benefit from a structured, consistent environment.
  - Difficulty recognizing and associating familiar objects: These patients may not recognize dangerous or hazardous objects, because they do not know

the purpose of the object. Assist these individuals with eating because they may not know the purpose of silverware. Monitor the environment for safety hazards and remove unsafe objects, such as scissors, from the bedside.

- Inability to orient self in space: These patients may require a restraint or wheelchair belt for support because they may not know if they are standing, sitting, or leaning.
- Misperception of own body and body parts: These patients may not perceive their foot or arm as being a part of their body. Teach them to concentrate on their body parts (e.g., by watching their feet carefully while walking).
- Impaired ability to recognize objects by means of the senses of hearing, vibration, or touch: These patients rely more on visual cues. Keep their environment simple to reduce sensory overload and enable concentration on visual cues. Remove distracting stimuli.

**Impaired verbal communication** related to aphasia secondary to cerebrovascular insult

*Desired outcome:* At a minimum of the 24-h period before hospital discharge, patient demonstrates improved self-expression and relates decreased frustration with communication.

---

**Note:** Aphasia is the partial or complete inability to use or comprehend language and symbols and may occur with dominant (left) hemisphere damage. It is not the result of impaired hearing or intelligence. There are many different types of aphasia. Generally the patient has a combination of types, which vary in severity. *Receptive aphasia* (e.g., Wernicke's, sensory) is characterized by inability to recognize or comprehend spoken words. It is as if a foreign language were being spoken or the patient has word deafness. The patient often is good at responding to nonverbal cues. *Expressive aphasia* (e.g., Broca's, motor) is characterized by difficulty expressing words or naming objects. Gestures, groans, swearing, or nonsense words may be used.

---

- Evaluate the nature and severity of the patient's aphasia. When doing so, avoid giving nonverbal cues. Assess patient's ability to point or look toward a specific object, follow simple directions, understand yes/no questions, understand complex questions, repeat both simple and complex words, repeat sentences, name objects that are shown, demonstrate or relate the purpose or action of the object, fulfill written requests, write requests, and read. When evaluating patient for aphasia, be aware that patient may be responding to nonverbal cues and may understand less than you think. Document this assessment with simple descriptions and specific examples of the patient's aphasia symptoms. Use it as the basis for a communication plan.
- Obtain a referral to a speech therapist or pathologist as needed. Provide therapist with a list of words that would enhance patient's independence and/or care. In addition, ask for tips that will help improve communication with patient.
- When communicating with the patient, try to reduce distractions in the environment, such as television or others' conversations. Because fatigue affects a person's ability to communicate, try to ensure that the patient is well rested.
- Communicate with patient as much as possible. General principles for patients who may not recognize or comprehend the spoken word include the following: face patient and establish eye contact, speak slowly and clearly, give patient time to process your communication and answer, keep messages short and simple, stay with one clearly defined subject, avoid questions with multiple choices but rather phrase questions so that they can be answered

"yes" or "no," and use the same words each time you repeat a statement or question (e.g., pill vs. medication, bathroom vs. toilet). If patient does not understand after repetition, try different words. Use gestures, facial expressions, and pantomime to supplement and reinforce your message. Give short, simple directions, and repeat as needed to ensure understanding. Use concrete terms (e.g., "water" instead of "fluid," "leg" instead of "limb").

- When helping patients regain use of symbolic language, start with nouns first, and progress to more complex statements as indicated, using verbs, pronouns, and adjectives. For continuity, keep a record at the bedside of words to be used (e.g., "pill" rather than "medication").

- Treat patient as an adult. It is not necessary to raise the volume of your voice unless the patient is hard of hearing. Be respectful.

- When patients have difficulty expressing words or naming objects, encourage them to repeat words after you for practice in verbal expression. Begin with simple words like "yes" or "no" and progress to others like "cup." Progress to more complex statements as indicated. Listen and respond to patient's communication efforts; otherwise patient may give up. Praise accomplishments. Be prepared for labile emotions because these patients become frustrated and emotional when faced with their impaired speech.

- When improvement is noted, let patient complete your sentence (e.g., "This is a _____"). Keep a list of words patient can say, and add to the list as appropriate. Use this list when forming questions patient can answer. Avoid finishing patient's sentences.

- Patients who have lost the ability to monitor their verbal output may not produce sensible language but may think they are making sense and not understand why others do not comprehend or respond appropriately to them. Avoid labeling patient "belligerent" or "confused" when the problem is aphasia and frustration. Listen for errors in conversation, and provide feedback.

- Patients who have lost the ability to recognize number symbols or relationships will have difficulty understanding time concept or telling time. Avoid instructing patient to "wait 5 minutes" because this may not be meaningful.

- Give practice in receiving word images by pointing to an object and clearly stating its name. Watch signals patient gives you.

- Patients with nondominant (right) hemisphere damage often have no difficulty speaking; however, they may use excessive detail, give irrelevant information, and get off on a tangent. Bring patient back to the subject by saying "Let's go back to what we were talking about."

- Provide a supportive and relaxed environment for those patients who are unable to form words or sentences or speak clearly or appropriately. If patient makes an error, do not criticize patient's effort but rather compliment it by saying "That was a good try." Do not react negatively to patient's emotional displays. Address and acknowledge patient's frustration over the inability to communicate. Maintain a calm and positive attitude. If you do not understand the patient, say so. Ask patient to repeat unclear words, ask for more clues, ask patient to use another word, or have patient point to the object. Observe for nonverbal cues, and anticipate patient's needs. Allow time to listen if patient speaks slowly. To validate patient's message, repeat or rephrase it aloud.

- Ensure that the call light is available and the patient knows how to use it.

- Dysarthria can complicate aphasia. For additional interventions for patients with dysarthria, see **Impaired verbal communication** in "General Care of Patients with Neurologic Disorders," p. 304.

**Knowledge deficit:** Cerebral artery bypass surgery

*Desired outcome:* Before the procedure, patient verbalizes understanding about the surgical procedure, including the purpose, risks, and anticipated benefits or outcome.

- After physician has explained the cerebral artery bypass surgery to the patient, determine patient's level of understanding. Reinforce information or clarify as indicated.

- As indicated, explain that cerebral artery bypass surgery connects an extra-cranial vessel to an intracranial vessel to bypass an obstruction and increase blood flow to the brain.
- Describe the following postoperative interventions, which may occur in the ICU during the immediate postoperative period:
  - VS and neurologic status checks are performed at least hourly: Patient will be asked to squeeze the examiner's hands, move extremities, answer questions, and extend the tongue. Emphasize the importance of performing these activities to the best of patient's ability and reporting any numbness, tingling, or weakness. Neurologic deficits, especially differences on either side of the body or face or indicators of IICP, will be reported to physician.
  - BP will be monitored frequently, and patient may require vasoactive medications to keep BP within prescribed parameters. Hypertension can cause bypass stretching and bleeding, with loss of anastomosis and graft. Hypotension may promote thrombosis, with loss of graft.
  - Strict bed rest usually is enforced for 24-48 h.
  - For patients with bypass surgery involving the temporal artery, prevention of impaired perfusion to the temporal area graft site is a key consideration. HOB probably will be elevated 30 degrees, and the head, neck, and body will be kept in good alignment to prevent neck flexion or hyperextension. It is critical that there be no pressure on the graft site. Explain that the patient will be positioned away from the operative side. Dressings will be kept loose to prevent constriction of the graft site. The patient can expect the elastic bands on nasal cannulas or $O_2$ masks to be taped to the face to ensure they do not constrict the head, neck, and graft. Eyeglasses are contraindicated unless the earpiece on the operative side is removed. These precautions with eyeglasses and other constrictive gear usually are in effect for 3 months after surgery.
  - The head dressing will be checked at frequent intervals for drainage and tightness. The scalp may swell after surgery, causing the dressing to tighten. The dressing should be loose enough to slip a finger beneath. Instruct patient to report any burning sensation on the scalp, which may indicate ischemia.
  - Graft patency will be assessed periodically either by palpation or using a Doppler probe on the temporal pulse.
  - The patient can expect anticoagulant and/or antiplatelet therapy for 3-6 months after the procedure.
  - Precautions are taken against IICP (see "General Care of Patients with Neurologic Disorders" for **Altered cerebral tissue perfusion** related to risk of IICP, p. 305). Teach these precautions to patient and significant others.
- For additional interventions, see this nursing diagnosis in Appendix One, "Caring for Preoperative and Postoperative Patients," p. 693).

**Knowledge deficit:**   Carotid endarterectomy procedure
***Desired outcome:***   Before surgery, patient verbalizes understanding of the carotid endarterectomy procedure, including the purpose, risks, expected benefits or outcome, and postsurgical care.

- After physician has explained the procedure to the patient, determine patient's level of understanding, and reinforce or clarify information as needed.
- As indicated, explain that carotid endarterectomy is the removal of plaque in the obstructed artery to increase blood supply to the brain.
- Describe the following postsurgical assessments, which will occur in the ICU during the immediate postsurgical period.
  - Monitoring of VS and neurologic status at least hourly. Explain that the

patient may be asked to swallow, move the tongue, smile, speak, and shrug shoulders to determine facial drooping, tongue weakness, hoarseness, dysphagia, shoulder weakness, or loss of facial sensation, which are signs of cranial nerve impairment. Stretching of the cranial nerves during surgery can occur, causing edema, and may leave a temporary deficit. The patient should report any numbness, tingling, or weakness, which may indicate occlusion of the carotid. In addition, the superficial temporal and facial pulses will be palpated for strength, quality, and symmetry to evaluate the patency of the external carotid artery.

- Periodic assessment of the neck for edema, hematoma, bleeding, or tracheal deviation. Explain that the patient should report immediately any respiratory distress, difficulty managing secretions, or sensation of neck tightness. Additional $O_2$ will most likely be supplied, even without respiratory distress or airway compromise, because manipulation of the carotid sinus may cause temporary loss of normal physiologic response to hypoxia.

- Frequent BP checks may be performed because temporary carotid sinus dysfunction may cause BP problems (usually hypertension). The patient may need vasoactive medications to keep BP within a specified range to maintain cerebral perfusion while preventing disruption of graft or sutures.

- HOB must be maintained in prescribed position (flat or elevated), and patient generally is positioned off the operative side.

- A drain may be indwelling in the neck for a few days, and the patient may have a leg incision if the graft was taken from the leg's saphenous vein.

- Anticoagulant/antiplatelet therapy (e.g., aspirin, warfarin) usually instituted for 3-6 months postprocedure.

- For additional interventions, see this nursing diagnosis in Appendix One, "Caring for Preoperative and Postoperative Patients," p. 693.

---

**Note:** See "Pulmonary Embolus" for **Altered protection** related to risk of prolonged bleeding or hemorrhage secondary to anticoagulant therapy, p. 17. See "Renal-Urinary Disorders" for related diagnoses for incontinence, retention, and neurogenic bladder. **Caution:** Credé's method and other interventions that increase intrathoracic or intraabdominal pressure are contraindicated until the risk of IICP is no longer a factor. See "Alzheimer's Disease" for **Sensory/perceptual alterations,** p. 219. See "Head Injury" for **High risk for disuse syndrome** related to prolonged inactivity, p. 256; and **Fluid volume excess** (related to SIADH), p. 256. For patients undergoing surgery see "Brain Tumors" for **Knowledge deficit:** Craniotomy procedure, p. 263. See "Seizure Disorders," p. 292, for related nursing diagnoses. See "General Care of Patients with Neurologic Disorders" for **High risk for trauma** related to unsteady gait, p. 298; **High risk for injury** related to impaired pain, touch, and temperature sensations, p. 299; **Impaired corneal tissue integrity,** p. 300; **Altered nutrition:** Less than body requirements, p. 300; **High risk for fluid volume deficit,** p. 301, **High risk for aspiration,** p. 302, **Self-care deficit,** p. 302; **Constipation,** p. 305; **Altered cerebral tissue perfusion,** p. 305; **Impaired swallowing,** p. 308; **Sensory/perceptual alterations** (visual), p. 307; and **Knowledge deficit:** Neurologic diagnostic tests, p. 311. See "Diabetes Insipidus," p. 346, for patients with this disorder or who are at risk. See "Pressure Ulcers," p. 687, and Appendix One, "Caring for Patients on Prolonged Bed Rest," p. 711, for nursing diagnoses and interventions related to immobility. Adjust interventions accordingly if patient has IICP or is at risk for this problem. See Appendix One, "Caring for Patients with Cancer and Other Life-Disrupting Illnesses," p. 753, for appropriate psychosocial nursing diagnoses.

PATIENT-FAMILY TEACHING AND DISCHARGE PLANNING

Give patient and significant others verbal and written information about the following:

- Importance of minimizing or treating the following risk factors: diabetes mellitus, hypertension, high cholesterol, high Na intake, obesity, inactivity, smoking, prolonged bed rest, and stressful life-style.
- Interventions that increase effective communication in the presence of aphasia or dysarthria.
- Referrals to the following as appropriate: public health nurse, visiting nurses association, psychologic therapy, vocational rehabilitation agency, home health agencies, and extended and skilled care facilities. Also provide the following address: National Stroke Association, 300 East Hampden Avenue, Suite 240, Englewood, CO 80110-2654, (303)-762-9922 or (800)-787-6537. For pamphlets, contact National Institute of Neurological Disorders and Stroke (NINDS), Building 31, Room 8A16, 9000 Rockville Pike, Bethesda, MD 20892, (301)-496-4188 or (800)-352-9424.
- For other information, see Patient-Family Teaching and Discharge Planning (third through tenth entries only), in "Multiple Sclerosis," p. 187.

# Section Six:    Seizure Disorders

Seizures result from an abnormal, uncontrolled, electrical discharge from the neurons of the cerebral cortex in response to a stimulus. If the activity is localized in one portion of the brain, the individual will have a partial seizure, but when it is widespread and diffuse, a generalized seizure occurs. Symptoms vary widely, depending on the involved area of the cerebral cortex.

Seizure threshold refers to the amount of stimulation needed to cause the neural activity. Although anyone can have a seizure if the stimulus is sufficient, the seizure threshold is lowered in some individuals and this may result in spontaneous seizures. Potential causes for lowered seizure threshold include congenital defects; head injury, particularly that from a penetrating wound; subarachnoid hemorrhage; intracranial tumors; infections, such as meningitis or encephalitis; exposure to toxins, such as lead; hypoxia; and metabolic and endocrine disorders, such as hypoglycemia, hypocalcemia, uremia, hypoparathyroidism, excessive hydration, and fever. Phenothiazide, tricyclic antidepressants, and alcohol usage increase the risk of seizure by lowering the seizure threshold. For susceptible individuals, "triggers" may include emotional tension or stress; physical stimulation, such as loud music or bright, flashing lights; lack of sleep or food; fatigue; menses or pregnancy; and excessive drug/alcohol use. If a trigger stimulus is identified, the individual has what is termed *reflex epilepsy.*

Although a seizure itself generally is not fatal, individuals can be injured by hitting their head or breaking bones if they lose consciousness and fall to the ground. Seizure activity increases cerebral $O_2$ consumption by 60% and cerebral blood flow by 250%. Instances of prolonged and repeated generalized seizures, *status epilepticus,* can be life-threatening because exhaustion, anoxia, respiratory arrest, and cardiovascular collapse can occur.

ASSESSMENT

There is a great variety of seizures (Table 4-4), but the following are the most serious or common:

**Generalized tonic-clonic (grand mal):**  Possible prodomal phase of increased irritability, tension, mood changes, or headache preceding the seizure by hours or days. Patient may experience the presence of an aura (a sensory

**T A B L E  4 - 4    International Classification of Epileptic Seizures**

I. Partial (seizure begun in a local area)
   A. Simple (consciousness not impaired)
      1. Motor (with or without Jacksonian march)
      2. Sensory or somatosensory
      3. Autonomic
      4. Psychic
   B. Complex (consciousness is impaired; may occur with or without automatisms)
      1. Simple partial onset—progresses to impaired consciousness
      2. Consciousness impaired at onset
   C. Secondarily generalized
      1. Simple partial onset—progresses to generalized seizure
      2. Complex partial onset—progresses to generalized seizure
      3. Simple partial to complex partial to generalized seizure
II. Generalized (all associated with loss of consciousness; may be convulsive or nonconvulsive)
   A. Absence (petit mal)
   B. Myoclonic
   C. Clonic
   D. Tonic-clonic (grand mal)
   E. Atonic (drop attacks)
III. Unclassified (because of inadequate or incomplete data)

Adapted from Commission on Classification and Terminology of the International League Against Epilepsy, 1981.

warning, such as a sound, odor, or a flash of light) immediately preceding the seizure by seconds or minutes. The seizure usually does not last more than 2-6 min and includes the following phases:

***Tonic (rigid/contracted):***  Often lasts only 15 sec, usually subsiding in less than a minute. Symptoms include loss of consciousness, clenched jaws (potential for tongue to be bitten), apnea (may hear cry as air is forced out of the lungs), and cyanosis. The patient may be incontinent, and the pupils may dilate and become nonreactive to light.

***Clonic (rhythmic contraction and relaxation of the extremities and muscles):***  May subside in 30 seconds but can last 2-5 min. The eyes roll upward, and excessive salivation results in foaming at the mouth. During this phase, the potential is greatest for biting the tongue.

***Stupor:***  May last 5 min. The individual is limp and unresponsive. The pupils react to light and return to their normal size.

***Postictal:***  In the period immediately after the seizure, the patient may be sleepy, semiconscious, confused, unable to speak clearly, uncoordinated, have a headache, complain of muscle aches, and have no recollection of the seizure event. Temporary weakness, dysphasia, or hemianopia lasting up to 24 h postseizure may be experienced.

**Generalized absence (petit mal):**  Patient has momentary loss of awareness with an abrupt cessation of voluntary muscle activity. The patient may appear to be daydreaming with a vacant stare. Patient may experience facial, eyelid, or hand twitching. The individual resumes previous activity when the seizure ends. There is usually no memory of the seizure, and the patient may have difficulty reorienting after the seizure event. This type of seizure can last 1-10 sec and may occur up to 100 times a day. This type of seizure usually resolves by puberty.

**Generalized myoclonic:**    Sudden, very brief contraction or jerking of muscles or muscle groups. The individual may have a very brief, momentary loss of consciousness with some postictal confusion.

**Partial simple motor (focal motor seizures):**    An irritative focus located in the motor cortex of the frontal lobe causes clonic movement in a particular part of the body, such as the hands or face. If the seizure activity spreads, or marches in an orderly fashion to an adjacent area (e.g., the hands to the arms to the shoulder), the seizure is termed a focal motor seizure with Jacksonian march. The seizure usually lasts several seconds to minutes. There is no loss of consciousness, and somatosensory symptoms (e.g., smells, sounds), autonomic symptoms (e.g., tachycardia, tachypnea, diaphoresis, and flushing), or psychic symptoms (e.g., fear, déja vu) may be experienced.

**Partial complex seizure (psychomotor):**    Generally lasts from 1-4 min. Usually there is loss of consciousness and a postictal state of confusion lasting several minutes. However, the individual does not fall to the ground. The patient is able to interact with the environment, exhibits purposeful but inappropriate movements or behavior, and has no memory of the event. The individual will perform such automatisms as lip sucking, chewing, facial grimacing, picking, or swallowing movements. These patients may experience and remember various sensory or emotional hallucinations or sensations that occur immediately before the seizure, such as smells, ringing or hissing sounds, or feelings of déja vu, fear, or pleasure.

**Status epilepticus:**    State of continuous or rapidly recurring seizures in which the individual does not completely recover baseline neurologic functioning between seizures. Individuals who suddenly stop taking their antiepilepsy medication are likely to develop this condition. This is a medical emergency, resulting in potential complications, such as cerebral anoxia and edema, aspiration, hyperthermia, and exhaustion. Irreversible damage may occur in 60 min. Death may result.

## DIAGNOSTIC TESTS

Because a variety of problems can precipitate seizures, testing may be extensive. Common tests include the following:

**Serum electrolytes:**    To rule out metabolic causes, such as hypoglycemia or hypocalcemia.

**EEG — both sleeping and awake:**    May reveal abnormal patterns of electrical activity, particularly with such stimuli as flashing lights or hyperventilation. Telemetry EEGs may also be performed. Generalized tonic-clonic shows up as high, fast voltage spikes in all leads.

**Positron emission tomography (PET):**    May find areas of cerebral glucose hypometabolism that correlate with the irritative seizure-causing focus. This test is useful in partial seizures.

**MRI:**    May show structural lesions causing partial seizures; also may reveal a space-occupying lesion such as a tumor or hematoma.

**CT scan:**    May reveal presence of a space-occupying lesion, such as a tumor or hematoma.

**Skull x-rays:**    To reveal fractures, tumors, calcifications, or congenital anomalies (pineal shift, ventricular deformity).

**Lumbar puncture (LP) and CSF analysis:**    To rule out IICP or infection, such as meningitis, as the source of the seizures.

---

**Note:**    See "General Care of Patients with Neurologic Disorders," **Knowledge deficit:** Neurologic diagnostic tests, p. 311, for care considerations for patients undergoing EEG, PET, MRI, CT scan, and LP.

## COLLABORATIVE MANAGEMENT

**Antiepilepsy drugs:**   To help prevent seizure activity.

*Hydantoin derivatives (e.g., phenytoin, mephenytoin, or ethotoin):*   For tonic-clonic, partial simple, and partial complex seizures.

*Carbamazepine:*   For tonic-clonic, partial simple, and partial complex seizures.

*Valproic acid:*   For absence, tonic-clonic, and mixed seizures types.

*Succinimide derivatives (e.g., ethosuximide):*   For absence seizures.

*Barbiturate derivatives (e.g., phenobarbital or primidone):*   May be used in conjunction with one of antiepilepsy drugs above or as monotherapy for tonic-clonic or partial seizures.

---

**Note:**   If the patient is seizure-free for 2-5 years, medication tapering over several months and then discontinuation may be attempted under physician supervision.

---

**Treatment of underlying causes:**   Such as metabolic disorder or infectious process.

**Stress management:**   Progressive relaxation training, diaphragmatic respiratory training, and biofeedback are used to reduce seizure frequency and severity by controlling stress or hyperventilation trigger stimulation.

**Nutrition:**   A balanced diet spaced evenly throughout the day is recommended to avoid hypoglycemia, which may trigger seizures. Patients are advised to avoid caffeine and alcohol products and to prevent overhydration, which also can precipitate seizure activity.

**Counseling or psychotherapy:**   For patients with poor self-concept or coping difficulties related to the diagnosis.

**Surgery:**   Brain tumors or hematomas may be evacuated if they are the source of seizure activity. For medically intractable seizures, excision of known epileptogenic areas may be attempted to obtain seizure control. These procedures may include cortical resection (e.g., temporal lobectomy for partial seizures) and corpus callostomy (for generalized seizures). To prevent increased or new neurologic deficits, extensive presurgical testing is done, possibly including CT scan and MRI to find structural abnormalities, angiograms to detect vascular abnormalities, 24-h EEG monitoring, invasive EEG monitoring with depth electrodes, and intracarotid sodium amytal test to determine hemispheric dominance and function. All these procedures require a craniotomy (see "Brain Tumors," p. 260).

**Management of status epilepticus**

*Respiratory management:*   $O_2$ therapy, oral airway suctioning, and intubation as needed to maintain airway and prevent hypoxia.

*Assessment of blood glucose and administration of IV glucose:*   If indicated, to reverse hypoglycemia.

*Serum laboratory studies:*   To evaluate for electrolyte (e.g., hyponatremia, hypocalcemia) or metabolic imbalances that may be causing seizures. Serum drug screens are performed to assess serum antiepilepsy drug level and determine the presence of alcohol or other drugs that may be causing the seizures.

*Slow administration of IV diazepam or lorazepam, 2 mg/min:*   Initially given bolus. If seizures continue, diazepam occasionally is given in a continuous IV drip (10-15 mg/h). **Note:** Monitor for signs of respiratory depression and hypotension.

*Administration of IV phenytoin:*   If diazepam is unsuccessful.

---

**Note:**   Do not mix phenytoin with other medications and most IV fluids; give it slowly, undiluted, IV push, at no more than 50 mg/min. It should be given only with normal saline IV fluids because it will precipitate in the presence of $D_5W$. Monitor for hypotension, apnea, and cardiac dysrhythmias.

---

*Administration of IV phenobarbital:*  If diazepam and phenytoin are unsuccessful. **Note:** Monitor for signs of respiratory depression.

*Administration of thiamine:*  If alcohol withdrawal occurs or is suspected.

*Administration of glucocorticosteroids (e.g., dexamethasone):*  To relieve cerebral edema.

*Administration of paraldehyde:*  May be given if other medications are unsuccessful. **Note:** Because the solution reacts negatively with plastic, use a glass syringe for IM and IV routes or a rubber catheter if it is given *via* retention enema. Occasionally lidocaine is administered.

*Intubation and general anesthesia with large doses of short-acting barbiturate (e.g., phenobarbital) or neuromuscular blocking agent:*  For severe cases. Neuromuscular blocking agents may stop the movement but will not stop brain activity.

*Search for the underlying cause:*  May include a wide variety of diagnostic tests (see diagnostic test section, above). Patients in status epilepticus are typically transferred to ICU.

## NURSING DIAGNOSES AND INTERVENTIONS

**High risk for trauma** related to oral, musculoskeletal, and airway vulnerability secondary to seizure activity

*Desired outcomes:*  Patient exhibits no signs of oral or musculoskeletal tissue injury or airway compromise after the seizure. Before hospital discharge, patient's significant others verbalize knowledge of actions necessary during seizure activity.

### Seizure precautions

- Pad side rails with blankets or pillows. Keep side rails up and the bed in its lowest position when the patient is in bed. Keep bed, wheelchair, or stretcher brakes locked.
- Tape a soft rubber oral airway to the bedside. Remove wooden tongue depressors (if used, they may splinter). Keep suction and oxygen equipment readily available. Consider a heparin lock for IV access for high-risk patient.
- Avoid using glass or other breakable oral thermometers when taking patient's temperature. If only breakable thermometers are available, take temperature *via* axillary or rectal route.
- Caution patients to lie down and push the call button if they experience a prodromal or aural warning. Encourage patient to empty the mouth of dentures or foreign objects. Keep call light within reach.
- Do not allow unsupervised smoking.
- Evaluate need for and provide protective headgear as indicated.

### During the seizure

- Remain with patient. Observe for, record, and report type, duration, and characteristics of seizure activity and any postseizure response. This should include, as appropriate, precipitating event, aura, initial location and progression, automatisms, type and duration of movement, changes in LOC, eye movement (e.g., deviation, nystagmus), pupil size and reaction, bowel and bladder incontinence, head deviation, tongue deviation, or teeth clenching.
- Prevent or break the fall, and ease patient to the floor if the seizure occurs while patient is out of bed. Keep patient in bed if the seizure occurs while there, and lower HOB to a flat position.
- If the patient's jaws are clenched, do not force an object between the teeth, because this can break teeth or lacerate oral mucous membrane. If able to do so safely and without damage to oral tissue, insert an airway. Tongue depressors should not be used, because they may splinter. A rolled washcloth may be used as an alternative. Never put your fingers in the patient's mouth.

- Protect patient's head from injury during seizure activity. A towel folded flat may be used to cushion the head from striking the ground. Be sure the head's position does not occlude the airway. Remove from the environment objects (e.g., chairs) that the patient may strike. Pad the floors to protect the patient's arms and legs. Remove patient's glasses.
- Do not restrain patient but rather guide the patient's movements gently to prevent injury.
- Roll patient into a side-lying position to promote drainage of secretions and maintain a patent airway. Use the head tilt, chin lift maneuver. Provide $O_2$ and suction as needed.
- Loosen tight clothing.
- Maintain patient's privacy. Clear nonessential people out of the room.
- Administer antiepilepsy drugs as prescribed.

*After the seizure*

- Reassure and reorient patient. Check neurologic status and VS; ask patient if an aura preceded the seizure activity. Record this information and postictal characteristics.
- Provide a quiet, calm environment because sounds and stimuli can be confusing to the awakening patient. Keep talk simple and to a minimum. Speak slowly and with pauses between sentences. Repeating may be necessary. Use room light that is behind, not above, patient to prevent additional seizures and for patient comfort. Do not offer food or drink until patient is fully awake.
- Check patient's tongue for lacerations and body for injuries. Monitor urine for red or cola color, which may signal rhabdomyolysis or myoglobinuria from muscle damage. Monitor for the presence of weakness or paralysis, dysphasia, or visual disturbances.
- Check blood fingerstick glucose and obtain serum lab tests as prescribed. Administer antiepilepsy medication as prescribed.
- Monitor for status epilepticus (i.e., state of continuous or rapidly recurring seizures in which the individual does not completely recover baseline neurologic functioning). This condition is life-threatening and can cause cerebral anoxia and edema, aspiration, hyperthermia, and exhaustion. Notify physician immediately.
- Provide significant others with verbal and written information for the preceding interventions.

**Impaired tissue integrity (or risk of same)** related to chemical irritation from IV phenytoin administration

*Desired outcome:* Patient's tissue surrounding the IV site remains undamaged as evidenced by absence of swelling, discoloration, discomfort, and blistering.

- If possible, avoid administering IV phenytoin through an insertion site in the wrist, hand, or foot. Ideally, IV phenytoin is administered through a central line. If a central line is not present, administer the drug through the largest-gauge needle possible.
- Monitor the insertion site for inflammation or infiltration before administering the drug. Check for line patency periodically during administration. Stop the injection immediately if there are any indicators of infiltration or inflammation.
- Flush the line with 0.9% NaCl before and after giving the drug to decrease the likelihood of irritation and prevent precipitation. Flush with enough solution to clear the line and tubing completely. Do not mix phenytoin with other medications. Phenytoin will precipitate in the presence of $D_5W$.
- Administer the drug undiluted and at a rate ≤50 mg/min. A more rapid administration rate will irritate the vein and also can cause hypotension, apnea, and cardiac dysrhythmias. For the older adult or a person with cardiovascular disease, a slower rate of 25 mg/min is recommended.

- After administration, inspect the insertion site often, for several hours. Monitor for swelling or discoloration. Instruct patient to report any pain at the site.
- Report any swelling or discoloration to the physician, and remove the vascular access device. Monitor for worsening discoloration, blistering, edema, or tissue sloughing. To control swelling, elevate patient's arm above the chest and, if prescribed, wrap the arm in warm compresses. Check circulation, sensation, and movement in the affected arm and hand, and report significant findings. Protect blisters with a sterile dressing.

**Knowledge deficit:** Life-threatening environmental factors and preventive measures for seizures

**Desired outcomes:** Before hospital discharge, patient verbalizes accurate information about measures that may prevent seizures and environmental factors that can be life-threatening in the presence of seizures. Patient exhibits health-care measures that reflect this knowledge.

- Assess patient's knowledge of measures that can prevent seizures and environmental hazards that can be life-threatening in the presence of seizure activity. Provide or clarify information as indicated.
- Advise patient to check into state regulations about automobile operation. Most states require 1-3 seizure-free years before an individual can obtain a driver's license.
- Caution patient to refrain from operating heavy or dangerous equipment, swimming, and possibly even tub bathing until he or she is seizure-free for the amount of time specified by physician. Teach patient never to swim alone, regardless of the amount of time he or she has been seizure-free. Caution patient to swim only in shallow water to make rescue easier if a seizure occurs.
- Advise patient to turn the temperature of hot water heaters down to prevent scalding if a seizure occurs in the shower.
- Encourage stress management, progressive relaxation techniques, and diaphragmatic respiratory training to control emotional stress and hyperventilation, which often trigger seizures.
- Advise patient that some activities, such as climbing or bicycle riding, require careful risk-benefit evaluation.
- Encourage vocational assessment and counseling. The patient's epilepsy may place others at risk in some occupations, such as bus driver or airline pilot.
- Advise female patients that seizure activity may change (increase or decrease) during menses or pregnancy. Tonic-clonic seizures have caused fetal death. Antiepilepsy drugs are associated with birth defects; however, 90% of women have normal pregnancies and normal children. Provide birth control information if requested.
- Teach patient that use of stimulants (e.g., caffeine) and depressants (e.g., alcohol) should be avoided. Withdrawal from stimulants and depressants can increase the likelihood of seizures.
- Teach patient that getting adequate amounts of rest, avoiding physical and emotional stress, and maintaining a nutritious diet may help prevent seizure activity. Meals should be spaced throughout the day to prevent hypoglycemia. Overhydration may precipitate seizure activity. If stimuli such as flashing lights or loud music appear to trigger seizures, advise patient to avoid environments that are likely to have these stimuli. Poorly adjusted TVs may trigger seizures and should be fixed.
- Encourage individuals who have seizures that occur without warning to avoid chewing gum or sucking on lozenges, which may be aspirated during a seizure.
- Encourage patient to wear a Medic-Alert bracelet or similar identification or to carry a medical information card.

**Knowledge deficit:** Purpose, precautions, and side effects of antiepilepsy medications

***Desired outcome:*** Before hospital discharge, patient verbalizes accurate information about the prescribed antiepilepsy medication.

- Stress the importance of taking the prescribed medication regularly and on schedule and not discontinuing the medication without physician guidance. Explain that missing a scheduled dose can precipitate a seizure several days later. Stress that abrupt withdrawal of any antiepilepsy medication can precipitate seizures and that discontinuing these medications is the most common cause of status epilepticus. Assist patients in finding methods that will help them remember to take the medication and monitor their drug supply to avoid running out. Drugs may be necessary for the rest of the patient's life. Medications cannot be taken prn, and lack of seizures does not mean the drug is unnecessary. Explain the concept of drug half-lives and steady blood levels.
- Reinforce prescribed drug dose instructions.
- Stress the importance of informing physician about side effects and keeping appointments for periodic lab work, which determines whether blood levels are therapeutic and assesses for side effects. Many antiepilepsy medications can cause blood dyscrasias or liver damage. Teach patient to report immediately any bruising, bleeding, or jaundice. Vitamin D, vitamin K, and folic acid supplements may be prescribed.
- Explain that antiepilepsy medications may make people drowsy. Advise patient to avoid activities that require alertness until his or her CNS response to the medication has been determined.
- Nausea and vomiting are common side effects of most antiepilepsy medications. Teach patient to take the drug with food or large amounts of liquid to minimize gastric upset. Patients taking valproic acid (Depakote) should not chew the medication, because it may irritate the oral mucous membrane. Also advise patients taking valproic acid that this drug may produce a false-positive test for urine ketones and that any visual change should be reported immediately because it may signal ocular toxicity.
- Instruct patient to notify physician if a significant weight gain or weight loss occurs because it may necessitate a change in dose or scheduling.
- Teach patient to avoid alcoholic beverages and OTC medications containing alcohol. Chronic alcohol use stimulates the body to metabolize phenytoin (Dilantin) more quickly, thus lowering the seizure threshold because of the decreased plasma phenytoin levels. Patients taking phenobarbital (Luminal) or primidone (Mysoline) should avoid alcohol, which potentiates central nervous system (CNS) depressant effects. Anticonvulsant agents are potentiated or inhibited by many other drugs, including aspirin and antihistamines, and may affect potency of other medications as well. Caution patient to avoid OTC medications.
- Other side effects common to antiepilepsy medications are ataxia, diplopia, nystagmus, and dizziness. Instruct patient to report these symptoms.
- Teach patients who take carbamazepine (Tegretol) or ethosuximide (Zarontin) to report immediately fever, mouth ulcers, sore throat, bruising, or bleeding.
- Advise patients taking phenytoin that this drug can cause gingival hypertrophy. The patient should perform frequent oral hygiene with gum massage and gentle flossing and brush teeth 3-4 times/day with a soft toothbrush. These patients also should report immediately any measlelike rash.
- Caution patients taking phenytoin that there are two types of this drug. Dilantin Kapseal is absorbed more slowly and is longer acting. It is important not to confuse this extended-release phenytoin with prompt-release phenytoin. Doing so may cause dangerous underdose or overdose. Generic phenytoin should not be substituted for Dilantin Kapseal.

**Noncompliance** with the therapy related to denial of the illness or perceived negative consequences of the treatment regimen secondary to social stigma, negative side effects of antiepilepsy medications, or difficulty with making necessary life-style change

***Desired outcome:***  Before hospital discharge, patient verbalizes knowledge about the disease process and treatment plan, acknowledges consequences of continued noncompliant behavior, explains the experience that caused patient to alter the prescribed behavior, describes the appropriate treatment of side effects or the appropriate alternatives, and exhibits health-care measures that reflect this knowledge, following an agreed-on plan of care.

- Assess patient's understanding of the disease process, medical management, and treatment plan. Explain or clarify information as indicated.
- Assess for causes of noncompliance, such as medication side effects or difficulty making significant life-style changes or following the medication schedule.
- Ensure awareness that stopping medications can be life-threatening (e.g., status epilepticus). Explain drug half-life and the concept of a steady blood level. Intermittent medication use may be informal experimentation or an effort to gain control. Explain the importance of physician guidance if medication is stopped for any reason.
- Evaluate patient's perception of his or her vulnerability to the disease process, and be alert to signs of denial of the illness. In addition, evaluate patient's perception of the effectiveness or noneffectiveness of treatment. Stress the importance of expressing feelings.
- Determine if a value, cultural, or spiritual conflict is causing noncompliance. Confront myths and stigmas. Provide realistic assessment of risks and counter misconceptions.
- Discuss methods of dealing with common problems, such as obtaining insurance, and job or workplace discrimination.
- Assess patient's support systems. Determine whether the presence of a family disruption pattern (whether or not it is caused by the patient's illness) is making compliance difficult and "not worth it."
- After the reason for noncompliance is found, intervene accordingly to ensure compliance. If it appears that changing the medical treatment plan (e.g., in scheduling medications) may promote compliance, discuss this possibility with physician. Provide patient with information about interventions that can minimize the drug side effects (e.g., taking the drug with food or large amounts of liquid to minimize gastric distress).
- Encourage involvement with support systems, such as local epilepsy centers and national organizations.

---

**Note:**   See "General Care of Patients with Neurologic Disorders" for **Knowledge deficit:** Neurologic diagnostic tests, p. 311. See Appendix One, "Caring for Patients with Cancer and Other Life-Disrupting Illnesses" for **Body image disturbance,** p. 760, **Ineffective individual coping,** p. 757, and **Altered family processes,** p. 763.

---

## PATIENT-FAMILY TEACHING AND DISCHARGE PLANNING

Give patient and significant others verbal and written information about the following:

- Reinforcement of knowledge of the disease process, pathophysiology, symptoms, and the precipitating or aggravating factors.
- Medications, including purpose, dosage, schedule, and potential side effects. See Table 4-5, "Common Antiepilepsy Drugs."
- Importance of follow-up care and keeping medical appointments. Stress that use of antiepilepsy drugs necessitates periodic monitoring of blood levels to ensure therapeutic medication levels and assessment for side effects. Instruct patient to keep emergency contact numbers for the physician.
- Environmental factors that can be life-threatening in the presence of seizures,

**T A B L E   4 - 5   Common Antiepilepsy Drugs**

| Name | Side effects | Precautions |
| --- | --- | --- |
| **phenytoin (Dilantin)** | Drowsiness, gingival hypertrophy, nausea, vomiting, increased body hair, rash, or blood dyscrasias. Signs of overdose include nystagmus, ataxia, slurred speech, confusion, and diplopia. | Ensure frequent oral hygiene, gum massage, and gentle flossing. Take drug with food or large amounts of liquid to decrease gastric upset. Periodic blood counts are necessary. Call MD if rash or jaundice appears. Vitamin K may be given to pregnant women 1 month before and during delivery to prevent neonatal hemorrhage. If prescribed, supplement with vitamins K and D and folic acid. |
| **carbamazepine (Tegretol)** | Blood dyscrasias, ataxia, rash, nystagmus, diplopia, nausea, vomiting, liver damage, drowsiness, and dizziness. | Check CBC frequently. Patient should report fever, mouth ulcers, sore throat, bruising, or bleeding immediately. Take drug with food. Liver and renal function tests should be performed periodically. Report jaundice to MD. |
| **phenobarbital (Luminal)** | Drowsiness, lethargy, dizziness, nausea, vomiting, constipation, ataxia, anemia, mild rash, depression. | Do not stop abruptly; this may cause withdrawal seizures. Avoid alcohol, which would potentiate CNS depressant effects. Vitamin D supplements are usually advised. Take with foods to prevent stomach upset. Vitamin K is usually given to pregnant women 1 month before and during labor to prevent neonatal hemorrhage. |
| **primidone (Mysoline)** | Drowsiness, emotional changes including depression and irritability, anemia, rash, nausea, vomiting, impotence. Incoordination, slurred speech, and blurred vision may be early signs of overdose. | Do not stop abruptly; it may cause withdrawal seizures. Take with food or large amounts of fluid. See information with phenobarbital above regarding alcohol avoidance and vitamin K. |
| **ethosuximide (Zarontin)** | Gastric distress, nausea, vomiting, dizziness, drowsiness, aplastic anemia, vaginal bleeding. | Take with food or large amounts of fluid. Follow-up lab studies are important for detecting anemia. Patient *Continued.* |

**T A B L E  4 - 5    Common Antiepilepsy Drugs—cont'd**

| Name | Side effects | Precautions |
|---|---|---|
| ethosuximide (Zarontin)— cont'd | | should immediately report fever, mouth ulcers, sore throat, bruising, and bleeding. |
| valproic acid (Depakote) | Sedation, dizziness, nausea, vomiting, anorexia, liver damage, transient alopecia, ataxia, and thrombocytopenia. Any visual change may signal ocular toxicity. | Do not chew; it may irritate mucous membranes. Take with food to prevent gastric upset. Patient should report any bleeding, bruising, or visual change immediately and monitor liver function studies *via* periodic lab tests. This drug may produce false-positive test for ketones in the urine. |

measures that may help prevent seizures, and safety interventions during seizures. Review state and local laws that apply to individuals with seizure disorders.
- Employment or vocational counseling as needed. Discuss the need to avoid overprotection and maintain, as possible, normal work and recreation.
- Risks of antiepilepsy drugs during pregnancy. Provide birth control information or genetic counseling referral as requested.

*In addition*
- Provide the following address as appropriate: Epilepsy Foundation of America, 4351 Garden City Drive, Suite 406, Landover, MD 20785, (301)-459-3700 and (800)-332-1000.

# Section Seven:    General Care of Patients with Neurologic Disorders

**High risk for trauma** related to unsteady gait secondary to sensorimotor deficit

*Desired outcomes:*   Patient is free of trauma caused by gait unsteadiness. Before hospital discharge, patient demonstrates proficiency with assistive devices, if appropriate.
- Evaluate patient's gait, and assess for motor deficits such as weakness, tremors, spasticity, or paralysis. Document baseline neurologic and physical assessments so that changes in status can be detected promptly.
- To minimize the risk of injury, assist patient as needed when unsteady gait, weakness, or paralysis is noted. Instruct patient to ask or call for assistance with ambulation. Check frequently on patients who may forget to call for assistance. Stand on patient's weak side to assist with balance and support. Use transfer belt for safety. Instruct patient to use stronger side for gripping railing when stair climbing.
- Orient patient to new surroundings. Keep necessary items (including water, snacks, telephone, and call light) within easy reach of patient. Assess pa-

tient's ability to use these items. The patient who is very weak or partially paralyzed may require a tap bell instead of a call light.

- Maintain an uncluttered environment with unobstructed walkways to mini-mize the risk of tripping. Ensure adequate lighting at night (e.g., a night light) to help prevent falls in the dark. In addition, keep side rails up and the bed in its lowest position with bed brakes on. Encourage patient to use any needed hearing aids and corrective lenses when ambulating.

- For unsteady, weak, or partially paralyzed patient, encourage use of low-heel, nonskid shoes for walking. Teach the use of a wide-based gait to pro-vide a broader base of support. Instruct patient to note foot placement when ambulating or transferring to ensure that the foot is flat and in a position of support. Teach, reinforce, and encourage use of assistive device, such as a cane, walker, or crutches, that provides patient with added stability. Teach exercises that strengthen arm and shoulder muscles for using walkers and crutches. Teach safe use of transfer or sliding boards. Teach patients in wheelchairs how and when to lock and unlock the wheels. Demonstrate how to secure and support weak or paralyzed arms to prevent subluxation and injury from falling into wheelchair spokes or wheels. Patients with poor sit-ting balance may need a seat or chest belt. Show how to get on and off elevators to prevent wheels from catching in the gaps. Keep wheelchair close to bed. Teach proper use of recliner mechanism or battery precautions on appropriate wheelchairs.

- Teach patients to maintain a sitting position for a few minutes before as-suming a standing position for ambulating. This procedure gives patients time to get their feet flat and under them for balance and minimizes any dizziness that may occur because of rapid position changes.

- Monitor spasticity, antispasmodic medications, and their effect on physical function. Uncontrolled or severe spasms may cause falls, while mild to mod-erate spasms can be useful in ADL and transfers if the patient learns to con-trol and trigger them.

- Review with patient and significant others potential safety needs at home, such as safety appliances (wall, bath, and toilet hand rails; elevated toilet seat; nonslip surface in bath tub or shower). Loose rugs should be removed to prevent slipping and falling. Temperatures on hot water heaters should be turned down to prevent scalding in the event of a fall in the shower or tub. Furniture in the home may need to be moved to provide clear path-ways. Strategically placed additional lighting also may be needed. The edges of steps in the home may require taping with a color strip to provide suffi-cient contrast that the edges can be recognized and more safely negotiated. Beds should be modified to prevent rolling. Activity should be balanced with rest periods because fatigue tends to increase unsteadiness and the potential for falls.

- Seek referral by physical therapist (PT) as appropriate.

**High risk for injury** related to impaired pain, touch, and temperature sensa-tions secondary to sensory deficit or decreased LOC

*Desired outcomes:* Patient is free of symptoms of injury caused by impaired pain, touch, and temperature sensations. Before hospital discharge, patient and significant others identify factors that increase the potential for injury.

- Assess patient for indicators of sensory deficits, such as decreased or absent vision and impaired temperature and pain sensation. Document baseline neu-rologic and physical assessments so that changes in status can be detected promptly.

- Protect patient from exposure to hot food or equipment that can burn the skin. Avoid use of heating pads.

- Always check the temperature of heating devices and bath water before pa-tient is exposed to them. Teach patient and significant others about these precautions.

- Inspect patient's skin bid for evidence of irritation. Teach coherent patient to perform self-inspection, and provide a mirror for inspecting posterior aspects of the body. The skin should be kept soft and pliable with emollient lotion.

- Teach patient to inspect placement of limbs with altered sensation to ensure that they are in a safe and supported position and to avoid placing ankles directly on top of each other. Pad the wheelchair seat, and teach patient to change position q15-30min by lifting self and shifting position side to side and forward to backward. Encourage frequent turning while in bed and, if tolerated and not contraindicated, periodic movement into the prone position. Have patient lift, not drag, self during transfers to prevent shearing damage.

- Give injections in muscles with tone, for better absorption and less risk of sterile abscess formation. Avoid injecting ≥1 ml into a flaccid muscle.

**Impaired corneal tissue integrity** related to irritation secondary to diminished blink reflex or inability to close the eyes

*Desired outcome:*   Patient's corneas remain clear and intact.

- Normally, blinking occurs every 5-6 sec. If patient has a diminished blink reflex and/or is stuporous or comatose, assess the eyes for irritation or the presence of foreign objects. Instill prescribed eye drops or ointment to prevent corneal irritation. Instruct coherent patients to make a conscious effort to blink the eyes several times a minute to help prevent corneal irritation. Indicators of corneal irritation include red, itchy, scratchy, or painful eye; sensation of foreign object in eye; scleral edema; blurred vision; or mucus discharge. Apply eye patches or warm, sterile compresses over closed eyes for relief.

- For patient who is unable to close the eyes completely, use caution in applying an eye shield or taping the eyes shut. Semiconscious patients may open eyes underneath and injure their corneas. Also consider use of moisture chambers (plastic eye bubble), protective glasses, soft contacts, or humidifiers.

- Teach patient to avoid exposing eyes to irritants such as talc or baby powder, wind, cold air, smoke, dust, sand, or bright sunlight. Instruct patient not to rub eyes; restrain patients who may be incoherent.

**Altered nutrition:**   Less than body requirements, related to inability to ingest food secondary to chewing and swallowing deficits, fatigue, weakness, paresis, paralysis, visual neglect, or decreased LOC

*Desired outcome:*   Patient experiences adequate nutrition as evidenced by maintenance of or return to baseline body weight by hospital discharge.

- Assess patient's alertness, ability to cough, and swallow and gag reflexes before all meals. Keep suction equipment at the bedside if indicated.

- Assess patient for type of diet that can be eaten safely. Request soft, semisolid, or chopped foods as indicated. Although a pureed diet may be needed eventually, this type of food can be unappealing to many people and may have a negative impact on patient's self-concept.

- To help patient focus on eating, reduce other stimuli in the room (e.g., turn off the TV or radio). Minimize conversation and other disruptions such as phone calls.

- Provide analgesics, if appropriate, before meals so that patient is comfortable and can concentrate on eating.

- Evaluate patient's food preferences and offer small, frequent servings of nutritious food. Encourage significant others to bring in patient's favorite foods if they are not contraindicated. Plan mealtimes for times when the patient is rested; use a warming tray or microwave oven to keep the food warm and appetizing until the patient is able to eat.

- Provide oral care before feeding to enhance the patient's ability to taste. Clean and insert dentures before each meal.

- Encourage liquid nutritional supplements, and try different methods to make them more palatable (e.g., making a milkshake, serving it over ice, or diluting with carbonated beverages).

- Cut up foods, unwrap silverware, and otherwise "set up" the food tray so that patients with a weak or paralyzed arm can manage the tray one-handed.
- For patient with visual neglect, place food within patient's unaffected visual field and return during the meal to make sure she or he has eaten from both sides of the plate. Turn the plate around so that any remaining food is in patient's visual field.
- Feed or assist very weak or paralyzed patients. If not contraindicated, position patient in a chair or elevate HOB as high as possible. Ensure that patient's head is flexed slightly forward to close the airway. Begin with small amounts of food. Do not hurry patient. Be sure that each bite is completely swallowed before giving another.
- If appropriate, provide assistive devices, such as built-up utensil handles, broad-handled spoons, spill-proof cups, rocker knife for cutting, wrist or hand splints with clamps to hold utensils, stabilized plates, sectionalized plates, and other devices that promote self-feeding and independence. Encourage eating of finger foods to promote independence and oral intake.
- Provide materials for oral hygiene after meals to minimize risk of aspiration of food particles. Good oral hygiene will also help maintain integrity of the mucous membranes to minimize risk of stomatitis, which may prevent adequate oral intake. Provide oral care for patients unable to do so for themselves.
- Document your assessment of the patient's appetite. Weigh patient regularly (at least weekly) to assess for loss or gain. If indicated, notify physician of the potential need for high-protein or high-calorie supplements. Obtain dietitian consultation. Patients unable to obtain adequate nutrition by eating may need enteral or parenteral nutrition. For additional information, see "Providing Nutritional Support," p. 665.
- For the weak, debilitated, or partially paralyzed patient, assess support systems, such as family or friends, who can assist patient with meals. Consider referral to an organization that will deliver a daily meal to patient's home.
- If appropriate for patient's diagnosis (e.g., multiple sclerosis [MS]) consider referral to a speech pathologist for exercises that enhance the ability to swallow.
- For patients with visual problems, assess their ability to see their food. Identify utensils and food and describe their location. Arrange foods in an established pattern to promote independence.
- For patients with chewing or swallowing difficulties, see interventions with **Impaired swallowing**, p. 308.

**High risk for aspiration** related to facial and throat muscle weakness, depressed gag or cough reflex, impaired swallowing, or decreased LOC

***Desired outcome:*** Patient is normovolemic as evidenced by balanced I&O, stable weight, good skin turgor, moist mucous membranes, BP within patient's normal range, HR ≤100 bpm, normothermia, and urinary output ≥30 ml/h.

- Assess patient's gag reflex, alertness, and ability to cough and swallow, before offering fluids. Keep suction equipment at the bedside if indicated.
- Monitor I&O to assess for fluid volume imbalance. Involve patient or significant others with the keeping of fluid intake records. Ensure that weight is measured daily if patient is at risk for sudden fluid shifts or imbalances. Patients with neurologic deficits may have great difficulty attaining adequate intake of fluids. Alert physician to a significant I&O imbalance, which may signal the need for enteral or IV therapy to prevent dehydration.
- Assess for and teach patient and significant others the indicators of dehydration, including thirst, poor skin turgor, decreased BP, increased pulse rate, dry skin and mucous membranes, increased body temperature, concentrated urine, and decreased urinary output. Advise them that conditions such as

fever or diarrhea increase fluid loss and place the patient at increased risk of dehydration.

- Evaluate patient's fluid type and temperature preferences, and offer fluids q1-2h. For nonrestricted patients, encourage a fluid intake of at least 2-3 L/day.

- Feed or assist very weak or paralyzed patients. If not contraindicated, assist patient into high-Fowler's position to facilitate oral fluid intake. Instruct patient to flex the head slightly forward, which closes the airway and helps prevent aspiration. Begin with small amounts of liquid. Instruct patient to sip rather than gulp fluids. Do not hurry patient.

- Provide periods of rest to prevent fatigue, which can contribute to decreased oral intake. Provide oral care as needed to enhance taste perception and prevent stomatitis, which may decrease oral intake.

- If appropriate, provide assistive devices such as spill-proof cups or straws, which promote independence. Teach patient with hemiparalysis or paresis to tilt the head toward the unaffected side to facilitate intake. The individual who is paralyzed (e.g., with spinal cord injury [SCI]) may be able to drink independently *via* an extra-long tubing/straw connected to a water pitcher.

- For patients at risk for IICP, maintain fluid restrictions.

- For patients with chewing or swallowing difficulties, see interventions with **Impaired swallowing**, p. 308.

**High risk for aspiration** related to facial and throat muscle weakness, depressed gag or cough reflex, impaired swallowing, or decreased LOC
*Desired outcomes:*  Patient is free of the signs of aspiration as evidenced by RR 12-20 breaths/min with normal depth and pattern (eupnea), normal color, normal breath sounds, normothermia, and absence of adventitious breath sounds. Following instruction and ongoing, patient or significant others relate measures that prevent aspiration.

- Monitor patient for the presence of dyspnea, pallor, restlessness, diaphoresis, and a change in the rate or depth of respirations. Auscultate lung fields for breath sounds. Note the presence of crackles (rales), rhonchi, or wheezes, and diminished breath sounds. Assess effectiveness of patient's cough and the quality, amount, and color of the sputum. Measure body temperature q4h. Often, a low-grade fever (100° F or less) is indicative of the need for aggressive pulmonary hygiene.

- Teach patient to deep-breathe and cough, and assist with repositioning at least q2h. If it is not contraindicated, maintain patient in a side-lying position with HOB elevated. **Caution:** Instruct patients at risk of IICP not to cough, because it increases intraabdominal and intrathoracic pressure, which in turn increase ICP. Explain that if sneezing is unavoidable, it should be done with an open mouth to minimize the increase in ICP.

- Assess swallow and gag reflexes. If poor or absent, withhold oral fluids and foods, and inform physician of the possible need for IV therapy or enteral or parenteral nutrition. Maintain adequate hydration to keep secretions thin.

- Keep HOB elevated after meals or assist patient into a right side-lying position to minimize the potential for regurgitation and aspiration. Provide oral hygiene after meals to prevent aspiration of food particles.

- For patients not at risk for IICP, assist with prescribed postural drainage, chest physiotherapy, and IPPB. Provide incentive spirometry as indicated.

- Keep $O_2$ and suction apparatus available as indicated. Assess patient frequently for the presence of obstructive material or secretions in the throat or mouth, and suction as needed. Anticipate the need for an artificial airway if secretions cannot be cleared. Teach significant others the Heimlich maneuver.

**Self-care deficit** related to spasticity, tremors, weakness, paresis, paralysis, or decreasing LOC secondary to sensorimotor deficits
*Desired outcome:*  At a minimum of 24 h before hospital discharge, patient performs care activities independently and demonstrates the ability to use adap-

tive devices for successful completion of ADL. (Totally dependent patients express satisfaction with activities that are completed for them.)

- Assess patient's ability to perform ADL.
- As appropriate, demonstrate use of adaptive devices, such as long- or broad-handled combs, brushes, and eating utensils, nonspill cups, and stabilized plates, all of which may assist the patient in maintaining independent care. For self-care interventions for oral hygiene, see this nursing diagnosis in "Stomatitis," p. 381.
- Set short-range, realistic goals with patient to decrease frustration and improve learning. Acknowledge progress, and encourage continued effort and involvement (e.g., in selection of meals, clothing).
- Provide care to the totally dependent patient, and assist those who are not totally dependent according to degree of disability. Encourage patient to perform self-care to the maximum ability as defined by the patient. Encourage autonomy. Allow sufficient time for patient to perform the task; do not hurry the patient. Involve significant others with care activity if they are comfortable with doing so. Ask for patient's input in planning schedules. Supervise activity until patient can safely perform the task without help.
- Provide privacy and a nondistracting environment. Place patient's belongings within reach. Set out items needed to complete self-care tasks in the order they are to be used. Apply any needed adaptive devices such as hand splints.
- Encourage patient to wear any prescribed corrective eye lenses or hearing aids.
- Provide analgesics to relieve pain, which can hinder self-care activity.
- Provide a rest period before self-care activity, or plan activity for a time when patient is rested, because fatigue will alter self-care ability.
- To facilitate dressing and undressing, encourage patient or significant others to buy shoes without laces, long-handled shoe horns, loose-fitting clothing, wide-legged pants, and clothing with front fasteners, zipper pulls, or Velcro closures. Lay out clothing in the order it will be put on.
- Place a stool in the shower if sitting down will enhance self-care with bathing. Bathrooms should have nonslip mats and grab bars for safety. Hand-held shower spray, long-handled bath sponge, or a washer mitt with a pocket that holds soap may promote autonomy.
- Provide a commode chair or elevated toilet seat or urinal if it will facilitate self-care with elimination. Teach self-transfer techniques that will enable patient to get to the commode or toilet. Keep the call light within patient's reach. Instruct patient to call as early as possible so that the staff will have time to respond and the patient will not have to rush because of urgency. Offer toileting reminders q2h, after meals, and before bed time.
- Some persons may have difficulty with perineal care after elimination. For many patients with limited hand or arm mobility, a long-handled reacher that can hold tissues or wash cloth may help patient maintain independence with perineal care.
- For patient with hemiparesis or hemiparalysis, teach use of the stronger or unaffected hand and arm for dressing, eating, bathing, and grooming. Instruct patient to dress the weaker side first.
- For patients with visual field deficit, avoid placing items on their blind side. Encourage these persons to scan their environment for needed items by turning their heads.
- Obtain a referral by occupational therapist (OT) if indicated to determine the best method for performing activity.
- Individuals with cognitive defects need simple visual or verbal cues, increased gesture use, demonstration, reminders of the next step, and gentle repetition. Provide a consistent caregiver and ADL routine.
- If indicated, teach patient self-catheterization, or teach the technique to the caregiver. At-home intermittent catheterization usually is done with clean,

not sterile, technique and equipment. The catheter is washed after use in warm, soapy water, rinsed, and place in a clean plastic sack. Crusted catheters are soaked in a solution of half-distilled vinegar and half water. Teach patient to monitor and notify health professional of cloudy, foul-smelling, or bloody urine; urine with sediment; chills or fever; pain in the lower back or abdomen; or a red or swollen urethral meatus.

- Discuss, as appropriate, changing the home environment to improve ADL and independence (e.g., with extended sinks, lower closet hooks, wheelchair-accessible shower, modified telephones, lowered mirrors, and lever door handles that operate with reduced hand pressure).
- Listen and provide opportunities for patient to express self, and communicate that it is normal to have negative feelings about changes in autonomy. Discuss with the health-care team ways to provide consistent and positive encouragement and strategies that increase independence progressively.

**Impaired verbal communication** related to facial/throat muscle weakness, intubation, or tracheostomy

*Desired outcome:*  Following intervention and ongoing, patient communicates effectively, either verbally or nonverbally, and relates decreasing frustration with communication.

- Assess patient's ability to speak, read, write, and comprehend.
- If appropriate, obtain referral to a speech therapist or pathologist to assist patient in strengthening muscles used in speech. Encourage patient to perform exercises that increase the ability to control the facial muscles and tongue. These exercises may include holding a sound for 5 sec, singing the scale, reading aloud, and extending the tongue and trying to touch the chin, nose, or cheek.
- Provide a supportive and relaxed environment for those patients who are unable to form words or sentences or who are unable to speak clearly or appropriately. Acknowledge patient's frustration over the inability to communicate, and explain that patience is needed for both the patient and caregiver. Maintain a calm, positive, reassuring attitude. Continue to speak to the patient using normal volume unless the patient's hearing is impaired. Maintain eye contact to promote focus. Provide enough time for the patient to articulate. Ask patient to repeat unclear words. Observe for nonverbal cues; watch patient's lips closely. Do not interrupt or finish sentences. Anticipate needs and phrase questions to allow simple answers, such as "yes" or "no." Provide continuity of care to decrease patient's frustration.
- Provide alternative methods of communication if patient is unable to speak (e.g., a language board, alphabet cards, flash cards, or pad and pencil). Other alternatives are systems that use eyeblinks or hand squeezes, bell signal taps, or gestures, such as hand signals, head nods, pantomine, or pointing. Use communication board for urgent situations. Document method of communication used.
- If patient's voice is weak and difficult to hear, reduce environmental noise to enhance listener's ability to hear words. Suggest that patient take a deep breath before speaking; provide a voice amplifier if appropriate for patient. Encourage patients to organize thoughts and plan what they will say before speaking. Encourage patients to express ideas in short, simple phrases or sentences. Remind patient to speak slowly, exaggerate pronunciation, and use facial expressions.
- If patient has swallowing difficulties that result in the accumulation of saliva, suction the mouth to promote clearer speech.
- For a patient with muscle rigidity or spasm, massage the facial and neck muscles before he or she attempts to communicate.
- If patient has a tracheostomy, ensure that a tap bell is within reach. Reassure patients with a temporary tracheostomy that they will regain the ability to speak. For patients with permanent tracheostomy, discuss learning alternate communication systems, such as sign language or esophageal speech.

Fenestrated tubes or covering the tracheostomy tube opening with a finger will enable speech.

- Establish a method of calling for assistance, and ensure that the patient knows how to use it. Keep the calling device where the patient can activate it (e.g., place call bell on unparalyzed side). Depending on the deficit, use a tap bell for weak patients, a pillow pad call light (triggered by arm or head movement), or a sip and puff device (triggered by mouth).
- For patients with the ability to write, encourage them to keep a diary or write letters as a means of ventilating feelings and expressing concerns. If patient has a weak writing arm, evaluate for the need of a splint that will enable patient to hold a pen or pencil. Felt-tip markers also are useful because they require minimal pressure for writing.

**Constipation** related to inability to chew and swallow a high-roughage diet, side effects of medications, immobility, and spinal cord involvement

*Desired outcome:* Within 2-3 days of intervention, patient passes soft, formed stools and maintains his or her normal bowel pattern.

- Although a high-roughage diet is ideal for the patient who is immobilized or on prolonged bed rest, the individual with chewing and swallowing difficulties may be unable to consume such a diet. For these patients, consuming a serving or two of cooked fruit or cooked bran cereal each day may be effective. Otherwise encourage use of natural fiber laxatives such as psyllium (e.g., Metamucil).
- A bowel elimination program may include the following elements: setting a regular time of day for attempting a bowel movement, preferably 30 min after eating a meal or drinking a hot beverage; using a commode instead of a bed pan for easier elimination; using a medicated suppository 15-30 min before a scheduled attempt; bearing down by contracting the abdominal muscles or applying manual pressure to the abdomen to help increase intraabdominal pressure; and drinking 4 oz of prune juice nightly. Abdominal and pelvic exercise also may be included in patient's morning and evening routine. Keep a call bell within patient's reach. Assess patient's sitting balance to ensure safety while up on commode. **Caution:** SCI patients with involvement at T-8 and above should use *extreme* caution if use of an enema or suppository is unavoidable, because either can precipitate life-threatening autonomic dysreflexia (AD). Liberal application of anesthetic jelly into the rectum should precede their use. In addition, instruct patient at risk of IICP not to bear down with bowel movements, because this action can cause increased intraabdominal pressure, which in turn increases ICP.
- If indicated by patient's diagnosis (e.g., MS), provide instructions for digital stimulation of the anus to promote reflex bowel evacuation. **Caution:** This intervention is contraindicated for SCI patients with involvement at T-8 or above because it can precipitate life-threatening AD.
- For other interventions, see **Constipation,** p. 716, in Appendix One, "Caring for Patients on Prolonged Bed Rest."

**Altered cerebral tissue perfusion** related to altered blood flow with risk of IICP and herniation secondary to positional factors, increased intrathoracic or intraabdominal pressure, fluid volume excess, hyperthermia, or discomfort

*Desired outcome:* Patient is free of symptoms of IICP and herniation as evidenced by stable or improving Glasgow Coma Scale score; stable or improving sensorimotor functioning; BP within patient's normal range; HR 60-100 bpm; pulse pressure 30-40 mm Hg (the difference between the systolic and diastolic BPs); orientation to person, place, and time; normal vision; bilaterally equal and normoreactive pupils; RR 12-20 breaths/min with normal depth and pattern (eupnea); normal gag, corneal, and swallowing reflexes; and absence of headache, nausea, nuchal rigidity, posturing, and seizure activity.

---

**Note:** ICP is the pressure exerted by brain tissue, CSF, and cerebral blood volume within the rigid, unyielding skull. An increase in any one of these components without a corresponding decrease in another will increase ICP. Normal ICP is 0-15 mm Hg; IICP is >15 mm Hg. Cerebral perfusion pressure (CPP) is the difference between systemic arterial pressure and ICP. As ICP rises, CPP may decrease. Normal CPP is 80-100 mm Hg. If CPP falls below 60, irreversible ischemia occurs. When CPP falls to 0, cerebral blood flow ceases. Cerebral edema and IICP usually peak 2-3 days after an injury and then decrease over 1-2 weeks.

- Monitor for and report any of the following indicators of IICP or impending/occurring herniation:
  - *Early indicators of IICP:* Declining Glasgow Coma Scale score, alterations in LOC ranging from irritability, restlessness, and confusion to lethargy; possible onset of or worsening of headache; beginning pupillary dysfunction, such as sluggishness; visual disturbances, such as diplopia or blurred vision; onset of or increase in sensorimotor changes or deficits, such as weakness; onset of or worsening of nausea. **Note:** The single most important indicator of early IICP is a change in LOC.
  - *Late indicators of IICP* (generally related to brain stem compression and disruption of cranial nerves and vital centers): Continuing decline in Glasgow Coma Scale score; continued deterioration in LOC leading to stupor and coma; projectile vomiting; hemiplegia; posturing; widening pulse pressure, decreased HR, and increased systolic BP; Cheyne-Stokes breathing or other respiratory irregularity; pupillary changes, such as inequality, dilatation, and nonreactivity to light; papilledema; and impaired brain stem reflexes (corneal, gag, swallowing).
  - *Brain herniation:* Deep coma, fixed and dilated pupils (first unilateral and then bilateral), posturing progressing to bilateral flaccidity, lost brain stem reflexes, and continuing deterioration in VS and respirations.
- If changes occur, prepare for possible transfer of patient to ICU. Insertion of ICP sensors for continuous ICP monitoring, CSF ventricular drainage, intubation, mechanical ventilation, neuromuscular blocking, or barbiturate coma therapy may be necessary.
- For patients at risk for IICP, prevention of hypoxia and $CO_2$ retention is essential for preventing vasodilatation of cerebral arteries. Preventive measures include ensuring a patent airway, delivering $O_2$ as prescribed, hyperventilating ("sighing" or bagging) patient before suctioning, and limiting suction to 10-15 sec. Reduce $Paco_2$ *via* hyperventilation by instructing conscious patients to take deep breaths on their own or by providing manual or machine hyperventilation when patient is intubated or has a tracheostomy. Monitor patient's ABG or pulse oximetry values.
- Promote venous blood return to the heart to reduce cerebral congestion by keeping HOB elevated at 15-30 degrees (unless otherwise directed); maintaining head-and-neck alignment to avoid hyperextension, flexion, or rotation; ensuring that tracheostomy and endotracheostomy ties or $O_2$ tubing do not compress the jugular vein; and avoiding Trendelenburg position for any reason. Ensure that pillows under the patient's head are flat so that the head is in a neutral rather than flexed position.
- Take precautions against increased intraabdominal and intrathoracic pressure in the following ways: Teach patient to exhale when turning. Provide passive ROM exercises rather than allow active or assistive exercises. Administer prescribed stool softeners or laxatives to prevent straining at stool; avoid enemas and suppositories because they can cause straining. Instruct patient not to move self in bed, because it requires a pushing movement; allow only passive turning; use a pull sheet. Instruct patient to avoid pushing or pulling against side rails or footboard. Avoid footboards; use high-top tennis shoes instead. Assist patient with sitting up and turning. Instruct patient to avoid coughing and sneezing or, if unavoidable, to do so with an open mouth; provide antitussive for cough as prescribed and antiemetic for vomiting. In-

struct patient to avoid hip flexion (increases intraabdominal pressure). Do not place patient in a prone position, and avoid using restraints (straining against them increases ICP). Rather than have patient perform Valsalva's maneuver to prevent an air embolism during insertion of a central venous catheter, physician should use a syringe to aspirate air from the catheter lumen.

- Help reduce cerebral congestion by enforcing fluid limitations as prescribed, typically to <1,500 ml/day. Administer IV fluids with a control device to prevent fluid overload. Keep accurate I&O records. When administering additional IV fluids (e.g., IV drugs) avoid using $D_5W$ because its hypotonicity can increase cerebral edema.

- Because fever increases metabolic requirements (10% for each 1° C) and aggravates hypoxia, help maintain patient's body temperature within normal limits by giving prescribed antipyretics, regulating temperature of the environment, limiting use of blankets, keeping patient's trunk warm to prevent shivering, and administering tepid sponge baths or hypothermia blanket to reduce fever. When using a hypothermia blanket, wrapping the patient's extremities in a blanket may prevent shivering. If prescribed, administer chlorpromazine to prevent shivering, which would increase ICP.

- Administer prescribed osmotic and loop diuretics to reduce cerebral edema and produce a state of dehydration. Administer glucocorticosteroids to reduce edema and inflammation. Administer BP medications as prescribed to keep BP within prescribed limits that will promote optimal cerebral blood flow without increasing cerebral edema. Because pain can increase BP and consequently increase ICP, administer prescribed analgesics promptly and as necessary. Barbiturates and narcotics are usually contraindicated because of the potential for masking the signs of IICP and causing respiratory depression.

- Administer antiepilepsy drugs as prescribed to prevent or control seizures, which would increase cerebral metabolism, hypoxia, and $CO_2$ retention, thereby increasing cerebral edema and ICP.

- Monitor bladder drainage tubes for obstruction or kinks because a distended bladder can increase ICP.

- Provide a quiet and soothing environment. Control noise and other environmental stimuli. Speak softly, use a gentle touch, and avoid jarring the bed. Try to limit painful procedures; avoid tension on tubes (e.g., urinary catheter); and consider limiting pain-stimulation testing. Avoid unnecessary touch (e.g., leave BP cuff in place for frequent VS); and talk softly, explaining procedures before touching in order to avoid startling patient. Try to avoid situations in which the patient may become emotionally upset. Do not say anything in the presence of the patient that you would not say if he or she were awake. Family discussions should take place outside the room. Limit visitors as necessary. Encourage significant others to speak quietly to patient because hearing a familiar voice may promote relaxation and decrease ICP. Listening to soft favorite music with earphones also may decrease ICP.

- Because multiple procedures and nursing care activities can increase ICP by increasing discomfort and anxiety, individualize care to ensure rest periods and optimal spacing of activities. Rousing patients from sleep has been shown to increase ICP. Plan activities and treatments accordingly so that patient can sleep undisturbed as often as possible.

**Sensory/perceptual alterations** (visual) related to diplopia
***Desired outcome:*** Following intervention, patient verbalizes that his or her vision has improved.

- Assess patient for the presence of diplopia.

- If patient has diplopia, provide an eye patch or eyeglasses with a frosted lens, which is a temporary means of eliminating this condition. Alternate the eye patch q4h.

- Orient the patient to his or her environment as needed.

- Advise patient of the availability of "talking books" (tapes) and large-type reading materials.
- Place a sign over patient's bed that indicates patient's visual impairment.
- Teach patient that depth perception will be altered and to use visual cues and scanning.

**Pain** related to spasms, headache, and photophobia secondary to neurologic dysfunction

*Desired outcomes:*   Within 1 h of intervention, patient's subjective perception of discomfort decreases, as documented by a pain scale. Objective indicators, such as grimacing, are absent or diminished.

- Assess characteristics (e.g., quality, severity, location, onset, duration, precipitating factors) of patient's pain or spasms. Devise a pain scale with patient, and document discomfort on a scale of 0 (no pain) to 10 (worst pain).
- Respond immediately to patient's complaints of pain. Administer analgesics and antispasmodics as prescribed. Consider scheduling doses of analgesia. Document effectiveness of the medication, using the pain scale. Monitor for untoward effects. Consult with physician if dose or interval change seems necessary. Teach patient and significant others about the importance of timing the pain medication so that it is taken before the pain becomes too severe and before major moves.
- Teach patient about the relationship between anxiety and pain, as well as other factors that enhance pain and spasms (e.g., staying in one position for too long, fatigue, and chilling).
- Instruct patient and significant others in the use of nonpharmacologic pain management techniques, such as repositioning; ROM; supporting painful extremity or part; back rubs, massage, warm baths, and other tactile distraction; auditory distraction such as listening to soothing music; visual distraction such as television; heat applications such as warm blankets or moist compresses; cold applications such as ice massage; guided imagery; breathing exercises; relaxation tapes and techniques; biofeedback; and a transcutaneous electrical nerve stimulation (TENS) device, as appropriate. See **Health-seeking behaviors:** Relaxation technique effective for stress reduction, p. 54.
- Encourage rest periods to facilitate sleep and relaxation. Fatigue tends to exacerbate the pain experience. Pain may result in fatigue, which in turn may cause exaggerated pain and further exhaustion. Try to provide uninterrupted sleep time at night.
- If patient has photophobia, provide a quiet and dark environment. Close the door and curtains; avoid artificial lights whenever possible.
- Pain in the SCI patient often is poorly localized and may be referred. Intrascapular area pain may be from the stomach, duodenum, or gall bladder. Umbilical pain may be from the appendix. Testicular or inner thigh pain may be from the kidneys (e.g., pyelonephritis). Evaluate patient for signs of infection or inflammatory process (e.g., tachycardia, restlessness, urinary incontinence when it was previously controlled, fever).
- If patient's present complaint of pain varies significantly from previous pain or if interventions are ineffective, notify physician.

**Impaired swallowing** related to decreased or absent gag reflex, decreased strength or excursion of muscles involved in mastication, perceptual impairment, or facial paralysis

*Desired outcome:*   Before oral foods and fluids are reintroduced, patient exhibits ability to swallow safely.

- Assess patient for factors that affect the ability to swallow safely, including LOC, gag and cough reflexes, and strength and symmetry of tongue, lip, and facial muscles. Monitor for signs of impaired swallowing, including regurgitation of food and fluid through the nares, drooling, food oozing from the lips, and food trapped in buccal spaces. The development of a weak or hoarse voice during or after eating may signal the potential for impaired swal-

lowing. Check the swallow reflex by first asking patient to swallow his or
her own saliva. If the larynx elevates with the attempt, a sign that the swallow reflex is intact, next ask the patient to swallow 3-5 ml plain water. Document your findings.

---

**Caution:**   The presence of the cough reflex is essential for the patient to relearn swallowing safely.

---

- Obtain a referral to a speech therapist for patients with a swallowing dysfunction. The act of swallowing is complex, and interventions vary according to the phase of swallowing that is dysfunctional. Video fluoroscopy may
  be used to evaluate swallowing. Encourage patient to practice any prescribed
  exercises (e.g., tongue and jaw ROM).
- Enteral or parenteral nutrition may be necessary for the patient who cannot
  chew or swallow effectively or safely. Alert physician to your findings. Be
  aware that an NG tube may desensitize the patient and impair the reflexive
  response to food bolus stimulus, thereby hindering the ability to relearn to
  swallow.
- Keep suction equipment and a manual resuscitation bag with face mask at
  patient's bedside. Suction secretions in the patient's mouth as necessary.
- Ensure that the patient is alert and responsive to verbal stimuli before attempting to swallow. Patients who are drowsy, inattentive, or fatigued have
  difficulty cooperating and are at risk of aspirating. To help minimize fatigue,
  provide a rest period before meals or swallowing attempts.
- Initial swallowing attempts should be made with plain water (see above) because of the risk of aspiration. Progressively add easy-to-swallow food and
  liquids as the patient's ability to swallow improves. Determine which foods
  and liquids are easiest for the patient to swallow. Generally, semisolid foods
  of medium consistency, such as puddings, hot cereals, and casseroles, tend
  to be easiest to swallow. Thicker liquids, such as nectars, tend to be better
  tolerated than thin liquids. Gravy or sauce added to dry foods often facilitates swallowing. Sticky, mucus-producing foods, such as peanut butter,
  chocolate, or milk, are often restricted or limited.
- To help the patient focus on swallowing, reduce stimuli in the room (e.g.,
  turn off the television, lower the radio volume, minimize conversation, and
  limit disruptions from phone calls). Caution patient not to talk while eating.
- Most patients will swallow best when in an upright position. Sitting in a
  straight-backed chair with feet on the floor is ideal. If the patient must remain in bed, use high-Fowler's position if possible. Support the shoulders
  and neck with pillows. Ensure that the head is erect and flexed forward
  slightly, with the chin at the midline and pointing toward the chest to promote movement of the food and fluid into the esophagus and minimize the
  risk that it will go into the airway. Stroking the neck lightly may help some
  patients swallow. Maintain patient in an upright position for at least 30-60
  min after eating to prevent regurgitation and aspiration.
- Teach patient to break down the act of chewing and swallowing. Encourage
  concentration and taking adequate time. Talk patient through the following
  steps:
  - Take small bites or sips.
  - Place food on the tongue.
  - Use the tongue to transfer food so that it is directly under the teeth on the
    unaffected side of the mouth.
  - Chew the food thoroughly.
  - Move the food to the middle of the tongue and hold it there.
  - Flex the neck and tuck the chin against the chest.
  - Hold the breath and think about swallowing.
  - Without breathing, raise the tongue to the roof of the mouth and swallow.
  - Swallow several times if necessary.

- When the mouth is empty, raise the chin, and clear the throat or cough purposefully once or twice.
- Start with small amounts of food or liquid. Feed slowly. Ensure that each previous bite has been swallowed. Check the mouth for pockets of food. After every few bites of solid food, provide a liquid to help clear the mouth. Avoid using a syringe because the force of the fluid, if sprayed, may cause aspiration.
- Teach patient who has food pockets in the buccal spaces to periodically sweep the mouth with the tongue or finger or clean these areas with a napkin.
- For patients who have a weak or paralyzed side, teach them to place food on the side of the face they can control. Tilting the head toward the stronger side will allow gravity to help keep the food or liquid on the side of the mouth they can manipulate. Some patients may find that rotating the head to the weak side will close the damaged side of the pharynx and facilitate more effective swallowing.
- Patients with loss of oral sensation may be unable to identify foods or fluids of tepid temperature by their tongue or oral mucosa, potentially resulting in tissue injury. Serve only warm or cool foods to these individuals. Verbal cues and use of a mirror may help ensure that these patients keep their mouths clear after swallowing.
- Patients with a rigid tongue (e.g., with Parkinsonism) have difficulty getting the tongue to move the bolus of food into the pharynx for swallowing. Encourage repeated swallowing attempts to facilitate movement of the food. Evaluate patient's swallowing ability at different times of the day. Reschedule mealtimes to times of the day when patient has improved swallowing, or, as appropriate, discuss with physician the possibility of changing the dose schedule of the patient's anti-Parkinson medication.
- If decreased salivation is contributing to the patient's swallowing difficulties, perform one of the following before feeding to stimulate salivation: swab the patient's mouth with a lemon-glycerin sponge; have the patient suck on a tart-flavored hard candy, dill pickle, or lemon slice; teach the patient to move the tongue in a circular motion against the inside of the cheek; or use artificial saliva. Moisten food with melted butter, broth or other soup, or gravy. Dip dry foods such as toast into coffee or other liquid to soften them. Rinse the patient's mouth as needed to remove particles and lubricate the mouth. Investigate medications the patient is taking for the potential side effect of decreased salivation.
- Tablets or capsules may be swallowed more easily when added to foods such as puddings or ice cream. Crushed tablets or opened capsules also mix easily into these types of foods. However, check with the pharmacist to ensure that crushing a tablet or opening a capsule does not adversely affect its absorption or duration.
- Teach significant others the Heimlich or abdominal thrust maneuver so that they can intervene in the event of choking.

**Altered body temperature** related to illness or trauma affecting temperature regulation and inability or decreased ability to perspire, shiver, or vasoconstrict

***Desired outcome:***  Following the intervention(s), patient is normothermic with core temperatures between 36.50° C and 37.78° C (97.8° F and 100° F).

---

**Note:**  Infection and hypothalamic dysfunction due to cerebral insult (trauma, edema) are two common causes of hyperthermia. The rapid development of spinal lesions (e.g., in SCI) breaks the connection between the hypothalamus and the sympathetic nervous system (SNS), causing an inability to adapt to environmental temperature. In spinal cord shock, temperatures tend to lower toward the ambient temperature. Inability to vasoconstrict and shiver makes heat conservation difficult; the inability to perspire prevents normal cooling.

---

- Monitor rectal, tympanic, or bladder core temperature q4h or, if patient is in spinal shock, q2h. Observe for signs of hypothermia: impaired ability to think, disorientation, confusion, drowsiness, apathy, and reduced HR and RR. Monitor for complaints of being too cold, goose bumps, and cool skin (in SCI patients, above the level of injury). Observe for signs of hyperthermia: flushed face, malaise, rash, respiratory distress, tachycardia, weakness, headache, and irritability. Monitor for complaints of being too warm, sweating, or hot and dry skin (in SCI patients, above the level of injury). Observe for signs of dehydration: parched mouth, furrowed tongue, dry lips, poor skin turgor, decreased urine output, and weak and fast pulse.
- *For hyperthermia:* Maintain a cool room temperature (20° C [68° F]). Provide a fan or air-conditioning to prevent overheating. Remove excess bedding, and cover patient with a thin sheet. Give tepid sponge baths. Place cool wet cloths at patient's head, neck, axilla, and groin. Administer antipyretic agent as prescribed. Use a padded hypothermia blanket. Provide cool drinks. Evaluate for potential infectious cause.
- *For hypothermia:* Increase environmental temperature. Protect patient from drafts. Provide warm drinks. Provide extra blankets. Provide warming (hyperthermia) blanket.
- Keep feverish patient dry. Change bed linens after diaphoresis. Provide careful skin care when patient is on a hypo- or hyperthermia blanket. Maintain adequate hydration. Consider insensible water loss from fever, which may affect total hydration, when measuring I&O. Increase caloric intake because of increased metabolic needs. Remember that steroids may mask fever or infection.

**Knowledge deficit:**   Neurologic diagnostic tests (EEG, positron emission tomography [PET], MRI, CT scan, lumbar puncture (LP), myelography, digital subtraction angiography [DSA], cerebral angiography, oculoplethysmography, EMG, nerve conduction velocity [NCV], and evoked potentials [EP])

*Desired outcome:*   Following explanation and before the procedure, patient verbalizes understanding about the prescribed diagnostic test, including purpose, risks, anticipated benefits, and expectations for the patient before, during, and after the test.

- After the physician has explained the diagnostic study to the patient, reinforce or clarify information as indicated. Adjust and simplify the information to what the patient can understand and repeat several times, as appropriate to the patient's cognitive dysfunction.
- If an EEG has been prescribed, explain that this test will indicate the amount of brain activity present and may reveal abnormal patterns of electrical activity, particularly with such stimuli as flashing lights or hyperventilation. Explain that an EEG may be performed while the patient is either asleep or awake and sometimes by telemetry. Cooperation is important, and the test may take 40-60 min. Alert EEG staff to medications the patient is taking. In addition, discuss the following as appropriate.
  - *Before the test:* Antiepilepsy medications, sedatives, and tranquilizers may be withheld 24-48 h before the test. The patient's hair should be thoroughly washed and dried, but sprays, creams, and oils must be avoided. If a sleep EEG has been prescribed, the patient will need to stay awake the night before the test. The patient usually is allowed a normal diet the morning of the test to prevent hypoglycemia, but caffeine-containing foods (e.g., chocolate) and beverages (e.g., coffee, tea, colas) are restricted.
  - *During the test:* Small electrode patches are attached to the patient's head. Reassure patient that he or she will not receive any electric shocks. The

patient may be asked to watch flashing lights or to hyperventilate to elicit electrical activity patterns in the brain.
- *After the test:* Hairwashing or acetone swabs will be provided to remove the paste used for attaching the electrodes. Medications probably will be reinstated at this time. If needle electrodes were used, avoid washing hair for 24 h.
- If PET has been prescribed, explain that this test may locate areas of cerebral glucose metabolism that correspond to the seizure-causing focus, distinguish tumor tissue from normal tissue by identifying abnormal metabolic activity of the tumor tissue, or identify areas of ischemia or low metabolism (e.g., Alzheimer's disease). In addition, discuss the following as appropriate.
  - *Before the test:* The procedure is contraindicated for pregnancy. Alcohol, caffeine, and tobacco may be restricted for 24 h to prevent skewing of test results. Because the test is based on tissue glucose metabolism, the patient should eat a meal 3-4 h before the test. If the patient has diabetes mellitus, the physician may give special instructions about insulin administration because insulin alters glucose metabolism. Generally, the patient will be allowed to take insulin before the pretest meal.
  - *During the test:* Explain that the test takes 60-90 min and the patient is required to be still during that time. Tranquilizers are contraindicated, however, because they alter glucose metabolism.
  - *After the test:* Encourage fluids if not contraindicated.
- If MRI has been prescribed, explain that this test may reveal biochemical changes caused by hypoxia or necrosis, degenerative disease, or by a mass such as a tumor, hemorrhage, tissue shift, or hydrocephalus. This test also may show structural lesions that may be responsible for symptoms such as seizures. MRI is more useful than CT scanning in evaluating pituitary tumors, acoustic neuromas, posterior fossa tumors, spinal cord tumors and trauma, demyelinating disease, cerebral atrophy, and situations in which the patient is allergic to contrast medium. In addition, discuss the following as appropriate.
  - *Before the test:* Confirm with patients that they do not have a pacemaker, surgical aneurysm clip, prosthetic heart valve, or umbrella filter for emboli and are not pregnant. Explain that the MRI is contraindicated during pregnancy, can deactivate pacemakers, and the strong magnetic field can move ferrous metal aneurysm clips and valve and umbrella filters within the body, putting the patient at obvious risk. The presence of these internal items makes the patient ineligible for MRI. The MRI also is not used on critically ill or unstable patients, because it is impossible to monitor cardiac rhythm and VS inside the scanner. The patient must be able to cope with confined spaces and the ability to lie motionless throughout the 15-90-min test. A soft, humming sound and on-off pulses will be heard. The physician may prescribe a sedative. The patient should void before the test and remove such items as jewelry, hair clips, clothing with metal fasteners, and glasses before entering the scanner.
- If a CT scan has been prescribed, explain that the test may detect masses from tumors, hemorrhage, tissue shift, and hydrocephalus. Serial scans may be performed to determine a tumor's response to therapy and detect a resolution or increase in a hemorrhage. CT scanning is more useful than MRI in evaluating acute trauma or hemorrhage, supratentorial enhancing tumors, and hydrocephalus; in predicting vasospasm; and when the patient has a pacemaker, internal ferrous metal objects, or is uncooperative. If contrast agents are not used, there are no known complications from CT scans. If a contrast agent is used, discuss the following with the patient as indicated.
  - *Before the test:* Allergies to iodine or iodine-containing substances such as shellfish or contrast medium must be reported to the physician. Food

and fluids may be restricted 4 h before the test. Remove hair pins. The test usually lasts 15-30 min, and the patient can expect to hear a clicking noise as the machine moves. The patient must lie still, and sedation may be prescribed.

- *During the test:* A warm flushed feeling or burning sensation is normal and may be felt with administration of the dye. The patient also may experience a salty taste with dye injection, nausea, vomiting, or a headache during or after the test. The patient may be asked to take and hold several deep breaths during the scanning.
- *After the test:* If it is not contraindicated, fluids are increased to ensure elimination of the contrast dye *via* the kidneys. The patient will be monitored for hives, rash, and itching, which may be delayed allergic reactions to the dye.
- If an LP has been prescribed, explain that it is performed to remove a sample of CSF for analysis and to determine CSF pressure. Typically, the CSF is evaluated for microorganisms, blood cells, and chemical analysis. Skin or bone infection at the puncture site is a contraindication. This procedure is performed with great caution in the presence of IICP. Uncooperation, severe degenerative joint disease, and anticoagulant therapy also may preclude its use. Also discuss the following as indicated:
  - *Before the test:* Assure patient that the needle will not enter the spinal cord. Explain that the patient should empty bladder at this time.
  - *During the test:* The patient will be assisted into a side-lying position, with the chin tucked into the chest and the knees drawn up to the abdomen. This position curves the spine and widens the intervertebral space for easier insertion of the spinal needle. The patient must lie still during the procedure, and a nurse will assist patient with maintaining the position. The patient should breathe normally during the test. There may be a short burning sensation when the local anesthetic is injected and some local transient pain when the spinal needle is inserted. The patient should report any pain or sensations that continue after or differ from these expected discomforts. The patient will be monitored for discomfort, elevated HR, pallor, and clammy skin during the procedure.
  - *After the test:* The patient will remain in bed with the HOB flat or raised slightly for a prescribed period of time, usually no more than 8 h; may turn from side to side during this time period; and should drink a large amount of fluids unless contraindicated. These measures will help prevent or minimize any postprocedure headache, which is the most common adverse effect of an LP. The patient should report any headache to the nurse so that analgesia, if prescribed, can be administered. The nurse will check the LP site periodically for redness, swelling, and drainage. The nurse also will check VS and neurologic status. The patient should report any neck stiffness, pain, numbness, or weakness.
- If myelography has been prescribed, explain that it is performed when other diagnostic tests are inconclusive to delineate or rule out blockage or disruption of the spinal cord. Radiopaque dye is injected into the subarachnoid space of the spine using a lumbar or cervical puncture. Discuss the following with the patient as indicated.
  - *Before the test:* Allergies or sensitivity to iodine, shellfish, and contrast medium; history of medications that could decrease the seizure threshold (e.g., phenothiazines, tricyclics, antidepressants, amphetamines) and epilepsy medication must be reported to the radiologist. Foods and fluids are withheld for a period of time, usually 4-8 h, before the test.
  - *During the test:* The patient may feel transient burning when the contrast dye is injected and a salty taste, headache, or nausea after the injection. With oil-based dyes, the table will tilt to facilitate flow of contrast dye to different parts of the spinal canal. With water-based dyes the patient will

need to sit quietly to enable the controlled upward dispersion of the dye. The patient may feel some discomfort during the procedure due to needle insertion, positions used, and removal of contrast dye (oil-based dyes) at the end of the procedure. Explain the importance of lying quietly during the 60-min procedure.

• *After the test:* VS and neurologic status will be monitored at frequent intervals. The patient should report any increased deficit from pretest status, chills, fever, neck stiffness, and redness or swelling at the puncture site. Headache, nausea, and vomiting are frequent side effects and should be reported so that comfort measures can be taken. Nonrestricted persons should drink extra fluids to replace the CSF lost during the test. The following positions may be used:

—If an oil-based dye was used (e.g., isophendylate): Patient must remain flat 6-24 h or as prescribed.

—If a water-based dye was used (e.g., metrizamide): HOB will be elevated to 60 degrees for 8 h to minimize irritation to the cranial nerves and structures. Seizures, hallucination, depression, confusion, speech problems, chest pain, and dysrhythmias may occur if metrizamide reaches the cranial vault.

• If DSA has been prescribed, explain that it is performed to help visualize cerebral blood flow and detect vascular abnormalities such as stenosis, aneurysm, and hematoma. Patients are expected to lie still for the 30-60-min procedure and hold their breath on command. This test is considered safer than angiography. Vein injection carries no risk of embolus and can be done on an outpatient basis. Vein injection (vs. arterial injection) requires more dye and carries increased risk of kidney damage. This test consists of two scans: one scan without contrast and the other with. The two images are then digitally subtracted from one another. Also discuss the following as indicated.

• *Before the test:* Patient will be assessed for good cardiac output to disperse the dye and good kidney function to excrete the dye. Allergies to iodine, shellfish, or radiopaque dye must be reported to the physician. Food and fluids usually are withheld 3-4 h before the procedure, although clear liquids sometimes are allowed. The patient may feel transient discomfort with insertion of the needle or catheter, as well as a headache, warm sensation, or metallic taste when the dye is injected.

• *After the test:* The patient will be required to drink large amounts of fluid, if not contraindicated, to promote dye excretion by the kidneys. Nurses will check the venipuncture site for redness and swelling. If an arterial route was used for injection, see the discussion of cerebral angiography, which follows.

• If cerebral angiography has been prescribed, explain that it enables visualization of the cerebral vasculature after injection of a contrast medium and determines the site, structure, and size of an aneurysm or arteriovenous malformation, the presence of vasospasm, and the site of rupture or obstructed blood flow. It also may show an abnormal perfusion pattern, which suggests presence of a tumor. Severe kidney, liver, or thyroid disease may contraindicate this test. Also discuss the following as indicated.

• *Before the test:* Allergies to iodine, shellfish, or radiopaque dyes must be reported to the physician. Foods and fluids are withheld for 8-10 h or as prescribed. Local anesthetic is used at the puncture site. Patient will feel a warm or burning sensation when the dye is administered and have a transient headache or metallic taste sensation. The proposed site may be shaved. If the femoral approach is used, pedal pulses will be checked and their location marked. If the carotid approach is used, the patient's neck circumference will be measured, marked, and recorded. Baseline neurologic status is checked and recorded for postprocedure comparison so that small changes can be detected early. Dentures and eyeglasses usually are removed.

- *After the test:* Patient will be on strict bed rest for 6-24 h, followed by a specified period of "bathroom privileges only." Patient's VS and pulse quality will be checked frequently. Patient should notify staff if signs of reaction to the dye occur, including respiratory distress, lightheadedness (hypotension), hives, or itching. Fluids will be encouraged to eliminate dye and protect from kidney damage. The puncture site will be checked frequently for bleeding or hematoma. The patient should not be alarmed if bleeding occurs. Manual pressure will be maintained until the bleeding stops. A pressure dressing may then be applied and the physician notified. The quality of distal pulses and the temperature, color, and sensation in the extremity will be monitored at frequent intervals. Weakening pulses, pallor, coolness, or cyanosis may signal thrombus formation and artery obstruction.
- —If the femoral approach was used, patient should keep the leg straight for the prescribed amount of time (usually 6-12 h) to minimize the risk of bleeding. Patients will use a bedpan or urinal and eat on their side during this time.
- —If the brachial approach was used, the patient's arm will be immobilized for 6-12 h or as prescribed. A sign will be posted over patient's bed that cautions against measuring BP or drawing blood in this arm.
- —If the carotid artery was the puncture site, the patient should report any difficulty swallowing or breathing or any weakness or numbness. The neck will be checked for increasing circumference or tracheal displacement, which may signal hematoma formation. Changes in LOC or neurologic deficits may indicate thrombus formation and arterial obstruction.
- If oculoplethysmography has been prescribed, explain that it will help detect and evaluate carotid occlusive disease by the indirect measurement of blood flow in the ophthalmic artery, which is the first major branch of the internal carotid artery. Also discuss the following as indicated.
- *Before the test:* A history of recent eye surgery (within 6 months), retinal detachment, or lens implantation, allergic reaction to local anesthetics, and current anticoagulant surgery should be reported to the physician. Contact lenses will be removed. Patients with glaucoma may take their usual eye medication. Anesthetic drops are instilled, and the patient's eyes may burn slightly for a short time after instillation.
- *During the test:* Small eye cups that resemble contact lenses are applied to the corneas and suction applied. The patient must be able to lie very still and resist blinking because constant blinking or nystagmus may cause an artifact, making the results difficult to interpret.
- *After the test:* Patient should not rub the eyes for at least 2 h because the eyes are susceptible to corneal abrasion from the local anesthetic. Patient should report symptoms of corneal abrasion, including pain and photophobia. As the eye drops wear off, the patient probably will experience mild burning. Patient should report the presence of severe burning. Patients who wear contact lenses should leave them out for 2 h to allow the anesthetic eye drops to wear off. A darkened room and sterile normal saline may sooth irritated eyes. A conjunctival hemorrhage may occur but will fade with time.
- EMG and NCV studies usually are performed together to diagnose and differentiate between peripheral nerve and muscle disorders.
- *Before the test:* Bleeding disorders or extensive skin infection may contraindicate the test. Explain that patient cooperation will be necessary during the 20-30-min test.
- *During the test:* There will be some discomfort as small needles are in-

serted into muscle. The muscle will twitch when electrical stimulus is applied, but this is not painful.
- *After the test:* Needle sites will be monitored to determine presence of hematomas or inflammation.
- EPs measure changes in the brain's electrical activity in response to sensory stimulation. Shampooing hair preprocedure is desired to remove oil and lotions from hair. Postprocedure shampooing is done to remove electrode paste. Also discuss the following:
  - *Visual evoked response:* Cooperation is needed. Electrodes are placed over the occipital region. Prescription glasses should be worn. Patterned and flashing lights will provide retinal stimulation. This test is good for diagnosing optic neuritis with MS.
  - *Somatosensory evoked response:* Peripheral nerve responses in upper or lower extremities help evaluate spinal cord function, sensory dysfunction with MS, and nerve root compression.
  - *Brain stem auditory evoked responses:* Used to evaluate brain stem function. Auditory stimulation *via* headphone is provided. A series of clicks will be heard, varying in rate, intensity, and duration. This test does not require patient cooperation. It can help diagnose brain stem lesion in MS, acoustic neuroma, brain stem lesions related to coma, and hearing loss. It also may be used to monitor cranial nerve VIII for surgical injury.
- After teaching, evaluate patient's level of understanding of the diagnostic test.

## Selected Bibliography

Adams BA, Clancey JK, Eddy M: Malignant glioma: current treatment perspectives, *J Neurosci Nurs* 23(1):15-19, 1991.

Andrus C: Intracranial pressure: dynamics and nursing management, *J Neurosci Nurs* 23(2):85-91, 1991.

Barker E: Brain tumor: frightening diagnosis, nursing challenge, *RN* 53(9):46-52, 1990.

Callanan M, Stowe AC: *Neurologic dysfunctions.* In Swearingen PL, Keen JH, editors: *Manual of critical care: applying nursing diagnoses to adult critical illness,* ed 2, St Louis, 1991, Mosby–Year Book.

Chipps E, Clanin N, Campbell V: *Neurologic disorders: Mosby's clinical nursing series,* St Louis, 1992, Mosby–Year Book.

Clevenger V: Nursing management of lumbar drains, *J Neurosci Nurs* 22(4):227-231, 1990.

Cook HA: Cerebral angioplasty: a new treatment for vasospasm secondary to subarachnoid hemorrhage, *J Neurosci Nurs* 22(5):319-321, 1990.

Cress NB, Owens BM, Hill FH: ImuVert therapy in the treatment of recurrent malignant astrocytomas: nursing implications, *J Neurosci Nurs* 23(1):29-33, 1991.

Edwards DK, Stupperich TK, Welsh DM: Hyperthermia treatment for malignant brain tumors: nursing managment during therapy, *J Neurosci Nurs* 23(1):34-38, 1991.

Emick-Herring B, Wood P: A team approach to neurologically based swallowing disorders, *Rehabilitation Nurs* 14(3):126-132, 1990.

Fickel VD: Acoustic neuroma: postoperative deficits and the role of the neuroscience nurse, *J Neurosci Nurs* 23(1):57-60, 1991.

Finocchiaro DN, Herzfeld ST: Understanding autonomic dysreflexia, *Am J Nurs* 90(9):56-69, 1990.

Fode NC: Carotid endarterectomy: nursing care and controversies, *J Neurosci Nurs* 22(1):25-31, 1990.

Goddard LR: Sexuality and spinal cord injury, *J Neurosci Nurs* 20(4):240-243, 1988.

Hall GR: This hospital patient has Alzheimer's, *Am J Nurs* 91(10):44-50, 1991.

Hart G: Strokes causing left vs. right hemiplegia: different effects and nursing implications, *Geriatr Nurs* 11(2):67-70, 1990.

Hickey JV: *The clinical practice of neurological and neurosurgical nursing,* ed 3, Philadelphia, 1992, JB Lippincott Co.

Interqual: The ISD-A review system with adult ISD criteria, August 1992, Northhampton, NH and Marlboro, MA, Interqual, Inc.

Jahnke H: Experimental ancrod (Arvin) for acute ischemic stroke: nursing implications, *J Neurosci Nurs* 23(6):386-389, 1991.

Kalbach LR: Unilateral neglect: mechanisms and nursing care, *J Neurosci Nurs* 23(2):125-129, 1991.

Kane-Carlsen PA: Managing patient with TIAs, *Nursing 92* 22(1):34-39, 1992.

Krause EA et al: Radiosurgery: a nursing perspective, *J Neurosci Nurs* 23(1):24-28, 1991.

Lederer JR et al: *Care planning pocket guide: a nursing diagnosis approach,* ed 5, Redwood City, Calif, 1993, Addison-Wesley.

Legion V: Health education for self-management by people with epilepsy, *J Neurosci Nurs* 23(5):300-305, 1991.

MacDonald E: Aneurysmal subarachnoid hemorrhage, *J Neurosci Nurs* 21(5):313-321, 1989.

Michael JE: Vagal nerve stimulation in treatment of intractable partial seizures: nursing implications, *J Neurosci Nurs* 24(1):19-23, 1992.

Mitchell M: *Neuroscience nursing: a nursing diagnosis approach,* Baltimore, 1989, Williams & Wilkins.

Mitchell PH et al: *AANN's neuroscience nursing: phenomena and practice, human responses to neurologic health problems,* Norwalk Conn, 1988, Appleton & Lange.

Morgan SP: A passage through paralysis, *Am J Nurs* 91(10):70-74, 1991.

Morgante LA, Madonna MG, Pokoluk R: Research and treatment in multiple sclerosis: implications for nursing practice, *J Neurosci Nurs* 21(5):285-289, 1989.

Neatherlin JS, Brent VA: The gamma knife: implications for nursing practice and patient education, *J Neurosci Nurs* 23(1):71-74, 1991.

North B, North C, Lee JL: Living in a halo, *Am J Nurs* 92(4):54-56, 1992.

Ohman K, Spaniol D: Halo immobilization: discharge planning and patient education, *J Neurosci Nurs* 22(6):351-357, 1990.

Paiva Z: Sundown syndrome: calming the agitated patient, *RN* 53(7):46-50, 1990.

Rancho Los Amigos Hospital, Inc., *Rehabilitation of the head-injured adult,* Downey, CA, 1980.

Raney DJ: Malignant spinal cord tumors: a review and case presentation, *J Neurosci Nurs* 23(1):44-49, 1991.

Ridgeway G, Like M: Demystifying tonic-clonic seizures, *Nursing 91* 21(11):62-64, 1991.

Rusy KL: Temporal lobectomy: a promising alternative, *J Neurosci Nurs* 23(5):320-324, 1991.

Samuels MA, editor: *Manual of neurology: diagnosis and therapy,* ed 4, Boston, 1991, Little, Brown & Co.

Snyder M: *A guide to neurological and neurosurgical nursing,* ed 2, Albany, NY, 1991, Delmar Publishers Inc.

Sosnowski C: Nimodipine: the use of calcium antagonist to prevent vasospasms following subarachnoid hemorrhage, *J Neurosci Nurs* 22(6):382-384, 1990.

Steinke GW: *Stages of Alzheimer's disease,* San Jose, Calif, 1987, Respite and Research for Alzheimer's Disease.

US Department of Health and Human Services: *Acute pain management: operative or medical procedures and trauma,* Public Health Service, Agency for Health Care Policy and Research, Rockville, MD, AHCPR 92-0032, 1992.

Vernon GM: Parkinson's disease, *J Neurosci Nurs* 21(5):273-282, 1989.

Volicer L et al: *Clinical management of Alzheimer's disease,* Rockville, MD, 1988, Aspen Publishers.

Wells T: Conquering incontinence, *Geriatr Nurs* 11(3):133-135, 1990.

Willis D: Intracranial astrocytoma: pathology, diagnosis and clinical presentation, *J Neurosci Nurs* 23(1):7-14, 1991.

# 5 ENDOCRINE DISORDERS

Section One   Disorders of the Thyroid Gland   319
   Hyperthyroidism   319
   Hypothyroidism   324
Section Two   Disorders of the Parathyroid Glands   329
   Hyperparathyroidism   329
   Hypoparathyroidism   334
Section Three   Disorders of the Adrenal Glands   336
   Addison's disease   337
   Cushing's disease   340
Section Four   Disorders of the Pituitary Gland   342
   Diabetes insipidus   343
   Pituitary and hypothalamic tumors   347
   Syndrome of inappropriate antidiuretic hormone   351
Section Five   Diabetes Mellitus   353
   General discussion   353
   Diabetic ketoacidosis   363
   Hyperosmolar hyperglycemic nonketotic syndrome   371
   Hypoglycemia   373
Selected Bibliography   376

## Section One:   Disorders of the Thyroid Gland

The thyroid gland produces three hormones: thyroxine ($T_4$), triiodothyronine ($T_3$), and thyrocalcitonin (calcitonin). Secretion of $T_3$ and $T_4$ is regulated by the anterior pituitary gland *via* a negative feedback mechanism. When serum $T_3$ and $T_4$ levels decrease, thyroid-stimulating hormone (TSH) is released by the anterior pituitary. This stimulates the thyroid gland to secrete more hormones until normal levels are reached. $T_3$ and $T_4$ affect all body systems by regulating overall body metabolism, energy production, and fluid and electrolyte balance and controlling tissue use of fats, proteins, and carbohydrates. Calcitonin inhibits mobilization of calcium from bone and reduces blood calcium levels.

### Hyperthyroidism

Hyperthyroidism is a clinical syndrome caused by excessive circulating thyroid hormone. Because thyroid activity affects all body systems, excessive thyroid hormone exaggerates normal body functions and produces a hypermeta-

**319**

bolic state. Family history of hyperthyroidism is a significant factor for development of this disorder. Hyperthyroidism also can be caused by nodular toxic goiters in which one or more thyroid adenomas hyperfunction autonomously.

*Graves' disease* (diffuse toxic goiter) accounts for approximately 85% of reported cases of hyperthyroidism. It is characterized by spontaneous exacerbations and remissions that appear to be unaffected by therapy. The cause of Graves' disease is unknown, but recent advances in diagnostic techniques have isolated an immunoglobulin known as long-acting thyroid stimulator in a majority of patients with this disorder, suggesting that Graves' disease is an autoimmune response.

The most severe form of hyperthyroidism is *thyrotoxic crisis,* or *thyroid storm,* which results from a sudden surge of large amounts of thyroid hormones into the bloodstream, causing an even greater increase in body metabolism. This is a *medical emergency.* Precipitating factors include infection, trauma, and emotional stress, all of which increase demands on body metabolism. Thyrotoxic crisis also can occur following subtotal thyroidectomy because of manipulation of the gland during surgery. Despite vigorous treatment, thyroid storm causes death in approximately 20% of affected patients.

## ASSESSMENT

**Signs and symptoms:**   Rapid pulse (usually noted by patient), menstrual irregularities, weight loss, fatigue, heat intolerance, increased perspiration, frequent defecation, anxiety, restlessness, tremor, and insomnia.

**Physical assessment:**   Tachycardia, palpitations, widened pulse pressure, hyperpyrexia, enlargement of the thyroid gland, muscle weakness, hyperreflexia, fine tremor, fine hair, thin skin, hypercholesterolemia, impaired glucose tolerance, and stare and/or lid dag. Occasionally males may present with gynecomastia.

**Thyrotoxic crisis (thyroid storm):**   Acute exacerbation of some or all the above signs, marked tachycardia, hyperpyrexia, central nervous system (CNS) irritability, and sometimes coma or heart failure.

## DIAGNOSTIC TESTS

**TSH test:**   Decreased in the presence of disease.

**Free thyroxine index and T$_3$:**   Elevated in the presence of disease.

**Thyrotropin-releasing hormone stimulation test:**   Failure of expected rise in TSH.

**Radioiodine ($^{123}$I) uptake and thyroid scan:**   Clarifies size of gland and detects presence of hot or cold nodules.

## COLLABORATIVE MANAGEMENT

### Pharmacotherapy

*Antithyroid agents:*   Propylthiouracil (PTU) and methimazole (Tapazole) are the first line of treatment. In milder cases methimazole is preferred because of its longer duration of action. The most severe side effect of these drugs is leukopenia. Patients should discontinue the drug at the first sign of infection and obtain a CBC. If the blood count is normal, medication is promptly resumed. Rash, another side effect, can be treated easily with antihistamines.

*Iodides:*   Usually reserved for the following indications: (1) failure to respond to antithyroid drugs, (2) relapse after 1-2 years of therapy, (3) toxic multinodular goiter, (4) solitary toxic nodules, and (5) noncompliant patients. Radioactive iodine ($^{131}$I) is the most commonly used agent. Its use usually results in hypothyroidism, which is controlled easily with replacement therapy.

*Beta-adrenergic blocking agent (e.g., propranolol [Inderal]):*   To relieve tachycardia, anxiety, heat intolerance, and tremor.

*Mild tranquilizers:*   To minimize anxiety and promote rest.

**Diet:**   If significant weight loss has occurred, a diet high in calories, protein, carbohydrates, and vitamins is recommended to restore a normal nutritional state.

**Subtotal thyroidectomy:**  Surgical removal of part of the gland often is the best treatment for patients with extremely enlarged glands or multinodular goiter. The patient is prepared with antithyroid agents until normal thyroid function is achieved (usually 6-8 weeks). The most frequent postoperative complication is hemorrhage at the operative site. The following complications are rare but can be extremely serious: hypoparathyroidism, laryngeal nerve injury, and tetany, owing to damage to the parathyroid glands.

## NURSING DIAGNOSES AND INTERVENTIONS

**Altered nutrition:**  Less than body requirements, related to hypermetabolic state and/or inadequate nutrient absorption

***Desired outcomes:***  By a minimum of 24 h before hospital discharge, patient has adequate nutrition as evidenced by stable weight and a positive nitrogen state. Within 24 h of the instruction, patient lists the types of foods that are necessary to restore a normal nutritional state.

- Provide foods high in calories, protein, carbohydrates, and vitamins. Teach patient about foods that will provide optimal nutrients. To maximize patient's consumption, provide between-meal snacks.
- Administer vitamin supplements as prescribed, and explain their importance to the patient.
- Administer prescribed antidiarrheal medications, which increase absorption of nutrients from the gastrointestinal (GI) tract.
- Weigh patient daily, and report significant losses to physician.

**Sleep pattern disturbance** related to accelerated metabolism

***Desired outcome:***  Within 48 h of hospital admission, patient relates the attainment of sufficient rest and sleep.

- Adjust care activities to patient's tolerance.
- Provide frequent rest periods of at least 90-min duration. If possible, arrange for patient to have bed rest in a quiet, cool room with nonexertional activities, such as reading, watching television, working crossword puzzles, or listening to soothing music.
- As necessary, assist patient with walking up stairs or other exertional activities.
- Administer short-acting sedatives (e.g., alprazolam [Xanax]) as prescribed to promote rest. After administering these agents, raise side rails, and caution patient not to smoke in bed.

**Altered protection** related to potential for thyrotoxic crisis (thyroid storm) secondary to emotional stress, trauma, infection, or surgical manipulation of the gland

***Desired outcomes:***  Patient is free of symptoms of thyroid storm as evidenced by normothermia; BP ≥90/60 mm Hg (or within patient's baseline range); HR ≤100 bpm; and orientation to person, place, and time. If thyroid storm occurs, it is noted promptly and reported immediately.

- Measure and report rectal or core temperature >38.3° C (101° F), because this often is the first sign of impending thyroid storm.
- In patients in whom thyroid storm is suspected, monitor VS hourly for evidence of hypotension and increasing tachycardia and fever.
- Monitor patient for signs of congestive heart failure, which occurs as an effect of thyroid storm: jugular vein distention, crackles (rales), decreased amplitude of peripheral pulses, peripheral edema, and hypotension. Immediately report any significant findings to physician, and prepare to transfer patient to ICU if they are noted.
- Provide a cool, calm, protected environment to minimize emotional stress. Reassure patient and explain all procedures before performing them. Limit the number of visitors.

- Ensure good handwashing and meticulous aseptic technique for dressing changes and invasive procedures. Advise visitors who have contracted or been exposed to a communicable disease either not to enter patient's room or to wear a surgical mask, if appropriate.

*In the presence of thyroid storm*

- As prescribed, administer acetaminophen to decrease temperature. **Caution:** Aspirin is contraindicated because it releases thyroxine from protein-binding sites and increases free thyroxine levels.
- Provide cool sponge baths, or apply ice packs to patient's axilla and groin areas to decrease fever. If high temperature continues, obtain a prescription for a hypothermia blanket.
- Administer PTU as prescribed to prevent further synthesis and release of thyroid hormones.
- Administer propranolol as prescribed to block sympathetic nervous system (SNS) effects.
- Administer IV fluids as prescribed to provide adequate hydration and prevent vascular collapse. Fluid volume deficit may occur because of increased fluid excretion by the kidneys or excessive diaphoresis. Carefully monitor I&O hourly to prevent fluid overload or inadequate fluid replacement. Decreasing output with normal specific gravity may indicate decreased cardiac output, whereas decreasing ouput with increased specific gravity can signal dehydration.
- Administer sodium iodide as prescribed, 1 h *after* administering PTU. **Caution:** If given before PTU, sodium iodide can exacerbate symptoms in susceptible persons.
- Administer small doses of insulin as prescribed to control hyperglycemia. Hyperglycemia can occur as an effect of thyroid storm because of the hypermetabolic state.
- Because $O_2$ demands are increased as the metabolism increases, administer prescribed supplemental $O_2$ as necessary.

**Anxiety** related to SNS stimulation

*Desired outcomes:*   Within 24 h of hospital admission, patient is free of harmful anxiety as evidenced by a HR ≤100 bpm, RR 12-20 breaths/min with normal depth and pattern (eupnea), and absence of or decrease in irritability and restlessness. Patient and significant others verbalize knowledge about the causes of the patient's behavior.

- Assess for signs of anxiety; administer short-acting sedatives (e.g., alprazolam [Xanax] or lorazepam [Ativan]) as prescribed.
- Provide a quiet, stress-free environment away from loud noises or excessive activity.
- Limit number of visitors and the amount of time they spend with patient. Advise significant others to avoid discussing stressful topics and refrain from arguing with the patient.
- Administer propranolol as prescribed to reduce symptoms of anxiety, tachycardia, and heat intolerance.
- Reassure patient that anxiety symptoms are related to the disease process and that treatment decreases their severity.
- Inform significant others that the patient's behavior is physiologic and should not be taken personally.

**Impaired corneal tissue integrity** related to dryness that can occur with exophthalmos in persons with Graves' disease

*Desired outcome:*   Within 24 h of admission, patient's corneas are moist and intact.

- Teach patient to wear dark glasses to protect the cornea.
- Administer lubricating eyedrops as prescribed to supplement lubrication and decrease SNS stimulation, which can cause lid retraction.
- If appropriate, apply eye shields or tape the eyes shut at bedtime.

- Administer thioamides as prescribed to maintain normal metabolic state and halt progression of exophthalmos.

**Body image disturbance** related to exophthalmos or surgical scar

*Desired outcome:*   Within the 24-h period before hospital discharge, patient verbalizes measures for disguising exophthalmos or surgical scar and exhibits self-acceptance.

- Encourage patient to communicate feelings of frustration.
- Advise patient to wear dark glasses to disguise exophthalmos.
- Suggest that patient wear customized jewelery, high-necked clothing such as turtlenecks, or loose-fitting scarves to disguise the scar.
- Suggest that after the incision has healed, patient can use makeup colored in his or her skin tone to decrease visibility of the scar.
- Caution patient that creams are contraindicated until the incision has healed completely, and even then may not minimize scarring. Patients are advised by some physicians to increase vitamin C intake up to 1 g/day to promote healing. Some surgeons also advise against direct sunlight to the operative site for 6-12 months to avoid hyperpigmentation of the incision. Instruct patient accordingly.
- For additional information, see this nursing diagnosis in Appendix One, p. 760.

**Knowledge deficit:**   Potential for side effects from iodides and thioamides or stopping thioamides abruptly

*Desired outcome:*   Within the 24-h period before hospital discharge, patient verbalizes knowledge about the potential side effects of prescribed medications, signs and symptoms of hypothyroidism and hyperthyroidism, and the importance of following the prescribed medical regimen.

- Explain the importance of taking antithyroid medications daily, in divided doses, and at regular intervals as prescribed.
- Teach patient the indicators of hypothyroidism (e.g., early fatigue, weight gain, anorexia, constipation, menstrual irregularities, muscle cramps, lethargy, inability to concentrate, hair loss, cold intolerance, and hoarseness), which may occur from excessive medication, and the signs and symptoms that necessitate medical attention, including cold intolerance, fatigue, lethargy, and peripheral or periorbital edema.
- Teach patient the side effects of thioamides and the symptoms that necessitate medical attention, including the appearance of a rash, fever, or pharyngitis, which can occur in the presence of agranulocytosis.
- Alert patients taking iodides to signs of worsening hyperthyroidism, including high body temperature, palpitations, rapid HR, irritability, anxiety, and feelings of restlessness or panic.

**Pain** related to surgical procedure

*Desired outcomes:*   Within 2 h of surgery, patient's subjective perception of pain decreases, as documented by a pain scale. Objective indicators, such as hesitation before turning or moving the head, are absent or diminished.

- Document the degree and character of the patient's pain, including precipitating events. Devise a pain scale with the patient, rating the pain on a scale of 0 (no pain) to 10 (worst pain).
- Inform patient that clasping the hands behind the neck when moving will minimize stress on the incision.
- After physician has removed surgical clips and drain, teach patient to perform gentle ROM exercises for the neck.
- For other interventions, see **Pain** in Appendix One, p. 694.

**Impaired swallowing (or high risk for same)** related to edema or laryngeal nerve damage resulting from surgical procedure

*Desired outcomes:*   Patient reports swallowing with minimal difficulty, has minimal or absent hoarseness, and is free of symptoms of respiratory dysfunction as evidenced by RR 12-20 breaths/min with normal depth and pattern (eupnea) and absence of inspiratory stridor. Laryngeal nerve damage, if it occurs, is detected promptly and reported immediately.

- Monitor respiratory status for signs of edema (dyspnea, choking, inspiratory stridor, inability to swallow). Also assess patient's voice. Although slight hoarseness is normal after surgery, hoarseness that persists is indicative of laryngeal nerve damage and should be reported to the physician promptly. If bilateral nerve damage is present, upper airway obstruction can occur.
- Elevate HOB 30-45 degrees to minimize edema and incisional stress. Support patient's head with flat or cervical pillows so that it is in a neutral position with the neck (does not flex or hyperextend).
- Keep tracheostomy set and $O_2$ equipment at the bedside at all times. Suction upper airway as needed, using gentle suction to avoid stimulating laryngospasm.
- To minimize pain and anxiety and enhance patient's ability to swallow, administer analgesics promptly and as prescribed.

---

**Note:** See nursing diagnoses and interventions in Appendix One, "Caring for Preoperative and Postoperative Patients," p. 693.

---

## PATIENT-FAMILY TEACHING AND DISCHARGE PLANNING

Provide patient and significant others with verbal and written information for the following:

- Diet high in calories, protein, carbohydrates, and vitamins. Inform patient that as a normal metabolic state is attained, the diet may change.
- Medications, including drug name, purpose, dosage, schedule, precautions, and potential side effects.
- Changes that can occur as a result of therapy, including weight gain, normalized bowel function, increased strength of skeletal muscles, and a return to normal activity levels.
- Importance of continued and frequent medical follow-up; confirm date and time of next appointment.
- Indicators that necessitate medical attention, including fever, rash, or sore throat (side effects of thioamides), and symptoms of hypothyroidism (see p. 325) or worsening hyperthyroidism.
- For patients receiving radioactive iodine, the importance of not holding children to the chest for 72 h following therapy, because they are more susceptible to the effects of radiation. Explain that there is negligible risk for adults.
- Importance of avoiding physical and emotional stress early in the recuperative stage and maximizing coping mechanisms for dealing with stress. See **Health-seeking behaviors:** Relaxation technique effective for stress reduction, p. 54.

# Hypothyroidism

Hypothyroidism is a condition in which there is an inadequate amount of circulating thyroid hormone, causing a decrease in metabolic rate that affects all body systems.

*Primary hypothyroidism* accounts for >90% of cases of hypothyroidism and is caused by pathologic changes in the thyroid itself. There are several possible causes, including dietary iodine deficiency, thyroiditis, thyroid atrophy or fibrosis of unknown cause, radiation therapy to the neck (e.g., with treatment for hyperthyroidism), surgical removal of all or part of the gland, drugs that suppress thyroid activity including propylthiouracil (PTU) and iodides, or a genetic dysfunction resulting in the inability to produce and secrete thyroid hormone. *Secondary hypothyroidism* is caused by dysfunction of the anterior pituitary gland, which results in decreased release of thyroid-stimulating hormone (TSH). It can be caused by pituitary tumors, postpartum necrosis of the pituitary gland, or hypophysectomy. *Tertiary hypothyroidism* is caused by a hypothalamic deficiency in the release of thyrotropin-releasing hormone (TRH).

When hypothyroidism is untreated, or when a stressor such as infection affects an individual with hypothyroidism, a life-threatening condition known as *myxedema coma* can occur. The clinical picture of myxedema coma is that of exaggerated hypothyroidism, with dangerous hypoventilation, hypothermia, hypotension, and shock. Coma and seizures can occur as well. Myxedema coma usually develops slowly, has a $>50\%$ mortality rate, and requires prompt and aggressive treatment.

## ASSESSMENT

Signs and symptoms can progress from mild early in onset to life-threatening.
**Signs and symptoms:**   Early fatigue, weight gain, anorexia, lethargy, cold intolerance, menstrual irregularities, depression, and muscle cramps.
**Physical assessment:**   Possible presence of goiter, bradycardia, hypothermia, deepened voice or hoarseness, hypercholesterolemia, and obesity. The skin may be dry, cool, and coarse and the hair may be thin, coarse, and brittle. The tongue may be enlarged (macroglossia), and the reflexes may be slowed.
**Myxedema coma:**   Hypoventilation, hypoglycemia, hypothermia, hypotension, bradycardia, and shock.

## DIAGNOSTIC TESTS

**TSH:**   Elevated unless the disease is longstanding or severe.
**TRH stimulation test:**   Elevated basal, with exaggerated rise in the presence of early hypothyroidism.
**Free thyroxine index (FTI) and thyroxine ($T_4$) levels:**   Decreased.
$^{131}I$ **scan and uptake:**   Will be $<10\%$ in a 24-h period. In secondary hypothyroidism, uptake increases with administration of exogenous TSH.
**Antimicrosomal antibodies:**   Positive test represents Hashimoto's thyroidism.

## COLLABORATIVE MANAGEMENT

**Oral thyroid hormone:**   Given early in treatment for primary hypothyroidism. To prevent hyperthyroidism caused by too much exogenous hormone, patients are started on low doses that are increased gradually, based on serial laboratory tests (TSH and $T_4$) and adjusted until the TSH is in a normal range. This therapy is continued for the patient's lifetime. For patients with secondary hypothyroidism, thyroid supplements can promote acute symptoms and therefore are contraindicated.
**Stool softeners:**   To minimize constipation owing to decreased gastric secretions and peristalsis.
**Diet:**   High in fiber and protein to help prevent constipation; restriction of sodium (Na) to decrease edema; and reduction in calories to promote weight loss.
### Treatment of myxedema coma
**Intubation and mechanical ventilation:**   To compensate for decreased ventilatory drive.
**IV thyroid supplements:**   Rapid IV administration of thyroid hormone can precipitate hyperadrenolism. This can be avoided by concomitant administration of IV hydrocortisone.
**Treatment of hypotension:**   Administration of IV isotonic fluids, such as normal saline and lactated Ringer's solution. Hypotonic solutions, such as 5% dextrose in water ($D_5W$), are contraindicated because they can decrease serum $Na^+$ levels further. Because of altered metabolism, these patients respond poorly to vasopressors.

**Treatment of hypoglycemia:**  IV glucose.
**Treatment of hyponatremia:**  Fluids are restricted, or hypertonic (3%) saline is administered, or both.
**Treatment of associated illnesses such as infections.**

---

**Caution:**  Because of alterations in metabolism, patients do not tolerate barbiturates and sedatives, and therefore central nervous system depressants are contraindicated. Also, external warming measures are contraindicated for hypothermia because they can produce vasodilation and vascular collapse.

---

## NURSING DIAGNOSES AND INTERVENTIONS

**Ineffective breathing pattern (or high risk for same)** related to upper airway obstruction occurring with enlarged thyroid gland and/or decreased ventilatory drive caused by greatly decreased metabolism
*Desired outcome:*  Patient has an effective breathing pattern as evidenced by RR 12-20 breaths/min with normal depth and pattern (eupnea), normal skin color, normal $SaO_2$ ($\geq 95\%$), and absence of adventitious breath sounds. Alternatively, if an ineffective breathing pattern occurs, it is detected, reported, and treated promptly.
- Assess rate, depth, and quality of breath sounds, and be alert to the presence of adventitious sounds (e.g., from developing pleural effusion) or decreasing or crowing sounds (e.g., from swollen tongue or glottis).
- Be alert to signs of inadequate ventilation, including changes in respiratory rate or pattern and circumoral or peripheral cyanosis. Immediately report significant findings to physician.
- Measure $SaO_2$ intermittently or continuously in patients with decreased ventilatory drive.
- Teach patient coughing, deep breathing, and use of incentive spirometer. Suction upper airway prn.
- For a patient experiencing respiratory distress, be prepared to assist physician with intubation or tracheostomy and maintenance of mechanical ventilatory assistance or transfer patient to ICU.

**Fluid volume excess** related to compromised regulatory mechanisms occurring with adrenal insufficiency
*Desired outcome:*  By a minimum of 24 h before hospital discharge, patient is normovolemic as evidenced by urinary output $\geq 30$ ml/h, stable weight, nondistended jugular veins, presence of eupnea, and peripheral pulse amplitude $\geq 2+$ on a 0-4+ scale.
- Monitor I&O hourly for evidence of decreasing output.
- Weigh patient at the same time every day, with the same clothing, and using the same scale. Report increasing weight gain to physician.
- Monitor patient for the following indicators of congestive heart failure (CHF): jugular vein distention, crackles (rales), SOB, dependent edema of extremities, and decreased amplitude of peripheral pulses. Report significant findings to physician.
- Restrict fluid and Na intake as prescribed. See Table 3-2, p. 115, for foods that are high in Na.
- Administer IV fluids using a rate control device to prevent accidental fluid overload.

**Activity intolerance** related to weakness and fatigue secondary to slowed metabolism and decreased cardiac output caused by pericardial effusions, atherosclerosis, and decreased adrenergic stimulation
*Desired outcome:*  During activity patient rates perceived exertion at $\leq 3$ on a 0-10 scale and exhibits cardiac tolerance to activity as evidenced by HR $\leq 20$ bpm over resting HR, systolic BP $\leq 20$ mm Hg over or under resting systolic

BP, warm and dry skin, and absence of crackles (rales), murmurs, chest pain, and new dysrhythmias.

- Monitor VS and apical pulse at frequent intervals. Be alert to hypotension, slow pulse, dysrhythmias, complaints of chest pain or discomfort, decreasing urine output, and changes in mentation. Ask patient to rate perceived exertion (see Appendix One, p. 711, for details). Promptly report significant changes to physician.
- Balance activity with adequate rest to decrease work load of the heart.
- As prescribed, administer IV isotonic solutions such as normal saline to help prevent hypotension.
- To prevent problems of immobility, assist patient with ROM and other in-bed exercises and consult with physician about the implementation of exercises that require greater cardiac tolerance. For detail, see Appendix One for **High risk for activity intolerance,** p. 711, and **High risk for disuse syndrome,** p. 713.

**High risk for infection** related to compromised immunologic status secondary to alterations in adrenal function

*Desired outcome:* Patient is free of infection as evidenced by normothermia, absence of adventitious breath sounds, normal urinary pattern and characteristics, and well-healing wounds.

- Be alert to early indicators of infection, including fever, erythema, swelling, or discharge from wounds or IV sites; urinary frequency, urgency, or dysuria; cloudy or malodorous urine; presence of adventitious sounds on auscultation of lung fields; and changes in color, consistency, and amount of sputum. Notify physician of significant findings.
- Minimize the risk of urinary tract infection by providing meticulous care of indwelling catheters.
- Use sterile technique when performing dressing changes and invasive procedures.
- Because open sores are sites of ingress for bacteria, provide good skin care to maintain skin integrity and prevent pressure ulcers.
- Advise visitors who have contracted or been exposed to a communicable disease not to enter patient's room or to wear a surgical mask, if appropriate.

**Altered nutrition:** More than body requirements of calories, related to slowed metabolism

*Desired outcomes:* Patient does not experience weight gain. Within the 24-h period before hospital discharge, patient verbalizes understanding of the rationale and measures for the dietary regimen.

- Provide a diet that is high in protein and low in calories. As prescribed, restrict or limit Na and foods high in Na content (see Table 3-2, p. 115) to decrease edema. Teach patient about foods to augment and limit or avoid.
- Provide small, frequent meals of appropriate foods the patient particularly enjoys.
- Encourage foods that are high in fiber content (e.g., fruits with skins, vegetables, whole grain breads and cereals, nuts) to improve gastric motility and elimination.
- Administer vitamin supplements as prescribed.

**Constipation** related to inadequate dietary intake of roughage and fluids, prolonged bed rest, and/or decreased peristalsis secondary to slowed metabolism

*Desired outcome:* Within 48-72 h of admission, patient relates the attainment of his or her normal pattern of bowel elimination.

- Query patient about current bowel function; document changes.
- Be alert to decreasing bowel sounds and the presence of distention and increases in abdominal girth, which can occur with ileus or an obstructive process.

- Encourage patient to maintain a diet with adequate roughage and fluids. Examples of foods high in bulk include fruits with skins, fruit juices, cooked fruits, vegetables, whole grain breads and cereals, and nuts. Ensure that fluid intake in persons without underlying cardiac or renal disease is at least 2-3 L/day.
- Administer stool softeners and laxatives as prescribed. **Caution:** Suppositories are contraindicated because of the risk of stimulating the vagus nerve, which would further decrease HR and BP.
- Advise patient to increase the amount of exercise to promote regularity.

**Sensory/perceptual alterations** related to altered sensory reception, transmission, or intregration secondary to cerebral retention of water

*Desired outcome:* Patient verbalizes orientation to person, place, and time. Alternately, if signs of myxedema coma appear, they are detected, reported, and treated promptly.

- Monitor patient's mental status at frequent intervals by assessing orientation to person, place, and time. Report increasing lethargy or confusion to physician because they can signal onset of myxedema coma.
- Reorient patient frequently. Have a clock and calendar visible, and use radio or television for orientation.
- Clearly explain all procedures to patient before performing them. Provide adequate time for patient to ask questions.
- If necessary, remind patient to complete ADL such as bathing and brushing hair.
- Encourage visitors to discuss topics of special interest to patient to enhance patient's alertness.
- Administer thyroid replacement hormones as prescribed to increase metabolic rate, which in turn will promote cerebral blood flow.

**Altered protection** (risk of myxedema coma) related to inadequate response to treatment of hypothyroidism or stressors such as infection

*Desired outcomes:* Patient is free of symptoms of myxedema coma as evidenced by HR $\geq$60 bpm, BP $\geq$90/60 mm Hg (or within patient's normal range), RR $\geq$12 breaths/min with normal depth and pattern (eupnea), and orientation to person, place, and time. Alternately, if myxedema coma occurs, it is detected, reported, and treated promptly.

- Monitor VS at frequent intervals and be alert to bradycardia, hypotension, or decrease in RR. Report systolic BP <90 mm Hg, HR <60 bpm, or RR <12 breaths/min.
- Monitor patient for signs of hypoxia (circumoral or peripheral cyanosis, decrease in LOC). Immediately report significant findings to physician.
- Double-check medication doses carefully before administration, especially barbiturates and sedatives, which may cause excessive sedation. Observe for signs of toxicity, such as decreased LOC and decreases in BP or ventilatory effort.
- Monitor serum electrolytes and glucose levels. Be especially alert to decreasing $Na^+$ (<137 mEq/L) and glucose (<80 mg/dl).
- In the presence of myxedema coma, implement the following:
  - Restrict fluids or administer hypertonic saline as prescribed to correct hyponatremia. Use an infusion control device to maintain accurate infusion rate of IV fluids.
  - As prescribed, administer IV thyroid replacement hormones with IV hydrocortisone and IV glucose to treat hypoglycemia.
  - Monitor patient for signs of CHF: jugular vein distention, crackles (rales), SOB, peripheral edema, weakening peripheral pulses, and hypotension. Notify physician of any significant findings.
  - Prepare to transfer patient to ICU. Keep an oral airway and manual resuscitator at the bedside in the event of seizure, coma, or the need for ventilatory assistance.

PATIENT-FAMILY TEACHING AND DISCHARGE PLANNING

Give patient and significant others verbal and written information about the following:

- Medications, including drug name, purpose, dosage, schedule, precautions, and potential side effects. Remind patient that thioamides, iodides, and lithium are contraindicated because they decrease thyroid activity. Be sure patient is aware that thyroid replacement medications are to be taken for life.
- Dietary requirements and restrictions, which may change as hormone replacement therapy takes effect.
- Expected changes that can occur with hormone replacement therapy: increased energy level, weight loss, and decreased peripheral edema. Neuromuscular problems should improve as well.
- Importance of continued, frequent medical follow-up; confirm date and time of next medical appointment.
- Importance of avoiding physical and emotional stress, and ways for patient to maximize coping mechanisms for dealing with stress. See **Health-seeking behaviors:** Relaxation technique effective for stress reduction, p. 54.
- Signs and symptoms that necessitate medical attention, including fever or other symptoms of upper respiratory, urinary, or oral infections and signs and symptoms of hyperthyroidism, which may result from excessive hormone replacement.

# Section Two:   Disorders of the Parathyroid Glands

The parathyroid glands regulate serum calcium and phosphorus levels *via* release of parathyroid hormone (PTH). This is accomplished by a negative-feedback mechanism: when serum calcium levels rise, PTH secretion is suppressed. PTH acts on bone to decrease calcium binding, and it stimulates the kidneys to increase resorption of calcium. The parathyroid glands affect serum phosphorus levels in two ways: directly, in that PTH causes increased renal excretion of phosphorus; and indirectly, in that phosphorus and calcium combine readily to form an insoluble salt, and increased serum phosphorus will facilitate this reaction, effectively lowering circulating calcium levels. PTH is also involved in the synthesis of a renal enzyme that catalyzes the formation of vitamin D, which in conjunction with PTH increases absorption of calcium from the GI tract.

## Hyperparathyroidism

Hyperparathyroidism is a clinical syndrome in which there is excessive secretion of PTH. *Primary hyperparathyroidism* is caused by pathology of one or more of the parathyroid glands. Approximately 80% of these cases are caused by a benign adenoma of one gland, another 10% by multigland involvement, and rare cases by carcinoma. In this disorder, excessive PTH acts on the skeletal, renal, and GI systems, and the overall effect is that of increased serum calcium levels and decreased phosphate levels.

Hyperparathyroidism is the second most common cause of hypercalcemia. The incidence of this diagnosis increases dramatically after age 50 and is much more prevalent in females. *Secondary hyperparathyroidism* is usually caused by renal insufficiency with decreased glomerular filtration. Although calcium and phosphorus are retained because of the lack of renal filtration, the high serum phosphate level depresses calcium concentration because phosphorus combines with calcium ions to form insoluble salts, resulting in hypocalcemia. In turn, the resulting hypocalcemia stimulates the parathyroid glands to release PTH in an effort to increase serum calcium levels. Bone resorption occurs because of increased PTH, but absorption of calcium from the GI tract is depressed because of calcium binding with high-phosphate GI secretions. The overall effect is that of decreased calcium levels and increased phosphate levels. *Tertiary hyperparathyroidism* occurs when secondary hyperparathyroidism progresses to a state in which excessive PTH is released independent of serum calcium levels.

## ASSESSMENT

**Signs and symptoms:**   Most individuals diagnosed with primary hyperparathyroidism are asymptomatic or have nonspecific symptoms such as muscular weakness, fatigue, personality disturbances, emotional lability, constipation, weight loss, renal calculi, nausea, vomiting, anorexia, polyuria, hematuria, drowsiness, stupor, and coma. In addition, the patient may have frequent kidney infections, anemia, arthralgia, pancreatitis, peptic ulcers, and pathologic fractures, as well as heart disease caused by calcium deposits in the tissues.
**Physical assessment:**   Hypotonic muscles, joint hyperextensibility, sensory loss, muscle weakness, tongue fasiculations, ataxic gait, and hardened fingernails. If the condition is severe, symptoms of postrenal (obstructive) failure may be present.

## DIAGNOSTIC TESTS

**Serum calcium:**   Elevated in primary hyperparathyroidism and low in secondary hyperparathyroidism. This test usually is repeated at least three times to confirm the diagnosis. Venous blood is drawn in the morning after the patient has been in a fasting state. Because calcium is bound to protein, the test results must be "corrected," based on a simultaneous test for albumin level. Serum calcium will change by 0.8 mg/dl for each 1 g/dl change in albumin level above or below normal. This represents the circulating calcium available for use by body cells and is considered the "true" calcium level. **Note:** To avoid venous stasis, which can produce erroneously high results, care must be taken not to apply the tourniquet too tightly or occlude the vessel for longer than necessary.
**Serum PTH:**   High or inappropriately high for serum calcium levels.
**Plasma phosphorus:**   Decreased in primary hyperparathyroidism and elevated in secondary hyperparathyroidism.
**24-h urine calcium:**   Elevated in primary hyperparathyroidism. This test is often used to rule out other causes of hypercalcemia.
**Skeletal x-rays:**   Will show diminution of bone mass in virtually all patients with hyperparathyroidism, as well as calcification of articular cartilage. X-rays of the hands will show subperiosteal resorption of the phalanges.
**ECG:**   May show shortened QT interval, which is reflective of hypercalcemia.

## COLLABORATIVE MANAGEMENT

*Surgical treatment for primary hyperparathyroidism*
The most effective form of treatment for primary hyperparathyroidism is surgical removal of one or more of the parathyroid glands (parathyroidectomy). The incision is somewhat wider than with a thyroidectomy, but the surgery is very similar. Only the affected gland or glands are removed, and in cases where all the parathyroid glands are enlarged, 3½ of the glands are removed. The remaining tissue is enough to provide normal calcium regulation. In addition to the postoperative complications potentially found with a thyroidectomy, abnormalities in serum calcium levels also may be found.

## Medical treatment for primary hyperparathyroidism

Medical treatment for primary hyperparathyroidism is reserved for patients who are poor surgical risks or who have only a mild form of the disease. The goals of treatment are to provide adequate hydration and reduce serum calcium levels. **Note:** Calcium levels >14 mg/dl are life-threatening and require vigorous and immediate treatment if the patient is to survive.

**Promotion of calcium excretion:**    Done in the absence of congestive heart failure or renal insufficiency. This is accomplished by forcing fluids orally or providing IV normal saline for patients who are stuporous or nauseated. Volumes up to 1,000 ml/h may be given for short periods.

**Increase in salt intake:**    *Via* either diet or salt tablets. Because $Na^+$ competes with calcium for excretion by the kidneys, increased $Na^+$ levels will cause the kidneys to excrete more calcium.

**Diet:**    Limitation of dietary calcium (e.g., milk, many cheeses, cottage cheese, mustard greens, kale, broccoli) intake to one serving per day.

**Pharmacotherapy**

*Diuretics:*    To prevent volume overload and maintain brisk diuresis. Loop diuretics (furosemide and ethacrynate sodium) are preferred because they increase urinary calcium excretion. Thiazide diuretics are contraindicated because they decrease calcium excretion.

*Oral phosphate supplements:*    For patients who have not been on recent glucocorticoid therapy, to help decrease bone resorption of calcium and bind calcium in the intestine to limit calcium absorption. Because they may cause precipitation of insoluble calcium-phosphate complexes in the soft tissues of the kidneys, lungs, and cardiac conductive system, they are given only to patients with a low serum phosphate level or to those who have normal kidney function. Diarrhea is a common side effect. IV phosphates are avoided except for extreme emergency (calcium >14 mg/dl).

*IM calcitonin:*    To decrease bone resorption of calcium and increase renal clearance. This has limited use, however, because it is short-acting and patients frequently become resistant.

*IV mithramycin:*    To inhibit bone resorption and lower serum and urine calcium levels. This is the drug of choice for treatment of *severe* hypercalcemia because it is more effective and works more rapidly than calcitonin. Effects usually are seen within 2 h. Side effects include bleeding abnormalities, hypocalcemia, and nausea.

*IV etidronate:*    As effective as mithramycin but has fewer side effects.

*Oral steroids:*    For their calciuric effect and to decrease calcium absorption in the presence of vitamin D intoxication. To avoid the immunosuppressive effects of these drugs, they are given in as small a dose as it takes to achieve therapeutic effects. This treatment usually is reserved for hypercalcemia associated with hematologic malignancies.

*PTH antagonists:*    Currently under investigation.

**Hemodialysis in a low-calcium bath:**    Sometimes prescribed for severe hypercalcemia to remove calcium ions from the plasma.

## Treatment for secondary hyperparathyroidism

**Reduction of dietary phosphorus:**    Helps prevent formation of insoluble salts, thus increasing the available circulating calcium ions (e.g., meat, poultry, fish, eggs, cheese, dried beans, and cereals may be limited).

**Oral calcium supplements:**    To increase serum calcium levels, which will help prevent further release of PTH.

**Aluminum-containing antacids (e.g., ALternaGel, Amphojel):**    For patients with chronic renal failure, to bind phosphorus in the intestine and prevent resorption.

**Oral vitamin D supplements:**    To correct deficiency.

## NURSING DIAGNOSES AND INTERVENTIONS

**Impaired physical mobility** related to neuromuscular weakness and joint pain secondary to increased serum calcium and altered phosphate levels

*Desired outcome:*  Within 2 days following treatment/interventions, patient demonstrates progression to his or her baseline or optimal level of mobiity with decreasing evidence of weakness or joint pain.

- Administer analgesics and antiinflammatory agents as prescribed to minimize discomfort and enhance the effectiveness of prescribed or necessary activity. Time exercise activity to coincide with the peak effectiveness of the medication.
- Adjust activity to patient's tolerance and provide rest periods at frequent intervals. Discuss the importance of activity with the patient, and set realistic short-term and long-term goals in clearly understood, empirical terms (e.g., "Ambulate the length of the hall 3 times, 4 times a day").
- Assist with ambulation as necessary. Provide a walker or cane if appropriate.
- For patients undergoing IV therapy, provide a stable rolling IV pole.
- Request physical therapy and occupational therapy consultations for gradually increasing the patient's muscular strength and endurance.

**High risk for fluid volume deficit** related to osmotic diuresis, vomiting, or diarrhea caused by oral phosphates

*Desired outcome:*  Patient remains normovolemic as evidenced by balanced I&O, urinary output ≥30 ml/h, good skin turgor, moist tongue and mucous membrane, brisk capillary refill (<2 sec), and BP ≥90/60 mm Hg or within patient's baseline.

- Monitor and document I&O. Be alert to indications of dehydration, including decreasing urinary output, dry mucous membranes, poor skin turgor, thirst, furrowed tongue.
- Monitor serum calcium levels. Decreasing levels signal correction of the dehydration. Normal range for calcium is 8.5-10.5 mg/dl.
- Be alert to the presence of hypotension, which can be further potentiated by oral phosphate supplements.
- Unless patient has coexisting renal or cardiac disease, encourage oral fluids to 3 L/day.
- Rehydrate with IV fluids (typically normal saline) as prescribed.
- Administer prescribed medications (e.g., calcitonin, mithramycin to decrease hypercalcemia; loop diuretics, steroids to increase urinary calcium excretion).

**High risk for trauma** (pathologic fractures) related to bone demineralization

*Desired outcome:*  Patient remains free of symptoms of pathologic fractures.

- Minimize the risk of pathologic fractures from falling by keeping the bed in its lowest position, keeping walkway free of clutter, and assisting patient with ambulation and any strenuous activity. Instruct unstable patient to request help when getting out of bed, promote the use of a cane or walker, and keep call light within patient's reach.
- Pad the side rails for patients with severe bone pathology.
- Apply chest restraints and/or mitts for patients who are severely confused and may attempt to leave the bed, or arrange for significant other to sit with patient.
- Assess each extremity daily for movement, pain, swelling, or deformity, which could signal pathologic fracture.
- Notify physician of patient complaints of back or chest pain, possibly signalling vertebral or rib fracture.

**Constipation** related to decreased peristalsis associated with increased serum calcium level

*Desired outcomes:*  After receiving instructions, patient verbalizes knowledge of measures that promote bowel elimination. Within 2-3 days of this intervention, patient relates the return of bowel elimination within his or her normal pattern.

- Auscultate bowel sounds in each abdominal quadrant for 2-3 min q shift. Report absence of bowel sounds.
- Monitor for physical indicators of constipation, such as abdominal pain and distention.
- Administer stool softeners, suppositories, laxatives, and enemas as prescribed.
- Teach patient to increase dietary fiber by adding dried fruits, whole grain cereals, nuts, fresh fruits, and vegetables to the diet.
- Inform patient that increasing fluid intake to 3 L/day will help promote bowel elimination. (This may be contraindicated for persons with underlying cardiac or renal disease.)
- Encourage as much activity as tolerated.

**Altered protection** related to high risk for hypercalcemia, hypocalcemia, tetany, and thyroid storm secondary to surgical procedure or manipulation of the gland

*Desired outcomes:* Optimally, patient remains free of symptoms of hypercalcemia, hypocalcemia, tetany, and thyroid storm as evidenced by RR 12-20 breaths/min with normal depth and pattern (eupnea); orientation to person, place, and time; absence of Chvostek's and Trousseau's signs; normal strength and motion in all extremities; HR 60-100 bpm; and normothermia. If hypercalcemia, hypocalcemia, tetany, or thyroid storm occur, they are detected and reported promptly.

- Be alert to the presence of hypercalcemia, which can be caused by an increased release of PTH secondary to surgical manipulation of the gland. Signs include nausea, vomiting, anorexia, abdominal pain, weakness, thirst, dyspnea, and coma.
- Monitor patient for numbness and tingling around the mouth, an early sign of hypocalcemia. Also be alert to indicators of tetany: muscle twitching, painful tonic muscle spasms, and grimacing facial spasms. Two tests to assess for tetany are Chvostek's and Trousseau's signs. Chvostek's sign is elicited by tapping the face just below the temple where the facial nerve emerges. The sign is positive if twitching occurs along the nose, lip, or side of the face. Trousseau's sign is tested by applying a BP cuff to the arm, inflating it to slightly higher than the systolic BP, and leaving it inflated for 1-4 min. Carpopedal spasms are indicative of hypocalcemia. Report significant findings to physician.
- Keep IV calcium readily available for prescribed treatment of hypocalcemia.
- Be alert to indicators of thyroid storm, including tachycardia, agitation, and hyperpyrexia. Immediately report the presence of these signs to physician. Although thyroid storm occurs rarely, it can be caused by a sudden release of excessive amounts of thyroid hormone into the bloodstream from manipulation of the gland during surgery.

**Pain** related to surgical procedure or arthralgia caused by bone demineralization

*Desired outcomes:* Within 1 h of intervention, patient's subjective perception of pain decreases, as documented by a pain scale. Objective indicators, such as grimacing, are absent or diminished.

- Monitor patient for pain, noting and documenting intensity, character, and precipitating factors. Devise a pain scale with patient that rates discomfort from 0 (no pain) to 10 (worst pain).
- Administer analgesics as prescribed, and document their effectiveness.
- Advise patient to notify staff as soon as discomfort occurs so that analgesics can be administered before pain becomes too severe.
- Administer analgesics 30-60 min before scheduled activities such as turning or ambulation.

- Teach patient to clasp hands behind the neck during postoperative moving to minimize stress on the incision.
- Teach gentle ROM exercises for the neck, as well as assisted or active ROM for painful joints.
- Provide comfort measures such as a foam mattress and a foot cradle to minimize pressure on the extremities.
- Provide backrubs, especially at bedtime, to reduce discomfort from prolonged bed rest and enhance relaxation.
- For additional pain interventions, see Appendix One, p. 694.

**Knowledge deficit:**   Potential side effects from steroids, phosphate supplements, and mithramycin

***Desired outcome:***   Following instructions, patient verbalizes knowledge of the side effects of prescribed medications and the importance of notifying physician if they occur.

- Teach patient the importance of monitoring for side effects of steroids. This includes frequent BP checks for hypertension, assessment for mental changes, daily weight measurement for evidence of weight gain, and blood tests for the presence of hyperglycemia.
- For patient taking phosphate supplements, explain that diarrhea is a common side effect.
- Teach patient to be alert to the following side effects of mithramycin: lower-extremity petechiae, which signal thrombocytopenia; jaundice, which signals hepatocellular necrosis; and tetany, which occurs with hypocalcemia. Explain that urinalysis results must be monitored for evidence of proteinuria.
- Explain the importance of notifying physician promptly if side effects occur.

---

**Note:**   See "Renal Calculi," p. 124, for nursing diagnoses and interventions for the care of patients with renal calculi. See "Hyperthyroidism" for **Impaired swallowing,** p. 323. As appropriate, see Appendix One, "Caring for Preoperative and Postoperative Patients," p. 693.

---

## PATIENT-FAMILY TEACHING AND DISCHARGE PLANNING

Give patient and significant others verbal and written information about the following:

- Diet, including calcium restriction, increased fluids, and possibly increased Na. As appropriate, arrange for a dietary consultation to help patient with meal planning and integration of individual restrictions into family meals.
- Importance of continued medical follow-up; confirm date and time of next medical appointment.
- Signs and symptoms of hypocalcemia and hypercalcemia (see **Altered protection,** p. 333), which necessitate medical attention if they occur.
- Medications to be taken at home, including drug name, purpose, dosage, schedule, precautions, and potential side effects.
- If surgery was performed, the indications of wound infection (e.g., erythema, local warmth, swelling, discharge, pain, or fever).

# Hypoparathyroidism

Hypoparathyroidism is a condition in which there is decreased production of parathyroid hormone (PTH). Most commonly, this disorder is iatrogenic, caused by damage to or accidental removal of the parathyroid glands during thyroid surgery or radioactive iodine treatment for hyperthyroidism. Damage can be temporary or permanent. If injury occurs in the absence of gland removal, the tissue generally recovers within a period of months and returns to normal function. Familial or autoimmune factors also can be significant in the development of hypoparathyroidism because of deficient PTH receptors in target tissues.

## ASSESSMENT

**Signs and symptoms:**   The main abnormality in hypoparathyroidism is hypocalcemia, so symptoms can include numbness and tingling around the mouth, fingertips, and sometimes in the feet; painful contractions or twitching of skeletal muscles; clonic and tonic spasms; grand mal seizures; laryngeal spasms; carpopedal spasm; nausea; vomiting; dysrhythmias; heart failure; cataracts (from calcium deposits); conjunctivitis; and photophobia.

**Physical assessment:**   Cardiorespiratory compromise with bronchial and/or laryngeal spasm, cardiac dysrhythmias, and prolonged QT and ST intervals on ECG. Neuropsychiatric signs of irritability and psychosis also may be present.

## DIAGNOSTIC TESTS

**Serum tests:**   Levels of ionized calcium will be decreased, phosphate will be increased, and PTH will be inappropriately low for the level of serum calcium.

**Skull and skeletal x-rays:**   May show evidence of increased density and calcification of basal ganglia.

## COLLABORATIVE MANAGEMENT

**Calcium supplements:**   Given either PO or IV, with dosage adjustments based on serum levels of calcium.

**PTH injections:**   To replace lost PTH.

**Vitamin D preparations:**   To facilitate absorption of calcium from the GI tract.

**Sedatives (phenobarbital) and magnesium sulfate:**   To minimize tetany and seizures.

**Aluminum hydroxide gels (e.g., ALternaGel, Amphojel):**   To bind phosphorus in the intestines and decrease serum phosphate levels.

**Diet:**   High in calcium (1 quart milk/day) and low in phosphorus (limit meat, poultry, fish, eggs, cheese, dried beans, and cereals). If hyperphosphatemia persists, it may be necessary to restrict dairy products and egg yolks and provide oral calcium supplements. Foods high in oxalate, which binds to calcium, also should be avoided. These include beets, figs, nuts, spinach, black tea, and chocolate.

## NURSING DIAGNOSES AND INTERVENTIONS

**Activity intolerance** related to weakness and fatigue secondary to decreased cardiac contractility

**Desired outcome:**   During activity, patient rates his or her perceived exertion at ≤3 on a 0-10 scale and exhibits cardiac tolerance to activity as evidenced by HR ≤20 bpm over resting HR, systolic BP ≤20 mm Hg over or under resting systolic BP, RR 12-20 breaths/min with normal depth and pattern (eupnea), normal skin color, warm and dry skin, and absence of crackles (rales), murmurs, chest pain, and new dysrhythmias.

- Monitor patient for signs of activity intolerance, and ask patient to rate his or her perceived exertion. See this nursing diagnosis in Appendix One, p. 711, for detail.
- Monitor patient for indicators of increasing cardiac failure, including hypotension, weak and thready pulse, tachycardia, SOB, pallor, or cyanosis. Report significant findings to physician.
- Provide adequate rest periods of at least 90 min in duration.

- Administer PO or IV calcium supplements as prescribed.
- Assist patient with ROM and other in-bed exercises to help prevent complications of inactivity. Consult with the physician about excercises that require increased cardiac tolerance. For guidelines, see Appendix One for **High risk for activity intolerance,** p. 711, and **High risk for disuse syndrome,** p. 713.

**Altered protection** related to potential for tetany, respiratory distress, and seizures secondary to hypocalcemia

*Desired outcome:*    Patient verbalizes orientation to person, place, and time and is free of symptoms of injury caused by tetany, respiratory distress, and seizures.

- Observe for early signs of hypocalcemia, such as tingling around the mouth and in the hands. Be alert to indicators of tetany, including muscle twitching, painful tonic muscle spasms, grimacing facial spasms, and positive Chvostek's and Trousseau's signs (see p. 333). Report significant findings to physician.
- Monitor for evidence of respiratory distress, including stridor, wheezing, and dyspnea; report significant findings to physician immediately.
- Monitor serum calcium levels, noting whether levels are increased or decreased. Either extreme will require a change in calcium therapy. Serum calcium levels <7mg/dl or >14 mg/dl (after being "corrected" with albumin level) are life-threatening. If they occur, notify physician immediately.
- Provide a restful, quiet environment away from loud noises and bright lights.
- Administer sedatives and anticonvulsant medications as prescribed.
- Keep side rails up at all times. Keep an oral airway at the bedside.
- Keep tracheostomy set, oxygen equipment, and IV calcium at the bedside.
- Also see "Seizure Disorders," p. 288, for nursing interventions for the care of patients who experience seizures.

## PATIENT-FAMILY TEACHING AND DISCHARGE PLANNING

Give patient and significant others verbal and written information about the following:

- Diet high in calcium, low in phosphorus, and low in oxalate (see p. 335). As appropriate, arrange for a dietary consultation so that patient's requirements and restrictions can be integrated into family meal planning.
- Medications, including drug name, purpose, dosage, schedule, precautions, and potential side effects.
- Signs and symptoms necessitating medical attention, including signs of worsening hypocalcemia (such as tetany) or signs of hypercalcemia, including weakness, fatigue, constipation, polyuria, and renal calculi.
- Importance of continued medical follow-up; confirm date and time of next appointment.

# Section Three:    Disorders of the Adrenal Glands

Each of the two adrenal glands is composed of two distinct parts: the adrenal cortex and the medulla. Adrenocortical hormones include glucocorticoids (cortisol is the primary glucocorticoid), which are responsible for regulation of protein, fat, and carbohydrate metabolism and affect the immunologic and inflammatory responses; mineralocorticoids (aldosterone), which affect $Na^+$, potassium ($K^+$), and water metabolism; and androgens, which affect sexual development. These hormones are released in response to serum levels of adrenocorticotropic hormone (ACTH), which functions *via* a negative-feedback mechanism: when serum cortisol levels decrease, ACTH release increases. The medulla secretes the catecholamines epinephrine and norepinephrine, which are released in response to sympathetic nervous system stimulation.

# Addison's disease

Addison's disease is a deficiency of adrenocortical hormones following destruction of the adrenal cortex, which can occur suddenly as a result of such stressors as trauma, infection, or surgery, but more commonly occurs gradually. As many as 80% of reported cases involve an autoimmune factor. *Primary Addison's disease* is a pathology of the adrenal glands themselves, while *secondary Addison's disease* is often caused by prior treatment with glucocorticoids, which inhibit pituitary ACTH release.

Deficiency of glucocorticoids retards the mobilization of tissue protein and inhibits the ability of the liver to store glycogen, which causes muscle weakness and hypoglycemia to occur. Wound healing is slowed, and these individuals become particularly susceptible to infection. There is a loss of vascular tone in the periphery as well as decreased vascular response to the catecholamines epinephrine and norepinephrine. Decreased secretion of aldosterone causes $Na^+$, $Cl^-$, and water loss from the kidneys and increased reabsorption of $K^+$.

The presence of acute symptoms in response to stressors is called *adrenal*, or *Addisonian, crisis*. It can be precipitated by any emotional stressor, simple infection, minor surgery, or trauma. Abrupt withdrawal of exogenous steroids also can precipitate a crisis. Unless treated rapidly and aggressively, this condition can lead to death within hours.

## ASSESSMENT

**Signs and symptoms:**  Apprehension, headache, nausea, anorexia, abdominal pain, diarrhea, confusion, and restlessness. In addition, individuals may have muscular weakness that becomes progressively worse throughout the day, anorexia, fatigue, weight loss, postural hypotension, and emotional instability.

**Physical assessment:**  Possible presence of cyanosis, fever, pallor, weak pulse, and tachypnea. Often there is emaciation with dehydration, generalized dark pigmentation of the skin with brown or black freckles, hypotension, and a small heart size.

**Addisonian crisis:**  Headache, nausea, vomiting, fever, intractable abdominal pain, and severe hypotension, which can lead to vascular collapse and shock.

**History of:**  Familial tendency, bilateral adrenalectomy, tuberculosis (TB), any kind of trauma or infection, damage to the pituitary gland.

## DIAGNOSTIC TESTS

**Cortrosyn (cosyntropic) stimulant test:**  Initially a blood sample is drawn to determine the baseline level of serum cortisol. Then, 250 mg cortrosyn is given IV push, at which time the patient may experience nausea and have a sudden urge to urinate, but these side effects resolve quickly. Additional blood samples are drawn 30 and/or 90 min later, or alternatively after 20 and 40 min to determine serum cortisol levels. Individuals with adrenal insufficiency will demonstrate a slight rise in serum cortisol, but not the peak values that would occur in individuals without adrenal insufficiency.

**Other blood studies:**  Will reveal elevated $K^+$; decreased plasma aldosterone, $Na^+$, and $Cl^-$ levels; and decreased blood sugar. Serum ACTH will be increased in primary Addison's disease and decreased in secondary Addison's disease.

**Urine $Na^+$ levels:**  Increased because of renal $Na^+$ wasting.

**Computerized axial tomography (CT) scan or magnetic resonance imaging (MRI):**  May show a decrease in adrenal or pituitary size, which signals glandular destruction.

## COLLABORATIVE MANAGEMENT

**Pharmacotherapy**

*Antibiotics or anti-TB therapy:*   If infection or TB is the cause.

*Maintenance doses of mineralocorticoids (e.g., cortisone); oral supplementary Na; and oral corticosteroids (usually hydrocortisone):*   The average daily replacement of hydrocortisone usually is 20 mg each morning and 10 mg each afternoon. Patients must take hormone replacement for life.

*Fludrocortisone acetate (Florinef acetate):*   For patients with primary adrenal insufficiency. A daily PO dosage of 0.1-0.2 mg is necessary, and it can be titrated appropriately based on monitoring of BP, serum $K^+$ levels, and plasma renin levels.

**Diet:**   High in calories, carbohydrates, proteins, and vitamins, and provided in small, frequent feedings to enhance nutritional state for these patients, who tend to be anorexic.

*For adrenal crisis*

**Replacement of fluids:**   To correct severe dehydration. 1-2 L $D_5NS$ is given over a brief period of time (e.g., 2 h).

**Hydrocortisone sodium succinate:**   To replace decreased cortisol. It is given 100 mg IV immediately and then q6h *via* infusion drip.

**Vasopressors:**   To maintain adequate BP.

**Continuous cardiac monitoring:**   For prompt identification of life-threatening dysrhythmias.

## NURSING DIAGNOSES AND INTERVENTIONS

**High risk for infection** related to compromised immunologic status secondary to decreased adrenal function

*Desired outcome:*   Patient is free of infection as evidenced by normothermia, WBC count $\leq$11,000 µl, clear and straw-colored urine, well-healing wounds, negative culture results, and absence of adventitious breath sounds and sore throat.

- Monitor for and report early signs of infection including fever; leukocytosis; frequency, urgency, dysuria, and cloudy or malodorous urine; persistent erythema, pain, swelling, or purulent discharge from wounds or the IV site; and complaints of sore throat and pharyngitis. Teach patient these indicators and the importance of reporting them to physician or staff promptly should they occur. As directed, culture any drainage.
- Monitor temperature q2-4h, and report significant elevation to physician.
- Use meticulous aseptic technique for all invasive procedures and when changing dressings. Ensure meticulous indwelling catheter care to help prevent urinary tract infection (UTI). Perform stringent handwashing technique before caring for these patients.
- Caution visitors who have contracted or been exposed to a communicable disease either not to enter room or to wear surgical masks when visiting patient.

**Altered protection** related to potential for Addisonian crisis

*Desired outcomes:*   Patient is free of symptoms of Addisonian crisis as evidenced by normothermia; BP $\geq$90/60 mm Hg (or within patient's baseline range); HR $\leq$100 bpm; RR 12-20 breaths/min with normal depth and pattern (eupnea); orientation to person, place, and time; and absence of abdominal pain, nausea, vomiting, and headache. If Addisonian crisis occurs, however, it is detected and reported promptly.

- Be alert to the following indicators of Addisonian crisis: headache, nausea, vomiting, fever, abdominal pain, and severe hypotension. Be aware that the profound hypotension can lead to vascular collapse and shock.
- Place patient in a quiet room away from loud noises and excessive activity. Caution staff and visitors not to discuss stress-provoking topics with patient.
- As prescribed, administer corticosteroids and prophylactic antibiotics, which help prevent Addisonian crisis from occurring.

- If Addisonian crisis is diagnosed, implement the following:
  - As prescribed, administer vasopressors to maintain BP and hydrocortisone sodium succinate to replace cortisol.
  - Administer IV fluids as prescribed to prevent circulatory collapse.
  - Monitor VS q15min until stable, then as prescribed. Report significant changes in BP, HR, or respiratory rate or pattern to physician.
  - Administer oxygen as prescribed.
  - Usually a continuous cardiac monitor is used if Addisonian crisis is diagnosed. Monitor for signs of hypokalemia (increased premature ventricular contractions, depressed T waves) or hyperkalemia (peaked T waves).
- Monitor for and report signs of Na retention and fluid volume excess (peripheral, pulmonary, and cerebral edema) caused by excessive doses of medications used to treat or prevent Addisonian crisis, including corticosteroids, Na, and fluids. Be alert to dependent edema, crackles (rales), weight gain, severe headache, irritability, and confusion. Teach these symptoms to patient and significant others, and stress the importance of reporting them promptly to physician or staff member.

**Activity intolerance** related to generalized weakness and fatigue secondary to decreased cardiac output

***Desired outcome:***   During activity, patient rates his or her perceived exertion at ≤3 on a 0-10 scale and exhibits cardiac tolerance to activity as evidenced by HR ≤20 bpm over resting HR, systolic BP ≤20 mm Hg over or under resting systolic BP, RR ≤20 breaths/min with normal depth and pattern (eupnea), warm and dry skin, and absence of crackles (rales), murmurs, chest pain, and new dysrhythmias.

- Monitor VS for evidence of activity intolerance, and ask patient to rate his or her perceived exertion (see this nursing diagnosis in Appendix One, p. 711, for detail). Also observe for and report indicators of impending circulatory collapse, such as hypotension, tachycardia, weak and thready pulse, pallor, and cyanosis.
- Gear activities to patient's tolerance. Provide frequent rest periods.
- To prevent complications of immobility, assist patient with ROM and other in-bed exercises. For details, see Appendix One for **High risk for activity intolerance,** p. 711, and **High risk for disuse syndrome,** p. 713.

**Fluid volume deficit** related to active loss secondary to diuresis

***Desired outcome:***   Patient becomes normovolemic within 24 h of hospital admission, as evidenced by balanced I&O, urinary output ≥30 ml/h, good skin turgor, stable weight, and moist tongue and oral mucous membranes.

- Monitor I&O and be alert to indicators of fluid volume deficit, including thirst, poor skin turgor, and furrowed tongue.
- If deficit is noted, encourage oral fluids.
- Administer maintenance doses of mineralocorticoids as prescribed to promote salt and water retention.
- If prescribed, administer supplementary Na to correct hyponatremia. As appropriate, advise patient to add salt to foods or eat foods relatively high in Na, such as meat, fish, poultry, eggs, and milk. See Table 3-2, p. 115, for a list of foods high in Na.

---

**Note:**  If the patient experiences Addisonian crisis, see psychosocial nursing diagnoses and interventions in Appendix One, "Caring for Patients with Cancer and Other Life-Disrupting Illnesses," p. 753.

---

## PATIENT-FAMILY TEACHING AND DISCHARGE PLANNING

Give patient and significant others verbal and written information about the following:

- Medications, including drug name, purpose, dosage, schedule, precautions,

and potential side effects. Ensure that patient understands the necessity of lifetime hormone replacement.
- Diet (e.g., foods to increase, such as those high in Na [see Table 3-2, p. 115]).
- Relationship between hormonal levels and stress. Instruct patient to seek medical help during periods of emotional or physical stress so that medication dosages can be adjusted accordingly.
- Signs and symptoms that necessitate medical attention. These include indicators of excessive adrenal hormones (e.g., weight gain, moon face, dependent edema, headache, weakness, irritability), adrenal insufficiency (e.g., progressive fatigue, nausea, vomiting, weakness, and postural hypotension), and infections (e.g., upper respiratory infection, wound, UTI, and oral).
- Methods for maximizing coping mechanisms to deal with stress, such as diversional activities and relaxation exercises. Explain the importance of avoiding physical or emotional stress. See **Health-seeking behaviors:** Relaxation technique effective for stress reduction, p. 54.
- Need for continued medical follow-up.
- Obtaining a Medic-Alert bracelet and identification card outlining the diagnosis and emergency treatment.

*In addition:*
- Prepare an emergency kit, including alcohol sponges and syringes with 100 mg of hydrocortisone to be carried and used in the event of Addisonian crisis. Teach technique for IM administration of the medication to patient and significant others.

# Cushing's disease

Cushing's disease is a spectrum of symptoms associated with prolonged elevated plasma concentration of adrenal steroids (e.g., cortisol). In individuals with normal functioning, the pituitary gland secretes adrenocorticotropic hormone (ACTH), which stimulates the adrenal glands to release the adrenal steroid hormones. This is regulated by a negative-feedback mechanism in which increasing levels of plasma cortisol suppress ACTH. In cases of pituitary pathology, this mechanism does not function and the pituitary gland continues to secrete excessive amounts of ACTH, with resultant abnormally high levels of adrenocortical hormones. This accounts for approximately 70% of reported cases and is termed *Cushing's disease. Cushing's syndrome,* on the other hand, is caused by pathology of the adrenal glands themselves, from ectopic ACTH-secreting tumors, or from iatrogenic causes, such as excessive ingestion of cortisol or ACTH.

Actions of excessive glucocorticoid (cortisol) secretion include the following: increased protein catabolism; increased production of glucose and glycogen, with resultant hyperglycemia; a rise in plasma lipid levels, which causes atherosclerotic changes in blood vessels; decreased bone formation and increased bone resorption, with resulting osteoporosis; and inhibition of the inflammatory response to tissue injury. Actions of excessive mineralocorticoid (aldosterone) include the following: $Na^+$ and water retention, increased renal excretion of $K^+$, and increased secretion of angiotensin II, a potent vasoconstrictor.

## ASSESSMENT

**Signs and symptoms:**  Weight gain; muscle weakness; kyphosis and back pain; generalized osteoporosis, especially in the vertebrae; pathologic fractures of the long bones; mental and emotional disturbances; easy bruising; arteriosclerotic changes in the heart, brain, and kidney; renal calculi; thirst and polyuria; menstrual changes; and impotence.

**Physical assessment:**  Patients exhibit "central obesity" with pendulous ab-

domens and thin legs and arms; moon face; fat deposits on the neck and supraclavicular area (buffalo obesity); edema; hypertension; and thin, transparent skin with multiple ecchymoses. Androgen excess is most noticeable in females, as evidenced by changes in menstruation, as well as virilism and hirsutism. Patients frequently have stretch marks with red and purple striae showing through the stretched skin. Patients with Cushing's syndrome have hyperpigmentation of facial skin secondary to ectopic ACTH-secreting tumors.
**History of:**  Excessive exogenous steroid ingestion, pituitary tumor.

## DIAGNOSTIC TESTS

**24-h urine sample for free cortisol levels:**  This test is highly accurate and is elevated in the presence of Cushing's disease.
**Overnight dexamethasone suppression test:**  The patient is given a 1-mg tablet of dexamethasone at 10 PM the evening before the test. For patients with Cushing's disease this dose should suppress plasma cortisol levels at 8 AM the following morning to <50% of baseline.
**Other blood tests:**  Blood glucose levels drawn after meals will be elevated in 80%-90% of patients with Cushing's disease. Serum $K^+$ levels will be decreased.
**CT scan or MRI:**  May show adrenal masses or abnormalities in the sella turcica, which are indicative of pituitary dysfunction.

## COLLABORATIVE MANAGEMENT

**Transsphenoidal pituitary surgery:**  The preferred treatment, this surgery offers a low rate of morbidity and postsurgical complications, although around 20% of patients develop diabetes insipidus (see p. 343).
**Adrenocortical inhibitors (e.g., metapyrone, aminoglutethimide, and cyproheptadine):**  To inhibit production of adrenocortical hormones. Exogenous steroids also may be given in conjunction with the adrenocortical inhibitors to prevent hypocorticolism. Adrenocortical inhibitors are used only short-term, however, because increased ACTH production quickly overcomes their effect.
**Irradiation of the pituitary gland:**  To decrease pituitary production of ACTH. It is used only in patients with a mild form of the disease or in those who are poor surgical candidates.
**Diet:**  Low in calories and carbohydrates to reduce hyperglycemia. Salt is restricted to reduce BP, and foods high in K (Table 3-4, p. 132) are given to raise serum $K^+$ levels.

## NURSING DIAGNOSES AND INTERVENTIONS

**Body image disturbance** related to hyperpigmentation, hair loss, and other physical changes associated with increased ACTH production
*Desired outcome:*  Within the 24-h period before hospital discharge, patient relates the attainment of self-acceptance and verbalizes knowledge that symptoms will abate with treatment.
- Encourage patient to verbalize feelings and frustrations.
- Reassure patient that symptoms should subside with adequate treatment of the disorder.
- Assist patient with measures to improve appearance, such as keeping hair well groomed, wearing own gown or pajamas if possible, and performing personal hygiene (e.g., bathing and brushing of teeth). Encourage use of cosmetics and toiletries as patient desires.
- See this nursing diagnosis in Appendix One, p. 760, for additional information.

**High risk for impaired skin integrity** related to thinning of skin and fragility of capillaries secondary to increased cortisol production
*Desired outcome:*  Patient's skin remains intact and nonerythematous.
- Ensure that patient on bed rest turns q2h. Establish and post a turning sched-

ule. Provide gentle massage with nonirritating, nonalcohol lotions to help prevent pressure ulcers.
- Place alternating air pressure mattress or other pressure-relief mattress or pad on the bed.
- Position foot cradle over the bed to prevent pressure areas on lower extremities by keeping bed linen off the feet.
- To protect the skin of confused patients, pad the siderails of the bed.

---

**Note:** See "Hyperparathyroidism" for **High risk for trauma** (pathologic fractures), p. 332. See "Addison's Disease" for **High risk for infection,** p. 338. See "Pituitary and Hypothalamic Tumors" for **Altered protection** (IICP, CSF leak, and diabetes insipidus) secondary to transsphenoidal hypophysectomy, p. 349. Also see Appendix One for nursing diagnoses and interventions in "Caring for Preoperative and Postoperative Patients," p. 693, and "Caring for Patients with Cancer and Other Life-Disrupting Illnesses," p. 753.

---

## PATIENT-FAMILY TEACHING AND DISCHARGE PLANNING

Give patient and significant others verbal and written information about the following:
- Diet, including foods to increase, such as those high in K (see Table 3-4, p. 132), and foods to restrict, including those high in Na (see Table 3-2, p. 115) or carbohydrates. Arrange for a dietary consultation to help patient with meal planning and integration of individual restrictions into family diet.
- Medications, including drug name, purpose, dosage, schedule, precautions, and potential side effects. Advise patient with bilateral adrenalectomy of the necessity for lifetime hormone replacement therapy.
- Importance of continued medical follow-up; confirm date and time of next medical appointment.
- Relationship between hormone levels and stress. Advise patient to seek medical assistance during periods of emotional or physical stress so that medications can be adjusted accordingly. Provide suggestions for patient to maximize coping mechanisms, such as relaxation exercises or diversional activities. See **Health-seeking behaviors:** Relaxation technique effective for stress reduction, p. 54.
- Indicators of *excessive adrenal hormone:* weight gain, thirst, polyuria, easy bruising, and muscle weakness; or *adrenal insufficiency:* easy fatiguability, weight loss, and abdominal pain; any of which necessitate medical attention.
- Signs and symptoms of urinary tract infection, upper respiratory infection, wound, and oral infections and the importance of seeking medical care should they occur.
- Importance of wearing a Medic-Alert bracelet and carrying an identification card to describe the disease and the necessary emergency measures.

*In addition:*
- For patients with bilateral adrenalectomy, provide an emergency kit with alcohol sponges and syringes filled with 100 mg of hydrocortisone for episodes of acute adrenal insufficiency. Teach patient and significant others the technique for IM administration of the medication for emergency treatment.

# Section Four:   Disorders of the Pituitary Gland

The pituitary (hypophysis) is composed of two lobes, the anterior pituitary (adenohypophysis) and posterior pituitary (neurohypophysis). The anterior lobe is larger, and its secretory activities are controlled by tropic hormones produced by and transmitted from the hypothalamus in response to negative-feedback mechanisms. It secretes seven of the nine pituitary hormones. These include (1) adrenocorticotropic hormone (ACTH), which stimulates adrenal cortical growth and secretion of adrenocortical hormones; (2) thyroid-stimulating hormone (TSH), or thyrotropic hormone, which stimulates thyroid growth and secretion of thyroid hormones; (3) follicle-stimulating hormone (FSH), which stimulates ovulation in females and sperm production in males; (4) luteinizing hormone (LH), called the interstitial cell-stimulating hormone (ICSH) in males, in whom it stimulates production of testosterone; in females it stimulates ovulation and development of ovarian follicles; (5) melanocyte-stimulating hormone (MSH), which causes pigmentation; (6) luteotropic hormone (LTH), also called prolactin, which stimulates secretion of milk in females; and (7) growth hormone (GH), or somatotropic hormone (STH), which accelerates body growth.

Posterior pituitary secretion is regulated by nerve impulses originating in the hypothalamus in response to stimuli from other parts of the body. It produces two hormones: antidiuretic hormone (ADH), or vasopressin, which acts on the renal tubules to increase reabsorption of water; and oxytocin, which stimulates milk "letdown" and contraction of the uterus. These hormones are synthesized in the hypothalamus and stored in secretory granules located in the nerve terminals of the posterior pituitary.

# Diabetes insipidus

Diabetes insipidus (DI) results from a defect in the synthesis of ADH by the hypothalamus or release from the posterior pituitary (neurogenic, or central, DI) or in the renal tubular response to ADH (nephrogenic DI) causing impaired renal conservation of water. The onset usually is insidious, with progressively increasing polydipsia and polyuria, but it can develop rapidly following an injury or infectious disease. Depending on the degree of injury, the condition can be either temporary or permanent. A rare form of DI, termed psychogenic diabetes insipidus, is associated with compulsive water drinking.

There are three phases associated with DI. The first phase, of polydipsia and polyuria, immediately follows the injury and lasts 4-5 days. In the second phase, which lasts about 6 days, the symptoms disappear; and in the third phase, the patient experiences permanent polydipsia and polyuria. The chief danger to these patients is dehydration from the inability to take in adequate fluids to balance the excessive output of urine. DI must be differentiated from other syndromes resulting in polyuria. History, physical, and simple laboratory procedures assist in diagnosis. Other causes of polyuria include recent lithium or mannitol administration, renal transplantation, renal disease, hyperglycemia, hyperosmolality (early), hypercalcemia, or $K^+$ depletion, including primary aldosteronism.

## ASSESSMENT
**Signs and symptoms:** Polydipsia, polyuria with dilute urine.
**Physical assessment:** Usually within normal limits, but patient may show signs of dehydration if fluid intake is inadequate. Individuals with cranial injury, disease, or trauma may exhibit impairment of neurologic status, including altered LOC and sensory or motor deficits.
**History of:** Cranial injury, especially basilar skull fracture; meningitis; primary or metastatic brain tumor; surgery in the pituitary area; cerebral hemorrhage; encephalitis; syphilis; or tuberculosis. Familial incidence rarely is a factor.

## DIAGNOSTIC TESTS
**Urine osmolality:** Decreased (<50-200 mOsm/kg) in the presence of disease.
**Specific gravity:** Decreased (<1.007) in the presence of disease.

**TABLE 5-1  Vasopressin Preparations**

| Generic name | Brand name | Onset | Duration | Usual dose | Advantages/ Disadvantages | Comments |
|---|---|---|---|---|---|---|
| *Nasal* | | | | | | |
| vasopressin | Pitressin (20 pressor U/ml) | within 1 h | 4-8 h | 5-10 U bid-tid | Action decreased by nasal congestion or discharge or atrophy of nasal mucosa | Administer by spray, cotton pledget, or dropper |
| desmopressin acetate | DDAVP (0.1 mg/ml) | within ½ h | 8-20 h | 0.1-0.4 ml qd in 1-3 doses (10-40 μg) | See vasopressin, above | Administer by spray or nasal tube system. Store in refrigerator at 4° C (39.2° F) |
| lypressin | Diapid (0.185 mg/ml) | within ½ h | 3-8 h | 7-14 μg qid (1 or 2 sprays into each nostril) | See vasopressin, above | Administer by spray |
| *Subcutaneous* | | | | | | |
| vasopressin | Pitressin (20 pressor U/ml) | ½-1 h | 2-8 h | 0.25-0.5 ml (5-10 U) q3-4h prn increased thirst or increased urine output | May be used as an alternative in patients for whom nasal route is contraindicated | Carbamazepine and chlorpropamide may potentiate the antidiuretic effects of all forms of vasopressin |

| | | Onset | Duration | Dose | Comments | Storage |
|---|---|---|---|---|---|---|
| desmopressin acetate | DDAVP | within ½ h | 1½–4 h | 0.5–1 ml (2–4 µg) qd in 2 divided doses | | Keep refrigerated at 4° C |
| **Intramuscular** vasopressin tannate in oil | Pitressin tannate in oil (5 pressor U/ml) | within 1–2 h | 36–48 h | 0.3–1 ml (1.5–5 U) q2–3 days for increased thirst or increased urine output | Longer duration of action and slower absorption than SC route. Response cumulative over 2–3 days | Store at 13–18° C (55–65° F). Roll vial between hands before withdrawing solution. Can warm vial by immersing in warm water |
| vasopressin | Pitressin (20 pressor U/ml) | ½–1 h | 2–8 h | 0.25–0.5 ml (5–10 U) q3–4h for increased thirst or increased urine output | | |
| **Intravenous** desmopressin acetate | DDAVP (4µg/ml) | within ½ h | 1½–4 h | 0.5–1.0 ml (2–4 µg) qd in 2 divided doses | Generally not for home use | Keep refrigerated at 4° C. Dilute in 10–50 ml 0.9% NaCl, and infuse over 15–30 min |

**Serum osmolality:** Increased ($\geq$300 mOsm/kg) in the presence of disease.
**Water deprivation test:** Baseline measurements of body weight, serum and urine osmolalities, and urine specific gravity are obtained. Fluids are not permitted, and the above measurements are repeated qh. The test is terminated when urine specific gravity exceeds 1.020 and osmolality exceeds 800 mOsm/kg (normal responses), urine specific gravity does not increase for 3 h (a positive result), or when 5% of body weight is lost. The latter is, in itself, an abnormal response, and the corresponding urine osmolality will be <400 mOsm/kg, which is diagnostic of DI. Because the most serious side effect of this test is severe dehydration, the test should be performed early in the day so the patient can be more closely monitored. Before a firm diagnosis of DI can be made from an abnormal water deprivation test, it is also necessary to demonstrate that the kidneys can respond to vasopressin (see below).
**Vasopressin SC or desmopressin nasal spray:** After administration of either drug (see Table 5-1), urine is collected q15min for 2 h. Quantity and specific gravity are then measured. Normally, individuals will show a concentration of urine but not as pronounced as that of persons with DI; a person with kidney disease will have a lesser response to vasopressin. **Note:** One serious side effect of this test is the precipitation of congestive heart failure in susceptible individuals.
**Hypertonic saline infusions:** 3% sodium chloride (NaCl) solution is infused IV to assess for subsequent water conservation. Although this test seldom is necessary for a diagnosis of DI, it does assist in documentation of changes in the osmotic threshold for ADH release.

## COLLABORATIVE MANAGEMENT
### For central, or neurogenic, DI
**Rehydration:** Lost water is replaced with IV hypotonic (e.g., 0.45% NaCl) solution. The initial replacement is rapid, necessitating close monitoring of BP, HR, and urine output.
**Administration of exogenous vasopressin (Pitressin):** Replacement therapy for ADH. There are several preparations available (Table 5-1), and it is important to read the package insert carefully to ensure proper administration. Potential side effects include hypertension secondary to vasoconstriction, myocardial infarction secondary to constriction of coronary vessels, uterine cramps, and increased peristalsis of the GI tract.
**Achieving a mild antidiuretic effect:** E.g., with chlorpropamide, clofibrate, carbamazepine, or other medication that increases the action or release of ADH.
### For nephrogenic DI
**Therapy with thiazide diuretics (e.g., hydrochlorothiazide 50-100 mg daily or chlorthalidone 50 mg daily):** Although it may seem antithetical to treat diuresis with a diuretic, one of the side effects of the thiazide diuretics is blocking of the kidneys' ability to excrete free water, which is the primary problem with DI.

## NURSING DIAGNOSES AND INTERVENTIONS
**Fluid volume deficit** related to active loss secondary to polyuria
*Desired outcomes:* Patient becomes normovolemic within 7 days of onset of symptoms as evidenced by stable weight, balanced I&O, good skin turgor, moist tongue and oral mucous membrane, BP $\geq$90/60 mm Hg (or within patient's normal range), HR $\leq$100 bpm, and CVP 2-6 mm Hg (or 5-12 cm $H_2O$).
- Monitor I&O, daily weight, and VS closely. Be alert to evidence of hypovolemia, including weight loss, inadequate fluid intake to balance output, thirst, poor skin turgor, furrowed tongue, hypotension, and tachycardia. If

available, monitor CVP for evidence of hypotension. Notify physician if any of the following occurs: (1) urinary output >200 ml in each of 2 consecutive hours, (2) urinary output >500 ml in any 2-h period, or (3) urine specific gravity <1.002.

- Provide unrestricted fluids. Keep water pitcher full and within easy reach of patient. Explain the importance of consuming as much fluid as can be tolerated.
- Administer vasopressin and antidiuretic agents (or thiazide diuretic for patient with nephrogenic DI) as prescribed.
- For unconscious patients, administer IV fluids as prescribed. Unless otherwise directed, for every ml of urine output, deliver 1 ml of IV fluid.

**Altered protection** related to potential for side effects of vasopressin

*Desired outcomes:*   Optimally, patient verbalizes orientation to person, place, and time and is free of signs of injury caused by side effects of vasopressin. As appropriate, patient and/or significant others demonstrate administration of coronary artery vasodilators by hospital discharge.

- Monitor VS and report significant changes such as systolic BP elevated >20 mm Hg over baseline systolic BP, or HR increased >20 bpm over baseline HR.
- Be alert to indicators of water intoxication, including changes in LOC, confusion, weight gain, headache, convulsions, and coma. If these develop, stop the medication, restrict fluids, and notify physician. Institute safety measures accordingly, and reorient patient as needed.
- For the older adult or persons with vascular disease, keep prescribed coronary artery vasodilators (i.e., nitroglycerine) at the bedside for use if angina occurs. Teach patient and significant others how to administer these medications.

## PATIENT-FAMILY TEACHING AND DISCHARGE PLANNING

Give patient and significant others verbal and written information about the following:

- Importance of continued medical follow-up; confirm date and time of next appointment.
- Indicators that necessitate medical attention (e.g., signs of dehydration or water intoxication).

## Pituitary and hypothalamic tumors

Lesions affecting pituitary function may be located in either the pituitary gland or the adjacent hypothalamus and include pituitary adenomas, craniopharyngiomas, metastatic tumors, primary pituitary cancer, and meningiomas. Undiagnosed, small pituitary adenomas have been reported in approximately 20%-30% of autopsies. Adenomas generally do not secrete anterior pituitary hormones, and patients manifest symptoms of hypopituitarism. Secreting tumors may produce any anterior pituitary hormone, but prolactin, adrenocorticotropic hormone (ACTH), and growth hormone (GH) secretion are found more often than thyroid-stimulating hormone (TSH) and gonadotropin secretion.

Hypopituitarism may result from primary pituitary disease or abnormal secretion of hormones by the hypothalamus and may be permanent or reversible. Gonadotropin or GH secretion generally are lost earlier in the disease process, followed by loss of TSH, ACTH, and prolactin at later stages. Loss of TSH secretion results in hypothyroidism (see p. 324), while loss of ACTH prompts adrenocortical insufficiency or Addison's disease (see p. 337). A small percentage of patients experience a mixture of both hypersecretion of some anterior pituitary hormones and hyposecretion of others.

## ASSESSMENT

**Altered neurologic status:**   Headache (dull, generalized) often unrelieved by analgesics, visual field changes (loss of peripheral vision, occasional double vision), and seizures and hydrocephalus (rare).

**Hypopituitarism:**   Delayed puberty and short stature (in preadolescents and adolescents); loss of libido and sexual characteristics; impotence; apathy; mental slowing; weakness; mild anemia; dry and scaly skin with pale, waxy complexion; increased wrinkling around the mouth and eyes; hypotension; orthostatic hypotension; occasional hypoglycemia; myxedema; sparse body hair; generalized sensitivity to coldness; decreased perspiration; and decreased resistance to colds, stress, and infections.

**Excessive prolactin (hyperprolactinemia):**   Males often present with impotence, decreased libido, infertility, and hypogonadism. Females often have amenorrhea, infertility, galactorrhea, reduced vaginal lubrication, dyspareunia, osteoporosis, and occasional hirsutism.

**Excessive GH:**   In growing children, excessive GH results in gigantism, and in adults, acromegaly. Symptoms of acromegaly include coarse facial features (i.e., large nose and thick lips), enlargement of hands and feet, oily skin, malodorous perspiration, chewing problems, need to change/refit dentures frequently, hoarseness, joint pain/deformities, cardiac enlargement, carpal tunnel syndrome, insulin resistance/hyperglycemia, headache, hypopituitarism, and salivary and thyroid gland enlargement.

**Excessive ACTH:**   See "Cushing's Disease," p. 340.

**Excessive TSH:**   See "Hyperthyroidism," p. 319.

**Excessive gonadotropin (luteinizing hormone [LH]/follicle-stimulating hormone [FSH]):**   Found most frequently in middle-aged males. Indicators include visual field changes, LH secretion alteration causing low testosterone level, or marked elevation in FSH.

## DIAGNOSTIC TESTS
*General*

**X-ray of skull:**   Will show enlarged pituitary gland, thickened skull, and distorted, enlarged pituitary fossa or sella turcica.

**CT scan or MRI:**   May reveal an abnormality of the sella turcica or extrasellar extension of the tumor.

**Skeletal x-rays:**   Will show thickening of long bones.

**Cerebral angiography:**   To exclude presence of aneurysm, extension of suprasellar and/or parasellar tumor, blood vessel involvement, and tumor blushes.

**Serum tests (in hyperpituitarism):**   May reveal elevated phosphate and postprandial blood glucose, prolactin, GH, ACTH, TSH, LH, and FSH levels.

**Insulin tolerance test and metapyrone test:**   Measures the ability of pituitary ACTH to increase in response to stress. These tests may be dangerous in elders and in individuals who are cardiac impaired or prone to seizures.

**Rapid ACTH stimulation test:**   Measures adrenal response to exogenous ACTH administration.

*For hypopituitarism*

**Urinary 17-ketosteroids, 17-hydroxycorticosteroids, and plasma cortisol:**   Decreased, but will rise slowly after administration of ACTH.

**Urinary and serum gonadotropins:**   Decreased.

**Plasma testosterone and estradiol:**   Decreased.

**Serum levels of ACTH, TSH, LH, FSH, and GH:**   Decreased.

## COLLABORATIVE MANAGEMENT

**Exogenous hormone replacements:**   As appropriate for syndromes of insufficiency secondary to hypopituitarism.

**Hormone suppression therapy:**   For hormone-secreting tumors. Dopamine agonists, such as bromocriptine (Parlodel), are used to inhibit synthesis and release of anterior pituitary hormones by the gland or adenoma. This therapy has proven effective in prolactin-, GH-, and ACTH-secreting tumors.

**X-ray and heavy-particle radiation therapy:**  For hormone-secreting tumors. Typically, the response with a return to normal is slow, but tumor progression is halted in most patients. Side effects can include malaise, nausea, serous otitis media, and hypopituitarism. For more information, see Appendix One, "Caring for Patients with Cancer and Other Life-Disrupting Illnesses," p. 719. Currently there are no chemotherapeutic agents that cure pituitary adenomas.

**Transsphenoidal hypophysectomy:**  Treatment of choice because it offers a more rapid cure with a low morbidity rate. An incision is made in the inner aspect of the upper lip, and the sella turcica is entered through the sphenoid process. Because an opening is created between the nose and upper airway, the patient is at increased risk for postoperative infection, necessitating preoperative use of nasal antibiotics. Postoperatively the patient will have periorbital ecchymosis. The pituitary is a highly vascular gland; therefore, hemorrhage at the operative site is a potential risk. Diabetes insipidus (DI) can result from pituitary destruction and removal. For larger tumors, a frontal craniotomy may be necessary. (See "Brain Tumors," p. 258.)

## NURSING DIAGNOSES AND INTERVENTIONS

**Altered protection** related to potential for increased intracranial pressure (IICP), DI, cerebrospinal fluid (CSF) leak, hemorrhage, and infection secondary to transsphenoidal hypophysectomy

***Desired outcomes:***  Optimally, patient verbalizes orientation to person, place, and time and is free of indicators of injury caused by complications of transsphenoidal hypophysectomy. Immediately after instruction, patient and significant others verbalize understanding of the importance of patient avoiding Valsalva-type maneuvers, describe the signs and symptoms of IICP, DI, and infection; and verbalize the importance of notifying staff of postnasal drip or excessive swallowing.

- Be alert to indicators of IICP, such as a change in LOC, sluggish or unequal pupils, and changes in respiratory rate or pattern. Monitor patient for decreased vision, eye muscle weakness, abnormal extraocular eye movement, double vision, and airway obstruction. Report significant findings to physician. A change in vision may necessitate a CT scan.
- Measure I&O hourly for 24 h and monitor urine specific gravity q1-2h. Report an output >200 ml/h for 2 consecutive h or a total of 500 ml/h. Specific gravity <1.007 is found with DI. Monitor weight daily for evidence of loss. Explain the signs of DI (see p. 343). DI often occurs as a result of the edema caused by manipulating the pituitary stalk and usually is transitory.
- Inspect nasal packing at frequent intervals for the presence of frank bleeding or CSF leakage. Note the number of times the mustache dressing is changed. Expect nasal packing removal in about 3-4 days. Test *non*sanguineous drainage for the presence of CSF fluid using a glucose reagent strip. If the drainage contains CSF, the test will be positive for the presence of glucose. Monitor patient for complaints of postnasal drip or excessive swallowing, which may signal CSF drainage down the back of patient's throat. **Caution:** Because the presence of CSF represents a serious breach in the integrity of the cranium, elevate the HOB to minimize the potential for bacteria entering the brain, and immediately report any suspicious drainage.
- Elevate the HOB 30 degrees to decrease ICP and swelling. Dexamethasone may be prescribed to reduce cerebral swelling.
- Explain to patient that coughing, sneezing, and other Valsalva-type maneuvers must be avoided because these actions can stress the operative site and increase ICP, causing CSF leakage. Teach patient to cough or sneeze with an opened mouth if either is unavoidable. Remind patient that nose-blowing should be avoided until the nasal mucosa is healed (about 1 month). Advise

patient about the importance of mouth breathing and the possibility of having a soft nasal airway. Obtain a prescription for a mild cathartic or stool softener to prevent straining with bowel movements if indicated.

- To prevent disturbance in the integrity of the operative site, do not allow patient to brush teeth. Provide mouthwash (e.g., hydrogen peroxide diluted with water to half strength) and sponge-tipped applicator for oral hygiene. Monitor for extreme erythema or swelling at the suture line. Remind patient that the front teeth should not be brushed until the incision has healed (about 10 days). Advise patient that the diet will be liquid initially but quickly will progress to soft.

- The patient may have periorbital edema, headache, and tenderness over the sinuses for 2-3 days, which may be helped with cold compresses to the eyes. The transsphenoidal donor site for fat or muscle packing usually is taken from the thigh or abdomen, and the patient should expect a small dressing there. Advise patient that the sense of smell usually returns in about 2-3 weeks.

- Be alert to and teach patient the following signs and symptoms of infection, which necessitate medical attention: fever, nuchal rigidity, headache, and photophobia.

**Sexual dysfunction** related to physiologic changes secondary to abnormal hormone levels

***Desired outcome:*** As appropriate, patient relates the attainment of satisfying sexual activity within 1 month following hospital discharge.

- Encourage patient to express feelings of anger and frustration and to communicate feelings to significant other.

- If appropriate, suggest alternatives other than sexual intercourse for pleasuring partner and self.

- Administer testosterone or estrogens as prescribed.

- Support physician's referral or suggest referral for psychotherapy related to loss of libido, sterility, impotence, or loss of self-esteem.

---

**Note:** See Appendix One for nursing diagnoses and interventions in "Caring for Preoperative and Postoperative Patients," p. 693.

---

## PATIENT-FAMILY TEACHING AND DISCHARGE PLANNING

Give patient and significant others verbal and written information about the following:

- Medications, including drug name, purpose, dosage, schedule, precautions, and potential side effects. Reinforce that following hypophysectomy, patient will be on lifetime hormone replacement therapy.

- Relationship between hormone levels and stress. Advise patient to seek medical help during times of emotional or physical stress so that dosages of medications can be adjusted accordingly.

- Measures for maximizing coping mechanisms to deal with stress, such as relaxation tapes, meditation, diversional activities. See **Health-seeking behaviors:** Relaxation technique effective for stress reduction, p. 54.

- Importance of continued medical follow-up; confirm time and date of next appointment.

- Indicators of *adrenal hormone excess:* weight gain, easy bruising, muscle weakness, moon face, thirst, and polyuria; *adrenal hormone insufficiency:* weight loss, easy fatigue, and adominal pain; *hypothyroidism:* weight gain, anorexia, apathy, slowed mentation, and cold intolerance; and *hyperthyroidism:* tachycardia, diaphoresis, and heat intolerance. All of these signs and symptoms necessitate medical attention.

- For patients requiring permanent vasopressin replacement therapy, the importance of obtaining a Medic-Alert bracelet and identification card outlining diagnosis and emergency treatment.

*For patients found to be acromegalic during hospitalization for another illness:*

- Role of GH excess in the development of hyperglycemia, diabetes mellitus, arthralgia, osteoarthritis, cardiac enlargement, headaches, sexual/reproductive dysfunction, dental problems, and change in physical appearance.
- Anatomy and physiology of the pituitary gland and hypothalamus, along with changes prompted by pituitary tumors.
- Management of pituitary tumors, including medical and surgical modalities.

## Syndrome of inappropriate antidiuretic hormone

Syndrome of inappropriate antidiuretic hormone (SIADH) is caused by excessive release of antidiuretic hormone (ADH) from the pituitary gland, resulting in excessive water retention and hyponatremia. The action of ADH increases reabsorption of water in the late-distal tubules and collecting ducts of the kidney. ADH secretion usually is stimulated by one of three mechanisms: (1) increased plasma osmolality; (2) decreased plasma volume; or (3) decreased BP. SIADH is a rare disorder that requires differential diagnosis from other problems that prompt elevation of vasopressin and resultant hyponatremia because of an appropriate response to hypovolemic or hypotensive stimuli.

In the presence of excessive ADH, water that normally would be excreted is reabsorbed into the circulation, resulting in water retention and eventually, water intoxication. The retained water expands extracellular fluid volume, causing serum osmolality and $Na^+$ to decrease because of dilutional effects. Decreased serum osmolality causes movement of water into the cells, which can result in cerebral edema. Further water retention results in an increased glomerular filtration rate and decreased aldosterone secretion, and more $Na^+$ is filtered out into the urine.

Water intoxication, cerebral edema, and severe hyponatremia cause altered neurologic/mental status, which if untreated may lead to death.

### ASSESSMENT

**Signs and symptoms:** Decreased urine output with concentrated urine. Signs of water intoxication may appear, including altered LOC, fatigue, headache, diarrhea, anorexia, nausea, vomiting, and seizures. **Note:** Because of the loss of $Na^+$, edema will not accompany the fluid volume excess.

**Physical assessment:** Weight gain without edema, elevated BP, altered mentation.

**History of:** Cancers of the lung, pancreas, duodenum, and prostate, which can secrete a biologically active form of ADH. Other common causes include pulmonary disease (e.g., tuberculosis, pneumonia, chronic obstructive pulmonary disease, empyema), head trauma, brain tumor, intracerebral hemorrhage, meningitis, and encephalitis. Positive pressure ventilation, physiologic stress, chronic metabolic illness, and a wide variety of medications (chlorpropamide, acetaminophen, oxytocin, narcotics, general anesthetic, carbamazepine, thiazide diuretics, tricyclic antidepressants, and cancer chemotherapy agents) all have been linked with SIADH.

### DIAGNOSTIC TESTS

**Serum $Na^+$ level:** Decreased to <137 mEq/L.
**Plasma osmolality:** Decreased to <275 mOsm/kg.
**Urine osmolality:** Elevated disproportionately in relation to plasma osmolality.
**Urine $Na^+$ level:** Increased to >200 mEq/L.
**Urine specific gravity:** >1.030.
**Plasma ADH level:** Elevated.

## COLLABORATIVE MANAGEMENT

**Fluid restriction:**   Based on urine output plus insensible losses.

**Isotonic (0.9%) or hypertonic (3%) NaCl:**   May be given if the patient has severe hyponatremia. Supplemental Na solutions may be administered with IV furosemide (Lasix) or bumetanide (Bumex) or osmotic diuretics, such as mannitol, to promote water excretion.

**Lithium or demeclocycline:**   Inhibits action of ADH on the distal renal tubules to promote water excretion.

**Treatment of underlying cause:**   SIADH associated with surgery, trauma, or drugs usually is temporary and self-limiting. In chronic situations the focus will be on treating the underlying cause *via* surgery (i.e., transsphenoidal hypophysectomy, craniotomy, thoracotomy), radiation therapy, or chemotherapy.

## NURSING DIAGNOSES AND INTERVENTIONS

**Fluid volume excess** related to compromised regulatory mechanisms resulting in increased serum ADH level, renal water reabsorption, and renal $Na^+$ excretion

*Desired outcome:*   Patient becomes normovolemic (and normonatremic) within 7 days of onset of symptoms, as evidenced by orientation to person, place, and time; intake that approximates output plus insensible losses; stable weight; CVP 2-6 mm Hg; BP within patient's normal range; and HR 60-100 bpm.

- Assess LOC, VS, and I&O at least q4h; measure weight daily. Be alert to decreasing LOC, elevated BP and CVP, urine output <30 ml/h, and weight gain. Promptly report significant findings or changes to physician.
- Monitor laboratory results, including those for serum $Na^+$, urine and serum osmolality, and urine specific gravity. Be alert to decreased serum $Na^+$ and plasma osmolality, urine osmolality elevated disproportionately in relation to plasma osmolality, and increased urine $Na^+$. Normal values are as follows: urine specific gravity 1.010-1.020, serum $Na^+$ 137-147 mEq/L, urine osmolality 300-1090 mOsm/kg, and serum osmolality 280-300 mOsm/kg. Report significant findings to physician.
- Maintain fluid restriction as prescribed. Explain necessity of this treatment to patient and significant others. Do not keep water or ice chips at the bedside. Ensure precise delivery of fluid administered intravenously by using a monitoring device.
- Elevate HOB no more than 10-20 degrees to enhance venous return and thus reduce ADH release.
- Administer demeclocycline, lithium, furosemide, or bumetanide as prescribed; carefully observe and document patient's response.
- Administer hypertonic NaCl as prescribed. Rate of administration usually is based on serial serum $Na^+$ levels. To minimize the risk of hypernatremia, make sure that specimens for laboratory tests are drawn on time and that results are reported to physician promptly.
- Institute seizure precautions to prevent patient injury in the event of seizure. These include padded side rails, supplemental oxygen, and oral airway at the bedside, as well as side rails up at all times when staff member is not present.

---

**Note:**   See "Diabetic Ketoacidosis" for **High risk for injury** related to altered cerebral function, p. 368. If the patient has undergone a transsphenoidal hypophysectomy, see "Pituitary and Hypothalamic Tumors" for **Altered protection** related to risk of IICP, DI, CSF leak, hemorrhage, and infection, p. 349.

---

## PATIENT-FAMILY TEACHING AND DISCHARGE PLANNING

Give patient and significant others verbal and written information about the following:

- Importance of fluid restriction for the prescribed period. Assist patient with planning permitted fluid intake (e.g., by saving liquids for social and recreational situations as indicated).
- How to safely enrich the diet with Na and K salts, particularly if ongoing diuretic use is prescribed.
- Obtaining daily weight measurements as an indicator of hydration status.
- Indicators of water intoxication and hyponatremia, including altered LOC, fatigue, headache, nausea, vomiting, and anorexia, any of which should be reported promptly to physician.
- Medications, including name, dosage, route, purpose, and potential side effects.
- Importance of continued medical follow-up; confirm date and time of next medical appointment.
- Procedure for obtaining a Medic-Alert bracelet/card identifying patient's diagnosis.

# Section Five:   Diabetes Mellitus

## General discussion

Diabetes mellitus (DM) is a chronic disease affecting 6% of the total population (12 million Americans) with metabolic, vascular, and neurologic disorders resulting from dysfunctional glucose transport into body cells. Insulin facilitates glucose transport into cells for oxidation and energy production. Food intake, glycogen breakdown, and gluconeogenesis increase the serum glucose level, which stimulates the beta islet cells of the pancreas to release the needed insulin for transport of glucose from the bloodstream into the cells. As glucose leaves the blood, serum levels return to normal (60-120 mg/dl).

Individuals with DM have impaired glucose transport owing to decreased or absent insulin secretion and/or ineffective insulin action. Carbohydrate, fat, and protein metabolism are abnormal, and patients are unable to store glucose in the liver and muscle as glycogen, store fatty acids and triglycerides in adipose tissue, and transport amino acids into cells normally. DM is classified into five types of disorders:

**Insulin-dependent diabetes mellitus (IDDM)/Type I:**   Complete lack of effective endogenous insulin, causing hyperglycemia and ketosis. Previously this was termed juvenile, or growth onset, diabetes because a majority of those affected are <30 years of age. This type of DM is precipitated by altered immune responses, genetic factors, and environmental stressors. It accounts for 10% of all DM. These individuals are dependent on insulin for survival and prevention of life-threatening diabetic ketoacidosis (DKA).

**Noninsulin-dependent diabetes mellitus (NIDDM)/Type II:**   Moderate to severe lack of effective endogenous insulin, causing severe hyperglycemia without ketosis. Previously it was termed adult, or maturity onset, diabetes, and it is precipitated by obesity and aging. Approximately 25% of individuals with Type II require periodic to regular insulin administration for blood glucose control. Oral hypoglycemia agents are used by 50% of these patients, while 25% control their blood glucose using only a structured American Diabetes Association (ADA) diet for maintenance of ideal body weight. This type accounts for 80%-90% of individuals with DM. Untreated hyperglycemia can result in hyperosmolar hyperglycemic nonketotic (HHNK) syndrome.

**Other types:**    Formerly termed secondary diabetes, these include:
- *Pancreatic diseases that destroy the beta islet cells:* E.g., pancreatitis, cystic fibrosis, hemochromatosis.
- *Drug-induced by insulin antagonists:* E.g., phenytoin (Dilantin), steroids (hydrocortisone, dexamethasone), hormones (estrogen).
- *Endocrine dysfunction/hormonal diseases:* E.g., acromegaly, Cushing's syndrome, pheochromocytoma.
- *Insulin resistance:* Caused by dysfunctional insulin receptors.
- *Genetic syndromes:* Those that predispose individuals to DM (e.g., human leukocyte antigen [HLA] genetic system defects).
- *Defective insulin molecule production:* Caused by mutation of the insulin gene.

**Gestational diabetes:**    Intolerance to glucose, which develops during pregnancy in 2%-3% of pregnant women, resulting in increased perinatal risk to the child and increased risk of the mother developing chronic DM during the next 10-15 years. This type does not include *previously* diabetic pregnant women.

**Malnutrition-related diabetes:**    Type of DM recently added by the World Health Organization (WHO) for a syndrome with onset in individuals 10-40 years of age in underdeveloped countries. This type requires insulin for control of blood glucose. Ketosis does not occur. The role of malnutrition as a cause currently is unknown.

Certain individuals may manifest chronic hyperglycemia without meeting other criteria for DM and are classified as having impaired glucose tolerance (IGT). IGT was formerly termed "borderline," "chemical," "latent," "subclinical," and "asymptomatic" diabetes. Of Americans >65 years of age, 10%-30% have IGT, and 1%-5% of individuals with IGT progress to DM annually. Other individuals may have a higher probability of developing glucose intolerance owing to previous abnormality or genetic predisposition. Genetically high-risk individuals often have never exhibited IGT and are classified as having potential abnormality of glucose tolerance.

## ASSESSMENT

**Metabolic:**    Fatigue, weakness, weight loss, mild dehydration, and symptoms of hyperglycemia (polyuria, polydipsia, and polyphagia). These indicators are seen in the early stages of illness.

**Impending Type I (IDDM) crisis:**    Profound dehydration and hyperglycemia, electrolyte imbalance, metabolic acidosis due to ketosis, altered mental status, Kussmaul respirations, acetone breath, possible hypovolemic shock (hypotension, weak and rapid pulse), abdominal pain, and possible strokelike symptoms.

**Impending Type II (NIDDM) crisis:**    Severe dehydration, hypovolemic shock (hypotension, weak and rapid pulse), severe hyperglycemia, shallow respirations, altered mental status, slight lactic acidosis or normal pH, possible strokelike symptoms.

## COMPLICATIONS

**Potential for acute crisis:**    *For Type I,* include DKA and hypoglycemia; *for Type II,* include HHNK and hypoglycemia. These complications should be preventable in individuals diagnosed with DM and will be discussed later in this section.

**Long-term complications:**    The most important factor in delaying progression to long-term complications is the stabilization of blood glucose levels to normal range.

*Macroangiopathy:*    Vascular disease affecting the coronary arteries and the larger vessels of the brain and lower extremities. Risk factors are hyperglycemia, hypertension, hypercholesterolemia, smoking, aging, and extended duration of DM. Macroangiopathy may result in myocardial infarction, cerebrovascular accident, and peripheral vascular disease.

*Microangiopathy:*  Thickening of capillary basement membranes resulting in retinopathy and nephropathy. Early symptoms include increased leakage of retinal vessels and microalbuminuria. Late manifestations are blindness and renal failure.

*Neuropathy:*  Affects the peripheral and autonomic nervous systems, resulting in impaired or slowed nerve transmission, e.g., numbness or lack of sensation, particularly in the feet (peripheral), and orthostatic hypotension, neurogenic bladder, and impaired gastric emptying (autonomic).

**Morning hyperglycemia:**  Blood glucose elevation found on awakening. Causes include:

*Insufficient insulin:*  The patient may need a higher dosage, a mixture of insulins, or longer-acting insulin.

*Dawn phenomenon:*  Glucose remains normal until approximately 3 AM, when the effect of nocturnal growth hormone may elevate glucose in Type I diabetes. It may be corrected by changing the time of the evening dose of intermediate-acting insulin injection to bedtime instead of dinnertime.

*Somogyi phenomenon:*  The patient becomes hypoglycemic during the night. Compensatory mechanisms to raise glucose levels are activated and result in overcompensation. It may be corrected by decreasing the evening dose of intermediate-acting insulin and/or eating a more substantial bedtime snack.

**Problems with insulin**

*Insulin resistance:*  A problem experienced by most individuals with DM and with other diseases at some point in the illness, when the daily insulin requirement exceeds 200 U to control hyperglycemia and prevent ketosis. Typically, it results from profound/complete insulin deficiency in Type I DM and obesity in Type II DM. It is characterized as one of the following anomalies:

—Prereceptor: Insulin abnormal or insulin antibodies present.

—Receptor: The number of insulin receptors is decreased, or insulin binding to the receptors is diminished.

—Postreceptor: Receptors not appropriately activated by insulin. This condition is treated by changing the insulin to a purer preparation or changing from an animal source (beef or pork) to human insulin.

*Local allergic reactions:*  Soreness, erythema, or induration at the insulin injection site within 2 h after injection. Reactions are decreasing in frequency with the evolution of more purified insulins.

*Systemic allergic reactions:*  Rare occurence that begins with a localized skin reaction, which evolves into generalized urticaria or anaphylaxis. Patients must be desensitized to insulin by progression from miniscule to more normal doses over the course of one day, using a series of SC injections.

*Lipodystrophy:*  Local disturbance in fat metabolism resulting in loss of fat (lipoatrophy) or development of abnormal fatty masses at the injection sites (lipohypertrophy). Lipoatrophy rarely has been seen since the development of $^{100}$U and human source insulins. Rotation of injection sites helps to prevent lipohypertrophy. Individuals experiencing lipohypertrophy should use alternate injection sites until the condition resolves. Treatment of lipoatrophy involves changing to $^{100}$U human source insulin and injecting subsequent scheduled doses into the periphery of the affected area(s).

## DIAGNOSTIC TESTS

WHO defines the following diagnostic criteria for DM in nonpregnant adults:

**Fasting blood sugar:**  A value >140 mg/dl is indicative of glucose intolerance if found on at least 2 occasions.

**Oral glucose tolerance test:**  The 2-h sample during the test is >200 mg/dl on at least 2 occasions.

**Random plasma glucose:**  Greater than 200 mg/dl on at least 2 occasions.

**Glycosylated hemoglobin (Hgb):**   Normal range is 4%-7%. Individuals with DM will have values >7%. This value is measured to assess control of blood glucose over a preceding 2-3 month period. The larger the percentage of glycosylated Hgb the poorer the blood glucose control.

## COLLABORATIVE MANAGEMENT

**Diet:**   The exchange programs of the ADA are the most commonly used methods of diet calculation and patient education. Dietary management is individually based on ideal body weight and adjusted to metabolic and activity needs. Typically the patient is put on a fixed ADA diet that is composed of 50%-60% carbohydrates, 12%-20% protein, and 20%-30% fat. The focus on weight reduction for individuals with Type II DM necessitates significant carbohydrate restriction if they are treated by diet alone. When treatment also includes oral hypoglycemic medications or insulin, increased amounts of carbohydrates are required to offset the hypoglycemic effects of these medications. Individuals with Type I DM require day-to-day consistency in diet and exercise to prevent hypoglycemia. Typically, three daily meals and an evening snack are prescribed. Some fat and protein should be present in all meals and snacks to slow down the elevation of postprandial blood glucose. Adding 10-15 g of fiber will slow the digestion of monosaccharides and disaccharides. For all types of diabetes, refined and simple sugars should be reduced, and complex carbohydrates (breads, cereals, pasta, beans) should be encouraged. Various artificial sweeteners are used in "diet" products. Some contribute calories, which must be accounted for in a calorie-restricted diet. Exchange lists commonly are used for meal planning.

**Monitoring of blood glucose:**   Control of blood glucose is facilitated by a glycohemoglobin monitoring device, which is designed to provide timely measurement of the glucose level from a small droplet of blood obtained by fingerprick. This simple technology affords the opportunity for closer monitoring and stabilization of glucose levels, which has been shown to decrease both the incidence and severity of long-term complications.

**Oral hypoglycemic medications (sulfonylureas):**   Used in individuals with Type II DM for whom diet alone cannot control hyperglycemia. Examples are found in Table 5-2. Their primary action is to increase insulin production by affecting existing beta-cell function. The most serious side effect is hypoglycemia, particularly with chlorpropamide (Diabenese), which has a 60-h duration and an average half-life of 36 h. Hypoglycemia involving the oral hypoglycemics can be severe and persistent. Nursing monitoring must be diligent. Oral hypoglycemics should be omitted several days before planned surgery. Any condition, situation, or medication that enhances the hypoglycemic ef-

**T A B L E   5 - 2   Sulfonylurea Oral Hypoglycemia Agents**

| Generic/trade name(s) | Usual dose (mg)/administration | Maximum dose (mg) | Duration of action (h) |
|---|---|---|---|
| tolbutamide/Orinase | 500-2,000/divided | 3,000 | 6-12 |
| chlorpropamide/Diabenese | 100-500/single | 750 | 60 |
| acetohexamide/Dymelor | 250-1,500/single or divided | 1,500 | 12-24 |
| tolazamide/Tolinase | 100-750/single or divided | 1,000 | 12-24 |
| glyburide/Micronase, Glynase, Diabeta | 1.25-10/single or divided | 20 | 12-24 |
| glypizide/Glucotrol | 5-25/single or divided | 40 | 10-24 |
| glibornuride | 12.5-75/single or divided | 100 | 12-24 |

**T A B L E  5 - 3  Types of Insulin***

| Insulin type | Examples | Onset of action (h)/SC injection | Peak action (h) | Duration (h) | Mixture compatibilities |
|---|---|---|---|---|---|
| ***Rapid-acting*** | | | | | |
| Regular | crystalline zinc insulin injection | 0.5-1 | 2-4 | 4-8 | All |
| Semilente | prompt insulin zinc suspension | 1.0-1.5 | 5-10 | 12-16 | Lente |
| ***Intermediate-acting*** | | | | | |
| NPH | isophane insulin suspension | 1.0-1.5 | 4-12 | 20-24 | Regular |
| Lente | insulin zinc suspension | 1.0-2.5 | 7-16 | 20-24 | Regular, Semilente |
| ***Long-acting*** | | | | | |
| Ultralente | extended insulin zinc suspension | 4.0-8.0 | 14-24 | >36 | Regular, Semilente |
| ***Intermediate/Rapid*** | | | | | |
| 70% NPH/30% regular | isophane insulin suspension, insulin injection | 0.5-1.0 | 4-8 | 20-24 | Premixed; do not mix |
| 50% NPH/50% regular | isophane insulin suspension, insulin injection | 0.5-1.0 | 2-4 | 18-24 | Premixed; do not mix |

*Source may be beef or pork, pancreatic extracts, or biosynthetic human insulin preparations

fects of these drugs requires close monitoring of blood glucose when symptoms of hypoglycemia arise. Common factors in the development of hypoglycemia are fasting for diagnostic purposes, skipping meals, malnourishment related to illness or nausea and vomiting, and other medication therapy (any of which adds to the hypoglycemic action of the oral hypoglycemics).

**Insulin:**  Examples of short-, intermediate-, and long-acting insulins are shown in Table 5-3.

- A split-dose (twice daily) regimen of insulin adminstration may be preferred because it allows for a higher level of blood glucose control. Daily insulin therapy usually consists of administering ⅔ of the total daily intermediate-acting insulin dose in the morning, with the remaining dose given in the evening. A rapid-acting insulin might be added to either or both doses, or a mixed insulin may be used. This regimen precludes the use of the longer-acting insulins, which are rarely used in a single dose because of the risk of nocturnal hypoglycemia.

- Multiple daily injection (MDI) (2-4 injections daily) permits better control of blood glucose for some individuals. Alteration in the quantity of food and timing of meals is a benefit to the patient who values flexibility. For the self-motivated individual who has control difficulties in spite of multidose therapy, portable insulin pumps can be helpful.

- The degree to which bovine and porcine sources of insulin deviate from the protein structure of human insulin affects the extent of their antigenic properties. Biosynthetic human insulins are less likely to produce allergic responses in susceptible individuals and are used most frequently. Beef, pork, and biosynthetic human insulin should not be combined or given to the same patient. The patient should receive only all pork, all beef, or all human biosynthetic insulin.

**Insulin delivery systems**

*Continuous subcutaneous insulin infusion/Portable insulin pumps:*  Devices that deliver a constant basal rate of insulin throughout the day and night with the capability of delivering a bolus of insulin at mealtime. The needle, which attaches to a syringe *via* a long strip of plastic tubing, remains indwelling in the subcutaneous tissue of the abdomen. Patients program their own pumps to deliver the optimal amount of insulin, based on self-monitoring of blood glucose. Patient should be alert to soreness and erythema at the insertion site, indicators of abscess or staphylococcal infection. Current literature reports a rare incidence of a toxic shocklike syndrome with these devices.

*Injection ports:*  Subcutaneous access ports inserted into the subcutaneous fat by the patient. These ports may remain in place for up to 3 days. They are constructed similarly to peripheral IV catheters, with introducer needles that are removed when the catheter is appropriately positioned. The device is secured by taping, and patients may use the port for dosage rather than puncturing the skin.

*Jet injectors:*  Deliver insulin in a fine, pressurized stream through the skin without use of a needle for injection. Absorption and peak and insulin levels may be altered by the injector, necessitating caution for the patient. Typically, onset and peak action occur earlier using these devices. Thorough training must be provided before allowing patients to use these devices independently.

*Insulin pens:*  Small, prefilled insulin cartridges, which are inserted into a penlike holder. After the attachment of a disposable needle, the insulin is injected by selecting a dose and/or depressing a button for either once each 1-2 U increment desired for the dosage (older device) or once for the entire selected dosage (newer device). Although patients must use needles for injection, there is no need for insulin to be drawn up from multidose vials, adding to the convenience and accuracy of administration.

**Patient teaching about drugs that potentiate hyperglycemia:**  These include estrogens, corticosteroids, thyroid preparations, diuretics, phenytoin, glucagon, and medications that contain sugar, such as cough syrup.

**Patient teaching about drugs that potentiate hypoglycemia:** These include salicylates, sulfonamides, tetracyclines, methyldopa, anabolic steroids, acetaminophen, MAO inhibitors, ethanol, haloperidol, marijuana. Propranolol and other beta adrenergic blocking agents mask the signs of and inhibit recovery from hypoglycemia.

**Exercise:** As important as diet and insulin in treating DM. It lowers blood glucose levels, helps maintain normal cholesterol levels, and increases circulation. These effects increase the body's ability to metabolize glucose and help reduce the therapeutic dose of insulin for most patients. The exercise program must be consistent and individualized (especially for individuals with Type I DM). Patients should be given a complete physical examination and encouraged to incorporate acceptable activities as part of their daily routine. **Note:** If blood glucose level is >250 mg/dl, exercise acts as a stressor, causing blood glucose to increase rather than decrease. Patients should monitor blood glucose levels with a monitoring device before beginning an exercise program.

**Transplantation:** Complete or partial pancreatic transplants have been performed on a small number of patients, usually in conjunction with kidney transplantation. Candidates must thoroughly evaluate the risks associated with antirejection medications vs. the benefits of pancreatic transplantation. Immunosuppression caused by the medications may promote development of opportunistic infections. Transplantation of only beta islet cells currently is being investigated as an alternative to other methods.

## NURSING DIAGNOSES AND INTERVENTIONS

**Altered peripheral, cardiopulmonary, renal, cerebral, and GI tissue perfusion (or high risk for same)** related to interrupted blood flow secondary to development and progression of macroangiopathy and microangiopathy

*Desired outcome:* Optimally, patient has adequate tissue perfusion as evidenced by warmth, sensation, brisk capillary refill time (<2 sec), and peripheral pulses >2+ on a 0-4+ scale in the extremities; BP within his or her optimal range; urinary output ≥30 ml/h; baseline vision; good appetite; and absence of nausea and vomiting.

- Compliance with the therapeutic regimen is essential for promoting optimal tissue perfusion. Check blood glucose before meals and at bedtime. Encourage patient to perform regular home blood glucose monitoring. Urine testing is less reliable and should not be used by patients with reduced renal function.

- Hypertension is a common complication of diabetes. Careful control of BP is critical in preventing or limiting the development of heart disease, retinopathy, or nephropathy. Check BP q4h. Alert physician about values outside of the patient's normal range. Administer antihypertensive agents as prescribed, and document the response.

- Patients may experience decreased sensation in the extremities because of peripheral neuropathy. In addition to sensation, assess capillary refill, temperature, peripheral pulses, and color. Protect patients with impaired peripheral perfusion from injury with sharp objects or heat (e.g., avoid use of heating pads). Teach patient to prevent venous stasis by avoiding pressure at the back of the knees (e.g., by not crossing the legs or "gatching" the bed under the knees) and avoiding constricting garments on the extremities and lower body. For additional information see **Impaired tissue integrity,** p. 361.

- Provide a safe environment for patients with diminished eyesight caused by diabetic retinopathy. Orient patient to the location of such items as water, tissues, glasses, and call light.

- Approximately half of all persons with Type I DM develop chronic renal failure (CRF) and end-stage renal disease. Monitor patients for changes in renal function (e.g., increases in blood urea nitrogen [BUN] [>20 mg/dl] and creatinine [>1.5 mg/dl] and altered urine output). Proteinuria (protein

>8 mg/dl in a random sample of urine) is an early indicator of developing CRF. Individuals with DM and with reduced renal function are at significant risk for dehydration or developing acute renal failure (ARF) after exposure to contrast medium. Observe these patients for indicators of ARF. (See "Acute Renal Failure," p. 129, and "Chronic Renal Failure," p. 135, for more information.) Insulin doses will decrease as renal function decreases.

- Be alert to indicators of hypoglycemia (e.g., changes in mentation, apprehension, erratic behavior, trembling, slurred speech, staggering gait, seizure activity). Treat hypoglycemia as prescribed (see discussion in "Collaborative Management," p. 374).

*In addition*
- Individuals with DM may experience multiple problems resulting from autonomic neuropathy, such as the following:
  - *Orthostatic hypotension:* Assist patients when getting up suddenly or after prolonged recumbency. Check BP while patient is lying down, sitting, and then standing to document presence of orthostatic hypotension. Alert physician to significant findings.
  - *Impaired gastric emptying with nausea, vomiting, and diarrhea:* Administer metoclopramide before meals, if prescribed. Keep a record of all stools. Nausea, vomiting, and anorexia can signal developing uremia in patients with progressive renal failure.
  - *Neurogenic bladder:* Encourage patients to void q3-4h during the day, using manual pressure (Credé's method) if necessary. Intermittent catheterization may be necessary in severe cases. Avoid use of indwelling urinary catheters because of the high risk of infection. For additional information see "Neurogenic Bladder," p. 167.

**High risk for infection** related to chronic disease process (e.g., hyperglycemia, neurogenic bladder, poor circulation)
*Desired outcome:* Patient is asymptomatic for infection as evidenced by normothermia, negative cultures, and WBC ≤11,000 µl.

---

**Note:**  Infection is the most common cause of DKA.

---

- Monitor temperature q4h. Alert physician to elevations.
- Maintain meticulous sterile technique when changing dressings, performing invasive procedures, or manipulating indwelling catheters.
- Monitor for indicators of infection (Table 5-4).
- Consult physician about obtaining culture specimens for blood, sputum, and urine during temperature spikes, or for wounds that produce purulent drainage.

---

**T A B L E  5 - 4  Infectious Processes Necessitating Medical Intervention**

| | |
|---|---|
| Upper respiratory infection: | Fever, chills, cough productive of sputum, crackles (rales), rhonchi, dyspnea, inflamed pharynx, sore throat |
| Urinary tract infection: | Burning or pain with urination, cloudy or malodorous urine, fever, chills, tachycardia, diaphoresis, nausea, vomiting, abdominal pain |
| Systemic sepsis: | Fever, chills, tachycardia, diaphoresis, nausea, vomiting, hypothermia, flushed skin, hypotension |
| Localized (IV sites): | Erythema, swelling, purulent drainage, warmth |

**Impaired tissue integrity (or high risk of same)** related to altered circulation and sensation secondary to peripheral neuropathy and vascular pathology
*Desired outcomes:* Patient's lower extremity tissue remains intact. Within the 24-h period before hospital discharge, patient verbalizes and demonstrates knowledge of proper foot care.

- Assess integrity of the skin and evaluate reflexes of the lower extremities by checking knee and ankle deep tendon reflexes, proprioceptive sensations, and vibration sensation (using a tuning fork on the medial malleolus). If sensations are impaired, anticipate patient's inability to respond appropriately to harmful stimuli. Monitor peripheral pulses, comparing the quality bilaterally. Be alert to pulses ≤2+ on a 0-4+ scale.
- Use foot cradle on bed, spaceboots for ulcerated heels, elbow protectors, and pressure-relief mattress to prevent pressure points and promote patient comfort.
- To alleviate acute discomfort yet prevent hemostasis, minimize patient activities and incorporate progressive passive and active exercises into daily routine. Discourage extended rest periods in the same position.
- Teach patient the following steps for foot care:
  - Wash feet daily with mild soap and warm water; check water temperature with water thermometer or elbow.
  - Inspect feet daily for the presence of erythema or trauma, using mirrors as necessary for adequate visualization.
  - Alternate between at least two pairs of properly fitted shoes to avoid potential for pressure points that can occur by wearing one pair only.
  - Prevent infection from moisture or dirt by changing socks or stockings daily and wearing cotton or wool blends.
  - Use gentle moisturizers to soften dry skin, avoiding areas between the toes.
  - Prevent ingrown toenails by cutting toenails straight across after softening them during bath. File nails with an emery board.
  - Do not self-treat corns or calluses; visit podiatrist regularly.
  - Attend to any foot injury immediately, and seek medical attention to avoid any potential complication.
  - Do not go barefoot indoors or outdoors.

**Knowledge deficit:** Proper insulin administration and dietary precautions for promoting normoglycemia
*Desired outcome:* Within the 24-h period before hospital discharge, patient verbalizes and demonstrates knowledge of proper insulin administration and the prescribed dietary regimen.

- Teach patient to check expiration date on insulin vial and to avoid using it if outdated. Also teach patient proper storage of insulin and the importance of avoiding temperature extremes.
- Explain that intermediate- and long-acting insulins require mixing (contraindicated for the intermediate/rapid). Demonstrate rolling the insulin vial between the palms to mix the contents. Caution patient that vigorous shaking produces air bubbles that can interfere with accurate dose measurement.
- Explain that insulin should be injected 30 min before mealtime.
- Explain that either making a change in insulin type or withholding a dose of insulin may be required for the following: when fasting for studies or surgery, when not eating because of nausea/vomiting, or when hypoglycemic. Remind patient that stress from illness or infection can increase insulin requirements (or necessitate insulin therapy for one who is normally controlled with oral hypoglycemics) and that increased exercise will necessitate additional food intake to prevent hypoglycemia when there is no change made in insulin dose. Adjustments are always individually based and require clarification with patient's physician.
- Provide patient with a chart that depicts rotation of the injection sites. Explain that injection sites should be at least 1 inch apart.
- Explain the importance of inserting the needle perpendicular to the skin

rather than at an angle to ensure deep SC administration of insulin. Very thin persons may use a 45-degree angle.

- Ensure that the patient understands and demonstrates the technique and timing for home monitoring of blood glucose using a commercial kit, which provides ongoing data reflecting the degree of control and may identify necessary changes in diet and medication before severe metabolic changes occur. This test also allows for patient's self-control and psychologic security.
- Caution patient about the importance of following a diet that is low in fat and high in fiber as an effective means of controlling blood fats, especially cholesterol and triglycerides. Stress that diet is the sole method of control for many individuals with Type II DM. Adequate nutrition and controlled calories are essential to maintaining normoglycemia in these persons.

---

**Note:**   As appropriate, see "Atherosclerotic Arterial Occlusive Disease," p. 96, and "Amputation," p. 564. Also see Appendix One, "Caring for Patients with Cancer and Other Life-Disrupting Illnesses," for psychosocial nursing diagnoses and interventions, p. 753.

---

## PATIENT-FAMILY TEACHING AND DISCHARGE PLANNING

Give patient and significant others verbal and written information about the following:

- Importance of carrying a diabetic identification card and wearing Medic-Alert bracelet or necklace.
- Recognizing warning signs of both hyperglycemia and hypoglycemia, treatment, and factors that contribute to both conditions. Remind patient that stress from illness or infection can increase insulin requirements (or necessitate insulin therapy for one who is normally controlled with oral hypoglycemics) and that increased exercise will necessitate additional food intake to prevent hypoglycemia when there is no change made in insulin dosage under normoglycemic conditions. Blood glucose at a level of >250 mg/dl at the beginning of exercise will make the exercise a stressor that elevates the glucose level rather than decreasing it.
- Home monitoring of blood glucose using commercial kits and possibly daily urine testing for glucose and ketones, which provide ongoing data reflecting the degree of control and may identify necessary changes in diet and medication before severe metabolic changes occur. These tests also provide a means for patient's self-control and psychologic security. Stress the need for careful control of blood glucose as a means of decreasing the risk of or minimizing long-term complications of DM.
- Importance of daily exercise, maintenance of normal body weight, and yearly medical evaluation.
- Diet that is low in fat and high in fiber as an effective means of controlling blood fats, especially cholesterol and triglycerides. Stress that diet is the sole method of control for many individuals with Type II. Adequate nutrition and controlled calories are essential to maintaining normoglycemia in these individuals.
- Necessity for individuals with Type I to use $^{100}$U syringes with $^{100}$U insulin. Various types/sources of insulin (beef, pork, biosynthetic) should not be mixed. When mixing various acting insulins, draw up the regular first, followed by the intermediate- or long-acting insulin.
- Availability of syringe magnifiers that can be used for patients with poor visual acuity. Other products that permit safe and accurate filling of syringes are also available.
- Necessity of rotating injection sites and injecting insulin at room temperature. Provide a chart showing possible injection sites, and describe the system for rotating the sites. Complications related to insulin injections, includ-

ing lipodystrophy, insulin resistance, and allergic reactions, should be discussed thoroughly.
- Importance of meticulous skin, wound, and foot care.
- Importance of annual eye examinations for early detection and treatment of retinopathy.
- Importance of regular dental checkups because periodontal disease poses a major problem for individuals with DM. The mouth often is the primary site of origination for low-grade infections.

*In addition*
- Explain the importance of inserting the needle perpendicular to the skin rather than at an angle to ensure deep SC administration of insulin. Individuals who are very thin may use a 45-degree angle.
- For any supplemental medications used, patient should be taught the name, purpose, dosage, schedule, precautions, and potential side effects.
- Assist patient with identifying available resources for ongoing assistance and information, including nurses, dietitian, patient's physician, and other individuals with DM in the patient care unit. Other resources include the local chapter of the ADA and the local library for free access to current materials on diabetes. The following are addresses of journals available to patients:
  - *Diabetes 93,* American Diabetes Association Subscription Department, 1660 Duke Street, Alexandria, VA 22314.
  - *Diabetes Forecast,* American Diabetes Association Membership Center, Box 2055, Harlan, IA 51593-0238.
  - *Diabetes in the News,* Ames Center for Diabetes Education, Miles Inc, Box 3105, Elkhart, IN 46515.
  - *Diabetes Self-Management,* Box 51125, Boulder, CO 80321-1125.
  - *Health-O-Gram,* SugarFree Center, 13725 Burbank Blvd, Van Nuys, CA 91401.
  - *Living Well with Diabetes,* Diabetes Center, 13911 Ridgedale Drive, Suite 250, Minnetonka, MN 55343.

# Diabetic ketoacidosis

Diabetic ketoacidosis (DKA) is a life-threatening condition caused by severe lack of effective insulin, resulting in abnormal carbohydrate, fat, and protein metabolism. The intracellular environment is unable to receive necessary glucose for oxidation and energy production without insulin to facilitate the transport of glucose from the bloodstream across the cell membrane. The impairment of glucose uptake results in hyperglycemia, while the intracellular environment continues to lack necessary nutrients. Glucagon secretion increases, causing available body stores of food substances to be broken down in an attempt to provide nourishment for the cells. Impaired amino acid transport, protein synthesis, and protein degradation facilitate protein catabolism with a resultant increase in serum amino acids, while the breakdown of fats results in elevated free fatty acids (FFA) and glycerol. The liver converts the newly available amino acids, fatty acids, and glycerol into glucose (gluconeogenesis) in an attempt to provide nourishment for the cells, but instead the hyperglycemia worsens because of the lack of insulin to transport glucose into the cells. The liver also produces ketone bodies from available FFA, causing mild to severe acidosis. Hyperglycemia acts as an osmotic diuretic, causing severe fluid and electrolyte losses, leading to hypovolemic shock if untreated. Individuals with severe DKA may lose nearly 500 mEq of $Na^+$, $Cl^-$, and $K^+$, along with approximately 7 L of water in 24 h.

## ASSESSMENT
See Table 5-5.

**TABLE 5-5  Comparisons of Diabetic Ketoacidosis, Hyperosmolar Hyperglycemic Nonketotic Syndrome, and Hypoglycemia**

| | DKA | HHNK | Hypoglycemia |
|---|---|---|---|
| *Diabetes type* | Usually Type I (IDDM) | Usually Type II (NIDDM) | |
| *Signs, symptoms/ physical assessment* | **Note:** Symptoms are a result mainly of hyperglycemia, intracellular hypoglycemia, hypotension or impending hypovolemic shock, and fluid-electrolyte imbalance with possible acid-base imbalance | | **Note:** Symptoms result from intracellular hypoglycemia and hypotension/ impending "insulin" shock (vasogenic) |
| *Neurologic* | Altered LOC (confusion, lethargy, irritability, coma); strokelike symptoms (unilateral/ bilateral weakness, paralysis, numbness, paresthesias); fatigue | Same as DKA, in addition to possible seizures and tremors | Tremors, trembling, shaking, confusion, apprehension, erratic behavior; may be same as DKA |
| *Respiratory* | Deep, rapid Kussmaul breathing | Shallow, rapid (tachypneic) breathing | Usually rapid (tachypneic) breathing |
| *Cardiovascular* | Tachycardia, hypotension, ECG changes | Same as DKA | Same as DKA, with possible diaphoresis |
| *Metabolic/GI/ endocrine* | Polyuria, polyphagia, polydipsia, fruity "acetone" breath, abdominal pain, weight loss, fatigue, generalized weakness, nausea, vomiting | Polyuria, polyphagia, polydipsia, fatigue, generalized weakness, nausea, vomiting | Hunger, nausea, eructation |
| *Integumentary* | Dry, flushed skin; poor turgor; dry mucous membranes | Same as DKA | Cool, clammy, pale skin |

| | | | |
|---|---|---|---|
| **VS monitoring** | BP: low (>20% below normal) HR: >100 bpm CVP: <2 mm Hg (<5 cm H$_2$O) Temperature: normal | BP: low (>20% below normal) HR: >100 bpm CVP: <2 mm Hg (<5 cm H$_2$O) Temperature: possibly elevated | BP: normal to low HR: >100 bpm CVP: usually unchanged |
| **Diagnostic tests/ laboratory values** | Values reflect dehydration/metabolic acidosis (ketosis) secondary to hyperglycemia, abnormal lipolysis, and osmotic diuresis. Fluid loss ≥6.5 L | Values reflect dehydration secondary to hyperglycemia, osmotic diuresis, and possible lactic acidosis from hypoperfusion. Fluid loss ≥9.0 L | Values reflect hypoglycemia with possible vasodilatation owing to insulin shock |
| Hgb/Hct | Elevated | Same as DKA | Unchanged to slightly decreased |
| Serum BUN/Creatinine | Elevated | Same as DKA | Normal |
| Serum electrolytes | Initially elevated, then decreased | Same as DKA | Usually unchanged |
| Serum glucose | 250-800 mg/dl (+ ketones) | 800-2000 mg/dl (− ketones) | 15-50 mg/dl |
| ABGs | pH 6.8-7.3; HCO$_3^-$ 12-20 mEq/L; CO$_2$ 15-25 mEq/L | pH 7.3-7.5; HCO$_3^-$ 20-26 mEq/L; CO$_2$ 30-40 mEq/L | pH 7.3-7.5; HCO$_3^-$ 20-26 mEq/L; CO$_2$ 30-40 mEq/L |
| Serum osmolality | 300-350 mOsm/L | >350 mOsm/L | <280 mOsm/L |
| Urine glucose/acetone | Positive/positive | Positive/negative | Negative/negative |

DKA = diabetic ketoacidosis; HHNK; = hyperosmolar hyperglycemic nonketotic syndrome; IDDM = insulin-dependent diabetes mellitus; NIDDM = non-insulin-dependent diabetes mellitus; DM = diabetes mellitus; CVA = cerebrovascular accident; MI = myocardial infarction.                                                    *Continued.*

**TABLE 5-5  Comparisons of Diabetic Ketoacidosis, Hyperosmolar Hyperglycemic Nonketotic Syndrome, and Hypoglycemia — cont'd**

|  | DKA | HHNK | Hypoglycemia |
|---|---|---|---|
| *Onset* | Hours to days | Same as DKA | Minutes to hours |
| *History/risk factors for development of crisis* | Undiagnosed DM<br>Infections<br><br>Acute pancreatitis<br>Uremia<br><br>Insulin resistance<br><br><br><br><br>*Medications:* digitalis intoxication; omission/reduction of insulin dosage; failure to increase insulin to compensate for stress of infections, injury, emotional problems, or surgery | Undiagnosed DM<br>Infections, especially gram negative<br><br>Acromegaly<br>Cushing's syndrome<br><br>Thyrotoxicosis, acute pancreatitis, hyper-alimentation<br>Pancreatic carcinoma<br>Cranial trauma/subdural hematoma<br>Uremia, hemodialysis, peritoneal dialysis<br>Burns, heat stroke<br>Pneumonia, MI, CVA<br>*Medications:* loop and thiazide diuretics (i.e., hydrochlorothiazide, chlorthalidone, furosemide); diazoxide; glucocorticoids (i.e., hydrocortisone, dexamethasone); propranolol (Inderal); phenytoin (Dilantin); sodium bicarbonate | Excessive dose of insulin<br>Excessive dose of sulfonylureas/oral hypoglycemic agents<br>Skipping meals<br>Too much exercise with controlled blood glucose without extra food intake<br><br><br><br><br><br><br><br><br>*Medications:* insulin, sulfonylureas (Table 5-2) |
| *Mortality rate* | ≤10% | 10%-25% | <0.1% |

DKA = diabetic ketoacidosis; HHNK: = hyperosmolar hyperglycemic nonketotic syndrome; IDDM = insulin-dependent diabetes mellitus; NIDDM = non-insulin-dependent diabetes; DM = diabetes mellitus; CVA = cerebrovascular accident; MI = myocardial infarction.

## DIAGNOSTIC TESTS
See Table 5-5.

## COLLABORATIVE MANAGEMENT

**Fluid replacement:** Usually, normal saline or 0.45% saline is administered until plasma glucose falls to 200-300 mg/dl. After that, dextrose-containing solutions usually are given to prevent rebound hypoglycemia. Initially, IV fluids are administered rapidly (i.e., 2,000 ml infused during the first 2 h of treatment and 200-300 ml/h thereafter).

**Rapid-acting insulin:** Usually given IV for rapid action and because poor tissue perfusion caused by dehydration makes SC route less effective. The initial dose may vary from 10-25 U, about 0.3 U/kg. Then the patient is maintained on 5-10 U/h, or 0.1 U/kg/h as a continuous infusion. Dosage is adjusted based on serial glucose levels and resolution of ketosis. When initiating the insulin administration, flush 50 ml of the IV insulin solution through the tubing to saturate adsorption sites, where the initial insulin molecules may adhere rather than be delivered to the patient.

**Restoration of electrolyte balance:** $Na^+$ and $Cl^-$ are replaced with IV normal saline. $K^+$ must be monitored and corrected carefully because $K^+$ returns to the intracellular compartment through accelerated transport into cells *via* insulin and following correction of acidosis, and therefore the patient is at risk for becoming hypokalemic. Use of phosphorus replacement is controversial, but if phosphorus levels remain low, potassium phosphate solutions can be used to assist with $K^+$ and phosphate replacement. Studies suggest that there is no difference in the outcome of patients who receive phosphorus replacement and those who do not.

**IV bicarbonate:** For pH <7.10. Its use is limited because acidosis will be corrected by insulin therapy. Excessive use of sodium bicarbonate can produce alkalosis, hyperosmolality, and respiratory depression.

**Insertion of gastric tube:** Prevents aspiration of gastric contents, particularly in comatose patients.

**Treatment of underlying cause:** E.g., infection is treated with appropriate antibiotics, and medications are evaluated along with diet and patient's habits.

**Treatment/prevention of complications:** E.g., arterial thrombosis, cerebrovascular accident, renal failure, adult respiratory distress syndrome, multiple organ failure, heart failure, cerebral edema, malignant dysrhythmias, death from irreversible hypovolemic shock.

## NURSING DIAGNOSES AND INTERVENTIONS

**Fluid volume deficit** related to failure of regulatory mechanisms or decreased circulating volume secondary to hyperglycemia with osmotic diuresis

***Desired outcome:*** Patient becomes normovolemic within 10 h of treatment, as evidenced by BP ≥90/60 mm Hg (or within patient's normal range), HR 60-100 bpm, CVP 2-6 mm Hg (5-12 cm $H_2O$), good skin turgor, moist and pink mucous membranes, balanced I&O, and urinary output ≥30 ml/h.

- Monitor VS q15min until stable for 1 h. Notify physician promptly of the following: HR >120 bpm, BP <90/60 or decreased ≥20 mm Hg from baseline, and CVP <2 mm Hg (or <5 cm $H_2O$).
- Monitor patient for physical indicators of dehydration, such as poor skin turgor, dry mucous membranes, sunken and soft eyeballs, tachycardia, and orthostatic hypotension.
- Weigh patient daily and measure I&O accurately. Decreasing urinary output may signal diminishing intravascular fluid volume or impending renal failure. Report to physician urine output <30 ml/h for 2 consecutive h.
- Administer IV fluids as prescribed to ensure adequate rehydration. Be alert to indicators of fluid overload, which can occur with rapid infusion of fluids: jugular vein distention, dyspnea, crackles (rales), CVP >6 mm Hg (>12 cm $H_2O$).

- Administer insulin as prescribed to correct or stabilize the existing hyperglycemia. Be aware that insulin, when added to IV solutions, may be absorbed by the container and plastic tubing. Before initiating treatment, flush the tubing with 50 ml of the insulin-containing IV solution to ensure that maximum adsorption of the insulin by the container and tubing has occurred before patient use.
- Monitor laboratory results for abnormalities. Serum $K^+$ should decline until it reaches normal levels. Promptly report to the physician serum $K^+$ levels <3.5 mEq/L. Serum $Na^+$ levels will increase gradually with appropriate IV saline replacement.
- Observe for clinical manifestations of the electrolyte, glucose, and acid-base imbalances associated with DKA as follows:
  - *Hyperkalemia:* Lethargy, nausea, hyperactive bowel sounds with diarrhea, numbness or tingling in extremities, muscle weakness.
  - *Hypokalemia:* Muscle weakness, hypotension, anorexia, drowsiness, hypoactive bowel sounds.
  - *Hyponatremia:* Headache, malaise, muscle weakness, abdominal cramps, nausea, seizures, coma.
  - *Hypophosphatemia:* Muscle weakness, progressive encephalopathy possibly leading to coma.
  - *Hypomagnesemia:* Anorexia, nausea, vomiting, lethargy, weakness, personality changes, tetany, tremor or muscle fasciculations, seizures, confusion progressing to coma.
  - *Hypochloremia:* Hypertonicity of muscles, tetany, depressed respirations.
  - *Hypoglycemia:* Headache, impaired mentation, agitation, dizziness, nausea, pallor, tremors, tachycardia, and diaphoresis.
  - *Metabolic acidosis:* Lassitude, nausea, vomiting, Kussmaul's respirations, lethargy progressing to coma.

**High risk for infection** related to inadequate secondary defenses (suppressed inflammatory response) secondary to protein depletion

*Desired outcome:*   Patient is free of infection as evidenced by normothermia, HR ≤100 bpm, BP within patient's normal range, WBC count ≤11,000 µl, and negative culture results.

- Monitor patient for evidence of infection (Table 5-4). Monitor laboratory results for increased WBC count, and culture purulent drainage as prescribed.
- Ensure good handwashing technique when caring for patient.
- Because patient is at increased risk of bacterial infection, use of invasive lines should be limited. Peripheral IV sites should be rotated q48-72h, depending on agency policy. Central lines should be discontinued as soon as feasible and when in place should be handled carefully. Schedule dressing changes according to agency policy, and inspect the site(s) for signs of local infection, including erythema, swelling, or purulent drainage. Document the presence of any of these indicators, and notify physician.
- Provide good skin care to maintain skin integrity. Use pressure-relief mattress on the bed to help prevent skin breakdown. Air circulation beds are recommended for severe skin breakdown.
- Use meticulous aseptic technique when caring for or inserting indwelling catheters to minimize the risk of bacterial entry *via* these sites. **Note:** Because of the increased risk of infection, limit use of indwelling urethral catheters to patients who are unable to void in a bedpan or when continuous assessment of urine output is essential.
- To help prevent pulmonary infection, provide incentive spirometry and encourage its use, along with deep-breathing and coughing exercises, hourly while patient is awake.

**High risk for injury** related to altered cerebral function secondary to dehydration or cerebral edema associated with DKA

*Desired outcome:*   Patient verbalizes orientation to person, place, and time;

normal breath sounds are auscultated over the patient's airway; and patient's oral cavity and musculoskeletal system remain intact and free of injury.
- Monitor patient's orientation, LOC, and respiratory status, especially airway patency, at frequent intervals. Keep an appropriately sized oral airway, manual resuscitator and mask, and supplemental oxygen at the bedside.
- Reduce the likelihood of injury due to falls by maintaining bed in lowest position, keeping side rails up at all times, and using soft restraints as necessary.
- Insert gastric tube in comatose patients, as prescribed, to decrease the likelihood of aspiration. Attach gastric tube to low, intermittent suction, and assess patency q4h.
- Elevate HOB to 45 degrees to minimize the risk of aspiration.
- Initiate seizure precautions. For details, see "Seizure Disorders," p. 288.

**Altered peripheral tissue perfusion (or high risk for same)** related to interrupted venous or arterial flow secondary to increased blood viscosity, increased platelet aggregation and adhesiveness, and patient immobility
*Desired outcomes:* Optimally, patient has adequate peripheral perfusion as evidenced by peripheral pulses >2+ on a 0-4+ scale; warm skin; brisk capillary refill (<2 sec); and absence of swelling, bluish discoloration, erythema, and discomfort in the calves and thighs. Alternatively, if signs of altered peripheral tissue perfusion occur, they are detected and reported promptly.
- Monitor hematocrit (Hct) results. Normal values are 40%-54% (male) or 37%-47% (female). With proper fluid replacement, results should return to normal within 24-48 h. Assess for a falling BUN value as an indicator of improved tissue perfusion and renal function. Normal BUN is 6-20 mg/dl.
- Assess peripheral pulses q2-4h. Report immediately any decrease in amplitude or absence of pulse(s) to physician.
- Be alert to indicators of deep vein thrombosis, such as erythema, pain, tenderness, warmth, swelling, or bluish discoloration or prominence of superficial veins in the extremities, especially the lower extremities. Arterial thrombosis may produce cyanosis with delayed capillary refill, mottling, and coolness of the extremity. Report significant findings to physician immediately.
- Assist with active or passive ROM exercises to all extremities q4h to increase blood flow to the tissues.
- Apply antiembolic hose, ace wraps, or pneumatic alternating pressure stockings to the lower extremities as prescribed to aid in the prevention of thrombosis.

**Knowledge deficit:** Cause, prevention, and treatment of DKA
*Desired outcome:* Within the 24-h period before hospital discharge, patient verbalizes understanding of the cause, prevention, and treatment of DKA.
- Determine patient's knowledge about DKA and its treatment. As needed, explain the disease process of diabetes mellitus (DM) and DKA and the common early symptoms of worsening hyperglycemia, including polyuria, polydipsia, polyphagia, dry and flushed skin, and increased irritability.
- Stress the importance of maintaining a regular diet, exercise, and insulin regimen for optimal control of serum glucose levels and prevention of adverse physical effects of DM, such as peripheral neuropathies and increased atherosclerosis.
- Explain the importance of testing urine ketone and blood glucose levels consistently and increasing the frequency of assessment during episodes of illness, injury, and stress. Blood glucose >200 mg/dl and the appearance of large amounts of urine ketones should be reported to the physician so that insulin dose can be increased. As indicated, review testing procedure with patient. Caution patient that DKA necessitates professional medical management and cannot be self-treated.
- Teach patient that insulin must be taken every day and that lifetime insulin therapy is necessary to achieve control of blood glucose. Explain that insu-

lin is administered 1-4 times a day as prescribed and that it may require adjustment during periods of illness or stress.

- Remind patient of the importance of maintaining an adequate oral fluid intake during illness. Anorexia or nausea may limit food intake, but patient should make every effort to continue fluid intake.

- Teach patient the indicators of *insulin excess (hypoglycemia)*, such as dizziness, impaired mentation, irritability, pallor, and tremors; and *insulin deficiency (hyperglycemia)*, such as increased polyuria and polydipsia and dry and flushed skin. Teach patient the importance of receiving prompt treatment if any of these indicators occurs.

- Explain the importance of dietary changes as prescribed by the physician. Typically the patient is put on a fixed-calorie American Diabetes Association (ADA) diet composed of 60% carbohydrates, 20%-30% fats, and 12%-20% proteins. Explain that the fats should be polyunsaturated and the proteins chosen from low-fat sources. Teach patient the importance of eating three meals a day at regularly scheduled times and a bedtime snack.

- Explain the causes for adjustments in insulin dose: (1) increased or decreased food intake; (2) any physical (e.g., exercise) or emotional stress. Teach patient that exercise and emotional stress increase release of glucose from the liver, which may increase insulin demand. Instruct patient to monitor blood glucose and urine ketone levels closely during periods of increased emotional stress and periods of increased or decreased exercise and to adjust insulin dose accordingly.

- Explain that persons with diabetes are susceptible to infection and that preventive measures, such as good hygiene and meticulous daily foot care, are necessary to prevent infection. Stress the importance of avoiding exposure to communicable diseases, and explain that the following indicators of infection necessitate prompt medical treatment: fever, chills, increased HR, diaphoresis, nausea, and vomiting. In addition, teach patient and significant others to be alert to wounds or cuts that do not heal, burning or pain with urination, and a productive cough.

- Instruct patient to implement the following therapy when becoming ill for any reason:
  - Do not alter insulin or sulfonylurea dosage unless physician has prescribed a supplemental regimen to be implemented by individuals with Type I DM for hyperglycemia secondary to illness.
  - Perform blood glucose monitoring and urine ketone checks q3h, and promptly report glucose >300 mg/dl and positive ketones to the physician.
  - Implement small, frequent meals of soft, easily digestible, nourishing foods if regular meals are not tolerated.
  - Maintain adequate hydration, particularly if diarrhea, vomiting, or fever is persistent.
  - Use a balance of regular sodas or juices and water to ensure adequate calories yet prevent hyperosmolality due to sugars in the beverages.
  - Report any of the above conditions to the physician to gain further insight into treatment modalities/prevention of dehydration.

- Provide the address of the ADA for acquisition of pamphlets and magazines related to the disease, its complications, and appropriate treatment: American Diabetes Association, Inc.,18 East 48th Street, New York, NY 10017.

---

**Note:**  Also see psychosocial nursing diagnoses and interventions in Appendix One, "Caring for Patients with Cancer and Other Life-Disrupting Illnesses," p. 753.

---

## PATIENT-FAMILY TEACHING AND DISCHARGE PLANNING
See **Knowledge deficit:** Cause, prevention, and treatment of DKA, above.

# Hyperosmolar hyperglycemic nonketotic syndrome

Hyperosmolar hyperglycemic nonketotic (HHNK) syndrome, also known as hyperosmolar coma, nonketotic hyperosmolar coma, hyperosmolar nonketotic syndrome, hyperosmolar hyperglycemic nonketotic coma, and nonketotic hyperglycemic hyperosmolar coma, is a life-threatening emergency resulting from a lack of effective insulin, which causes severe hyperglycemia. Usually patients are elderly, with undiagnosed or inadequately treated Type II diabetes mellitus (DM). Often HHNK is precipitated by a stressor, such as trauma or infection, that increases insulin demand. It is believed that enough insulin is present to prevent lipolysis and the formation of ketone bodies, thereby preventing acidosis, but not enough to prevent hyperglycemia. Without adequate insulin to facilitate transport into cells, glucose molecules accumulate in the bloodstream, causing serum hyperosmolality with resultant osmotic diuresis and simultaneous loss of electrolytes, most notably $K^+$, $Na^+$, and phosphate. Patients may lose up to 25% of their total body water. Fluids are pulled from individual body cells by increasing serum hyperosmolality and extracellular fluid loss, causing intracellular dehydration and body cell shrinkage. Neurologic deficits (i.e., slowed mentation, confusion, seizures, strokelike symptoms, or coma) can occur as a result. Loss of extracellular fluid stimulates aldosterone release, which facilitates $Na^+$ retention and prevents further loss of $K^+$. However, the aldosterone cannot halt severe dehydration. As extracellular volume decreases, blood viscosity increases, causing slowing of blood flow. Thromboemboli are common because of increased blood viscosity, enhanced platelet aggregation and adhesiveness, and possibly patient immobility. Cardiac work load is increased and may lead to myocardial infarction (MI). Renal blood flow is decreased, potentially resulting in renal impairment or failure. Cerebrovascular accident (CVA) may result from thromboemboli or decreased cerebral perfusion. These severe complications, in addition to the initial precipitating disorder, contribute to a mortality rate of 10%-25%.

Unlike diabetic ketoacidosis (DKA), in which acidosis produces severe symptoms requiring fairly prompt hospitalization, symptoms of HHNK develop more slowly and frequently are nonspecific. The cardinal symptoms of polyuria and polydipsia are noted first, but may be ignored by elders or their families. Neurologic deficits may be mistaken for signs of impending CVA or senility. The similarity of these symptoms to those of other disease processes common to this age group may delay differential diagnosis and treatment, allowing progression of pathophysiologic processes with resultant hypovolemic shock and multiple organ failure.

## ASSESSMENT

See Table 5-5. **Note:** Patients with HHNK usually are >50 years of age and may have preexisting cardiac or pulmonary disorders. Assessment results often cannot be evaluated based on accepted normal values. Evaluate results based on what is normal or optimal for the individual patient. CVP, HR, and BP should be evaluated in terms of deviations from the patient's baseline and concurrent clinical status.

## DIAGNOSTIC TESTS

- *Serum electrolytes:* Serum values change as osmotic diuresis progresses. At the late stages, the patient may reflect the following electrolyte values/losses:
  - $Na^+$: 125-160 mEq/L. Although the patient has lost large quantities of $Na^+$, osmotic diuresis causes abnormally high blood concentration. The $Na^+$ value may appear high despite probable $Na^+$ deficits.
  - $K^+$: <3.5 mEq/L.
  - $Cl^-$: <95 mEq/L.
  - Phosphorus: <1.7 mEq/L.
  - Magnesium: <1.5 mEq/L.

- *Serum osmolality:* Will be >350 mOsm/L. A quick bedside calculation of serum osmolality can be obtained by using this formula:

$$2(Na^+ + K^+) + \frac{BUN(mg/dl)}{2.8} + \frac{glucose\ (mg/dl)}{18} = mOsm/L$$

*For example:* $Na^+ = 140$; $K^+ = 4.5$; BUN = 20; glucose = 120

$$2\ (140 + 4.5) + \frac{20}{2.8} + \frac{120}{18} = 2\ (144.5) + 7 + 6.7$$

$$289 + 7 + 6.7 = 302.7\ mOsm/L$$

- See Table 5-5 for a discussion of other diagnostic tests.

## COMPLICATIONS

Complications of HHNK include arterial thrombosis, CVA, renal failure, heart failure, multiple organ failure, cerebral edema, malignant dysrhythmias, and gram negative sepsis (from infection that may have caused the problem to ensue).

## COLLABORATIVE MANAGEMENT

**Fluid replacement:**    Usually 0.9% normal saline or 0.45% saline is administered at 200-300 ml/h until the plasma glucose is 200-300 mg/dl. For the first 2 h of fluid infusion, >1,000 ml/h may be initiated to correct the hypovolemia and hypotension; 6-20 L may be given in the first 24 h. Dextrose solutions (i.e., $D_5W$ with 0.45% saline or $D_5W$ with 0.9% saline) are administered when blood glucose reaches 200-300 mg/dl. CVP measurements, coupled with thorough cardiovascular and pulmonary physical assessments, can be used to guide therapy and assess tolerance to the rapid fluid infusion.

**Rapid-acting insulin:**    Initial dose of 10-25 U (0.3 U/kg) followed by continuous infusion of 5-10 U/h (0.1 U/kg/h) of regular insulin until blood glucose level is lowered to 200-250 mg/dl, at which time the infusion should be decreased to 2-3 U/h. SC administration is less predictable if the patient is hypotensive, because tissue perfusion is decreased throughout the body, sometimes profoundly to the skin. Dosage is adjusted based on serial glucose levels and resolution of ketosis. When initiating insulin by continuous solution, 50 ml of the insulin IV solution should be flushed through the tubing to saturate adsorption sites, where the initial insulin molecules may adhere rather than be delivered to the patient. If the insulin is ineffective in reducing blood glucose, consider a possible insulin resistance.

**Restoration of electrolyte balance:**    $Na^+$ and $Cl^-$ are replaced with IV normal saline, and $K^+$ is replaced with 10-40 mEq of KCl or potassium phosphate if the patient also needs phosphorus replacement. All electrolytes are replaced carefully because fluid and electrolytes will be shifting between fluid compartments as the fluids are replaced and insulin is administered.

**Bicarbonate therapy for management of acidosis:**    50 mEq (1 Bristojet) of bicarbonate given for pH <7.10. Lactic acidosis begins to resolve *via* insulin, oxygen/ventilation, and fluid therapies. Bicarbonate may be administered *via* continuous infusion or bolus therapy, using ABG values to guide therapy.

**Supportive care:**    Protective measures are instituted for the neurologically impaired or patients in a coma. These include seizure precautions, endotracheal intubation, placement of indwelling urinary catheter, insertion of a gastric tube, pressure-relieving mattress, specialty bed, and possibly restraints for patients who are confused or agitated.

## NURSING DIAGNOSES AND INTERVENTIONS

**Knowledge deficit:**   Causes, prevention, and treatment of HHNK
*Desired outcome:*   Within the 24-h period before hospital discharge, patient verbalizes understanding of the causes, prevention, and treatment of HHNK.

- Determine patient's understanding of HHNK and its treatment. Enable patient to verbalize fears and feelings about the diagnosis; correct any misconceptions. As needed, explain the disease process of DM and HHNK and the common early symptoms of worsening diabetes, including polyuria, polydipsia, polyphagia, dry and flushed skin, and increased irritability.
- Teach the importance of testing urine acetone and blood glucose levels qid or as prescribed before meals and at bedtime. Explain that blood glucose >200 mg/dl should be reported to the physician so that insulin dose can be increased. As indicated, review testing procedure with patient.
- Stress the importance of dietary changes as prescribed by the physician. Typically the person with Type II DM is obese and will be on a reduced-calorie diet with fixed amounts of carbohydrate, fat, and protein. Explain that the fats should be polyunsaturated and the proteins chosen from low-fat sources. Teach patient the importance of eating three meals a day at regularly scheduled times and a bedtime snack. Explain that increased or decreased food intake will necessitate an adjustment in insulin dosage. Provide a referral to a dietitian as needed.
- Caution patient about the importance of taking oral hypoglycemic agents as prescribed. In addition, explain that exogenous insulin may be required during periods of physical and emotional stress and that blood glucose levels should be monitored closely during these times.
- For patients with Type II DM, explain the benefits of regular exercise for maintaining blood glucose levels. Exercise increases insulin effectiveness and reduces serum triglyceride and cholesterol levels, thus also decreasing the risk of atherosclerosis. Aerobic exercises, such as walking or swimming, are most effective in lowering blood glucose levels. Caution patient always to monitor blood glucose level before exercise. A level >250 mg/dl is indicative of abnormal metabolism. In this case exercise would be a stressor, resulting in further elevation of blood glucose.
- Explain the need for measures to prevent infection, such as good hygiene and meticulous daily foot care. Stress the importance of avoiding exposure to communicable diseases. Explain that the following indicators of infection necessitate prompt medical treatment: fever, chills, tachycardia, diaphoresis, and nausea and vomiting. In addition, teach patient and significant others to be alert to wounds or cuts that do not heal, burning or pain with urination, and cough that is productive of sputum.
- Provide booklets or pamphlets from the American Diabetes Association or pharmaceutical companies about diabetes and appropriate treatment.

---

**Note:**  See "Seizure Disorders" for **High risk for trauma** related to musculoskeletal, oral, and airway vulnerability secondary to seizure activity, p. 292. See "Diabetic Ketoacidosis" for **Fluid volume deficit,** p. 367; **High risk for infection,** p. 368; and **Altered peripheral tissue perfusion,** p. 369. For psychosocial nursing diagnoses and interventions, see Appendix One, "Caring for Patients with Cancer and Other Life-Disrupting Illnesses," p. 753.

---

PATIENT-FAMILY TEACHING AND DISCHARGE PLANNING
See **Knowledge deficit:** Causes, prevention, and treatment of HHNK, p. 372.

# Hypoglycemia

Hypoglycemia is a lowering of blood glucose caused by an excessive dose of insulin or oral hypoglycemic agents, skipping meals, or too much exercise without a concomitant increase in food intake. Unlike diabetic ketoacidosis and hyperosmolar hyperglycemic nonketotic syndrome, hypoglycemia can have a sudden onset, and its course is precipitous if it is left untreated. Typically, hypoglycemia occurs during the time of the peak action of the insulin/ hypoglycemic agent, particularly at night when the patient is asleep and has not eaten an adequate bedtime snack.

The patient usually becomes symptomatic when blood glucose is <50 mg/dl or there is a relatively significant drop in blood glucose (e.g., when an elder's blood glucose drops to 90 mg/dl from 180-200 mg/dl). Alcohol consumption also can cause hypoglycemia because it depletes glycogen stores, resulting in increased insulin levels. **Caution:** Mentation changes caused by severe hypoglycemia can be indistinguishable from those caused by alcoholic stupor. If hypoglycemic symptoms are misdiagnosed as alcoholic stupor and an individual with hypoglycemic is left to "sleep it off," death can ensue.

## ASSESSMENT
See Table 5-5.

## COLLABORATIVE MANAGEMENT
**Administration of rapid-acting sugar:**   10-15 g of a fast-acting sugar (e.g., 4-6 oz fruit juice or nondiet soda, 2-3 tsp honey or table sugar, 5-10 Lifesavers or small hard candies, or 2-4 commercially manufactured glucose tablets) are given by mouth. If symptoms persist for >15 min, the treatment is repeated. After resolution of the event, the patient should continue to consume a protein/complex carbohydrate snack, such as cheese or peanut butter on crackers/whole grain bread, or milk with crackers/bread.
**Glucagon:**   For patients unable to swallow, 1 mg glucagon is injected SC or IM. Glucagon stimulates the liver to break down stored glycogen into glucose and usually results in the patient regaining consciousness in 15-30 min, at which time the patient should be given a fast-acting sugar followed by the snack described above. Patients and their significant others are instructed in glucagon administration as a part of their diabetes education. Glucagon is used rarely in the hospital setting.
**50% dextrose:**   Hospitalized patients may receive an IV injection of 25-50 ml of 50% dextrose ($D_{50}$), which usually revives the unconsconscious individual in <10 min. Patients may experience hyperglycemia and headache after $D_{50}$, particularly if given 50 ml. These individuals may benefit from a protein or complex carbohydrate snack once consciousness is regained unless blood glucose has been elevated to >200 mg/dl. If the patient has frequent episodes of hypoglycemia, an alteration in dietary composition or insulin administration should be evaluated.

## NURSING DIAGNOSES AND INTERVENTIONS
**Altered protection** related to potential for brain damage or death secondary to hypoglycemia
*Desired outcome:*   Within 10-30 min of intervention, patient is alert and verbalizes orientation to person, place, and time.

---

**Caution:**   Hypoglycemia requires immediate intervention because, if severe, it can lead to brain damage and death. When the cause of coma in a person with diabetes mellitus (DM) is unknown, immediately draw a blood sample for evaluation of glucose and prepare to administer IV $D_{50}$.

---

- Administer a fast-acting carbohydrate: 2-3 tsp sugar; 4-6 oz fruit juice or nondiet soda; or 6-10 lifesavers (or 2-4 commercially manufactured glucose tablets). Notify physician if patient is incoherent, unresponsive, or incapable of taking carbohydrates by mouth. If any of these indicators occur, an IV access is required and you should prepare to administer prescribed 50 ml $D_{50}$ by IV push. Consciousness should be restored within 10 min.

- Using an appropriate reagent strip, continue to monitor blood glucose levels q30-60min to identify recurrence of hypoglycemia.
- Once the patient is alert, question him or her about the most recent food intake. Any situation preventing food intake, such as nausea, vomiting, dislike of hospital food related to cultural preferences, or fasting for a scheduled test, should be determined and addressed immediately.
- If food intake has been adequate, consult with physician about a reduction in patient's daily dose of antihyperglycemic medication.

---

**Note:** Sometimes hypoglycemia leads to rebound hyperglycemia (Somogyi phenomenon). If hypoglycemia goes undetected, the rebound hyperglycemia may be inappropriately treated with increased insulin. Suspect the Somogyi phenomenon if there are wide fluctuations in blood glucose over several hours. Notify the physician if these changes are observed or if the patient is experiencing nocturnal hypoglycemia.

---

**Altered protection** related to neurosensory alterations with risk of seizures secondary to hypoglycemia
***Desired outcome:*** Within 4 h of the event, patient verbalizes orientation to person, place, and time and is free of signs of trauma caused by seizures or altered LOC. Alternatively, if patient experiences a seizure, it is detected, reported, and treated promptly.
- Monitor LOC at frequent intervals. Anticipate seizure potential in presence of severe hypoglycemia, and have airway, protective padding, and suction equipment at bedside. Keep all side rails raised.
- Notify physician of any seizure activity; do not leave patient unattended if a seizure occurs.
- Place call light within patient's reach, and have patient demonstrate its proper use every shift. The patient's inability to use the call light properly necessitates assessments at least q30min. If necessary, consider moving patient to a room next to the nurses' station for close monitoring.
- Keep all potentially harmful objects, such as knives, forks, and hot beverages, out of patient's reach.
- If necessary to prevent patient from wandering and causing self-injury, obtain a prescription for soft restraints. Explain these safety precautions to patient and significant others.
- For other information, see "Seizure Disorders," p. 288.

**Knowledge deficit:** Disease process, diagnostic testing, indicators of hypoglycemia, and therapeutic regimen
***Desired outcome:*** Within the 24-h period before hospital discharge, patient verbalizes knowledge about DM, including testing and management, indicators of hypoglycemia, and therapeutic regimen.
- Assess patient's knowledge about DM, including diagnostic testing and management. Provide information or clarify as appropriate.
- Review the indicators and immediate interventions for hypoglycemia with the patient.
- Evaluate current diet for adequate nutritional requirements, caloric content, and patient satisfaction. Assist patient in making acceptable and realistic changes. Consider patient's activity level and need for changes to achieve normoglycemia. Refer patient and significant others to dietitian as needed.
- Review with patient the onset, peak action, and duration of the hypoglycemic medication. Advise patient to avoid drugs that contribute to hypoglycemia (salicylates, sulfonamides, methyldopa, anabolic steroids, acetaminophen, ethanol, haloperidol, marijuana).
- Stress the importance of testing blood glucose at the time symptoms of hypoglycemia occur.

- Explain that injection of insulin into a site that is about to be exercised heavily (e.g., a jogger's thigh) will result in quicker absorption of the insulin and possible hypoglycemia.
- Inform patient that a change in the type of medication may require a change in dose to prevent hypoglycemia. Caution patient about the need to follow prescription directions precisely.

---

**Note:**    Also see "General Discussion," p. 353.

---

## PATIENT-FAMILY TEACHING AND DISCHARGE PLANNING

See **Knowledge deficit,** above. Also see "General Discussion," p. 353, for general care of patients with DM.

### Selected Bibliography

American Diabetes Association: Buyer's guide to diabetes products, *Diabetes Forecast* 43(10): 34-74, 1990.

American Diabetes Association: Clinical practice recommendations, *Diabetes Care* 14(suppl 2): S1-S80, 1991.

American Hospital Formulary Service: *Drug information 92,* Bethesda, Md, 1992, American Society of Hospital Pharmacists.

Booth DE, Morris CL: Hyperparathyroidism: the overlooked disorder, *J Gerontol Nurs* 5(1): 16-119, 1990.

Bromelow I: Transformed by thyroxine, *Nurs Times* 88(8): 40-42, 1992.

Cagno J: Nursing care plan: diabetes insipidus, *Crit Care Nurs* 9(6): 86-93, 1989.

Davidson MB: *Diabetes mellitus: diagnosis and treatment,* ed 3, New York, 1991, Churchill Livingstone.

Francis B: Hypothyroidism, *Adv Clin Care* 5(2): 29-31, 1990.

Fritz ME: Periodontal disease and diabetes, *Clin Diabetes* 7(5): 80-84, 1989.

Greenspan FS: *Basic and clinical endocrinology,* ed 3, Norwalk, Conn, 1991, Appleton & Lange.

Griffiths RD, Moses RG: Implementing a holistic approach to diabetes care, *Diabetes Educator* 17(2): 125-128, 1991.

Gumowski J et al: Endocrinopathies of hyperfunction: Cushing's syndrome and aldosteronism, *AACN Clinical Issues Crit Care Nurs* 3(2): 331-349, 1992.

Hoops S: Renal and retinal complications in insulin dependent diabetes mellitus: the art of changing the outcome, *Diabetes Educator* 16(3): 221-231, 1990.

Horne MM, Swearingen PL: *Pocket guide to fluid, electrolyte, and acid-base balance,* ed 2, St Louis, 1993, Mosby–Year Book.

Huzar J: Diabetes now: preventing acute complications, *RN* 52(8): 34-40, 1989.

Interqual: The ISD-A review system with adult ISD criteria, August 1992, Northhampton, NH and Marlboro, MA, Interqual, Inc.

Kim MJ, McFarland GK, McLane AM: *Pocket guide to nursing diagnoses,* ed 5, St Louis, 1993, Mosby–Year Book.

Majzoub JA: *Disorders of the posterior pituitary.* In Kelley WN, editor: *Textbook of internal medicine,* ed 2, Philadelphia, 1992, JB Lippincott.

Marshall JC, Barkan AL: *Disorders of the hypothalamus and anterior pituitary.* In Kelley WN, editor: *Textbook of internal medicine,* ed 2, Philadelphia, 1992, JB Lippincott.

Poe CM, Taylor LM: Syndrome of inappropriate antidiuretic hormone: assessment and nursing implications, *Oncol Nurs Forum* 16(3): 373-381, 1989.

Robertson C: Coping with chronic complications, *RN* 52(9): 34-43, 1989.

Rosenberg C: Wound healing in the patient with diabetes mellitus, *Nurs Clin North Am* 25(1): 247-261, 1990.

Sabo C, Michael S: Managing DKA and preventing a recurrence, *Nursing 89* 19(2):50-56, 1989.

Saltiel-Berzin R: Managing a surgical patient who has diabetes, *Nursing 92* 22(4): 34-41, 1992.

Sands J: *Endocrinologic dysfunctions*. In Swearingen PL, Keen JH, editors: *Manual of critical care: applying nursing diagnoses to critical illness*, ed 2, St Louis, 1991, Mosby–Year Book.

Sanford SJ: *Endocrine crises and patient care*. In Kinney MR, Packa DR, Dunbar SB, editors: *AACN's clinical reference for critical care nursing*, ed 2, New York, 1988, McGraw-Hill.

Schultz PN: Hypopituitarism in patients with a history of irradiation to the head and neck area: diagnoses and nursing implications, *Oncol Nurs Forum* 16(6): 823-826, 1989.

Selam J, Charles M: Devices for insulin administration, *Diabetes Care* 13(9): 955-979, 1990.

Smeltzer SC, Bare BG: *Brunner and Suddarth's textbook of medical-surgical nursing*, ed 7, Philadelphia, 1992, JB Lippincott.

Yeates S, Blaufuss J: Managing the patient in diabetic ketoacidosis, *Focus Crit Care* 17(3): 240-248, 1990.

# 6 GASTRO-INTESTINAL DISORDERS

Section One   Disorders of the Mouth and Esophagus   379
   Stomatitis   379
   Hiatal hernia and reflux esophagitis   382
   Achalasia   386
Section Two   Disorders of the Stomach and Intestines   389
   Peptic ulcers   389
   Malabsorption/Maldigestion   394
   Obstructive processes   398
   Hernia   402
   Peritonitis   404
   Appendicitis   407
   Hemorrhoids   411
Section Three   Intestinal Neoplasms and Inflammatory Processes   414
   Diverticulosis/Diverticulitis   414
   Colorectal cancer   417
   Polyps/Familial adenomatous polyposis   420
   Ulcerative colitis   421
   Crohn's disease   428
   Fecal diversions   434
Section Four   Abdominal Trauma   439
Section Five   Hepatic and Biliary Disorders   449
   Hepatitis   450
   Cirrhosis   457
   Cholelithiasis and cholecystitis   465
Section Six   Pancreatic Disorders   470
   Pancreatitis   470
   Pancreatic tumors   476
Selected Bibliography   479

# Section One:   Disorders of the Mouth and Esophagus

## Stomatitis

Inflammatory and infectious diseases of the mouth are commonly overlooked in the debilitated hospitalized patient. Typically, they occur secondary to systemic disease and infection, nutritional and fluid deficiencies, poorly fitting dentures, neglect of oral hygiene, and as side effects of irritants and drugs. Stomatitis (inflammation of the mouth and mucous membrane) is the term generally applied to a variety of mouth disorders characterized by mucosal cell destruction and disruption of the mucosal lining. It is one of the major side effects of cancer chemotherapy, occurring in over 30% of this population. It also is seen frequently in ICU patients, as well as in individuals with human immunodeficiency virus (HIV).

## ASSESSMENT

**Signs and symptoms:**   Oral pain; sensitivity to hot, spicy foods; foul taste; oral bleeding or drainage; fever; xerostomia (dry mouth); difficulty chewing or swallowing; poorly fitting dentures.

**Physical assessment:**   The oral mucosa will appear swollen, red, and ulcerated; the lymph glands may be swollen; and the breath is often foul-smelling. The lips may have cracks, fissures, blisters, ulcers, and lesions; the tongue may appear dry and cracked, and contain masses, lesions, or exudate.

## DIAGNOSTIC TESTS

In most incidences, diagnosis of the offending organism is made by physical exam. However, the following may be used in selected patients:

**Culture:**   May be taken of the lesion or drainage to identify the offending organism. The most common organism is *Candida albicans,* followed by herpes simplex virus I.

**Platelet count:**   Done if any bleeding is present.

## COLLABORATIVE MANAGEMENT

The treatment varies, depending on the type of impairment and its cause.

**Identification and attempt to control or remove causative factor(s):**   If appropriate (e.g., if poor nutrition is the cause of stomatitis, the goal is to improve nutrition and follow through with other treatments that may be necessary, such as antibiotics).

**Oral hygiene/mouth irrigations:**   The accepted mouthwash, in particular for immunosuppressed patients with stomatitis, is sodium bicarbonate with normal saline. A typical solution is made with 500 ml normal saline and 15 ml sodium bicarbonate. Oral hygiene should be repeated 4-5 times a day or even more frequently, depending on the degree of oral mucosal impairment.

**Pharmacotherapy**

*Local/systemic analgesics and local anesthetics:*   For relief of pain.

*Topical/systemic steroids:*   To reduce inflammation and promote healing.

*Antibiotics, antifungals, and antiviral agents:*   To combat infection.

*Vitamins:*   To correct deficiencies (e.g., vitamin C to strengthen connective tissue in the gums, and niacin and riboflavin to promote efficient cellular growth).

**Dietary management:**   Typically, a diet high in protein to promote wound healing, high in calories for protein sparing, and high in vitamins to correct the specific deficiency. Usually, hot and spicy foods are restricted, and the consistency of the food ranges from liquid to regular, as tolerated. Fluids are encouraged.

**Cauterization of ulcerations:**   If required.

**Dental restoration and repair:**   If needed.

**Adequate rest:**   For optimal tissue repair.

## NURSING DIAGNOSES AND INTERVENTIONS

**Altered oral mucous membrane** (stomatitis) related to ineffective oral hygiene, dehydration, irritants, or pathologic condition

*Desired outcomes:*   Patient demonstrates knowledge about oral hygiene interventions and complies with the therapeutic regimen within 12-24 h of instruction. Patient's oral mucosal condition improves, as evidenced by intact mucous membrane, moist and intact tongue and lips, and absence of pain and lesions.

- Inspect the mouth 3 times a day for inflammation, lesions, and bleeding. Record observations, and report significant findings to physician.
- Administer analgesics; corticosteroids; anesthetics, such as xylocaine jelly, diphenhydramine (Benadryl), and Maalox (or other antacid); and mouthwashes (described below) as prescribed. Avoid commercial mouthwashes, which are high in alcohol. For mild stomatitis, provide mouth care after every meal and before bedtime. For moderate stomatitis, provide mouth care q4h; for severe stomatitis, provide mouth care q2h or even hourly if indicated.
- Prepare a solution containing 15 ml sodium bicarbonate and 500 ml normal saline. Instruct patient to rinse the mouth with the solution (as often as indicated by assessments described above) to provide local relief and promote healing.
- Instruct patient to brush teeth after meals and at bedtime, using a soft-bristled toothbrush and nonabrasive toothpaste. Patients with severe stomatitis who have dentures should remove them until the oral mucosa has healed. Dietary alterations may be necessary (e.g., changing to a full liquid or pureed diet). A dietary or nutritional consultation may be necessary.
- Advise patient to floss teeth *gently* every day, using unwaxed floss.
- Advise patient to keep the lips moist with emollients, such as lanolin or any nonpetroleum surgical lubrication.
- Advise patient to avoid irritants, including smoking and foods that are hot, spicy, and rough in texture.
- Offer ice or popsicles to help anesthetize the mouth.

**Self-care deficit:** Oral hygiene, related to sensorimotor deficit or decreased LOC
***Desired outcome:*** Patient or significant other demonstrates ability to perform patient's oral care by the day of hospital discharge.

- Assess patient's ability to perform mouth care. Identify performance barriers such as sensorimotor or cognitive deficits.
- If the patient has decreased LOC or is at risk for aspiration, remove dentures and store them in a water-filled denture cup.
- If the patient cannot perform mouth care, cleanse the teeth, tongue, and mouth at least 2 times a day with a soft-bristled toothbrush and nonabrasive toothpaste. If the patient is unconscious or at risk for aspiration, turn the patient to a side-lying position. Swab the mouth and teeth with a sponge-tipped applicator or gauze pad moistened with the mouthwash solution described earlier, and irrigate the mouth with a syringe. If the patient cannot self-manage the secretions, use only a small amount of liquid at a time, using a suction catheter or Yankeur tonsil suction catheter to remove the secretions. This regimen should be performed at least q4h. As appropriate, teach the procedure to significant others.
- For patients with physical disabilities, the following toothbrush adaptations can be made:
  - *For patients with limited hand mobility:* Enlarge the toothbrush handle by covering it with a sponge hair roller or aluminum foil, attaching with an elastic band; or by attaching a bicycle handle grip with plaster of Paris.
  - *For patients with limited arm mobility:* Extend the toothbrush handle by overlapping another handle or rod over it and taping them together.

**Knowledge deficit:** Disease process, treatment, and factors that potentiate oral bleeding
***Desired outcome:*** Within the 24-h period before hospital discharge, patient verbalizes knowledge about the cause, preventive measures, and treatment of stomatitis and the factors that potentiate oral bleeding.

- Describe the causes of the patient's stomatitis, and remind patient that the best treatment is prevention.
- Explain the importance of meticulous, frequent oral hygiene and periodic dental examinations.
- Advise patient to avoid irritating foods and substances (e.g., alcohol; tobacco; and hot, spicy, and rough foods).
- Teach the importance of discontinuing flossing when the platelet count drops below 50,000 μl, or as suggested by physician, and discontinuing brushing when the count drops below 30,000 μl, or per physician's instructions, to avoid possible bleeding. Instead, instruct patient to perform oral hygiene using the mouth irrigation technique described in **Altered oral mucous membrane,** gently swabbing the mouth, teeth, and lips with a sponge-tipped applicator moistened in a sodium bicarbonate and normal saline solution.

**Altered nutrition:** Less than body requirements related to inability to ingest food secondary to discomfort with chewing and swallowing

*Desired outcome:* At a minimum of 24 h before hospital discharge, patient exhibits optimal nutrition as evidenced by stable weight, serum protein 6-8 g/dl, serum albumin 3.5-5.5 g/dl, and a balanced or positive nitrogen (N) state.

- Assess the patient's ability to chew and swallow.
- Monitor I&O. Unless contraindicated, ensure that patient has optimal hydration (at least 2-3 L/day) and a diet that is high in protein, calories, and essential vitamins and minerals. Alert physician if the need for IV or nasogastric (NG) tube feedings becomes apparent.
- Provide any special equipment to facilitate ingestion, such as straws, nipples, or syringes.
- If the patient's mouth is very painful, encourage intake of soft foods (e.g., cooked cereals, soups, gelatin, ice cream). Drinks that are high in calories and protein are especially helpful. Consider adding Polycose to beverages, and powdered milk or protein powder to food preparations.
- Encourage mouth care after every meal or more frequently to minimize the risk of infection due to the nonintact oral mucosa.

## PATIENT-FAMILY TEACHING AND DISCHARGE PLANNING

Give patient and significant others verbal and written information about the following:

- Essentials of diet, medications, and oral hygiene; adaptations that may be required at home; and the importance of monitoring for changes of LOC, which will necessitate precautions to prevent aspiration during oral hygiene (see **Self-care deficit,** p. 381).
- Importance of notifying physician if any of the following recur or worsen: oral pain, fever, drainage, continuous bleeding, or inability to eat or drink.
- Necessity of follow-up care; reconfirm date and time of next medical appointment.
- Importance of visiting the dentist at least twice a year.

# Hiatal hernia and reflux esophagitis

Hiatal hernia is defined as a herniation of a portion of the stomach into the chest through the esophageal hiatus of the diaphragm. Hernias are classified as (1) rolling or esophageal and (2) sliding or direct. When there is an increase in intraabdominal pressure, a portion of the lower esophagus and stomach may rise up into the chest. Causative factors include degenerative changes (aging), trauma, kyphoscoliosis (a curvature of the spine), and surgery. Increased intraabdominal pressure can occur with coughing, straining, bending, vomiting, obesity, pregnancy, trauma, constricting clothing, ascites, and severe physical exertion. Complications of hiatal hernia include aspiration of reflux contents, ulceration, hemorrhage, stricture, gastritis, and in severe cases, strangulation of the hernia.

The diagnosis of diaphragmatic hernia is often suspected on the basis of reflux symptoms. However, gastroesophageal reflux disease is not caused by any one abnormality. The multiple factors that determine whether or not reflux esophagitis is present include (1) efficacy of the antireflux mechanism, (2) volume of gastric contents (in the stomach), (3) potency of refluxed material, (4) efficiency of esophageal clearance, and (5) resistance of the esophageal tissue to injury and the ability for tissue repair. By definition, however, the patient must have several episodes of reflux for reflux disease to be present. Reflux esophagitis is the result of an incompetent lower esophageal sphincter that allows regurgitation of acidic gastric contents into the esophagus.

The most common type of hiatal hernia is the sliding hernia, which accounts for 90% of adult hiatal hernias. It is characterized by the upper portion of the stomach and esophageal junction sliding up into the chest when the individual assumes a supine position, and sliding back into the abdominal cavity when sitting or standing. The incidence of hiatal hernia increases with age. Women and obese individuals are more often affected.

## ASSESSMENT

Many individuals are asymptomatic unless esophageal reflux is present.

**Signs and symptoms:** Reflux esophagitis often occurs 1-4 h after eating, possibly aggravated by reclining, stress, and increased intraabdominal pressure. Heartburn, belching, regurgitation, vomiting, retrosternal or substernal chest pain (dull, full, heavy), hiccups, mild or occult bleeding found in vomitus or stools, mild anemia, and dysphagia also can occur. The older adult often presents with symptoms of pneumonitis caused by aspiration of reflux contents into the pulmonary system. Peptic stricture of the esophagus is a serious sequela of aggressive reflux esophagitis.

**Physical assessment:** Auscultation of peristaltic sounds in the chest, presence of palpitations, abdominal distention. **Note:** These findings are not diagnostic, nor are they usually helpful in making the diagnosis.

## DIAGNOSTIC TESTS

For most patients with reflux, obtaining a complete history is sufficient for starting therapy without the necessity of comprehensive diagnostic tests.

**Barium swallow:** This is the most specific diagnostic test for revealing hernias and gastroesophageal and diaphragmatic abnormalities. With fluoroscopy, a hiatal hernia will appear as a barium-containing outpouching at the lower end of the esophagus, and gastric barium will move into the esophagus with reflux. It may be necessary for the patient to be in Trendelenburg's position for the hernia to appear on x-ray.

**Chest x-ray:** Will reveal large hernias that look like air bubbles in the chest; infiltrates will be seen in the lower lobes of the lungs if aspiration has occurred.

**Upper endoscopy and biopsy:** Aid in differentiating between hiatal hernia and gastroesophageal lesion.

**Esophageal motility studies:** Identify primary and secondary motor dysfunction before surgical repair of the hernia is performed. Included are manometry, which graphically records swallowing waves; pH probe, which will be low (acidic) in the presence of gastroesophageal reflux; and Bernstein test (acid perfusion), which attempts to reproduce the symptoms of reflux by instilling hydrochloric acid into the esophagus.

**Gastric analysis:** To assess for bleeding, which can occur if ulceration is present.

**CBC:** May reveal an anemic condition if bleeding ulcers are present.

**Stool occult blood test:** Will be positive if bleeding has occurred.

**ECG:** To rule out cardiac origin of pain.

## COLLABORATIVE MANAGEMENT

Conservative medical management, which is successful in 90% of the cases, is preferred over surgical intervention. The goals are to prevent or reduce gastric reflux caused by increased intraabdominal pressure and increased gastric acid production.

**Limitation of activities that increase intraabdominal pressure:**  E.g., coughing, bending, straining, and heavy lifting.

**Restriction or limitation of gastric acid stimulants:**  E.g., caffeine and nicotine.

**Dietary management:**  Small, frequent meals; bland foods; weight reduction for obese individuals; food restriction 2-3 h before reclining; refraining from fatty foods, acidic foods, chocolate, and alcohol.

**Elevation of HOB:**  Using 4- to 10-inch blocks to prevent postural reflux at night, depending on the severity of the reflux; the more severe, the higher the blocks.

**Restriction of tight, waist-constricting clothing.**

**Pharmacotherapy**

*Antacids:*  To neutralize gastric acid.

*Histamine $H_2$-receptor blockers:*  For example, ranitidine and cimetidine to suppress acid secretion.

*Sucralfate (Carafate):*  Binds to the esophageal mucosa and acts as a physical barrier that prevents mucosal injury.

*Gastrointestinal stimulators:*  E.g., metaclopromide to augment gastric emptying and increase lower esophageal sphincter (LES) pressure.

*Selective anticholinergics and selective prokinetics:*  E.g., pirenzepine and bethanechol to promote gastric motility and prevent reflux.

*Antiemetics, cough suppressants, and stool softeners:*  To prevent increased intraabdominal pressure from vomiting, coughing, and straining with bowel movements.

**Surgery:**  To restore gastroesophageal integrity and prevent reflux if symptoms do not resolve and complications (obstruction, bleeding, aspiration) occur. The most common procedure is a fundoplication, in which a portion of the upper stomach is wrapped around the distal esophagus and sutured to itself to prevent reflux from recurring. Typically, an abdominal rather than a thoracic approach is used.

**Postsurgical management:**  Includes chest physiotherapy to prevent respiratory complications, administration of IV fluids and electrolytes until bowel sounds are present, a gradual increase in diet as tolerated after the return of peristalsis, and in some cases, gastric tubes for decompression and feeding.

## NURSING DIAGNOSES AND INTERVENTIONS

**Knowledge deficit:**  Disease process and treatment for hiatal hernia and reflux esophagitis

*Desired outcome:*  Within the 24-h period before hospital discharge, patient verbalizes knowledge about the cause and therapeutic regimen for hiatal hernia and reflux esophagitis.

---

**Note:**   The cornerstone for many patients with reflux is a change in life-style.

---

- Assess patient's knowledge about the disorder, its treatment, and the methods used to prevent symptoms and their complications. Provide instructions as appropriate.
- Explain the following methods of dietary management: eating a low-fat, high-protein diet; eating small, frequent meals; eating slowly; chewing well to avoid reflux; avoiding extremely hot or cold foods; limiting stimulants of gastric acid, such as alcohol, caffeine, chocolate, spices, fruit juices, and nicotine; and losing weight, if appropriate.

- Advise the patient to drink water after eating to cleanse the esophagus of residual food, which can be irritating to the esophageal lining.
- Explain the following alterations in body positions and activities: avoiding the supine position 2-3 h after eating; sleeping on the right side with the HOB elevated on 4-10 inch blocks to promote gastric emptying; and avoiding bending, coughing, lifting heavy objects, straining with bowel movements, strenuous exercise, and clothing that is too tight around the waist.
- Stress the importance of the following pharmacologic regimen: antacids after meals; histamine H$_2$-receptor blockers on a regular basis, even if symptoms no longer are persistent; and sucralfate 3-4 times a day, 1 h after antacids are taken.

**Pain,** nausea, and feeling of fullness related to gastroesophageal reflux and increase in intraabdominal pressure

***Desired outcomes:*** Patient's subjective perception of discomfort decreases within 1 h of intervention, as documented by a pain scale. Objective indicators, such as grimacing, are absent or diminished.

- Assess and document the amount and character of the discomfort. Devise a pain scale with patient, rating discomfort from 0 (no pain) to 10 (worst pain).
- Administer medications as prescribed. Document their effectiveness, using the pain scale.
- Encourage the patient to follow dietary and activity restrictions.
- If prescribed, insert an NG tube and connect it to suction to reduce pressure on the diaphragm and relieve vomiting.
- Determine whether a position change would improve symptoms (e.g., raise the HOB or have the patient turn from side to side).
- For additional information, see this nursing diagnosis in Appendix One, p. 694.

## For patients with a fundoplication

**Ineffective breathing pattern** related to guarding secondary to pain of thoracic incision or chest tube insertion

***Desired outcome:*** Patient's RR is 12-20 breaths/min with normal depth and pattern (eupnea) within 1 h following pain-relieving intervention.

- If a thoracic rather than an abdominal approach was used, chest tubes may be present. Assess the insertion site and suction apparatus for integrity, patency, function, and character of drainage. Tape all chest tube insertion sites. **Caution:** Be alert to the following indications of a pneumothorax: dyspnea, cyanosis, sharp chest pain. (See "Pneumothorax/ Hemothorax," p. 19, for care of the patient with a chest tube.)
- Encourage and assist patient with coughing, deep breathing, incentive spirometry, and turning q2-4h, and note quality of breath sounds, cough, and sputum.
- Facilitate coughing and deep breathing by teaching patient how to splint incision with hands or pillow.
- To enhance compliance with the postoperative routine, medicate patient about ½ h before major moves such as ambulation and turning. If patient-controlled analgesia is available, advise its use accordingly. Be aware that narcotics will depress respirations.
- Reassure patient that sutures will not break and tubes will not fall out with coughing and deep breathing.

**Altered protection** related to risk of obstruction, recurring reflux, esophageal tear, or perforation, which can occur secondary to surgery

***Desired outcomes:*** Patient is free of gastrointestinal (GI) complications, as evidenced by presence of bowel sounds 24-72 h after surgery; bowel movements 48-72 h after surgery; a soft and nondistended abdomen; absence of reflux and severe midsternal pain; ease with swallowing and burping; BP, RR, and HR within patient's baseline limits; and normothermia.

- Assess the abdomen for the presence of distention, tenderness, and bowel sounds; document all findings. Bowel sounds normally reappear within 24-72 h and bowel movements within 48-72 h after surgery.

- Instruct patient to report reflux, a symptom that should *not* be present after fundoplication, and which may signal that the surgical wraparound is too loose. Also have the patient alert you to difficulty with swallowing or burping, which may be indicative of a wraparound that is too tight and may lead to obstruction.
- Patient will have an NG tube after surgery, which often will remain in place until the esophagus has healed. Assess for patency immediately after surgery, hourly for 6 h, and then q2-3h for 24 h. Generally the surgeon will prescribe a specific irrigating solution. If a specific irrigating solution has not been prescribed, check for patency by instilling 10 ml normal saline and aspirating the same amount. Do not leave the tube connected to low intermittent suction unless specifically prescribed, because this may lead to ulceration. If suction is prescribed, check settings q8h: low is ≤20 cm suction. **Caution:** Do not attempt to replace or manipulate the NG tube, because esophageal perforation can occur. It may be necessary to restrain the hands of patients who attempt to remove or reposition the tube.
- Take measures to decrease intraabdominal pressure, which may cause disruption of the suture line: Control nausea and vomiting; prohibit the use of straws, which can cause aerophagia; and introduce food and fluids gradually and in small amounts because the stomach will have decreased storage capacity. When fluids are allowed, administer them in amounts <60 ml/h, and be alert to indicators of esophageal tear (see following).
- An esophageal tear or perforation can be a complication of the surgery. Be alert to and report the following indicators: severe midsternal pain, a drop in BP, and increases in TPR.
- Teach patient the signs and symptoms of the potential complications, and stress the importance of reporting them to staff member promptly if they occur.

---

**Note:**  See "Providing Nutritional Support," p. 669, for information regarding administering NG tube feedings. See Appendix One for nursing diagnoses and interventions in "Caring for Preoperative and Postoperative Patients," p. 693.

---

## PATIENT-FAMILY TEACHING AND DISCHARGE PLANNING

Give patient and significant others verbal and written information about the following:

- Importance of dietary management and activity restrictions (see **Knowledge deficit,** p. 384).
- Medications, including drug name, dosage, schedule, purpose, precautions, and potential side effects.
- Indicators that signal recurrence of hernia or reflux (which happens only rarely following surgery): dysphagia, hematemesis, and increased pain.
- Importance of follow-up care; reconfirm date and time of next medical appointment.
- Care of incision, including dressing changes. Ensure that the patient can verbalize indicators of infection (e.g., increasing pain, local warmth, fever, purulent drainage, swelling, and foul odor).
- Procedure for enteral feedings and care of tubes, if appropriate.

# Achalasia

Achalasia (cardiospasm) is a chronic, progressive motor disorder that affects the lower two-thirds of the esophagus. It is characterized by ineffective peristalsis, a hypertonic lower esophageal sphincter (LES) that does not relax in response to swallowing, and esophageal dilatation. The exact cause of achalasia is unknown, but evidence indicates there is an impairment in the innervative response of the esophagus to parasympathetic activity. Complications of achalasia include esophagitis with edema and hemorrhage, respiratory complications caused by aspiration of esophageal contents, malnutrition, and a probable predisposition for esophageal carcinoma. On occasion, a gastric carcinoma may mimic achalasia (pseudoachalasia).

## ASSESSMENT

As the disease progresses, symptoms increase in severity and frequency.

**Signs and symptoms:** Dysphagia; halitosis; feeling of fullness in the chest; weight loss; and retrosternal pain during or after meals, which can radiate to the back, neck, and arms. In addition, regurgitation of esophageal contents can occur when the patient is horizontal, and nocturnal choking can occur during the later stages of the disorder.

## DIAGNOSTIC TESTS

Barium swallow, esophageal motility studies, and upper endoscopy usually are performed. See "Hiatal Hernia," p. 383 for a description of these tests. In addition, computerized tomography (CT) scan and endoscopic ultrasonography may be employed. Some researchers have suggested that endoscopic ultrasonography may be superior to CT scanning for staging esophageal malignancies, and therefore this technique may help differentiate between achalasia and pseudoachalasia.

## COLLABORATIVE MANAGEMENT

Medical management strives toward relieving symptoms caused by the LES obstruction and emptying esophageal contents.

**Activity/positional alterations:** The patient is instructed to remain upright after meals, wait 2-4 h after a meal before lying down, and sleep with the HOB elevated or raised on 4-10 inch blocks. In addition, to help increase hydrostatic pressure and thereby facilitate swallowing, patients are taught to arch their backs, flex their chins toward their chests, and strain (Valsalva's maneuver) while swallowing.

**Dietary management:** Small, frequent meals are recommended. The patient is taught to eat and drink slowly in a relaxed environment; avoid rough foods and foods that can cause discomfort, such as spices, stimulants, and cold fluids; and drink fluids with meals to enhance movement of food into the stomach.

**Pharmacotherapy:** Salicylates and nonsteroidal antiinflammatory agents are contraindicated because they can cause ulceration.

*Antacids:* To reduce the amount of gastric acid and relieve pain. However, reflux esophagitis rarely is a problem because the LES is often closed, preventing any significant reflux.

*Nitrates:* For direct relaxation of the smooth muscle fibers of the LES and improvement of esophageal emptying. Nitrates may cause headaches in a third of the individuals who use them.

*Calcium channel blockers:* Nifedipine and diltiazem also relax the LES muscle.

*Vitamins and iron supplements:* To treat malnutrition and anemia.

**Mechanical esophageal dilatation:** Achieved by the insertion of a graduated instrument or inflatable tube into the esophagus. Balloon dilatation with sudden distention of the LES can rupture some muscle fibers and thus facilitate passage of food. This procedure is successful in in 60%-80% of patients.

**Presurgical interventions:** To correct preexisting conditions, such as anemia, malnutrition, and fluid and electrolyte disturbances. Esophageal lavage may be necessary to remove food residue in preparation for surgery or balloon dilatation.

**Surgical interventions:** Required in approximately 20%-25% of cases. The most common procedure is an esophagomyotomy or cardiomyotomy, in which an incision is made through the muscle fibers that surround the narrowed area of the esophagus. This allows the mucosa under the muscular layers to expand, enabling food to pass into the stomach unobstructed. Often, an antireflux procedure, such as a fundoplication (see "Hiatal Hernia," p. 384), is performed as well.

## NURSING DIAGNOSES AND INTERVENTIONS

**Altered nutrition:** Less than body requirements, related to decreased intake secondary to dysphagia or surgery

***Desired outcome:*** Before hospital discharge, patient has adequate nutrition as evidenced by maintenance of desired body weight, serum protein 6-8 g/dl, albumin 3.5-5.5 g/dl, and a balanced or positive N state.

- Monitor I&O; document weight daily.
- Administer local anesthetics, analgesics, and other medications (e.g., nifedipine) before meals, as prescribed, to relax the esophagus and aid ingestion.
- Monitor for and document substances patient can and cannot swallow.
- Provide oral hygiene before and after meals and at bedtime.
- During the nonacute phase, provide foods that increase LES pressure (e.g., proteins and complex carbohydrates).
- Restrict or limit (as prescribed) foods and substances that decrease LES pressure, such as fats and refined carbohydrates, as well as stimulants, such as chocolate, peppermint, alcohol, and tobacco.
- Restrict or limit (as prescribed) foods that can irritate the esophageal lining (e.g., coffee, citrus juices, and tomato juice, as well as all other foods known to cause patient distress).
- Administer vitamin and iron supplements if prescribed.
- If advised by physician, have the patient drink water and perform Valsalva's maneuver with swallowing to promote ingestion.

**Knowledge deficit:** Disease process and therapeutic regimen for achalasia

***Desired outcome:*** Patient verbalizes knowledge about the disease process and therapeutic regimen for achalasia before hospital discharge.

- Assess patient's knowledge about the disorder, its treatment, and measures used to prevent symptoms and complications. Provide information as appropriate.
- Instruct patient to avoid or limit intake of foods and substances that decrease LES pressure, irritate the esophageal lining, and cause distress. Provide patient with lists of foods to eat and foods to restrict or limit. See **Altered nutrition,** above, for additional information.
- Advise patient to avoid smoking and constrictive clothing.
- Emphasize the importance of increased nutritional intake and precautions to take while eating. Teach patient to eat small, frequent meals; chew thoroughly; eat slowly; and dine in a relaxed atmosphere.
- Instruct patient to remain upright after meals, wait 2-4 h after meals before reclining, and sleep with HOB elevated.
- Instruct patient to avoid salicylates and nonsteroidal antiinflammatory agents, which may result in ulceration and bleeding.
- If the patient is scheduled for a balloon dilatation, provide only clear liquids the day before the procedure, and instruct patient to remain NPO the morning of the procedure.

---

**Note:** See Appendix One for nursing diagnoses and interventions in "Caring for Preoperative and Postoperative Patients," p. 693.

---

## PATIENT-FAMILY TEACHING AND DISCHARGE PLANNING

Give patient and significant others verbal and written information about the following:

- Prescribed alterations in dietary patterns.

- Activity restrictions/alterations.
- Medications, including drug name, dosage, schedule, purpose, precautions, and potential side effects.
- Need for follow-up care; confirm date and time of next medical appointment.

# Section Two:  Disorders of the Stomach and Intestines

## Peptic ulcers

Peptic ulcers are erosions of the upper GI tract mucosa. They may occur anywhere the mucosa is exposed to the erosive action of gastric acid and pepsin. Commonly ulcers are gastric or duodenal, but the esophagus, surgically created stomas, and other areas of the upper GI tract may be affected. Autodigestion of mucosal tissue and ulceration are associated with an increase in acidity of the stomach juices or an increased sensitivity of the mucosal surfaces to erosion. Erosions can penetrate deeply into the mucosal layers and become a chronic problem; or they can be more superficial and manifest as a more acute problem as a result of severe physiologic or psychologic trauma, infection, or shock (stress ulceration of the stomach or duodenum). Both duodenal and gastric ulcers can occur in association with high-stress life-style, smoking, use of irritating drugs, presence of *Campylobacter pylori,* and secondary to other disease states. Ulceration may occur as a part of Zollinger-Ellison syndrome, in which gastrinomas (gastrin-secreting tumors) of the pancreas or other organs develop. Gastric acid hypersecretion and ulceration subsequently occur.

Serious and disabling complications, such as hemorrhage, GI obstruction, perforation, peritonitis, or intractable ulcer pain are common. With treatment, ulcer healing usually occurs within 4-6 weeks (gastric ulcers can take up to 12-16 weeks to heal), but there is potential for recurrence in the same or another site.

### ASSESSMENT

**Signs and symptoms:**  Postprandial epigastric pain (e.g., burning, gnawing, dull ache). Discomfort occurs more frequently between meals and at night. With duodenal ulcer, eating usually alleviates discomfort; with gastric ulcer, pain often worsens after meals. GI bleeding, if present, is evidenced by hematemesis or melena.

**Physical assessment:**  Tenderness over the involved area of the abdomen. With perforation, there will be severe pain (see "Peritonitis" for more information).

**History of:**  Chronic or acute stress; smoking; coffee drinking (even decaffeinated coffee can increase acidity); use of irritating agents such as caffeine, alcohol, steroids, salicylates, reserpine, indomethacin, nonsteroidal antiinflammatory drugs (NSAIDs), or phenylbutazone; disorders of the endocrine glands, pancreas, or liver; and hypersecretory conditions, such as Zollinger-Ellison syndrome.

### DIAGNOSTIC TESTS

**Barium swallow (upper GI series, small bowel series):**  Uses contrast agent (usually barium) to detect abnormalities. Patient should be kept NPO and not smoke for at least 8 h before the test. Postprocedure care involves administration of prescribed laxatives and enemas to facilitate passage of the barium and prevent constipation and fecal impaction.

**Endoscopy:**    Allows visualization of the stomach (gastroscopy), duodenum (duodenoscopy), or both stomach and duodenum (gastroduodenoscopy), or the esophagus, stomach, and duodenum (esophagogastroduodenoscopy) *via* passage of a lighted, flexible tube. Patient is kept NPO 8-12 h before the procedure, and written consent is required. Before the test a sedative is administered to relax the patient, a narcotic analgesic is given to prevent pain, and atropine is administered to decrease GI secretions and prevent aspiration. Local anesthesic may be sprayed into the posterior pharynx to ease passage of the tube. A biopsy may be performed as part of the endoscopy procedure. Postprocedure care involves maintaining NPO status for 2-4 h, administering throat lozenges or analgesics as prescribed, ensuring return of the gag reflex before allowing the patient to eat (if local anesthetic was used), and monitoring for complications, such as bleeding or perforation (e.g., hematemesis, pain, dyspnea, tachycardia).

**Gastric secretion analysis:**    Helpful in differentiating gastric ulcer from gastric cancer. An NG tube is passed, and the stomach contents are aspirated and analyzed for the presence of blood and free hydrochloric acid. Achlorhydria (absence of free hydrochloric acid) is suggestive of gastric cancer, while mildly elevated levels suggest gastric ulcer. Excessive elevation of free hydrochloric acid occurs with Zollinger-Ellison syndrome. A tubeless gastric analysis involves administration of a gastric stimulant followed by a resin dye. A urine specimen is obtained 2 h later and analyzed for the presence of dye. Absence of dye indicates achlorhydria. The patient is kept NPO for at least 8 h before either test.

**CBC:**    Reveals a decrease in hemoglobin (Hgb), hematocrit (Hct), and RBCs when acute or chronic blood loss accompanies ulceration.

**Stool for occult blood:**    Positive if bleeding is present.

## COLLABORATIVE MANAGEMENT

Conservative management is preferred over surgical intervention, with the therapy aimed at decreasing hyperacidity, healing the ulcer, relieving symptoms, and preventing complications.

**Activity as tolerated with adequate rest:**    So that tissue repair can occur. The patient who is anemic from bleeding ulcers will require activity limitations and more assistance with ADL owing to fatigue.

**Dietary management:**    Well-balanced diet with avoidance of foods that are not tolerated. Three meals a day are recommended, with elimination of bedtime snacks. Consumption of coffee and alcohol should be reduced or eliminated. For acute episodes of upper GI hemorrhage, the patient will be NPO and given IV fluid and electrolyte replacement, with foods and fluids introduced orally after bleeding subsides.

**Pharmacotherapy (generally short-term and given in combination) (see Table 6-1):**

*Histamine H_2-receptor blockers* (e.g., Tagamet, Zantac, Axid, Pepcid):    Administered PO or IV to suppress secretion of gastric acid and facilitate ulcer healing. They also can be used prophylactically for limited periods of time, especially in patients susceptible to stress ulceration. These medications should be administered with meals at least an hour apart from antacids, since antacids can reduce their absorption.

*Sucralfate (Carafate):*    An antiulcer agent that coats the ulcer with a protective barrier so that healing can occur. This drug must be taken before meals and at bedtime. It should not be taken within 30 min of antacids, since acid facilitates adherence of sucralfate to the ulcer.

*Antacids:*    Administered orally or through an NG tube to provide symptomatic relief, facilitate ulcer healing, and prevent further ulceration; or they might be administered prophylactically in patients who are especially prone to ulceration. They are administered after meals and at bedtime, or are given periodically *via* NG tube for patients who are intubated. **Note:** Because of the effec-

**T A B L E  6 - 1  Peptic Ulcer Medications**

| | Anticholinergics (e.g., atropine, propantheline) | Antacids (e.g., Maalox, Mylanta, Riopan) | Sucralfate (Carafate) | H₂ blockers (e.g., cimetidine, ranitidine, famotidine, nizatidine) | Misoprostol (Cytotec) | Omeprazole (Prilosec) |
|---|---|---|---|---|---|---|
| Mechanism of action | Block secretion of acid | Neutralize acid | Coats mucosa | Block secretion of acid | Enhances mucosal protection; decreases acid secretion | Inhibits proton pump |
| Relative efficacy | + | ++ | ++ | ++ | ++ | +++ |
| Drug interactions | Few | Many | Some | Many with cimetidine; some with others | Few | Some |
| Comments | Many side effects; not first-line therapy; not for gastric ulcers | Inconvenient; magnesium-containing cause diarrhea; aluminum-containing cause constipation. Usually given prn for pain | Give 30 min before meal or at hs | Single daily dose often given at hs. Cimetidine may cause impotence and other undesired effects with long-term use | Used for NSAID-induced ulcers; causes diarrhea. May cause abortion; do not give in pregnancy | Very potent; may completely inhibit gastric-acid secretion; not for long-term use |

tiveness of histamine $H_2$-receptor blockers, these drugs rarely are given.

*Omeprazole (Prilosec):*  Deactivates the enzyme system that pumps hydrogen ions ($H^+$) from the parietal cells, thus inhibiting gastric acid secretion; used for short-term treatment of active duodenal and gastric ulcers and for long-term treatment of hypersecretory conditions.

*Misoprostol (Cytotec):*  Synthetic prostaglandin $E_1$ analog that enhances the body's normal mucosal protective mechanisms and decreases acid secretion. The drug is used in the healing and prevention of NSAID-induced ulcers.

**NG tube with gastric lavage:**  For acute, severe GI bleeding, to clear blood from the stomach before endoscopy and to prevent accumulation of clotted blood. For this procedure the patient should be in a semi-Fowler's position or higher. A large-bore NG tube or an Ewald tube is inserted. Gastric contents are aspirated, followed by the instillation of 100-250 ml room temperature normal saline or tap water, as prescribed, and the contents are then aspirated. The process is repeated until returns are clear or light pink and clot-free. Vasopressin may be administered IV to diminish uncontrolled bleeding before surgery.

**Surgical interventions:**  Indicated for hemorrhage, intractable ulcers, GI obstruction, and perforation. Common surgical procedures include the following, singly or in combination:

*Pyloroplasty:*  Enlargement of the pyloric opening to relieve obstruction.

*Vagotomy:*  Severing of the branches of the vagus nerve to inhibit gastric acid secretion.

*Subtotal gastrectomy:*  Removal of part of the stomach with anastomosis to the duodenum (Billroth I for gastric ulcer) or removal of part of the stomach and the duodenum with anastomosis to the jejunum (Billroth II for duodenal ulcer). Vagotomy may accompany subtotal gastrectomy.

*Total gastrectomy:*  Removal of the entire stomach (rarely performed).

**Postsurgical care:**  Involves temporary GI decompression with NG tube; analgesics for pain; IV fluid and electrolyte replacement; symptomatic relief of dumping syndrome (rapid gastric emptying characterized by abdominal fullness, weakness, diaphoresis, fatigue, tachycardia, palpitations, dizziness) with a low-carbohydrate, high-fat, high-protein diet, small meals without liquids, and supine position after meals; treatment of pernicious anemia (decreased production of intrinsic factor secondary to removal of that part of the stomach that contains the parietal cells) with $B_{12}$ injections; and treatment with iron supplements for iron-deficiency anemia (which might occur secondary to loss of blood or iron-absorbing surface in the GI tract). Prevention of hypoventilation and subsequent atelectasis and hypoxemia is especially important in patients who have had abdominal surgery. Deep-breathing exercises are imperative (see "Atelectasis," p. 2).

**Life-style alterations:**  Such as smoking cessation, decreased consumption of alcohol, avoidance of irritating drugs, and stress reduction therapies.

---

**Note:**  See "Obstructive Processes" for treatment of GI obstruction secondary to inflammatory edema or scar tissue formation with ulcer healing. See "Peritonitis" for care of the patient with peritonitis due to perforation.

---

## NURSING DIAGNOSES AND INTERVENTIONS

**Pain** related to gastric or duodenal lesions secondary to increased secretions

*Desired outcomes:*  Patient's subjective perception of pain decreases within 24 h of admission and is absent at time of hospital discharge, as documented by a pain scale. Objective indicators, such as grimacing, are absent or diminished.

- Assess for and document presence of pain, including its severity, character, location, duration, precipitating factors, and methods of relief. Devise a pain scale with patient, rating discomfort on a scale of 0 (no pain) to 10 (worst pain).

- Administer histamine $H_2$-receptor blockers, sucralfate, and other medications as prescribed. If antacids are administered *via* NG tube, use a 14 Fr or larger tube because antacids frequently plug smaller feeding tubes. Rate the degree of relief obtained using the pain scale.
- Advise patient to avoid irritating foods and drugs, especially those associated with the symptoms.
- Advise patient to eat three balanced meals per day and to avoid bedtime snacks.
- Offer nonpharmacologic methods of pain control, such as distraction, back rub, massage, and guided imagery.
- Promote prevention and control of anxiety by encouraging self-helping behaviors and expression of feelings.
- Encourage stress reduction techniques. See **Health-seeking behaviors:** Relaxation technique effective for stress reduction, p. 54.

**Altered protection** related to potential for bleeding, obstruction, and perforation secondary to ulcerative process
*Desired outcome:* Patient is free of signs and symptoms of bleeding, obstruction, perforation, and peritonitis as evidenced by negative results for occult blood testing, passage of stool and flatus, soft and nondistended abdomen, good appetite, and normothermia.

- Assess for indicators of bleeding, including hematemesis and melena. Check all stools for occult blood. Report positive findings. Be alert to Hct <40% (male) or <37% (female) and Hgb <14 g/dl (male) or <12 g/dl (female).
- If indicated, insert gastric tube to evacuate blood from the stomach and to administer gastric lavage as prescribed.
- Monitor and note indicators of obstruction, including abdominal pain, distention, anorexia, nausea, vomiting, and the inability to pass stool or flatus. For more information, see "Obstructive Processes."
- Be alert to indicators of perforation and peritonitis, such as sudden or severe abdominal pain, distention and abdominal rigidity, fever, nausea, and vomiting. Notify physician immediately of significant findings. See "Peritonitis" for more information.
- Teach patient the signs and symptoms of GI complications and the importance of reporting them promptly to the staff or physician if they occur.

**Impaired tissue integrity** related to exposure to chemical irritants (gastric acid and pepsin)
*Desired outcomes:* Patient verbalizes knowledge of the necessary life-style alterations within the 24-h period before hospital discharge and demonstrates compliance with medical recommendations for peptic ulcer throughout the hospital stay. Gastric and duodenal mucosal tissue heal and remain intact as evidenced by reduced or absent pain and absence of bleeding.

- Encourage patient to avoid foods that seem to cause pain or increase acid secretion. The response is highly individual.
- Advise patient to avoid foods and drugs that are associated with increased acidity and GI erosions: coffee, caffeine, alcohol, aspirin, and ibuprofen and other NSAIDs.
- Recommend strategies for smoking cessation.
- Stress the importance of taking medications at the prescribed intervals, not just for symptomatic relief of pain.
- Refer patient to community resources and support groups for assistance in smoking cessation or abstinence from drinking.

**Pain,** abdominal fullness, weakness, and diaphoresis after meals related to postgastrectomy dumping syndrome
*Desired outcome:* Within the 24-h period before hospital discharge, patient verbalizes preventive measures for discomfort and relates the absence of discomfort after meals.

- Advise patient to avoid high-carbohydrate meals, which precipitate an osmotic pull of fluids into the GI tract and contribute to symptoms.
- Instruct patient to avoid fibrous foods and to chew all food thoroughly.
- Advise patient to avoid taking liquids with meals and to lie supine after meals to discourage the rapid gastric emptying that occurs with dumping syndrome.

---

**Note:**   If the patient has a gastric obstruction, see related discussion in "Obstructive Processes," p. 398. Also see Appendix One for nursing diagnoses and interventions in "Caring Preoperative and Postoperative Patients," p. 693.

---

### PATIENT-FAMILY TEACHING AND DISCHARGE PLANNING

Give patient and significant others verbal and written information about the following:

- Importance of following the prescribed diet to facilitate ulcer healing, prevent exacerbation or recurrence, or control postsurgical dumping syndrome. If appropriate, arrange a consultation with a dietitian.
- Medications, including drug name, rationale, dosage, schedule, precautions, and potential side effects.
- Signs and symptoms of exacerbation, recurrence, and potential complications.
- Care of the incision line and dressing change technique, as necessary. Teach patient about the signs of wound infection, including persistent redness, swelling, purulent drainage, local warmth, fever, and foul odor.
- Role of life-style alterations in preventing exacerbation or recurrence of ulcer, including smoking cessation, stress reduction (see **Health-seeking behavior:** Relaxation technique effective for stress reduction, p. 54), decreasing or eliminating consumption of alcohol, and avoidance of irritating foods and drugs. In addition, the histamine $H_2$-receptor blockers are more effective in individuals who are nonsmokers.
- Referral to a health-care specialist for assistance with stress reduction, as necessary.

## Malabsorption/Maldigestion

Malabsorption or maldigestion refers to a condition in which a specific nutrient or a variety of nutrients are inadequately digested or absorbed from the GI tract. The causes of malabsorption are varied and can include the following.
**Postgastrectomy malabsorption:**   Frequently seen in individuals following subtotal gastrectomy, because of rapid gastric emptying and decreased intestinal transit time.
**Inadequate presence of digestive substances in the GI tract:**   Examples are lactase enzyme deficiency, which is characterized by an inability to digest and absorb lactose, a disaccharide found in milk and dairy products; bile deficiency secondary to liver and gallbladder disease and biliary tract obstruction, which is characterized by inability to digest and absorb fats and fat-soluble vitamins; and pancreatic secretion deficiency secondary to pancreatic insufficiency or obstruction to the flow of pancreatic secretions as seen with pancreatic disorders or cystic fibrosis.
**Inadequate absorptive space in the GI tract** secondary to GI surgery (especially ileal resection) and characterized by general nutrient malabsorption (short bowel syndrome).
**Mucosal lesions that impair absorption:**   Mucosal changes occur secondary to intestinal invasion of microorganisms endemic to tropical islands (tropical sprue) or ingestion of gluten in the diet (celiac disease, nontropical sprue, gluten-induced enteropathy). Gluten-containing foods include malt, rye, bar-

ley, oats, and wheat. With Whipple's disease, which is a rare disorder, a small bowel lipodystrophy occurs, resulting in impaired absorption.

**Inflammatory conditions of the GI tract** such as ulcerative colitis (see p. 421) and Crohn's disease (see p. 428), which involve significant diarrhea and malabsorption and deficiencies of various nutrients. Inflammation and mucosal ulceration secondary to chemotherapy also can impair digestion and absorption.

**Use of drugs that alter intestinal fluids or mucosa** (and subsequently affect absorption of specific nutrients). These include antacids, mineral oil, broad-spectrum antibiotics, hypocholesterolemic agents, antiinflammatory agents, oral hypoglycemics, and oral potassium chloride (KCl).

**Overgrowth of microbes in the GI tract** secondary to diverticula (outpouchings) of the small intestine, inadequate gastric acid secretion (e.g., secondary to total or partial gastrectomy or aggressive antisecretory therapy), immunologic defects, gastroenteritis, blind loop syndrome, and intestinal obstruction.

**Excessive use of enemas or cathartics:**    Nutrients pass too rapidly through the intestinal tract to be absorbed. Complications can include specific or generalized malnutrition, fluid and electrolyte imbalances, and acid-base imbalances, any of which may necessitate hospitalization.

## ASSESSMENT

**Signs and symptoms:**    Symptoms will vary, depending on the specific nutrients that are not absorbed. Patient might have unexplained weight loss with muscle atrophy, despite normal or increased appetite; diarrhea; steatorrhea (greasy, pale, foul-smelling stools); bloating; excessive flatus; abdominal cramping; and indicators of specific nutrient deficiencies (e.g., anemia with iron or $B_{12}$ deficiency; tetany and paresthesias with calcium deficiency; bleeding or easy bruising with vitamin K deficiency).

**History of:**    GI surgery; excessive use of enemas or cathartics; diseases that cause diarrhea; immunologic defects; diverticulosis; liver, pancreatic, or gallbladder disease; inflammatory/infectious disorders of the intestinal tract; medications that increase GI motility and cause diarrhea; chemotherapy.

## DIAGNOSTIC TESTS

**72-h fecal fat test:**    Increased when steatorrhea characterizes malabsorption.

**Stool culture:**    May be diagnostic of bacterial overgrowth.

**Schilling's test:**    Analysis of a 24-h urine specimen collected after ingestion of radioactive $B_{12}$ followed by an IM injection of nonradioactive $B_{12}$ will reveal below-normal levels of $B_{12}$. Further testing, during which intrinsic factor is administered, will facilitate diagnosis of pernicious anemia from malabsorption or renal disease.

**D-xylose tolerance test:**    Will show inadequate presence of xylose (an easily absorbed monosaccharide) in a 5-h collection of urine after oral administration.

**Serum tests:**    Will show depressed levels of carotene, calcium, magnesium, and other electrolytes and minerals, depending on specific malabsorption problem. In addition, serum albumin, total iron-binding capacity, and transferrin may be decreased owing to protein depletion.

**Lactose tolerance test:**    Will show failure of fasting blood glucose levels to rise and the presence of abdominal symptoms after ingestion of lactose. These signs are diagnostic of lactase deficiency (lactose intolerance).

**Hydrogen breath test:**    Will show an increase in hydrogen after ingestion of lactose. Because unabsorbed lactose is converted to hydrogen, this test is diagnostic of lactase deficiency.

**Lactulose breath test:**    Assesses for presence of bacterial overgrowth. Nonabsorbent lactulose is administered, and the breath is tested for hydrogen. With the abnormal presence of bacteria in the proximal intestine, lactulose is hydrolyzed earlier than normal.

**Barium swallow:**  Facilitates diagnosis of the specific cause of malabsorption (e.g., diverticula of the small intestine). For a description, see "Peptic Ulcers," p. 389.

**Abdominal x-ray:**  Facilitates diagnosis of the specific cause of malabsorption (e.g., pancreatic calcifications might be noted, which are suggestive of pancreatic source).

**Ultrasound of the abdomen:**  Facilitates diagnosis of the specific cause of malabsorption (e.g., abnormalities of specific organs such as pancreas, gallbladder, or liver might be noted). Patient usually is NPO 8-12 h before the procedure and will be required to lie still in the supine position during the procedure, which lasts 30-60 min.

**CT scan of the abdomen:**  Facilitates diagnosis, especially for pancreatic involvement. Patients are NPO 3-4 h before the procedure. To minimize flatus, a low-residue diet may be prescribed for 48 h before the testing. Patients should be assessed ahead of time for allergy to iodine (as well as to shellfish if patient is not knowledgeable about iodine allergy). For this procedure an iodine dye is injected, and scanning is done over a period of 1½ h. A warm flushed feeling or burning sensation and nausea may be felt with administration of the dye, and patients are required to hold several deep breaths during scanning. Oral or IV fluids should be adequate to ensure elimination of the dye *via* the kidneys after the procedure.

**Endoscopy with or without biopsy:**  The small (duodenoscopy) or large (colonoscopy) bowel is visualized through a lighted, flexible tube (endoscope) that is inserted through the mouth (duodenoscopy) or rectum (colonoscopy). The patient is NPO before the procedure. Written consent is required. Sedation may be prescribed to relax the patient, and atropine may be administered to decrease GI secretions. Specimens of tissue may be taken for biopsy or cytologic evaluation. Hemorrhage is a potential complication after biopsy, and VS should be monitored closely for 4-8 h after the procedure.

**Endoscopic retrograde cholangiopancreatography (ERCP):**  Involves passage of an endoscope into the duodenum to the ampulla of Vater (distal end of the pancreatic and common bile duct drainage system) for visualization. A contrast medium is injected into the scope, and x-rays are taken. This test is diagnostic for pancreatic disease. Patient is NPO for 8-12 h before the test and must be assessed for allergies to iodine (and/or to shellfish) before undergoing the test. Written consent is required. Oral or IV fluids should be adequate to ensure elimination of dye *via* the kidneys after the procedure.

**Hormonal stimulation test:**  Checks for pancreatic insufficiency. A collecting tube is passed into the duodenum of the NPO patient. IV secretin and/or cholecystokinin is given, and the duodenal secretions are collected and analyzed for bicarbonate and trypsin levels, which are decreased with pancreatic insufficiency. Written consent is required.

## COLLABORATIVE MANAGEMENT

Management will vary, depending on the specific cause of malabsorption and the nutrient deficiencies that are exhibited.

**Activity as tolerated:**  Patient may be fatigued and require limited activity as a consequence of diarrhea and malnutrition.

**Dietary management:**  Will vary, depending on the specific disorder that is precipitating the malabsorption. A *low-residue* diet may be useful for controlling diarrhea. For lactase deficiency, a *low-lactose diet* (avoidance of milk and milk products) is prescribed, and for nontropical sprue, a *gluten-free diet* is prescribed (see Table 6-2). Until specific problems (such as liver or gallbladder disorders) are corrected, dietary intake of fats is avoided. Any specific nutrient deficiencies are corrected. For the seriously malnourished patient, parenteral nutrition may be necessary (see "Providing Nutritional Therapy," p. 673).

## TABLE 6-2 Sample Diet Plans

**Low-residue diet**

Encourage intake of enriched/refined breads and cereals; rice and pasta dishes

Avoid fruits, vegetables, whole wheat products (cereals and breads)

**Gluten-free diet**

Avoid cereals and bakery goods made from wheat, malt, barley, rye, and oats. Also avoid the following if they contain any of the above grain products: coffee substitutes, sauces, commercially prepared luncheon meats, gravies, noodles, macaroni, spaghetti, flour tortillas, crackers, cakes, cookies, pastries, puddings, commercial ice cream, and alcoholic beverages

**High-residue diet**

Encourage intake of fruits, vegetables, large amounts of fluid, whole grain breads and cereals

Avoid highly refined cereals and pasta (e.g., white rice, white bread, spaghetti noodles, and ice cream)

Use the following (if allowed): rice, corn, eggs, potatoes; breads made from rice flours, cornmeal, soybean flour, gluten-free wheat starch, and potato starch; cereals made from corn or rice (grits, corn meal mush, cooked Cream of Rice, puffed rice, rice flakes); pasta made from rice or corn flour; homemade ice cream; tapioca pudding

**Pharmacotherapy:** Will vary, depending on the specific disorder that has precipitated malabsorption and the specific nutrient deficiencies.

**Mineral, vitamin, and electrolyte supplements:** To correct specific deficiencies.

**Antibiotics:** For treatment of bacterial overgrowth.

**Cholestyramine (an antihyperlipidemic agent):** May be given to control diarrhea when it is associated with ileal resection.

**IV fluids and electrolytes:** As necessary to rehydrate and correct electrolyte imbalances.

**Surgical intervention:** May be necessary to correct specific disorders that precipitate malabsorption, such as biliary tract obstruction.

## NURSING DIAGNOSES AND INTERVENTIONS

**Diarrhea,** bloating, excessive flatus, and abdominal cramping related to malabsorption in the bowel

**Desired outcome:** Patient is free of discomfort from diarrhea and other symptoms of malabsorption a minimum of 24 h before hospital discharge, as evidenced by passage of normal stools (soft, semiformed) and absence of excessive flatus and cramping.

- Assess and document presence of GI discomfort and symptoms, including the onset and duration of symptoms and the precipitating and palliative factors. Instruct patient to avoid foods associated with symptoms.
- Teach patient the importance of dietary compliance in the treatment for some malabsorptive disorders (e.g., dietary restriction, such as a low-lactose diet with lactase intolerance or a gluten-free diet with nontropical sprue, may be necessary to prevent symptoms). Have patient plan a 3-day menu that includes and excludes foods from the lists in Table 6-2 as appropriate.

**High risk for fluid volume deficit** related to excessive loss with diarrhea

**Desired outcome:** Patient is normovolemic as evidenced by good skin tur-

gor, moist mucous membranes, urinary output $\geq 30$ ml/h, HR $\leq 100$ bpm, absence of orthostatic systolic BP changes, and absence of thirst.
- Assess patient for evidence of fluid volume deficit: weight loss, hypotension, poor skin turgor, dry skin and mucous membranes, and thirst.
- Ensure precise maintenance and documentation of fluid I&O records.
- Administer IV fluids and parenteral nutrients appropriately and at prescribed rate.
- Encourage prescribed dietary compliance for relief of symptomatic diarrhea.
- Administer medications, and teach patient self-administration of medications, to control diarrhea or treat underlying condition.

---

**Note:** For assessment of nutrient deficiencies, see "Providing Nutritional Support," p. 665.

---

## PATIENT-FAMILY TEACHING AND DISCHARGE PLANNING
Give patient and significant others verbal and written information about the following:
- Use of medications (vitamins, antibiotics), including drug name, purpose, dosage, schedule, precautions, and potential side effects.
- Prescribed dietary replacement of deficiency nutrients and dietary management of symptoms, if appropriate.
- Problems that necessitate medical attention: nutrient deficiencies (see "Providing Nutritional Support," p. 665), fluid volume deficit, and acid-base imbalances.

# Obstructive processes

Obstruction of the GI tract is a condition in which the normal peristaltic transport of GI contents does not take place. Therefore the digestion and absorption of foods and fluids and the elimination of wastes are impaired or totally blocked. Furthermore, GI fluids become hypertonic, precipitating osmotic fluid loss from the body into the GI lumen. Subsequently, nutritional and fluid and electrolyte status are compromised and distention occurs. Increased pressure in the GI tract also can result in perforation and peritonitis or necrosis of the GI mucosa. Obstruction can occur anywhere along the GI tract, but most commonly it occurs at the pyloric area of the stomach or in the small bowel owing to adhesions in the ileum. Obstruction can occur as a result of the inflammation and edema that accompany GI disease (peptic ulcers, diverticulitis, colitis, gastroenteritis, trauma); GI surgery with subsequent edema and possibly adhesions (gastrectomy, appendectomy, colon resection); growths (polyps, tumors); adynamic (paralytic) ileus secondary to peritoneal insult, such as surgery or peritonitis; diminished GI motility owing to uremia, diabetes mellitus (DM), or use of narcotics, diuretics, or anticholinergic drugs; volvulus; or incarcerated hernia.

## ASSESSMENT
**Signs and symptoms:**   Severe and crampy pain, abdominal distention, vomiting, back pain, restlessness, hiccoughs, belching, and inability to pass stool or flatus (accompanied by a feeling of "fullness"). Symptoms vary, depending on the type and site of obstruction (Table 6-3).
**Physical assessment:**   Abdominal distention, abdominal tenderness, high-pitched and intermittent bowel sounds above the point of obstruction. Bowel sounds are absent or diminished with paralytic ileus. Patients may have decreased urinary output, poor skin turgor, and dry skin and mucous membranes associated with dehydration owing to pathophysiology of the obstruction. Bleeding may be noted on rectal exam if strangulation or tumor is present.

**T A B L E  6 - 3    Assessment of Patients with Obstructive Processes**

|  | Small bowel obstruction | Large bowel obstruction | Paralytic ileus |
|---|---|---|---|
| Pain* | Severe, episodic | Moderate, more continuous | Not prominent |
| Vomiting | Occurs early; may be projectile | Occurs late; feculent (if duodenal valve is incompetent) | Not prominent |
| Abdominal distention | Occurs late | Pronounced | Present |
| Passage of stool/flatus | None, except with partial obstruction of the large bowel, with which "pencil" stools may be passed | | |

*Note:  With obstruction associated with intestinal strangulation, pain always is severe, vomiting is present, and the abdomen is distended, rigid, and tender.

**History of:**    Abdominal hernia, recent or past abdominal surgery, GI inflammation or perforation secondary to various disease processes, DM, chronic renal failure, or use of narcotics, diuretics, or anticholinergics.

## DIAGNOSTIC TESTS

**WBC count:**    Usually elevated in the presence of strangulation or obstruction secondary to inflammatory process.

**X-ray of abdomen:**    Will reveal distention of bowel loops with air and fluid proximal to the obstruction. The presence of free air under the diaphragm suggests intestinal perforation.

**Barium swallow/barium enema:**    Facilitates quick assessment to determine presence and location of obstruction. Barium enema (to exclude colon obstruction) should precede barium swallow. Barium will not advance past the site of obstruction. For more information, see "Peptic Ulcer," p. 389.

**Aspiration of fecal matter from NG/intestinal tube:**    Fecal matter, which is identified by its characteristic foul odor, is an indication of obstruction.

## COLLABORATIVE MANAGEMENT

The specific cause of the obstruction must be identified quickly so that the appropriate treatment can be instituted and complications prevented. In the interim, management is supportive and aimed at maintaining nutritional and fluid and electrolyte balance and promoting comfort.

**Activity as tolerated:**    With paralytic ileus, the patient is encouraged to ambulate to enhance return of peristalsis. With other forms of obstruction, activity may be limited because of pain or complications.

**Dietary management:**    Patient will be NPO until obstruction is resolved (or bowel sounds are returned in paralytic ileus).

**GI decompression:**    Accomplished *via* gastric or intestinal tube connected to low, intermittent suction. See Table 6-4.

**IV fluid and electrolyte support:**    Lactated Ringer's or isotonic saline solutions (or isotonic dextrose/saline combinations) are commonly prescribed. Volume of IV fluid required often is dependent on the amount of gastric or intestinal tube drainage (replacement fluids often prescribed ml for ml). K is added to IV fluids to prevent hypokalemia. Total parenteral nutrition (TPN) may be indicated to meet nutritional needs if obstruction/recovery is prolonged.

**Pharmacotherapy:**    May include the following.

*Antibiotics:*    To prevent infection.

**T A B L E  6 - 4    Gastric/Intestinal Tubes Used in Obstructive Processes**

| Tube | Obstructive process | Purpose |
|------|---------------------|---------|
| Gastric tube* | Pyloric obstruction, small bowel obstruction, paralytic ileus | Decompresses the GI tract of retained fluids, alleviates abdominal distention, relieves edema in the intestinal wall, prevents vomiting, and promotes comfort |
| Intestinal tube*† (e.g., single-lumen Cantor or Harris tube or double-lumen Miller-Abbott tube) | Small or large bowel obstruction, paralytic ileus | See gastric tube, above. Presence of tube may promote return of peristalsis in paralytic ileus. Tube may relieve edema sufficiently to relieve obstruction, thereby avoiding need for surgery |

*In some cases, gastric and intestinal tubes are used together.
†Long intestinal tubes primarily are indicated when obstruction is partial.

*Analgesics:*  For pain relief. However, they can mask symptoms and interfere with diagnosis. Narcotics, such as morphine, can decrease intestinal motility and increase nausea and vomiting.
*Antiemetic agents (e.g., prochlorperazine [Compazine]):*  For relief of nausea and vomiting.
*GI stimulants (e.g., metoclopramide [Reglan], dexpanthenol [Ilopan]):*  Used perioperatively to minimize paralytic ileus. Metoclopramide is used with diabetic gastric stasis.
*Surgical intervention:*  Indicated for obstruction that does not subside. In some cases, inflammatory processes subside and obstruction resolves without surgery. Paralytic ileus generally resolves in 2-3 days without any treatment. In most other cases, surgery is indicated to identify and relieve the source of obstruction. Exploratory laparotomy is performed when diagnosis is uncertain. When diagnosis is known, the indicated surgery is performed (e.g., pyloroplasty for pyloric obstruction or bowel resection with or without colostomy for removal of tumor or adhesions).

## NURSING DIAGNOSES AND INTERVENTIONS

**Pain,** nausea, and distention related to obstructive process or malfunction of gastric or intestinal drainage tube
*Desired outcomes:*  Patient's subjective perception of discomfort decreases within 8 h of admission and is absent by hospital discharge, as documented by a pain scale. Objective indicators, such as grimacing, are absent or diminished.
- Assess the degree of the patient's discomfort. Devise a pain scale with patient, rating discomfort from 0 (no discomfort) to 10 (worst discomfort). Be alert to characteristics of pain, vomiting, and distention, depending on the type of obstructive process (see Table 6-3).
- Implement comfort measures to provide pain relief: distraction, backrubs,

conversation, relaxation therapy. See **Health-seeking behaviors:** Relaxation technique effective for stress reduction, p. 54.
- Administer prescribed analgesics and antiemetic agents as indicated. Assess and document the degree of relief obtained, using the pain scale. Be aware that opioid analgesics contribute to intestinal hypomotility.
- Maintain patency and proper functioning of the gastric or intestinal tube.
  - Maintain connection to low, intermittent suction or as prescribed.
  - Irrigate tube with 30 ml normal saline prn or as prescribed.
  - Keep gastric tube properly positioned in stomach by securing it with tape or other adhesive.
  - Avoid occlusion of the vent side of sump suction tubes because this may result in vacuum occlusion of the tube and excessive suction to gastric mucosa.
  - Advance intestinal tube slowly, 2-3 inches at a time or as prescribed, until it reaches the desired location. Positioning patient in various positions (right side-lying, supine, left side-lying) may facilitate passage of the tube. Do not tape the tube to the patient's skin until it reaches the desired location.
- Keep HOB elevated 30-45 degrees as permitted, to promote comfort and facilitate ventilation. A slightly Trendelenburg, right side-lying position may reduce gas pains in patients with paralytic ileus.
- Encourage turning in bed and activity as permitted to promote peristalsis.
- Provide oral care at frequent intervals. Frequent brushing of teeth and rinsing of the mouth will alleviate dryness. Provide lubricant for lips.
- Provide mouth rinses at frequent intervals to alleviate pharyngeal discomfort from tube. Apply water-soluble lubricant to naris to alleviate discomfort. Apply viscous lidocaine solution to naris or back of throat, as prescribed, to alleviate discomfort from the tube.

**High risk for fluid volume deficit** related to *excessive loss* secondary to obstructive process and subsequent vomiting or gastric decompression of large volumes of GI fluids; and *decreased intake* secondary to fluid restrictions
*Desired outcome:* Patient is normovolemic as evidenced by good skin turgor, moist mucous membranes, urinary output ≥30 ml/h, stable weight, HR ≤100 bpm, absence of orthostatic systolic BP changes, and absence of thirst.
- Ensure precise measurement and documentation of fluid I&O. Weigh patient daily.
- Take special note of the amount and character of GI aspirate. Check GI aspirate for electrolyte loss or pH as prescribed.
- Administer appropriate IV fluids at the prescribed rate. Replace volume of GI fluids aspirated by suction, if prescribed.
- Measure abdominal girth q8h.
- For other interventions, see this nursing diagnosis in the appendix, p. 703.

---

**Note:** For nursing diagnoses and interventions for the delivery of enteral and parenteral nutrition, see "Providing Nutritional Support," p. 673. If surgery was performed, see Appendix One, "Caring for Preoperative and Postoperative Patients," p. 693.

---

## PATIENT-FAMILY TEACHING AND DISCHARGE PLANNING

Give patient and significant others verbal and written information about the following:
- Specific disease process that precipitated the obstruction and methods to prevent recurrence, such as compliance with prescribed therapies.
- Symptoms of recurring obstruction to report to physician.
- Medications, including drug name, purpose, dosage, schedule, precautions, and potential side effects.

# Hernia

A hernia is a protrusion of an organ (usually the intestine) through the abdominal wall. Although a hernia can occur secondary to a congenital weakness in the abdominal wall, most commonly it occurs as a consequence of disease, age-related weakening of the abdominal wall, increased abdominal pressure, or disruption of the abdominal wall secondary to trauma or surgery (incisional hernia). Hernias can develop at the umbilicus, inguinal opening (most common), femoral ring, or at a previous surgical or trauma site. They can be precipitated or aggravated by those factors related to an increase in intraabdominal pressure, such as lifting, sneezing, coughing, straining at stool, pregnancy, ascites, and obesity. Potential complications include incarceration (hernia is irreducible in that it cannot be replaced manually in its normal position) with subsequent intestinal obstruction; and strangulation (hernia is incarcerated and blood supply to the bowel is compromised) with subsequent infection or necrosis.

## ASSESSMENT

**General signs and symptoms:**   Tenderness and bulging at herniation site; pain with straining.

**Obstruction secondary to incarceration:**   Abdominal pain and distention, nausea, vomiting (may be feculent), hiccoughs, back pain, sensation of constipation, and inability to pass stool or flatus. See "Obstructive Processes," p. 398.

**Infection or necrosis secondary to strangulation:**   Fever and possibly peritonitis (see "Peritonitis," p. 404).

**Physical assessment:**   Bulge with straining will be noted on inspection; palpation of herniation site will reveal a soft and tender mass or bulge. In men, the scrotum should be examined whenever a hernia is diagnosed or suspected because herniation at the inguinal area can cause herniation of bowel into the scrotum. See "Obstructive Processes" or "Peritonitis" if these complications are present.

## DIAGNOSTIC TESTS

**X-ray:**   May reveal presence of a hernia or incarceration. However, diagnosis is made primarily through physical exam.

**WBC count:**   Will be elevated in the presence of strangulation.

## COLLABORATIVE MANAGEMENT

Management is aimed at reduction of the hernia (placement of herniated area back through the abominal wall) and prevention of strangulation and incarceration.

**Activity as tolerated:**   With restriction of stretching and straining, and emphasis on proper body mechanics.

**Manual reduction:**   Return of the herniated area to its anatomically correct position. The patient is usually placed in Trendelenburg's position and given sedatives/relaxants to facilitate the procedure.

**Truss (firm support):**   Might be prescribed for applying pressure to the herniated area to maintain correct anatomic position. A truss is especially important with ambulation and activity.

**High-residue diet:**   To prevent constipation and straining with stools.

**Laxatives:**   Bulk-producing (e.g., methylcellulose, psyllium), surfactant (e.g., docusate), or stimulant (e.g., bisacodyl) laxatives may be prescribed to prevent constipation and straining.

**Antibiotics:**   Usually prescribed in the presence of strangulation and infection. Also see discussion with "Peritonitis," if peritonitis is present.

**With incarceration:**   Care of the patient with an obstructive process will apply (see "Obstructive Processes").

**Herniorrhaphy:**   Surgery performed when the hernia is irreducible by other means, or when strangulation or incarceration occurs. It is performed under general or regional anesthetic. Inguinal hernia repairs often are done with local or spinal anesthetic on an outpatient basis. Hernias in the upper abdomen usually are repaired under general anesthetic with hospitalization.

## NURSING DIAGNOSES AND INTERVENTIONS

**Pain** (especially with straining) related to hernia condition or surgical intervention

*Desired outcomes:*   Within 1 h of intervention, patient's subjective perception of discomfort decreases, as documented by a pain scale. Objective, indicators, such as grimacing, are absent or diminished.

- Assess and document presence of pain: severity, character, location, duration, precipitating factors, and methods of relief. Devise a pain scale with patient, rating discomfort from 0 (no pain) to 10 (worst pain). Report presence of severe, persistent pain, which can signal complications.
- Advise patient to avoid straining, stretching, coughing, and heavy lifting. Teach patient to splint incision manually or with a pillow during coughing episodes. This procedure is especially important during the early postoperative period and for up to 6 weeks after surgery.
- Teach patient the use of a truss, if prescribed, and advise its use as much as possible, especially when out of bed. **Note:** Apply truss before patient gets out of bed.
- Apply or teach patient application of scrotal support or ice packs, which often are prescribed to limit edema and control pain after inguinal hernia repair.
- Administer prescribed analgesics as indicated, especially before postoperative activities. Use comfort measures as well: distraction, verbal interaction to enhance expressions of feelings and reduction of anxiety, backrubs, and stress reduction techniques, such as relaxation exercises. Document the degree of relief obtained using the pain scale.
- For additional information, see this nursing diagnosis in the appendix, p. 694.

**Urinary retention (or risk of same)** related to pain, trauma, and use of anesthetic during lower abdominal surgery

*Desired outcomes:*   Patient voids without difficulty within 8-10 h of surgery. Urine output is ≥100 ml for each voiding and is adequate (approximately 1,000-1,500 ml) over a 24-h period.

- Assess for and document presence of suprapubic distention or patient verbalizations of inability to void.
- Monitor urinary output. Document and report frequent voidings of <100 ml at a time.
- Facilitate voiding by implementing interventions in "Urinary Retention," p. 166.

**Knowledge deficit:**   Potential for GI complications associated with presence of a hernia and measures that can prevent their occurrence

*Desired outcome:*   Following instruction, patient verbalizes knowledge about the signs and symptoms of GI complications and complies with the prescribed measures for prevention.

- Teach patient to be alert to and report severe and persistent pain, nausea and vomiting, fever, and abdominal distention, which can herald onset of incarceration or strangulation.
- Encourage patient to comply with medical regimen: use of a truss or other support and avoidance of straining, stretching, constipation, and heavy lifting.
- Teach patient to consume a high-residue diet or dietary fiber supplements to prevent constipation (see list of foods in Table 6-2). Encourage intake of at least 2-3 L/day of fluids to promote soft consistency of stools.

- Teach patient proper body mechanics for moving and lifting.

---

**Note:**   Altered sexual function may occur in men after repair of inguinal hernia, because of decreased blood supply to the testes. See nursing diagnoses **Body image disturbance, Altered sexuality patterns,** and **Sexual dysfunction,** as appropriate, in other sections of this book. Also see Appendix One for nursing diagnoses and interventions in "Caring for Preoperative and Postoperative Patients," p. 693.

---

## PATIENT-FAMILY TEACHING AND DISCHARGE PLANNING

Give patient and significant others verbal and written information about the following:

- Care of incision and dressing change technique, if appropriate. Teach patient the signs of infection at the incision site, which require medical intervention: fever, persistent redness, swelling, local warmth, tenderness, purulent drainage, and foul odor.
- Symptoms of hernia recurrence and postsurgical complications.
- Postsurgical activity limitations as directed: usually heavy lifting (>10 lb) and straining are contraindicated for about 6 weeks. Anticipate return to work in 2 weeks for office workers and 6 weeks for heavy laborers.
  - Importance of proper body mechanics to prevent recurrence, especially when lifting and moving.
  - Prevention of constipation and straining with stools, (e.g., by following a high-residue diet [see Table 6-2] and using laxatives when needed). Caution against frequent and long-term use of stimulants.
  - Medications, including drug name, purpose, dosage, schedule, precautions, and potential side effects.

# Peritonitis

Peritonitis is the inflammatory response of the peritoneum to offending chemical and bacterial agents invading the peritoneal cavity. The inflammatory process can be local or generalized and acute or chronic, depending on the pathogenesis of the inflammation. Common causes include intraoperative and abdominal trauma; postoperative leakage into the peritoneal cavity; ischemia; ruptured or inflamed organs; poor aseptic techniques (e.g., with peritoneal dialysis); and direct contamination of the bloodstream. The peritoneum responds to invasive agents by attempting to localize the infection, which results in tissue edema, the development of fibrinous exudate, and hypermotility of the intestinal tract. As the disease progresses, paralytic ileus occurs, and intestinal fluid, which then cannot be reabsorbed, leaks into the peritoneal cavity. As a result of the fluid shift, cardiac output and tissue perfusion are reduced, and this leads to impaired cardiac and renal function. If the infection continues, respiratory failure and shock can ensue. Peritonitis is frequently progressive and can be fatal. It is the most common cause of death following abdominal surgery.

## ASSESSMENT

**Signs and symptoms:**   Abdominal pain with any movement, nausea, vomiting, fever, malaise, weakness, prostration, hiccoughs, diaphoresis, abdominal rigidity.

**Physical assessment:**   Presence of tachycardia, hypotension, and shallow and rapid respirations caused by abdominal distention and discomfort. Often, the patient assumes a supine position with the knees flexed. On abdominal exam, palpation usually reveals distention, abdominal rigidity with general or localized tenderness, and rebound tenderness. Auscultation findings include hyperactive bowel sounds during the gradual development of peritonitis and an absence of bowel sounds during later stages if paralytic ileus occurs. Mild ascites may be present as well.

**History of:** Abdominal disease, peptic ulcer, ruptured appendix, cholecystitis, trauma, surgery, peritoneal dialysis.

## DIAGNOSTIC TESTS

**Serum tests:** May reveal the presence of leukocytosis, hemoconcentration, and electrolyte imbalance, particularly hypokalemia. Hypoalbuminemia also can occur.

**ABG values:** May reveal the presence of hypoxemia ($Pao_2$ < 80 mm Hg) or acidosis (pH < 7.40).

**Urinalysis:** Often performed to rule out genitourinary involvement.

**Peritoneal aspiration with culture and sensitivity:** May be performed to determine the presence of blood, bacteria, bile, pus, and amylase content and identify the causative organism.

**Abdominal x-rays:** May be performed to determine the presence of abnormal levels of fluid and gas, which usually collect in the large and small bowel in the presence of a perforation. "Free air" under the diaphragm also may be visualized.

## COLLABORATIVE MANAGEMENT

**Bed rest:** With patient in semi- or high-Fowler's position to promote fluid shift to the lower abdomen, which will reduce pressure on the diaphragm and allow for deeper and easier respirations.

**NG or intestinal tube:** Inserted to reduce or prevent GI distention, nausea, and vomiting.

**IV fluids, electrolyte therapy, and parenteral feedings:** To correct fluid, electrolyte, and nutritional disorders. Daily measurements of serum electrolytes and calculations of fluid volume are performed to determine the necessary types of fluids and electrolyte replacement. Plasma, protein, and blood may be administered to correct hypovolemia, hypoproteinemia, and anemia. Patient is NPO during the acute phase, and oral fluids are not resumed until the patient has passed flatus and the gastric tube has been removed. Total parenteral nutrition (TPN) usually is initiated in the early stages to promote nutrition and protein replacement.

**CVP catheter:** May be inserted to monitor circulatory status in the critically ill patient. CVP values should be maintained at 2-6 mm Hg (5-12 cm $H_2O$). A pulmonary artery (i.e., Swan-Ganz) catheter may be inserted if the patient develops hypovolemic shock.

**Parenteral antibiotic therapy.**

**$O_2$:** Often prescribed to treat hypoxia.

**Narcotics and sedatives:** To relieve severe pain and discomfort once the diagnosis has been confirmed.

**Surgical intervention:** May be required to remove the source of infection or drain the abscess and accumulated fluids. This can include the removal of an organ, such as the appendix or gallbladder. Drains usually are inserted to remove purulent drainage and excessive fluids. Intestinal decompression may be employed to decrease massive abdominal distention. Intraoperative and postoperative irrigation may be indicated if bowel contents have grossly contaminated the peritoneal cavity.

**Peritoneal lavage:** May be used if the patient does not respond to the above interventions and is a surgical risk. Rapid dialysis exchanges may be performed along with antibiotic lavages.

## NURSING DIAGNOSES AND INTERVENTIONS

**Pain,** abdominal distention, and nausea related to inflammatory process, fever, and tissue damage

*Desired outcomes:*   Patient's subjective perception of pain decreases within 1 h of intervention, as documented by a pain scale. Objective indicators, such as grimacing and abdominal guarding, are absent or diminished.

- Assess and document the character and severity of the discomfort q1-2h. Devise a pain scale with the patient, rating discomfort on a scale of 0 (no pain) to 10 (worst pain).
- After the diagnosis has been made, administer narcotics, analgesics, and sedatives as prescribed to promote comfort and rest. Document the relief obtained, using the pain scale.
- Keep patient on bed rest to minimize pain, which can be aggravated by activity; provide a restful and quiet environment.
- Keep patient in a position of comfort, usually semi-Fowler's position.
- Explain all procedures to patient to help minimize anxiety, which can exacerbate discomfort.
- Offer mouth care and lip moisturizers at frequent intervals to help relieve discomfort/nausea from continuous or intermittent suction, dehydration, and NPO status.
- See "Stomatitis," p. 380, for mouth care interventions.

**Ineffective breathing pattern** related to decreased depth of respirations secondary to guarding with abdominal pain or distention

*Desired outcomes:*   Patient has an effective breathing pattern as evidenced by absence of adventitious breath sounds, $Pao_2 \geq 80$ mm Hg, oxygen saturation $\geq 95\%$, $BP \geq 90/60$ mm Hg (or within patient's baseline range), $HR \leq 100$ bpm, and orientation to person, place, and time. Eupnea occurs within 1 h following pain-relieving intervention.

- Monitor ABG results, and be alert to indicators of hypoxemia, including low oxygen saturation and $Pao_2$, and to the following clinical signs: hypotension, tachycardia, hyperventilation, restlessness, central nervous system (CNS) depression, and possibly cyanosis.
- Auscultate lung fields to assess ventilation and detect pulmonary complications. Note and document the presence of adventitious breath sounds.
- Keep patient in semi-Fowler's or high-Fowler's position to aid respiratory effort; encourage deep breathing to enhance oxygenation.
- Administer oxygen as prescribed.

**Altered protection** related to potential for worsening/recurring peritonitis or development of septic shock secondary to inflammatory process

*Desired outcome:*   Patient is free of symptoms of worsening/recurring peritonitis or septic shock as evidenced by normothermia, $BP \geq 90/60$ mm Hg (or within patient's normal range), $HR \leq 100$ bpm, presence of eupnea, urinary output $\geq 30$ ml/h, CVP 2-6 mm Hg (5-12 cm $H_2O$), decreasing abdominal girth measurements, and minimal tenderness to palpation.

- Assess the abdomen q1-2h during the acute phase and q4h once the patient is stabilized. Monitor for increasing distention by measuring abdominal girth, and auscultate bowel sounds to assess motility. Bowel sounds often are frequent during the beginning phase of peritonitis, but are absent in the presence of paralytic ileus. *Lightly* palpate the abdomen for evidence of increasing rigidity or tenderness, which is indicative of disease progression. If the patient experiences more pain on removal of your hand, rebound tenderness is present. Notify physician of significant findings.
- If prescribed, insert gastric tube and connect it to suction to prevent or decrease distention.
- Monitor VS at least q2h and more frequently if the patient's condition is unstable. Be alert to signs of septic shock: increased temperature, hypotension, tachycardia, shallow and rapid respirations, urine output $< 30$ ml/h, and CVP $< 2$ mm Hg (or $< 5$ cm $H_2O$). In the early (warm) stage of shock, the skin usually is warm, pink, and dry secondary to peripheral venous pooling, and the BP and CVP begin to drop. In the late (cold) stage of shock,

the extremities become pale and cool because of the decreasing tissue perfusion.
- Administer antibiotics as prescribed.
- Monitor CBC count for the presence of leukocytosis, which signals infection, and hemoconcentration (increased Hct and Hgb), which occurs with a decrease in plasma volume. Normal values are as follows: WBC: 4,500-11,000 μl; Hgb: 14-18 g/dl (male) or 12-16 g/dl (female); and Hct: 40%-54% (male) or 37%-47% (female). With peritonitis, WBC count usually will be greater than 20,000 μl. Notify physician of significant findings.
- Maintain sterile technique with dressing changes and all invasive procedures.
- Teach patient the signs and symptoms of recurring peritonitis and the importance of reporting them promptly if they occur: fever, chills, abdominal pain, vomiting, and abdominal distention.

**Altered nutrition:** Less than body requirements, related to vomiting and intestinal suctioning

*Desired outcome:* By a minimum of 24 h before hospital discharge, patient has adequate nutrition as evidenced by stable weight, balanced or positive N state, and serum albumin 3.5-5.5 g/dl.
- Keep patient NPO as prescribed during acute phase of the disorder. If the patient has an ileus, an NG tube will be inserted to decompress the abdomen. Reintroduce oral fluids gradually once motility has returned, as evidenced by presence of bowel sounds, decreased distention, and passage of flatus.
- As prescribed, support patient with peripheral parenteral nutrition (PPN) or TPN, depending on the duration of the acute phase (usually by day 3).
- Administer replacement fluids, electrolytes, and vitamins as prescribed.

---

**Note:** See "Providing Nutritional Support," p. 669, for the care of patients on enteral or parenteral feedings. See Appendix One for nursing diagnoses and interventions in "Caring for Preoperative and Postoperative Patients," p. 693. Also see Appendix One, "Caring for Patients on Prolonged Bed Rest" for **High risk for activity intolerance,** p. 711, and **High risk for disuse syndrome,** p. 713.

---

## PATIENT-FAMILY TEACHING AND DISCHARGE PLANNING

Give patient and significant others verbal and written information about the following:
- Medications, including the drug name, dosage, schedule, purpose, precautions, and potential side effects.
- Activity alterations as prescribed by physician, such as avoiding heavy lifting (>10 lb), resting after periods of fatigue, getting maximum amounts of rest, and gradually increasing activities to tolerance.
- Notifying physician of the following indicators of recurrence: fever, chills, abdominal pain, vomiting, abdominal distention.
- If patient has undergone surgery, indicators of wound infection: fever, pain, chills, incisional swelling, persistent erythema, purulent drainage.
- Importance of follow-up medical care; confirm date and time of next medical appointment.

# Appendicitis

Appendicitis is the most commonly occurring inflammatory lesion of the bowel and one of the most frequent reasons for abdominal surgery. The appendix is a blind, narrow tube that extends from the inferior portion of the cecum and does not serve any useful function. Appendicitis is usually caused by obstruction of the appendiceal lumen by a fecalith (hardened bit of fecal material), inflammation, a foreign body, or a neoplasm. Obstruction prevents drainage of secretions that are produced by epithelial cells in the lumen, thereby increasing intraluminal pressure and compressing mucosal blood vessels. This tension causes impaired viability, which can lead to necrosis and perforation. Inflammation and infection result from normal bacteria invading the devitalized wall. Mild cases of appendicitis can heal spontaneously, but severe inflammation can lead to a ruptured appendix, which can cause local or generalized peritonitis.

## ASSESSMENT

Signs and symptoms will vary because of differences in anatomy, size, and age.

**Early stage:**  Abdominal pain (either epigastric or umbilical) that may be vague and diffuse; nausea and vomiting; fever; and sensitivity over the appendix area.

**Intermediate, "acute" stage:**  Pain that shifts from epigastrium to RLQ at McBurney's point (approximately 2 inches from the anterior superior iliac spine on a line drawn from the umbilicus) and is aggravated by walking or coughing. The pain may be accompanied by a sensation of constipation ("gas stoppage" sensation). Anorexia, malaise, occasionally diarrhea, and diminished peristalsis also can occur.

**On physical assessment,** the patient will experience pain in the RLQ elicited by *light* palpation of the abdomen; presence of rebound tenderness; RLQ guarding, rigidity, and muscle spasms; tachycardia; low-grade fever; absent or diminished bowel sounds; and pain elicited with rectal exam. A palpable, tender mass may be felt in the peritoneal pouch if the appendix lies within the pelvis.

**Acute appendicitis with perforation:**  Increasing, generalized pain; and recurrence of vomiting.

**On physical assessment,** the patient usually will exhibit temperature increases >38.5° C (101.4° F) and generalized abdominal rigidity. Typically, the patient remains rigid with flexed knees. Presence of abscess can result in a tender, palpable mass. The abdomen may be distended.

## DIAGNOSTIC TESTS

**WBC with differential:**  Will reveal presence of leukocytosis and an increase in neutrophils. A shift to the left with more than 75% neutrophils is found in about 90% or more cases.

**Urinalysis:**  To rule out genitourinary conditions mimicking appendicitis; may reveal microscopic hematuria and pyuria.

**Abdominal x-ray:**  May reveal presence of a fecalith. If perforation has occurred, the presence of free air will be noted.

**Intravenous pyelogram:**  May be performed to rule out ureteral stone or pyelitis.

**Abdominal ultrasound:**  May be done to rule out appendicitis or conditions that mimic it, such as Crohn's disease, diverticulitis, or gastroenteritis.

**Abdominal CT scan:**  May reveal an appendiceal abscess or acute appendicitis.

## COLLABORATIVE MANAGEMENT

*Preoperative care*

**Bed rest:**  For observation.

**NPO status:**  Parenteral fluids are begun if surgery is imminent.

**Pharmacologic therapy:**  Narcotics are avoided until diagnosis is certain because they mask clinical signs and symptoms.

*Antibiotics:*  To prevent systemic infection.

*Tranquilizing agents:* For sedation.
**Gastric tube:** Inserted for gastric suction and lavage, if needed.

---

**Note:** Cathartics and enemas are contraindicated because they increase peristalsis and can cause perforation.

---

## Surgery
**Appendectomy:** Performed as soon as the diagnosis is confirmed and fluid imbalance and systemic reactions have been controlled. The appendix is removed through an incision made over McBurney's point or through a right paramedial incision. In the presence of abscess, rupture, or peritonitis, an incisional drain is inserted.

*Laparoscopic appendectomy* incidental to gynecologic procedures (e.g., endometriosis involving the appendix) or for acute or chronic appendicitis (in the absence of rupture or signs of peritonitis) is gaining in popularity and is performed using from 1 umbilical puncture to 3 or 4 abdominal punctures. Advantages to this technique over traditional surgery include earlier ambulation and hospital discharge, decreased risk of wound infection, improved cosmesis, and less pain.

## Postoperative care
**Activities:** Ambulation begins either the day of surgery or the first postoperative day. The patient may be hospitalized for 3-5 days. Normal activities are resumed 2-3 weeks after surgery.

**Diet:** Advances from clear liquids to soft solids during the second through fifth postoperative day; parenteral fluids are continued if required.

**Pharmacotherapy**

*Antibiotics:* Continued in the presence of infection.

*Mild laxatives:* Given if necessary, but enemas continue to be contraindicated during the first few postoperative weeks until adequate healing has occurred and bowel function has been restored.

*Analgesics:* For postoperative pain.

## NURSING DIAGNOSES AND INTERVENTIONS

**High risk for infection** related to inadequate primary defenses (risk of rupture, peritonitis, and abscess formation) secondary to inflammatory process

*Desired outcomes:* Patient is free of infection as evidenced by normothermia, HR ≤ 100 bpm, BP ≥ 90/60 mm Hg, RR 12-20 breaths/min with normal depth and pattern (eupnea), soft and nondistended abdomen, and bowel sounds 5-34/min in each abdominal quadrant. Following instruction, patient verbalizes the rationale for not administering enemas or laxatives preoperatively and enemas postoperatively and demonstrates compliance with the therapeutic regimen.

- Assess and document quality, location, and duration of pain. Be alert to pain that becomes accentuated and generalized or to the presence of recurrent vomiting, and note whether patient assumes side-lying or supine position with flexed knees. Any of these signs can signal worsening appendicitis, which can lead to rupture. Be alert to pain that worsens and then disappears—a signal that rupture may have occurred.
- Monitor VS for elevated temperature, increased pulse rate, hypotension, and shallow/rapid respirations; and assess the abdomen for presence of rigidity, distention, and decreased or absent bowel sounds, any of which can occur with rupture. Report significant findings to physician.
- Caution patient about the danger of preoperative self-treatment with enemas and laxatives because they increase peristalsis, which increases the risk of perforation. If constipation occurs postoperatively, physician may prescribe hs laxatives/stool softeners after the third day. Remind patient that enemas

should be avoided until approved by physician (usually several weeks after surgery).

- Teach patient about postoperative incisional care, as well as care of drains if patient is to be discharged with them.
- Provide instructions about prescribed antibiotics if patient is to be discharged with them.
- See "Peritonitis" for more information.

**Pain** and nausea related to the inflammatory process

*Desired outcomes:*   Within 1-2 h of pain-relieving intervention, patient's subjective perception of pain decreases, as documented by a pain scale. Objective indicators, such as grimacing, are absent or diminished.

- Assess and document quality, location, and duration of pain. Devise a pain scale with patient, rating discomfort from 0 (no pain) to 10 (worst pain). Be aware of the characteristics of discomfort during the following stages of appendicitis:

*Early stage:*   Abdominal pain (either epigastric or umbilical) that may be vague and diffuse; nausea and vomiting; fever; and sensitivity over the appendix area.

*Intermediate (acute) stage:*   Pain that shifts from the epigastrium to the RLQ at McBurney's point (approximately 2 inches from the anterior superior iliac spine on a line drawn from the umbilicus) and is aggravated by walking or coughing. The pain may be accompanied by a sensation of constipation ("gas stoppage" sensation). Anorexia, malaise, occasional diarrhea, and diminished peristalsis also can occur.

*Acute appendicitis with perforation:*   Increasing, generalized pain; recurrence of vomiting; increasing abdominal rigidity.

- Medicate patient with antiemetics, sedatives, and analgesics as prescribed; evaluate and document patient's response, using the pain scale.
- Keep patient NPO before surgery; after surgery, nausea and vomiting usually disappear. If prescribed, insert gastric tube for decompression.
- Teach technique for slow, diaphragmatic breathing to reduce stress and help relax tense muscles.
- Help position patient for optimal comfort. Many patients find comfort from a side-lying position with the knees bent, while others find relief when supine with pillows under the knees. Avoid pressure on the popliteal area.

---

**Note:**   See Appendix One for nursing diagnoses and interventions in "Caring for Preoperative and Postoperative Patients," p. 693.

---

## PATIENT-FAMILY TEACHING AND DISCHARGE PLANNING

Give patient and significant others verbal and written information about the following:

- Medications, including drug name, dosage, purpose, schedule, precautions, and potential side effects.
- Care of incision, including dressing changes and bathing restrictions, if appropriate.
- Indicators of infection: fever, chills, incisional pain, redness, swelling, and purulent drainage.
- Postsurgical activity precautions: avoid lifting heavy objects (>10 lb) for the first 6 weeks or as directed, be alert to and rest after symptoms of fatigue, get maximum rest, gradually increase activities to tolerance.
- Importance of avoiding enemas for the first few postoperative weeks. Caution patient about the need to check with physician before having an enema.

# Hemorrhoids

Traditionally, both internal and external hemorrhoids were believed to be varicosities of the hemorrhoid veins, caused by conditions that precipitate increased intraabdominal pressure or obstruct venous return (e.g., pregnancy, chronic constipation, physical exertion, portal hypertension, infiltrating carcinoma, infection, ulcerative colitis). However, a more current concept is that internal hemorrhoids are normal vascular cushions containing a rich arteriovenous network. They may be present at birth and can narrow the anal lumen, thereby contributing to continence. These vascular cushions project into the lumen, where they are subjected to downward pressure during defecation. The muscular fibers that anchor the cushions become attenuated, and the hemorrhoids slide, become congested, bleed, and eventually prolapse. Internal hemorrhoids are found proximal to the anal sphincter and are not visible unless they become large enough to protrude through the anus. External hemorrhoids are distal to the anal sphincter and can become thrombosed if the vein ruptures.

## ASSESSMENT

**Signs and symptoms:**   Hemorrhoids may be manifested by rectal bleeding (fresh, bright red blood, especially on the toilet paper or surface of the stool), prolapsed tissue, pain in the presence of thrombosis, and pruritus. Chronic blood loss can cause iron deficiency.

**Physical assessment:**   External hemorrhoids are visible as bluish protrusions in the subcutaneous perianal tissue. They appear grapelike on inspection. Internal hemorrhoids may require anoscopy, since they are rarely palpated on digital examination unless they are thrombosed.

**Risk factors:**   Diet low in fiber; obesity; long-term constipation and straining; life-style or career that requires constant sitting or standing; portal hypertension; and pregnancy.

## DIAGNOSTIC TESTS

**Stool occult blood test:**   To assess for the presence of blood.

**CBC:**   To assess for anemia from chronic blood loss.

**Anoscopy or flexible sigmoidoscopy:**   To confirm the diagnosis and rule out neoplastic or inflammatory disease that may be responsible for the symptoms.

**Colonoscopy and barium enema:**   May be necessary to exclude other causes of rectal bleeding.

## COLLABORATIVE MANAGEMENT

**Regulation of bowel movements:**   Bulk cathartic, stool softener, high-fiber diet, exercise, augmenting fluid intake, avoiding prolonged sitting.

**Treatment of pain and itching:**   Warm or cold compresses and warm sitz baths.

**Pharmacotherapy:**   *Topical anesthetics,* such as dibucaine hydrochloride (Nupercainal) ointment; *astringents,* such as witch hazel (Tucks) pads; and *antiinflammatory preparations,* such as hydrocortisone ointment, to relieve pain and itching and shrink mucous membranes.

**Manual reduction of prolapsed and strangulated hemorrhoids:**   Returning hemorrhoid to rectum with a lubricated, gloved finger.

**Sclerosing agent:**   Injection into the submucosal tissue surrounding the hemorrhoids to produce an inflammatory response, which leads to tissue shrinkage and fixation of the hemorrhoid. This is a palliative and temporary measure. Usually 5% phenol in vegetable oil is the sclerosing agent.

**Rubber band ligation:**   Nonsurgical method of constricting the blood circulation of the hemorrhoid, causing tissue necrosis, separation, and sloughing to occur. Sepsis is a potential complication of this technique if it is done improperly, because of the necrosing and sloughing of the tissue. Observe for the following triad of symptoms, which necessitates prompt medical attention: anal pain, urinary retention, and fever.

**Incision and drainage:**    To remove clots from thrombosed hemorrhoids. This is performed on an outpatient basis using a local anesthetic.

**Coagulation techniques:**    Use of infrared coagulation, bipolar electrode therapy, and direct current electrotherapy of the hemorrhoids. Infrared photocoagulation is a relatively new procedure, causing fibrosis of the hemorrhoid. There is a very high cost associated with laser therapy, and results are similar to those obtained with injections and ligation.

**Hemorrhoidectomy:**    Removal by cautery, clamp, or excision of hemorrhoids that do not respond to the above therapies.

## NURSING DIAGNOSES AND INTERVENTIONS

**Constipation** related to less than adequate dietary fiber, fluid intake, or physical activity; or pain with defecation

*Desired outcome:*    Within 1-3 days of initiation of treatment patient reports bowel movements of soft stools without straining or pain.

- Teach patient about high-fiber diet and the need for adequate fluid intake (>2-3 L/day unless contraindicated).
- Administer prescribed stool softeners and bulk cathartics. Teach this regimen to the patient.
- Teach patient about use of therapeutic measures such as sitz baths, warm/cold compresses, topical anesthetics, prescribed antiinflammatory preparations (e.g., hydrocortisone creams or suppositories), astringent pads, exercise, and avoidance of prolonged sitting while attemping a bowel movement.
- Instruct patient to respond to the urge to defecate as quickly as possible to prevent pressure buildup in the rectum.
- For other interventions, see **Constipation,** in Appendix One, "Caring for Patients on Prolonged Bed Rest," p. 716.

**Pain** and itching related to hemorrhoidectomy

*Desired outcomes:*    Patient's subjective perception of discomfort decreases within 1-2 h following pain-relieving intervention, as documented by a pain scale. Objective indicators, such as grimacing, are absent or diminished.

- Monitor patient for the presence of pain. Devise a pain scale with patient, rating discomfort on a scale of 0 (no pain) to 10 (worst pain). Administer topical anesthetics, astringents, and antiinflammatory preparations as prescribed. Rate the degree of relief obtained, using the pain scale.
- Administer cold or warm compresses to rectal area. Provide warm sitz baths 3-4 times a day, or as prescribed. **Caution:** Be alert to hypotension, which can be caused by the dilatation of pelvic blood vessels.
- Administer narcotics for severe postoperative pain as prescribed.
- Ensure that the patient takes stool softeners during the early postoperative period in preparation for the first bowel movement.
- If indicated, position a flotation pad under the buttocks for comfort. Doughnut-shaped cushions are contraindicated because they can increase rather than decrease pressure at the operative site.
- Provide warm sitz baths after each bowel movement to minimize discomfort and promote healing.

**Constipation** related to fear of pain with postoperative defecation

*Desired outcomes:*    Patient has bowel movements without straining during the early postoperative period. Following instruction, patient verbalizes the rationale for the importance of postoperative bowel movements and complies with the therapeutic regimen.

- Explain to patient that discomfort is common with the first bowel movements after surgery.
- Administer stool softeners and bulk cathartics as prescribed. Administer analgesic ½-1 h before the patient attempts defecation.

- Encourage ambulation the day of surgery or first postoperative day to enhance peristalsis.
- In nonrestricted patients, encourage fluid intake of at least 2-3 L/day to help soften stools and promote elimination.
- Document the first bowel movement, which should occur by the third or fourth postoperative day. Stay with the patient or stand just outside the bathroom door because dizziness and fainting are common at this time owing to dilatation of the pelvic blood vessels. Record the amount and character of the stool and the patient's response.
- If the patient avoids having a bowel movement after surgery because of anticipated pain, explain that a normal postsurgical bowel movement will prevent complications, such as constriction of the anal lumen.

**Altered pattern of urinary elimination** (anuria or dysuria) related to local swelling or presence of rectal packing secondary to hemorrhoidectomy
*Desired outcome:*    Patient relates the resumption of his or her normal voiding pattern 6-8 h following surgery.
- If patient has difficulty voiding in the early postoperative period because of local swelling or rectal packing, encourage patient to get out of bed to void.
- Encourage sitz baths or warm showers, which stimulate the voiding reflex.
- If patient is unable to void, evaluate for the need for urinary catheterization, and consult with physician accordingly.

**High risk for fluid volume deficit** related to postoperative bleeding caused by slipped ligatures
*Desired outcome:*    Patient is normovolemic as evidenced by BP within patient's baseline range, HR $\leq$ 100 bpm, RR $\leq$ 20 breaths/min with normal depth and pattern (eupnea), and $\leq$2 saturated dressings/8 h.
- Hemorrhage can result from a slipped ligature, and bleeding easily can go undetected. Be alert to the presence of pallor, diaphoresis, hypotension, and increasing pulse and respiration rates. Orthostatic hypotension and BP and pulse changes are early signs of hypovolemia. If bleeding occurs, be prepared to assist physician with insertion of a Foley catheter (22-28 Fr) into the rectum and inflation of balloon to provide pressure to the bleeding site.
- Assess for rectal bleeding. After surgery and into the first or second postoperative day, the patient will have rectal packing. Inspect the perianal area for evidence of fresh bleeding. After physician removes the packing, replace the perianal dressing (typically a sanitary napkin) as necessary. Be alert to excess bleeding, as evidenced by >2 saturated pads/8 h. Query patient about the presence of a frequent, unrelieved urge to defecate, which can signal sequestered hemorrhage.
- Advise patient to avoid straining or sitting on the toilet longer than necessary. Instruct patient to avoid positions that increase pressure, such as prolonged sitting, standing, or squatting.
- Instruct patient to keep perianal area clean but to avoid vigorous wiping after bowel movement. *Moist* perineal wipes should be used to cleanse the area. Encourage sitz baths after every bowel movement to cleanse the rectal area and relieve local irritation. Be alert to hypotension, which can be caused by dilatation of pelvic blood vessels.
- As appropriate, advise the patient to abstain from anal intercourse until proper healing has taken place and it is approved by physician.
- Explain to patient that some bleeding can be expected about 8-12 days postoperatively when the sutures begin to dissolve.
- Be alert to the potential for sepsis, which is a rare but possible complication of the rubber band ligation technique.

**Knowledge deficit:**    Potential for recurrence of hemorrhoids and measures that help prevent it
*Desired outcome:*    Within the 24-h period before hospital discharge, patient verbalizes knowledge about the potential for recurrence of hemorrhoids and can list preventive measures.

- Advise patient to use mild bulk cathartics or stool softeners if constipation recurs and to avoid straining with defecation.
- Encourage a high-fiber diet, such as whole grain products (breads, cooked grains, and cereals), apples, peas, and kidney and other dried beans.
- For nonrestricted patients, explain that a minimum fluid intake of 2-3 L/day is necessary to soften the stool and promote elimination.
- Encourage daily exercise, which enhances peristalsis and promotes elimination. Advise patient to avoid prolonged standing and sitting.

---

**Note:**   See Appendix One for nursing diagnoses and interventions in "Caring for Preoperative and Postoperative Patients," p. 693

---

### PATIENT-FAMILY TEACHING AND DISCHARGE PLANNING

Give patient and significant others verbal and written information about the following:
- Medications, including drug name, dosage, schedule, purpose, precautions, and potential side effects.
- Importance of avoiding straining, and methods for preventing constipation, such as exercise, diet high in fiber content, augmenting fluid intake, and taking stool softeners or mild bulk cathartics if necessary.
- Postoperative activity precautions as directed: avoid fatigue, get maximum rest, and gradually increase activities to tolerance.
- Awareness that some bleeding can occur about 8-12 days postoperatively, when sutures begin to dissolve.

# Section Three:   Intestinal Neoplasms and Inflammatory Processes

## Diverticulosis/Diverticulitis

*Diverticulosis* is acquired small pouches or sacs (diverticula) in the colon formed by the herniation of mucosal and submucosal linings through the muscular layers of the intestine. Although diverticula can be found anywhere in the colon, they are seen most frequently in the sigmoid colon because it is the narrowest part of the colon, harbors the firmest stool, and, as a result, must generate higher pressures than the rest of the colon. It is theorized that diverticula develop secondary to a low-residue diet and increased intracolonic pressure, such as that created with straining to have a bowel movement.

*Diverticulitis* is a complication of diverticulosis. It is an inflammatory process, and it is theorized that it begins with a single diverticulum, usually in the sigmoid colon, and is caused by the irritating presence of trapped fecal material within the diverticulum. When the obstructing fecal plug remains and bacteria proliferate, the inflammation can spread from the thin wall at the apex of the diverticulum to peridiverticular tissue. The resulting inflammation and infection can be localized or be more extensive (as in peritonitis) and life-threatening.

### ASSESSMENT

**Diverticulosis:**   Lower GI bleeding or symptoms of irritable bowel syndrome such as steady or crampy abdominal pain in the LLQ, associated with consti-

pation or diarrhea and increased flatulence. The patient may be asymptomatic.
**Diverticulitis:** See the above indicators. In addition, fever, nausea, vomiting, and obstipation can be present if obstruction or peritonitis occurs. Fistulas to the bladder, vagina, or skin, and gas or stool elimination from the involved site also may be present.

**Physical assessment:** Presence of tender, palpable mass, usually in the LLQ; rebound tenderness secondary to infection or abscess formation; abdominal distention; hypoactive or hyperactive bowel sounds; and possibly, absence of stool felt on rectal examination. Tachycardia, hypotension, and shallow respirations can be present if there is severe abdominal discomfort. Often the patient assumes a side-lying position with the knees flexed to relieve pain.

## DIAGNOSTIC TESTS
### Diverticulosis
**Barium enema:** To determine presence and number of diverticula.
**CBC:** To determine if anemia is present.
**Sigmoidoscopy:** To reveal presence of diverticula and thickening of bowel wall.
### Diverticulitis
**Abdominal x-rays:** To determine presence of abnormal gas and fluid levels, which collect in the intestine above the affected area of the colon, indicating the presence and degree of bowel obstruction or ileus; and reveal the presence of free air in the peritoneal cavity, signalling noncontainment of diverticular perforation. These films also may show the presence of air in the urinary bladder if a colovesical fistula is present.
**CBC with differential:** Usually reveals leukocytosis with a shift to the left and an increase in neutrophils, indicating presence of infection.
**Blood culture:** May reveal presence of bacteremia in severely ill patients.
**Urinalysis:** To rule out bladder involvement; may show presence of red and white cells in the presence of colovesical fistula.
**Barium enema:** To support the diagnosis of diverticulitis by demonstrating the presence of barium outside the lumen of the colon or outside of a diverticulum, a fistula or fistulas leading from the colon, or a paracolic mass. This exam should be deferred during the acute phase of illness if perforation is suspected. Water-soluble agents can be used if risk of perforation is great or fistula formation is suspected.
**CT scan:** To demonstrate diverticula, changes in the wall of the colon that are indicative of diverticulitis, and related abscesses and fistulas. Since this exam is noninvasive, it can be used in acutely ill or septic individuals for whom barium enema studies can be hazardous.

## COLLABORATIVE MANAGEMENT
### Diverticulosis
The goal of medical therapy for uncomplicated disease is to relieve symptoms and prevent or postpone complications.
**High-residue diet:** Including fruits and vegetables and the use of wheat bran in the form of 100% bran cereal or 2 tbsp/day of unprocessed bran to increase moisture content of the stool, thus softening it to promote elimination and reduce intracolonic pressure. Also see Table 6-2.
**Pharmacotherapy:** Commercial *bulk laxative,* such as psyllium (Metamucil), 1-2 tsp PO bid, which can replace bran in the diet.
### Diverticulitis
The goal of medical therapy is to "rest" the bowel, resolve infection and inflammation, and prevent or decrease the severity of complications.
**Bed rest and NPO status:** To promote physical, emotional, and bowel rest.
**Gastric suction:** To relieve nausea, vomiting, or abdominal distention, if present.

**Parenteral replacement of fluids, electrolytes, and blood products:** As indicated by laboratory test results to maintain intravascular volumes, electrolyte and acid-base balance, urinary output, and caloric intake.

**Pharmacotherapy**

*Parenteral antibiotics:* To limit secondary infection.

*Analgesics:* To relieve pain. Meperidine (Demerol) is the agent of choice. In addition to producing analgesia, it also decreases GI motility and spasm. Pentazocine (Talwin) also reduces sigmoid activity in analgesic doses. It should be used with caution in elders since it may cause confusion, disorientation, and hallucinations. The use of morphine and other opiates is contraindicated since they increase intraluminal pressure in the sigmoid colon, thus potentially increasing the risk of perforation.

**Emergency diverting colostomy:** With or without resection of the affected bowel segment. This is the therapy of choice for most surgeons. Once inflammation has subsided (after approximately 6 weeks), the affected bowel segment is surgically resected if this was not done with the colostomy. After surgical anastomoses have healed, as documented by x-ray (3-6 weeks later), a third surgery is performed. The colostomy is taken down and the continuity of the GI tract is restored.

## NURSING DIAGNOSES AND INTERVENTIONS

*For diverticulitis* treated by emergency surgical intervention with diverting temporary colostomy: See "Fecal Diversions" for **Bowel incontinence,** p. 436, **Body image disturbance,** p. 437, and **High risk for impaired peristomal skin integrity** *and* **impaired stomal tissue integrity,** p. 435. See Appendix One for nursing diagnoses and interventions in "Caring for Preoperative and Postoperative Patients," p. 693, and "Caring for Patients with Cancer and Other Life-Disrupting Illnesses," p. 719.

## PATIENT-FAMILY TEACHING AND DISCHARGE PLANNING

Give patient and significant others verbal and written information about the following:

- Medications, including the name, rationale, dosage, schedule, precautions, and potential side effects.
- Signs and symptoms that necessitate medical attention, including fever; nausea or vomiting; cloudy or malodorous urine; diarrhea or constipation; change in stoma color from the normal bright and shiny red; peristomal skin irritation; and incisional pain, drainage, swelling, or redness.
- Importance of a normal diet that includes all four food groups (meat, eggs, and fish; fruits and vegetables; milk and cheese; cereal and breads) and drinking adequate fluids (at least 2-3 L/day). Also teach the patient to add fiber to the diet in the form of fruits and vegetables, and whole grain cereals with the addition of bran in the form of 100% bran cereal or 2 tbsp/day of coarse, unprocessed bran that can be taken with milk or juice or sprinkled over cereal. Because bran initially may cause abdominal distention and excessive flatus, instruct the patient to begin with 1 tbsp/day and increase gradually. Caution patient to avoid nuts and berries and foods with seeds.
- Gradual resumption of ADL, excluding heavy lifting (>10 lb), pushing, or pulling for 6 weeks to prevent development of incisional herniation.
- Care of incision, dressing changes, and permission to take baths or showers once sutures/drains are removed.
- Care of stoma and peristomal skin; use of ostomy skin barriers, pouches, and accessory equipment; and method for obtaining supplies.
- Referral to community resources, including enterostomal therapy (ET) nurse, home health care agency, and the United Ostomy Association.
- Importance of follow-up care with physician or ET nurse; confirm date and time of next appointment.

# Colorectal cancer

Colorectal cancer is second only to lung cancer and nonmelanoma skin cancer in the annual number of newly diagnosed cancer cases. It is estimated that 150,000-160,000 new cases of colorectal cancer are reported each year in the United States. Over 90% of colorectal cancers are adenocarcinomas, of which 50% are located in the rectum, 20% in the sigmoid colon, 6% in the descending colon, 8% in the transverse colon, and 16% in the cecum and ascending colon. Many arise from malignant degeneration of benign adenomatous polyps. Metastatic disease occurs through lymph nodes, direct extension to adjacent tissues, and the bloodstream.

The cause of colorectal cancer is unknown, but risk factors include a high-fat, low-fiber diet, age >40 years, a personal history of colorectal polyps or colorectal carcinoma, a family history of polyposis syndromes (i.e., familial polyposis coli, Gardner's syndrome, Turcot's syndrome, Muir's syndrome, Peutz-Jeghers' syndrome, familial juvenile polyposis from adenomas), first-degree relatives with colorectal cancer, and a personal history of inflammatory bowel disease (i.e., chronic ulcerative colitis, Crohn's colitis).

## ASSESSMENT

**Right colon cancer:**  Vague, dull abdominal pain. The patient may be asymptomatic.

**Physical assessment:**  Possible presence of a palpable mass in the RLQ, black or dark-red stools, and presence of abdominal distention. The patient also may appear anemic.

**Left colon cancer:**  Increasing abdominal cramping ("gas pains"), change in bowel elimination patterns, decrease in caliber of stools (pencil- or ribbon-shaped), constipation, vomiting, obstipation, and acute large bowel obstruction causing progressive increase in abdominal pain. Patient may be asymptomatic.

**Physical assessment:**  Possible absence of stool felt on rectal examination, presence of bright red blood coating the surface of the stool, and abdominal distention.

**Rectal cancer:**  Sensation of incomplete evacuation, tenesmus, perineal or sacral pain owing to local invasion of surrounding nerves, bladder, or vaginal wall. Pain is a late manifestation. The patient may be asymptomatic.

**Physical assessment:**  Potential presence of palpable mass; bright red blood coating surface of the stool.

**History of** (for all types of colorectal cancer): Blood on or in stools, change in stool elimination pattern, vague abdominal discomfort or pain.

## DIAGNOSTIC TESTS

**Occult blood test of 3 serial stool specimens:**  To detect presence of blood associated with tumor mass bleeding.

**Proctosigmoidoscopy or colonoscopy:**  To examine areas of intestine visually. Because rectal and sigmoid lesions sometimes are difficult to diagnose radiologically, proctosigmoidoscopy should be used to complement air contrast barium enemas (ACBaE). If a neoplasm is detected radiographically or on sigmoidoscopy or if the patient is at high risk because of personal or family history, a full colonoscopic examination should be performed.

**Biopsy:**  To confirm diagnosis.

**ACBaE:**  To detect colon irregularities suspicious of tumor. ACBaE exams are more accurate than single contrast barium enemas in diagnosing cancers and detecting small neoplastic lesions.

**CT scan and MRI:**  To identify metastatic colon cancer by imaging tissue outside the rectal wall and distant metastases. However, since these techniques are unable to discriminate the individual layers of the rectal wall, they are not very conclusive for early stage disease.

**Endorectal ultrasound:**  To identify lesions confined to the layers of the bowel wall and to distinguish involved lymph nodes. This technique is useful in early stage disease.

**Carcinoembryonic antigen (CEA):**  Serum elevation can be indicative of intestinal tumor. CEA is not useful as a screening test, because of its lack of sensitivity in detecting early colorectal cancer. However, CEA may be useful in preoperative staging and postoperative follow-up to identify early recurrence. Other serologic tumor markers currently are being examined for sensitivity for early detection and diagnosis of colorectal cancer; their effectiveness for screening is still undetermined.

## COLLABORATIVE MANAGEMENT

**Surgery:**  Resection of tumor mass and lymph nodes that drain the area, with reanastomosis of colon. If bowel ends cannot be reanastomosed, a colostomy is created. The exact extent of the colonic resection is determined by the distribution of regional lymph nodes and by the blood supply. The margins of the resection should be at least 2-5 cm from either side of the tumor. Surgical treatment includes right hemicolectomy for lesions located in the right colon, left hemicolectomy for lesions located in the left colon, a subtotal or total colectomy for synchronous right- and left-sided lesions, low anterior resection for lesions in the rectosigmoid and upper rectum, and abdominoperineal resection (APR) with colostomy for lesions in the mid-rectum and low rectum. With the development of end-to-end stapling devices, APR is being replaced by low anterior resection with reanastomosis for lesions of the mid-rectum and even for low rectal lesions, if a distal margin of at least 2 cm of normal bowel can be resected below the lesion. At present, there appears to be no significant difference in survival and recurrence rates with low anterior resection when compared with APR as long as a 2-5 cm distal margin is preserved. Alternatives to radical operations are being investigated for lesions confined to a local site. These methods used to ablate tumors locally include local excision, electrofulguration with tumor destruction by burning *via* electrocautery, cryotherapy with liquid nitrogen probes, thermal destruction by laser, and endocavitary irradiation (delivering a large dose of radiation [i.e., 9,000-15,000 cGy] to a limited field).

**Radiation therapy:**  To eliminate cancer cells, reduce tumor mass, or decrease pain from advanced disease. As a method of treatment of colorectal cancer, radiation therapy generally is ineffective. It may provide palliation of pelvic pain or rectal or vaginal bleeding secondary to tumor invasion in advanced rectal disease. It is used mainly as an adjuvant therapy to surgery. Preoperatively it is used to reduce tumor mass, converting unresectable large tumors and tumors fixed to pelvic organs to resectable lesions. It also is used preoperatively or postoperatively to decrease local recurrence in patients at high risk (penetration of bowel wall and positive lymph nodes) or in a combined preoperative-postoperative "sandwich" technique.

**Chemotherapy:**  For advanced disease, usually fluorouracil (5-FU), alone or in combination with other agents, such as levamisole, to eliminate cancer cells and provide relief from pain with advanced disease. Generally it is used as adjuvant therapy, combined with surgery or with both surgery and radiation therapy. For more information, see Appendix One "Caring for Patients with Cancer and Other Life-Disrupting Illnesses," p. 719.

**Nutritional management:**  May include elemental fluid supplements and/or parenteral nutrition if oral intake is inadequate. For further details, see "Providing Nutritional Therapy," p. 665.

## NURSING DIAGNOSES AND INTERVENTIONS

**Health-seeking behaviors:**  Recommendations for follow-up diagnostic care after colon resection or polypectomy for malignant polyps

***Desired outcome:*** Before hospital discharge, patient verbalizes accurate information about recommendations for follow-up diagnostic care.

*For patients who have had colorectal cancer resections:*

- Teach patient that colonoscopy is recommended 6-12 months after surgery, followed by yearly colonoscopy for 2 consecutive years; if the aforementioned are negative, colonoscopy or ACBaE plus proctosigmoidoscopy is performed every 3 years.
- Explain that fecal occult blood testing is performed every year.
- Remind patient that serum CEA levels are measured at regular intervals (3 times at 6-month intervals, then 5 times at yearly intervals).

*For postpolypectomy patients with malignant polyps:*

- Teach patient that a colonoscopy is performed within 6 months of polypectomy; if this second examination is negative, colonoscopy is performed every 2 years. However, if the second examination is positive, colonoscopy is performed at yearly intervals until negative, then colonoscopy at 2-year intervals.
- Explain that fecal occult blood testing is performed between colonoscopies.

---

**Note:** See "Fecal Diversions" for **Bowel incontinence,** p. 436, **Body image disturbance,** p. 437, **High risk for impaired peristomal skin integrity,** *and* **Impaired stomal tissue integrity,** p. 435, and **Knowledge deficit:** Colostomy irrigation procedure, p. 438. See Appendix One for nursing diagnoses and interventions in "Caring for Preoperative and Postoperative Patients," p. 693, and "Caring for Patients with Cancer and Other Life-Disrupting Illnesses," p. 719.

---

## PATIENT-FAMILY TEACHING AND DISCHARGE PLANNING

Give patient and significant others verbal and written information about the following:

- Medications, including drug name, rationale, dosage, schedule, precautions, and potential side effects.
- Signs and symptoms that necessitate medical attention, including fever, nausea and vomiting, diarrhea, or constipation.
- If an intestinal stoma is present, the importance of reporting change in stoma color from the normal bright and shiny red; presence of peristomal skin irritation; and incisional pain, drainage, swelling, or redness.
- Importance of a normal diet that includes all four food groups (meat, eggs, and fish; fruits and vegetables; milk and cheese; cereal and breads) and drinking adequate fluids (at least 2-3 L/day).
- Enteral or parenteral feeding instructions if patient is to supplement diet or is NPO.
- Gradual resumption of ADL, excluding heavy lifting (>10 lb), pushing, or pulling for 6 weeks to prevent incisional herniation.
- Care of incision and perianal wounds, including dressing changes, and bathing once sutures/drains are removed. Sitz baths may be recommended for perianal wound.
- If stoma is present, care of stoma and peristomal skin; use of ostomy skin barriers, pouches, and accessory equipment; and method for obtaining supplies.
- Referral to community resources, including home health-care agency, American Cancer Society and, if appropriate, to ET nurse and United Ostomy Association.
- Importance of follow-up care with physician (or ET nurse if appropriate); confirm date and time of next appointment.
- Recommendations for follow-up diagnostic care after colon resection or polypectomy: See **Health-seeking behaviors,** p. 418.

## Polyps/Familial adenomatous polyposis

Of the single, multiple, sessile, and pedunculated polypoid colon tumors, the adenomatous polyp is the most common. The practical significance of these polyps is their tendency to become malignant (see "Colorectal Cancer"). *Familial adenomatous polyposis* (FAP) is characterized by, but distinct from, frequent colon polyp formation. This disorder is also known as multiple familial adenomatosis, adenomatosis coli, and hereditary multiple polyposis. In this disorder the glandular epithelia of the colon and rectum undergo excessive proliferation throughout the mucous membranes, which leads to the formation of sessile or pedunculated polyps. These are soft and red or purplish-red in color, vary in size from a few millimeters to several centimeters, and range in number from a few to several thousand. They can be found anywhere along the entire length of the colon, but the rectum is almost always involved. Every individual with untreated familial polyposis will develop cancer because at some point in time one or more of these polyps will undergo malignant degeneration. This is a hereditary disease passed from generation to generation as an autosomal dominant trait, and it appears most often during late childhood through the early 30s. The incidence of FAP is estimated at approximately 1 in 8,300 births.

### ASSESSMENT

**FAP:**   Mild, early symptoms, such as diarrhea or melena, although many patients remain asymptomatic for years. Once malignant degeneration has begun, these symptoms become more pronounced and there can be intermittent or constant colicky pain. Tenesmus and a frequent urge to defecate also can be present. If blood loss is significant, anemia, weight loss, loss of appetite, and fatigue can occur.

**Physical assessment:**   In the presence of a well-developed malignant growth, a mass can be palpated on abdominal exam. Digital rectal examination may detect presence of polyps.

**History of:**   FAP, mild colicky abdominal discomfort with or without diarrhea, presence of blood in stools.

### DIAGNOSTIC TESTS

**Proctosigmoidoscopy or colonoscopy:**   For visualization of polyposis.

**Biopsy:**   To confirm diagnosis. Histopathologically, the criteria for malignant potential are polyp size, histologic type, and degree of dysplasia.

**X-ray examination with barium enema and air contrast:**   To determine extent of the disease.

**CBC:**   To detect presence of anemia.

### COLLABORATIVE MANAGEMENT

Because colorectal cancer is inevitable, appearing approximately 10-15 years after the onset of the polyposis if the colon is not removed, surgical resection is the treatment of choice for FAP. Once the diagnosis has been made, it is not advisable to delay surgery.

**Proctocolectomy:**   Surgical cure *via* removal of colon and rectum with continent (Kock) ileostomy, conventional (Brooke) ileostomy, or ileoanal reservoir for fecal diversion (see "Fecal Diversions," p. 434).

**Colectomy with preservation of rectum and ileorectal anastomosis:**   After this procedure, follow-up proctoscopies are necessary at frequent intervals to assess the rectum for further evidence of the disease or malignant changes.

**Radiation or chemotherapy:**   May be indicated as adjuvant therapy or for advanced malignant disease.

## NURSING DIAGNOSES AND INTERVENTIONS

**Note:** See "Colorectal Cancer" for **Health-seeking behaviors:** Recommendations for follow-up diagnostic care following colon resection or polypectomy for malignant polyps, p. 418. See "Fecal Diversions" for **Bowel incontinence,** p. 436, **Body image disturbance,** p. 437, and **High risk for impaired peristomal skin integrity** *and* **impaired stomal tissue integrity,** p. 435. See Appendix One for nursing diagnoses and interventions in "Caring for Preoperative and Postoperative Patients," p. 693, and "Caring for Patients with Cancer and Other Life-Disrupting Illnesses, p. 719.

## PATIENT-FAMILY TEACHING AND DISCHARGE PLANNING

Give patient and significant others verbal and written information about the following:
- Importance of informing all close members of the family that because familial polyposis is inherited, periodic examinations of the rectum and colon are essential.
- For other guidelines, see this section in "Colorectal Cancer," p. 419.

# Ulcerative colitis

Ulcerative colitis is a nonspecific, chronic inflammatory disease of the mucosa and submucosa of the colon. Generally the disease begins in the rectum and sigmoid colon, but it can extend proximally and uninterrupted as far as the cecum. In some instances, a few cm of distal ileum are affected. This is sometimes referred to as "backwash ileitis," and it occurs in only about 10% of patients with ulcerative colitis involving the entire colon. The cause of ulcerative colitis is unknown, but theories include infection, allergy, immunologic abnormalities, psychosomatic factors, and heredity. Individuals with ulcerative colitis develop colonic adenocarcinomas at 10 times the rate of the general population.

## ASSESSMENT

**Signs and symptoms:**   Bloody diarrhea (the cardinal symptom). The clinical picture can vary, from acute episodes with frequent discharge of watery stools mixed with blood, pus, and mucus, accompanied by fever, abdominal pain, rectal urgency, and tenesmus, to loose or frequent stools, to formed stools coated with a little blood. However, nearly two-thirds of patients have cramping abdominal pain and varying degrees of fever, vomiting, anorexia, weight loss, and dehydration. Remissions and exacerbations are common. Extracolonic manifestations also can occur, including polyarthritis, skin lesions (erythema nodosum, pyoderma gangrenosum), liver impairment, and ophthalmic complications (iritis, uveitis). Also see Tables 6-5 and 6-6.

**Physical assessment:**   With severe disease, the abdomen will be tender, especially in the LLQ; and distention and a tender and spastic anus also may be present. With rectal examination, the mucosa might feel gritty, and the examining gloved finger may be covered with blood, mucus, or pus.

**Risk factors:**   Duration of active disease greater than 10 years, pancolitis, and family history of colonic cancer.

## DIAGNOSTIC TESTS

**Stool examination:**   Reveals the presence of frank or occult blood. Stool cultures and smears rule out bacterial and parasitic disorders. **Note:** Collect specimens *before* barium enema is performed.

**T A B L E   6 - 5    Comparison of Gross Physiologic Features of Ulcerative Colitis and Crohn's Disease**

| Pathologic features | Ulcerative colitis | Crohn's disease |
| --- | --- | --- |
| Thickened mesentery | Rare | Common |
| Enlarged mesenteric lymph nodes | Rare | Common |
| Shortening of colon | Frequent | Rare |
| Small bowel involvement | Never | May occur |
| Serositis | Not present | Common |
| Thickening of intestinal wall | Rare | Common |
| Segmental disease | Never | Frequent |
| Strictures | Never | Frequent |
| Abdominal wall and internal fistulas | None | Frequent |
| Cobblestoning of mucosa | Rare | Common |
| Mucosal ulcerations | Diffuse | Normal mucosa between ulcers |
| Pseudopolyps | Frequent | Rare |

From Broadwell DC, Jackson BS: *Principles of ostomy care,* St Louis, 1982, Mosby–Year Book, Inc.

**T A B L E   6 - 6    Comparison of Clinical Features of Inflammatory Bowel Disease**

| Clinical features | Ulcerative colitis (mucosal) | Crohn's disease (transmural) |
| --- | --- | --- |
| Age | Young to middle age | Young |
| Sex distribution | Equal | Equal |
| Diarrhea | Remission | More constant |
| Tenesmus | Constant | Occurs |
| Fever (intermittent) | Occurs | Common |
| Weight loss | Common | Severe |
| Abdominal cramping pains | Occurs | Severe |
| Gross bleeding | Common | Infrequent |
| Fistulas | Rare | Common |
| Perforation | Common | Rare |
| Abdominal mass | Rare | Occurs |
| Anal lesions | Occurs | Common |
| Toxic megacolon | Common | Occurs |
| Carcinoma | Common | Occurs |
| Proctoscopic findings | Rectum involved in most cases | Rectum may be spared |
| Extracolonic complications: arthralgia, ocular (uveitis), skin disorders (erythema nodosum, pyoderma gangrenosum) | Frequent | Common |

From Broadwell DC, Jackson BS: *Principles of ostomy care,* St Louis, 1982, Mosby–Year Book, Inc.

**Sigmoidoscopy:** Reveals red, granular, hyperemic, and extremely friable mucosa; strips of inflamed mucosa undermined by surrounding ulcerations, which form pseudopolyps; and thick exudate composed of blood, pus, and mucus. **Note:** Enemas should not be given before the examination because they can produce hyperemia and edema and may cause exacerbation of the disease.

**Colonoscopy:** Will help determine the extent of the disease and differentiate ulcerative colitis from Crohn's disease. However, colonoscopy usually is unnecessary during diagnostic evaluation of ulcerative colitis because sigmoidoscopy and double-contrast barium enema usually will provide sufficient information for making a correct diagnosis. **Note:** This test may be contraindicated in patients with acute disease because of the risk of perforation or hemorrhage.

**Rectal biopsy:** Will aid in differentiating ulcerative colitis from carcinoma and other inflammatory processes.

**Barium enema:** Reveals mucosal irregularity from fine serrations to ragged ulcerations, narrowing and shortening of the colon, presence of pseudopolyps, loss of haustral markings, and the presence of spasms and irritability. A double-contrast technique may facilitate detection of superficial mucosal lesions. With a double-contrast technique, barium is instilled into the colon as with a conventional barium enema, but most of the barium is then withdrawn and the colon is inflated with air, which causes a thin coating of barium to line the intestinal wall. **Note:** Irritant cathartics and enemas should not be given before the examination, since they produce hyperemia and edema and may cause exacerbation of the disease.

**Blood tests:** Anemia, with hypochromic microcytic red blood indices in severe disease, usually is present because of blood loss, iron deficiency, and bone marrow depression. WBC count may be normal to markedly elevated in severe disease. Sedimentation rate is usually increased according to the severity of illness. Hypoalbuminemia and negative N state occur in moderately severe to severe disease and result from decreased protein intake, decreased albumin synthesis in the debilitated condition, and increased metabolic needs. Electrolyte imbalance is common; hypokalemia is often present because of colonic losses (diarrhea) and renal losses in patients on high doses of corticosteroids. Bicarbonate may be decreased because of colonic losses and may signal metabolic acidosis.

## COLLABORATIVE MANAGEMENT

Medical therapy is symptomatic. The goals are to terminate the acute attack, reduce symptoms, and prevent recurrences.

**Parenteral replacement of fluids, electrolytes, and blood products:** To maintain acutely ill patient, as indicated by laboratory test results.

**Physical and emotional rest:** Including bed rest and limitation of visitors.

**Pharmacotherapy**

*Sedatives and tranquilizers:* To promote rest and reduce anxiety.

*Hydrophilic colloids* (e.g., kaolin and pectin mixture) and *anticholinergics and antidiarrheal preparations* (e.g., tinctures of belladonna and opium, **diphenoxylate hydrochloride, loperamide, and codeine phosphate**)*:* To relieve cramping and diarrhea. **Note:** Opiates and anticholinergics should be administered with extreme caution since they contribute to the development of toxic megacolon.

*Antiinflammatory agents:* Corticosteroids to reduce mucosal inflammation. Dosage and routes of administration vary with the severity and extent of the disease. In patients with mild disease limited to the rectum and sigmoid colon, rectal instillation of steroids (enema or suppository) may induce or maintain remission. In patients with more extensive (pancolonic) or more active disease, oral corticosteroid therapy with prednisone or prednisolone usually is initiated. In severely ill patients, IV corticosteroids are given. Once clinical remission is achieved, IV and oral corticosteroids are tapered until discontinuation since these medications have not been shown to prolong remission or prevent future exacerbations.

*Sulfasalazine:*  To help maintain remissions. This drug generally is effective in the treatment of mild to moderate attacks of ulcerative colitis and appears to decrease the frequency of subsequent relapse. Sulfasalazine is considered inferior to corticosteroids in the treatment of severe attacks of disease; once remission has been attained by use of corticosteroid therapy, sulfasalazine appears to be superior to systemic corticosteroids in the maintenance of remission.

When administered orally, sulfasalazine is broken down by colonic bacteria into its two constituents: 5-aminosalicylic acid (5-ASA), which is considered the active therapeutic component, and sulfapyridine, which is the carrier and responsible for the side effects experienced by more than a third of the individuals treated with this therapy. When administered as an enema, 5-ASA alone has been providing encouraging results for individuals with ulcerative colitis limited to the left colon and is proving more effective than hydrocortisone enemas during initial attacks and for subsequent relapses. Investigations are ongoing regarding administration of oral forms of 5-ASA *via* a time-release capsule or according to pH of the contents of the GI tract.

*Immunosuppressive therapy:*  To reduce inflammation in patients not responding to steroids and sulfasalazine and who are unwilling or unable to undergo colectomy. Azathioprine has been used alone and in combination with

---

**T A B L E  6 - 7**   **Most Common Drug Therapies for Ulcerative Colitis and Crohn's Disease***

| Drug | Ulcerative colitis | Crohn's disease |
| --- | --- | --- |
| Sulfasalazine | Valuable for mild to moderate disease, definitely helpful in maintaining remissions and in chronic disease | Valuable for acute and chronic disease; perhaps of most value for disease of large bowel |
| Corticosteroids | Definitely valuable for acute and severe cases; not valuable for maintaining remissions | Definitely valuable for acute and chronic cases; most valuable for disease limited to the ileum |
| Antidiarrheals | Valuable for symptomatic treatment in chronic cases | Valuable for symptomatic treatment in chronic cases |
| Antimicrobials | Possibly beneficial in acute cases | Possibly beneficial in acute cases |
| Immunosuppressives | May have a steroid-sparing effect | May have a steroid-sparing effect |
| Hyperalimentation | Most often indicated as preparation for surgery; possibly of value in severe, acute phase | May be of value in adjunctive treatment; perhaps of most value in patients with moderately severe disease or acute disease and in children |

From Broadwell DC, Jackson BS: *Principles of ostomy care*, St Louis, 1982, Mosby–Year Book, Inc.

*See text for more detail on newer medications.

**Note:** There is no current treatment that will reduce relapse rate.

steroids. It may have a steroid-sparing effect, thus enabling steroid dosages to be reduced. When used as standard therapy, it may have little to offer in most cases of ulcerative colitis.

*Antibiotics:* To limit secondary infection. Antibiotics are not indicated in the management of mild to moderate disease, since infectious agents generally are not thought to be responsible for ulcerative colitis. In the patient with acute pancolitis or toxic megacolon, broad-spectrum IV antibiotic therapy is recommended since secondary bacterial infection of deeply inflamed colonic mucosa is likely. See Table 6-7.

**Nutritional management:** Varies with patient's condition. In severely ill patients, total parenteral nutrition (TPN) along with NPO status is prescribed to replace nutritional deficits while allowing complete bowel rest and improving patient's nutritional status before surgery. For less severely ill patients, low-residue elemental diet provides good nutrition with low fecal volume to allow bowel rest. A bland, high-protein, high-calorie, low-residue diet with vitamin and mineral supplements and excluding raw fruits and vegetables provides good nutrition and decreases diarrhea. Milk and wheat products are restricted to reduce cramping and diarrhea in patients with lactose and gluten intolerances. See Table 6-2 for sample diet plans.

**Referral to mental health practitioner:** As indicated for supportive psychotherapy for patient who has difficulty dealing with any type of chronic or disabling illness.

**Surgical interventions:** Indicated only when the disease is intractable to medical management or when the patient develops a disabling complication. *Total proctocolectomy* cures ulcerative colitis and results in construction of a permanent fecal diversion, such as Brooke ileostomy, continent (Kock pouch) ileostomy, or ileoanal reservoir. See "Fecal Diversions," p. 434, for additional details.

*Postoperative management:* Includes routine chest physiotherapy to prevent respiratory complications; IV fluid and electrolyte replacement or TPN as the patient's condition warrants; gastric tube for decompression until bowel sounds are present and the patient is eliminating flatus or stool; gradual resumption of diet as tolerated following NG tube removal and return of bowel function; aseptic incisional care to prevent infection; and fecal diversion care and teaching.

## NURSING DIAGNOSES AND INTERVENTIONS

**Fluid volume deficit** related to active loss secondary to diarrhea and gastrointestinal bleeding/hemorrhage

*Desired outcome:* Patient is normovolemic within 24 h of admission as evidenced by balanced I&O, urine output $\geq$ 30 ml/h, good skin turgor, moist mucous membranes, stable weight, BP $\geq$ 90/60 mm Hg (or within patient's normal range), and RR 12-20 breaths/min.

- Monitor I&O; weigh patient daily; and monitor laboratory values to evaluate fluid, electrolyte, and hematologic status. Optimal values are serum $K^+$ $\geq$3.5 mEq/L, Hct 40%-54% (male) and 37%-47% (female), Hgb 14-18 g/dl (male) and 12-16 g/dl (female), and RBCs 4.5-6.0 million/$\mu$l (male) and 4.0-5.5 million/$\mu$l (female).
- Monitor frequency and consistency of stool. Assess and record presence of blood, mucus, fat, and undigested food.
- Monitor patient for indicators of dehydration: thirst, poor skin turgor (may not be a reliable indicator of hydration in the older adult), dryness of mucous membranes, fever, and concentrated and decreased urinary output.
- Monitor patient for signs of hemorrhage: hypotension, increased HR and RR, pallor, diaphoresis, and restlessness. Assess stool for quality (e.g., is it grossly bloody and liquid?) and quantity (e.g., is it mostly blood or mostly stool?). Report significant findings to physician.
- If the patient is acutely ill, maintain parenteral replacement of fluids, electrolytes, and vitamins as prescribed.

- Administer blood products and iron as prescribed to correct existing anemia and losses due to hemorrhage.
- When patient is taking food by mouth, provide bland, high-protein, high-calorie, and low-residue diet, as prescribed. Assess tolerance to diet by determining incidence of cramping, diarrhea, and flatulence.

**Altered protection** related to risk of perforation secondary to deeply inflamed colonic mucosa

*Desired outcome:*   Patient is free of signs of perforation as evidenced by normothermia; HR 60-100 bpm; RR 12-20 breaths/min with normal depth and pattern (eupnea); normal bowel sounds; absence of abdominal distention, tympany, or rebound tenderness; negative culture results; and orientation to person, place, and time.

---

**Note:**   Patients with severe ulcerative colitis can have markedly elevated WBC counts: >20,000/μl, and occasionally as high as 50,000/μl.

---

- Monitor patient for fever, chills, increased respiratory and heart rates, diaphoresis, and increased abdominal discomfort, which can occur with perforation of the colon and potentially result in localized abscess or generalized fecal peritonitis and septicemia. **Note:** Systemic therapy with corticosteroids and antibiotics can mask the development of this complication.
- Report any evidence of sudden abdominal distention associated with the preceding symptoms because they can signal toxic megacolon. Factors contributing to the development of this complication include hypokalemia, barium enema examinations, and use of opiates and anticholinergics.
- If patient has a sudden temperature elevation, culture blood and other sites as prescribed. Monitor culture reports, notifying physician promptly of any positive cultures.
- Administer antibiotics as prescribed and in a timely fashion.
- Evaluate patient's orientation and LOC q2-4h.

**Pain,** abdominal cramping, and nausea related to intestinal inflammatory process

*Desired outcomes:*   Within 4 h of intervention, patient's subjective perception of discomfort decreases as documented by a pain scale. Objective indicators, such as grimacing, are absent or diminished.

- Monitor and document characteristics of discomfort, and assess whether it is associated with ingestion of certain foods or medications or with emotional stress. Devise a pain scale with patient, rating discomfort from 0 (no pain) to 10 (worst pain). Eliminate foods that cause cramping and discomfort.
- As prescribed, maintain patient on NPO or TPN to provide bowel rest.
- Provide nasal and oral care at frequent intervals to lessen discomfort from NPO status or presence of gastric tube.
- Keep patient's environment quiet, and plan nursing care to provide maximum periods of rest.
- Administer sedatives and tranquilizers as prescribed to promote rest and reduce anxiety.
- Administer hydrophilic colloids, anticholinergics, and antidiarrheals as prescribed to relieve cramping and diarrhea.
- Document the degree of relief obtained, rating it according to the pain scale.
- Observe for intensification of symptoms, which can indicate the presence of complications. Notify physician of significant findings.

**Diarrhea** related to inflammatory process of the intestines

*Desired outcome:*   Patient's stools become normal in consistency, and frequency is lessened within 3 days of admission.

- Monitor and record the amount, frequency, and character of patient's stools.

- Provide covered bedpan, commode, or bathroom that is easily accessible and ready to use at all times.
- Empty bedpan and commode to control odor and decrease patient anxiety and self-consciousness.
- Administer hydrophilic colloids, anticholinergics, and antidiarrheals as prescribed to decrease fluidity and number of stools.
- Administer topical corticosteroid preparations and antibiotics *via* retention enema, as prescribed, to relieve local inflammation. If patient has difficulty retaining the enema for the prescribed amount of time, consult with physician about the use of corticosteroid foam, which is easier to retain and administer.
- Monitor serum electrolytes, particularly $K^+$, for abnormalities. Alert physician to $K^+ < 3.5$ mEq/L.

**High risk for impaired perineal/perianal skin integrity** related to persistent diarrhea
*Desired outcome:* Patient's perineal/perianal skin remains intact with no erythema.
- Provide materials or assist patient with cleansing and drying of perineal area after each bowel movement.
- Apply protective skin care products such as skin preparations, gels, or barrier films, *only* to normal, unbroken skin. Petrolatum emollients, moisture barrier ointments, and vanishing creams also can be used to prevent irritation from frequent liquid stools.
- Administer hydrophilic colloids, anticholinergics, and antidiarrheals as prescribed to decrease fluidity and number of stools.

---

**Note:** See "Fecal Diversions" for **Bowel incontinence,** p. 436, **Body image disturbance,** p. 437, and **High risk for impaired peristomal skin integrity** *and* **impaired stomal tissue integrity,** p. 435. If surgery is performed, see Appendix One for nursing diagnoses and interventions in "Caring for Preoperative and Postoperative Patients, p. 693, and "Caring for Patients with Cancer and Other Life-Disrupting Illnesses," p. 753.

---

## PATIENT-FAMILY TEACHING AND DISCHARGE PLANNING

Give patient and significant others verbal and written information about the following:
- Medications, including name, rationale, dosage, schedule, route of administration, precautions, and potential side effects. **Note:** For patients on high-dose steroid therapy, caution them about abrupt discontinuation of steroids to prevent precipitation of adrenal crisis. Withdrawal symptoms include weakness, lethargy, restlessness, anorexia, nausea, and muscle tenderness. Instruct patient to notify physician if these symptoms occur.
- Signs and symptoms that necessitate medical attention, including fever, nausea and vomiting, diarrhea or constipation, and any significant change in appearance and frequency of stools, any of which can signal exacerbation of the disease.
- Dietary management to promote nutritional and fluid maintenance and prevent abdominal cramping, discomfort, and diarrhea.
- Importance of perineal care after bowel movements.
- Enteral or parenteral feeding instructions if patient is to supplement diet or is NPO.
- Referral to community resources, including Crohn's and Colitis Foundation of America.
- Importance of follow-up medical care, particularly in patients with long-standing disease, since so many of them develop colonic adenocarcinoma.

- Referral to a mental health specialist if recommended by registered nurse or physician.

*In addition, if patient has a fecal diversion:*

- Care of incision, dressing changes, and permission to take baths or showers once sutures/drains are removed.
- Care of stoma, peristomal/perianal skin, or perineal wound; use of ostomy equipment; and method for obtaining supplies. Sitz baths may be indicated for perineal wound.
- Medications that are contraindicated (e.g., laxatives) or that may not be well tolerated or absorbed (e.g., antibiotics, enteric-coated tablets, or long-acting tablets).
- Gradual resumption of ADL, excluding heavy lifting (>10 lb), pushing, or pulling for 6-8 weeks to prevent incisional herniation.
- Referral to community resources, including home health-care agency, ET nurse, and the local chapter of United Ostomy Association.
- Importance of reporting signs and symptoms that require medical attention, such as change in stoma color from the normal bright and shiny red; peristomal or perianal skin irritation; diarrhea; incisional pain, drainage, swelling, or redness; signs and symptoms of fluid and electrolyte imbalance; and signs and symptoms of mechanical or functional obstruction.

# Crohn's disease

Crohn's disease, also known as regional enteritis, granulomatous colitis, or transmural colitis, is a chronic inflammatory disease that can involve any part of the GI tract from the mouth to the anus. Usually the disease occurs segmentally, demonstrating discontinuous areas of disease with segments of normal bowel in between. The terminal ileum is the most frequent site of involvement, followed by the colon. The disease affects all layers of the bowel: the mucosa, submucosa, circular and longitudinal muscles, and serosa. A family history of this disease or ulcerative colitis occurs in 15%-20% of affected patients. The cause is unknown, but theories include infection, immunologic factors, environmental factors, and genetic predisposition.

During the past 20 years, the incidence of Crohn's disease has increased dramatically, while that of ulcerative colitis has not changed. This rise may reflect increased diagnostic awareness rather than a real change in frequency in Crohn's disease.

## ASSESSMENT

**Signs and symptoms:**   Clinical presentation varies as a direct reflection of the location of the inflammatory process, its extent, severity, and relationship to contiguous structures. Sometimes the onset is abrupt and the patient can appear to have appendicitis, ulcerative colitis, intestinal obstruction, or a fever of obscure origin. Acute symptoms include RLQ pain, tenderness, spasm, flatulence, nausea, fever, and diarrhea. A more typical picture is insidious onset with more persistent but less severe symptoms, such as vague abdominal pain, unexplained anemia, and fever. Diarrhea—liquid, soft, or mushy stools—is the most common symptom. The presence of gross blood is rare. Abdominal pain is a frequent symptom, and it may be colicky or crampy, initiated by meals, centered in the lower abdomen, and relieved by defecation because of the chronic partial obstruction of the small intestine, colon, or both. As the disease progresses, anorexia, malnutrition, weight loss, anemia, lassitude, malaise, and fever can occur in addition to fluid, electrolyte, and metabolic disturbances. See Tables 6-4 and 6-5 for comparisons of ulcerative colitis and Crohn's disease.

**Physical assessment:**   In the early stages the exam is often normal but might demonstrate mild tenderness in the abdomen over the affected bowel. In more advanced disease, a palpable mass may be present, especially in the RLQ with terminal ileum involvement. Persistent rectal fissure, large ulcers, perirectal abscess, or rectal fistula is the first indication of disease in 15%-25% of patients with small bowel involvement and in 50%-75% of patients with colonic involvement. Rectovaginal, abdominal, and enterovesical fistulas also can occur. Extraintestinal manifestations characteristic of ulcerative colitis do occur, but less frequently (10%-20%).

## DIAGNOSTIC TESTS

**Stool examination:**  Usually reveals the presence of occult blood; frank blood may be noted in stools of patients with colonic involvement or with ulcerations and fistulas of the rectum. A few patients present with bloody diarrhea. Stool cultures and smears rule out bacterial and parasitic disorders. Specimens are also examined for presence of fecal fat.

**Sigmoidoscopy:**  To evaluate possible colonic involvement and obtain rectal biopsy. The finding of granulomas on mucosal biopsy argues strongly for the diagnosis of Crohn's disease. However, since granulomas are more numerous in the submucosa, suction biopsy of the rectum provides deeper, larger, and less traumatized specimens for a better diagnostic yield than mucosal biopsy obtained through an endoscope.

**Colonoscopy:**  May help differentiate Crohn's disease from ulcerative colitis. Characteristic patchy inflammation (skip lesions) rules out ulcerative colitis. However, colonoscopy usually does not add useful diagnostic information in the presence of positive findings from sigmoidoscopy or radiologic examination. When the diagnosis is unclear and there is a question of malignancy, colonoscopy provides the means of directly visualizing mucosal changes and obtaining biopsies, brushings, and washings for cytologic examination. Colonoscopy also may assist in planning for surgery by documenting the extent of colonic disease. **Note:** This procedure may be contraindicated in patients with acute phases of Crohn's colitis or when deep ulcerations or fistulas are known to be present because of the risk of perforation.

**Barium enema and upper GI series with small bowel follow-through:**  Contribute to the diagnosis of Crohn's disease. Involvement of only the terminal ileum or segmental involvement of the colon or small intestine is almost always indicative of Crohn's disease. Thickened bowel wall with stricture (string sign) separated by segments of normal bowel, cobblestone appearance, and presence of fistulas and skip lesions are common findings. A double-contrast barium enema technique may increase sensitivity in detecting early or subtle changes. **Note:** Barium enema may be contraindicated in patients with acute phases of Crohn's colitis because of the risk of perforation. Upper GI barium series is contraindicated in patients in whom intestinal obstruction is suspected.

**Blood tests:**  Are nonspecific for the diagnosis of Crohn's disease but help determine whether or not the inflammatory process is active and evaluate the patient's overall condition. Anemia may be present and may be (1) microcytic owing to iron deficiency from chronic blood loss and bone marrow depression secondary to chronic inflammatory process, or (2) megaloblastic owing to folic acid or $B_{12}$ deficiency (usually seen only in patients with extensive ileitis causing malabsorption). Increased WBC count and sedimentation rate reflect disease activity and inflammation. Hypoalbuminemia corresponds with the disease activity and results from decreased protein intake, extensive malabsorption, and significant enteric loss of protein. Hypokalemia is seen in patients with chronic diarrhea; hypophosphatemia and hypocalcemia are seen in patients with significant malabsorption. Liver function studies may be abnormal secondary to pericholangitis.

**Urinalysis and urine culture:**  May reveal urinary tract infection secondary to enterovesicular fistula.

**Tests for malabsorption:**  Since patients with active, extensive disease (especially when it involves the small intestine) may develop malabsorption and malnutrition, the following tests are clinically significant: D-xylose tolerance test (for upper jejunal involvement); Schilling's test (for ileal involvement); serum albumin, carotene, calcium, and phosphorus levels; and fecal fat (steatorrhea).

## COLLABORATIVE MANAGEMENT

The initial treatment is nonoperative, and it is individualized and based on symptomatic relief. Medical treatment is more likely to be successful early in the course of the disease, before permanent structural changes have occurred.

**Parenteral replacement of fluids, electrolytes, and blood products:** Maintenance therapy for acute exacerbation as indicated by laboratory test results.

**Physical and emotional rest:**   Complete bed rest and assistance with ADL during acute phases.

**Pharmacotherapy:**   It has not been proven that drugs, singly or in combination, can prolong remission and prevent relapse of Crohn's disease.

*Sedatives and tranquilizers:*   To promote rest and reduce anxiety.

*Antidiarrheals:*   To decrease diarrhea and cramping. Codeine or loperamide often reduces diarrhea with a concomitant decrease in abdominal cramping. Anticholinergics are not recommended, because they may mask obstructive symptoms and precipitate toxic megacolon. For these reasons, antidiarrheals should be administered with caution. If a patient does not respond appropriately to standard antidiarrheals and mild sedation, the presence of obstruction, bowel perforation, or abscess formation is suspected.

*Sulfasalazine:*   To treat acute exacerbations of colonic and ileocolonic disease. It appears to be more effective in patients with disease limited to the colon than in those with disease limited to the small bowel. Since it has not been shown to prevent recurrence, the goal of management is to discontinue the drug gradually following remission of active Crohn's colitis (Crohn's disease limited to the colon). **Note:** Because sulfasalazine impairs folate absorption, patients receive folic acid supplements during treatment.

*Corticosteroids:*   To reduce the active inflammatory response, decrease edema, and control exacerbations. Prednisone is effective in diminishing activity of the disease process, but is more beneficial in patients with small bowel involvement than it is in those with disease limited to the colon. As active disease subsides, prednisone is tapered with the goal of eliminating the drug. However, many Crohn's disease patients become steroid-dependent, meaning they are symptomatic with low-dose therapy (5-15 mg/day) or with total discontinuation of the drug. In some cases of chronic disease, continuous corticosteroid therapy may be necessary.

*Immunosuppressive agents:*   To reduce inflammation when corticosteroids have failed, or in combination with corticosteroids to allow dosage reduction of corticosteroids. Because they are toxic agents with serious side effects and there is a lack of consensus about their benefits, immunosuppressives such as azathioprine and 6-mercaptopurine are considered only when persistent severe disease does not respond to standard therapy or when reduction of steroid dosage is required but otherwise unattainable.

*Antibiotics:*   To control suppurative complications. Patients with bacterial overgrowth of the small bowel may be treated with broad-spectrum antibiotics. See Table 6-7. In patients who are allergic, intolerant, or unresponsive to sulfasalazine, metronidazole (Flagyl) appears to be effective in colonic disease and in healing perianal disease.

**Nutritional management:**   A major component of therapy. During acute exacerbations, total parenteral nutrition and NPO status can be used to replace nutritional deficits and allow complete bowel rest. Elemental diets that are free of bulk and residue, low in fat, and digested in the upper jejunum provide good nutrition with low fecal volume to allow bowel rest in selected patients.

Bland diets low in residue, roughage, and fat but high in protein, calories, carbohydrates, and vitamins provide good nutrition and reduce excessive stimulation of the bowel. A diet free of milk, milk products, gas-forming foods, alcohol, and iced beverages reduces cramping and diarrhea. When remission occurs, a less restricted diet can be tailored to the individual patient, excluding foods known to precipitate symptoms. Patients with involvement of the small intestine frequently require supplementation of vitamins and minerals, especially calcium, iron, folate, and magnesium secondary to malabsorption or to compensate for foods excluded from the diet. Patients with extensive ileal disease or resection frequently require vitamin $B_{12}$ replacement, and if bile salt deficiency exists, cholestyramine and medium-chain triglycerides might be needed to control diarrhea and reduce fat malabsorption and steatorrhea.

**Referral to mental health practitioner for supportive psychotherapy:** If indicated, because of the chronic and progressive nature of Crohn's disease.

**Surgical management:** Because surgery is not a cure for Crohn's disease, it is reserved for complications rather than used as a primary form of therapy. Common indications for surgery include bowel obstruction, internal and enterocutaneous fistulas, intraabdominal abscesses, and perianal disease. Conservative resection of the affected bowel segments with restoration of bowel continuity, preserving as much of the intestine as possible, is the preferred surgical approach. If fecal diversion using an ostomy is required, the type of diversion used will depend on the location and amount of intestinal segment(s) to be resected. (For details, see "Fecal Diversions," p. 434.)

## NURSING DIAGNOSES AND INTERVENTIONS

**Fluid volume deficit** related to active loss secondary to diarrhea or presence of GI fistula

*Desired outcomes:* Patient is normovolemic within 24 h of admission as evidenced by balanced I&O, urinary output $\geq 30$ ml/h, BP $\geq 90/60$ mm Hg (or within patient's normal range), RR 12-20 breaths/min, stable weight, good skin turgor, and moist mucous membranes. Patient reports that diarrhea is controlled.

- Monitor I&O, weigh patient daily, and monitor laboratory values to evaluate fluid and electrolyte status. Optimal values are serum $K^+$ 3.5-5.0 mEq/L, serum $Na^+$ 137-147 mEq/L, and serum $Cl^-$ 95-108 mEq/L.
- Monitor frequency and consistency of stools. Assess and record presence of blood, mucus, fat, or undigested food.
- Monitor patient for indicators of dehydration: thirst, poor skin turgor, dryness of mucous membranes, fever, and concentrated and decreased urinary output.
- Maintain patient on parenteral replacement of fluids, electrolytes, and vitamins as prescribed to promote anabolism and healing.
- When the patient is taking food by mouth, provide bland, high-protein, high-calorie, low-residue diet, as prescribed. Assess tolerance to diet by determining incidence of cramping, diarrhea, and flatulence. Modify diet plan accordingly.

**High risk for infection/altered protection** related to potential for complications caused by intestinal inflammatory disorder

*Desired outcome:* Patient is free from indicators of infection and intraabdominal injury as evidenced by normothermia; HR 60-100 bpm; RR 12-20 breaths/min; normal bowel sounds; absence of abdominal distention, rigidity, or localized pain and tenderness; absence of nausea and vomiting; negative culture results; and orientation to person, place, and time.

- Monitor patient for indicators of intestinal obstruction, including abdominal rigidity and increased episodes of nausea and vomiting. **Note:** Contributing factors to the development of this complication include use of opiates and the prolonged use of antidiarrheals.

- Monitor patient for fever, increased RR and HR, chills, diaphoresis, and increased abdominal discomfort, which can occur with intestinal perforation, abscess or fistula formation, or generalized fecal peritonitis and septicemia. **Note:** Systemic therapy with corticosteroids and antibiotics can mask development of these complications.
- Evaluate patient's orientation and LOC q2-4h.
- If the patient has a sudden temperature elevation, obtain cultures of blood, urine, fistulas, or other possible sources of infection, as prescribed. Abscesses or fistulas to the abdominal wall, bladder, or vagina are common in Crohn's disease, as well as abscesses or fistulas to other loops of small bowel and colon. Monitor culture reports and notify physician promptly of any positive results.
- If draining fistulas or abscesses are present, change dressings or irrigate tubes or drains as prescribed. Note color, character, and odor of all drainage. Report the presence of foul-smelling or abnormal drainage or the loss of tube/drain patency.
- Administer antibiotics as prescribed and in a timely manner.
- Prevent the transmission of potentially infectious organisms by good handwashing technique before and after caring for the patient and by disposing of dressings and drainage using Body Substance Isolation (see Appendix, p. 777).

**Pain,** abdominal cramping, and nausea related to intestinal inflammatory process

***Desired outcomes:*** Patient's subjective perception of discomfort decreases within 4 h of intervention, as documented by a pain scale. Objective indicators, such as grimacing, are absent or diminished.

- Monitor and document characteristics of discomfort, and assess whether it is associated with ingestion of certain foods or with emotional stress. Devise a pain scale with patient, rating discomfort from 0 (no discomfort) to 10 (worst discomfort). Eliminate foods that cause cramping and discomfort.
- As prescribed, keep patient NPO and provide parenteral nutrition to provide bowel rest.
- Administer antidiarrheals and analgesics as prescribed to reduce abdominal discomfort.
- Provide nasal and oral care at frequent intervals to lessen discomfort from NPO status and presence of gastric tube.
- Administer antiemetic medications before meals to enhance appetite when nausea is a problem.
- Document relief obtained, using the pain scale.
- For additional information, see this nursing diagnosis in Appendix One, p. 694.

**Diarrhea** related to intestinal inflammatory process

***Desired outcome:*** Patient reports a reduction in frequency of stools and a return to more normal stool consistency within 3 days of hospital admission.

- If the patient is experiencing frequent and urgent passage of loose stools, provide covered bedpan or commode, or be sure the bathroom is easily accessible and ready to use at all times.
- Empty the bedpan and commode promptly to control odor and decrease patient anxiety and self-consciousness.
- Administer antidiarrheals as prescribed to decrease fluidity and number of stools.
- If bile salt deficiency (because of ileal disease or resection) is contributing to diarrhea, administer cholestyramine as prescribed to control diarrhea.
- Eliminate or decrease fat content in the diet because it can increase diarrhea in individuals with malabsorption syndromes. Also, restrict foods and beverages that can precipitate diarrhea and cramping, such as raw vegetables and fruits, whole grain cereals, condiments, gas-forming foods, alcohol, iced

and carbonated beverages, and, in lactose-intolerant patients, milk and milk products.

**Activity intolerance** related to generalized weakness secondary to intestinal inflammatory process

*Desired outcome:* Patient adheres to prescribed rest regimen and sets appropriate goals for self-care as the condition improves (optimally within 3-7 days of admission).

- Keep patient's environment quiet to facilitate rest.
- Because adequate rest is necessary to sustain remission, assist patient with ADL and plan nursing care to provide maximum rest periods.
- As prescribed, administer sedatives and tranquilizers to promote rest and reduce anxiety.
- As the patient's physical condition improves, encourage self-care to the greatest extent possible, and assist patient with setting realistic, attainable goals.
- For additional information, see **High risk for activity intolerance,** p. 711, in Appendix One.

---

**Note:** *If surgery is performed,* see "Fecal Diversions" for **Bowel incontinence,** p. 436, **Body image disturbance,** p. 437, and **High risk for impaired peristomal skin integrity** *and* **impaired stomal tissue integrity,** p. 435. See Appendix One for nursing diagnoses and interventions in "Caring for Preoperative and Postoperative Patients," p. 693, and "Caring for Patients with Cancer and Other Life-Disrupting Illnesses," p. 753.

---

## PATIENT-FAMILY TEACHING AND DISCHARGE PLANNING

Give patient and significant others verbal and written information about the following:

- Medications, including name, rationale, dosage, schedule, route of administration, precautions, and potential side effects.
- Signs and symptoms that necessitate medical attention, including fever, nausea and vomiting, abdominal discomfort, any significant change in appearance and frequency of stools, passage of stool through the vagina, or stool mixed with urine, any of which can signal recurrence or complications of Crohn's disease.
- Importance of dietary management to promote nutritional and fluid maintenance and prevent abdominal cramping, discomfort, and diarrhea.
- Importance of perineal/perianal skin care after bowel movements.
- Importance of balancing activities with rest periods, even during remission, because adequate rest is necessary to sustain remission.
- Referral to community resources, including National Foundation for Ileitis and Colitis.
- Importance of follow-up medical care, including supportive psychotherapy, because of the chronic and progressive nature of Crohn's disease.

*In addition, if the patient has a fecal diversion:*

- Care of incision, dressing changes, and bathing.
- Care of stoma and peristomal skin, use of ostomy equipment, and method for obtaining supplies.
- Gradual resumption of ADL, excluding heavy lifting ($>10$ lb), pushing, or pulling for 6-8 weeks to prevent incisional herniation.
- Referral to community resources, including home health-care agency, ET nurse, and local chapter of United Ostomy Association.
- Importance of reporting signs and symptoms that require medical attention, such as change in stoma color from the normal bright and shiny red; lesions of stomal mucosa that may indicate recurrence of the disease; peristomal

skin irritation; diarrhea or constipation, fever, chills, abdominal pain, distention, nausea, and vomiting; and incisional pain, drainage, swelling, or redness.

# Fecal diversions

**Note:**   For a discussion of diverticulitis, see p. 414; colorectal cancer, see p. 417; polyps/familial adenomatous polyposis, see p. 420; ulcerative colitis, see p. 421; and Crohn's disease, see p. 428.

## SURGICAL INTERVENTIONS

It is sometimes necessary to interrupt the continuity of the bowel because of intestinal disease or its complications. The resulting fecal diversion can be located anywhere along the bowel, depending on the location of the diseased or injured portion; and it can be permanent or temporary. The most common sites for fecal diversion are the colon and ileum.

**Colostomy:**   Created when the surgeon brings a portion of the colon to the abdominal skin surface. An opening in the exteriorized colon permits elimination of flatus and stool through the stoma. The continuity of the colon can be interrupted anywhere along its length.

*Transverse colostomy:*   This is the most frequently created stoma to divert the fecal stream on a temporary basis. Surgical indications include relief of bowel obstruction before definitive surgery for tumors or diverticulitis and colon perforation secondary to trauma. Stool is usually soft, unformed, and eliminated unpredictably. A temporary colostomy may be double-barrelled, with a proximal stoma through which stool is eliminated and a distal stoma adjacent to the proximal stoma called a mucous fistula. More commonly, a loop colostomy is created with a supporting rod placed beneath it until the exteriorized loop of colon becomes affixed to the skin.

*Descending or sigmoid colostomy:*   This is usually a permanent fecal diversion. Cancer of the rectum is the most common cause for surgical intervention. Stool is usually formed, and some individuals may have stool elimination at predictable times. In a permanent colostomy, the surgeon brings the severed end of the colon to the abdominal skin surface. To mature the stoma, the colon above the skin surface is cuffed back on itself and sutured to the skin so that the mucosal surface of the intestine is exposed.

*Cecostomy or ascending colostomy:*   Uncommon. The procedure done most often is a temporary diverting stoma, which eliminates unformed, soft or liquid, and unpredictable stool. Surgical intervention is similar to that with transverse colostomies.

**Ileostomy**

*Conventional (Brooke) ileostomy:*   Created by bringing a distal portion of the ileum up and out onto the surface of the skin of the abdominal wall. A permanent ileostomy is matured by the same procedure discussed with a permanent colostomy. Surgical indications include ulcerative colitis, Crohn's disease, and familial adenomatous polyposis (FAP) requiring excision of the entire colon and rectum.

*Temporary ileostomy:*   Usually a loop stoma with or without a supporting rod in place beneath the loop of the ileum until the exteriorized loop of ileum becomes affixed to the skin. The purpose is to divert the fecal stream away from a more distal anastomosis site or fistula repair site until healing has occurred. Output is usually liquid or pastelike, contains digestive enzymes, and is eliminated continually. A collection pouch is worn over the stoma on the abdomen to collect gas and fecal discharge.

*Continent (Kock pouch) ileostomy:*   An intraabdominal pouch constructed from approximately 30 cm of distal ileum. A 10-cm portion of ileum is intussuscepted to form an outlet valve from the pouch to the skin of the abdomen, where a stoma is constructed flush with the skin. The intraabdominal pouch is continent for gas and fecal discharge and is emptied approximately qid by inserting a catheter through the stoma. No external pouch is needed, and a Band-Aid or small dressing is worn over the stoma to collect mucus. Surgical indications include ulcerative colitis and FAP requiring removal of the colon and rectum. Crohn's disease is generally a contraindication for this procedure because the disease can recur in the pouch, necessitating its removal.

**Ileoanal reservoir:**   A two-staged surgical procedure developed to preserve fecal continence and prevent the need for a permanent ileostomy. During the first stage following total colectomy and removal of the rectal mucosa, an ileal reservoir is constructed just above the junction of the ileum and anal canal; the ileal outlet from the reservoir is brought down through the cuff of the rectal muscle and anastomosed to the anal canal. The anal sphincter is preserved, and the resulting ileal reservoir provides a storage place for feces. A temporary diverting ileostomy is required for 2-3 months to allow healing of the anastomosis. The second stage occurs when the diverting ileostomy is taken down and fecal continuity is restored. Initially, the patient experiences fecal incontinence and 10 or more bowel movements a day. After 3-6 months, the patient experiences a decrease in urgency and frequency with 4-8 bowel movements per day. This procedure is an option for patients requiring colectomy for ulcerative colitis or FAP. It is contraindicated in patients with Crohn's disease and incontinence problems.

## NURSING DIAGNOSES AND INTERVENTIONS

**High risk for impaired peristomal skin integrity** related to exposure to effluent or sensitivity to appliance material; *and*
**Impaired stomal tissue integrity (or risk of same)** related to improperly fitted appliance resulting in impaired circulation
***Desired outcome:***   Patient's stomal and peristomal skin and tissue remain intact.

*After colostomy or conventional ileostomy (permanent or temporary)*

- Apply a pectin, methylcellulose-based, solid-form skin barrier around the stoma to protect the peristomal skin from contact with stool, which would cause irritation.
  - Cut an opening in the skin barrier the exact circumference of the stoma, remove the release paper, and apply the sticky surface directly to the peristomal skin.
  - Remove the skin barrier and inspect the skin q2-3days. Peristomal skin should look like other abdominal skin. Changes such as erythema, erosion, serous drainage, bleeding, or induration signal the presence of infection, irritation, or sensitivity to materials placed on the skin and should be documented and reported to the physician because topical medication may be required. Irritating materials should be discontinued and other materials substituted. Patch-test the patient's abdominal skin to determine sensitivity to suspected materials.
  - Because stomas become less edematous for some weeks after surgery, the opening in the skin barrier must be recalibrated each time it is changed so that it is always the exact circumference of the stoma to prevent contact of stool with the skin.
- Apply a two-piece pouch system or a pouch with access cap so that the stoma can be inspected for viability q12-24h. A matured stoma will be red in color with overlying mucus. A nonmatured stoma will be red and moist where the mucous membrane is exposed, but can be a darker, mottled, grayish-red with a transparent or translucent film of serosa elsewhere.
- When removing the skin barrier and pouch for routine care, cleanse the patient's skin with mild soap and water, rinse well, and dry it so that the skin

retains its normal integrity and the skin barrier and pouch materials adhere well to the skin.

- To maintain a secure pouch seal, empty the pouch when it is ⅓ to ½ full of stool or gas.

### After a continent ileostomy (Kock pouch)

- A catheter is inserted through the stoma and into the pouch and sutured to the peristomal skin. Avoid stress on the suture, and monitor for erythema, induration, drainage, or erosion. Report significant findings to physician. As prescribed, maintain catheter on low, continuous suction or gravity drainage to prevent stress on the nipple valve, and maintain pouch decompression so that suture lines are allowed to heal without stress or tension.
- Check the catheter q2h for patency, and irrigate with sterile saline (30 ml) to prevent obstruction. Notify physician if unable to instill solution, if there are no returns per suction catheter, or if leakage of irrigating solution or pouch contents appears around the catheter.
- To prevent peristomal skin irritation, change 4×4 dressing around the stoma q2h or as often as it becomes wet. The drainage will be serosanguineous at first and mixed with mucus. Report presence of frank bleeding to physician.
- Assess stoma for viability with each dressing change. It should be red in color and wet and shiny with mucus. A stoma that is pale or dark purple to black or dull in appearance can indicate circulatory impairment and should be reported to physician immediately and documented.

### After ileoanal reservoir

- Perform routine care for diverting ileostomy (see earlier).
- After the first stage of the operation, the patient may have incontinence of mucus. Maintain perineal/perianal skin integrity by irrigating the mucus out of the reservoir daily with 60 ml water, or gently cleansing the area with water and cotton balls or soft tissues. (**Note:** Pouch irrigation to remove mucus rarely is indicated now because of new reservoir configurations that allow sponatenous emptying of the reservoir.) Avoid soap, which can cause itching or irritation. Use an absorbent pad at night to absorb incontinence of mucus.
- After the second stage of operation (when the ileostomy is taken down), expect the patient to experience frequency and urgency of defecation.
- Wash perineal/perianal area with warm water or commercial perianal/perineal cleansing solution, using a squeeze bottle, cotton balls, or soft tissues. Do not use toilet paper, because it can cause irritation. If desired, dry the area wtih a hair dryer on a cool setting.
- Provide sitz baths to promote comfort and help clean the perineal/perianal area.
- Apply protective skin sealants or ointments. Skin sealants should not be used on irritated or eroded skin because of the high alcohol content, which would cause a painful burning sensation.

**Bowel incontinence** related to disruption of normal function with fecal diversion

***Desired outcomes:*** Within 2-4 days after surgery, patient has bowel sounds and eliminates gas and stool *via* the fecal diversion. Within 3 days after teaching has been initiated, patient verbalizes understanding of measures that will maintain normal elimination pattern and demonstrates care techniques specific to the fecal diversion.

### After colostomy and conventional ileostomy (permanent and temporary)

- Empty stool from the bottom opening of the pouch, and assess the quality and quantity of stool to document return of normal bowel function.
- If the colostomy is not eliminating stool after 3-4 days and bowel sounds have returned, gently insert a gloved, lubricated finger into the stoma to determine presence of stricture at the skin or fascial levels and note presence of any stool within reach of the examining finger. To stimulate elimination

of gas and stool, physician may prescribe colostomy irrigation. (For procedure, see **Knowledge deficit:** Colostomy irrigation procedure, p. 438.)

## After continent ileostomy (Kock pouch)

- Monitor I&O, and record color and consistency of output.
- Expect aspiration of bright red blood or serosanguinous liquid drainage from the Kock pouch during the early postoperative period.
- As GI function returns after 3-4 days, expect the drainage to change in color from blood-tinged to greenish-brown liquid. When ileal output appears, suction is discontinued and the pouch catheter is placed to gravity drainage.
- As the patient's diet progresses from clear liquids to solid food, the ileal output thickens. Check and irrigate the catheter q2h and as needed to maintain patency. If the patient reports abdominal fullness in the area of the pouch along with decreased fecal output, check placement and patency of the catheter.
- When the patient is alert and taking food by mouth, teach catheter irrigation procedure, which should be performed q2h; demonstrate how to empty the pouch contents through the catheter into the toilet.
- Before hospital discharge, teach patient how to remove and reinsert the catheter.

## After ileoanal reservoir

- Monitor I&O, observing quantity, quality, and consistency of output from diverting ileostomy and reservoir. Monitor patient for elevation of temperature accompanied by perianal pain and discharge of purulent, bloody mucus from drains and anal orifice. Report significant findings to physician.
- If drains are present, irrigate them as prescribed to maintain patency, decrease stress on suture lines, and decrease incidence of infection.
- After the first stage of the operation, patient may experience incontinence of mucus. Advise patient to wear small pad to avoid soiling of outer garments.
- After the second stage of the operation (when the ileostomy is taken down), expect incontinence and 15-20 bowel movements per day with urgency when patient is on a clear-liquid diet. Assist patient with perianal care, and apply protective skin care products. To decrease incontinence at night, the catheter can be placed in the reservoir and connected to gravity drainage bag.
- Expect the number of bowel movements to decrease to 6-12/day and the consistency to thicken when the patient is on solid foods.
- Administer hydrophilic colloids and antidiarrheals as prescribed to decrease frequency and fluidity of stools.
- Provide diet consultation so that patient will be able to avoid foods that cause liquid stools (spinach, raw fruits, highly seasoned foods, green beans, broccoli, prune and grape juice, alcohol) and increase intake of foods that cause thick stools (cheese, ripe bananas, applesauce, creamy peanut butter, jello, pasta).
- Reassure patient that frequency and urgency are temporary and that as the reservoir expands and absorbs fluid, bowel movements should become thicker and less frequent.

**Body image disturbance** related to presence of fecal diversion

***Desired outcome:*** Within 5-7 days after surgery, patient demonstrates actions that reflect beginning acceptance of the fecal diversion and incorporates changes into self-concept as evidenced by acknowledging body changes, viewing the stoma, and participating in the care of the fecal diversion.

- Expect the following fears, which may be expressed by patients experiencing a fecal diversion: physical, social, and work activities will be curtailed significantly; rejection, isolation, and feelings of uncleanliness will occur; everyone will know about the altered pattern of fecal elimination; and loss of voluntary control may occur (many patients view incontinence as a return to infancy).

- Encourage patient to discuss feelings and fears; clarify any misconceptions. Involve family members in the discussions because they, too, may have anxieties and misconceptions.
- Provide a calm and quiet environment for patient and significant others to discuss the surgery. Initiate an open and honest discussion. Monitor carefully for and listen closely to expressed or nonverbalized needs because each patient will react differently to the surgical procedure.
- Encourage acceptance of fecal diversion by having patient participate in care. Assure patient that education offers a means of control.
- Assure patient that physical, social, and work activities will not be affected by the presence of a fecal diversion.
- Expect the patient to have fears about sexual acceptance, although these fears usually are not expressed overtly. Concerns center on change in body image; fears about odor and the ostomy appliance interfering with intercourse; conception, pregnancy, and discomfort from perianal wound and scar in women; and impotence and failure to ejaculate in men, especially after more radical dissection of the pelvis in the patient with cancer. If you are uncomfortable talking about sexuality with patients, be aware of these potential concerns and arrange for a consultation with someone who can speak openly and honestly about these problems.
- Consult with patient's surgeon about a visit by another ostomate. Patients gain reassurance and build positive attitudes by seeing a healthy, active person who has undergone the same type of surgery.

**Knowledge deficit:**   Colostomy irrigation procedure
***Desired outcome:***   Within 3 days after initiation of teaching, patient demonstrates proficiency with the procedure for colostomy irrigation.

---

**Note:**   Teach prescribed colostomy irrigation to patient with permanent descending or sigmoid colostomy. Colostomy irrigation is performed daily or every other day so that wearing a pouch becomes unnecessary. An appropriate candidate is a patient who has 1-2 formed stools each day at predictable times (same as normal stool elimination pattern before illness). In addition, the patient must be able to manipulate the equipment, remember the technique, and be willing to spend approximately an hour a day performing the procedure. It may take 4-6 weeks for the patient to have stool elimination regulated with irrigation.

---

*Instruct patient about the following steps:*
- Position an irrigating sleeve over the colostomy and hold it in place with an adhesive disk or belt. Place the distal end in the toilet.
- Fill an enema container with 500-1,000 ml warm water. With the patient in a sitting position, place the container so that the bottom surface is at the patient's shoulder level. Flush the tubing with the water to remove air from the tubing. Allow the water to slowly enter the colostomy from the container through tubing that has either a lubricated cone attachment or a shield on a lubricated catheter, which keeps the irrigating water in the colostomy. Hold the cone snugly against the stoma. It should take 3-5 min for fluid to enter the colon.
- After water has entered the colon, advise the patient to wait 30-40 min for the water to be eliminated along with the stool in the colon.
- Remove the irrigation sleeve, and cleanse and dry the peristomal area.
- Apply a small dressing or security pouch over the colostomy between irrigations.

---

**Note:**   See Appendix One for nursing diagnoses and interventions in "Caring for Preoperative and Postoperative Patients," p. 693, and "Caring for Patients with Cancer and Other Life-Disrupting Illnesses," p. 719.

## PATIENT-FAMILY TEACHING AND DISCHARGE PLANNING

Give patient and significant others verbal and written information about the following:

- Medications, including name, rationale, dosage, schedule, route of administration, precautions, and potential side effects.
- Importance of dietary management to promote nutritional and fluid maintenance.
- Care of incision, dressing changes, and permission to take baths or showers once sutures/drains are removed.
- Care of stoma, peristomal, and perianal skin; use of ostomy equipment; and method for obtaining supplies.
- Gradual resumption of ADL, excluding heavy lifting (>10 lb), pushing, or pulling for 6-8 weeks to prevent development of incisional herniation.
- Referral to community resources including home health-care agency, ET nurse, and local chapter of United Ostomy Association.
- Importance of follow-up care with physician and ET nurse; confirm date and time of next appointment.
- Importance of reporting signs and symptoms that require medical attention, such as change in stoma color from the normal bright and shiny red; peristomal or perianal skin irritation; any significant changes in appearance, frequency, and consistency of stools; fever, chills, abdominal pain, or distention; and incisional pain, drainage, swelling, or redness.

# Section Four:   Abdominal Trauma

Injury to abdominal contents is related to the nature of the force applied and the consistency of the affected structures. Forces involved are classified as blunt (e.g., those caused by falls, physical assault, motor vehicle collisions, crush injury) or penetrating (e.g., stab, gunshot wounds). Organs are categorized as solid (e.g., liver, spleen, pancreas) or hollow (e.g., stomach, intestine). Blunt abdominal trauma typically results in injury to solid viscera because hollow viscera tend to be more compressible. However, hollow organs may rupture, especially when full, if there is a sudden increase in intraluminal pressure. Usually injury inflicted by stab wounds follows a more predictable pattern and involves less tissue destruction than injury from gunshot wounds, although stab wounds to major vascular structures and organs can be fatal. Removing penetrating objects can result in additional injury, so attempts at removal are made only in a controlled surgical environment. High-velocity weapons (e.g., rifles) not only cause injury to tissue in the direct path of the missile but to adjacent organs as well because of energy shock waves that surround the missile path. Tissue destruction is not as great with low-velocity pistols. The rate of complications and death increases greatly if injury to multiple abdominal organs is sustained.

Abdominal trauma results in direct injury to organs, blood vessels, and supporting structures. Other pathophysiologic changes associated with abdominal trauma include (1) fluid shifts related to tissue damage, blood loss, and shock; (2) metabolic changes mediated by the CNS and macro/microendocrine systems; (3) coagulation problems associated with massive hemorrhage and multiple transfusions; (4) inflammation, infection, and abscess formation due to release of GI secretions and bacteria into the peritoneum; and (5) nutritional and electrolyte alterations that develop as a consequence of disruption of GI tract integrity. The following is a brief overview of common injuries.

**Spleen:** The organ most frequently injured following blunt trauma. Massive hemorrhage from splenic injury is common. All efforts are made to repair the spleen since total splenectomy increases the long-term risk of sepsis, especially in children and young adults.

**Liver:**　Because of its size and location, it is the organ most frequently involved in penetrating trauma and often is affected with blunt injury, as well. Control of bleeding and bile drainage are major concerns with hepatic injury.

**Lower esophagus and stomach:**　Occasionally the lower esophagus is involved in penetrating trauma. Because the stomach is flexible and readily displaced, it is usually not injured with blunt trauma but may be injured by direct penetration. Any serious injury to the lower esophagus and stomach results in the escape of irritating gastric fluids and the release of free air below the level of the diaphragm.

**Pancreas and duodenum:**　Although traumatic pancreatic or duodenal injury occurs relatively infrequently, it is associated with high morbidity and mortality rates because of the difficulty of detecting these injuries and the likelihood of massive injury to nearby organs. These organs are retroperitoneal, and clinical indicators of injury often are not obvious for several hours.

**Small intestine and mesentery:**　These injuries are common and may be caused by penetrating or nonpenetrating forces. Compromised intestinal blood flow with eventual infarction is the consequence of undetected mesenteric damage. Perforations or contusions can result in release of bacteria and intestinal contents into the abdominal cavity, causing serious infection.

**Colon:**　Injury most frequently caused by penetrating forces, although lap belts, direct blows, and other blunt forces cause a small percentage of colonic injuries. Because of the high bacterial content, infection is always a serious concern. Many patients with colon injury require a temporary colostomy (see "Fecal Diversions").

**Major vessels:**　Injuries to the abdominal aorta and inferior vena cava are most often caused by penetrating trauma but also occur with deceleration injury. Hepatic vein injuries frequently are associated with juxtahepatic vena caval injury and result in rapid hemorrhage. Blood loss after major vascular injury is massive, and survival depends on rapid prehospital transport and immediate surgical intervention.

**Retroperitoneal:**　Tears in retroperitoneal vessels associated with pelvic fractures or damage to retroperitoneal organs (pancreas, duodenum, kidney) can cause bleeding into the retroperitoneum. Even though the retroperitoneal space can accommodate up to 4 L of blood, detection of retroperitoneal hematomas is difficult, and sophisticated diagnostic techniques may be required.

## ASSESSMENT

**Signs and symptoms:**　A wide variation can occur. Mild tenderness to severe abdominal pain may be present, with the pain either localized to the site of injury or diffuse. Blood or fluid collection within the peritoneum causes irritation resulting in involuntary guarding, rigidity, and rebound tenderness. Fluid or air under the diaphragm may cause referred shoulder pain. Kehr's sign (left shoulder pain caused by splenic bleeding) also may be noted, especially when the patient is recumbent. Nausea and vomiting may be present, and the conscious patient who has sustained blood loss often complains of thirst, an early sign of hemorrhagic shock. Symptoms of abdominal injury may be minimal or absent in the patient who is intoxicated or has sustained head or spinal cord injury. **Note:** The absence of signs and symptoms does not exclude the presence of major abdominal injury.

**Physical assessment:**　Abdominal assessment is highly subjective, and serial evaluations by the same examiner are strongly recommended in order to detect subtle changes.

*Inspection:* Abrasions and ecchymoses are suggestive of underlying injury (e.g., ecchymosis over LUQ suggests splenic rupture; ecchymotic areas on the flank are suggestive of retroperitoneal bleeding; and erythema and ecchymosis across the lower abdomen suggest intestinal injury due to lap belts). Ecchymoses may take hours to days to develop, depending on the rate of blood loss.

*Auscultation:* It is important to auscultate before palpation and percussion

**T A B L E  6 - 8  Signs and Symptoms Suggestive of Peritoneal Irritation**

Generalized abdominal pain or tenderness
Involuntary guarding of the abdomen
Abdominal wall rigidity
Rebound tenderness
Abdominal pain with movement or coughing
Decreased or absent bowel sounds

because these maneuvers can stimulate the bowel and confound assessment findings. Bowel sounds are likely to be decreased or absent with abdominal organ injury, intraperitoneal bleeding, or recent surgery. However, the presence of bowel sounds does not exclude significant abdominal injury. Bowel sounds should be auscultated frequently, especially in the first 24-48 h after injury. Absence of bowel sounds is expected immediately after surgery. Failure to auscultate bowel sounds within 24-48 h after surgery is suggestive of ileus, possibly caused by continued bleeding, peritonitis, or bowel infarction.

*Palpation:* Tenderness or pain to palpation strongly suggests abdominal injury. Blood or fluid in the abdomen can result in signs and symptoms of peritoneal irritation (see Table 6-8).

*Percussion:* Tympany suggests the presence of gas. Unusually large areas of dullness may be percussed over ruptured blood-filled organs (e.g., a fixed area of dullness in the LUQ suggests a ruptured spleen).

**Vital signs and hemodynamic measurements:**  Ventilatory excursion often is diminished because of pain, thoracic injury, or limited diaphragmatic movement due to abdominal distention. Initial compensatory tachycardia and vasoconstriction secondary to blood loss usually maintain a normal BP until blood loss becomes major. At that point, BP rapidly deteriorates.

**History:**  Details regarding circumstances of the accident and mechanism of injury are invaluable in detecting the possibility of specific injuries. In addition, ascertain time of patient's last meal, previous abdominal surgeries, and use of safety restraints (if appropriate). If possible, determine current medications and allergies, particularly to contrast material, antibiotics, and tetanus toxoid. The history may be difficult to obtain because of alcohol or drug intoxication, head injury, breathing difficulties, or impaired cerebral perfusion. In such cases, family members may be valuable sources of information.

## DIAGNOSTIC TESTS

**Hct:**  Serial levels reflect the amount of blood lost. If drawn immediately after the injury, Hct may be normal, but serial levels will reveal dramatic decreases during resuscitation and as extravascular fluid mobilizes during the recovery phase.

**WBC count:**  Leukocytosis is expected immediately after injury. Splenic injuries, in particular, result in the rapid development of a moderate to high WBC count. A later increase in WBCs or a shift to the left reflects an increase in the number of neutrophils, which signals an inflammatory response and possible intraabdominal infection. In the patient with abdominal trauma, ruptured abdominal viscera must be considered as a potential source of infection.

**Platelet count:**  Mild thrombocytosis is seen immediately following traumatic injury. After massive hemorrhage, thrombocytopenia may be noted. Platelet transfusion usually is not required unless spontaneous bleeding is present.

**Glucose:**  Initially elevated because of catecholamine release and insulin resistance associated with major trauma. Glucose metabolism is abnormal following major hepatic resection, and patients should be monitored in order to prevent hypoglycemic episodes.

**Amylase:** Elevated serum levels are associated with pancreatic or upper small bowel injury, but values may be normal even with severe injury to these organs.

**Serum glutamic-oxaloacetic transaminase (SGOT), serum glutamic-pyruvic transaminase (SGPT), lactic dehydrogenase (LDH):** Elevations of these enzymes reflect hepatic dysfunction due to liver ischemia during prolonged hypotensive episodes or direct traumatic damage. Fluctuations in these enzymes during the postoperative period can be used to detect evidence of liver necrosis.

**X-rays:** Initially, flat and upright chest x-rays exclude chest injuries (frequently associated with abdominal trauma) and establish a baseline. Subsequent chest x-rays aid in detecting complications, such as atelectasis and pneumonia. In addition, chest, abdominal, and pelvic x-rays may reveal fractures, missiles, free intraperitoneal air, hematoma, or hemorrhage.

**Occult blood:** Gastric contents and stool should be tested for blood in the initial and recovery periods because GI bleeding can occur as a result of both direct injury and later complications.

**Diagnostic peritoneal lavage (DPL):** Involves insertion of a peritoneal dialysis catheter into the peritoneum to check for intraabdominal bleeding. DPL is indicated for confirmed or suspected blunt abdominal trauma for the following patients: (1) those in whom signs and symptoms of abdominal injury are obscured by intoxication, head or spinal cord trauma, narcotic administration, or unconsciousness; (2) those about to undergo general anesthesia for repair of other injuries (e.g., orthopedic, facial); and (3) any patient with equivocal assessment findings. DPL is unnecessary for patients who have obvious intraabdominal bleeding or other indications for immediate laparotomy (see "Surgical Considerations," below).

**CT scan:** Can detect intraperitoneal and retroperitoneal bleeding and free air (associated with rupture of hollow viscera). It is most useful in assessing injury to solid abdominal organs. This procedure also is helpful in detecting abscesses and other complications. **Caution:** Because of the risk of rapid deterioration, patients with recent injuries (24-48 h) or in unstable condition should be accompanied by a nurse during the CT scan. Appropriate monitoring and resuscitation equipment must be readily available.

**Angiography:** Performed selectively with blunt trauma to evaluate injury to spleen, liver, pancreas, duodenum, and retroperitoneal vessels when other diagnostic findings are equivocal. **Caution:** Because of the large amount of contrast material used during this procedure, ensure adequate hydration and monitor urine output closely for several hours for a possible decrease.

Abdominal injuries often are associated with multisystem trauma. Also see diagnostic test discussions in "Pneumothorax/Hemothorax," p. 20, "Head Injury," p. 250, and "Spinal Cord Injury," p. 234.

## COLLABORATIVE MANAGEMENT

**Oxygen:** Individuals sustaining abdominal trauma are likely to be tachypneic, with the potential for poor ventilatory effort. Supplemental $O_2$ is delivered until patient's ABG values while breathing room air are acceptable.

**Fluid management:** Massive blood loss is frequently associated with abdominal injuries. Restoration and maintenance of adequate volume is essential. Initially, Ringer's lactate or similar balanced salt solution is given. Colloid solutions, such as albumin, are helpful in the postoperative period if the patient is hypoalbuminemic. Typed and cross-matched fresh blood is the optimal fluid for replacement of large blood losses. However, since fresh whole blood is rarely available, a combination of packed cells and fresh frozen plasma most often is used. For the hemodynamically stable patient, balanced crystalloid solutions with additional K are used until the patient is able to tolerate enteral or oral feedings.

**Gastric intubation:** Gastric tube permits gastric decompression, aids in removal of gastric contents, and prevents accumulation of gas or air in the GI tract. Aspirated contents can be checked for blood to aid in the diagnosis of lower esophageal, gastric, or duodenal injury. The tube usually remains in place until bowel function returns.

**Urinary drainage:** An indwelling catheter is inserted soon after admission to obtain a specimen for urinalysis, monitor hourly urine output, and aid in the diagnosis of genitourinary trauma.

**Pharmacotherapy**

*Antibiotics:* Abdominal trauma is associated with a high incidence of intraabdominal abscess, sepsis, and wound infection, particularly injury to the terminal ileum and colon. Individuals with suspected intestinal injury are started on parenteral antibiotic therapy immediately. Broad-spectrum antibiotics are continued postoperatively and stopped after several days unless there is evidence of infection.

*Analgesics:* Because narcotics alter the sensorium, making evaluation of the patient's condition difficult, they are used cautiously in the early stages of trauma. Small doses of IV analgesics are preferred because absorption from IM sites may be prolonged and erratic. Narcotic analgesics are used in the immediate postoperative period to relieve pain and promote ventilatory excursion. They may be delivered intermittently by the nurse or *via* patient-controlled pumps. As the severity of pain lessens, alternate analgesics such as NSAIDs (e.g., ketorolac, ibuprofen) may be prescribed. The risk of excessive bleeding and gastric stress ulcers must be weighed against the potential benefit of NSAIDs.

*Tetanus prophylaxis:* Tetanus immune globulin and tetanus toxoid are considered, based on Centers for Disease Control recommendations (see Table 6-9).

**Nutrition:** Patients with abdominal trauma have complex nutritional needs owing to the hypermetabolic state associated with major trauma and traumatic or surgical disruption of normal GI function. Often infection and sepsis contribute to negative N state and increased metabolic needs. Prompt initiation of parenteral feedings in patients unable to accept enteric feedings and the administration of supplemental calories, proteins, vitamins, and minerals are essential for healing. For more information, see "Providing Nutritional Support," p. 665.

**Surgical considerations for penetrating abdominal injuries:** The issue of

---

**T A B L E  6 - 9**  **Tetanus Prophylaxis in Routine Wound Management— United States**

| History of adsorbed tetanus toxoid (doses) | Clean, minor wounds | | All other wounds* | |
|---|---|---|---|---|
| | Td† | TIG | Td† | TIG |
| Unknown or < three | Yes | No | Yes | Yes |
| ≥three‡ | No§ | No | No‖ | No |

Adapted from Centers for Disease Control: *Morbidity Mortality Weekly Report* 34(27):422, 1985.

*Such as, but not limited to, wounds resulting from missiles, crushing, burns, and frostbite.

†For children <7 years old; DPT (DT, if pertussis vaccine is contraindicated) is preferred to tetanus toxoid alone. For persons 7 years old and older, Td is preferred to tetanus toxoid alone.

‡If only three doses of *fluid* toxoid have been received, a fourth dose of toxoid, preferably an adsorbed toxoid, should be given.

§Yes, if >10 years since last dose.

‖Yes, if more than 5 years since last dose. (More frequent boosters are not needed and can accentuate side effects.)

mandatory surgical exploration vs. observation and selective surgery, especially with stab wounds, remains controversial. Patients without obvious injury or peritoneal signs generally are observed for positive peritoneal signs and stability of VS. Indications for laparotomy include one or more of the following: (1) penetrating injury suspected of invading the peritoneum; (2) positive peritoneal signs (Table 6-8); (3) shock; (4) GI hemorrhage; (5) free air in the peritoneal cavity as seen on x-ray; (6) evisceration; (7) massive hematuria; or (8) positive DPL. **Note:** Recently injured or preoperative patients should be evaluated for peritoneal signs at hourly intervals by the same professional. Notify surgeon immediately if the patient develops peritoneal signs, evidence of shock, gastric or rectal bleeding, or gross hematuria.

**Surgical considerations for nonpenetrating abdominal injuries:**   Physical examination usually is reliable in determining the necessity for surgery in alert, cooperative, unintoxicated patients. Additional diagnostic tests such as DPL or CT scan are necessary to evaluate the need for surgery in the patient who is intoxicated, unconscious, or who has sustained head or spinal cord trauma. Immediate laparotomy for blunt abdominal trauma is indicated under the following circumstances: (1) clear signs of peritoneal irritation (see Table 6-8); (2) free air in the peritoneum; (3) hypotension due to suspected abdominal injury or persistent and unexplained hypotension; (4) positive DPL; (5) GI aspirate or rectal smear positive for blood; or (6) other positive diagnostic tests such as CT scan or arteriogram. Carefully evaluated stable patients with blunt abdominal trauma may be admitted to critical care for observation. These patients should be evaluated in the same manner as that described for penetrating abdominal injuries, above. It is important to note that damage to retroperitoneal organs, such as the pancreas and duodenum, may not cause significant signs and symptoms for 6-12 h or longer. Relatively slow bleeding from abdominal viscera may not be clinically apparent for 12 h or longer after the initial injury. In addition, the nurse should be aware that complications, such as bowel obstruction, may develop days or weeks after the traumatic event. The need for vigilant observation in the care of these patients cannot be overemphasized.

## NURSING DIAGNOSES AND INTERVENTIONS

**Fluid volume deficit** related to active loss secondary to bleeding/hemorrhage; related to GI fluid loss through vomiting; diarrhea; or gastric, intestinal, incisional, or other drainage tube; or related to presence of enterocutaneous fistulas

*Desired outcomes:*   Within 4 h of admission or upon definitive repair (e.g., surgery), patient is normovolemic as evidenced by systolic BP $\geq$ 90 mm Hg (or within patient's baseline range), HR 60-100 bpm, CVP 2-6 mm Hg or 5-12 cm $H_2O$, urinary output $\geq$30 ml/h, warm extremities, brisk capillary refill ($<$2 sec), distal pulses $>$2+ on a 0-4+ scale, and absence of orthostasis.

- *In recently injured patients,* monitor BP hourly, or more frequently in the presence of obvious bleeding or unstable VS. Be alert to increasing diastolic BP and decreasing systolic BP. Even a small but sudden decrease in systolic BP signals the need to notify physician, especially with the trauma patient in whom the extent of injury is unknown. Most trauma patients are young, and excellent neurovascular compensation results in a near normal BP until there is a large intravascular volume depletion. In the *stable postoperative patient,* perform routine VS assessment.
- Be alert to the clinical indicators of fluid volume deficit (see Table 6-10), and report them accordingly.
- Monitor HR and cardiovascular status hourly until the patient's condition is stable. Note and report sudden increases or decreases in HR, especially if associated with indicators of fluid volume deficit, as noted above.
- Monitor for physical indicators of fluid volume deficit, including diaphore-

**T A B L E  6 - 1 0    Indicators of Fluid Volume Deficit**

Increasing diastolic BP (early)
Decreasing systolic BP (later)
Tachycardia (>100 bpm)
Tachypnea (>20 breaths/min)
Anxiety (early)
Altered/depressed mental status (later)
Delayed capillary refill (≥2 seconds)
Cool, pale skin
Low or decreasing central venous pressure
Low urinary output (<30 ml/hr)

---

sis, cool extremities, delayed capillary refill (≥2 sec), and absent or decreased strength of distal pulses.
- In the patient with evidence of volume depletion or active blood loss, administer prescribed fluids rapidly through one or more large-caliber (16-gauge or larger) IV catheters. **Caution:** Evaluate patency of IV catheters frequently during rapid volume resuscitation. Monitor patient closely to avoid fluid volume overload and complications such as heart failure (see p. 60) and pulmonary edema (see p. 85).
- Measure CVP q1-4h if indicated. Be alert to low or decreasing values. Report sudden decreases in CVP, especially if associated with other indicators of fluid volume deficit, as noted above.
- Measure urinary output q4h (or when patient voids). Be alert to decreasing urinary output and to infrequent voidings. Low urine output usually reflects inadequate intravascular volume in the abdominal trauma patient. Before administering diuretics, evaluate patient for evidence of fluid volume deficit, as noted above.
- Estimate ongoing blood loss. Measure all bloody drainage from tubes or catheters, noting drainage color (e.g., coffee ground, burgundy, bright red). Note the frequency of dressing changes due to saturation with blood to estimate amount of blood loss *via* wound site. Note and report signficant increases in the amount of drainage, especially if it is bloody.

**Pain** related to irritation caused by intraperitoneal blood or secretions, actual trauma or surgical incision, and manipulation of organs during surgery
*Desired outcomes:*   Within 4 h of admission, patient's subjective perception of pain decreases, as documented by a pain scale. Objective indicators, such as grimacing, are absent or diminished.
- Evaluate patient for presence of preoperative and postoperative pain. Devise a pain scale with patient, rating discomfort from 0 (no pain) to 10 (worst pain). Preoperative pain is anticipated and is a vital diagnostic aid. The nature of postoperative pain also can be important. Incisional and some visceral pain can be anticipated, but intense or prolonged pain, especially when accompanied by other peritoneal signs (see Table 6-8) can signal bleeding, bowel infarction, infection, or other complications. Recognize that the autonomic nervous system response to pain can complicate assessment of abdominal injury and hypovolemia. For details, see **Pain,** p. 694, in Appendix One.
- Administer narcotics and other analgesics as prescribed. Avoid administering analgesics preoperatively until the patient has been evaluated thoroughly by a trauma surgeon. Administer postoperatively prescribed analgesics on a continual or regular schedule promptly with additional analgesia as needed,

or provide patient with patient-controlled analgesia (PCA). Analgesics are helpful in relieving pain as well as aiding in the recovery process by promoting greater ventilatory excursion. Be aware that intoxication often is involved in traumatic events; therefore, victims may be drug or alcohol users, with a higher-than-average tolerance for narcotics. These same individuals may suffer symptoms of alcohol or narcotic withdrawal that need recognition and treatment. In addition, recognize that narcotic analgesics can decrease GI motility and may delay return to normal bowel function. Document the degree of relief obtained, using the pain scale.

- Monitor PCA, if prescribed, and document effectiveness, using the pain scale.
- Supplement analgesics with nonpharmacologic maneuvers (e.g., positioning, backrubs, distraction) to aid in pain reduction.

**High risk for infection** related to inadequate primary defenses secondary to disruption of the GI tract (particularly of the terminal ileum and colon) and traumatically inflicted open wound; related to multiple indwelling catheters and tubes; and related to compromised immune state due to blood loss and metabolic response to trauma

***Desired outcome:*** Patient is free of infection as evidenced by core or rectal temperature <37.8° C (100° F); HR ≤ 100 bpm; orientation to person, place, and time; and absence of unusual erythema, warmth, or drainage at surgical incisions or wound sites.

- Monitor VS for evidence of infection, noting temperature increases and associated increases in heart and respiratory rates. Notify surgeon of sudden temperature elevations.

## T A B L E 6 - 1 1  Characteristics of Gastrointestinal Drainage

| Source | Composition and usual character |
|---|---|
| Mouth and oropharynx | Saliva; thin, clear, watery; pH 7.0 |
| Stomach | Hydrochloric, gastrin, pepsin, mucus; thin, brownish to greenish; acidic |
| Pancreas | Enzymes and bicarbonate; thin, watery, yellowish-brown; alkaline |
| Biliary tract | Bile, including bile salts and electrolytes; bright yellow to brownish-green |
| Duodenum | Digestive enzymes, mucus, products of digestion; thin, bright yellow to light brown, may be greenish; alkaline |
| Jejunum | Enzymes, mucus, products of digestion; brown, watery with particles |
| Ileum | Enzymes, mucus, digestive products, greater amounts of bacteria; brown, liquid, feculant |
| Colon | Digestive products, mucus, large amounts of bacteria; brown to dark brown, semiformed to firm stool |
| Postoperative (GI surgery) | Initially drainage expected to contain fresh blood; later drainage mixed with old blood and then approaches normal composition |
| Infection present | Drainage cloudy, may be thicker than usual; strong or unusual odor, drain site often erythematous and warm |

- Evaluate orientation and LOC q8h. Note mental confusion or deterioration from baseline LOC.
- Ensure patency of all surgically placed tubes or drains. Irrigate or attach to low-pressure suction as prescribed. Promptly report unrelieved loss of tube patency.
- Evaluate incisions and wound sites for evidence of infection: unusual erythema, warmth, delayed healing, and purulent or unusual drainage.
- Note amount, color, character, and odor of all drainage (Table 6-11). Report the presence of foul-smelling or abnormal drainage. Test drainage for pH and the presence of blood; compare to expected characteristics.
- Administer antibiotics in a timely fashion. Reschedule parenteral antibiotics if a dose is delayed for more than 1 h. Recognize that failure to administer antibiotics on schedule may result in inadequate blood levels and treatment failure.
- As prescribed, administer pneumococcal vaccine in patients with total splenectomy to minimize the risk of postsplenectomy sepsis.
- Administer tetanus immune globulin and tetanus toxoid as prescribed.
- Change dressings as prescribed, using aseptic technique. Prevent cross-contamination from various wounds by changing one dressing at a time.
- If patient has or develops evisceration, do not reinsert tissue or organs. Place a sterile, saline-soaked gauze over the evisceration and cover with a sterile towel until the evisceration can be evaluated by the surgeon.

**Ineffective breathing pattern** related to pain from injury or surgical incision; chemical irritation of blood or bile on pleural tissue; and diaphragmatic elevation due to abdominal distention

*Desired outcome:* Within 24 h of admission or surgery, patient is eupneic with RR 12-20 breaths/min and clear breath sounds.

- Administer supplemental oxygen as prescribed. Monitor and document effectiveness.
- Administer analgesics at dose and frequency that relieves pain and associated impaired chest excursion.
- For additional interventions, see this nursing diagnosis in Appendix One, p. 703, "Caring for Preoperative and Postoperative Patients."

**Altered gastrointestinal (GI) tissue perfusion (or high risk for same)** related to interrupted blood flow to abdominal viscera secondary to vascular disruption or occlusion, or related to moderate to severe hypovolemia caused by hemorrhage

*Desired outcomes:* Patient has adequate GI tissue perfusion as evidenced by normoactive bowel sounds; soft, nondistended abdomen; and return of bowel elimination. Gastric secretions, drainage, and excretions are negative for occult blood.

- Auscultate for bowel sounds hourly for recently injured patients and q8h during the recovery phase. Report prolonged or sudden absence of bowel sounds because these signs may signal bowel ischemia or infarction. Anticipate absent or diminished bowel sounds for up to 72 h after surgery.
- Evaluate patient for peritoneal signs (see Table 6-8), which may occur acutely secondary to injury or may not develop until days or weeks later if complications due to slow bleeding or other mechanisms occur.
- Ensure adequate intravascular volume (see discussion in **Fluid volume deficit,** p. 444).
- Evaluate laboratory data for evidence of bleeding (e.g., serial Hct) or organ ischemia (e.g., SGPT, SGOT, LDH). Optimal values are Hct > 30%; SGOT 5-40 IU/L; SGPT 5-35 IU/L; and LDH 90-200 ImU/ml.
- Document amount and character of GI secretions, drainage, and excretions. Note changes suggestive of bleeding (presence of frank or occult blood), infection (e.g., increased or purulent drainage), or obstruction (e.g., failure to eliminate flatus or stool within 72 h after surgery).

**High risk for impaired skin integrity** related to exposure to irritating GI drainage; *and*

**Impaired tissue integrity (or risk of same)** related to direct trauma and surgery, catabolic posttraumatic state, and altered circulation

***Desired outcome:*** Patient exhibits wound healing by time of hospital discharge, and the skin remains clear and unbroken.

- Promptly change all dressings that become soiled with drainage or blood.
- Protect the skin surrounding tubes, drains, or fistulas, keeping the areas clean and free from drainage. Gastric and intestinal secretions and drainage are irritating and can lead to skin excoriation. If necessary, apply ointments, skin barriers, or drainage bags to protect the surrounding skin. Apply reusable dressing supports such as Montgomery straps to protect the surrounding skin. Consult ostomy nurse for complex or involved cases.
- Inspect wounds, fistulas, and drain sites for signs of irritation, infection, and ischemia.
- Identify infected and devitalized tissue. Aid in their removal by irrigation, wound packing, or preparing patient for surgical debridement.
- Ensure adequate protein and calorie intake for tissue healing (see **Altered nutrition,** below).
- For more information, see "Managing Wound Care," p. 681.

**Altered nutrition:** Less than body requirements, related to decreased intake secondary to disruption of GI tract integrity (traumatic or surgical) and increased need secondary to hypermetabolic posttrauma state

***Desired outcome:*** By a minimum of 24 h before hospital discharge, patient has adequate nutrition as evidenced by maintenance of baseline body weight and positive or balanced N state.

- Collaborate with physician, dietitian, and pharmacist to estimate patient's metabolic needs, based on type of injury, activity level, and nutritional status before injury.
- Consider patient's specific injuries when planning nutrition (e.g., expect patients with hepatic or pancreatic injury to have difficulty with blood sugar regulation; patients with trauma to the upper GI tract may be fed enterally, but feeding tube must be placed distal to the injury; disruption of the GI tract may require feeding gastrostomy or jejunostomy; patients with major hepatic trauma may have difficulty with protein tolerance).
- Ensure patency of gastric or intestinal tubes to maintain decompression and encourage healing and return of bowel function. Avoid occlusion of the vent side of sump suction tubes because this may result in vacuum occlusion of the tube and excessive suction to gastric mucosa. Use caution when irrigating NG or other tubes that have been placed in or near recently sutured organs.
- Do not start enteral feeding until bowel function returns (i.e., bowel sounds are present, patient experiences hunger).
- Recognize that narcotics decrease GI motility and may contribute to nausea, vomiting, abdominal distention, and ileus. Consider administration of prescribed nonnarcotic analgesics (e.g., ketorolac).
- For more information, see "Providing Nutritional Support," p. 665.

**Posttrauma response** related to life-threatening accident or event resulting in trauma

***Desired outcomes:*** By a minimum of 24 h before hospital discharge, patient verbalizes that the psychosocial impact of the event has decreased and does not exhibit signs of severe stress reaction, such as display of inconsistent affect, suicidal or homicidal behavior; or extreme agitation or depression. Patient cooperates with treatment plan.

---

**Note:** Many victims of major abdominal trauma sustain life-threatening injury. The patient is often aware of the situation and fears death. Even after the physical condition stabilizes, the patient may have a prolonged or severe re-action triggered by recollection of the trauma.

- Evaluate mental status at systematic intervals. Be alert to indicators of se-vere stress reaction, such as display of affect inconsistent with statements or behavior, suicidal or homicidal statements or actions, extreme agitation or depression, and failure to cooperate with instructions related to care.
- Consult with specialists such as psychologist, psychiatric nurse clinician, or pastoral counselor if patient displays signs of severe stress reaction as de-scribed previously.
- Consider organic causes that may contribute to posttraumatic response (e.g., severe pain, alcohol intoxication or withdrawal, electrolyte imbalance, met-abolic encephalopathy, or impaired cerebral perfusion).
- For other pyschosocial interventions, see Appendix One, "Caring for Pa-tients with Cancer and Other Life-Disrupting Illnesses," p. 753.

**Note:**   As appropriate, see nursing diagnoses and interventions in "Fecal Di-versions," p. 435; "Caring for Preoperative and Postoperative Patients," p. 693; "Caring for Patients on Prolonged Bed Rest," p. 711; and "Caring for Patients with Cancer and Other Life-Disrupting Illnesses," p. 719.

## PATIENT-FAMILY TEACHING AND DISCHARGE PLANNING

Anticipate extended physical and emotional rehabilitation for the patient and significant others. Provide verbal and written information about the following:
- Probable need for emotional care, even for patients who have not required extensive physical rehabilitation. Provide referrals to support groups for trauma patients and family members.
- Availability of rehabilitation programs, extended care facilities, and home health agencies for patients unable to accomplish self-care on hospital dis-charge.
- Availability of rehabilitation programs for substance abuse, as indicated. Im-mediately following the traumatic event, the patient and family members are very impressionable, making this period an ideal time for the substance abuser to begin to resolve the problem.
- Medications, including drug name, purpose, dosage, schedule, precautions, and potential side effects. Encourage patients on antibiotics to take the med-ications for the prescribed length of time, even though they may be asymp-tomatic. If patient received tetanus immunization, ensure that he or she re-ceives a wallet-sized card documenting the immunization.
- Wound and catheter care. Have patient or caregiver describe and demon-strate proper technique before hospital discharge.
- Importance of seeking medical attention if indicators of infection or bowel obstruction occur (e.g., fever, severe or unusual abdominal pain, nausea and vomiting, unusual drainage from wounds or incisions, or a change in bowel habits).
- Injury prevention. Immediately following a traumatic injury, the patient is especially likely to respond to injury prevention education. Provide instruc-tions on proper seat-belt applications (across the pelvic girdle rather than across soft tissue of the lower abdomen), safety for infants and children, and other factors suitable for the individuals involved.

# Section Five:   Hepatic and Biliary Disorders

The liver lies directly beneath the diaphragm and occupies most of the RUQ of the abdomen. It has many functions, among them the storage of vitamins, synthesis of blood proteins, destruction of worn-out red blood cells, removal of toxic substances from the body, and management of the formation and secretion of bile.

The gallbladder, which lies directly beneath the right lobe of the liver, and the hepatic, cystic, and common bile ducts make up the biliary system. The biliary duct system transports bile from the liver to the gallbladder. Bile is concentrated and stored in the gallbladder and released to the small intestine (duodenum), where it facilitates the absorption of fats, fat-soluble vitamins, and certain minerals, and also activates the release of pancreatic enzymes. If an obstructive lesion is present in the biliary ducts, the flow of bile is blocked, resulting in hemoconcentration. When this occurs, a variety of clinical manifestations can surface, including obstructive jaundice, dark-amber urine, and clay-colored stools. Pruritus occurs because of the deposition of bile salts in skin tissue. Steatorrhea and bleeding tendencies result from the inability of the duodenum to absorb fats and fat-soluble vitamins A, D, E, and K. Vitamin K is necessary for adequate clotting of the blood.

# Hepatitis

Viral hepatitis may be caused by one of five viruses that are capable of infecting the liver: A, B, C, D, or E. Although symptomatology is similar, immunologic and epidemiologic characteristics are different (Table 6-12). When hepatocytes are damaged, necrosis and autolysis can occur, which in turn lead to abnormal liver functioning. Generally these changes are completely reversible after the acute phase. In some cases, however, massive necrosis can lead to liver failure and death.

*Chronic hepatitis* is inflammation of the liver for more than 6 months in duration. The term is used to describe a spectrum of inflammatory liver diseases ranging from mild chronic persistent hepatitis to severe chronic active hepatitis. Forms of chronic hepatitis are associated with infection from hepatitis B, C, or D viruses; viral infections such as cytomegalovirus (CMV); excessive alcohol consumption; inflammatory bowel disease; and autoimmunity (chronic active lupoid hepatitis). *Alcoholic hepatitis* occurs as a result of tissue necrosis caused by alcohol abuse. Generally it is a precursor to cirrhosis (see p. 457), but it may be simultaneous with cirrhosis.

Jaundice may be seen in any patient with impaired hepatic function. It is classified as prehepatic (hemolytic), caused by increased production of bilirubin; hepatic (hepatocellular), caused by the dysfunction of the liver cells; or posthepatic (obstructive), caused by an obstruction of the flow of bile out of the liver.

## ASSESSMENT

**Signs and symptoms:**  Nausea, vomiting, malaise, anorexia, muscle or joint aches, fatigue, irritability, slight to moderate temperature increases, epigastric discomfort, dark urine, clay-colored stools, pruritus, aversion to smoking.

**Acute hepatic failure:**  Nausea, vomiting, and abdominal pain tend to be more severe. Jaundice is likely to appear earlier and deepen more rapidly. Neurologic alterations, coma, seizures, ascites, sharp rise in temperature, significant leukocytosis, coffee-ground emesis, GI hemorrhage, purpura, shock, oliguria, and azotemia all may be present.

**Physical assessment:**  Presence of jaundice; palpation of lymph nodes and abdomen may reveal lymphadenopathy, hepatomegaly, and splenomegaly. Liver size usually is small with acute hepatic failure.

**History of:**  Clotting disorders, multiple blood transfusions, excessive alcohol ingestion, injecting drug use, exposure to hepatotoxic chemicals or medications, travel to developing countries.

**T A B L E  6 - 1 2  Comparison of Characteristics of Viral Hepatitis Types**

| | Hepatitis A virus | Hepatitis B virus | Hepatitis C virus | Hepatitis D virus | Hepatitis E virus |
|---|---|---|---|---|---|
| Likely modes of transmission | Fecal-oral. Food-borne most common; parenteral transmission rare | Contact with blood or serum, sexual contact, perinatal. Often transmitted by chronic carriers | Contact with blood or serum. Perinatal transmission rare unless coexistent HIV infection in mother. Often transmitted by chronic carriers | Similar to HBV; can only cause infection in presence of HBV | Fecal-oral, food, or water-borne routes |
| Population most often affected | Children; individuals in areas with poor sanitation | Injecting drug users, health-care and public safety workers with exposure to blood, clients and staff of institutions for the developmentally disabled, homosexual men, men and women with multiple heterosexual partners, young children of infected mothers, recipients of certain blood products, hemodialysis patients | Injecting drug users, recipients of blood products prior to 1991. Potential risk to health-care and public safety workers exposed to blood | Only infects individuals with HBV infection. Injecting drug users, hemophiliacs, and recipients of multiple blood transfusions | Individuals living in or traveling to parts of Asia, Africa, and Mexico where there is poor sanitation |

HAV = hepatitis A virus; HBV = hepatitis B virus; HCV = hepatitis C virus; HDV = hepatitis D virus; HEV = hepatitis E virus; IgG = immunoglobuline; HBsAg = hepatitis B surface antigen; HBeAg = hepatitis Be antigen; IgM = immunoglobulin M; HBIG = hepatitis B immune globulin; CDC = Centers for Disease Control

*Continued.*

**TABLE 6-12  Comparison of Characteristics of Viral Hepatitis Types—cont'd**

| | Hepatitis A virus | Hepatitis B virus | Hepatitis C virus | Hepatitis D virus | Hepatitis E virus |
|---|---|---|---|---|---|
| Incubation | 2-6 weeks | 6 weeks to 6 months | 6-11 weeks | | |
| Serum markers of acute disease | Antibody to HAV (anti-HAV). IgG class antibody to HAV (IgG anti-HAV) also indicates immunity present | HBsAg, HBeAg, IgM class antibody to HBcAg (IgM anti-HBc) | Only available test is antibody to HCV (anti-HCV), which detects chronic, not acute, cases | Antibody to HDV (anti-HDV) | As for HAV |
| Measures for reducing exposure | Handwashing; good personal hygiene; sanitation; Body Substance Isolation (see appendix) | Handwashing; good personal hygiene; Body Substance Isolation (see appendix); autoclaving all nondisposable items; avoidance of used needles; careful handling of needles and sharps | As for HBV | As for HBV | |

| | | | | Effectiveness of IG manufactured in US is unknown |
|---|---|---|---|---|
| Prophylaxis | IG before exposure or 1-2 weeks after exposure | Immunization of all health-care workers with blood contact, as well as risk groups identified above. HBIG for known exposure to HBsAg-contaminated material. Routine immunization of all children recommended by CDC | IG before exposure or 1-2 weeks after exposure (controversial) | Immunization against HBV |
| Comments | Symptoms usually mild. Rarely causes fulminant hepatic failure | HBsAg persists in carrier state. Chronic hepatitis may develop. Fulminany hepatic failure may ensue | Carrier state and chronic hepatitis may develop. Fulminant hepatic failure may ensue | Increased risk of serious complications (including fulminant hepatic failure) and death. Carrier state and chronic hepatitis may develop | Disease not endemic in US or Western Europe. Also known as enterically transmitted non-A, non-B hepatitis |

HAV = hepatitis A virus; HBV = hepatitis B virus; HCV = hepatitis C virus; HDV = hepatitis D virus; HEV = hepatitis E virus; IgG = immunoglobulin G; IG = immune globuline; HBsAg = hepatitis B surface antigen; HBeAg = hepatitis Be antigen; IgM = immunoglobulin M; HBIG = hepatitis B immune globulin; CDC = Centers for Disease Control

## DIAGNOSTIC TESTS

**Hematologic tests:**   Anti-HAV IgM will be present with hepatitis A, as will HBsAg with hepatitis B. Anti-HCV will be present approximately 15 weeks after infection with hepatitis C. SGOT (frequently called serum aspartate transaminase, AST) and SGPT will be elevated initially and then drop. Total bilirubin will be elevated, and prothrombin time (PT) will be prolonged. Differential WBC count will reveal leukocytosis, monocytosis, and atypical lymphocytes; gamma globulin levels will be increased.

**Urine tests:**   Will reveal elevation of urobilinogen, mild proteinuria, and mild bilirubinuria.

**Liver biopsy:**   Performed for differential diagnosis.

## COLLABORATIVE MANAGEMENT

**Monitoring of activity level:**   Bed rest may be indicated when symptoms are severe, with a gradual return to normal activity as symptoms subside.

**Diet:**   In general, dietary management consists of giving palatable meals as tolerated without overfeeding. If oral intake is substantially decreased, parenteral or enteral nutrition may be initiated. Na or protein restrictions may be indicated in the presence of fluid retention or encephalopathy. All alcoholic beverages are strictly forbidden. Vitamins usually are given, and folic acid may be indicated in alcoholic hepatitis.

**Management of pruritus:**   Alkaline soaps are restricted; emollients and lipid creams (i.e., Eucerin) are prescribed. Antihistamines and tranquilizers, if used, are administered with caution and in low doses because they are metabolized by the liver. See Table 6-13, which lists hepatotoxic drugs.

**Pharmacotherapy**

*Parenteral vitamin K:*   For those patients with prolonged PT.

*Antihistamines (e.g., diphenhydramine):*   For symptomatic relief of pruritus. However, they may cause excessive sedation.

*Antiemetics:*   For patients with nausea. Avoid phenothiazines such as prochlorperazine (Compazine) because it causes excessive sedation.

*IG:*   Given routinely to all close personal contacts of patients with hepatitis A and to individuals traveling to or residing in endemic regions.

*HBIG:*   Recommended for individuals exposed to HBsAg-contaminated material.

*HB vaccines:*   Developed for prevention of hepatitis, they reduce the incidence of HBV by approximately 92%. Recombinant HB vaccine is indicated for all except immunocompromised (e.g., hemodialyzed) patients. Immunization is recommended for all health-care workers with risk of exposure to blood and body secretions.

*Corticosteroids:*   Used in some patients to control symptomatology and reduce abnormal liver function.

*Recombinant interferon:*   An antiviral agent that inhibits viral replication.

**Restriction of hepatotoxic drugs:**   See Table 6-13.

## NURSING DIAGNOSES AND INTERVENTIONS

**Fatigue** related to decreased metabolic energy production secondary to liver dysfunction, which causes faulty absorption, metabolism, and storage of nutrients

*Desired outcome:*   By a minimum of 24 h before hospital discharge, patient relates the lessening of fatigue and the attainment of increasing amounts of energy.

- Take a diet history to determine food preferences. Encourage significant others to bring in desirable foods, if permitted.
- Monitor and record intake.
- Encourage small, frequent feedings and provide emotional support during meals.
- Obtain prescription for vitamin and mineral supplements, if appropriate.

---

## T A B L E  6 - 1 3   Drugs with the Potential for Hepatotoxicity

acetaminophen*
alcohol*
allopurinol
amiodarone
androgenic steroids
aspirin and other salicylates*
carbamazepine
carmustine (BCNU)
chlorpromazine (CPZ)
cyclosporine
dantrolene
diazepam
erythromycin
glucocorticoids
haloperidol
halothane and related anesthetics
isoniazid (INH)
ketoconazole
mercaptopurine (6-MP)
methotrexate (MTX)
methyldopa
mitomycin
monoamine oxidase (MAO) inhibitors
NSAIDs
oral contraceptives
oxacillin
phenindione
phenylbutazone
phenytoin sodium
rifampin
sulfonamides
vitamin A*

---

*Available without prescription.

- Provide rest periods of at least 90 min before and after activities and treatments.
- Keep frequently used objects within easy reach.
- Promote rest and sleep by decreasing environmental stimuli, providing back massage and relaxation tapes, and speaking with patient in short, simple terms.
- Administer antacids, antiemetics, antidiarrheals, and cathartics as prescribed to minimize gastric distress and promote absorption of nutrients.

**Knowledge deficit:**  Causes of hepatitis and modes of transmission
*Desired outcome:*  Within the 24-h period before hospital discharge, patient verbalizes knowledge about the causes of hepatitis and measures that help prevent transmission.

- Assess patient's knowledge about the disease process, and educate as necessary. Make sure patient knows you are not making moral decisions about alcohol/drug use or sexual behavior.

- Teach patient and significant others the importance of good handwashing and of wearing gloves if contact with feces is possible.
- If appropriate, advise patients with HAV that crowded living conditions with poor sanitation should be avoided to prevent recurrence.
- Remind patients with HBV and HCV that they should modify sexual behavior as directed by physician. Explain that blood donation is no longer possible.
- Advise patients with HBV that their sexual partners should receive HB vaccine.
- Refer patient to drug treatment programs as necessary.

**High risk for impaired skin integrity** related to pruritus secondary to hepatic dysfunction
*Desired outcome:*  Patient's skin remains intact.

- Keep patient's skin moist by using tepid water or emollient baths, avoiding alkaline soap, and applying emollient lotions at frequent intervals.
- Encourage patient not to scratch skin and to keep nails short and smooth. Suggest use of the knuckles if patient must scratch. Wrap or place gloves on patient's hands (especially comatose patients).
- To prevent infection, treat any skin lesion promptly.
- Administer antihistamines as prescribed; observe closely for excessive sedation.
- Encourage patient to wear loose, soft clothing; provide soft linens (cotton is best).
- Keep the environment cool.
- Change soiled linen as soon as possible.

**Body image disturbance** related to presence of jaundice
*Desired outcome:*  Within the 24-h period before hospital discharge, patient verbalizes knowledge about measures for enhancing appearance and demonstrates an interest in daily grooming.

- Encourage patient and significant others to verbalize feelings, concerns.
- Encourage patient to maintain daily grooming.
- Explain that wearing yellow and green intensifies yellow skin tone. Suggest wearing bright reds and blues or black instead.
- Provide privacy as necessary.
- For additional information, see this nursing diagnosis in Appendix One, p. 760.

**Altered protection** related to increased risk of bleeding secondary to decreased vitamin K absorption
*Desired outcome:*  Patient is free of bleeding as evidenced by negative tests for occult blood in the feces and urine, absence of ecchymotic areas, and absence of bleeding at the gums and injection sites.

- Monitor PT levels daily. The optimal range is 10.5-13.5 sec.
- Handle patient gently (e.g., when turning or transferring).
- Minimize IM injections. Rotate sites, and use small-gauge needles. Apply moderate pressure after an injection, but do not massage the site. Administer medications orally or intravenously when possible.
- Observe for ecchymotic areas. Inspect the gums and test the urine and feces for bleeding. Report significant findings to physician.
- Teach patient to use electric razor and soft-bristled toothbrush.
- Administer vitamin K as prescribed.

## PATIENT-FAMILY TEACHING AND DISCHARGE PLANNING

Give patient and significant others verbal and written information about the following:

- Importance of rest and getting adequate nutrition.
- Importance of avoiding hepatotoxic agents, including OTC drugs (see Table 6-13).

- Prescribed medications (e.g., multivitamins), including name, purpose, dosage, schedule, potential side effects, and precautions.
- Importance of informing physicians, dentists, and other health-care workers of hepatitis diagnosis.
- Potential complications, including delayed healing, skin injury, and bleeding tendencies.
- Importance of avoiding alcohol during recovery.
- Referral to alcohol/drug treatment programs as appropriate.

## Cirrhosis

Cirrhosis is a chronic, serious disease in which normal configuration of the liver is changed, resulting in cell death. When new cells are formed, the resulting scarring causes disruption of blood and lymph flow. Although pathologic changes do not occur for many years, structural changes gradually lead to total liver dysfunction. Manifestations of cirrhosis are related to hepatocellular necrosis and portal hypertension. Complications caused by cellular failure are similar to those of acute hepatitis and include inability to metabolize bilirubin and the presence of jaundice; difficulty producing serum proteins, including albumin and some clotting factors; hyperdynamic circulation and decreased vasomotor tone; pulmonary changes (V/Q mismatch) and sometimes cyanosis; changes in N metabolism (e.g., inability to convert ammonia to urea); and difficulty metabolizing some hormones. Complications related to portal hypertension include development of ascites, bleeding esophageal and gastric varices, portal-systemic collaterals, encephalopathy, and splenomegaly.

**Alcoholic cirrhosis:**   Associated with chronic alcohol abuse and accounts for 50% of all cases. Changes in liver structure due to cirrhosis are irreversible, but compensation of liver function can be achieved if the liver is protected from further damage by alcohol cessation.

**Postnecrotic cirrhosis:**   Associated with history of viral hepatitis or hepatic damage from drugs or toxins; accounts for 20% of all cases. This type appears to predispose the patient to the development of a hepatoma.

**Biliary cirrhosis:**   Associated with posthepatic biliary obstruction and accounts for 15% of all cases.

### ASSESSMENT

**Signs and symptoms:**   Weakness, fatigability, weight loss, fever, anorexia, nausea, occasional vomiting, abdominal pain, menstrual abnormalities, impotence, loss of libido, sterility, hematemesis. Urine may be dark because of the presence of bilirubin and stools may be light because of its absence.

**Physical assessment:**   Jaundice, hepatomegaly, ascites, peripheral edema, and fetor hepaticus (a musty, sweetish odor on the breath). There may be slight changes in personality and behavior, which can progress to coma (a result of hepatic encephalopathy); spider angiomas, testicular atrophy, gynecomastia, pectoral and axillary alopecia (a result of hormonal changes); splenomegaly; hemorrhoids (a result of portal hypertension complications); spider nevi; and palmar erythema.

**History of:**   Excessive alcohol ingestion; hepatitis B, C, or D infection; exposure to hepatotoxic drugs (see Table 6-13) or chemicals; biliary or metabolic disease; poor nutrition.

### DIAGNOSTIC TESTS

**Hematologic:**   RBCs will be decreased in hypersplenism and decreased with hemorrhage. WBCs will be decreased with hypersplenism and increased with infection.

**Serum biochemical tests**

*Bilirubin levels:*   Elevated because of failure in hepatocyte metabolism and obstruction in some instances. Very high or persistently elevated levels are considered a poor prognostic sign.

*Alkalkine phosphatase levels:*   Normal to mildly elevated.

*SGOT and SGPT levels:*   Usually elevated >300 U with acute failure. Normal or mildly elevated with chronic failure. SGPT is more specific for hepatocellular damage.

*Albumin levels:*   Reduced, especially with ascites. Persistently low levels suggest a poor prognosis.

*$Na^+$ levels:*   Normal to low. Na is retained but is associated with water retention, which results in normal serum $Na^+$ levels or even a dilutional hyponatremia. Often severe hyponatremia is present in the terminal stage and is associated with tense ascites and hepatorenal syndrome.

*$K^+$ levels:*   Slightly reduced unless patient has renal insufficiency, which would result in hyperkalemia. Chronic hypokalemic acidosis is common in patients with chronic alcoholic liver disease.

*Glucose levels:*   Hypoglycemia sometimes occurs owing to impaired gluconeogenesis and glycogen depletion in patients with severe or terminal liver disease.

*BUN levels:*   May be slightly decreased because of failure of Krebs' cycle enzymes in the liver; or elevated because of bleeding or renal insufficiency.

*Ammonia levels:*   Elevation is expected because of inability of the failing liver to convert ammonia to urea and shunting of intestinal blood *via* collateral vessels. GI hemorrhage or an increase in intestinal protein from dietary intake will increase ammonia levels. **Note:** Keep patient NPO except for water for 8 h before the drawing of the ammonia level. Notify lab of all antibiotics taken by patient because they may lower the ammonia level.

**Coagulation:**   Prothrombin time (PT) will be prolonged and, in severe liver disease, unresponsive to vitamin K therapy.

**Urine tests:**   Urine bilirubin will be increased; urobilinogen will be normal or increased.

**Liver biopsy:**   Obtains a specimen of liver for microscopic analysis and diagnosis of cirrhosis, hepatitis, or other liver disease. After local anesthetic is administered and the patient's skin is prepared, a large needle is inserted into the eighth or ninth intercostal space in the midaxillary line. It is critical that patients hold their breath at the end of expiration in order to elevate the liver maximally. Patient movement or failure to sustain expiration can result in puncture through the lung rather than liver. Type and cross-matching sometimes is performed before the procedure in anticipation of hemorrhagic complications. Percutaneous liver biopsy is contraindicated in patients with markedly prolonged PT or very low platelet counts because of the risk of hemorrhage. In these patients a transvenous biopsy *via* the jugular and hepatic vein may be attempted instead. (See Table 6-14 for care of patients undergoing liver biopsy.)

**Barium swallow:**   Used in nonemergency situations (i.e., for patients without active bleeding) to verify the presence of gastroesophageal varices. **Note:** The patient should be NPO from midnight until completion of the test. Because of the constipating effects of barium, enemas should be given upon the patient's return from the procedure.

**Radiologic studies:**   Ultrasound differentiates hemolytic and hepatocellular jaundice from obstructive jaundice and shows hepatomegaly and intrahepatic tumors. CT scan of the liver/spleen is done to evaluate size and location of tumors and to rule out gallbladder disease. Percutaneous transhepatic cholangiography reveals the extent of obstruction *via* contrast dye. Endoscopic retrograde cholangiopancreatography is a fiberoptic technique used to show pancreatic causes of jaundice. Liver scans enable visualization of the spleen and

**T A B L E  6 - 1 4    Nursing Care of the Patient Undergoing Liver Biopsy**

*Prebiopsy*

Explain the procedure to patient and significant others.

*Intrabiopsy*

Assist patient with remaining motionless.

Coach patient in sustaining exhalation during puncture (or manually ventilate intubated
  patient to prevent lung inflation during puncture) to prevent pneumothorax.

*Postbiopsy*

Auscultate breath sounds immediately after the procedure and at 1-2 h intervals for
  6-8 h after the procedure to detect pneumothorax or hemothorax (unlikely but serious
  complications). Diminished sounds on the right side and tachypnea suggest pneumothorax or hemothorax.

Position patient on the right side for several hours after the biopsy to tamponade the
  puncture site.

Enforce bed rest for 8-12 h postbiopsy to minimize the risk of hemorrhage from the
  puncture site.

Administer analgesics as prescribed. Avoid NSAIDs (Table 8-1, p. 519), which may
  affect clotting, and hepatotoxins (Table 6-13).

Monitor patient for indicators of peritonitis or intraperitoneal bleeding, which can occur as a result of puncture of blood vessels or major bile duct: severe abdominal
  pain, abdominal distention and rigidity, rebound tenderness, nausea, vomiting,
  tachycardia, tachypnea, pallor, decreased BP, and rising temperature.

---

liver *via* injection of radioisotopes. **Note:** After injection of the dye, the patient may experience nausea, vomiting, and transient elevated temperature.
**Angiographic studies:**  Establish patency of the portal vein and visualize the
portosystemic collateral vessels to determine cause and effective treatment for
variceal bleeding. Portal venous anatomy must be established before such operations as portal systemic shunt or hepatic transplantation. In patients with
previously constructed surgical shunts, loss of patency may be confirmed as a
factor leading to the present bleeding episode. Loss of shunt patency is a cause
of variceal bleeding in these patients. See Table 6-15 for nursing implications
of angiographic studies.

- The most common procedure is portal venography by indirect angiography.
  The femoral artery is catheterized, and contrast material is injected into the
  splenic artery. Contrast material flows through the spleen into the splenic
  and portal veins.
- Hepatic vein wedge pressure is measured by introducing a balloon catheter
  into the femoral vein and threading it into a hepatic vein branch.
- Direct access to the portal vein may be achieved through transhepatic portography. During this procedure, varices may be obliterated by injection of
  thrombin or gel foam into veins that supply the varices. **Note:** Transhepatic
  portography involves a direct puncture through the liver and has many of
  the same risks as does liver biopsy. Patients returning from this procedure
  should be positioned on their right side and monitored closely.

**Esophagoscopy:**  Visualizes the esophagus and stomach directly *via* a fiberoptic esophagoscope. Varices in the esophagus and upper portion of the
stomach are identified, and attempts are made to identify the exact source of
bleeding. Variceal bleeding may be treated by sclerotherapy during the endoscopic procedure (see "Collaborative Management," p. 461). See Table 6-16
for nursing implications of esophagoscopy.

---

**T A B L E  6 - 1 5    Nursing Care for the Patient Undergoing Angiographic Studies**

---

*Preprocedure*

Explain procedure to patient and significant others.

Maintain NPO status for 8 h before the procedure.

Verify patency of IV catheter.

Note allergies to seafood, iodine, and contrast material.

Administer sedatives as prescribed. Be aware that dosage usually is reduced if cirrhosis or hepatitis is diagnosed.

*Intraprocedure*

Assist radiology personnel with positioning and draping patient.

Monitor VS q15min or more often for evidence of anaphylaxis or hemorrhagic shock.

*Postprocedure*

Check VS q15min initially and q1-2h once patient's condition has stabilized.

Maintain patient in supine position.

Keep pressure dressing and sandbag over puncture site for 6-8 h.

Evaluate distal pulses and perfusion in affected extremity q1-2h for 8 h. Arterial thrombosis and large hematomas that compromise femoral blood flow may develop as a result of manipulation of the artery and clotting abnormalities associated with liver disease.

Monitor urine output q1-2h, and report volume <30 ml/hr.

---

**T A B L E  6 - 1 6    Nursing Care for the Patient Undergoing Esophagoscopy**

---

*Preprocedure*

Explain procedure to patient and significant others.

Maintain NPO status for 8 h before procedure.

Clear stomach of blood and gastric contents immediately before endoscope is passed.

Verify patency of two large-bore IV catheters, which are used for rapid administration of fluids and medications.

Administer sedatives as prescribed. Be aware that dosage usually is reduced if cirrhosis or hepatitis is diagnosed.

*Intraprocedure*

Maintain patient in side-lying position to reduce likelihood of aspiration.

Have pharyngeal and tracheal suction readily available.

*Postprocedure*

Maintain side-lying position until patient is fully alert.

Note evidence of change in rate of hemorrhage.

Be alert for immediate complications, such as aspiration pneumonia (evidenced by difficulty breathing, diminished breath sounds, coarse crackles, and rhonchi) and perforation (rare— evidenced by severe retrosternal pain and bleeding).

---

**EEG:**   Traces the electrical impulses of the brain to detect or confirm encephalopathy. EEG changes occur very early, usually before behavioral or biochemical alterations.

**Psychometric testing:**   Evaluates for hepatic encephalopathy. A common test is the Reitan number connection (trail-making) test. The patient's speed and accuracy at connecting a series of numbered circles is evaluated at intervals. A daily handwriting test is an easy check of intellectual deterioration or improvement.

## COLLABORATIVE MANAGEMENT

**Treatment of underlying causes:** E.g., exposure to hepatotoxins, use of alcohol, biliary obstruction.

**Pharmacotherapy**

*Diuretics:* To reduce edema. K-sparing diuretics (e.g., spironolactone) often are used. If indicated, teach patient to avoid excessive ingestion of K-rich foods (see Table 3-4, p. 132) or salt substitutes.

*Antibiotics:* To control intestinal flora that aggravate encephalopathy.

*Hematinics (iron preparations such as ferrous sulfate):* To control anemia. They are used to replace iron after abnormal blood loss.

*Blood coagulants and vasopressors:* To control bleeding.

*Laxatives and stool softeners:* To prevent straining and rupture of varices.

*Antidiarrheals:* As necessary to control diarrhea.

*Antihistamines (e.g., diphenhydramine):* For pruritus.

*Topical anesthetics:* For hemorrhoids.

*Supplemental vitamins and minerals:* Such as folic acid for macrocytic anemia and vitamin K for prolonged PT.

---

**Note:** Narcotics and sedatives, which are metabolized by the liver, are contraindicated. Small doses of IV oxazepam (Serax) may be administered if absolutely necessary. See Table 6-13 for a list of hepatotoxic drugs.

---

**Dietary management:** With fluid retention and ascites, Na and fluids are restricted. Usually half the calories are supplied as carbohydrates. Protein is restricted in hepatic coma or precoma because the action of intestinal bacteria on protein increases blood ammonia levels, which causes or worsens the coma state. Parenteral or enteral nutrition is administered in the presence of bleeding or coma.

**Bed rest:** In the presence of fever, infection.

**Treatment of complications**

*Hemorrhage from esophageal varices:* Usually, a 4-lumen Minnesota sump tube or 3-lumen Sengstaken-Blakemore tube is used for immediate tamponade, followed by endoscopic sclerosis or surgery. Surgical procedures include portocaval shunt (anastomosis of portal vein and vena cava) or a splenorenal shunt (anastomosis of splenic vein and left renal vein). Both shunts divert blood from the portal system to the vena cava; however the portocaval shunts are associated with a high incidence of disabling encephalopathy.

Hemorrhage may be controlled temporarily by administering infusions of vasopressin to promote arterial vasoconstriction and lower portal pressure. It usually is given IV but may be administered intraarterially *via* the superior mesenteric artery.

During endoscopy, varices are injected with a sclerosing solution (endoscopic scleropathy), such as sodium tetradecyl sulfate, to cause variceal obliteration *via* fibrosis. This treatment is used both to control acute bleeding and to manage long-term or chronic bleeding *via* serial injections. Chronic sclerotherapy limits additional bleeding in many patients, but emergency surgery is necessary if rebleeding becomes uncontrollable. A serious complication of sclerotherapy is esophageal ulceration (see Table 6-17 for other complications). Ulcer prophylaxis with antacids, histamine $H_2$-receptor blockers, or sucralfate may be initiated.

*Ascites:* Dietary management may include Na and fluid restrictions. Diuretics, usually aldosterone antagonists, are often given to minimize fluid collection. If indicated, surgical management includes a peritoneovenous shunt

**T A B L E  6 - 1 7    Side Effects and Complications of Esophageal Sclerotherapy**

*Anticipated mild side effects*
Mild retrosternal pain
Transient fever
Diminished breath sounds
Transient dysphagia
Local ulcerations

*Serious side effects/complications*
Bleeding from remaining varices or ulcers
Stricture formation evidenced by prolonged dysphagia
Perforation evidenced by bleeding, severe pain, or fever
Pulmonary problems, including aspiration pneumonia, pleural effusion, mediastinitis
Bacteremia evidenced by fever, tachycardia, positive blood culture results

(LeVeen or Denver), which provides a route for reinfusion of ascitic fluid into the venous system. Monitor for these potential complications: cardiac or renal overload (see "Heart Failure," p. 60, "Pulmonary Edema," p. 85, "Pulmonary Hypertension," p. 44), shunt occlusion, disseminated intravascular coagulation (DIC, see p. 504), hemorrhage, infection, and extravasation of ascitic fluid from the incisions. Paracentesis is usually not indicated unless there is severe respiratory distress or discomfort or if it is essential for diagnosis of a tumor or bacterial peritonitis.

*Hepatic encephalopathy (hepatic coma):*   Dietary management includes restriction of protein from the diet to decrease blood ammonia levels, giving sweetened fruit juices to provide the necessary carbohydrates for energy, and administering parenteral/enteral nutrition if the patient is comatose. Pharmacologic management includes antibiotics to inhibit intestinal bacteria and magnesium sulfate or enemas to cleanse the intestines after GI bleeding. Lactulose is administered to produce 1-2 soft stools/day, which aids in decreasing blood ammonia levels, which in turn improves mentation. The following drugs are contraindicated: barbiturates and narcotics (because of the liver's inability to detoxify them), K-depleting diuretics (aldosterone antagonists are the first-line choice since edema is related to inadequate detoxification of aldosterone), and ammonia-containing medications or food, which would cause or worsen hepatic coma.

*Spontaneous bacterial peritonitis:*   Occurs in cirrhotic patients with ascites. Abdominal pain, worsening ascites, fever, and progressive encephalopathy suggest peritonitis. Mortality rate is high. See "Peritonitis," p. 405, for treatment.

*Irreversible end-stage liver disease:*   Individuals with irreversible liver failure due to chronic active hepatitis, primary biliary cirrhosis, sclerosing cholangitis, alcoholic cirrhosis, metabolic liver disease, acute fulminant hepatic necrosis, and other conditions may be considered for transplantation. Severe failure is manifested by serum bilirubin >10 mg/dl, albumin <2.5 g/dl, and prothrombin time >5 sec beyond the control. The patient must be refractory to all medical and other surgical treatments and have no absolute contraindications to transplantation (e.g., active substance abuse, metastatic disease). Patients are referred to specialized medical centers where they receive extensive preoperative evaluation and preparation. Survival rates at 1 and 5 years are 70% and 60% respectively (Coleman, 1991).

## NURSING DIAGNOSES AND INTERVENTIONS

**Altered nutrition:** Less than body requirements, related to anorexia, nausea, or malabsorption

*Desired outcome:* By 24 h before hospital discharge, patient verbalizes knowledge about foods that are permitted and restricted and develops a 3-day menu that includes or excludes these foods appropriately.

- Encourage foods that are permitted within patient's dietary restrictions. Remember that Na and fluids are restricted. If the ammonia level rises (normal levels are whole blood 70-200 μg/dl and plasma 56-150 μg/dl), protein and foods high in ammonia also will be restricted. Explain dietary restrictions to the patient. Foods high in Na are listed in Table 3-2, p. 115.
- Monitor I&O; weigh patient daily.
- Encourage small, frequent meals to ensure adequate nutrition.
- Encourage significant others to bring in desirable foods as permitted.
- Have nourishing foods available to patient at night.
- Administer vitamin and mineral supplements, as prescribed.
- Administer the following prescribed medications to decrease gastric distress: antacids, antiemetics, antidiarrheals, cathartics.
- Promote bed rest to reduce metabolic demands on the liver.
- Provide soft diet if patient has esophageal varices that are not bleeding. Patients with bleeding esophageal varices are NPO.
- Discuss need for feeding supplements and enteral or parenteral nutrition (see "Providing Nutritional Support," p. 665) with physician if appropriate.

**Impaired gas exchange** related to altered oxygen supply secondary to shallow breathing occurring with ascites or pleural effusion; altered oxygen-carrying capacity of the blood secondary to erythrocytopenia; and possible intrapulmonary shunting

*Desired outcome:* Within 24 h of admission, patient has adequate gas exchange as evidenced by $Paco_2 \leq 45$ mm Hg, $Pao_2 \geq 80$ mm Hg, $O_2$ saturation $\geq 95\%$, and RR 12-20 breaths/min with normal depth and pattern (eupnea).

- During complaints of dyspnea or orthopnea, assist patient into semi-Fowler's or high Fowler's position to promote gas exchange.
- Administer oxygen as prescribed.
- Monitor ABG values and pulse oximetry ($O_2$ saturation); notify physician of significant findings.
- Encourage patient to change positions and deep-breathe at frequent intervals to promote gas exchange. If secretions are present, ensure that the patient coughs frequently.
- Notify physician of indicators of respiratory infection, such as spiking temperatures, chills, diaphoresis, and adventitious breath sounds.
- Obtain baseline abdominal girth measurement, and measure girth either daily or every shift. Measure around the same circumferential area each time; mark the site with indelible ink. Report significant findings to physician.

**Altered protection** related to increased risk of esophageal bleeding secondary to portal hypertension and altered clotting factors

*Desired outcomes:* Patient is free of esophageal bleeding as evidenced by BP $\geq 90/60$ mm Hg; HR $\leq 100$ bpm; warm extremities; distal pulses $>2+$ on a 0-4+ scale; brisk capillary refill ($<2$ sec); and orientation to person, place, and time.

- Monitor VS q4h (or more frequently if VS are outside of patient's baseline values). Be alert to hypotension and increased HR, as well as to physical indicators of hypovolemia and hemorrhage, including cool extremities, delayed capillary refill, decreased amplitude of distal pulses, and decreasing LOC.
- Teach patient to avoid swallowing foods that are chemically or mechanically irritating (e.g., rough or spicy foods, hot foods, hot liquids, alcohol) and, therefore, injurious to the esophagus.

- Instruct patient to avoid actions that increase intraabdominothoracic pressure, such as coughing, sneezing, lifting, or vomiting.
- Administer stool softeners as prescribed to help prevent straining with defecation.
- Inspect stools for presence of blood, which would signal bleeding within the GI tract; perform stool occult blood test as indicated.
- As appropriate, instruct patient about alcohol's role in causing esophageal varices.
- Monitor PT for abnormality (normal range is 10.5-13.5 sec), and assess patient for signs of bleeding such as altered VS, irritability, air hunger, pallor, weakness, melena, and hematemesis.
- As appropriate, encourage intake of foods rich in vitamin K (e.g., spinach, cabbage, cauliflower, liver) to help decrease the PT.
- As often as possible, avoid invasive procedures such as giving injections and taking rectal temperatures.
- Monitor the patient undergoing injection sclerotherapy for evidence of perforation, including increased HR, decreased BP, pallor, weakness, and air hunger. If signs of perforation occur, notify physician immediately, keep the patient NPO, and prepare for gastric suction. Administer antibiotics as prescribed to prevent infection. For more information see Table 6-17.

**Altered protection** related to increased risk of neurosensory changes secondary to hepatic coma occurring with cerebral accumulation of ammonia or GI bleeding

***Desired outcome:***   Patient verbalizes orientation to person, place, and time; exhibits intact signature; and is free of symptoms of injury caused by neurosensory changes.

- Perform a baseline assessment of patient's personality characteristics, LOC, and orientation. Enlist the aid of significant others to help determine slight changes in personality or behavior.
- Have patient demonstrate his or her signature daily. If the writing deteriorates, ammonia levels may be increasing. Be alert to generalized muscle twitching and asterixis (flapping tremor induced by dorsiflexion of wrist and extension of fingers). Report significant findings to physician.
- Remind patient to avoid protein and foods high in ammonia such as gelatin, onions, and strong cheeses. The diseased liver is unable to convert ammonia to urea, and the buildup of ammonia adds to the progression of hepatic encephalopathy.
- Monitor for indicators of GI bleeding, including melena or hematemesis. GI bleeding can precipitate hepatic coma. Report bleeding promptly to physician, and obtain prescription for cleansing enemas if indicated.
- Protect patient against injury that can be precipitated by confused state (e.g., keep the side rails up and the bed in its lowest position, and assist patient with ambulation when need is determined).
- Use caution when administering sedatives, antihistamines, and other agents affecting the central nervous system. Avoid opiate analgesics and phenothiazines.

**Fluid volume excess** related to compromised regulatory mechanism with sequestration of fluids secondary to portal hypertension and hepatocellular failure

***Desired outcome:***   By a minimum of 24 h before hospital discharge, patient is normovolemic as evidenced by stable or decreasing abdominal girth, RR 12-20 breaths/min with normal depth and pattern (eupnea), HR ≤ 100 bpm, edema ≤ 1+ on a 0-4+ scale, and absence of crackles (rales).

- Obtain baseline abdominal girth measurement. Place patient in the supine position and mark abdomen with indelible ink to ensure serial measurements from the same circumferential site. Measure girth daily or every shift as appropriate.
- Monitor weight and I&O. Output should be equal to or exceed input. Weight

loss should not exceed 0.23 kg/day (½ lb). Assess the degree of edema, from 1+ (barely detectable) to 4+ (deep, persistent pitting), and document accordingly.
- Be alert to clinical indicators of pulmonary edema, including dyspnea, basilar crackles that do not clear with coughing, orthopnea, and tachypnea.
- Give frequent mouth care, and provide ice chips to help minimize thirst.
- Monitor serum $Na^+$ and $K^+$ values and report abnormalities to physician. Optimal values are serum $Na^+$ 137-147 mEq/L and serum $K^+$ 3.5-5.0 mEq/L. Restrict Na and replace K as prescribed.
- Remind patient to avoid food (Table 3-2, p. 115) and nonfood items that contain Na, such as antacids, baking soda, and some mouthwashes.
- Elevate extremities to decrease peripheral edema. Apply TED support stockings as prescribed.
- Bear in mind that rapid increases in intravascular volume can precipitate variceal hemorrhage in susceptible patients. Monitor for hemorrhage accordingly (see **Altered protection,** above).
- If a LeVeen peritoneovenous or Denver shunt is in place, teach the patient to inhale against resistance, using a blow bottle to facilitate the flow of ascitic fluid through the shunt. Inhaling against resistance raises intraperitoneal pressure sufficiently to enable ascitic fluid to flow through the shunt. In addition, provide instructions about the following: importance of life-style changes such as low-Na diet (Table 3-2, p. 115), abstinence from alcohol, practicing breathing exercises, obtaining daily weight and abdominal girth measurements, and monitoring I&O and edema.

---

**Note:** See "Hepatitis" for **Knowledge deficit:** Causes of hepatitis and modes of transmission, p. 455, and **Body image disturbance,** p. 456

---

## PATIENT-FAMILY TEACHING AND DISCHARGE PLANNING

Give patient and significant others verbal and written information about the following:
- Medications, including drug name, purpose, dosage, schedule, precautions, and potential side effects.
- Dietary restrictions, in particular that of Na (see Table 3-2, p. 115), protein, and ammonia.
- Potential need for life-style changes, including cessation of alcoholic beverages. Stress that alcohol cessation is a major factor in survival of this disease. Include appropriate referrals (e.g., to Alcoholics Anonymous, Al-Anon, and Al-Ateen). As appropriate, provide referrals to community nursing support agencies.
- Awareness of hepatotoxic agents (see Table 6-13), especially OTC drugs, including acetaminophen and aspirin.
- Importance of breathing exercises (see p. 463) when ascites is present.
- Indicators of variceal bleeding/hemorrhage (i.e., vomiting of blood, change in LOC) and the need to inform physician should they occur.

# Cholelithiasis and cholecystitis

*Cholelithiasis* is characterized by the presence of stones in the gallbladder. Gallstones may cause pain or other symptoms or remain asymptomatic for years. *Choledocholithiasis* is the term used to describe gallstones in the common bile duct. Gallstones are classified as cholesterol or pigment stones. Cholesterol stones are more common in the United States. Black-pigment stones are composed mainly of calcium bilirubinate and are associated with cirrhosis and chronic hemolysis. Brown-pigment stones are the predominant type found in native Asians and may be associated with bacterial infection of the bile.

Precipitating factors for stone formation include disturbances in metabolism, biliary stasis, obstruction, and infection. Gallstones are especially prevalent in women who are multiparous, on estrogen therapy, or who use oral contraceptives. Other risk factors include obesity, dietary intake of fats, sedentary lifestyle, and familial tendencies. The incidence increases with age, and it is estimated that one out of every three persons who reach age 75 have gallstones. Cholelithiasis is frequently seen in such disease states as diabetes mellitus, regional enteritis, and certain blood dyscrasias. Usually, cholelithiasis is asymptomatic until a stone becomes lodged in the cystic tract. If the obstruction is unrelieved, biliary colic (intermittent painful episodes) and cholecystitis can ensue.

*Cholecystitis* is most commonly associated with cystic duct obstructions due to impacted gallstones; however, it also may result from stasis, bacterial infection, or ischemia of the gallbladder. Cholecystitis involves acute inflammation of the gallbladder and is associated with pain, tenderness, and fever. With obstruction, structural changes can occur, such as hypertrophy of the gallbladder and a swelling and thickening of the gallbladder walls. If the edema is prolonged, the walls become scarred and fibrosed, and the constant presssure of bile can lead to mucosal irritation. As a complication of the impaired circulation and edema, pressure ischemia and necrosis can develop, resulting in gangrene or perforation. With chronic cholecystitis, stones almost always are present, and the gallbladder walls are thickened and fibrosed.

## ASSESSMENT

**Cholelithiasis:**   History of intolerance to fats and occasional discomfort after eating. As the stone moves through the duct or becomes lodged, a sudden onset of mild, aching pain will occur in the midepigastrium after eating and increase in intensity during a colic attack, potentially radiating to the RUQ and right subscapular region. Nausea, vomiting, tachycardia, and diaphoresis also can occur. Many individuals with gallstones are entirely asymptomatic.

**Cholecystitis:**   History of intolerance to fats and discomfort after eating, including regurgitation, flatulence, belching, epigastric heaviness, indigestion, heartburn, chronic upper abdominal pain, and nausea. Amber-colored urine, clay-colored stools, pruritus, jaundice, steatorrhea, and bleeding tendencies can be present if there is bile obstruction. Symptoms may be vague. An acute attack may last for 7-10 days, but it usually resolves in several hours.

**Physical assessment**

*Cholelithiasis:* Palpation of RUQ will reveal a tender abdomen during colic attack. Otherwise, between attacks, the examination is usually normal.

*Cholecystitis:* Palpation will elicit tenderness localized behind the inferior margin of the liver. With progressive symptoms, a tender, globular mass may be palpated behind the lower border of the liver. With the patient taking a deep breath, palpation over the RUQ will elicit Murphy's sign (pain and inability to inspire when the examiner's hand comes in contact with the gallbladder).

## DIAGNOSTIC TESTS

**Ultrasonography:**   An abdominal ultrasound is the preferred test for confirming the presence of gallstones, as well as their number and size. Ultrasonography of the gallbladder and biliary tract may be used to determine the location of gallstones and detect tumors.

**Radiologic studies:**   Tests such as oral cholangiogram, IV cholangiogram, nuclear scans, and percutaneous transhepatic cholangiogram may be performed to determine the patency of the biliary or cystic ducts and help rule out other conditions that mimic cholelithiasis or cholecystitis. Chest, abdominal, upper GI, and barium enema x-rays often are used to rule out pulmonary or other GI disorders.

**Oral cholecystogram:** Measures gallbladder function and demonstrates the number and size of gallstones. This test requires ingestion of iodine-based tablets (i.e., Telepaque) for 2 consecutive nights, with x-ray films taken the following morning. Failure to visualize the gallbladder indicates a nonfunctioning gallbladder, usually owing to complete obstruction of the cystic duct or chronic irritation of the gallbladder wall. Diarrhea may be caused by the iodine tablets and sometimes results in nonvisualization of the gallbladder.
**CT scan:** To detect dilated bile ducts and the presence of gallbladder cysts or tumors.
**Endoscopic retrograde cholangiopancreatography (ERCP):** Visualization and evaluation of the biliary tree to rule out or treat common duct stones.
**ECG:** To rule out cardiac disease.
**CBC with differential:** To assess for presence of infection or blood loss.
**Prothrombin time:** To assess for a prolonged clotting time secondary to faulty vitamin K absorption.
**Bilirubin tests (serum and urine) and urobilinogen tests (urine and fecal):** To differentiate between hemolytic disorders, hepatocellular disease, and obstructive disease. Usually there is an increase of bilirubin in the plasma and urine with biliary disease.
**Serum liver enzyme test:** Usually normal in cholecystitis but often becomes abnormal in the presence of prolonged cholecystitis or common duct stones.

## COLLABORATIVE MANAGEMENT

### Pharmacologic therapy

*Analgesics:* Generally opioid analgesics, which may be delivered IM on a scheduled or as needed basis. For the postoperative patient, epidural, continuous IV, and patient-controlled infusions are used with increasing frequency and superior efficacy (see **Pain,** p. 694, in the appendix for more information).
*Antacids:* To neutralize gastric hyperacidity and reduce associated pain.
*Antibiotics:* For infection.
*Antiemetics:* For nausea and vomiting.
*Bile sequestrant therapy:* Cholestyramine (Questran) and colestipol (Colestid) bind with bile salts in the intestine to facilitate their excretion and may be given to provide relief from pruritus caused by prolonged obstructive jaundice.
*Gallstone solubilizing agents:* Ursodeoxycholic acid (also known as UDCA or ursodiol [Actigall]) or, rarely, chenodeoxycholic acid (also known as CDCA or chenodiol [Chenix]) may be used in selected patients with relatively small, uncalcified (cholesterol) stones to reduce size and eventually dissolve them. Treatment duration ranges from months to years with variable results. Patients should be advised of the many potential drug interactions, serious side effects, and need for careful follow-up treatment.
**Chemical dissolution of cholesterol gallstones with a solvent:** May be used in patients with a functioning gallbladder and an unobstructed biliary tract. The solvent is infused *via* a T-tube or endoscopically placed catheter. Agents such as monoctanoin are used in carefully selected patients. Oral solubilizing agents (see above) are administered after chemical dissolution to prevent recurrence of stones.
**Dietary management:** Varies according to the patient's condition. During an acute attack, NPO status with IV fluids may be instituted. With severe nausea and vomiting, a gastric tube is inserted and attached to low, intermittent suction. Diet advances to patient's tolerance, and small, frequent feedings of a low-fat diet are recommended for both the acute and chronic conditions.
**ERCP:** The common bile duct may be cannulated, and if a stone is present, an endoscopic sphincterotomy (a technique that cuts the opening of the bile duct) can be performed with stone extraction *via* a snare or balloon catheter.

**Nonoperative biliary stone removal:** One method of stone extraction, which is performed under fluoroscopy in the radiology department. The stone is removed with a basket that is inserted *via* a catheter or T-tube through the sinus tract into the common duct. If this technique is unsuccessful, forceps are used to manipulate the stone. A cholangiogram is done before and after the procedure. If the x-ray is normal after the procedure, the T-tube is removed; if stones are still present, a new T-tube or catheter is inserted and the patient returns the following day for the same procedure. This technique may be ideal for an individual who is not a good surgical candidate.

**Lithotripsy:** Gallstones, like kidney stones, can be fragmented by exposure to extracorporeal shock waves. The stones are broken up into small granules that can be passed through the intestine or dissolved with ursodiol. Patients are carefully selected and evaluated before therapy. During the approximately 1-h procedure the patient is mildly sedated and may feel some RUQ tenderness immediately after the procedure.

**Surgical interventions:** Usually required for relief of long-term symptoms of cholelithiasis and acute cholecystitis. Surgery is the best treatment choice for patients with frequent or severe episodes of biliary pain, cholecystitis, diabetes, or suspected gallbladder cancer. The type of surgery depends on the severity and length of illness, site of obstruction, and condition of the patient. The following procedures may be performed:

*Cholecystectomy (removal of the gallbladder):* The most commonly performed procedure for biliary disease. A right subcostal incision is made. The stones are removed and a T-tube may be inserted to maintain patency of the common duct and drain bile. The gallbladder is then excised from the liver; the cystic duct, vein, and artery are ligated. Often a drain (usually Penrose) is inserted and brought out through a stab wound for drainage of blood, serum, and bile.

*Laparoscopic cholecystectomy:* Relatively new operation in which a surgical team skilled in this technique inserts a laparoscope through a small abdominal incision and removes the gallbladder using small, specialized instruments. Surgical complications are fewer and postoperative recovery is more rapid than with conventional cholecystectomy.

*Cholecystostomy:* Opening and draining the gallbladder of gallstones.

*Choledochotomy:* Opening the common bile duct to remove stones.

*Choledochoduodenostomy:* Anastomosis of the common bile duct to the duodenum.

*Choledochojejunostomy:* Anastomosis of the common bile duct to the jejunum.

## NURSING DIAGNOSES AND INTERVENTIONS

**Pain,** spasms, nausea, and itching related to obstructive or inflammatory process

*Desired outcomes:* Patient's subjective perception of discomfort decreases within 1 h of intervention, as documented by a pain scale. Objective indicators, such as grimacing, are absent or diminished.

- Monitor patient for the presence of pain or other discomfort. Devise a pain scale with patient, rating discomfort on a scale of 0 (no pain) to 10 (worst pain).
- Explain to patient that a low-Fowler's position will minimize pressure in the RUQ.
- Teach patient to avoid fatty and rough or fibrous foods to prevent nausea and spasms.
- Administer bile salt binding agent (e.g., cholestyramine) as prescribed for itching.
- Help control itching by providing cool Alpha Keri baths and cold water or ice for topical application and using soft linens on the bed.

- For additional interventions, see **Pain** in the appendix, p. 694.

**Altered protection** related to use of T-tube or recurrence of biliary obstruction

***Desired outcomes:*** Patient is free of symptoms of postsurgical perforation as evidenced by <1,000 ml/day of dark brown drainage (with gradual diminishment) and the presence of a soft and nondistended abdomen. Patient is free of symptoms of recurring biliary obstruction as evidenced by normal skin color, brown-colored stools, and straw-colored urine.

- When the patient returns from surgery, mark the T-tube at the skin line with a narrow strip of sterile tape to provide a baseline for position assessment.
- Tape the tube securely to the abdomen with adhesive tape, avoiding any tension on the tube.
- Note and record the color, amount, odor, and consistency of drainage q2h on the day of surgery and at least every shift thereafter. Initially the drainage will be dark brown with small amounts of blood and can amount to 500-1,000 ml/day. Report greater amounts of blood or drainage to physician. The amount should subside gradually as the swelling diminishes in the common duct and drainage into the duodenum normalizes. Typically the tube is removed within 6 days of surgery.
- Be alert to abdominal distention, rigidity, and complaints of diaphragmatic irritation along with a cessation or significant decrease in the amount of drainage. If these occur, notify physician immediately and anticipate tube replacement with a 14 Fr catheter.
- When the patient ambulates with a T-tube, attach a small drainage collection container to the distal end, position it in a robe pocket, and ensure that it is below the level of the common duct to prevent reflux.
- Monitor the color of the skin, sclera, urine, and stool. If obstruction recurs and bile is forced back into the bloodstream, jaundice will be present, the urine will be amber, and the stools will be clay-colored. (Clay color is normal if bile is drained *via* the tubes.) The brown color should return to the stools once bile begins to drain normally into the duodenum.

---

**Note:** See "Hepatitis" for **High risk for impaired skin integrity** related to pruritus, p. 456 Also see Appendix One for nursing diagnoses and interventions in "Caring for Preoperative and Postoperative Patients," p. 693.

---

## PATIENT-FAMILY TEACHING AND DISCHARGE PLANNING

Give patient and significant others verbal and written information about the following:

- Notifying physician if the following indicators of recurrent biliary obstruction occur: dark urine, pruritus, jaundice, clay-colored stools. Inform patient that loose stools may occur for several months as the body adjusts to the continuous flow of bile.
- Medications, including drug name, dosage, schedule, purpose, precautions, and potential side effects.
- Care of dressings and tubes if patient is discharged with them, and monitoring the incision and drain sites for signs of infection (e.g., persistent redness, pain, purulent discharge, swelling, and local warmth).
- Importance of maintaining a diet low in fat and eating frequent, small meals for medically managed patients.
- Importance of follow-up appointments with physician; reconfirm time and date of next appointment.
- Avoiding alcoholic beverages during the first 2 postoperative months to minimize the risk of pancreatic involvement.
- Necessity of postsurgical activity precautions: Avoid lifting heavy objects

(>10 lb) for the first 4-6 weeks or as directed, rest after periods of fatigue, get maximum amounts of rest, and gradually increase activities to tolerance.

# Section Six:  Pancreatic Disorders

The pancreas serves both exocrine (nonhormonal) and endocrine functions. The exocrine portion comprises 98% of tissue mass. Its function is the secretion of potent enzymes that act to reduce proteins, fats, and carbohydrates into simpler chemical substances. Pancreatic lipase acts on fats to produce glycerides, fatty acids, and glycerol; pancreatic amylase acts on starch to produce disaccharides. The pancreas also secretes sodium bicarbonate to neutralize the strongly acidic gastric contents as they enter the duodenum. The resultant mixture of acids and bases provides an optimal pH for the activation of pancreatic enzymes.

## Pancreatitis

Pancreatitis occurs when pancreatic ductal flow becomes obstructed and digestive enzymes escape from the pancreatic duct into surrounding tissue. Self-destruction of the pancreas produces edema, hemorrhage, and necrosis of pancreatic and surrounding tissue. Biochemical abnormalities and disruption of cardiopulmonary, renal, metabolic, and GI function are likely. Triggering factors include biliary obstruction, alcoholism, and direct physical trauma.

Pancreatitis is characterized by varying degrees of pancreatic insufficiency, which results in decreased production of enzymes and bicarbonate and malabsorption of fats and proteins. The digestion of fat is affected most severely. As a result, a high fat content in the bowel stimulates water and electrolyte secretion, which produces diarrhea. The action of bacteria on fecal fat produces flatus, fatty stools (steatorrhea), and abdominal cramps. Often diabetes mellitus occurs as a result of chronic pancreatitis because of damage to the insulin-producing beta cells and resultant deficient insulin production.

Complications of pancreatitis include pancreatic abscess, hemorrhage, pancreatic pseudocyst, fistula formation, and diabetes. Acute, life-threatening complications include renal failure, septicemia, acute respiratory distress syndrome (ARDS), shock, and disseminated intravascular coagulation (DIC).

### ASSESSMENT

**Acute pancreatitis:**  Sudden onset of constant, severe epigastric pain, often following a large meal or alcohol intake. The pain frequently radiates to the back or left shoulder and is somewhat relieved by a sitting position. Nausea and vomiting, sometimes with persistent retching, usually occur. Jaundice suggests biliary tree obstruction. Extreme malaise, restlessness, respiratory distress, and diminished urinary output may be present.

**Physical assessment:**  Diminished or absent bowel sounds, suggesting presence of ileus; mild to moderate ascites; generalized abdominal tenderness; tachypnea, crackles (rales) at the lung bases related to atelectasis, and interstitial fluid accumulation; diminished ventilatory excursion related to splinting and guarding with pain; low-grade fever (37.8-100°-102° F) or pronounced fever with abscess or sepsis; and agitation, confusion, and altered mental status may occur owing to electrolyte/metabolic abnormalities or acute alcohol withdrawal. Grey-blue discoloration of the flank (Grey Turner's sign) or around the umbilicus (Cullen's sign) sometimes is present with pancreatic hemorrhage.

**Chronic pancreatitis:**  Constant, dull epigastric pain; steatorrhea (greasy, foul-smelling stools) resulting from malabsorption of fats and protein; severe weight loss; and onset of symptoms of diabetes mellitus: polydipsia, polyuria, polyphagia. In addition, chemical addiction is often seen because of the chronic pain.

**History of:**  Biliary tract disease, chronic excessive alcohol consumption, physicial trauma to the abdomen (especially in young people), duodenal ulcer, coxsackie virus, mumps, hypothermia, and use of estrogen-containing oral contraceptives, glucocorticoids, sulfonamides, chlorothiazides, and azothioprine.

## DIAGNOSTIC TESTS

**Serum amylase:**  When significantly elevated (>500 U/100 ml), rules out acute abdomen conditions, such as cholecystitis, appendicitis, bowel infarction/obstruction, and perforated peptic ulcer, and confirms presence of pancreatitis. These levels return to normal 48-72 h after the onset of acute symptoms, even though clinical indicators may continue.

**Serum lipase:**  Levels rise more slowly than serum amylase and persist longer. Both lipase and amylase levels reflect the degree of necrotic pancreatic tissue.

**Serum calcium and magnesium:**  Levels may be lower than normal. On ECG, hypocalcemia is evidenced by prolonged QT segment with a normal T wave.

**CBC:**  Elevated WBCs owing to inflammatory process. Polymorphonuclear bodies may increase if bacterial peritonitis is present secondary to duodenal rupture.

**Urinalysis:**  May show presence of glycosuria, which can signal the onset of diabetes mellitus. Elevated urine amylase levels are useful diagnostically when serum levels have dropped off. An elevated specific gravity reflects the presence of dehydration.

**Hyperglycemia:**  Occurs because of interference with beta-cell function. It is transient with acute pancreatitis but common with chronic pancreatitis, during which diabetes mellitus is likely to develop.

**Abdominal x-rays:**  May show dilatation of the small or large bowel and presence of pancreatic calcification in chronic pancreatitis.

**GI x-rays:**  May reveal an edematous pancreatic head that exerts pressure on the duodenum or stomach.

**Endoscopic retrograde cholangiopancreatography (ERCP):**  A combined endoscopic-radiographic tool that is used to study the degree of pancreatic disease *via* assessment of biliary-pancreatic ductal systems. It allows direct visualization of the ampulla of Vater, diagnoses biliary stones and duct stenosis, and distinguishes cancer of the pancreas from pancreatic calculi. This test is also used for patients with bleeding tendencies for whom PTHC (see below) is contraindicated; it is not performed until the acute episode has subsided.

**Percutaneous transhepatic cholangiogram (PTHC):**  To rule out obstructive vs. nonobstructive jaundice. Bleeding complications are possible, and the patient must be assessed carefully after the procedure (see "Liver Biopsy," p. 458).

## COLLABORATIVE MANAGEMENT

Medical goals are to reduce stimuli for pancreatic secretion and rehydrate with fluids.

### For acute pancreatitis

**Fluid and electrolyte replacement:**  To maintain adequate circulating blood volume (e.g., parenteral solutions that do not stimulate the pancreas, such as glucose or free amino acids, and blood volume expanders, such as albumin and plasma protein fraction).

**Bed rest:**  To reduce metabolic demands on the body and thereby minimize need for pancreatic activity.

**Pharmacotherapy**

*Meperidine, morphine:*  For pain. **Note:** Both morphine and meperidine may

## T A B L E  6 - 1 8   Histamine H₂-Receptor Antagonists

| Generic name | Trade name | Usual dosage | Comments |
|---|---|---|---|
| cimetidine | Tagamet | 800-1,200 mg/day* | Reduces hepatic blood flow; inhibits metabolism of some drugs in the liver |
| ranitidine | Zantac | 150-300 mg/day* | 5 to 12 times more potent than cimetidine; fewer drug interactions than with cimetidine |
| famotidine | Pepcid | 40-120 mg/day* | 30 to 100 times more potent than cimetidine |
| nizatidine | Axid | 150-300 mg/day† | |

From Keen JH. In Swearingen PL, Keen JH: *Manual of critical care, ed 2,* St Louis, 1991, Mosby–Year Book.
*PO, IM, or IV administration or continuous IV infusion titrated to gastric pH value.
†Available in oral form only.

cause spasms at the sphincter of Odi, although meperidine may be less likely to do so. Response varies with the individual. Atropine may be given to prevent this from occurring.

**Broad spectrum antibiotics:**  For infection or abscess if present or suspected.

**Steroids:**  To reduce inflammation in certain types of pancreatitis when infection is not a problem.

**Anticholinergics:**  To impede impulses that stimulate pancreatic secretions.

**Histamine H₂-receptor blockers:**  To reduce gastric acid secretion, which stimulates pancreatic enzymes (see Table 6-18).

**Antacids:**  To neutralize gastric acid and reduce associated pain.

**NPO status and NG suction:**  Initiated early in the course of illness to decrease stimulus for pancreatic secretions and alleviate pressure in the GI tract.

**Ruling out of underlying factors (e.g., hyperparathyroidism and hyperlipoproteinemia)** that can contribute to the development of pancreatitis.

**Peritoneal lavage:**  Removes toxic factors present in peritoneal exudate and can result in immediate clinical improvement. The procedure is similar to peritoneal dialysis. A soft lavage catheter is positioned in the peritoneum, and continual lavage is instituted for 2-7 days, depending on the patient's clinical course.

**Surgery:**  In general, nonsurgical management of acute pancreatitis is preferred. Surgical interventions may not improve the patient's condition, and the risk of respiratory and other complications is great. Because symptoms of acute pancreatitis are easily confused with those of other acute abdominal emergencies that require urgent surgery, exploratory laparotomy is necessary for some patients. For unstable patients with severe acute pancreatitis, prompt surgical debridement sometimes is necessary to limit vessel erosion, bleeding, and abscess formation. Surgery in these patients carries a high mortality rate, and complications are numerous.

### For chronic pancreatitis

**For exacerbations:**  See treatment for acute pancreatitis.

**Alcohol rehabilitation:**  If alcoholism is the cause of pancreatitis.

**Long-term pain management:**  With lowest effective dose of analgesic (e.g., meperidine). Nerve blocks that interfere with transmission of pain sensations along visceral nerve fibers are effective in the relief of pancreatic pain. Bilateral splanchnic nerve or left celiac ganglion blocks may be performed.

**Oral enzyme supplements (e.g., pancreatin and pancrelipase):** To treat malabsorption.

**Diet:** High in carbohydrates and protein and low in fat; avoidance of spicy foods, caffeine, and nicotine.

**Insulin therapy:** May be required to ensure adequate carbohydrate metabolism if endocrine function is impaired. Lab values of fasting blood sugar and bedside monitoring of blood glucose will reveal abnormalities in blood glucose levels and direct the appropriate insulin therapy. (See "Diabetes Mellitus," p. 358, for more information.)

**Surgical interventions:** Indicated when pancreatitis is due to an obstructive process, such as gallstone formation or cancer. When gallstones are the cause of the pancreatitis, surgical removal of the stone(s) and usually the gallbladder is performed (see "Cholelithiasis/Cholecystitis," p. 468). The surgery is performed when the acute symptoms of pancreatitis have abated. A common bile duct exploration may be done at the time of surgery to uncover and retrieve all stones. See "Pancreatic Tumors," p. 477, for a discussion of total pancreatectomy and other surgical procedures performed if cancer of the pancreatic head is present.

## NURSING DIAGNOSES AND INTERVENTIONS

**Fluid volume deficit** related to active loss secondary to NG suctioning, vomiting, diaphoresis, or pooling of fluids in the abdomen and retroperitoneum

*Desired outcome:* Patient is normovolemic within 8 h of admission as evidenced by HR 60-100 bpm, CVP 2-6 mm Hg (5-12 cm $H_2O$), brisk capillary refill ($<2$ sec), peripheral pulse amplitude $>2+$ on a 0-4+ scale, urinary output $\geq30$ ml/h, and stable weight and abdominal girth measurements.

- Monitor VS q2-4h and be alert to falling BP and increasing tachycardia, which can occur with moderate to severe fluid loss.
- Measure I&O and CVP, if available, q2-4h. Because fluid loss requires immediate replacement to prevent shock and circulatory collapse, be alert to and report I&O imbalances. CVP $<2$ mm Hg ($<5$ cm $H_2O$) can occur with volume-related hypotension. Measure orthostatic VS initially and q8h in patients without CVP catheters. Be alert to decreasing BP and increasing HR on standing, which suggests the need for crystalloid and/or colloid volume expansion.
- Administer plasma volume expanders as prescribed. For high volumes, use volume control pump to prevent sudden fluid shifts caused by excessive osmotic pressure, which can result in fluid overload.
- Administer electrolytes ($K^+$, calcium [$Ca^{2+}$]) as prescribed to prevent cardiac dysrhythmias and tetany.
- Be alert to indicators of hypocalcemia, such as muscle twitching, tetany, or irritability, which can occur with electrolyte loss.
- Monitor values of the following for irregularities: Hct, Hgb, $Ca^{2+}$, glucose, BUN, and $K^+$. Normal values are as follows: Hct 40%-54% (male) and 37%-47% (female); Hgb 14-18 g/dl (male) and 12-16 g/dl (female); $Ca^{2+}$ 8.5-10.5 mg/dl [4.3-5.3 mEq/L]; glucose $<145$ mg/dl (2 h postprandial) and 65-110 mg/dl (fasting); BUN 6-20 mg/dl; and $K^+$ 3.5-5.0 mEq/L.

**Pain** related to inflammatory process of the pancreas

*Desired outcomes:* Within 6 h of intervention, patient's subjective perception of discomfort decreases, and it is controlled within 24 h, as documented by a pain scale. Objective indicators, such as splinting of abdominal muscles, are absent or diminished.

- Assess for and document the degree and character of the patient's discomfort. Devise a pain scale with the patient, rating the discomfort on a scale of 0 (no pain) to 10 (worst pain).
- To minimize pancreatic secretions and pain and to maximize needed rest, ensure that patient maintains bed rest.
- Maintain NPO status to minimize stimulation of pancreatic secretions.

- Administer analgesics, histamine H-$_2$ receptor antagonists, and anticholinergics as prescribed; be alert to patient's response to medications, using the pain scale. If analgesia is ineffective, notify physician because patient may require a nerve block or other intervention. Optimally, analgesics are administered *via* patient-controlled pumps. Small, frequent doses of IV opiates usually are more effective than IM injections. Avoid IM injections in individuals with clotting or bleeding complications.
- Assist patient in attaining a position of comfort. A sitting or supine position with knees flexed often helps to relax abdominal muscles.
- Emphasize nonpharmacologic pain interventions (e.g., relaxation techniques, distraction, guided imagery, massage). These interventions are especially important for patients who develop chronic pancreatitis and are prone to chemical dependence. See **Health-seeking behaviors:** Relaxation technique effective for stress reduction, p. 54.
- Pancreatitis can be very painful. Prepare significant others for personality changes and behavioral alterations associated with extreme pain and narcotic analgesia. Family members sometimes misinterpret patient's lethargic or unpleasant disposition and may even blame themselves. Reassure them that these are normal responses.
- Monitor patient's respiratory pattern and LOC closely because both may be depressed by the large amount of narcotics usually required to control pain. If epidural analgesia is used, monitor patient closely for respiratory compromise. Continuous pulse oximetry will alert you to decreasing oxygen saturation associated with hypoventilation. **Note:** Narcotic analgesics decrease intestinal motility and delay return to normal bowel function.
- For additional pain interventions, see **Pain** in the appendix, p. 694.

**Impaired gas exchange (or high risk for same)** related to alveolar-capillary membrane changes secondary to atelectasis and pulmonary fluid accumulation
*Desired outcome:* Patient has adequate gas exchange as evidenced by RR 12-20 breaths/min with normal depth and pattern (eupnea); oxygen saturation ≥95%; orientation to person, place, and time; and breath sounds that are clear and audible throughout the lung fields.

- Monitor and document RR q2-4h as indicated by patient's condition. Note pattern, degree of excursion, and whether patient uses accessory muscles of respiration. Report significant deviations from baseline.
- Auscultate both lung fields q4-8h. Note presence of abnormal (crackles, rhonchi, wheezes) or diminished breath sounds.
- Be alert to early signs of hypoxia, such as restlessness, agitation, and alterations in mentation.
- Monitor oxygen saturation by pulse oximetry q8h or as indicated. Monitor ABG results as available. Be alert to decreasing oxygen levels.
- Administer oxygen as prescribed. Check oxygen delivery system q4-8h.
- Maintain body position that optimizes ventilation and oxygenation. Elevate HOB 30 degrees or higher, depending on patient comfort. If pleural effusion or other defect is present on one side, position patient with the unaffected lung dependent to maximize the ventilation-perfusion relationship.
- Avoid overaggressive fluid resuscitation.

**High risk for infection** related to tissue destruction with resulting necrosis secondary to release of pancreatic enzymes
*Desired outcome:* Patient remains free of infection as evidenced by body temperature <37.8° C (<100° F); negative culture results; HR 60-100 bpm; RR 12-20 breaths/min; BP within patient's normal range; and orientation to person, place, and time.

- Check patient's temperature q4h for increases. Be aware that hypothermia may preceed hyperthermia in some individuals.
- If there is a sudden elevation in temperature, obtain specimens for culture of blood, sputum, urine, wound, drains, and other sites as indicated. Monitor culture reports, and report findings promptly.

- Evaluate patient's orientation and LOC q4-8h. Document and report significant deviations from baseline.
- Monitor BP, HR, and RR q4h. Be alert to increases in HR and RR associated with temperature elevations.
- Administer parenteral antibiotics in a timely fashion. Reschedule antibiotics if a dose is delayed for >1 h. Recognize that failure to administer antibiotics on schedule can result in inadequate blood levels and treatment failure.
- Observe all secretions and drainage for changes in appearance or odor that may signal infection.
- Prevent transmission of potentially infectious agents by using good hand-washing technique before and after caring for the patient and by disposing of dressings and drainage carefully.

**Altered nutrition:** Less than body requirements, related to anorexia, dietary restrictions, and digestive dysfunction

***Desired outcomes:*** Patient maintains baseline body weight and exhibits a positive or balanced N state on N studies by 24 h before hospital discharge.

- Initiate parenteral nutrition and adjust insulin amounts according to blood glucose levels, as prescribed.
- Provide oral hygiene at frequent intervals to enhance appetite and minimize nausea.
- Monitor blood sugar levels for presence of hyperglycemia, and be alert to dysphagia, polydipsia, and polyuria, which occur with DM. These indicators reflect the need for medical evaluation and intervention to ensure proper metabolism of carbohydrates.
- When the gastric tube is removed, provide diet as prescribed (e.g., small high-carbohydrate meals at frequent intervals [6/day] with protein added according to patient's tolerance). Keep diet bland to minimize pancreatic stimulation, and instruct patient to avoid stimulants that increase enzyme secretion, such as coffee, tea, alcohol, and nicotine.
- Weigh patient daily to assess gain or loss. Weight loss may signal the need to change the diet or provide enzyme replacement therapy.
- Note amount and degree of steatorrhea (foamy, foul-smelling stools high in fat content) as an indicator of fat intolerance. As prescribed, administer pancreatic enzyme supplements, which are given before introducing fat into the diet.
- If prescribed, administer other dietary supplements that support nutrition and caloric intake. These may include products that consist of medium-chain triglycerides (MCTs) such as Isocal or MCT oil. These supplements do not require pancreatic enzymes for absorption.
- Avoid administering pancreatin with hot foods or drinks, which will deactivate enzyme activity.
- To help alleviate the bloating, nausea, and cramps experienced by some patients, provide meals in small feedings throughout the day.

---

**Note:** See Appendix One for nursing diagnoses and interventions in "Caring for Preoperative and Postoperative Patients," p. 693.

---

## PATIENT-FAMILY TEACHING AND DISCHARGE PLANNING

Give patient and significant others verbal and written information about the following:

- Cause for current episode of pancreatitis, if known, so that recurrence may be avoided.
- Alcohol consumption, which can cause or exacerbate chronic pancreatitis.
- Availability of chemical dependency programs to prevent/treat drug dependence, which is a common occurrence with chronic pancreatitis; or to treat alcoholism.

- Diet: frequent, small meals that are high in carbohydrates and protein. Food should be bland until gradual return to normal diet is prescribed. Remind patient to avoid enzyme stimulants, such as coffee, tea, nicotine, and alcohol.
- Medications, including drug name, purpose, dosage, schedule, precautions, and potential side effects.
- Signs and symptoms of diabetes mellitus, including fatigue, weight loss, polydipsia, polyuria, and polyphagia.
- Necessity of medical follow-up; confirm time and date of next medical appointment.
- Potential for recurrence of steatorrhea as evidenced by foamy, foul-smelling stools that are high in fat content. Steatorrhea can indicate recurrence of disease process or ineffectiveness of drug therapy and should be reported to physician.
- Weighing daily at home; importance of reporting weight loss to physician.
- If surgery was performed, the indicators of wound infection: redness, swelling, discharge, fever, pain, or local warmth.

# Pancreatic tumors

Pancreatic tumors, either benign (adenoma) or malignant (carcinoma), can develop anywhere within the pancreas. The most frequent site for pancreatic tumors is the pancreatic head, particularly in the region around the ampulla of Vater. These are malignant tumors (adenocarcinomas), whose detection is difficult and for which the prognosis is poor. Because of vague, ill-defined symptoms that appear early in the disease process with pancreatic cancer, metastasis often occurs before a diagnosis can be made. A tumor that develops at the islet cells is called an insulinoma and is characterized by hypersecretion of insulin. Usually it is treated surgically with a subtotal pancreatectomy.

## ASSESSMENT

**Signs and symptoms:**   Progressive, unexplained, rapid weight loss; upper or midabdominal pain that radiates to the back, can be aggravated by eating, and is not related to posture or activity. The patient also may have clay-colored stools, dark urine, pruritus, anorexia, nausea, vomiting, steatorrhea caused by fat and protein malabsorption, bleeding tendencies, malnutrition, and electrolyte disturbances. In addition, diabetes mellitus (DM) symptoms often appear as early indicators of the disorder (see "Diabetes Mellitus," p. 353).

**Physical assessment:**   Jaundice caused by obstruction of the flow of bile from the liver, mild ascites, abdominal tenderness, muscle wasting, generalized bruising and ecchymosis, generalized weakness, and poor skin turgor.

## DIAGNOSTIC TESTS

**Serum alkaline phosphatase:**   Elevated with obstructive bile duct disease.

**Serum bilirubin:**   Elevated if the pancreatic tumor obstructs the flow of bile from the liver. Levels >3 mg/100 ml will result in jaundice; levels >25 mg/100 ml are common with this condition.

**Prothrombin time (PT):**   Prolonged because of vitamin K deficiency. Vitamin K is required for synthesis of prothrombin in the liver, and it is absorbed poorly in the presence of pancreatic insufficiency because it is a fat-soluble vitamin.

**GI x-rays:**   May show displacement of visceral organs by the enlarged pancreatic tumor.

**CT scan of pancreas:**   To delineate pancreatic mass.

**Endoscopic retrograde cholangiopancreatography (ERCP):**   Permits direct visualization of the ampulla of Vater *via* injection of a radiopaque dye into the pancreatic and biliary ducts. In patients with marked bleeding tendencies, neither ERCP nor PTHC (see below) is performed.

**Percutaneous transhepatic cholangiogram (PTHC):**   To determine the level of biliary obstruction and confirm the presence of cholelithiasis. There is a risk of postprocedure bleeding (see "Liver Biopsy," p. 458), and it is contraindicated for patients with bleeding tendencies.

**5-hour glucose tolerance test:**   Helps confirm diagnosis of insulinoma.

**Cytologic examination of duodenal contents:**   Reveals malignant cells, if present.

**Ultrasound:**   To rule out presence of cystic lesions and metastases.

**Fine-needle aspiration biopsy:**   To confirm diagnosis. It may be CT-scan guided.

## COLLABORATIVE MANAGEMENT

Pancreatic cancer frequently results from metastasis; and even when the pancreas is the primary site, diagnosis and interventions are thwarted by the vague symptomatology and insidious onset of this disease. The medical and surgical approaches will vary depending on the status of the tumor found with the initial exploratory surgery (exploratory laparotomy).

**Whipple procedure (pancreatoduodenectomy):**   A surgical attempt to cure cancer of the pancreatic head when the tumor is judged to be resectable (e.g., it has not metastasized and is not interfering with major blood vessels). This extensive surgery involves resection of the head of the pancreas and duodenum and three anastomoses of the following: common bile duct to the jejunum (choledochojejunostomy); the remainder of the pancreas to the jejunum (pancreaticojejunostomy); and the stomach to the jejunum (gastrojejunostomy).

**Vagotomy** (dividing the vagus nerve branches to the stomach): May be done in addition to the Whipple procedure to minimize gastric secretions.

**Total pancreatectomy:**   May be performed for patients with chronic pancreatitis or cancer of the pancreatic head. The location of the surgical incision will vary with the extent of the surgery; however, whether it is vertical or oblique, the incision usually extends high into the abdomen. The patient will have one or two drains, depending on the extent of the surgery. A Penrose drain may exit from the abdomen; a T-tube, sump tube, or portable wound drainage system also may be present. For patients who have undergone a total pancreatectomy, the resultant pancreatic endocrine and exocrine deficiency requires treatment with insulin, pancreatic enzymes, and a diabetic diet that is low in fat.

**Palliative measures:**   Initiated when the tumor is not resectable (90% of the cases). Although the tumor is left intact, the gallbladder may be anastomosed to the duodenum to permit bile from the liver to bypass the tumor and flow directly into the duodenum. Another approach is the percutaneous biliary drain, which is used for inoperable liver, pancreatic, or bile duct carcinoma. This tube or catheter, which is perforated with holes at the distal end, is inserted percutaneously through the liver, past the obstructed common bile and pancreatic ducts, and into the duodenum. The catheter collects fluid from the surrounding tissues and permits their passage into the duodenum for excretion. It is a palliative measure to prolong life and minimize discomfort. The catheter must be changed q6-8 weeks and flushed qod with small amounts of saline to maintain patency.

**Postoperative chemotherapy:**   Sometimes used for further palliation after patient has recovered from surgery.

---

**Note:**   Postoperative prognosis is extremely poor: patients usually survive <1 year, and the 5-year survival rate is 2%.

---

## NURSING DIAGNOSES AND INTERVENTIONS

**High risk for fluid volume deficit** related to postsurgical hemorrhage (due to vascularity of surgical site or multiple anastomosis sites) or fluid shift to third-space (interstitial) compartments

*Desired outcome:*  Patient is normovolemic as evidenced by BP $\geq$ 90/60 mm Hg (or within patient's baseline range), HR $\leq$100 bpm, RR $\leq$20 breaths/min with normal depth and pattern (eupnea), good skin turgor, brisk capillary refill ($<$2 sec), balanced I&O, urinary output $\geq$30 ml/h, stable weight, and moist mucous membranes.

- Monitor BP, HR, and RR, and check capillary refill in nailbeds at frequent intervals. Tachycardia, hypotension, increased respirations, and slow capillary refill can signal the presence of dehydration and hypovolemia, which can lead to shock. Also be alert to cool, clammy skin, which can occur with hemorrhage and a low urinary output ($<$30-40 ml/h for 2 consecutive h). Report significant findings to physician.

- Administer crystalloids and colloids (e.g., albumin) as prescribed. Large amounts of fluid may be necessary because of fluid sequestration, surgical loss, and loss from incisions or drains. Fluid often is prescribed as a baseline amount with additional amounts according to previous 8-h drainage.

- Prevent increased pressure on suture lines by keeping all tubes patent and free of kinks. *Gently* irrigate NG tube with air or saline q4h or as needed. Keep gravity drains dependent to the wound site, and secure all connections with tape.

- Note and document the amount and character of drainage from the tubes. Drainage from the surgical incision or drains may be profuse. Increasing amounts of fluid from the surgical incision or drains can suggest infection or fistula formation. Note the amount, consistency, color, and odor, and inform the surgeon accordingly. Persistent, bloody drainage in steady or increasing amounts signals active bleeding. Report significant findings to physician.

- Monitor blood study results, including PT, for clotting factor and Hct and Hgb, which can fall with blood loss. Optimal values are as follows: PT 11-15 sec, Hct 40%-54% (male) and 37%-47% (female), and Hgb 14-18 g/dl (male) and 12-16 g/dl (female).

- Monitor serum protein levels (normal range for random specimen is 2-8 mg/dl), and be alert to weight gain, which may signal interstitial spacing of fluids. Monitor I&O; note if intake exceeds output. Preoperatively most of these patients are protein deficient. Low serum protein alters serum colloid osmotic pressure, resulting in fluid shift from intravascular to interstitial compartments (third spacing of body fluids). **Note:** Intravascular fluid loss can occur despite adequate fluid replacement.

- Monitor lab study results for evidence of electrolyte imbalances, especially $K^+$ and $Na^+$. Normal $K^+$ range is 3.5-5.0 mEq/L, and normal $Na^+$ range is 137-147 mEq/L.

**High risk for impaired skin integrity** related to wound drainage or pressure on incision

*Desired outcome:*  Patient's skin remains intact, with evidence of good wound healing.

- Promote adequate drainage from drainage tubes to prevent pressure from fluid collection around wound site. Evaluate proper functioning of the wall suction and drains. Do not occlude the air port of the sump drainage devices, which could result in excessive suction. Be certain to protect surrounding skin by using Karaya or other nonirritating adhesive disks and stoma pouches over the drain or wound sites. Consult ET nurse or wound specialist as available.

- Assess and document condition of incision and quality/quantity of wound drainage. Fistula formation is a major complication of Whipple's procedure, so it is important to monitor periincisional skin carefully for signs of irrita-

tion. If irritation occurs or a fistula does form, cover site with a pectin wafer skin barrier (and stoma pouch for fistula).
- Keep patient in semi-Fowler's position to minimize pressure on the incision. Use pressure-relief mattress to minimize potential for skin breakdown.
- When regular diet is resumed after surgery, provide small, frequent meals that are high in protein, vitamins, and calories, and low in fat. Administer pancreatic enzyme replacements and insulin, as prescribed, for patient who has had a total pancreatectomy. These interventions will help ensure optimal tissue repair, as well.
- For more information, see "Managing Wound Care," p. 681.

**Pain** related to major abdominal surgery
***Desired outcomes:*** Patient's subjective perception of discomfort decreases within 1 h of intervention, as documented by a pain scale. Objective indicators, such as splinting of abdominal muscles, are absent or diminished.
- Assess the degree and quality of the patient's discomfort. Devise a pain scale with the patient, rating discomfort from 0 (no pain) to 10 (worst pain).
- Physical dependence on narcotics is of minimal importance in patients who are terminally ill. Administer analgesics liberally. Document the degree of pain relief obtained, using the pain scale.
- Note and report patient's failure to respond to analgesics, because peritonitis and pancreatitis are potential postoperative complications.
- Because intraabdominal pressure may be a source of the patient's discomfort, ensure proper drainage from tubes.
- For additional pain interventions, see **Pain** in the appendix, p. 694.

---

**Note:** See "Hepatitis" for **High risk for impaired skin integrity** related to pruritus, p. 456, **Body image disturbance** related to jaundice, p. 456, and **Altered protection** related to increased risk of bleeding secondary to decreased vitamin K absorption, p. 456. See Appendix One for nursing diagnoses and interventions in "Caring for Preoperative and Postoperative Patients," p. 693, and "Caring for Patients with Cancer and Other Life-Disrupting Illnesses," p. 719.

---

## PATIENT-FAMILY TEACHING AND DISCHARGE PLANNING

Give patient and significant others verbal and written information about the following:
- For patients with DM, a review of insulin action, dosage, and administration; diabetic diet; and signs and symptoms of hyperglycemia and hypoglycemia. See "Diabetes Mellitus," p. 353, for more information.
- Wound care, such as cleansing, dressing changes, and care of drains if patient is discharged with them; indicators of wound infection, such as drainage, warmth along incision line, persistent incisional redness, swelling, fever, and pain.
- Medications, including drug name, purpose, dosage, schedule, precautions, and potential side effects.
- Arrangements for community services in home care, such as Visiting Nurse Association, or placement in hospice facility.

### Selected Bibliography

Boggs RL: Multiple-system trauma: nursing implications, *J Adv Med Surg Nurs* 2(1):1-6, 1989.
Broadwell DC, Jackson BS: *Principles of ostomy care,* St Louis, 1982, The CV Mosby Co.
Brown A: Acute pancreatitis: pathophysiology, nursing diagnoses, and collaborative problems, Focus Crit Care 18(2):121-130, 1991.
Centers for Disease Control: *Morbidity Mortality Weekly Report* 34(27):422, 1985.

Center for Prevention Services, Division of Quarantine: *Health information for international travel,* Atlanta, 1991, Centers for Disease Control.

Coellen D: Understanding diverticular disease. *J Enterostomal Ther* 16(4):176-180, 1989.

Coleman J et al: Liver diseases that lead to transplantation, *Crit Care Nurs Quart* 13(4):41-50, 1991.

Committee on Trauma: *Advanced trauma life support instructor manual,* Chicago, 1989, American College of Surgeons.

Dudley SL, Starin RB: Cholelithiasis: diagnosis and current therapeutic options, *Nurse Pract* 16(3):12-24, 1991.

Finne CO: Advances in colorectal cancer, *J Enterostomal Ther* 18(3):82-89, 1991.

Fitzsimmons L, Hadley S: The metabolic response to injury in the surgical/trauma patient, *Dimens Crit Care Nurs* 10(1):4-12, 1991.

Hampton BG, Bryant PA: *Ostomies and continent diversions,* St Louis, 1992, Mosby–Year Book.

Herrera L et al: Perspectives in colorectal cancer, *J Surg Oncol Suppl* 2:92-103, 1991.

Huggins B: Trauma physiology, *Nurs Clin North Am* 25(1):1-10, 1990.

Interqual: ISD-A review system with adult ISD criteria, August 1992, Northhampton, NH, and Marlboro, MA, Interqual, Inc.

Jackson MM, McPherson DC: Hepatitis A through E—current and future trends, *Inside OR* 13(10):7-12, 1991.

Jeffres C: Complications of acute pancreatitis, *Crit Care Nurs* 9(4):38-48, 1989.

Katz SL: Hepatitis B virus: a comprehensive strategy for eliminating transmission in the United States through universal childhood vaccination, *Morbid & Mortal Weekly Rep* 40(RR-13):1-25, Nov 22, 1991.

Kedzierski M: Management of viral hepatitis, *Nurs Stand* 5(42):29-32, 1991.

Keen JH: *Gastrointestinal disorders.* In Swearingen PL, editor: *Pocket guide to medical-surgical nursing,* St Louis, 1992, Mosby–Year Book, Inc.

Keen JH: *Gastrointestinal dysfunctions.* In Swearingen PL, Keen JH, editors: *Manual of critical care: applying nursing diagnoses to adult critical illness,* ed 2, St Louis, 1991, Mosby–Year Book.

Kim MJ, McFarland GK, McLane AM: *Pocket guide to nursing diagnoses,* ed 5, St Louis, 1993, Mosby–Year Book.

Koda-Kimble MA et al: *Applied therapeutics: the clinical use of drugs,* ed 5, Vancouver, Wash, 1992, Applied Therapeutics.

Loogman E: *Therapies for acid peptic disease,* Society of Gastroenterology Nurses and Associates, 198-201, Spring 1991.

Nowzaradan Y et al: Laparoscopic appendectomy for acute appendicitis: indications and current use, *J Laparoendoscopic Surg* 1(5):247-257, 1991.

Nyhus LM: Inguinal hernia repairs, *AORN J* 52(2):292-304, 1990.

Semonin-Holleran R: Critical nursing care for abdominal trauma, *Crit Care Nurs* 8(3):48-59, 1988.

Sherlock S: *Diseases of the liver and biliary system,* ed 9, Oxford, 1992, Blackwell.

Shindo M et al: Decrease in serum hepatitis C viral RNA during alpha-interferon therapy for chronic hepatitis C, *Ann Intern Med* 115(9):700-704, 1991.

Sleisenger MH, Fordtran JS: *Gastrointestinal disease: pathophysiology, diagnosis, and management,* Philadelphia, 1989, WB Saunders.

Smith A: When the pancreas self destructs, *Am J Nurs* 91(8):38-48, 1991.

Smith S, Ciferni M: Liver transplantation, *Crit Care Nurs Clin North Am* 4(1):131-148, 1992.

Stanley M: Ascites in alcoholic cirrhosis: choosing the optimal level of treatment, *J Crit Ill* 7(4):529-535, 1992.

Stanley M: Peritovenous shunting: patient selection and management, *J Crit Ill* 7(4):529-535, 1992.

Swearingen PL: *Addison-Wesley's photo-atlas of nursing procedures,* ed 2, Redwood City, Calif, 1991, Addison-Wesley.

Tepper JE: Role of radiation therapy in the treatment of carcinoma of the rectum, *J Surg Oncol Suppl* 2:51-53, 1991.

Toole M: Advanced assessment of the abdomen and gastrointestinal problems, *Nurs Clin North Am* 25(4):773, 1990.

Trunkey D, Lewis FR, editors: *Current therapy of trauma,* ed 2, vol 2, Philadelphia, 1990, Mosby–Year Book.

US Department of Health and Human Services: *Acute pain management: operative or medical procedures and trauma,* 1992, Public Health Service, Agency for Health Care Policy and Research, Rockville, MD, AHCPR 92-0032.

Wagner MM: The patient with abdominal injuries, *Nurs Clin North Am* 25(1):45-56, 1990.

Wolenski M, Markus E, Pelosi MA: Laparoscopic appendectomy incidental to gynecologic procedures, *Today's OR Nurse* 13(12):12-18, 1991.

Wyngaarden JB et al: *Cecil textbook of medicine,* ed 19, Philadelphia, 1992, WB Saunders.

# 7 HEMATOLOGIC DISORDERS

Section One   Disorders of the Red Blood Cells   483
   Iron deficiency anemia   483
   Pernicious anemia   485
   Hemolytic anemia   488
   Hypoplastic (aplastic) anemia   491
   Polycythemia   497
Section Two   Disorders of Coagulation   499
   Thrombocytopenia   500
   Hemophilia   502
   Disseminated intravascular coagulation   504
Section Three   Neoplastic Disorders of the Hematopoietic System   508
   Lymphomas   508
   Acute leukemia   510
   Chronic leukemia   513
Selected Bibliography   514

## Section One:   Disorders of the Red Blood Cells

The erythrocyte, or RBC, is the transport mechanism for hemoglobin (Hgb), which carries $O_2$ from the heart and lungs to the tissues, exchanges it for $CO_2$, and then returns to the heart and lungs. RBCs are very flexible and capable of bending, elongating, and squeezing through tiny capillaries. Normal RBCs can travel under high pressure and speed, are extremely active metabolically, and have an average life of 120 days. The bone marrow produces and replaces RBCs every day and can respond to an increased need for RBCs by increasing production. However, with increased production, immature RBCs (reticulocytes) often are released into the circulation; a high or abnormally low level of reticulocytes often aids in the diagnosis of RBC disorders.

*Anemia* is a common hematopoietic disorder, defined as a reduced RBC volume (hematocrit [Hct]) or a reduced concentration of Hgb. The general effects of anemia result from a deficiency in the $O_2$-carrying mechanism, although some effects are related to varied pathogenesis. Four basic types of anemias are discussed in this section: iron deficiency, pernicious, hemolytic, and hypoplastic.

### Iron deficiency anemia

Iron deficiency anemia, the most common type of anemia, is classified as microcytic and hypochromic. That is, the RBCs are small in size (microcytic) and low in Hgb content (hypochromic). The RBC lacks sufficient Hgb to mature into $O_2$-carrying RBCs. Iron is required for the formation of Hgb, and when there is a deficiency because of either decreased intake (dietary) or increased need (pregnancy or secondary to gastrointestinal [GI] bleeding), anemia occurs.

## ASSESSMENT

**Chronic indicators:**   The patient may be asymptomatic or have brittle hair and nails. In the presence of severe and chronic disease, dysphagia, stomatitis, and inflammation of the tongue may be present.

**Acute indicators:**   Fatigue, decreased ability to concentrate, cold sensitivity, menstrual irregularities, and loss of libido.

**Physical assessment:**   Tachycardia, palpitations, tachypnea, exertional dyspnea, pale mucous membranes, pale nailbeds, vertigo.

## DIAGNOSTIC TESTS

**Blood count:**   Usually RBCs and Hgb are decreased; Hct usually is low because the percentage of RBCs in the total blood volume is decreased.

**Peripheral blood smear to examine RBC indices:**   Mean corpuscular volume (MCV) is low because the amount of Hgb is low and cell volume is decreased; mean corpuscular hemoglobin concentration (MCHC) is low because low Hgb is seen as a "pale" cell.

**Total iron-binding capacity:**   Increased in iron-deficient states because it measures the amount of iron with which transferrin can bind.

**Reticulocyte count:**   High if the marrow is functioning. A reticulocyte is an immature RBC and can be used to differentiate causes of anemia.

## COLLABORATIVE MANAGEMENT

**Correct the underlying cause:**   E.g., increase dietary intake of iron, or treat GI bleeding.

**Iron replacement:**   May be done orally or parenterally. The oral route is preferred, and the drugs of choice are ferrous sulfate and ferrous gluconate.

## NURSING DIAGNOSES AND INTERVENTIONS

**Activity intolerance** related to imbalance between oxygen supply and demand secondary to decreased oxygen-carrying capacity of the RBCs

*Desired outcome:*   Following treatment, patient rates perceived exertion at ≤3 on a 0-10 scale and exhibits tolerance to activity as evidenced by RR 12-20 breaths/min with normal depth and pattern (eupnea), HR ≤100 bpm, and absence of headache and dizziness.

- Monitor patient during activity. Be alert to indications of decreased oxygenation, including dyspnea, dizziness, palpitations, headaches, and verbalizations of increased perceived exertion level (see description, p. 711).
- Provide frequent rest periods between care activities, allowing 90 min for undisturbed rest.
- Monitor for and report chest pain.
- Monitor HR during activity, noting strength. Report an increase in HR and a decrease in strength of the beat.
- Monitor Hgb and Hct for evidence of severity of anemia. Report decreases in these values.
- Administer packed RBCs as prescribed to increase the blood's oxygen-carrying capacity.
- Administer iron as prescribed. Use Z-track method to administer iron intramuscularly. For oral iron, use the following guidelines:
  - Administer with meals to maximize absorption.
  - Do not give with milk, which would decrease absorption.
  - Increase vitamin C intake, which will help increase iron absorption.

- If the iron is liquid, have patient take it through a straw and rinse mouth after administration to minimize tooth staining.

---

**Note:** Also see "Pernicious Anemia" for **High risk for infection,** p. 486, **Altered nutrition,** p. 487, and **Diarrhea** *or* **Constipation,** p. 487.

---

## PATIENT-FAMILY TEACHING AND DISCHARGE PLANNING
Give patient and significant others verbal and written information about the following:
- Importance of a well-balanced diet, especially iron intake, which is found in foods such as red meat, green vegetables, and raisins.
- Special instructions for taking iron, depending on type prescribed.
- Benefits of eating 6 small meals/day rather than trying to get all nutrition in 3 meals.

# Pernicious anemia

Vitamin $B_{12}$ is supplied by dietary intake of such foods as liver, milk, and eggs and stored in the liver to be used for maturation of RBCs. Deficiency of this vitamin leads to the development of immature erythrocytes, a chronic condition known as pernicious anemia. Decreased dietary intake of animal products, increased need for this vitamin with pregnancy or a tumor, presence of parasites, and surgery involving the small intestine where the vitamin is absorbed are conditions that can lead to vitamin $B_{12}$ deficiency. The most common condition is a decrease in production by the gastric mucosa of the microprotein *intrinsic factor,* which when combined with vitamin $B_{12}$ facilitates absorption and use of the vitamin by body cells, particularly in the bone marrow, GI tract, and nervous system. Anemias related to vitamin $B_{12}$ are called megaloblastic anemias because they are characterized by RBCs that are large and immature (megaloblasts). Altered production of one bone marrow element usually will cause altered or decreased production of the other elements, including leukocytes and thrombocytes.

## ASSESSMENT
**Chronic indicators:** Brittle nails, smooth tongue, numbness and tingling of the extremities, fatigue, and dysphagia. However, because of slow progression, many patients remain asymptomatic. Anorexia, weight loss, jaundice from destruction of malformed erythrocytes, and gingivitis from absence of vitamin $B_{12}$ also can occur.
**Acute indicators:** Dyspnea on exertion, irritability, palpitations, and dizziness in the presence of severe deficiency. In addition, because the nervous system is particularly sensitive to the lack of vitamin $B_{12}$, degenerative changes of the cerebral cortex and spinal cord can occur, seen mainly in the form of paresthesias.
**Physical assessment:** Presence of oral lesions (e.g., glossitis) and gingivitis, tachycardia, unsteady gait, and clumsiness.

## DIAGNOSTIC TESTS
**Peripheral blood smear:** Will demonstrate oval macrocytes, hypersegmented neutrophils, and possibly giant platelets.
**Schilling's test:** Patient is given radioactive tagged vitamin $B_{12}$, then urine concentration of tagged $B_{12}$ is measured. Normally, $B_{12}$ is absorbed and excreted in the urine. In the presence of pernicious anemia, $B_{12}$ is not absorbed and urine levels will be low ($<3\%$).

**Trial administration of vitamin B$_{12}$:**   May be given to evaluate the patient's response. In the presence of pernicious anemia, symptoms will be relieved.
**Hematologic studies:**   Hgb, erythrocytes, leukocytes, and thrombocytes will be decreased.
**Bone marrow aspiration:**   Will reveal hyperplasia with increased numbers of large-sized megaloblasts.
**Gastric analysis:**   Will reveal decreased volume of gastric secretions. Atrophic gastritis is characteristic of pernicious anemia.
**Folate level:**   Will be low because of decreased absorption in the upper small intestine.

## COLLABORATIVE MANAGEMENT

**Vitamin B$_{12}$ replacement:**   Replacement therapy is required for life. Dosage will depend on the individual and the response to treatment (e.g., 100 mg cyanocobalamin may be given IM qd × 7 days; if improvement occurs, it is given qod × 7 days and then q3-4 days × 2-3 weeks). **Note:** Increasing the dietary intake of vitamin B$_{12}$ will not be effective in individuals with intrinsic factor deficiency.
**Concurrent treatment of underlying disorder:**   If present (e.g., gastric mucosal problem).
**Serial measurements of reticulocytes:**   To determine effectiveness of treatment.
**O$_2$:**   To maximize arterial O$_2$ content.

## NURSING DIAGNOSES AND INTERVENTIONS

**Activity intolerance** related to imbalance between oxygen supply and demand secondary to decreased oxygen-carrying capacity of the blood due to immature RBCs
*Desired outcome:*   Following treatment, patient rates his or her perceived exertion at ≤3 on a 0-10 scale and exhibits tolerance to activity as evidenced by RR 12-20 breaths/min with normal depth and pattern (eupnea), HR ≤100 bpm, and absence of headache and dizziness.
- As patient performs ADL, be alert to indicators of decreased tissue oxygenation, such as dyspnea on exertion, dizziness, palpitations, headaches, and verbalization of increased perceived exertion level (see description, p. 711).
- Provide frequent rest periods between care activities, allowing time for at least 90 min of undisturbed rest.
- Reassure patient that symptoms usually are relieved and tolerance for activity is increased with therapy.
- As patient's condition improves, encourage increase in activities to tolerance. Set specific goals with patient (e.g., "Today I would like you to walk from your room to the nurses' station and back 3 [or appropriate number, depending on patient's tolerance] times").
- Administer oxygen as prescribed to elevate arterial oxygen content.
- Teach patient the necessity of vitamin B$_{12}$ replacement for life, even when symptoms resolve.
  - Teach the technique for administering vitamin B$_{12}$, or arrange for monthly clinic visits for injection.
  - For injections performed by patient or significant other, provide information about how to obtain vitamin B$_{12}$, 22-gauge needles, 3-ml syringes, and alcohol sponges. Teach patient the proper method for disposing of needles and syringes, including where to obtain an appropriate receptacle for disposal.

**High risk for infection** related to inadequate secondary defenses secondary to leukopenia (associated with decrease in all blood elements)
*Desired outcome:*   Patient is free of infection as evidenced by normothermia;

RR 12-20 breaths/min with normal depth and pattern (eupnea); urine that is straw-colored, clear, and of characteristic odor; absence of adventitious breath sounds; and absence of unusual erythema, warmth, or drainage at any wound sites.

- Maintain strict asepsis when performing invasive procedures. Wash hands well before caring for patient.
- Teach patient and significant others the technique for effective handwashing.
- Be alert to the following indicators of respiratory infection and report to physician: cough; changes in the amount, color, and consistency of sputum; increased RR; and presence of crackles (rales), rhonchi, and fever. Teach these indicators to patient and significant others, along with the indicators of other common infections as described in "Care of the Renal Transplant Recipient," p. 141.
- To prevent stasis of secretions in the lung, which can lead to infection, teach patient how to perform effective coughing and deep breathing.

**Altered nutrition:** Less than body requirements, related to decreased intake secondary to fatigue, impairment of oral mucosa, or anorexia

*Desired outcome:* By a minimum of 24 h before hospital discharge, patient exhibits adequate nutrition as evidenced by maintenance of or return to baseline body weight.

- Weigh patient daily and document patient's dietary intake.
- If patient is easily fatigued, encourage small, frequent meals; document intake.
- Monitor for oral lesions or soreness of the gums, tongue, and esophagus. If oral lesions or cracks are present, encourage soft and bland foods. For more information, see "Stomatitis," p. 379.
- For patient with decreased appetite, encourage significant others to bring in patient's favorite foods and stay with patient during meals to encourage eating.
- Administer vitamins and minerals as prescribed.

**Altered protection** related to neurosensory alterations secondary to inability to absorb and use vitamin $B_{12}$

*Desired outcome:* Patient verbalizes orientation to person, place, and time and is free of symptoms of injury caused by neurosensory deficit.

- Assess for sensory deficit (i.e., paresthesias), and protect patient from extremes of heat and cold if deficit is noted.
- Assess patient's orientation to person, place, and time. As needed, orient patient to all activities and surroundings at frequent intervals.
- Assess muscle strength and motor ability before allowing patient to ambulate unassisted.
- Teach patient and significant others the signs and symptoms of neurologic deficit and the importance of reporting them to staff or physician promptly. Reassure patient that neurologic deficit usually reverses with therapy.

**Diarrhea** *or* **constipation** related to gastrointestinal mucosal atrophy secondary to reduced Hct

*Desired outcome:* By a minimum of 24 h before hospital discharge, patient relates the return of soft, formed stools.

- If the patient is constipated, implement the following:
  - Assist patient with establishing a regular bowel pattern (e.g., by increasing fluids [to at least 2-3 L/day] and dietary fiber and initiating a regular exercise program).
  - For other interventions, see Appendix One for **Constipation,** p. 716, in "Caring for Patients on Prolonged Bed Rest."
- If diarrhea occurs, teach patient to avoid high-roughage foods, and encourage increased intake of fluids to prevent dehydration.
- Administer antidiarrheal medications as prescribed.

## PATIENT-FAMILY TEACHING AND DISCHARGE PLANNING

Give patient and significant others verbal and written information about the following:

- Necessity of vitamin $B_{12}$ replacement for life, even when symptoms resolve.
- Technique for administering vitamin $B_{12}$ or arrangement for monthly clinic visits for injection.
- For injections that will be performed by patient or significant other, the need for a supply of vitamin $B_{12}$, 22-gauge needles, 3-ml syringes, and alcohol sponges. Teach patient the proper method for disposing of needles, and provide an appropriate receptacle for needle and syringe disposal.
- Importance of regular medical follow-up, including serial monitoring of blood levels.

# Hemolytic anemia

Hemolytic anemia is characterized by abnormal or premature destruction of RBCs. Hemolysis can be intrinsic or result from such conditions as infection or radiation. *Sickle cell anemia* is a form of chronic hemolytic anemia characterized by abnormal, crescent-shaped, rigid, and elongated erythrocytes. These "sickle" RBCs interfere with circulation because they cannot get through the microcirculation and are destroyed in the process. Sickle cell anemia can affect almost every body system through decreased $O_2$ delivery, decreased circulation caused by occlusion of the vessels by RBCs, and inflammatory process. This disorder occurs when the gene is inherited from both parents (homozygous); a carrier state exists when it is inherited from one parent (heterozygous). Medical treatment has improved the prognosis for this disorder, which is seen predominantly in blacks.

*Acquired hemolytic anemia* is usually the result of an abnormal immune response that causes premature destruction of RBCs. Hemolysis can occur because of a foreign antigen, as from a transfusion reaction, or an autoimmune reaction in which the hemolytic agent is intrinsic to the patient's body. Other possible causes include exposure to radiation and ingestion of such drugs as sulfisoxazole (e.g., Gantrisin), phenacetin, and methyldopa (e.g., Aldomet).

**Hemolytic crisis:**   Individuals with chronic hemolytic anemia may do relatively well for a period of time, but many factors can precipitate a hemolytic crisis or acute hemolysis (i.e., an individual with mild hemolytic anemia can become severely anemic with an acute infectious process or with any other physiologic or emotional stressor, including surgery, trauma, or emotional upset). Widespread hemolysis causes an acute decrease in $O_2$-carrying capacity of the blood, resulting in decreased $O_2$ delivery to the tissues. Organ congestion from the hemolyzed blood cells occurs, and this affects organ function and precipitates a shock state.

## ASSESSMENT

**Chronic indicators:**   Pallor (e.g., conjunctival), fatigue, dyspnea on exertion, and intermittent dizziness, all of which depend on the severity of the anemia. With chronic hemolytic anemia, the individual sometimes will exhibit jaundice, arthritis, renal failure, and skin ulcers because of hemolysis and chronic organ damage.

**Acute indicators:**   Fever, visual blurring, temporary blindness, abdominal pain, back and joint pain, palpitations, SOB, chills, splenomegaly, hepatomegaly, headache, lymphadenopathy, and decreased urinary output (signs and symptoms of hemolytic crisis). Peripheral nerve damage can result in paralysis or paresthesias, vomiting, and chills.

## DIAGNOSTIC TESTS

**Sickle cell test:**   To screen for sickle cell anemia.

**Hgb and Hct:** Decreased because of RBC destruction.

**Serum tests:** Lactate dehydrogenase (LDH) will be elevated because of the release of this enzyme when the red blood cell is destroyed. Bilirubin will be elevated because the liver cannot process the excess that occurs from rapid RBC destruction.

**Urine and fecal urobilinogen:** Levels are increased. These are more sensitive indicators of RBC destruction than serum bilirubin levels.

**Bone marrow aspiration:** Will reveal erythroid hyperplasia, especially with chronic hemolytic anemia.

**Hgb electrophoresis:** Will diagnose Hgb AS, a sickle cell trait, and may show sickled Hgb.

**Reticulocyte count:** Will be elevated because of the rapid destruction of RBCs.

**Serum haptoglobin:** Decreased because the Hgb released from hemolyzed RBCs is bound to haptoglobin.

## COLLABORATIVE MANAGEMENT

**Elimination or discontinuation of causative factor:** If possible (e.g., chemical, drug, incompatible blood).

**Volume replacement:** For hypovolemic individuals to prevent decreased organ perfusion owing to hemolysis.

**$O_2$ therapy:** For patients who are hypoxemic.

**Supportive therapy for shock state:** If it occurs.

**Transfusion:** If circulatory failure or severe anemic anoxia occurs.

**Erythrocytapheresis (RBC exchange):** A relatively new procedure that removes abnormal RBCs and infuses healthy RBCs to correct the anemia.

*Patient assessment during erythrocytapheresis:*
- Monitor for symptom relief following one RBC exchange.
- Monitor arterial $Pao_2$ for evidence of improvement, optimally $\geq 80$ mm Hg.
- Monitor Hct. Values $\geq 30\%$ are necessary to prevent bone marrow stimulation.

**Corticosteroids:** To help stabilize cell membranes and decrease the inflammatory response. Usually 50-100 mg prednisone is given with antacids.

**Folic acid:** To help prevent hemolytic crisis by increasing the production of RBCs in individuals with chronic hemolytic anemias.

**Splenectomy:** To provide relief, depending on the cause of the anemia. The spleen is the site of RBC destruction.

## NURSING DIAGNOSES AND INTERVENTIONS

**High risk for impaired skin integrity _or_ impaired tissue integrity** related to altered circulation (occlusion of the vessels), resulting in impaired oxygen transport to the tissues and skin

*Desired outcome:* Patient's skin and tissue remain nonerythematous and intact.
- Assess the patient's skin, especially that over bony prominences and extremities, noting changes in integrity, such as erythema, increased warmth, and blisters.
- Use a bed cradle to keep pressure of bed linen and blankets off patient's tissue and skin.
- Keep extremities warm to promote circulation. Also encourage moderate exercises or ROM to promote circulation.

---

**Caution:** Avoid any activity or exercise if the signs and symptoms of hemolytic crisis are present (see "Patient-Family Teaching and Discharge Planning," below).

---

- Caution patient about the importance of avoiding trauma or injury to the skin and tissues.
- Apply dry, sterile dressings or dressing materials such as Op-Site and Tegaderm to areas of tissue breakdown. Use aseptic technique to help prevent infection. See "Managing Wound Care," p. 681, for more information.

**Altered renal tissue perfusion** related to interrupted blood flow secondary to hemolytic obstruction

*Desired outcome:*  Following intervention/treatment, patient has adequate renal perfusion as evidenced by equal I&O and urinary output ≥30 ml/h.

- Monitor I&O. Report urine output <30 ml/h in the presence of adequate intake.
- In the absence of renal or cardiac failure, encourage fluid intake to maintain adequate glomerular blood flow.
- Deliver IV fluid as prescribed to maintain fluid balance and renal perfusion.

**Altered peripheral and cardiopulmonary tissue perfusion** related to interrupted blood flow secondary to inflammatory process and occlusion of blood vessels with RBCs

*Desired outcome:*  Following treatment, patient has adequate peripheral and cardiopulmonary perfusion as evidenced by systolic BP ≤10 mm Hg lower than baseline systolic BP, peripheral pulses >2+ on a 0-4+ scale, HR ≤100 bpm, RR 12-20 breaths/min with normal depth and pattern (eupnea), and normal skin color.

- Assess BP at frequent intervals, and report significant drops (>10 mm Hg from baseline systolic readings).
- Assess amplitude of peripheral pulses as an indicator of peripheral perfusion. Be alert to pulses ≤2+ amplitude.
- Be alert to signs of cardiac depression, including decreased BP, increased HR, decreased pulse amplitude, dyspnea, and decreased urine output.
- Assess for and report indicators of hypoxia or respiratory dysfunction, such as increased RR, dyspnea, SOB, and cyanosis.
- Administer oxygen as prescribed if hypoxemia is present.
- Assist patient with ROM exercises to enhance tissue perfusion as well as increase joint mobility.

---

**Caution:**  Exercise should be avoided if any early signs of hemolytic crisis appear (see "Patient-Family Teaching and Discharge Planning," p. 491) because exercise can aggravate hemolysis.

---

- Report significant findings to patient's physician.

**Altered protection** related to neurosensory alterations secondary to peripheral nerve hypoxia resulting from erythrocytopenia

*Desired outcomes:*  Patient is free of symptoms of injury caused by neurosensory deficit. Visual disturbances, which can signal hemolytic crisis, are detected and reported promptly to patient's physician.

- Monitor motor strength and coordination, and report changes in peripheral sensation. Protect patient from extremes of heat and cold if impaired sensation is noted.
- Accompany patient during ambulation; provide physical support as necessary.
- Assess patient for visual disturbances. Report immediately the presence of blurred vision or blindness, which are indicators of hemolytic crisis.
- Teach patient and significant others the indicators of sensorimotor dysfunction, including gait unsteadiness, incoordination, paresthesias, and paralysis. Instruct them to report these indicators promptly if they occur.

**Pain** related to joint hemolysis secondary to hemolytic crisis

*Desired outcomes:*  Within 1 h of intervention, patient's subjective percep-

tion of discomfort decreases, as documented by a pain scale. Objective indicators, such as grimacing, are absent or diminished.
- Monitor for the presence of pain. Devise a pain scale with the patient, rating the discomfort on a scale of 0 (no pain) to 10 (worst pain). Administer pain medications as prescribed, and document effectiveness using the pain scale.
- Reassure patient that pain will subside when acute hemolytic episode is over.
- Elevate extremities to promote comfort.
- Apply moist heat packs to the joints to increase circulation and decrease pain. Use heat cautiously, especially for patients with decreased peripheral sensations (see **Altered protection,** p. 490).
- Apply elastic stockings or wraps, if prescribed, to support joints and promote circulation.

---

**Note:** See "Pernicious Anemia" for **Activity intolerance,** p. 486, and **High risk for infection,** p. 486.

---

## PATIENT-FAMILY TEACHING AND DISCHARGE PLANNING

Give patient and significant others verbal and written information about the following:
- Side effects of steroids, if prescribed, including weight gain, headache, and increased appetite.
- Support groups available for sickle cell anemia and thalassemia.
- Indicators of hemolytic crisis, including jaundice, dyspnea, SOB, joint or abdominal pain, decreasing BP, and increased HR; and factors that precipitate hemolytic crisis, such as emotional stress, physical stress, infection, trauma, chemicals, and toxic drug reactions (e.g., to penicillin, methyldopa, sulfonamides, quinine).
- Importance of maintaining a calm environment for the patient. Teach patient stress reduction techniques, such as meditation and relaxation exercises. See **Health-seeking behaviors:** Relaxation technique effective for stress reduction, p. 54.
- Importance of avoiding infectious processes, such as upper respiratory infections, and getting prompt medical attention should infection occur.
- Medications, including drug name, purpose, schedule, dosage, precautions, and potential side effects.
- Importance of medical follow-up.

## Hypoplastic (aplastic) anemia

This type of anemia results from inability of erythrocyte-producing organs, specifically the bone marrow, to produce erythrocytes. The causes of hypoplastic anemia are varied but can include use of antineoplastic or antimicrobial agents, infectious process, pregnancy, hepatitis, and radiation. Approximately half the patients with hypoplastic anemia have had exposure to drugs or chemical agents, while the remaining half have had immunologic disorders. Hypoplastic anemia most often involves pancytopenia, the depression of production of all three bone marrow elements: erythrocytes, platelets, and granulocytes. Usually the onset of hypoplastic anemia is insidious, but it can evolve quickly in some cases. Prognosis usually is poor for these individuals.

## ASSESSMENT

**Chronic indicators:**   Weakness, fatigue, pallor, dysphagia, and numbness and tingling of the extremities.
**Acute indicators:**   Fever and infection (because of decreased neutrophils);

**T A B L E   7 - 1    Commonly Used Blood Products**

| Product | Approximate volume | Indications | Precautions/comments |
|---|---|---|---|
| Whole blood | 500–510 ml (450 WB; 50–60 anticoagulants) | Acute, severe blood loss; hypovolemic shock. Increases both red cell mass and plasma | Must be ABO and Rh compatible. Do not mix with dextrose solutions; always prime tubing with normal saline. Observe for dyspnea, orthopnea, cyanosis, and anxiety as signs of circulatory overload; monitor VS |
| Packed RBCs | 250 ml | Increase RBC mass and $O_2$-carrying capacity of the blood | Must be ABO and Rh compatible. Leukocyte-depleted RBCs may be used to reduce the risk of antibody formation and nonhemolytic reactions. Irradiated RBCs may be used to prevent graft vs. host disease in patients who are immunocompromised. Packed RBCs have less volume than WB, thus reducing the risk of fluid overload |
| Fresh frozen plasma | 250 ml | Treatment of choice for combined coagulation factor deficiencies and factor V and XI deficiencies; alternate treatment for factor VII, VIII, IX, and X deficiencies when concentrates are not available | Must be ABO compatible. Supplies clotting factors. Usual dose is 10–15 ml/kg body weight. Transfuse within 24 h of thawing. Do not use if patient needs volume expansion |

| | | |
|---|---|---|
| Random donor platelet concentrate | 50 ml (usual adult dose is 5-6 U) | Treatment of choice for thrombocytopenia. Also used for leukemia and hypoplastic anemia | Usual dose is 0.1 U/kg body weight to increase platelet count to 25,000/μl. Administer as rapidly as tolerated. ABO compatibility is preferable. Effectiveness is decreased by fever, sepsis, and splenomegaly. Febrile reactions are common. Use special platelet tubing and filter. Special filters are available for removing leukocytes and thus decrease the risk of alloimmunization to HLA. Platelets must be infused within 4 h of initiation |
| Platelet concentrate by platelet pheresis (single donor platelets) | 200 ml, but may vary | Treatment for thrombocytopenic patients who are refractory to random donor platelets | Involves removing donor's venous blood, removing the platelets by differential centrifuge, and returning the blood to donor. Approximately 3-4 L of whole blood are processed to obtain a therapeutic dose of platelets. May use special donors who are HLA matched to the patient |
| Cryoprecipitate (factor VIII) | 10-25 ml | Routine treatment for hemophilia (factor VIII deficiency) and fibrinogen deficiency (factor XIII deficiency) | Made from fresh frozen plasma. Infuse immediately upon thawing |

**Note:** DNA recombinant technology may decrease complications from factor concentrates.

*These products carry no risk of disease transmission.

**Note:** When administering blood products it is important to recognize that most blood products have risk associated with delivery. Risks include transmission of human immunodeficiency virus, hepatitis B, hepatitis C, cytomegalovirus, and HTLV-I.

WB = whole blood; HLA = human leukocyte antigen.

*Continued.*

**T A B L E  7 - 1　Commonly Used Blood Products—cont'd**

| Product | Approximate volume | Indications | Precautions/comments |
|---|---|---|---|
| AHG (factor VIII) concentrates | 20 ml | Alternative treatment for hemophilia A | Allergic and febrile reactions occur frequently. Administer by syringe or component drip set. Can store at refrigerator temperature, making it convenient for hemophiliacs during travel |
| Factor II, VII, IX, X concentrate | 20 ml | Treatment of choice for hemophilia B and factor IX deficiencies | Can precipitate clotting. Allergic and febrile reactions occur occasionally. Contraindicated in liver disease |
| Albumin* | 50 or 250 ml | Hypovolemic shock, hypoalbuminemia, protein replacement for burn patients | Osmotically equal to 5× its volume of plasma. Used as a volume expander in conjunction with crystalloids. Also used in hypoalbuminemic states. Commercially available |
| Plasma protein fraction* | 250 ml (83% albumin with some alpha and beta globulins) | Volume expansion | Commercially available; expensive. Certain lots reported to have caused hypotension, possibly related to vasoactive amines used in preparation |
| Granulocyte transfusion (collected from a single apheresis donor) | 200 ml, but may vary | Leukemia with granulocytopenia related to treatment | Not a common treatment. Febrile and allergic symptoms are frequent. Must be ABO compatible |

**Note:** DNA recombinant technology may decrease complications from factor concentrates.

*These products carry no risk of disease transmission.

**Note:** When administering blood products it is important to recognize that most blood products have risk associated with delivery. Risks include transmission of human immunodeficiency virus, hepatitis B, hepatitis C, cytomegalovirus, and HTLV-I.
WB = whole blood; HLA = human leukocyte antigen.

bleeding (because of thrombocytopenia); and dizziness, dyspnea on exertion, progressive weakness, and oral ulcerations.

**History of:** Exposure to chemical toxins or radiation; use of antibiotics, such as chloramphenicol; viral infections, such as hepatitis C.

## DIAGNOSTIC TESTS

**CBC with differential:** Low levels of Hgb, WBCs, and RBCs; however, RBCs usually appear to be normal morphologically.

**Platelet count:** Low.

**Bleeding time:** Prolonged.

**Bone marrow aspiration:** Will reveal hypocellular or hypoplastic tissue with a fatty and fibrous appearance and depression of erythroid elements.

**Reticulocyte count:** This test, which is a determinant of bone marrow function, will show a marked decrease because of the bone marrow's inability to respond.

**Peripheral blood smear:** Will show nucleated RBCs and immature granulocytes.

**Cultures:** If infection is suspected.

## COLLABORATIVE MANAGEMENT

**Determination of the cause of anemia.**

**Transfusion with packed RBCs or frozen plasma:** See Table 7-1. **Note:** Because of the potential for antibody formation, patients considered candidates for bone marrow transplants should be given leukocyte-poor and cytomegalovirus (CMV)-negative blood products.

**Transfusion with concentrated platelets:** To keep platelet count >20,000/mm$^3$. Hemorrhage occurs less frequently when platelet count is above this level (Table 7-1).

**Bone marrow transplantation (BMT):** In this procedure, 500-700 ml of bone marrow are aspirated from the pelvic bones of the donor and then filtered and infused into the patient. Optimally, the donated marrow is antigen-compatible (known as human leukocyte antigen [HLA] matched), and for that the donor should be an identical twin or sibling. However, only about one-third of potential BMT recipients have an HLA-matched sibling donor. The use of unrelated donors is an area of research and potential benefit.

**Treatment with antilymphocyte globulin:** To cause immunosuppression before BMT.

**Antibiotic therapy:** If infection is found.

**Steroid therapy:** To stimulate granulocyte production, although results with adults are not always successful.

**O$_2$:** If anemia is severe.

**Granulocyte transfusion:** See Table 7-1. Although rarely used today, the following are indications for use: documented infection, fever unresponsive to antibiotics, WBC <500/mm$^3$, and expectations for bone marrow regeneration.

**Androgen therapy:** An attempt to stimulate bone marrow activity.

## NURSING DIAGNOSES AND INTERVENTIONS

**High risk for infection** related to inadequate secondary defenses secondary to leukopenia with granulocytopenia

*Desired outcome:* Patient is free of infection as evidenced by normothermia, HR ≤100 bpm, RR 12-20 breaths/min with normal depth and pattern (eupnea), and absence of erythema, warmth, and drainage at any invasive or wound sites.

- Perform meticulous handwashing before patient contact.
- If appropriate, maintain protective/reverse isolation, using gloves, gown, and masks; make sure that visitors follow the same protocol. Discourage delivery of plants and flowers to the room.
- Report any signs of systemic infection (e.g., fever); obtain prescription for

blood, wound, and urine cultures as indicated. Administer antibiotics as prescribed.

- Monitor for and report any signs of local infection, such as sore throat or erythematous or draining wounds. **Note:** With decreased or absent granulocytes, pus may not form; therefore it is important to look for other signs of infection.
- Provide oral care at frequent intervals to prevent oral lesions, which may result in bleeding and infection.
- Provide and encourage adequate perianal hygiene to prevent rectal abscess. Avoid giving medications or taking temperature rectally.
- Avoid invasive procedures, if possible.
- Encourage ambulation, deep breathing, turning, and coughing to prevent problems of immobility, which can result in pneumonia and skin breakdown.
- Arrange for patient to have a private room when possible.
- Institute reverse isolation if granulocyte count is <200/mm$^3$. Discuss with the patient granulocyte transfusion and BMT if appropriate.
- Teach patient and significant others signs and symptoms of infection and the importance of notifying staff or physician promptly if they are noted.

**Knowledge deficit:**   Potential for bleeding (caused by low platelet count) and measures that can help prevent it
*Desired outcome:*   After patient-teaching, patient verbalizes knowledge about the potential for bleeding and the measures that can prevent it.

- Teach patient about the potential for bleeding and the importance of monitoring for hematuria, melena, frank bleeding from the mouth, epistaxis, or coughing up blood and notifying staff promptly if they occur.
- Teach patient to use an electric razor and soft-bristled toothbrush.
- Explain the importance of maintaining regularity with bowel movements to prevent straining and potential bleeding.
- Teach patient to avoid potentially traumatic procedures, such as enemas and rectal temperatures.
- Caution patient to avoid using aspirin and aspirin products, which decrease platelet aggregation and further increase the potential for bleeding.
- Explain that concentrated platelets usually are transfused to keep the platelet count >20,000 μl. Hemorrhage occurs less frequently when the platelet count is maintained above this level.

**Activity intolerance** related to imbalance between oxygen supply and demand secondary to decreased oxygen-carrying capacity of the blood, which occurs with decreased production of erythrocytes
*Desired outcome:*   By a minimum of 24 h before hospital discharge, patient rates perceived exertion at ≤3 on a 0-10 scale and exhibits tolerance to activity as evidenced by RR 12-20 breaths/min with normal depth and pattern (eupnea), HR ≤100 bpm, and absence of dizziness and headaches.

- Monitor for signs of activity intolerance, and ask patient to rate perceived exertion (see this nursing diagnosis in Appendix One, p. 711, for detail).
- Plan frequent and undisturbed rest periods of at least 90 min.
- Administer oxygen as prescribed, and encourage deep breathing to augment oxygen delivery to the tissues.
- Administer blood components (usually RBCs) as prescribed. Double-check typing with a colleague, and monitor for and report signs of transfusion reaction.
- Encourage gradually increasing activities to tolerance as patient's condition improves. Set mutually agreed on goals with patient (e.g., "Let's plan this morning's activity goals. Do you feel you could walk up and down the hall once, or twice?" or appropriate amount, depending on patient's tolerance).

**Altered protection** related to neurosensory and musculoskeletal alterations secondary to tissue hypoxia occurring with decreased production of erythrocytes
*Desired outcome:*   Patient verbalizes orientation to person, place, and time

and is free of symptoms of injury caused by neurosensory alterations.

- Perform neurologic checks and assess patient's orientation as indicators of cerebral perfusion. If signs of decreasing cerebral perfusion occur, establish precautionary measures (e.g., keeping side rails up and the bed in the lowest position) to protect patient from injury. Request restraints, if indicated.
- Assess sensorimotor status to help evaluate nervous system oxygenation. Be alert to paresthesias, decreased muscle strength, and altered gait.
- Prevent injury from heat or cold applications for patients with paresthesias.
- Do not allow patient to ambulate unassisted if muscle or gait alterations are present.
- Administer oxygen as prescribed.
- Teach patient deep-breathing exercises, which may increase oxygenation by augmenting gas exchange.
- Report promptly indicators of a worsening condition to patient's physician.

---

**Note:**  See "Pernicious Anemia" for **Altered nutrition,** p. 487.

---

## PATIENT-FAMILY TEACHING AND DISCHARGE PLANNING

Give patient and significant others verbal and written information about the following:

- Medications, including drug name, purpose, dosage, schedule, precautions, and potential side effects.
- Indicators of systemic infection, including fever, malaise, fatigue, as well as signs and symptoms of upper respiratory infection, urinary tract infection, and wound infection (see p. 141, 681).
- Importance of avoiding exposure to individuals known to have acute infections; preventing trauma, abrasions, and breakdown of the skin; and maintaining good nutritional intake to enhance resistance to infections.
- Signs of bleeding/hemorrhage, which necessitate medical attention: melena, hematuria, epistaxis, ecchymosis, and bleeding of gums.
- Measures to prevent hemorrhage, such as using electric razor and soft-bristled toothbrush and avoiding activities that can traumatize the tissues.
- Importance of reporting general symptoms of anemia, including fatigue, weakness, paresthesias.
- Importance of avoiding aspirin and aspirin products in the presence of a bleeding disorder.

# Polycythemia

Polycythemia is a chronic disorder characterized by excessive production of RBCs. As the number of RBCs increases, blood volume, blood viscosity, and Hgb concentration increase, causing excessive work load for the heart and congestion of such organ systems as the liver and kidney.

*Secondary polycythemia* results from an abnormal increase in erythropoietin production (e.g., because of hypoxia that occurs with chronic lung disease), or it can occur inappropriately, as with renal tumors. *Polycythemia vera* is a primary disorder of unknown cause, resulting in increased RBC mass, leukocytosis, and slight thrombocytosis. Because of the increased viscosity and decreased microcirculation, mortality rate is high if the condition is left untreated. In addition, there is a potential for this disorder to evolve into other hematopoietic disorders, such as leukemia.

## ASSESSMENT

**Signs and symptoms:**  Headache, dizziness, visual disturbances, dyspnea, thrombophlebitis, joint pain, pruritus, night sweats, fatigue, chest pain, and a feeling of "fullness," especially in the head.

**Physical assessment:**    Hypertension, crackles (rales), cyanosis, ruddy complexion, hepatosplenomegaly.

## DIAGNOSTIC TESTS

**CBC:**    Increased RBC mass (8-12 million/mm$^3$), Hgb, and leukocytes; overproduction of thrombocytes.
**Platelet count:**    Elevated as a result of increased production.
**Bone marrow aspiration:**    Will reveal RBC proliferation.
**Uric acid levels:**    May be increased because of increased nucleoprotein, an end product of RBC breakdown.

## COLLABORATIVE MANAGEMENT

**Phlebotomy:**    Blood withdrawn from the vein to decrease blood volume (and decrease Hct to 45%). Usually 500 ml are removed every 2-3 days until the Hct is 40%-45%. For the older adult, 250-300 ml are removed.
**Myelosuppressive agents such as radiophosphorus:**    To inhibit proliferation of RBCs.
**Alkylating (myelosuppressive) agents (e.g., busulfan and chlorambucil):**    To decrease bone marrow function.

## NURSING DIAGNOSES AND INTERVENTIONS

**Pain** related to headache, angina, and abdominal and joint discomfort secondary to altered circulation occurring with hyperviscosity of the blood
*Desired outcomes:*    Within 1 h of intervention, patient's subjective perception of discomfort decreases, as documented by a pain scale. Objective indicators, such as grimacing, are absent or diminished.
- Assess patient for the presence of headache, angina, abdominal pain, and joint pain. Devise a pain scale with the patient, rating discomfort from 0 (no pain) to 10 (worst pain).
- In the presence of joint pain, elevate the extremity; apply moist heat to ease discomfort.
- Administer analgesics as prescribed.
- Encourage use of nonpharmacologic pain control, such as relaxation and distraction.
- Document the degree of pain relief, using the pain scale.
- Be alert to indicators of peripheral thrombosis, such as calf pain and tenderness.
- Report significant findings to patient's physician.
**Altered renal, peripheral, and cerebral tissue perfusion** related to interrupted blood flow secondary to hyperviscosity of the blood
*Desired outcome:*    Following treatment, patient has adequate renal, peripheral, and cerebral perfusion as evidenced by urinary output ≥30 ml/h, peripheral pulses >2+ on a scale of 0-4+, distal extremity warmth, adequate/baseline muscle strength, and orientation to person, place, and time.
- Monitor I&O; report urine output <30 ml/h in the presence of adequate intake, which can signal congestion and decreased perfusion.
- In the absence of signs of cardiac and renal failure, encourage fluid intake to decrease viscosity.
- Monitor peripheral perfusion by palpating peripheral pulses. Be alert to amplitude ≤2+ and coolness in the distal extremities.
- Encourage patient to exercise and ambulate to tolerance to enhance circulation.
- Monitor patient for indicators of impending neurologic damage, such as muscle weakness and decreases in sensation and LOC. If these indicators are present, protect patient by assisting with ambulation or raising side rails on the bed, depending on the degree of deficit.
- Administer myelosuppressive agents, as prescribed, to inhibit proliferation of RBCs.

- Report significant findings to patient's physician.

**Altered nutrition:** Less than body requirements, related to anorexia secondary to feelings of fullness occurring with organ system congestion

***Desired outcome:*** By a minimum of 24 h before hospital discharge, patient exhibits adequate nutrition as evidenced by maintenance of or return to baseline body weight.

- Weigh patient daily for trend.
- Encourage patient to eat small, frequent meals. Document intake.
- Request that significant others bring in patient's favorite foods if they are unavailable in the hospital.
- Advise patient to avoid spicy foods and to eat mild foods, which are better tolerated.
- Teach patient to avoid intake of iron to help minimize abnormal RBC proliferation.

**Altered cerebral and cardiopulmonary tissue perfusion (or risk of same)** related to hypovolemia secondary to phlebotomy

***Desired outcome:*** Patient has adequate cerebral and cardiopulmonary perfusion as evidenced by orientation to person, place, and time; HR ≤100 bpm; BP ≥90/60 mm Hg (or within patient's baseline range); absence of chest pain; and RR ≤20 breaths/min.

- During procedure, keep patient recumbent to prevent dizziness or hypotension.
- Assess for tachycardia, hypotension, chest pain, or dizziness during procedure; notify patient's physician of significant findings.
- After the procedure, assist patient with sitting position for 5-10 min before ambulation to prevent orthostatic hypotension. For more information about orthostatic hypotension, see this same nursing diagnosis in Appendix One, "Caring for Patients on Prolonged Bed Rest," p. 715.
- Teach patient about the potential for orthostatic hypotension and the need for caution when standing for at least 2-3 days after the phlebotomy.

## PATIENT-FAMILY TEACHING AND DISCHARGE PLANNING

Give patient and significant others verbal and written information about the following:

- Need for continued medical follow-up, including potential for phlebotomy every 1-3 months.
- Medications, including drug name, purpose, dosage, schedule, precautions, and potential side effects.
- Importance of augmenting fluid intake to decrease blood viscosity.
- Signs and symptoms that necessitate medical attention: angina, muscle weakness, numbness and tingling of extremities, decreased tolerance to activity, and joint pain.
- Nutrition: importance of maintaining a balanced diet to increase resistance to infection, and limiting intake of iron to help minimize abnormal RBC proliferation.

# Section Two:  Disorders of Coagulation

The formation of a visible fibrin clot is the conclusion of a complex series of reactions involving different clotting factors in the blood that are identified by Roman numerals I to XIII. All are plasma proteins except factor III (thromboplastin) and factor IV (calcium ion). When a vessel injury occurs, these factors interact to form the end product, a clot. The clots that are formed are eventually dissolved by the fibrinolytic system.

Platelets play a role in coagulation by releasing substances that activate the clotting factors. At the time of vascular injury, platelets migrate to the site and adhere to each other to form a temporary plug to stop the bleeding.

# Thrombocytopenia

Thrombocytopenia is a common coagulation disorder that results from a decreased number of platelets. It can be congenital or acquired, and it is classified according to cause. Common causes include deficient formation of thrombocytes, as occurs with bone marrow disease or destruction; accelerated platelet destruction, loss, or increased use, as in hemolytic anemia, diffuse intravascular coagulation, or damage by prosthetic heart valves; and abnormal platelet distribution, as in hypersplenism and hypothermia. Potential triggers include autoimmune disorder, severe vascular injury, and spleen malfunction. In addition, thrombocytopenia can occur as a side effect of certain chemotherapeutic agents and antibiotics. Regardless of the cause or trigger, the disorder affects coagulation and hemostasis. With chemical-induced thrombocytopenia, prognosis is good after withdrawal of the offending drug. Prognosis for other types is dependent on the form of thrombocytopenia and the individual's response to treatment.

*Thrombotic thrombocytopenic purpura (TTP)* is a very acute, often fatal disorder. The cause is presumed to be the absence of a factor in the plasma or the presence of a platelet-stimulating factor. Platelets become sensitized and clump in blood vessels, occluding them. *Idiopathic thrombocytopenic purpura* (ITP) is believed to be an immune disorder specifically involving antiplatelet immunoglobulin G (IgG), which destroys platelets. The acute form is most often seen in children (2-6 years of age) and may be related to a previous viral infection. The chronic form is seen more often in adults (18-50 years of age) and is of unknown origin.

## ASSESSMENT

**Chronic indicators:**   Long history of mild bleeding or hemorrhagic episodes. Increased bruising, gum bleeding, and petechiae also may be noted.

**Acute indicators:**   Fever, splenomegaly, acute and severe bleeding episodes, weakness, lethargy, malaise, hemorrhage into mucous membranes, gum bleeding, and GI bleeding. Prolonged bleeding can lead to a shock state with tachycardia, SOB, and decreased LOC. Intracranial hemorrhage also can occur.

**Note:** With TTP, the individual may exhibit signs associated with platelet thrombus formation and ischemic organs, such as decreased renal function or neurologic changes.

**History of:**   Recent infection; recent vaccination; use of chlorothiazide, digitalis, quinidine, rifampin, sulfisoxazole, chloramphenicol, phenytoin.

## DIAGNOSTIC TESTS

**Platelet count:**   Can vary from only slightly decreased to nearly absent. Less than $100,000/\mu l$ is significantly decreased; $<20,000/\mu l$ results in a serious risk of hemorrhage.

**Peripheral blood smear:**   Will reveal megathrombocytes (large platelets), which are present during premature destruction of platelets.

**CBC:**   Low Hgb and Hct levels because of blood loss; WBC count usually is within normal range.

**Bleeding time:**   Increased owing to decreased platelets.

**Bone marrow aspiration:**   Will reveal increased number of megakaryocytes (platelet precursors) in the presence of ITP, but may be decreased with certain causes of thrombocytopenia.

**Platelet antibody screen:**   May be positive owing to the presence of IgG antibodies.

## COLLABORATIVE MANAGEMENT

**Treatment of underlying cause or removal of precipitating agent.**

**Platelet transfusion:** Unless platelet destruction is the cause of the disorder (see Table 7-1).

**Corticosteroids:** To enhance vascular integrity or diminish platelet destruction.

**Splenectomy:** Removal of an organ responsible for platelet destruction. This is considered viable treatment unless patient has acute bleeding, a severe deficiency of platelets, or a cardiac disorder that contraindicates surgery.

**Plasma exchange *via* apheresis:** Removes the antibody or immune complex; used for short-term therapy.

## NURSING DIAGNOSES AND INTERVENTIONS

**Altered protection** related to increased risk of bleeding secondary to decreased platelet count

***Desired outcomes:*** Patient is free of the signs of bleeding as evidenced by secretions and excretions negative for blood, BP ≥90/60 mm Hg or within patient's baseline range, HR ≤100 bpm, RR 12-20 breaths/min with normal depth and pattern (eupnea), and absence of bruising.

- Monitor patient for hematuria, melena, epistaxis, hematemesis, or severe ecchymosis. Teach patient to be alert to and report these indicators promptly.
- When appropriate, protect patient from injury by padding and keeping up side rails.
- When possible, avoid venipuncture. If performed, apply pressure on site for 5-10 min or until bleeding stops.
- Avoid IM injections. If performed, use small-gauge needle when possible.
- Monitor platelet count daily. Optimal range is 150,000-400,000/μl.
- Advise patient to avoid straining at stool or coughing, which increases intracranial pressure and can result in intracranial hemorrhage. Obtain prescription for stool softeners, if indicated, to prevent constipation. Teach patient anticonstipation routine as described in **Constipation,** p. 716, in Appendix One, "Caring for Patients on Prolonged Bed Rest."
- Administer corticosteroids as prescribed to help minimize platelet destruction.
- Teach patient to use electric razor and soft-bristled toothbrush.
- Administer platelets as prescribed and be alert to indicators of transfusion reaction, including chills, back pain, dyspnea, hives, and wheezing.
- Alert patient's physician to significant findings.

**Altered cerebral, peripheral, and renal tissue perfusion (or risk of same)** related to interrupted blood flow secondary to presence of thrombotic component, which results in sensitization and clumping of platelets in the blood vessels

***Desired outcome:*** Patient's cerebral, peripheral, and renal perfusion are adequate as evidenced by orientation to person, place, and time; normoreactive pupillary responses; absence of headaches, dizziness, and visual disturbances; peripheral pulses >2+ on a 0-4+ scale; and urine output ≥30 ml/h.

- Assess patient for changes in LOC and pupillary responses.
- Monitor for headaches, dizziness, or visual disturbances.
- Palpate peripheral pulses. Be alert to pulses ≤2+.
- Assess urine output. Adequate perfusion is reflected by urine output ≥30 ml/h for 2 consecutive h.
- Monitor I&O. The patient should be well hydrated (2-3 L/day) to increase perfusion of the small vessels.

**Pain** related to joint discomfort secondary to hemorrhagic episodes or blood extravasation into the tissues

***Desired outcomes:*** Within 1 h of intervention, patient's subjective perception of discomfort decreases, as documented by a pain scale. Objective indicators, such as grimacing, are absent or diminished.

- Monitor patient for the presence of fatigue, malaise, and joint pain. Devise a pain scale with patient, rating discomfort on a scale of 0 (no pain) to 10 (worst pain).
- Maintain a calm, restful environment; provide periods of undisturbed rest.
- Elevate legs to minimize joint discomfort in the lower extremities. Support legs with pillows. Avoid gatching the bed at the knee, which could occlude popliteal vessels.
- Use a bed cradle to decrease pressure on the tissues of the lower extremities.
- Administer analgesics as prescribed. Document relief obtained, using the pain scale. **Caution:** Aspirin and other nonsteroidal antiinflammatory drugs are contraindicated because of their antiplatelet action.

**High risk for fluid volume deficit** related to postsplenectomy bleeding/hemorrhage

*Desired outcome:*   Patient is normovolemic as evidenced by BP ≥90/60 mm Hg (or within patient's normal range), HR ≤100 bpm, RR 12-20 breaths/min with normal depth and pattern (eupnea), soft and nondistended abdomen, and absence of frank bleeding.

- Monitor postoperative VS for changes that may indicate bleeding (e.g., decreasing BP and increasing HR). Be alert to restlessness as well.
- Inspect abdomen for presence of distention, and question patient about abdominal pain or tenderness, any of which can signal internal bleeding.
- Inspect operative site for the presence of frank bleeding.
- Monitor postoperative platelet count. Approximately 60%-70% of postsplenectomy patients have increased platelet counts. Optimal range for these patients is 200,000-300,000/μl.
- Report significant findings to patient's physician.

---

**Note:**   If surgery is performed, see nursing diagnoses and interventions in Appendix One, "Caring for Preoperative and Postoperative Patients," p. 693.

---

## PATIENT-FAMILY TEACHING AND DISCHARGE PLANNING

Give patient and significant others verbal and written information about the following:

- Importance of preventing trauma, which can cause bleeding.
- Seeking medical attention for *any* signs of bleeding or infection. Review the signs and symptoms of common infections, such as upper respiratory infection, urinary tract infection, and wound infection. Signs and symptoms of common infections are described in **High risk for infection** in "Care of the Renal Transplant Recipient," p. 141. Also teach patient to assess for hematuria, melena, hematemesis, oozing from mucous membranes, and petechiae.
- Importance of regular medical follow-up for platelet counts.
- If discharged on corticosteroids, the potential side effects that necessitate medical attention: acne, moon face, buffalo hump, hypertension, gastric upset, weight gain, thinning of arms and legs, edema, and mood changes. Stress the importance of *not* discontinuing steroids unless directed by patient's physician.
- Other medications, including drug name, dosage, purpose, schedule, precautions, and potential side effects.

# Hemophilia

Hemophilia is a type of hereditary bleeding disorder characterized by a deficiency of one or more clotting factors. Classic hemophilia is caused by deficiency of factors VIII (hemophilia A) and IX (hemophilia B).

Both types of hemophilia are sex-linked inherited disorders. Individuals affected are usually males, whereas their mothers and sisters are asymptomatic carriers. This disorder also can occur in females if it is inherited from an affected male and a female carrier or if it is due to X chromosome inactivation during embryologic development. Intracranial hemorrhage is the most common cause of death.

## ASSESSMENT

**Chronic indicators:** Bruising after minimal trauma, joint pain.
**Acute indicators:** Acute bleeding episodes after minimal trauma. Hemarthrosis is the most common and debilitating symptom, causing painful and swollen joints. Large ecchymoses can occur, as well as bleeding from the gums, tongue, GI tract, urinary tract, or from cuts in the skin. Shock can result from severe bleeding.

## DIAGNOSTIC TESTS

**Partial thromboplastin time:** Prolonged.
**Bleeding time:** Prolonged.
**Platelet count:** Usually normal.
**Activated clotting time:** Prolonged.
**Assays of factors VIII and IX:** Will reveal low activity.

## COLLABORATIVE MANAGEMENT

**Factor transfusion:** For hemophilia B (see Table 7-1).
**Transfusion of fresh frozen plasma:** See Table 7-1.
**Cryoprecipitate:** For infusion of factor VIII with classic hemophilia A (see Table 7-1). **Note:** Commercially prepared, heat-treated factor VIII is also being used to decrease the risk of disease and contamination. A product called monoclonal antibody–derived factor VIII currently is demonstrating no risk of disease transmission. However, its use is limited by cost and availability.
**Agents such as desmopressin (DDAVP) and aminocaproic acid (Amicar):** To enhance intrinsic mechanisms and decrease the need for factor replacement.

## NURSING DIAGNOSES AND INTERVENTIONS

**Altered protection** related to increased risk of bleeding secondary to clotting factor deficiency
*Desired outcome:* Patient is free of bleeding as evidenced by systolic BP ≥90 mm Hg (or within patient's baseline range), HR ≤100 bpm, RR 12-20 breaths/min with normal depth and pattern (eupnea), and secretions and excretions negative for blood.
- Monitor VS for signs of bleeding, including hypotension and increased HR. Also be alert to patient restlessness.
- Monitor patient for evidence of bleeding, including swollen joints, abdominal pain, hematuria, hematemesis, melena, and epistaxis.
- If signs of bleeding occur, elevate the affected area if possible, and apply cold compresses and gentle pressure to the site.
- When indicated, institute measures to minimize the risk of bleeding from trauma, such as keeping side rails up and padded, assisting with ambulation, and limiting invasive procedures if possible.
- Teach patient to use electric razor and soft-bristled toothbrush.
- Do not administer aspirin; caution patient about its anticoagulant action.
- Administer clotting factors as prescribed.
- Teach patient the importance of lifetime medical follow-up and regular factor transfusions. For patient in whom factor VIII prophylaxis is used, teach patient or significant other the procedure for intravenous administration of factor VIII as appropriate.

**High risk for impaired skin integrity** *and* **impaired tissue integrity** related to altered blood circulation to the tissues secondary to bleeding

*Desired outcome:*   Patient's skin and tissue remain intact with absence of bruising and swelling.
- Inspect patient's skin at least q4h, being alert to bruising, pressure areas, and swelling.
- Apply ice or pressure over sites of intradermal bleeding to promote vaso-constriction.
- Handle patient gently to minimize the risk of tissue trauma.
- To enhance joint mobility and perfusion to the tissues, assist patient with ROM exercises daily. However, avoid exercise for 48 h after bleeding to prevent recurrence.
- To promote circulation to the tissues, assist patient with ambulation when it is tolerated.

**Pain** related to swollen joints (hemarthrosis)

*Desired outcomes:*   Within 1 h of intervention, patient's subjective perception of discomfort decreases, as documented by a pain scale. Objective indicators, such as grimacing, are absent or diminished.
- Monitor patient for the presence of joint discomfort. Devise a pain scale with the patient, rating discomfort on a scale of 0 (no pain) to 10 (worst pain).
- Apply splints or other supportive devices to joints; immobilize joints in slight flexion.
- Elevate or position pillows under affected joints to promote comfort.
- Administer analgesics as prescribed; avoid aspirin because of its anticoagulant action. Document pain relief achieved, using the pain scale.
- Assist patient with ambulation as needed.
- As needed, use ice for its topical analgesia and ability to constrict the vessels, which will decrease swelling. **Caution:** Avoid use of warm thermotherapy for these patients because it will increase swelling.
- Discuss with patient the importance of frequent assessment of joint function to enable rapid identification and treatment of hemophilic arthritis.

## PATIENT-FAMILY TEACHING AND DISCHARGE PLANNING

Give patient and significant others verbal and written information about the following:
- Importance of avoiding trauma, and necessity of seeking medical attention for any bleeding.
- Phone numbers to call in the event of emergency.
- Procedure in case of bleeding: application of cold compresses and gentle, direct pressure; elevation of affected part if possible; seeking medical attention promptly.
- Importance of notifying physician if dental procedures need to be done.
- Importance of lifetime medical follow-up and regular factor transfusions.
- Importance of frequent assessment of joint function to allow rapid identification and treatment of hemophilic arthritis.

*In addition*
- In patients for whom factor VIII prophylaxis is used, patient or significant other will require instruction in the IV administration of factor VIII.

# Disseminated intravascular coagulation

Disseminated intravascular coagulation (DIC) is an acute coagulation disorder characterized by paradoxical clotting and hemorrhage. The sequence usually progresses by massive clot formation, depletion of the clotting factors, and activation of diffuse fibrinolysis, followed by hemorrhage (see Figure 7-1). DIC occurs secondary to widespread coagulation factors in the bloodstream caused by extensive surgery, burns, shock, neoplastic diseases, and abruptio placentae; extensive destruction of blood vessel walls caused by eclampsia,

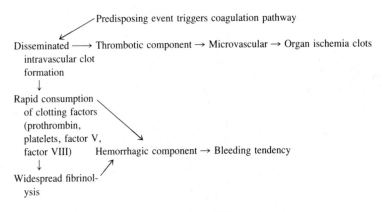

**Figure 7-1:**   Overview of DIC syndrome.

anoxia, and heat stroke; or damage to blood cells caused by hemolysis, sickle cell disease, and transfusion reactions (see Table 7-2). DIC is also associated with sepsis. Prompt assessment of the disorder can result in a good prognosis. Usually affected patients are transferred to ICU for careful monitoring and aggressive therapy.

## ASSESSMENT

**Clinical indicators:**   Bleeding of abrupt onset, oozing from venipuncture sites or mucosal surfaces; bleeding from surgical sites; the presence of hematuria, blood in the stool, bruising, pallor, or mottled skin. The patient also may bleed from the vagina, nose, and mucous membranes. Joint pain may signal bleeding into the joints. Symptoms of hypoperfusion can occur, including decreased urine output and abnormal behavior.

**Physical assessment:**   Abdominal assessment may reveal signs of GI bleeding, such as guarding and a rigid, boardlike abdomen.

**Risk factors:**   Infection, burns, trauma, hepatic disease, hypovolemic shock, severe hemolytic reaction, obstetric complications, and hypoxia. See Table 7-2.

## DIAGNOSTIC TESTS

**Serum fibrinogen:**   Low because of abnormal consumption of clotting factors in the formation of fibrin clots.

**Platelet count:**   Will be $<250,000/\mu l$ because of platelet's role in clot formation.

**Fibrin split products (FSP), also known as fibrin degradation products (FDP):**   Increased, indicating widespread dissolution of clots. Fibrinolysis produces FSPs as an end product.

**Prothrombin time (PT):**   Increased because of depletion of clotting factors.

**Partial thromboplastin time (PTT):**   High because of depletion of clotting factors.

**Peripheral blood smear:**   Will show fragmented RBCs.

**Bleeding time:**   Prolonged because of decreased platelets.

## COLLABORATIVE MANAGEMENT

**Identification and treatment of primary disorder:**   See Table 7-2.

**Anticoagulant therapy:**   Although this therapy is controversial, heparin may be administered. Heparin interferes with the coagulation process and minimizes

**TABLE 7 - 2   Clinical Conditions that Can Activate Disseminated Intravascular Coagulation**

| Obstetric | GI disorders | Tissue damage | Infections | Hemolytic processes | Vascular disorders | Miscellaneous |
|-----------|--------------|---------------|------------|---------------------|--------------------|----------------|
| Abruptio placentae | Cirrhosis | Surgery | Viral | Transfusion reaction | Shock | Fat or pulmonary embolism |
| Toxemia | Hepatic necrosis | Trauma | Bacterial | Acute hemolysis secondary to infection or immunologic disorder | Aneurysm | Snake bite |
| Amniotic fluid embolism | Pancreatitis | Burns | Rickettsial | | Giant hemangioma | Neoplastic disorder |
| Septic abortion | Peritoneovenous shunts | Prolonged extracorporeal circulation | Protozoal | | | Acute anoxia |
| Retained dead fetus | Necrotizing enterocolitis | Transplant rejection | | | | |
| | | Heat stroke | | | | |

consumption of the coagulation factors and activation of the fibrinolytic system. Heparin dose is regulated and determined by the PTT.

**Compartment replacement of platelets and clotting factors:** Replacement of clotting factors by administering fresh frozen plasma, packed RBCs, and platelets may counteract deficiencies. Blood replacement also supports blood volume (see Table 7-1).

**Epsilon-aminocaproic acid (Amicar):** Disrupts the fibrinolysis process, and may be administered to stop bleeding.

## NURSING DIAGNOSES AND INTERVENTIONS

**Altered cardiopulmonary, peripheral, renal, and cerebral tissue perfusion** related to interrupted blood flow secondary to coagulation/fibrinolysis processes

*Desired outcome:* Following treatment, patient has adequate cardiopulmonary, peripheral, renal, and cerebral perfusion as evidenced by BP ≥90/60 mm Hg and HR ≤100 bpm (or within patient's baseline range); peripheral pulse amplitude >2+ on a 0-4+ scale; urinary output ≥30 ml/h; equal and normoreactive pupils; normal/baseline motor function; and orientation to person, place, and time.

- Monitor VS. Be alert to and report decreased BP, increased HR, or decreased amplitude of peripheral pulses, which signal that coagulation is occurring.
- Monitor I&O; report output <30 ml/h in the presence of adequate intake, which is another indicator of the coagulation process.
- Perform neurologic checks, including orientation, pupil function, and motor response, and assess LOC to evaluate cerebral perfusion. If signs of impaired cerebral perfusion occur, protect patient from injury by instituting measures such as keeping bed in the lowest position and side rails up.
- Monitor for hemorrhage from surgical wounds, GI tract, and mucous membranes, which can occur after fibrinolysis.
- Monitor laboratory work for values suggestive of DIC, including low serum fibrinogen (<200 mg/dl), low platelet count (<250,000/μl), increased fibrin split products (>8μ/ml), increased PT (>11-15 sec), and increased PTT (>40-100 sec).
- Report significant findings to patient's physician; prepare for transfer to ICU if condition worsens.

**Altered protection** related to increased risk of bleeding secondary to hemorrhagic component of DIC

*Desired outcome:* Patient is free of signs of bleeding as evidenced by systolic BP ≥90 mm Hg, HR ≤100 bpm (or within patient's normal range); RR 12-20 breaths/min with normal depth and pattern (eupnea); urinary output ≥30 ml/h; secretions and excretions negative for blood; stable abdominal girth measurements; and orientation to person, place, and time.

- Monitor VS and LOC at frequent intervals; report significant changes. Be alert to hypotension, tachycardia, dyspnea, and disorientation, which can signal hemorrhage. **Note:** Be cautious of the pressure used with BP cuffs. Frequent BP readings may cause bleeding under the cuff.
- Monitor coagulation studies, being alert to PTT >40-100 sec.
- Use a reagent stick to check stool, urine, emesis, and nasogastric drainage for blood.
- Monitor for internal bleeding by measuring abdominal girth q8h. Also assess for abdominal pain and a boardlike abdomen, other signs of GI bleeding.
- Assess puncture sites regularly for oozing or bleeding.
- Be alert to other signs of bleeding, including joint pain and headache. Visual changes may signal retinal hemorrhage.
- Avoid giving IM injections or performing venipunctures for blood drawing.
- Administer blood products and IV fluids as prescribed.
- Teach patient to use electric shavers and soft-bristled toothbrushes.

**High risk for impaired skin integrity** *or* **impaired tissue integrity** related to altered circulation secondary to hemorrhage and thrombosis
*Desired outcome:* Patient's skin and tissue remain intact.
- Assess patient's skin, noting changes in color, temperature, and sensation, which may signal decreased perfusion and can lead to tissue damage.
- Eliminate or minimize pressure points by ensuring that the patient turns q2h and by using sheepskin on elbows and heels. Do not pull on extremities when turning patient.
- Keep patient's extremities warm to prevent tissue hypoxia.
- If patient has areas of breakdown, see "Managing Wound Care," p. 681.

---

**Note:** See "Pulmonary Embolus" for **Altered protection** related to increased risk of bleeding or hemorrhage secondary to anticoagulant therapy, p. 17.

---

PATIENT-FAMILY TEACHING AND DISCHARGE PLANNING
See patient's primary diagnosis.

# Section Three:    Neoplastic Disorders of the Hematopoietic System

WBCs, also called leukocytes, are the blood cells responsible for both immunity and the body's response to infectious organisms. WBCs are classified according to structure, specialized function, and response to dye in the laboratory. The three main classifications of WBCs are granulocytes, lymphocytes, and monocytes, all of which may undergo malignant transformations. The bone marrow has a reserve of approximately 10 times the number of circulating WBCs, and these are released into the circulation during an infectious process.

## Lymphomas

Lymphomas are disorders that cause neoplastic proliferation of lymphoid cells and tissue (e.g., lymph nodes and spleen). This results in abnormal functioning of the lymph cells responsible for immunity and eventually results in system obstruction. Lymphomas are classified as Hodgkin's lymphoma and non-Hodgkin's lymphoma.

*Hodgkin's lymphoma* is a tumor of the lymph tissue. It is distinguished from other lymphomas by the presence of large, variable cells called Reed-Sternberg cells, which proliferate and invade normal lymph tissue throughout the body. Lymph tissue is found in the spleen, liver, bone marrow, lymph nodes, and lymph channels, which connect virtually all tissues. Clinical presentation depends on the degree of malignant cell growth, extent of the invasion, and the tissues affected. Hodgkin's disease frequently affects young people, and it can be treated successfully, particularly with early diagnosis and intervention. The cause of the disorder is unclear, but a hereditary component has been implicated. Although no infectious organism has been identified, infection has been suggested as a potential cause. Long-term survival (20 years) is now possible.

*Non-Hodgkin's lymphomas* are characterized by disseminated spread, often with extranodal infiltration. They can appear in the GI tract, bone marrow, and testes. They tend to affect individuals around the age of 50 and are more common than Hodgkin's lymphomas. This disorder involves an abnormal, malignant lymphocytic invasion of the lymph nodes; Reed-Sternberg cells are not involved in the malignancy.

## ASSESSMENT

**Chronic indicators:**   Nonspecific symptoms, such as persistent fever, night sweats, malaise, weight loss, and pruritus (termed *B symptoms* [symptomatic] for staging).

**Acute indicators:**   Worsening of the above symptoms, in addition to unexplained pain in the lymph nodes after drinking alcohol. In addition, individuals with non-Hodgkin's lymphoma may experience GI symptoms, including nausea, vomiting, and abdominal pain.

**Physical assessment:**   Enlarged (painless) lymph nodes in the cervical area; possible splenomegaly and hepatomegaly.

## DIAGNOSTIC TESTS

**CBC:**   Decreased Hgb and Hct (confirming anemia); increased, decreased, or normal levels of WBCs. Neutrophilic leukocytosis may occur, and lymphocyte levels will be low.

**Platelet count:**   May be low.

**Lymph node biopsy:**   May reveal presence of characteristic Reed-Sternberg cells.

**Lymphangiogram:**   To determine extent of involvement. Cannulas are inserted into the lymph vessels, and contrast medium is injected. Before the procedure, assessment must be made regarding patient allergy to contrast medium. This procedure is less useful in non-Hodgkin's lymphoma since it does not allow visualization of mesenteric nodes, which often are involved.

**Biopsy of the bone marrow, lung, liver, pleura, or bone:**   May be performed to determine involvement.

**Serum alkaline phosphatase:**   If elevated, will indicate liver or bone involvement.

**Erythrocyte sedimentation rate:**   Will be elevated.

**Staging laparotomy with splenectomy and liver biopsy:**   To determine extent of the disease and plan of care.

**Chest x-ray or abdominal computerized axial tomography (CT) scan:**   To help determine presence of nodal involvement.

**Bone scan:**   To detect bone involvement.

## COLLABORATIVE MANAGEMENT

**Staging:**   To determine extent of the disease. A simplified description of staging follows (based on Ann Arbor Staging Classification):

*Stage I:*   Limited to a single lymph node region or a single extralymphatic organ.

*Stage II:*   Involves two or more lymph node regions on the same side of the diaphragm or localized involvement of an extralymphatic organ.

*Stage III:*   Involves lymph node regions on both sides of the diaphragm, accompanied by involvement of an extralymphatic region and/or the spleen.

*Stage IV:*   Diffuse involvement of one or more extralymphatic regions or tissues.

**Radiation therapy to lymph node regions:**   For stages I and II. Whole body radiation may be used for individuals with lymphoma who are symptomatic.

**Chemotherapy in combination with radiation:**   For stages III and IV. One common combination of chemotherapeutic agents includes mechlorethamine hydrochloride (nitrogen mustard), vincristine, prednisone, and procarbazine. For non-Hodgkin's lymphoma, a variety of antineoplastic drugs currently are being used, including cytoxan, vincristine, prednisone, procarbazine, doxorubicin, and bleomycin. **Note:** Adults with non-Hodgkin's lymphoma often have central nervous system involvement, and therefore intrathecal chemotherapy may be administered. For more information, see Appendix One, "Caring for Patients with Cancer and Other Life-Disrupting Illnesses," p. 719.

**Interferon, monoclonal antibodies, and autologous bone marrow transplant:**   Research currently is being conducted regarding efficacy.

## NURSING DIAGNOSES AND INTERVENTIONS

**Note:** See "Pernicious Anemia" for **Activity intolerance,** p. 486, and **Altered nutrition:** Less than body requirements, p. 487. See "Hypoplastic Anemia" for **High risk for infection,** p. 495. See "Disseminated Intravascular Coagulation" for **Altered protection** related to increased risk of bleeding, p. 507. See Appendix One, "Caring for Preoperative and Postoperative Patients," p. 693, and "Caring for Patients with Cancer and Other Life-Disrupting Illnesses," p. 719.

## PATIENT-FAMILY TEACHING AND DISCHARGE PLANNING

Give patient and significant others verbal and written information about the following:

- For patients in stage I or II, the resumption of normal life-style with minor adjustments, as prescribed.
- Continuing radiation or chemotherapy, if prescribed, which is given on an outpatient basis; confirm date and time of next appointment.
- Signs and symptoms that necessitate medical attention: persistent fever, weight loss, enlarged lymph nodes, malaise, and decreased exercise tolerance.
- Importance of preventing infection and avoiding exposure to individuals with infection, which is essential because of alterations in WBC count and patient's decreased resistance to infection secondary to therapy. Teach patient the indicators of common infections, such as urinary tract infection, upper respiratory infection, and wound infection. See **High risk for infection,** p. 141, in "Care of the Renal Transplant Recipient."
- Importance of maintaining good nutritional habits to increase resistance to infection.
- Referral to American Cancer Society and local support groups.
- Avoiding trauma, which can cause bruising, especially in the presence of thrombocytopenia, which can occur secondary to chemotherapy.
- If appropriate, measures for assisting patient with ADL.

# Acute leukemia

Acute leukemia is an abnormal, malignant proliferation of WBC precursors, also called *blasts*. These abnormal cells accumulate in bone marrow, body tissues, and blood vessels and eventually cause malfunction by encroachment, hemorrhage, or infection. In addition, they function inappropriately in response to infection and prevent normal WBC maturation. Moreover, the accumulation of WBCs in the bone marrow alters and decreases the production of RBCs and platelets. The two most common types of acute leukemia are *myelocytic* (arising from the myeloblast, which matures into a neutrophil) and *lymphocytic* (arising from the lymphoblast, which matures into a lymphocyte). Untreated acute leukemia invariably is fatal, and even with treatment the prognosis varies. Acute lymphocytic leukemia (ALL) most often affects children under 15 years old, while acute myelocytic leukemia usually affects individuals older than 20 years.

## ASSESSMENT

**Chronic indicators:**  Fever, pallor, chills, and weakness, which can be present for days, weeks, or months before acute crisis occurs. Gingivitis, easy bruising, and prolonged menstruation also may occur.

**Acute indicators:**  High fever, diffuse petechiae, ecchymosis, epistaxis, anorexia, nausea, vomiting, headaches, visual disturbances, weakness, feeling of abdominal fullness, lethargy, and seizures.

**Physical assessment:**   Sternal and bone tenderness on palpation, splenomegaly, hepatomegaly, palpable lymph nodes, pallor, papilledema, cranial nerve disorders, and diffuse bleeding of mucous membranes.

## DIAGNOSTIC TESTS

**CBC:**   Hgb will be decreased; WBC count usually is high (often >50,000/µl) and will include many immature cells.
**Bone marrow aspiration:**   Will reveal increased numbers of myeloblasts or lymphoblasts.
**Platelet count:**   Will be decreased.
**Prothrombin time and partial thromboplastin time:**   May be increased owing to clotting deficiencies.
**Uric acid:**   Increased secondary to rapid cell destruction.

## COLLABORATIVE MANAGEMENT

The goal is complete remission or reduction in the number of malignant cells and increased number of normal leukocytes by normal hematopoiesis. Secondary management goals are to return the erythrocyte index and thrombocyte count to normal.
**Chemotherapy/pharmacotherapy:**   Used in combination to produce remission (less than 5% blast cells and no identifiable leukemic cells in the bone marrow). Treatment may be continued for 1½-2 years after remission occurs.
**Note:** For children with ALL, treatment may last up to 3 years.
*For ALL:*   Vincristine sulfate and prednisone and daunorubicin with or without L-asparaginase and methotrexate may be given intrathecally for central nervous system prophylaxis.
*For acute myelocytic leukemia:*   Daunorubicin hydrochloride, cytarabine, and thioguanine.

---

**Note:**   For lymphocytic leukemias, therapeutic lymphocytapheresis or leukocytapheresis may be performed to decrease tumor load before and at the start of chemotherapy. Usually this is performed when the WBC count is >100,000/µl and the individual has signs of decreased circulation.

---

**Transfusion of packed RBCs:**   To restore erythrocytes. Leukocyte-poor packed RBCs are preferable to whole blood because febrile reactions to WBCs or platelet antibodies are prevented. Because of possible antibody formation and increased transfusion reactions over time, transfusions are given conservatively, especially in individuals for whom long-term transfusions of platelets and granulocytes are anticipated. Therefore patients may need to tolerate a certain degree of anemia. (See Table 7-1.)
**Platelet transfusion:**   To restore platelet levels to >20,000/mm³. (See Table 7-1.)
**Bone marrow transplantation:**   Available in specialized centers. See discussion in "Hypoplastic Anemia," p. 495.

## NURSING DIAGNOSES AND INTERVENTIONS

**High risk for infection** related to inadequate secondary defenses secondary to myelosuppression from disease process or therapy
*Desired outcome:*   Patient is free of infection as evidenced by normothermia, negative culture results, absence of adventitious breath sounds, HR ≤100 bpm, and the presence of well-healing wounds.
• Monitor patient's temperature frequently. In the presence of any suspected infections, obtain prescription for a culture. Report temperature >38° C (100.4° F) that lasts for >24 h and occurs concurrently with chills and/or HR >100 bpm.
• Be aware that as the neutrophil count decreases, the risk of infection in-

creases. When the patient becomes neutropenic, perform reverse (protective) isolation using a gown, mask, and gloves; provide a private room.
- Perform meticulous handwashing before caring for patient.
- Avoid all invasive procedures (e.g., catheterization) unless absolutely necessary. When such procedures are performed, use strict asepsis.
- Assist patient with ambulation when possible. Institute turning, coughing, and deep breathing at frequent intervals to help prevent problems of immobility that can result in infection, such as skin breakdown and respiratory dysfunction.
- Provide oral hygiene and perianal care at frequent intervals.
- Monitor I&O, and maintain adequate hydration by encouraging 3 L/day of fluids unless contraindicated.
- Administer antibiotic therapy if prescribed.
- Administer transfusion of granulocytes if prescribed.

**Altered protection** related to increased risk of bleeding secondary to decreased platelet count

*Desired outcomes:*   Patient is free of symptoms of bleeding as evidenced by BP ≥90/60 mm Hg, HR ≤100 bpm (or within patient's baseline range), and excretions and secretions negative for blood.
- Monitor platelet counts. Counts <50,000/µl dramatically increase the risk of bleeding. Monitor Hct and Hgb values for levels that are suggestive of bleeding. Report values outside of the following normal ranges: Hct 40%-54% (male) and 37%-47% (female); Hgb 14-18 g/dl (male) and 12-16 g/dl (female).
- Request that patient alert staff members to oozing of blood from the gums.
- Inspect patient's skin, mouth, nose, urine, feces, sputum, emesis, and IV sites for signs for bleeding. Test all excretions for the presence of occult blood.
- Monitor VS at frequent intervals, and be alert to signs of bleeding such as hypotension and increased HR.
- Limit invasive procedures to those that are absolutely necessary.
- Use small-gauge needle when possible. Maintain gentle pressure on injection site until bleeding stops.
- If bleeding occurs, elevate the affected part, if possible, and apply cold compresses and gentle pressure.
- Pad side rails to prevent trauma.
- Administer stool softeners as prescribed to minimize risk of rectal bleeding.
- Teach patient the signs and symptoms of bleeding and the importance of notifying staff promptly if they occur.
- Teach patient to use soft-bristled toothbrushes or sponge-tipped applicators and electric shavers.

**Activity intolerance** related to imbalance between oxygen supply and demand secondary to decreased oxygen-carrying capacity of the blood due to erythrocyte destruction

*Desired outcome:*   Following treatment, patient rates his or her perceived exertion at ≤3 on a 0-10 scale and exhibits tolerance to activity as evidenced by HR ≤100 bpm, RR ≤20 breaths/min, and absence of headache and dizziness.
- Monitor patient's response to activity, and ask patient to rate his or her perceived exertion. See **High risk for activity intolerance** in Appendix One, p. 711, for a description.
- If prescribed, administer packed RBCs to restore normal erythrocyte level.
- Assist patient with ADL as necessary.
- Provide periods of undisturbed rest.
- Minimize restlessness, which increases oxygen use, by providing frequent comfort measures such as backrubs.
- Administer oxygen if prescribed. Encourage deep-breathing exercises, which may promote oxygenation by enhancing gas exchange.
- As patient's condition improves, encourage activities to tolerance. Set mu-

tually agreed on goals (e.g., "Can you walk the length of the hall 2 or 3 times [or appropriate number, depending on tolerance] this morning?"). Be alert to and document activity intolerance as evidenced by pallor, weakness, headache, and dizziness. Discontinue activity and assist patient with getting back into bed if these symptoms occur.

**Altered renal tissue perfusion** related to interrupted blood flow secondary to destruction of RBCs and their precipitation in the kidney tubules

***Desired outcome:*** By a minimum of 24 h before hospital discharge, patient has adequate renal perfusion as evidenced by balanced I&O, urinary output ≥30 ml/h, and stable weight.

- Monitor for and report signs of renal insufficiency, including positive fluid balance, weight gain, and urinary output <30 ml/h in the presence of adequate intake.
- Maintain adequate hydration of at least 2-3 L/day (unless contraindicated) to enhance urinary flow.
- Encourage ambulation or in-bed exercises to patient's tolerance to promote renal circulation.
- Alert patient's physician to significant findings.

---

**Note:** See Appendix One for nursing diagnoses and interventions in "Caring for Patients with Cancer and Other Life-Disrupting Illnesses," p. 719.

---

## PATIENT-FAMILY TEACHING AND DISCHARGE PLANNING

Give patient and significant others verbal and written information about the following:

- Importance of avoiding infections and bleeding and measures to prevent same, including the following: Avoid exposure to individuals with infection, maintain good hygiene, avoid situations with high risk of trauma or injury, and report any signs of infection to patient's physician (e.g., fever, chills, and malaise).
- Side effects of chemotherapy: constipation, alopecia, nausea and vomiting, anorexia, diarrhea, stomatitis, skin rash, nail changes, hyperpigmentation of the skin, weight gain from steroid use, ecchymosis, and cystitis. For more information, see "Caring for Patients with Cancer and other Life-Disrupting Illnesses," p. 719.
- Importance of good nutrition, eating small and frequent meals, consuming 2-3 L/day of fluids (unless contraindicated by cardiac or renal disorder), and using soft-bristled toothbrush and electric razor.
- Referrals to American Cancer Society, Leukemia Society of America, local support groups, and home care or hospice groups, if appropriate.

# Chronic leukemia

Chronic leukemias are characterized by malignant proliferation of abnormal immature WBCs. These abnormal cells eventually infiltrate body tissues and organs and prevent maturation of normal WBCs, thus preventing usual and necessary WBC function. The proliferation of abnormal WBCs in the bone marrow inhibits the formation of other bone marrow elements, including RBCs and platelets. Chronic leukemic cells are a more mature form than is seen in acute leukemias, and they accumulate much more slowly. The two most common types of chronic leukemia are *chronic myelocytic* (sometimes called *granulocytic*—involves the myelocyte, precursor of the neutrophil) and *chronic lymphocytic* (involves the lymphocyte). Causes of chronic leukemia are unclear, although chromosomal abnormality is suspected in many cases of myelogenous leukemia. Also implicated are hereditary factors and immunologic defects.

## ASSESSMENT

**Chronic indicators:**   Fatigue, anorexia, weight loss, gingivitis, prolonged menstruation, sensation of heaviness in the spleen area, malaise, unexplained low-grade fever, and lymph node enlargement.

**Acute indicators:**   High fever, diffuse petechiae, ecchymosis, epistaxis, anorexia, headaches, visual disturbances, weakness, sensation of abdominal fullness, and lethargy.

## DIAGNOSTIC TESTS

**CBC with differential:**   Elevated WBC; decreased Hgb and neutrophils.
**Platelet count (thrombocytes):**   Low.
**Bone marrow aspiration:**   Usually identifies abnormal distribution or increased number of cells.

## COLLABORATIVE MANAGEMENT

*For chronic lymphocytic leukemia*
**Chemotherapy:**   Chlorambucil or cyclophosphamide and prednisone to produce remission.
**Local irradiation of spleen and lymph nodes:**   Performed when drug therapy has failed. This procedure is associated with decreasing peripheral leukocyte counts.
*For chronic myelocytic leukemia*
**Bone marrow transplantation:**   Uses matched sibling donors and is the treatment of choice. Marrow grafting using unrelated donors is a potentially beneficial treatment.
**Chemotherapy**
*Busulfan and hydroxyurea:*   During the stable chronic phase.
*Daunorubicin, cytarabine, vincristine, prednisone, and thioguanine:*   During the acute phase.
**Splenectomy:**   May be necessary if the spleen is destroying platelets.
**Whole brain irradiation or leukopheresis:**   May be done during an acute crisis for rapid reduction of WBCs.

## NURSING DIAGNOSES AND INTERVENTIONS

See "Acute Leukemia," p. 511.

---

**Note:**   Although patients survive longer and the severity of symptoms is less with chronic leukemias, the same principles and nursing interventions apply. Also see Appendix One, "Caring for Preoperative and Postoperative Patients," p. 693, if splenectomy is performed, and "Caring for Patients with Cancer and Other Life-Disrupting Illnesses," p. 719.

---

## PATIENT-FAMILY TEACHING AND DISCHARGE PLANNING

See this section in "Acute Leukemia," p. 513.

### Selected Bibliography

Baird SB et al: *A cancer source book for nurses,* ed 6, Atlanta, 1991, American Cancer Society.

Beatty PG: The use of unrelated bone marrow transplantation in the treatment of chronic myelogenous leukemia, *Transfus Sci* 12(3):119-122, 1991.

Beaurling-Harbury C, Shade SG: Platelet activation during pain crisis in sickle cell anemia patients, *Am J Hematol* 31(4):237-241, 1989.

Brown RG: Normocytic and macrocytic anemias, *Postgrad Med* 89(8):125-136, 1991.

Brown RG: Determining the cause of anemia, *Postgrad Med* 89(6):161-164, 1991.

Francis RB: Elevated fibrin D-dimer fragment in sickle cell anemia: evidence for activation of coagulation during the steady state as well as in painful crisis, *Haemostasis* 19(2):105-111, 1989.

Horne MM, Swearingen PL: *Pocket guide to fluid, electrolyte, and acid-base balance,* ed 2, St Louis, 1993, Mosby–Year Book.

Howard MR: Unrelated donor marrow transplantation for severe aplastic anemia, *Transfus Sci* 12(3):123-134, 1991.

Interqual: The ISD-A review system with adult ISD criteria, August 1992, Northhampton, NH, and Marlboro, MA, Interqual, Inc.

Jordan KS, Mackey D, Garvey E: Case review: a 39-year old man with acute hemolytic crisis secondary to IV injection of hydrogen peroxide, *JEN* 17(1):8-10, 1991.

Kim MJ, McFarland GK, McLane AM: *Pocket guide to nursing diagnoses,* ed 5, St Louis, 1993, Mosby–Year Book.

Miller K: *Hematologic dysfunctions.* In Swearingen PL, Keen JH, editors: *Manual of critical care: applying nursing diagnoses to adult critical illness,* ed 2, St Louis, 1991, Mosby–Year Book.

National Blood Resource Education Program's Nursing Education Working Group: Choosing blood components and equipment, *Am J Nurs* 91(6):42-56, 1991.

Perez WE: Transfusion and coagulation, Part I: Blood banking and transfusion practices, *Nurs Anesthesia* 1(3):149-161, 1990.

Schardin KE: Case management of the anemic patient, *ANNA* 17(6):468-469, 1990.

Vietz JL, Yawn DH: Transfusion and coagulation, Part II: Pharmacologic adjuncts, cell salvages, alternatives in blood donation, *Nurs Anesthesia* 1(4):206-220, 1990.

Section One   Inflammatory Disorders   517
    Osteoarthritis   518
    Gouty arthritis   522
    Rheumatoid arthritis   525
Section Two   Muscular and Connective Tissue Disorders   529
    Ligamentous injuries   529
    Dislocation/Subluxation   532
    Meniscal injuries   535
    Torn anterior cruciate ligament   536
    Ischemic myositis (compartment syndrome)   538
Section Three   Skeletal Disorders   542
    Osteomyelitis   542
    Fractures   546
    Benign neoplasms   553
    Malignant neoplasms   555
    Osteoporosis   557
    Paget's disease (osteitis deformans)   560
Section Four   Musculoskeletal Surgical Procedures   562
    Bunionectomy   562
    Amputation   564
    Tendon transfer   569
    Bone grafting   570
    Repair of recurrent shoulder dislocation   571
    Total hip arthroplasty   573
    Total knee arthroplasty   577
Selected Bibliography   579

## Section One:   Inflammatory Disorders

Arthritis is inflammation of a joint. There are many forms, including osteoarthritis, gouty arthritis, rheumatoid arthritis, Reiter's syndrome, ankylosing spondylitis, systemic lupus erythematosus, and psoriatic arthritis. Osteoarthritis, gouty arthritis, and rheumatoid arthritis are frequently seen in hospitalized patients and therefore are discussed in this section.

# Osteoarthritis

Osteoarthritis (OA), also known as degenerative joint disease (DJD), is an extremely prevalent disorder. It is a chronic, progressive disease characterized by increasing pain, deformity, and loss of function. About 20 million Americans exhibit signs of OA; 90% of all people show radiographic evidence of OA by age 40. Incidence increases with age, but it can be found in any age group, usually following trauma or as a complication of congenital malformation. OA is characterized by hypertrophy of bone at articular margins and degeneration of cartilage. True joint inflammation seldom is present (except in the distal interphalangeal joints). Hereditary and mechanical factors are suspected to be the primary causes of this process. OA may be classified as idiopathic or secondary.

*Ideopathic osteoarthritis* may be localized or generalized and occurs in the distal interphalangeal (DIP), proximal interphalangeal (PIP), metacarpophalangeal (MCP), and carpometacarpal (CMC) joints of the thumb, hip, knee, first metatarsophalangeal (MTP) joint, the cervical and lumbosacral spine, or other single joints. Generalized OA involves 3 or more joints listed under localized. *Secondary arthritis* can occur in any joint and usually follows some form of intraarticular injury or extraarticular change that affects joint dynamics. Examples include posttraumatic, congenital (e.g., Legg-Calve-Perthes), or developmental (e.g., scoliosis) processes; calcium deposition disease; other bone or joint disorders (e.g., septic arthritis, osteitis deformans); and other diseases (e.g, endocrine, neuropathic arthropathy, frost bite).

## ASSESSMENT

Involvement can range from incidental findings on x-ray to pervasive disease that affects the patient's independence in the performance of ADL.

**Signs and symptoms:** Onset is insidious, beginning with joint stiffness, especially early morning stiffness lasting <15 min. It evolves into joint pain, which worsens with activity and is relieved with rest. Signs of local inflammation usually are absent, except occasionally in the DIP, PIP, and CMC joints. There are no systemic signs or symptoms.

**Physical assessment:** Characteristic findings include limited joint motion, Heberden's nodes (enlargement of the DIP joint), Bouchard's nodes (enlargement of the PIP joint), varus or valgus deformity of the knee, bony enlargement of the joint, and flexion contracture of the knee. Frequently crepitation is found.

## DIAGNOSTIC TESTS

There are no characteristic laboratory studies associated with this disorder. Erythrocyte sedimentation rate and WBC counts may be assessed to rule out other arthropathic conditions (e.g., rheumatoid arthritis or infection).

**X-ray studies:** May reveal narrowing of the joint space, osteophytosis (bony projections) of the joint margins, bone cysts, sharpened articular margins, and dense subchondral bone.

## COLLABORATIVE MANAGEMENT

**Rest:** The principal therapy for preventing progression. The patient is advised to avoid activities that will stress the joint further. Use of ambulatory assistive devices, splints, or orthotics may be prescribed to allow rest or decreased stress on affected joints, and the patient is instructed in methods that prevent postural strain. Regular rest periods of 30-60 min often are advised for patients prone to overworking.

**Weight reduction:** For patients for whom excessive weight contributes to the pathology.

**Local moist heat:** To decrease stiffness and provide some subjective pain relief. Hydrotherapy with warm water is especially useful in aiding ROM exercises. Patients who cannot afford to purchase a device to supply moist heat may be required to use a traditional heating pad. Some patients find greater subjective relief from cold packs than from moist heat.

**ROM and muscle-strengthening exercises:**    May be useful in selected cases to increase joint function and supplement joint strength. Exercises may include passive ROM, active ROM, active-assisted ROM, and isometric and isotonic exercises. The maxim that is followed for the appropriate amount of exercise is that pain that lasts until the next exercise period (or several hours) indicates the exercise was too strenuous.

**Intraarticular steroids:**    Used by some physicians to provide transient relief of symptoms. However, they do not halt the progression of the disease and run the risk of introducing refractory infections.

**Pharmacotherapy:**    Includes the use of analgesics and antiinflammatory agents. Analgesics may be necessary to combat the pain associated with DJD. Aspirin, acetaminophen, and the nonsteroidal antiinflammatory drugs (NSAIDs [Table 8-1]) usually are satisfactory, but occasionally narcotic analgesics may be required for short periods following physical therapy or surgical interventions. Antiinflammatory agents may be used as maintenance therapy to control or reduce symptoms.

**Surgical interventions:**    Various orthopedic surgeries may be used to correct underlying congenital anomalies or defects created by trauma. Arthroplastic surgery allows damaged joint surfaces to be augmented, repaired, or replaced; while periarticular tissues may be repaired to improve joint strength. Joint replacement has been used to replace most joints, but the greatest suc-

---

**T A B L E  8 - 1    Nonsteroidal Antiinflammatory Drugs**

| Generic name | Common brand names | Usual daily dosage (mg) |
|---|---|---|
| acetylsalicylic acid | Aspirin | 650-1,300 q4h |
| choline magnesium trisalicylate | Trilisate | 1,000-1,250 bid |
| choline salicylate | Arthropan | 650 q4-6h |
| diclofenac sodium | Voltaren | 100-150 bid or tid |
| diflunisal | Dolobid | 500-1,000 qd or divided q12h |
| etodolac | Lodine | 600-1,200 bid, tid, or qid |
| fenoprofen calcium | Nalfon | 300-600 qid |
| flurbiprofen | Ansaid | 200-300 bid, tid, or qid |
| ibuprofen | Motrin, Advil, Nuprin | 200-400 qid |
| indomethacin | Indocin | 20-50 tid |
| ketoprofen | Orudis | 25-75 q6-8h |
| magnesium salicylate | Mobidin | 600-1,200 tid or qid |
| meclofenamate sodium | Meclomen | 50 tid or qid |
| mefenamic acid | Ponstel | 250 qid |
| nabumetone | Relafen | 1,000-2,000 qd or divided bid |
| naproxen | Naprosyn | 250-375 qid |
| naproxen sodium | Anaprox | 275 q6-8h |
| oxyphenbutazone | Oxalid | 100-200 tid |
| piroxicam | Feldene | 20 qd |
| salsalate | Disalcid | 500 q4h |
| sulindac | Clinoril | 150-200 bid |
| tolmetin sodium | Tolectin | 200-400 tid |

cess has been found with the hip (see p. 573) and knee (see p. 577) implant arthroplasties. In joints that are chronically infected or not amenable to standard or implant arthroplasties, an arthrodesis (joint fusion) may provide joint stability and permit some function. Arthroscopy may be used to debride osteoarthritic joints of loose bodies, osteophytes, frayed cartilage, and hypertrophied synovium. Valgus osteotomy has been successful in transferring the weight-bearing stresses of the proximal tibia from the medial compartment to the usually less diseased lateral compartment.

**Splints and orthotic devices:**   May be used to supplement joint strength or protect the joint from excessive strain.

**Assistive devices:**   A great variety have been developed to help patients perform ADL independently, even in cases of significant joint function loss. Examples include stocking helpers, built-up eating utensils, pickup sticks, and raised toilet seats.

## NURSING DIAGNOSES AND INTERVENTIONS

**Pain** related to joint changes and corrective therapy

*Desired outcomes:*   Within 1-2 h of intervention, patient's subjective perception of pain decreases, as documented by a pain scale. Objective indicators, such as grimacing, are absent or diminished. Patient demonstrates ability to perform ADL without complaints of discomfort.

- Devise and help patient use a rating system to evaluate pain and analgesic relief on a scale of 0 (no pain) to 10 (worst pain).
- Administer analgesics and antiinflammatory agents as prescribed (or 30 min before strenuous activity), and document their effectiveness, using the pain scale. As appropriate, teach patient about the function of epidural anesthesia or patient-controlled analgesia.
- Teach patient use of nonpharmacologic methods of pain control, including guided imagery; graduated breathing (as in Lamaze); enhanced relaxation; massage; biofeedback; cutaneous stimulation (*via* a counterirritant, such as oil of wintergreen); a transcutaneous electrical nerve stimulation (TENS) device; warm or cool thermotherapy; music therapy; and tactile, auditory, visual, or verbal distractions.
- Use traditional nursing interventions to counteract the pain, including backrubs, repositioning, and encouraging the patient to verbalize feelings.
- Incorporate rest, local warmth or cold, and elevation of the affected joints, when possible, to help control discomfort.
- Advise patient to coordinate the time of peak effectiveness of the antiinflammatory agent with periods of exercise or mandatory use of arthritic joints.
- Instruct patient in the use of moist heat and hydrotherapy, which will help reduce long-term discomfort.
- For additional interventions, see this nursing diagnosis in the appendix, p. 694.

**Knowledge deficit:**   Use of a heating device

*Desired outcome:*   Within 24 h of instruction, patient verbalizes and demonstrates proper use of the heating device.

- Assess patient's baseline knowledge in the use of a heating device.
- As appropriate, provide patient with instructions for the proper use of moist or dry heat. Because older individuals may have decreased neuronal function and skin that is more easily traumatized, instruct them in the use of a thermometer (with adequate-size numbers for reading) or a controlled warming device.
- Caution patients about the potential for increasing their tolerance to heat. This can occur when the heat has been used for long periods of time and may cause the patient to feel the need for a higher degree of heat than that which is safe.

**Impaired physical mobility** related to musculoskeletal impairment and adjustment to a new walking gait with an assistive device
*Desired outcomes:*    By hospital discharge, patient demonstrates adequate upper body strength for use of an assistive device. Patient demonstrates appropriate use of the assistive device on flat and uneven surfaces.
- Before ambulation, ensure the necessary strength of the patient's upper extremities for using the assistive device by incorporating the interventions listed in **High risk for disuse syndrome,** p. 713, in Appendix One. Triceps muscle strength is especially important for ambulation with crutches or a walker. Having patients push down on the bed as they extend their arms to lift their buttocks off the bed will strengthen the triceps muscles.
- Provide a thorough discussion with a demonstration to teach the patient how the assistive device is used.
- When fitting crutches, ensure that the patient is wearing flat-heeled, properly fitting, supportive shoes. With the patient standing and with his or her elbows slightly flexed at 10-30 degrees, be sure that the crutch tops rest 1-1.5 inches (or the width of two fingers) below the axillae. Be aware that complaints of upper extremity paresthesias may indicate improperly fitted crutches. Ensure that the crutches have rubber tips to prevent slipping, and rubber axillary pads to reduce pressure at the axillae.
- Once the assistive device is in position, repeat the instructions, and then supervise the ambulation. Ambulation should begin in small increments on level ground and eventually progress to all surfaces the patient is expected to encounter after hospital discharge.
- Ensure that before discharge, the patient is able to demonstrate independence in ambulation with the assistive device on level surfaces and stairs and with getting in and out of a car.

---

**Note:**    See "Gouty Arthritis" for **Knowledge deficit:** Disease process and medication regimen, p. 523. See "Ligamentous Injuries" for **Knowledge deficit:** Potential for joint weakness, and the techniques for applying external supports and assessing neurovascular status, p. 532. See "Fractures" for **Knowledge deficit:** Potential for infection, p. 552. See Appendix One for nursing diagnoses and interventions in "Caring for Patients on Prolonged Bed Rest," p. 711, and "Caring for Preoperative and Postoperative Patients" (if surgery is performed), p. 693.

---

## PATIENT-FAMILY TEACHING AND DISCHARGE PLANNING

Give patient and significant others verbal and written information about the following:
- Medications, including drug name, dosage, purpose, schedule, precautions, and potential side effects.
- Importance of systemic rest as well as rest of the affected joints.
- Weight reduction, if it is appropriate for the patient.
- Proper use of moist heat.
- Necessity of ROM and muscle-strengthening exercises.
- Use of splints or orthotics, including care and cleansing and where to get replacements.
- Use, care, and replacement of assistive device.
- If surgery was performed, the precautions related to the procedure, wound care (see "Wounds Closed by Primary Intention," p. 681), indicators of wound infection (i.e., persistent redness, swelling, increasing pain, wound drainage, local warmth, and fever), or complications of surgery.
- Importance of follow-up care and the date of the next appointment; a phone number to call should any questions arise.

# Gouty arthritis

Gout is the most prevalent form of crystal-induced synovitis, a disorder that results from an abnormal amount of urates. *Primary gout*, an inherited metabolic disorder, is caused by either excess production or underexcretion of urates. Most patients (90%) are male over the age of 30 years. *Secondary gout* results from other conditions in which uric acid is retained or excessively produced, such as lead poisoning, use of thiazide diuretics, chronic renal disease, myeloproliferative disease, psoriasis, lymphoproliferative disease, hemoglobinopathies, cancer chemotherapy, or multiple myeloma. The pathophysiology involves the formation of tophus (nodular deposition of monosodium urate monohydrate crystals), which causes a pronounced inflammatory response. Tophi may be found in synovial tissues, cartilage, periarticular tissues, tendon, bone, and the kidneys. There appears to be a relationship between rapid fluctuations in the level of serum uric acid and an acute gouty attack. Uric acid renal calculi, nephrosclerosis, and gouty nephritis can accompany this process.

## ASSESSMENT

**Chronic indicators:**   Joint changes similar to those of osteoarthritis (see p. 518). Uncontrolled or untreated gout results in a progressive, chronic disorder that causes severe joint deformity and loss of function. Hypertension, uric acid nephrolithiasis, renal failure, and obesity are associated with this process.

**Acute indicators:**   Sudden onset, acute inflammation, and an excruciatingly painful joint that presents with erythema, joint effusion, restricted motion, warmth, and tenderness. Systemic indicators include tachycardia, anorexia, fever, headache, and malaise. Although usually it is monoarticular, polyarticular attacks have been noted with this disorder.

**Physical assessment:**   Tophi may be noted as subcutaneous nodules on the hands, feet, olecranon bursa, prepatellar bursa, and ears. The most commonly affected joint (90% of cases) is the metatarsophalangeal joint of the great toe, but the tarsal joints, ankles, and knees also are commonly affected.

**History of:**   Recent surgery, trauma, oral intake high in purines, alcoholic excess, infection, use of diuretics, increased stress, or severe medical illness (e.g., cerebrovascular accident or myocardial infarction).

## DIAGNOSTIC TESTS

**Serum tests:**   Normal values for serum uric acid are 2.0-7.5 mg/dl for men and 2.0-6.5 mg/dl for women. Uric acid frequently is elevated above normal during an acute attack unless the patient is taking medications that depress the serum levels of uric acid (large doses of ASA, methyldopa, phenothiazines, x-ray contrast agents, warfarin, sulfinpyrazone, or clofibrate). There also will be leukocytosis and an elevated sedimentation rate, reflecting an inflammatory process.

**Joint fluid aspiration:**   For examination of wet smears to reveal presence of monosodium urate (MSU) crystals.

**Tophus aspiration:**   Provides identification of typical MSU crystals.

**X-ray:**   Will demonstrate no change early in the disease, but with chronic disease there will be radiolucent urate tophi (which look like punched-out areas on the x-ray) adjacent to soft tissue tophi. During acute attacks there is radiographic evidence of periarticular or intra-articular soft tissue swelling.

## COLLABORATIVE MANAGEMENT

### Pharmacotherapy

*NSAIDs:*   May be used for chronic or acute forms of the disease; have become the drug of choice in acute attacks (see Table 8-I). Indomethacin commonly is being used.

*Colchicine:*   This agent is believed to mediate the inflammatory response caused by the urate crystals. Usual dosage is 0.5 mg qh or 1 mg q2h until either the pain is controlled or side effects appear. Side effects include nausea, vomiting, abdominal cramping, and diarrhea. Colchicine is contraindicated in patients with inflammatory bowel disorders, significant hepatic disease, or renal disease.

*Corticosteroids:* May control acute attacks. Because septic arthritis may coexist with gouty arthritis, joint aspirate should be sent for Gram stain before initiation of steroid therapy.

*Analgesics (e.g., acetaminophen with codeine or oxycodone preparations):* To control the pain of gout, which is usually excruciating. Agents containing aspirin should be avoided because they may contribute to hyperuricemia.

**Joint rest:** Mandatory in acute phases and should include complete bed rest with elevation of the inflamed joint. Sometimes topical cooling (ice applications to the joint) is prescribed to aid in reducing inflammation.

**Management between attacks:** May be accomplished with the following:

*Colchicine:* Prophylactic or interim use. Usual dosage is 0.6 mg bid.

*Uricosuric agents (e.g., probenecid or sulfinpyrazone):* Dosage is determined by the patient's serum uric acid levels. Nonrestricted patients should maintain a fluid intake of at least 2-3 L/day or use an alkalinizing agent, such as sodium bicarbonate, which maintains urinary pH above 6.0 to prevent uric acid calculi. Gastrointestinal (GI) side effects occur in 10% of patients; rash and fever may occur in 5%.

*Allopurinol, a xanthine oxidase inhibitor:* Lowers serum uric acid, decreases the concentration of uric acid in the urine, and mobilizes the uric acid crystals in tophi. Dosage varies, depending on serum uric acid levels. Because hepatotoxicity and renal calculi can occur, the drug is used cautiously in patients with renal and hepatic disease. The most common side effect is pruritic rash.

**Diet therapy:** Complete restriction of purines (metabolic precursors to uric acid) seldom is prescribed because purines are found in most protein foods, and rigid dietary restriction would be unhealthy; however, visceral meats generally are high in purines and should be avoided. Alcoholic beverage intake should be limited because of its connection with the precipitation of acute attacks. Fluid intake should be high enough to ensure urinary output of >2 L/day. Obesity should be avoided.

**Avoidance of hyperuricemic agents:** These include diuretics, low-dose aspirin, and nicotinic acid.

**Surgical intervention:** Gouty tophi are excised when they erode through the skin or cause mechanical impairment. Chronic joint involvement may require surgical procedures discussed in "Osteoarthritis," p. 519.

## NURSING DIAGNOSES AND INTERVENTIONS

**Knowledge deficit:** Disease process and medication regimen

*Desired outcome:* Within 24 h of instruction, patient verbalizes knowledge about the disease process, medication regimen, and potential drug side effects.

- Assess patient's knowledge of the disease process, medication regimen, and potential side effects of the drugs. As appropriate, teach the pathophysiology of the disease. In addition, when secondary gout is suspected, inform patient about the primary disease causing the gout.
- Provide thorough instructions for the medication therapy, including rationale, dose, schedule, precautions, and potential side effects.
- When initiating colchicine treatment for an acute attack, assess patient carefully for preexisting bowel, liver, or renal disease. Instruct patient to notify the staff promptly when pain has abated or when nausea, vomiting, abdominal cramping, or diarrhea occurs. Colchicine doses usually are decreased or terminated at the onset of any of these indicators.
- For patients taking uricosuric agents, stress the potential for the development of uric acid renal calculi and the need for at least 2-3 L/day of fluid in nonrestricted patients or the use of an alkaline ash diet or an alkalinizing

agent, such as sodium bicarbonate, to ensure that the urine pH remains >6. Teach these patients how to use a test tape that checks urine pH.

- Caution patients taking allopurinol of the potential for renal and hepatic complications.
- Caution patients taking narcotic analgesics of the potential for altered sensorium, and advise them to avoid using machinery, driving, or performing other activities requiring alertness.

**Knowledge deficit:**   Proper care of inflamed joints

*Desired outcomes:*   Within 12 h of instruction, patient verbalizes knowledge of the importance of resting the joint during periods of inflammation and demonstrates elevation of the joint, assisted ROM, and use of thermotherapy.

- Assess patient's knowledge about care of inflamed joints.
- As appropriate, teach patient the importance of elevating the inflamed joint with pillows above the level of the heart. Explain the rationale to the patient.
- Perform passive ROM of the joints bid (or have patient perform assisted ROM). Avoid weight-bearing on inflamed joints.
- Instruct patient to increase joint ROM as the inflammation subsides, following the process described under the nursing diagnosis **High risk for disuse syndrome,** p. 713, in Appendix One.
- Advise patient to use thermotherapy (usually applications of ice) as prescribed, using care to ensure adequate protection of the involved skin. (See **Knowledge deficit:** Use of a heating device, p. 520.)

**Knowledge deficit:**   Assessments and preventive measures for uric acid renal calculi

*Desired outcome:*   Within 24 h of instruction, patient verbalizes knowledge of the assessments and preventive measures for uric acid renal calculi.

- Assess patient's knowledge about the assessments and preventive measures for uric acid renal calculi.
- As appropriate, teach patient the indicators of renal calculi (e.g., severe renal colic, costovertebral angle tenderness, chronic urinary tract infection, urinary retention, nausea, vomiting, and pain located in the flank, side, lower back, suprapubic area, groin, labia, or scrotum). Instruct patient to alert physician if any of these signs and symptoms occur after hospital discharge.
- Ensure that patient is knowledgable about preventive measures, including a fluid intake of at least 2-3 L/day in nonrestricted patients, alkalinating measures to ensure urinary pH >6, and use of pH test tape to monitor urinary pH.
- For additional information, see "Renal Calculi," p. 123.

**Altered nutrition:**   More of purine or alcohol than the body can process

*Desired outcome:*   By the 24-h period before hospital discharge, patient demonstrates knowledge about the prescribed dietary regimen by planning 3 meals a day for 3 successive days.

- In severe disease forms, it may be necessary to restrict the patient's intake of purine-containing foods. High-purine-content foods include bouillon, broth, consommé, gravy, organ meats, mackerel, yeast, poultry, meats, fish, shellfish, scallops, asparagus, beans, lentils, mushrooms, peas, and spinach. Ensure that the patient receives diet consultation with both verbal and written instruction in the dietary regimen.
- Inform patient that excessive use of alcohol has been known to precipitate gout attacks.

---

**Note:**   See "Osteoarthritis" for **Pain,** p. 520. See Appendix One for nursing diagnoses and interventions in "Caring for Preoperative and Postoperative Patients," p. 693, and "Caring for Patients on Prolonged Bed Rest," p. 711

## PATIENT-FAMILY TEACHING AND DISCHARGE PLANNING

Give patient and significant others verbal and written information about the following:

- Pathophysiology of the patient's form of gout.
- Medications, including drug name, purpose, dosage, schedule, precautions, and potential side effects.
- Indicators of renal calculi (see "Renal Calculi," p. 123).
- Diet therapy if appropriate, and the importance of avoiding excessive alcohol consumption.
- Use of therapeutic local and systemic rest.

# Rheumatoid arthritis

Rheumatoid arthritis (RA) is the most common inflammatory arthritis. It has a prevalence of 1%-2% in the general population, with females outnumbering males 3:1. This systemic disease is characterized by remissions and exacerbations of inflammation of the connective tissue throughout the body. Although many connective tissues have potential for involvement (heart, blood vessels, lungs, spleen, and kidney) and generalized systemic effects may be noted, this discussion centers on the arthritic aspects of this process. RA most commonly affects the synovial joints, but the effects of this disease are highly variable. Recent research into the pathogenesis of RA indicates that the chronic inflammatory reaction in the rheumatoid synovial membrane is the result of active immune response. Susceptibility to RA is determined genetically. The originating stimulus of this response is still unknown but it has been speculated to be food allergies; hereditary deficit; or infections by parvovirus, Epstein-Barr virus, and rubella. The disease onset and progression can be rapid and fulminating or slow and chronic.

The inflammatory process results in chronic synovitis with the formation of pannus, an inflammatory exudate that accumulates over the surface of the synovial membrane, eventually eroding cartilage, bone, ligaments, and tendons. Involvement of connective periarticular tissues results in loss of support structures and leads to characteristic joint changes, which further contribute to the pathology.

## ASSESSMENT

Specific criteria have been developed by the American College of Rheumatology to enable a more accurate diagnosis of this process. These include morning stiffness, arthritis of ≥3 joints, arthritis of the hand joints, symmetrical arthritis, rheumatoid nodules, serum rheumatoid factor, and radiologic changes.

**Acute indicators:** Morning stiffness lasting >60 min, symmetrical joint involvement, joint effusion, periarticular edema, pain, local warmth, and erythema. Joint stiffness usually is worsened by stress placed on the joint, and it can follow periods of inactivity as well. Involvement of the proximal interphalangeal (PIP) and metacarpophalangeal (MCP) joints, wrists, knees, ankles, and toes occurs frequently. Prodromal signs and symptoms may incude malaise, weight loss, vague periarticular pain, low-grade fever, and vasomotor disturbances resulting in paresthesias and Raynaud's phenomenon. Sometimes an acute exacerbation is related to stress, such as infection, surgery, trauma, emotional strain, or the postpartum period.

**Chronic indicators:** Progressive thickening of the periarticular tissues, subluxation, fibrous ankylosis, atrophy of skin and muscle, severe limitation of ROM with progressive loss of function, joint and muscle contractures, juxta-articular and generalized osteoporosis, synovial cysts (ganglion on the dorsum of the wrist or Baker's cyst in the popliteal space), tendon rupture, nerve entrapment (carpal or tarsal tunnel syndrome), dryness of the eyes and mucous membranes, subluxation of the cervical vertebra, swan neck, boutonnière deformity of the fingers, ulnar deviation of the wrist and joints of the hands and fingers, and subcutaneous nodules. Some patients develop splenomegaly and enlarged lymph nodes.

## DIAGNOSTIC TESTS

**Serologic studies:**    Many are performed to detect certain macroglobulins.

***Rheumatoid factor (an immunoglobulin M [IgM] antibody directed against other globulins):***    Positive in 75% of the individuals with RA. Higher titers are associated with more severe clinical disease. Because false positives are common, a definite diagnosis cannot be made on this test alone.

***Antinuclear antibodies:***    May appear in 20% of cases, but titers are lower in RA than in systemic lupus erythematosus.

***Erythrocyte sedimentation rate:***    If elevated, is an indicator of inflammation.

***Gamma globulins, especially IgM and immunoglobulin G (IgG):***    If elevated, strongly suggest an autoimmune process as the cause of RA.

***Normocytic hypochromic anemia:***    Usually present secondary to long-standing inflammation.

**WBC count:**    Usually normal or slightly elevated, but leukopenia can be present, especially in the presence of splenomegaly.

**Joint fluid aspiration from the involved joint:**    May reveal synovial fluid greater in volume than normal, opaque and cloudy yellow in appearance, glucose level lower than serum level, and elevated WBC and polymorphonuclear leukocytes in the presence of RA.

**X-ray studies of the involved joints:**    In the early phases will illustrate soft tissue swelling, erosion of joint surfaces normally covered by articular cartilage, and osteoporosis of adjacent bone. In long-standing disease, the joint will show instability, subluxation, joint space narrowing, bone cyst formation, and concurrent osteoarthritic changes. Special attention is paid to upper cervical vertebrae, where subluxation of C-1 or C-2 can result in life-threatening neurologic complications.

**Radionuclide joint scanning:**    To identify inflamed synovium in patients with appropriate symptoms.

## COLLABORATIVE MANAGEMENT

**Systemic rest:**    Mandatory throughout all phases of this disease. In exacerbations, bed rest may be required until significant clinical joint findings have decreased for 2 weeks. During this period, proper joint positioning is essential to prevent contractures. Concurrent physical therapy is prescribed to put joints through passive ROM at least once a day. During remissions, the patient should receive 8 h of sleep each night and 1-2 h rest at midday. Any increase in symptomatology necessitates increasing the amount of rest.

**Emotional support:**    To lessen stress and help patients deal with fear, feelings of helplessness, disability, and the many losses they will incur. Patients need to be introduced to the concept of chronic disease control through multiple methods that will change in response to the disease progression.

**Rest of inflamed joints:**    Imperative. Unstable joints should be splinted or braced to provide support and put through passive ROM at least daily while inflamed. Reduction of inflammation in affected joints is aided by articular rest. Relaxing hip and knee muscles to prevent contractures is best performed by prone positioning for at least 15 min tid. Sitting is not an effective method of joint rest and should be avoided for prolonged periods.

**Joint exercise:**    Essential to maintain joint function and muscle strength, with the amount increasing as inflammation decreases. A graded exercise program should include the following: passive ROM, active-assisted ROM, active ROM, and resistive ROM with gradually increasing levels of resistance. Isometric exercise is used to maintain muscle strength during active joint inflammation. Any signs of increasing joint inflammation are cause for regression to a less stressful exercise until joint inflammation has again decreased. Inflamed weight-bearing joints should be protected from stress by orthotics and ambulatory adjuncts (cane, crutches, and walker, or a wheelchair if imperative).

**Thermotherapy:**   To relax muscles and reduce pain. Cold therapy is used during inflammatory stages to reduce pain. Moist heat (especially warm tub baths) is useful for exercising stiffened joints because the heat and buoyancy aid motion. When submersion is not possible, use of moist warm cloths before exercise will decrease the patient's discomfort. Caution must be employed to avoid thermal injury to atrophied skin over affected joints. Paraffin baths may be used to provide heat to involved small joints (e.g., in the hands and feet).

**Assistive devices:**   E.g., stocking helpers, raised toilet seats, pickup sticks.

**Antiinflammatory agents:**   See Table 8-1. Aspirin (ASA) is the mainstay of pharmacotherapy in RA. Dosage is determined by the ability to provide adequate symptom relief without toxic reactions. Adult dosages may reach 4-6 g, producing serum levels of 20-30 mg/dl. Tinnitus and GI upset are prodromal signs of toxicity, indicating a need to reduce dosages until these symptoms clear. GI upset may be decreased by taking ASA with food or antacids or using enteric coated forms. **More potent antiinflammatory agents** also used in the treatment of RA include the slow-acting antirheumatic drugs (SAARDs). Early treatment with the SAARDs may prevent irreversible joint damage. However, the SAARDs are associated with significant, possibly life-threatening, side effects. SAARDs include:

*Antimalarials (chloroquine phosphate, 250 mg/day; or hydroxychloroquine sulfate, 200 mg/day):*   Result in long-term control of symptoms for some patients. Side effects include keratitis and retinitis, necessitating periodic ophthalmic examinations for early assessment of complications.

*Chrysotherapy (use of medicinal gold salts):*   Benefits up to 60% of patients with RA through an unknown mechanism of action. Contraindications include severe drug allergies, previous gold toxicity, hepatotoxicity, renal toxicity, or hematologic pathology. It is administered by weekly injections of increasing dosage (up to 50 mg/week) until clinical results are noted or toxic reactions encountered. Usual dosage of auranofin (an oral agent) is 3 mg bid. A significant antiinflammatory effect often takes several months of therapy. Potential toxic reactions include exfoliative dermatitis, thrombocytopenia, bone marrow depression, stomatitis, and nephritis. Before each injection and periodically for oral forms, the patient should have a urinalysis (for proteinuria and microscopic hematuria) and CBC with differential for hemoglobin (Hgb), platelet levels, and WBC count. The patient also should be assessed for skin or mucous membrane lesions. Periodic hepatic function tests should be done, and the patient should be advised to avoid direct sunlight.

*Corticosteroids:*   To control the symptoms of RA, but they do not substantially alter the progression of the disease. Cessation of the steroid frequently results in exacerbation of symptoms, so steroids usually are used only to carry the patient through a severe flareup or to control concurrent connective tissue disease (e.g., eye lesions or pericarditis). They are used cautiously at the lowest dose possible (i.e., 8-10 mg qod) to control signs of inflammation. Deflazacort is a new corticosteroid with bone-sparing properties for RA patients with significant osteoporosis. Intra-articular steroids may be used on occasion (no more than 4 times a year) for especially troublesome joints.

*Penicillamine:*   Used *only after* all other methods have been ineffective in controlling symptoms; 50% of patients taking this drug will develop side effects, including stomatitis, skin rashes, thrombocytopenia, leukopenia, aplastic anemia, nephrotic syndrome, and immune complex disease (myasthenia gravis). This medication is taken between meals to aid absorption.

*Methotrexate:*   This drug is believed to be the agent most useful for RA that is refractory to NSAIDs and gold. Common side effects are gastric irritation and stomatitis. Pneumonitis and hepatotoxicity occur less frequently. Cytopenia and infection also may occur.

**Surgical interventions**

*Synovectomy:*   To remove the inflamed synovium and prevent pannus formation. This may be performed by either surgical excision or instillation of a radioactive solution to "burn" the synovium.

*Arthroplasty:*   To correct periarticular weakness, which in turn will correct subluxation and external stressors on the diseased joint.

*Osteotomy:*   To correct disruptive force vectors placed on the joint surfaces or to correct bony malalignments.

*Carpal tunnel release, tarsal tunnel release, ganglionectomy, tendon repair, and removal of Baker's cyst:*   Examples of surgeries performed to correct concurrent connective tissue defects associated with RA.

*Implant arthroplasty:*   Significantly increases functional capabilities for selected RA patients. Used for many joints, but greatest success has been seen with the hip and knee. The rate of success is dependent on the joint, patient's general condition, stage of disease, and rate of compliance with therapy.

*Arthroscopy:*   May be used for diagnosis or treatment. Bodies may be excised, plica (redundant tissue) incised, and cartilage abraded (or "shaved") through an arthroscope.

*Arthrodesis:*   Although less often used since the advent of implant arthroplasty, joint fusion allows for a stable, painless joint in severely affected joints with pronouncedly weakened periarticular tissues and muscle atrophy.

**Experimental therapies under trial in the United States:**   Include additional NSAIDs, an anthelmintic agent (Levamisole), cyclophosphamide, azathioprine, sulphasalazine, chlorambucil, chondroprotective agent (e.g., Rumalon), a bovine bone marrow and cartilage extract that affects the growth and metabolism of articular cartilage), plasmapheresis, leukapheresis, lymphocytapheresis, and irradiation of the lymph nodes. Experimental surgeries include various new implant designs and joint transplantation.

## NURSING DIAGNOSES AND INTERVENTIONS

**Fatigue** related to state of discomfort, psychoemotional demands, and the effects of prolonged immobility

*Desired outcome:*   Within 24 h of admission, patient verbalizes a reduction in fatigue.

- Assess the time the fatigue occurs, its relationship to required activities, and activities that relieve or aggravate the symptoms.
- Investigate the patient's sleep pattern and intervene as appropriate to ensure adequate rest (see **Sleep pattern disturbance** in Appendix One, p. 756).
- Assess for dietary and physiologic sources of fatigue, and intervene to correct as needed.
- Determine whether patient's pain is adequately controlled, and intervene with pharmacologic and nonpharmacologic treatments as indicated.
- Assess patient for stress or psychoemotional distress; intervene as necessary or seek assistance from an appropriate clinical specialist in psychiatric nursing.
- Discuss the rationale for a graded exercise regimen to increase endurance and strength (see Appendix One for **High risk for activity intolerance,** p. 711, and **High risk for disuse syndrome,** p. 713). Encourage patient to set realistic goals and post these goals to facilitate participation of associated health-care professionals.
- Pace activities and intersperse rest periods of at least 90 min in duration.
- Teach patient use of adjunctive and assistive devices.

---

**Note:**   See "Intervertebral Disk Disease" for **Health-seeking behavior:** Pain control measures, p. 228. See "Osteoarthritis" for **Pain,** p. 520, **Knowledge deficit:** Use of heating device, p. 520, and **Impaired physical mobility** related to musculoskeletal impairment and adjustment to new walking gait, p. 521. See "Gouty Arthritis" for **Knowledge deficit:** Disease process and medication regimen, p. 523, and **Knowledge deficit:** Proper care of inflamed joints, p. 524. See "Ligamentous Injuries" for **Knowledge deficit:** Need for elevation of the involved extremity, use of thermotherapy, and prescribed exercise, p. 530, **Knowledge deficit:** Care and assessment of the casted extremity, p. 531, and **Knowledge deficit:** Potential for joint weakness, and the techniques for applying external supports and assessing neurovascular status, p. 532. See "Fractures" for **Self-care deficit,** p. 550, and **Knowledge deficit:** Potential for disuse osteoporosis, p. 551. See "Amputation" for **Knowledge deficit:** Postsurgical exercise regimen, p. 566. See "Total Hip Arthroplasty" for **Knowledge deficit:** Potential for infection caused by foreign body reaction to the endoprosthesis, p. 575. See "Total Knee Arthroplasty" for **High risk for fluid volume deficit** related to postsurgical hemorrhage or hematoma formation, p. 578. See Appendix One for nursing diagnoses and interventions in "Caring for Preoperative and Postoperative Patients," p. 693, and "Caring for Patients on Prolonged Bed Rest," p. 711. For psychosocial nursing interventions, see Appendix One, "Caring for Patients with Cancer and Other Life-Disrupting Illnesses," p. 753.

## PATIENT-FAMILY TEACHING AND DISCHARGE PLANNING

Give patient and significant others verbal and written information about the following:

- Treatment regimen, including physical therapy, systemic rest, rest of inflamed joints, exercise, and thermotherapy. For more information, see "Ligamentous Injuries" for **Knowledge deficit:** Need for elevation of the involved extremity, use of thermotherapy, and prescribed exercise, p. 530.
- Medications, including drug name, dosage, schedule, precautions, and potential side effects.
- Potential complications of the disease and therapy and the need to recognize and seek medical attention promptly should they occur.
- Potential concurrent pathology, such as pericarditis (see p. 63) and ocular lesions, and the need to report them promptly to health-care professional.
- Use and care of splints and orthotics, including return demonstration.
- Use of adjunctive aids as appropriate, such as pickup sticks, long-handled shoe horn, crutches, walker, and cane, including return demonstration.
- As necessary, referral to visiting or public health nurses for ongoing care after discharge.
- Phone numbers to call should questions or concerns arise about therapy or disease after discharge. In addition, many cities have local arthritis support groups.
- Treatment and facilities available for these patients, which can be obtained by writing to Arthritis Foundation, 1314 Spring Street NW, Atlanta, GA 30309.

# Section Two:   Muscular and Connective Tissue Disorders

## Ligamentous injuries

Ligaments are collections of fascial tissues that connect bone to bone, thereby supplementing joint stength. Ligament tears usually result from direct trauma or transmission of a force to the joint. The degree of trauma incurred will vary with the strength of the involved ligament and the force applied (e.g., strong ligaments will require more force before tearing than will a ligament weakened by previous injury or disease.) Tears can be longitudinal, transverse, tangential, complete, or partial and can involve avulsion fractures of their origin or insertion.

## ASSESSMENT

**Signs and symptoms:**   Localized ecchymosis, edema, tenderness, weakness, pain, joint effusion, limited ROM, or joint instability. A diagnosis is based primarily on consideration of the patient's complaints, the mechanism of the injury, and the physical assessment.

Ankle sprains may be graded for severity, from Grade 1, least severe, to Grade 3, most severe. Grading is based on edema/hemorrhage, point tenderness, decreased function, decreased ligament strength, anterior drawer test (anterior joint instability), and talar tilt test (mediolateral joint instability).

## DIAGNOSTIC TESTS

**X-ray studies:**   Stressing the weakened joint during x-ray exam may reveal an enlarged joint space.

**Arthrogram (instillation of a radiopaque dye or radiolucent gas into the joint):**   To identify torn or weakened ligaments.

**Arthroscopy:**   To rule out concurrent intra-articular pathology or trauma.

## COLLABORATIVE MANAGEMENT

**Treatment for uncomplicated ligamentous injuries:**   RICE is a useful acronym for treatment of ligamentous injuries: **R**est, **I**ce, **C**ompression, and **E**levation. Rest is accomplished *via* not actively using the joint and/or splinting, casting, or bracing. Cryotherapy is well established as a means of controlling inflammation from trauma. Compression *via* elastic wraps prevents swelling and supports joints. Elevation aids resolution of edema. NSAIDs are used for analgesic and antiinflammatory effects.

**Surgical repair:**   For injuries resulting in grossly unstable joints. The surgery involves removal of the nonviable ligament and suture repair or reefing of the stretched ligament, using strong, absorbable suture material. An avulsion injury (tearing away of a bony insertion) without fracture may be reinserted onto its bony insertion site by using bone staples or passing a suture through holes drilled into the bony insertion site. Additional procedures may involve use of prosthetic devices to stent, temporarily replace, or augment ligament repairs.

**ROM and muscle-strengthening exercises:**   Begun after an appropriate period of immobilization of the injured area (a minimum of 3 weeks).

## NURSING DIAGNOSES AND INTERVENTIONS

**Knowledge deficit:**   Need for elevation of the involved extremity, use of thermotherapy, and prescribed exercise

*Desired outcome:*   Within 8 h of instruction, patient verbalizes understanding about the rationale for treatment and returns a demonstration of the exercise regimen and the use of elevation and thermotherapy.

- Teach patient the pathophysiology of the injury and the concomitant inflammatory response.
- Instruct patient to keep the injured extremity elevated until edema no longer is a problem (usually 3-7 days). Explain that the involved extremity should be kept above the level of the heart, with each successively distal joint elevated above the level of the preceding joint.
- Explain that ice usually is applied for the first 48 h to prevent excessive edema. Ice is contraindicated for patients with suspected compartment syndrome or those with peripheral vascular disease, decreased local sensation,

coagulation disorders, or similar pathology that increases the potential for thermal injury. Advise the patient to apply thermotherapy with at least two thicknesses of terry cloth to protect the skin from injury.
- Explain each prescribed exercise in detail, including the rationale. The optimal method is to teach it to the patient, demonstrate it, and then have the patient return the demonstration. Provide written instructions that describe the exercises and list the frequency and number of repetitions for each. Include a phone number in case the patient has questions after hospital discharge.

**Knowledge deficit:**    Care and assessment of the casted extremity

***Desired outcome:***    Within 12 h of instruction, patient verbalizes understanding about the care of the casted extremity and knowledge of self-assessment of neurovascular status and returns a demonstration of the use of ambulatory aids, exercise, and general cast care.

- Explain the function of the patient's cast.
- Instruct patient in the rationale and procedure for neurovascular checks of the casted extremity. Explain that they should be performed q2-4h for the first 2 days, and then 4 times a day until the cast is removed. Advise patient to be alert to and promptly report pallor, cyanosis, coolness, decreased pulse or capillary refill, increasing pain, decreasing sensation, and paralysis of the distal portion of the casted limb.
- Ensure that the patient demonstrates independence in ADL and ambulation before discharge. If ambulatory aids (crutches, walker, cane) are used, be sure the patient demonstrates independent use on all surfaces likely to be encountered and that the patient understands and verbalizes precautions. Be sure patient will have adequate assistance or is independent in self-care before discharge. If necessary, initiate a referral for home care.
- Instruct patient to exercise the parts of the extremity that are not immobilized by the cast (e.g., wiggling the toes or fingers and putting the most proximal joints through complete ROM) unless doing so is contraindicated by the injury or the physician. Isometric exercises for muscles beneath the cast will be prescribed for some patients. When prescribed, provide patient with the rationale and instructions for these exercises, including written instructions that review the information and list the frequency and number of repetitions of each exercise.
- Provide patient with a phone number for the appropriate person to call if problems or questions arise after hospital discharge.
- Instruct patient in the basic components of cast care:

*With plaster of Paris cast:*
- Use plastic bags while showering or in the rain to avoid getting cast wet. Damp cloths can be used to clean soiled cast surfaces, but saturation must be avoided.
- Use white shoe polish *sparingly* to cover stains.
- Petal the cast edges with tape if they are rough or if cast crumbs are falling into the cast. If the edges continue to irritate the skin, they can be padded with moleskin, sheepskin, or foam rubber. Notify the physician if irritation continues.
- Avoid putting anything beneath the cast because skin under the cast is more susceptible to injury.
- Report any pain, burning, changes in sensation, drainage on the cast, or foul odor because they can signal the presence of pressure necrosis.

*With synthetic cast material:*
- Immersion in water may be permitted by physician, depending on the materials used, the type of injury, and whether surgery was performed. If immersion is permitted, it is necessary to dry the cast thoroughly (using a hair dryer on a cool setting) to prevent skin maceration.
- If permitted, dirt or sand can be rinsed from the cast.

- Avoid overexercising the casted extremity; perform exercises within the prescribed range.
- Avoid putting anything under the cast because skin under the cast is more susceptible to injury.
- Report any pain, burning, changes in sensation, drainage on the cast, or foul odor because they can indicate the presence of pressure necrosis.

**Knowledge deficit:**   Potential for joint weakness, and the techniques for applying external supports and assessing neurovascular status

*Desired outcome:*   Within 8 h of the instruction, patient verbalizes understanding about the potential for joint weakness and returns a demonstration of applying external supports and self-checking neurovascular status.

- Advise patient about the potential for joint weakness and the need for limiting or omitting activities that aggravate the condition.
- If the physician has prescribed elastic wraps, elastic supports, or orthotic devices to supplement joint strength until exercise has compensated for the joint laxity, explain and demonstrate their use and application. Show the patient how to apply elastic wraps diagonally from the distal to proximal areas with an overlap of two-thirds to one-half the width of the wrap for each successive layer.
- Teach patient how to self-check neurovascular status 15 min after application and to rewrap the joint if a deficit is found. For detail, see **Knowledge Deficit:** Care and assessment of the casted extremity, above.
- Ensure that the patient receives two wraps, supports, or orthotic devices to allow for cleaning. These devices typically are washed with mild soap and water and allowed to air dry without stretching (or see manufacturer's recommendations).

---

**Note:**   If surgery was performed, see "Total Knee Arthroplasty" for **High risk for fluid volume deficit** related to postsurgical hemorrhage or hematoma formation, p. 578. See Appendix One for nursing diagnoses and interventions in "Caring for Preoperative and Postoperative Patients," p. 693

---

## PATIENT-FAMILY TEACHING AND DISCHARGE PLANNING

Give patient and significant others verbal and written information about the following:

- Prescribed therapies, such as rest, ice, compression, elevation, cast care, exercise, and external supports.
- Potential complications, including subluxation/dislocation (see below), wound infection (i.e., local warmth, persistent redness, swelling, wound drainage, foul odor from within the cast, sensation of burning from within the cast, drainage from the cast, and fever), and neurovascular deficit (see above), all of which necessitate immediate medical attention.
- ADL and ambulation. Ensure that patient demonstrates independence before hospital discharge.
- Medications, including drug name, rationale, dosage, schedule, precautions, and side effects.

# Dislocation/Subluxation

A dislocation occurs when the joint surfaces are completely out of contact. A subluxation is an incomplete dislocation in that some of the joint surfaces remain in contact. Most dislocations and subluxations are the result of trauma and can involve significant periarticular damage, including fractures. Some subluxations are associated with pronounced connective tissue disease, such as ulnar deviation of the phalanges and metacarpals, which is seen with severe rheumatoid arthritis.

## ASSESSMENT

**Signs and symptoms:**   Vary with the joint involved. Although any joint can dislocate, some joints are more prone than others. One finding common to most forms of dislocation is limb shortening. Usually there is significant pain, ecchymosis, loss of normal bony contour, edema, and loss or limitation of joint ROM. Complications include recurrent dislocation, joint contracture, neurovascular injury, and eventual traumatic arthritis.

## DIAGNOSTIC TESTS

**X-rays:**   Both anterior/posterior and lateral views commonly are used. Occasionally an oblique view or other special approach is required. Because muscle spasms frequently force the dislocated bones back into normal alignment, it is sometimes necessary to stress the joint to permit visualization of the injury (called a *stress film*). Computerized axial tomography (CT) scans or magnetic resonance imaging (MRI) may be necessary to aid in diagnosis.

**Bone scans:**   May demonstrate nondisplaced avulsion fractures, areas of recent excessive stress, or bony insertions of joint ligaments following dislocation.

**Arthrogram:**   Use of radiopaque dye or radiolucent gas for outlining the joint cavity to visualize injured ligaments, capsule, or intra-articular structures, such as the menisci.

**Arthroscopy:**   May be used to rule out injury to joint surfaces or intra-articular structures.

## COLLABORATIVE MANAGMENT

Interventions vary with the degree of subluxation or dislocation and the joint involved. Many patients are discharged from the hospital with instructions for the use of thermotherapy, elevation, and pain medication.

**Dislocation of the sternoclavicular joint:**   Usually reduced manually with local anesthesia. After reduction, the joint is immobilized with a clavicular strap (figure-of-8 bandage) for 2-6 weeks. Occasionally, an open reduction with internal fixation (ORIF) using screws, pins, or wire is necessary to maintain reduction.

**Uncomplicated subluxation or dislocation of the acromioclavicular (AC) joint:**   May be classified as Type I (least severe) to Type III (most severe). The AC joint may be immobilized with a clavicular strap, brace, or harness or might require ORIF. After satisfactory joint stability has been achieved, the patient is started on a regimen of progressively more rigorous exercise to regain muscle strength and ROM.

**Dislocation of the shoulder:**   Careful assessment should be made for complications of nerve injury, fractures, and rotator cuff tears. This dislocation is reduced under anesthesia or strong sedation and then immoblized in a Velpeau bandage, sling and swathe binder, or spica cast of the shoulder; all of which support the arm while immobilizing the shoulder. Immobilization usually is continued for 3-6 weeks, followed by progressive exercises to regain muscle strength and ROM. Surgical procedures usually include reefing (taking up redundant ligament with sutures) of the articular capsule and transferring or shortening the subcapsular muscle to tighten the periarticular tissues. Also see "Repair of Recurrent Shoulder Dislocation," p. 571.

**Dislocation of the elbow:**   Frequently associated with fractures of the humerus, ulna, or radius. The elbow and fractures are carefully reduced, usually under general anesthesia, and the area is immobilized in a posterior splint at approximately 90-degree flexion for 2-4 weeks. ORIF may be required. Because of the area of the injury, these patients are at risk for nerve injury and Volkmann's ischemic contracture (ischemic myositis), and therefore the extremity must be monitored carefully for evidence of neurovascular deficit. (See "Ischemic Myositis," p. 538.) Progressive exercises are used to regain muscle strength and ROM.

**Dislocation of the radioulnar or radiocarpal joints:**    Frequently involves fractures. This dislocation is usually reduced using regional anesthesia and then immobilized in a posterior splint or long arm cast for 2-6 weeks. However, an ORIF may be performed. Progressive exercise is used to regain muscle strength and ROM.

**Dislocation of the finger:**    Usually reduced using regional or digital block anesthesia. The finger may be immobilized with a metal splint or taped to an adjacent finger, followed by progressive mobilization. Surgery might be performed to reef the stretched periarticular tissues, followed by transfixion of the joint during the healing period, usually 10-14 days.

**Dislocation of the metacarpophalangeal joint of the thumb:**    Surgery usually is indicated owing to the importance of this joint for hand grip strength and function. Surgical repair includes suturing torn ligaments, repair of avulsion injuries, and transfixion of the joint with a K-wire to maintain joint stability in slight (15-degree) flexion. A thumb spica cast immobilizes the joint for 4 weeks, followed by an orthoplast splint, which is used intermittently for an additional 4 weeks, during which ROM exercises are instituted gradually.

**Dislocation of the hip:**    Usually requires general anesthesia with significant muscle relaxation for reduction. Typically immobilization is accomplished *via* balanced suspension traction for 3-6 weeks, followed by progressive ambulation, mobilization of the joint, and muscle-strengthening exercises. Open reduction with surgical repair of the torn capsule and ligaments might be required for severe or recurrent dislocations. A fractured acetabulum may require internal fixation or replacement *via* total hip arthroplasty.

**Dislocation of the patella:**    Often self-limiting, in that the patella usually reduces itself. Immobilization may be accomplished with a knee immobilizer, posterior splint, cylinder cast, or long leg cast for 10-21 days, followed by progressive mobilization and quadriceps setting exercises. Surgery may be required to reef the periarticular tissues or reinsert the insertion of the patellar tendon to overcorrect distorted joint vectors that cause recurrent dislocation.

**Dislocation of the ankle:**    Commonly associated with malleolar fractures. This dislocation is usually reduced under regional or general anesthesia. The joint is immobilized in a long leg plaster cast for 6-12 weeks. Surgery may be necessary to reef stretched periarticular tissues. Progressive mobilization and exercises are used to regain motion and strength.

**Dislocation of the toe:**    Usually reduced using regional anesthesia. Often the toe is immobilized for 3-5 days, using an adjacent toe as a splint (taping the toes together).

## NURSING DIAGNOSES AND INTERVENTIONS

See "Osteoarthritis" for **Pain,** p. 520, and **Impaired physical mobility** related to musculoskeletal impairment and adjustment to a new walking gait, p. 521. See "Ligamentous Injury" for **Knowledge deficit:** Need for elevation of the involved extremity, use of thermotherapy, and prescribed exercise, p. 530, and **Knowledge deficit:** Care and assessment of the casted extremity, p. 531. See "Fractures" for **Self-care deficit,** p. 550. See "Bunionectomy" for **High risk for peripheral neurovascular dysfunction** related to interrupted arterial flow secondary to compression from circumferential casts or dressings, p. 563. If surgery was performed, see "Total Knee Arthroplasty" for **High risk for fluid volume deficit** related to postsurgical hemorrhage or hematoma formation, p. 578. See Appendix One for nursing diagnoses and interventions in "Caring for Preoperative and Postoperative Patients," p. 693, and "Caring for Patients on Prolonged Bed Rest," p. 711

## PATIENT-FAMILY TEACHING AND DISCHARGE PLANNING

Give patient and significant others verbal and written information about the following:

- Therapy that will be used at home, including thermotherapy, elevation, and exercises (see "Ligamentous Injuries," p. 530), use of immobilization devices, cast care (see p. 531), and medications.
- Potential complications that should be observed for at home, such as recurrent dislocations, neurovascular deficit (see "Ligamentous Injuries," p. 531), or wound infection (i.e., persistent redness, swelling, fever, local warmth, increasing pain, wound discharge, foul odor from within the cast, burning sensation from within the cast, and drainage from the cast).
- Precautions that should be taken at home, including activity limitations (as directed by physician), monitoring for changes in neurovascular status qid, and following the guidelines described for cast, splint, or orthotic care.
- Medications, including drug name, rationale, dosage, schedule, precautions, and potential side effects.

# Meniscal injuries

Meniscal injuries involve the intra-articular fibrocartilages on the medial or lateral side of the knee's tibial plateau. These half-moon–shaped cartilages facilitate joint motion, while also absorbing some of the stress placed on the joint. There are a variety of cartilage injuries that can occur, and all involve a tear to varying degrees. Most commonly, a meniscal injury is the result of trauma to the knee or, less frequently, degeneration of the joint secondary to arthritis. Medial meniscus injuries are the most common and usually follow a knee movement involving internal rotation. Injuries to the lateral meniscus are more commonly associated with external rotation that occurs while the knee is partially flexed.

## ASSESSMENT

**Chronic indicators:**   Same as those seen with arthritis because arthritis will follow untreated or severe meniscal injuries. There may be weakness and atrophy of the quadriceps muscle group from disuse caused by joint pain.

**Acute indicators:**   Occur after knee trauma that causes joint effusion (distention with fluid) and limited ROM. If the tear is large enough, it may result in locking, which is the inability to fully extend the joint. Joint pain or pain along the joint margins will occur. It may be possible to delineate point tenderness along the joint margin in the area of the tear.

## DIAGNOSTIC TESTS

**McMurray's test for a torn medial meniscus:**   With the patient's leg fully flexed, the foot externally rotated, and the leg abducted, the examiner's index finger and thumb are positioned along the joint margins of the knee. The knee is then gradually extended. Clicks or pops accompanied by patient complaints of pain as the leg is extended are indicative of a medial meniscal tear. A lateral meniscal tear is tested for by placing the thumb and index finger along the joint margin of the knee with the patient's leg flexed and adducted and the foot internally rotated. Clicks or pops, with patient complaints of pain as the leg is extended, are indicative of lateral meniscus injury.

**Apley grinding test:**   Performed with the patient prone and the knee flexed at 90 degrees. With one hand, the examiner forces the foot and lower leg down on the femur while rotating the foot internally and externally. The examiner's other hand is positioned to palpate the joint margins as described in McMurray's test. Grinding or crepitus is usually indicative of a meniscal injury.

**Arthrogram:**   Involves injection of radiopaque dye and radiolucent gas (usually air) into the joint to outline the area of injury and provide diagnosis of a meniscal tear as evidenced by absence of normal contour.

**Arthroscopy:**   To diagnose and treat meniscal injuries. Under sterile conditions, the arthroscope is introduced into the joint to allow direct visualization of the meniscus. The patient is given local, regional, or general anesthesia for this procedure.

## SURGICAL INTERVENTIONS

**Arthroscopic surgery:**   Preferred over the outdated knee arthrotomy for partial meniscectomy or suture repair because it is the least traumatic and allows more normal joint function and a more rapid return to normal level of health. The patient usually is discharged the same evening of surgery and placed on weight-bearing as tolerated for 5-21 days using some form of external support for the knee, either an elastic wrap or knee immobilizer. Weight-bearing may be permitted with the knee in full extension by some physicians. Patients with sutured meniscal tears may be maintained on nonweight-bearing for 4-6 weeks, after which they begin a slow progression of partial weight-bearing to full weight-bearing. Knee exercises (quadriceps setting and leg lifts) are prescribed for regaining muscle strength, usually with a brace for 1-3 months.

## NURSING DIAGNOSES AND INTERVENTIONS

See "Osteoarthritis" for **Pain,** p. 520, and **Impaired physical mobility** related to musculoskeletal impairment and adjustment to new walking gait, p. 521. See "Ligamentous Injury" for **Knowledge deficit:** Need for elevation of the involved extremity, use of thermotherapy, and prescribed exercise, p. 530. See "Bunionectomy" for **High risk for peripheral neurovascular dysfunction** related to interrupted arterial flow secondary to compression from circumferential casts or dressing, p. 563. See "Total Knee Arthroplasty" for **High risk for fluid volume deficit** related to postsurgical hemorrhage or hematoma formation, p. 578. See Appendix One, "Caring for Preoperative and Postoperative Patients," p. 693.

## PATIENT-FAMILY TEACHING AND DISCHARGE PLANNING

Give patient and significant others verbal and written information about the following:

- Use of elevation, thermotherapy, and exercise (see "Ligamentous Injuries," p. 530) as prescribed.
- Use of external support devices (elastic wraps, knee immobilizer, or brace), including care of the device, care of the skin beneath the device, and monitoring for areas of irritation and neurovascular deficit (see "Ligamentous Injuries," p. 531).
- Cast care (see p. 531).
- Prescribed medications, including drug name, rationale, dosage, schedule, precautions, and potential side effects.
- Indicators of wound infection, which necessitate medical attention: erythema, edema, joint effusion, purulent discharge, local warmth, pain, and fever.
- Ambulation and use of assistive device. Ensure that patient is independent with ambulation, using the assistive device on level surfaces and stairs before hospital discharge (see "Osteoarthritis," p. 521).

# Torn anterior cruciate ligament

The anterior cruciate ligament (ACL) prevents excessive forward motion and internal rotation of the tibia. Injury to this ligament can result in strain, with microtears, partial tears, complete tears, or avulsion of the tibial or femoral attachments. Stresses that can result in tears include forceful contraction of the quadriceps muscles combined with restricted extension, "clipping" injuries incurred in football, forced pivoting on the knee, or excessive forward motion of the tibia, which can occur when stopping quickly while running.

## ASSESSMENT

**Acute indicators:** Sensation of the knee giving way, joint effusion, restricted ROM, joint instability and pain.

**Chronic indicators:** Untreated tears of the ACL result in gross instability, which eventually can cause osteoarthritis (see assessment for osteoarthritis, p. 518).

## DIAGNOSTIC TESTS

**Lachman test:** Positive if the ACL is torn. The patient's knee is partially flexed at 10-15 degrees, and the foot is planted flat on the examining table. The examiner then pulls the tibia forward while holding the femur stable. Excessive forward movement of the tibia is evidenced by a convex curve of the patellar tendon, and this is indicative of an ACL tear.

**Drawer test:** Performed with the knee flexed at 60 degrees and the foot planted flat on the table. The tibia is pulled forward as the femur is stabilized. Excessive forward movement compared to the other knee indicates a tear. The test is then repeated with the foot externally rotated 15 degrees to assess concurrent injury of medial joint structures (meniscus or periarticular ligaments). Finally, the test is repeated with the foot internally rotated 30 degrees to assess concurrent lateral joint injury.

**Arthrography:** Outlines tears *via* injection of radiopaque dye and radiolucent gas.

**Radiography of the knee (including anterior/posterior, lateral, tunnel, and skyline views, with and without stress on the joint):** Evaluates for the presence of abnormal joint contours.

**Arthroscopy:** Allows direct visualization of the ACL injury to determine degree of injury and assess need for surgery.

## COLLABORATIVE MANAGEMENT

The type of therapy is determined by the type of injury, length of time since the original injury, concurrent joint pathology, and the patient's age and functional goals.

**Bracing:** To provide primary support for an incompletely torn ACL or to supplement adjunctive joint support structures (posterior oblique ligament, collateral ligaments, lateral capsular ligament, and the menisci). Functional braces provide support and immobilization following reconstruction and allow control of ROM in rehabilitation. Any of several commercial braces can be used to provide anteroposterior, lateral, and rotational stability of the joint. Concurrent physiotherapy is provided to strengthen periarticular structures and muscles.

**Primary ACL repair:** Involves direct suturing of the torn ligament *via* an arthrotomy or arthroscopy. The suture is heavy and nonabsorbable and is used in repairing tears that are less than 6 weeks old.

**ACL reconstruction:** Involves use of either anatomic grafts (autograft or allograft) or prosthetics. Regardless of the surgical procedure used, an arthrotomy requires prolonged knee immobilization (6-12 weeks in flexion in a long leg cast and/or a splint), followed by extensive physiotherapy and bracing. Physical therapy (PT) is continued until the knee is functionally normal. In addition, many patients return from surgery with a closed wound drainage system consisting of a wound drain, tubing, and a reservoir. Most surgeons bring the drainage tubing out through the area using a separate stab wound. Arthroscopic ACL repair or reconstruction allows for less joint trauma, earlier hospital discharge (1-3 days), more rapid initiation of PT (1-3 days), and excellent long-term results.

## NURSING DIAGNOSES AND INTERVENTIONS

See "Intervertebral Disk Disease" for **Health-seeking behavior:** Pain control measures, p. 228. See "Osteoarthritis" for **Pain,** p. 520, and **Impaired phys-**

**ical mobility** related to musculoskeletal impairment and adjustment to new walking gait, p. 521. See "Ligamentous Injury" for **Knowledge deficit:** Need for elevation of the involved extremity, use of thermotherapy, and prescribed exercise, p. 530, and **Knowledge deficit:** Potential for joint weakness, and the techniques for applying external supports and assessing neurovascular status, p. 532. See "Fractures" for **Self-care deficit,** p. 550. See "Bunionectomy" for **High risk for peripheral neurovascular dysfunction** related to interrupted arterial flow secondary to compression from circumferential casts or dressings, p. 563. See Appendix One for nursing diagnoses and interventions in "Caring for Preoperative and Postoperative Patients," p. 693

## PATIENT-FAMILY TEACHING AND DISCHARGE PLANNING

Give patient and significant others verbal and written information about the following:

- Telephone number of appropriate person for patient's questions after hospital discharge.
- Use of external support devices (elastic wraps, knee immobilizer, or orthosis), including care of the device, care of the skin beneath the device, and monitoring for areas of irritation and neurovascular deficit (see "Ligamentous injuries," p. 531).
- Prescribed exercise regimen, including rationale, how it is performed, number of repetitions, and frequency.
- Prescribed medications, including drug name, rationale, dosage, schedule, precautions, and potential side effects.
- Indicators of wound infection, which necessitate medical attention: erythema, edema, joint effusion, purulent discharge, local warmth, pain, and fever.
- Ambulation with assistive device, including patient's demonstration of independence on level and uneven ground and stairs (see "Osteoarthritis," p. 521).

# Ischemic myositis (compartment syndrome)

Ischemic myositis is a progressive degeneration of muscle that occurs because of a severe interruption in blood flow to an area. Volkmann's ischemic contracture of the forearm and anterior tibial compartment syndrome are associated with this process. Edema within an anatomic compartment eventually can occlude arterial blood supply and cause ischemic myositis. Similarly, impaired venous return from a compartment can lead to edema, which can impinge on arterial blood supply. Arterial injury, from fracture fragments or the mechanism of injury, with resultant reflex vasospasm, also has been implicated as a potential cause of this process. Elevation and application of ice may aggravate the process by contributing to decreased blood supply.

An iatrogenic compartment syndrome can result from any circumferential cast or dressing that adversely affects the circulation of tissues. This syndrome is most commonly seen in trauma or surgery involving the elbow, wrist, knee, or ankle. Additional causes include bleeding disorders (hemophilia), major vascular surgery, thermal injuries (especially circumferential burns or frostbite), snakebites, and infiltration of IV infusions into deep veins. Systemic hypotension increases the risk of compartment syndrome. Because muscle tissue requires large amounts of blood to meet the muscle's demands, necrosis will occur rapidly if the blood supply is inadequate. If not corrected quickly, ischemic myositis can result in a severely contracted, functionally useless, and disfiguring limb distal to the area of injury. Complications of ischemic myositis include infection, renal failure from excessive release of myoglobin, hyperkalemia owing to potassium ($K^+$) loss from injured muscle cells, and metabolic acidosis due to loss of built-up lactic acid in injured muscle.

## ASSESSMENT

**Signs and symptoms:**   The mnemonic six *p*'s: **p**ain, **p**aresthesias, **p**allor, **p**olar, **p**aralysis, and **p**ulselessness (the latter two may be late findings). Pain is especially diagnostic because it increases in severity, exceeds that expected for the incurred trauma, and might not be controlled by narcotics. Passive movement of the involved distal extremity, especially movement that stretches the muscles of the involved compartment, will result in severe pain. Paresthesias may include sensations of numbness, decreased sensation, or burning. Sensory deficit may be an early finding. Pallor and polar (coolness) are associated with decreased circulation through the compartment; while slowed capillary refill and impaired venous return can be prodromal signs. Progressive edema may be noted as tenseness or swelling along the length of the compartment. Weakness of involved muscle groups generally precedes frank paralysis. Paralysis may be pseudoparalysis because of the patient's avoidance of movements that stress the involved compartment, or frank paralysis of muscle that is enervated by injured nerves in the involved compartment. Pulselessness usually is a late finding.

## DIAGNOSTIC TESTS

**Compartment pressure:**   Can be measured *via* a variety of devices (e.g., slit, wick, or large-bore catheter) that are introduced into the compartment and attached to a saline-primed manometer or transducer. Normal tissue pressures are <15 mm Hg; sustained pressures >30 mm Hg are considered significantly elevated above normal. Continuous monitoring of high-risk patients may be necessary to warn of impending ischemic myositis. Patients with low blood pressure are at increased risk and may develop compartment syndrome with lower tissue pressures. In such patients, the delta pressure should be determined. Delta pressure equals the mean arterial pressure minus the compartment tissue pressure. Delta pressure ≤30 for 6 h or ≤40 for 8 h should be reported promptly to the physician.

**Arteriogram and venogram:**   To rule out vasospasm, thrombus, embolus, or arterial trauma, which can result in ischemic myositis, especially in patients with supracondylar fractures of the humerus.

**MRI:**   May show muscle ischemia.

## COLLABORATIVE MANAGEMENT

**Conservative measures:**   Used initially when ischemic myositis is suspected. The constriction limiting the swelling (e.g., cast, splint, or circumferential dressing) is loosened down to skin level. However, if a fracture is involved, adequate immobilization should not be compromised. After a fracture the limb is elevated to enhance venous return, and ice is applied to cause vasoconstriction in the area of the injury and inhibit further edema formation. However, if compartment syndrome is suspected, ice and elevation are contraindicated because they may contribute to decreased vascular supply. Often, larger-than-normal levels of narcotics with potentiation such as aspirin, acetaminophen, promethazine (Phenergan), or hydroxyzine (Vistaril) are required for pain control.

**Fasciotomy:**   Necessary if conservative measures fail to control the progressive symptoms. Fasciotomy is the surgical incision of the fascia for the entire length of the involved compartment to remove any restriction to swelling. After several days the fasciotomy is closed primarily or the area is grafted with skin.

**Surgical repair of a lacerated artery:**   Performed if the cause is arterial injury. If vasospasm is the suspected cause, some surgeons will expose the involved artery and apply topical papaverine to control the problem; if unsuccessful, resection of the involved artery with reanastomosis frequently is necessary.

## NURSING DIAGNOSES AND INTERVENTIONS
*For patients at risk for ischemic myositis*
**High risk for peripheral neurovascular dysfunction** related to interruption of capillary blood flow secondary to increased pressure within the anatomic compartment

*Desired outcomes:* Patient has adequate peripheral neurovascular function in the involved limb as evidenced by brisk (<2 sec) capillary refill; peripheral pulse amplitude >2+ on a 0-4+ scale; normal tissue pressures (<15 mm Hg); and absence of edema, tautness, and the mnemonic six *p*'s over the compartment. Patient verbalizes understanding about the importance of reporting symptoms indicative of impaired neurovascular status.

- Monitor neurovascular status of injured extremity with each VS check (at least q2h). Monitor for sluggish capillary refill, increasing limb edema, and tautness over individual compartments. Also assess for the mnemonic six *p*'s: **p**ain (especially on passive digital movement and with pressure over the compartment), **p**aresthesias, **p**aralysis, **p**olar, **p**allor, and **p**ulselessness.
- Report deficits in neurovascular status promptly. Apply ice when appropriate (see p. 539), and loosen all circumferential dressings as indicated. **Caution:** When compartment syndrome is suspected, ice and elevation are contraindicated because they may compromise vascular supply further.
- Teach patient the symptoms that necessitate prompt reporting: increasing pain, paresthesias (diminished sensation, hyperesthesia, or anesthesia), paralysis, and coolness.
- Monitor tissue pressures on a continuous basis if an intracompartmental pressure device is present. Alert physician to pressures higher than normal. Be aware that pressures >30 mm Hg may be significantly elevated above normal.
- Ensure that fluid resuscitation is accomplished as necessary to ensure adequate circulation to the involved compartments.
- In patients with lowered systemic BP, monitor delta pressure (mean arterial pressure minus compartment tissue pressure). Report delta pressure ≤30 mm Hg for 6 hrs or ≤40 mm Hg for 8 h.

*For patients who are experiencing ischemic myositis*
**Pain** related to tissue ischemia secondary to compartment syndrome

*Desired outcomes:* Within 8 h of treatment, patient's subjective perception of discomfort decreases as documented by a pain scale. Nonverbal indicators of discomfort, such as grimacing, are absent or diminished. Patient verbalizes understanding of the need to report uncontrolled or increasing pain.

- Assess the patient's complaints of pain for onset, duration, progression, and intensity. Devise a pain scale with patient, rating discomfort from 0 (no pain) to 10 (worst pain).
- Determine if passive stretching of digits and pressure over limb compartments increase the pain because both are likely to occur with compartment syndrome.
- Adjust the medication regimen to the patient's needs; document medication effectiveness.
- Prevent pressure on involved compartment and neurovascular structures. When not contraindicated by evidence of impaired circulation, apply ice if it has been prescribed.
- If patient has had a fasciotomy, be aware that if the pain does not subside after this procedure, it could signal an incomplete fasciotomy. Pain that increases several days after a fasciotomy may signal compartmental infection
- Continue to monitor neurovascular function with each VS check to assess for recurring compartment syndrome or infection.

**High risk for infection** related to inadequate primary defenses secondary to necrotic tissue, wide compartmental fasciotomy, and open wound

*Desired outcome:* Patient is free of infection as evidenced by normothermia, WBC count ≤11,000 µl, erythrocyte sedimentation rate (ESR) ≤20 mm/h (fe-

male) or ≤15 mm/h (male), and absence of wound erythema and other clinical indicators of infection.
- Monitor patient for fever, increasing pain, and laboratory data indicative of infection (e.g., increased WBC count, increased ESR).
- Assess exposed wounds and dressings for erythema, increasing wound drainage, purulent wound drainage, increasing wound circumference, edema, and localized tenderness.
- Monitor distal neurovascular status (see **High risk for peripheral neurovascular dysfunction** in "Bunionectomy," p. 563) for deficit, which may be indicative of infection or pressure on these structures caused by nearby deep infection.
- After primary closure or grafting of wound, continue to assess wound for signs of infection (see above).
- Be aware of and assess for chronic infection and osteomyelitis as potential complications after compartment syndrome. Teach patient about the increased potential for infection with this type of wound and that chronic infection and osteomyelitis are late complications after compartment syndrome has occurred.
- Use aseptic technique when changing dressings and providing wound care. As indicated, teach aseptic technique to patient before hospital discharge.
- Notify physician promptly of significant findings.

**Body image disturbance** related to physical changes secondary to large, irregular fasciotomy wound and skin grafted scar; loss of function and cosmesis of an extremity; or amputation

***Desired outcomes:*** By the 24-h period before hospital discharge, patient acknowledges body changes and demonstrates movement toward incorporating changes into self-concept. Patient does not exhibit maladaptive response (e.g., severe depression) to wound or functional loss.
- Encourage questions about compartment syndrome, therapeutic interventions, and long-term effects.
- Provide time for verbalization of feelings about change in appearance and function. Encourage discussion of these feelings with patient's significant other.
- Identify and emphasize patient's strengths to facilitate adaptation to cosmetic and functional loss. Help patient set realistic goals for recovery.
- Facilitate patient's progression through the grieving process, as appropriate.
- Recognize individuality in adjustment; enable patient to determine when to view or discuss the injury.
- If the extremity will be amputated, collaborate with physician about a visit by an amputee who has successfully adapted and who can serve as patient's role model.
- Encourage maximum self-care. Provide necessary adjunctive aids (e.g., built-up utensils, button hooks, orthotics) to facilitate independence.
- For additional interventions, see this nursing diagnoses in Appendix One, p. 760.

---

**Note:** See "Osteoarthritis" for **Pain,** p. 520. See "Ligamentous Injuries" for **Knowledge deficit:** Need for elevation of the involved extremity, use of thermotherapy, and prescribed exercise, p. 530. See "Bunionectomy" for **High risk for peripheral neurovascular dysfunction** related to interrupted arterial flow secondary to compression from circumferential casts or dressings, p. 563. If surgery was performed, see Appendix One for nursing diagnoses and interventions in "Caring for Preoperative and Postoperative Patients," p. 693.

---

## PATIENT-FAMILY TEACHING AND DISCHARGE PLANNING
Give patient and significant others verbal and written information about the following:

- Phone number of appropriate person to call for questions after hospital discharge.
- Instructions regarding the process of ischemic myositis, use of elevation and ice, and loosening of restrictive dressings.
- Discharge instructions for patients with fractures (see "Fractures," p. 553).
- Importance of seeking medical attention promptly if signs and symptoms of wound infection occur.
- Importance of monitoring for vascular changes in patients who have undergone vascular surgery (exploration or resection). Teach patient to be alert to color changes (pallor, cyanosis, duskiness), coolness, pulselessness, or decreased or absent capillary refill. Caution patient about the importance of reporting these findings promptly.

# Section Three:    Skeletal Disorders

## Osteomyelitis

Osteomyelitis is an acute or chronic infection involving a bone. Patients at risk for osteomyelitis include those who are undernourished, the elderly, and individuals with diabetes mellitus (DM) and chronic obstructive pulmonary disease. *Primary osteomyelitis* is a direct implantation of microorganisms into bone *via* compound fractures, penetrating wounds, diagnostic bone marrow aspiration, or surgery. *Secondary or acute hematogenic osteomyelitis* is an infection of bone that occurs through its own blood supply or by infection from contiguous soft tissues (especially ischemic, diabetic, or neurotrophic ulcers), IV drug abuse, or joints involved with septic arthritis. Although osteomyelitis often remains localized, it can spread through the marrow, cortex, and periosteum. Conditions favoring the development of osteomyelitis include recent bone trauma or bone with low $O_2$ tension, such as that found in sickle cell anemia. Acute hematogenic osteomyelitis is most frequently caused by *Staphylococcus aureus* (90%-95%), but it also can result from *Escherichia coli*, *Pseudomonas* species, *Klebsiella, Enterobacter, Proteus, Salmonellae, Streptococcus* (groups A, B, and G), and *Hemophilus influenzae*. Chronic osteomyelitis is comparatively rare and is characterized by persistent, multiple, draining sinus tracts.

### ASSESSMENT

**Acute osteomyelitis:**   Abrupt onset of pain in the involved area, fever, malaise, and limited motion. Pseudoparalysis is especially indicative of osteomyelitis in children who refuse to move an adjacent joint because of pain.

**Chronic osteomyelitis:**   Bone infection that persists intermittently for years, usually flaring up after minor trauma to the area or lowered systemic resistance. Edema and erythema over the involved bone, weakness, irritability, and generalized signs of sepsis can occur. Sometimes the only symptom is persistent purulent drainage from an old pocket or sinus tract. With implant arthroplasty osteomyelitis, the symptoms involve loosening and pain 3-5 months postoperatively.

**History of:**   Total joint replacement, compound fracture, use of external fixator, vascular insufficiency (e.g., with DM), recurrent urinary tract infections, sickle cell disease.

### DIAGNOSTIC TESTS

**CBC:**   Will reveal leukocytosis and anemia in the presence of osteomyelitis.
**Erythrocyte sedimentation rate:**   Elevated in the presence of osteomyelitis.

**Bone biopsy:** Will provide infectious material for accurate culture and sensitivity studies. This study is limited to large bones because of the risk of fracture in small bones.

**Blood or sequestrum cultures:** To identify the causative organism *via* Gram stain and culture and sensitivity. Sequestrum is a piece of necrotic bone that is separated from surrounding bone as a result of osteomyelitis.

**X-rays:** May reveal subtle areas of radiolucency (osteonecrosis) and new bone formation. No x-ray changes will be evident until the disease has been active at least 5 days in infants, 8-10 days in children, and 2-3 weeks in adults.

**Radioisotope scanning:** Methods include bone scans with technetium-99 and gallium-67 and leukocyte scans with indium-111. These scans may reveal areas of increased vascularity (called *hot spots*), which may be indicative of osteomyelitis. False-positive results occur frequently with these tests, and they are used cautiously for this reason. Negative bone scan results do not guarantee that osteomyelitis is not present.

**CT and MRI scans:** CT scans may demonstrate bone damage and soft tissue inflammation. MRI will not reveal bone changes, but it is an excellent means for identifying pockets of purulence, especially intramedullar infections.

## COLLABORATIVE MANAGEMENT

**IV antimicrobial therapy:** Continued for at least 6 weeks. Once instructed in proper technique, selected patients are discharged on IV antibiotics.

**Bed rest.**

**Immobilization of affected extremity:** With splint, cast, or traction to relieve pain and decrease the potential for pathologic fracture.

**Blood transfusions:** To correct any accompanying anemia.

**Removal of internal fixation device or endoprosthesis, if present:** To help control the infection.

**Surgical decompression of infected bone:** May be followed by primary closure, myocutaneous flaps to cover the denuded bone, or leaving the area open to drain and heal by secondary intention or with secondary closure.

**Drains:** May be inserted into the affected bone to drain the site or act as ingress-egress tubes to funnel topical antibiotics directly into the area of infection. This system may incorporate suction to aid drainage.

**Topical antibiotics:** May be used *via* continuous or intermittent infusion into the wound and are continued until 3 successive drain cultures have been negative. As an alternative, acrylic beads with antibiotics may be packed into affected sites for 2-4 weeks, after which the wound is reopened, the beads are removed, and bone graft is packed in the deficit.

**Long-term antibiotic therapy:** May be continued for 3-6 months. Cefonicid is an effective agent for IV or deep IM route, and enoxacin has been shown effective in treating osteomyelitis as an oral agent.

**Hyperbaric $O_2$:** May be used in selected patients with accessible areas of involvement to improve local $O_2$ supply.

**Amputation:** Although rarely performed, it may be required for extremities in which persistent infection severely limits function.

## NURSING DIAGNOSES AND INTERVENTIONS

**High risk for infection** *(for others)* related to risk of cross-contamination; *(for patient)* related to disease chronicity

**Desired outcomes:** At the time of patient's hospital discharge, patient, other patients, and staff members are free of symptoms of infection as evidenced by normothermia and WBC count $\leq 11,000/\mu l$. Within 24 h of instruction, patient verbalizes knowledge of the potential chronicity of the disease and the importance of strict adherence to the prescribed antibiotic therapy.

- When appropriate for the infecting organism, isolate the patient from other patients, especially those with orthopedic disorders.

- Ensure that the patient's drainage system is properly handled, using Body Substance Isolation (BSI), and that careful handwashing is observed between patients by all staff members to prevent cross-contamination.
- Teach patient about the disease and potential for chronic infection. Stress the importance of adherence to the prescribed antibiotic therapy.
- Follow BSI (i.e., use of gloves) when performing irrigations, changing dressings, or handling contaminated dressings (see Appendix Two, p. 777). Wash hands well between patients.

**Knowledge deficit:**  Side effects from prolonged use of potent antibiotics
*Desired outcome:*  Within 24 h of instruction, patient verbalizes knowledge about potential side effects of antibiotic therapy and precautions that must be taken.

*Aminoglycoside antibacterials:* Gentamicin sulfate, kanamycin sulfate, neomycin, streptomycin, and tobramycin are used to combat gram-negative organisms. Potential toxic reactions include ototoxicity (exhibited by dizziness, vertigo, tinnitus, and decreased auditory acuity); nephrotoxicity (evidenced by rising blood urea nitrogen [BUN] and serum creatinine levels, from progressive renal tubular necrosis, which can progress to renal failure if untreated); and superimposed infections, which occur because of loss of normal body flora protection against bacterial overgrowth.

- Teach patient about the potential complications and the need to report symptoms as early as possible.
- Advise patient that with long-term therapy, a baseline audiogram with weekly audiograms should be performed to identify potential hearing deficit; serum creatinine and BUN should be drawn weekly while patient is on aminoglycosides; and weight should be checked daily to help assess for fluid retention (patients should report weight gain of ≥2 lb/day). Monitor I&O during patient's hospitalization to help assess renal function.
- Advise patient to observe for superimposed infections, especially fungal infections, by assessing for fever, black or furry tongue, nausea, diarrhea, oral monilial growth, or vaginal monilial growth. If a venous access device is used for antibiotic administration, the infusion site should be closely monitored for indicators of irritation that do not respond to usual treatments with topical antibiotics. During hospitalization, consult with physician about culturing suspicious areas of inflammation.

*Penicillins:* Ampicillin, carbenicillin, cyclacillin, methacillin, mezlocillin, oxacillin, and piperacillin are used to combat organisms that demonstrate sensitivity to them. Potential toxic reactions include anemia, hypersensitivity reactions, and overgrowth of nonsusceptible organisms.

- Teach patient about the potential complications and the need to report symptoms promptly.
- Use penicillin cautiously in patients with allergies or allergic pathologies such as asthma, hay fever, or dermatitis. Erythematous, maculopapular rash; urticaria; and anaphylaxis can occur. Caution patient about these potential reactions.
- Instruct patient to seek medical attention if rash, fever, chills, or signs of infection/inflammation develop.

*Cephalosporins:* Cefadroxil, cefamandole, cefazolin, cefoperazone, cefotetan, cefoxitin, ceftazidine, ceftriaxone, cefuroxime, cephalothin, cephapirin, cephradine, and tazicef are used in the treatment of susceptible organisms. Potential toxic reactions include overgrowth of nonsusceptible organisms, photosensitivity, increased BUN, hepatotoxicity, and pseudomembranous colitis.

- Advise patient about the potential complications, which necessitate prompt medical attention.
- Explain that patients with suspected renal or hepatic disease should have baseline and serial (weekly) serum liver enzymes (lactate hydrogenase [LDH], serum glutamic-oxaloacetic transminase [SGOT], serum glutamic-pyruvic transminase [SGPT]), BUN, and serum creatinine evaluations. I&O

should be monitored along with daily weight to determine hydration status. Scleral and skin icterus, as well as darkening of the urine (from increased urobilinogen), should be noted. Persistent diarrhea (>3 liquid stools or liquid stools for >2 days) should be reported promptly to the health care provider.

- Advise patient to avoid direct sunlight or ultraviolet light sources. Suggest the use of sunscreening agents to help prevent photosensitivity reactions.
- When oral medications are used, instruct patient to avoid concurrent intake with dairy or iron products because they can inhibit absorption from the gut.

   ***Sulfonamides:*** Sulfadiazine, sulfamethoxazole, sulfapyridine, and sulfisoxazole can cause toxic reactions, including disruption of intestinal flora, which results in decreased production of metabolically active vitamin K and hemorrhagic tendencies; agranulocytosis; nephrotoxicity; and crystalluria.

- Teach patient about the potential complications and the importance of seeking prompt medical attention if they occur.
- Advise patients on long-term therapy of the need to have baseline BUN and serum creatinine level determination along with weekly levels to rule out nephrotoxicity. Baseline and serial (weekly) granulocyte determinations also should be performed. Agranulocytosis can manifest as lesions of the throat, mucous membranes, GI tract, and skin. Daily weight and I&O evaluation should be watched to help assess hydration status.
- Teach patient how to monitor for bleeding, especially epistaxis, bleeding gums, hemoptysis, hematemesis, melena, hematuria, prolonged bleeding from wounds, and ecchymosis. During patient's hospitalization, hematest suspicious secretions, or send them to the lab if prescribed, to determine if blood is present. Teach patient to control bleeding with ice, pressure, or elevation and to seek medical assistance promptly if unable to control hemorrhage.
- Advise patient to consume at least 2-3 L/day of fluids (unless contraindicated by cardiac or renal disease) to prevent crystalluria. Teach the indicators of urinary calculi and the importance of getting medical attention should they occur: hematuria, pyuria, retention, frequency, urgency, and pain in the flank, lower back, perineum, thighs, groin, labia, or scrotum.

**Knowledge deficit:**    Potential for infection and air embolus related to use of Hickman catheter or other venous access device for long-term intermittent antibiotic therapy

***Desired outcome:***    By a minimum of the 24-h period before hospital discharge, patient demonstrates care of the catheter and verbalizes knowledge about the indicators of infection and air embolus.

- Teach patient how to care for the catheter and monitor the entry site for indicators of infection or inflammation if therapy is to be continued at home. Use sterile technique for dressing changes, following hospital protocol for the procedure, which usually includes defatting the skin with acetone or alcohol, applying povidone-iodine, and covering the site with an air-occlusive dressing. Have patient or significant other return the demonstration before hospital discharge. If appropriate, arrange for a visit by a home health-care nurse.
- Caution patient about the importance of keeping the tubing clamped unless he or she is aspirating or injecting solutions into the catheter. Teach patient and significant others to be alert to indicators of air embolism: labored breathing, cyanosis, cough, chest pain, and syncope. Explain that if air embolism is suspected, the patient should be rolled immediately to the left side and placed in Trendelenburg's position while reclamping the catheter, and medical assistance should be obtained as rapidly as possible.
- Teach patient the importance of preventing inadvertent puncture or breakage of the tubing and checking for kinks or cracks daily. Explain the necessity of taping all tube junctures to prevent accidental separation and positioning the clamp over tape tabs to minimize stress on the tubing.

**Note:** See "Intervertebral Disk Disease" for **Health-seeking behavior:** Pain control measures, p. 228. See "Osteoarthritis" for **Pain,** p. 520. See "Fractures" for **Self-care deficit,** p. 550. See Appendix One for nursing diagnoses and interventions in "Caring for Preoperative and Postoperative Patients," p. 693. "Caring for Patients on Prolonged Bed Rest," p. 711, and "Caring for Patients with Cancer and Other Life-Disrupting Illnesses," p. 719.

## PATIENT-FAMILY TEACHING AND DISCHARGE PLANNING

Give patient and significant others verbal and written information about the following:

- Necessary patient care after hospital discharge (e.g., dressing changes, warm soaks, ROM exercises). Involve significant others in patient care during hospitalized period to familiarize them with care activities after discharge.
- When parenteral antibiotic therapy is to be given at home (usually *via* a Hickman catheter, Portacath, or similar long-term vascular access device), the method of administering medications and care of the device used.
- Medications, including drug name, route, dosage, purpose, schedule, precautions, and potential side effects.
- Involving a public health, visiting nurse, or similar home health-care service professional to ensure adequate follow-up at home.
- Indicators of potential complications, such as recurring infection, pathologic fracture, joint contracture, pressure necrosis, and medication reactions or toxic effects.

# Fractures

A fracture is a break in the continuity of a bone. It occurs when stress is placed on the bone that exceeds the bone's biologic loading capacity. Most commonly the stress is the result of trauma. *Pathologic fractures* are the result of decreased biologic loading capacity so that even normal stress can result in a break.

## ASSESSMENT

**Chronic indicators:**   These are rare. Osteoporotic fractures of the vertebral column may be found incidental to an x-ray in an asymptomatic patient or in a patient who complains of back discomfort. Delayed union is a failure of the bone to unite within the normally accepted timeframe for that bone's healing, and a chronic fracture may result. Nonunion is demonstrated by nonalignment and lost function secondary to lost bony rigidity. Pseudoarthrosis is a state in which the fracture fails to heal and a false joint forms at the fracture site. Avascular necrosis occurs when the fracture interrupts the blood supply to a segment of bone, which then eventually necroses. Reflex sympathetic dystrophy is an incompletely understood process that results in pain, reduced function, joint stiffness, and trophic changes in soft tissues and skin following fracture. Other complications can include altered sensation, limb length descrepancies, and chronic lymphatic or venous stasis.

**Acute indicators:**   Sudden pain, which usually is associated with trauma or physical stress, such as jogging or strenuous exercise. In pathologic fractures, the patient may describe signs and symptoms associated with the underlying pathology (see "Benign Neoplasms," p. 553, and "Malignant Neoplasms," p. 555).

**Physical assessment:**   Loss of normal bony or limb contours, edema, ecchymosis, limb shortening, decreased ROM of adjacent joints, false motion (movement that occurs outside of a joint), and crepitus, which should not be elicited purposely because of the risk of injury to surrounding soft tissues.

Complicated and complex fractures can present with signs and symptoms of perforated viscus (internal organ), neurovascular deficit, joint effusion, or excessive joint laxity. Compound fractures involve a break in the skin and will demonstrate a wound in the area of suspected fracture, or bone may be exposed in the wound.

---

**Note:** Any patient with a suspected fracture should be treated as though a fracture is present until it is ruled out. Interventions should include immobilization and elevation of the involved area, application of ice, and careful monitoring of the neurovascular status distal to the injury.

---

## DIAGNOSTIC TESTS

Most fractures are identified easily with standard anterior-posterior (A-P) and lateral x-rays. MRI may be useful in evaluating complicated fractures; its usefulness in identifying different bone densities is limited. Occasionally it is necessary to involve special techniques, such as the mortise view to demonstrate bimalleolar ankle fractures or x-rays through the open mouth to identify fractures of the odontoid process. Bone scans, tomograms, CT scans, stereoscopic films, and arthrograms also can be used. Intra-articular fractures sometimes may be diagnosed with arthroscopy.

## COLLABORATIVE MANAGEMENT

The choice of treatment varies with the complexity of the fracture and with the patient's age, concurrent health problems, and functional goals. The goal of treatment is to provide immobilization of the bone until healing occurs. The length of time for immobilization varies with the type of fracture. The following is a brief overview of common examples of treatment interventions.

**Bed rest:** May be all that is required to maintain reduction for simple, uncomplicated fractures, such as those of the posterior elements of the vertebrae and some pelvic fractures.

**Traction**

*Cervical fractures:* Skeletal traction *via* Turner, Cone, Vinke, or Crutchfield tongs, which are inserted into the outer plate of the cranial vault. An alternative is the halo vest, which allows the insertion of four pins into the outer plate of the cranium. The pins are attached to a halo device that is connected to four metal posts encompassed within a body jacket, cast, or orthosis. This "four-posted" jacket allows exposure of the head and neck yet maintains immobilization of the fracture. Cervical collars and a wide variety of orthotics can be used to provide support for some simple fractures or to maintain stability of more complex fractures following therapy with traction or ORIF.

*Humeral fractures:* Dunlop's side arm or overhead 90/90 traction. Skeletal traction may be applied with a Kirschner wire through the proximal ulna.

*Pelvic fractures:* Balanced suspension, pelvic sling, or pelvic belt may be used for nondisplaced fractures, while skeletal traction with pins in the ilium or femur may be required for displaced fractures.

*Femoral fractures:* Skin traction (Buck's extension, Bohler-Braun, Russell's, or balanced suspension traction) may be applied until skeletal traction can be used or the fracture is internally or externally fixated. Skeletal traction may involve a Steinmann pin or Kirshner wire positioned through the distal femur or proximal tibia. When skeletal traction is used, it is provided in combination with balanced suspension or Russell's traction and is used for 1-4 months.

*Tibial fractures:* Temporary traction can be accomplished with Buck's extension, or for longer periods of time with a pin placed through the distal tibia or calcaneus, augmented with balanced suspension, Bohler-Braun, or Russell's traction.

**Immobilization devices**
*Uncomplicated, simple fractures of the cervical vertebrae:*   A variety of orthotics, soft or hard cervical collars, or a minerva jacket cast for less stable fractures.
*Dorsal and lumbar vertebral fractures:*   Plaster of Paris body cast or a variety of orthotic devices.
*Clavicular fractures:*   Figure-of-8 dressing, modified Velpeau dressing (a wrap that holds the arm against the thorax with the elbow flexed at 90 or 45 degrees), sling and swathe shoulder immobilizer, clavicular straps.
*Humeral fractures:*   Velpeau cast, shoulder spica cast (which abducts or extends the upper arm), or Caldwell's hanging plaster cast, which is a long arm cast with additional layers of plaster of Paris that provide weight to distract fracture fragments and aid in alignment. Patients in Caldwell's casts should be instructed to allow the cast to be dependent, which will help ensure adequate fracture distraction. A coaptation splint may be used to immobilize midshaft humeral fractures. The coaptation splint consists of a long plaster splint applied over a thick layer of padding, beginning at the medial aspect of the upper arm in the axilla and extending around the elbow and up the outside of the upper arm. An elastic wrap secures the splint. Posterior splints may immobilize distal shaft fractures temporarily. Posterior or coaptation splints accommodate progressive edema, reducing the potential for compartment syndrome. Undisplaced, stable fractures may require immobilization only, with a sling and swathe shoulder immobilizer or functional bracing. Prefabricated polypropylene sleeves have been used successfully to immobilize fractures of the lower half of the humerus.
*Ulnar or radial fractures:*   Long arm casts for proximal fractures or short arm casts for distal fractures. In the presence of significant edema, a sugar tong splint may be used to provide immobilization while accommodating progressive edema. This is applied over heavy padding and consists of one long plaster splint that extends from the back of the wrist, bends around the elbow, covers the underside of the forearm to the wrist, and is held in place with an elastic wrap. Some fractures are immobilized in a posterior splint for 3-7 days before casting to allow for the edema to subside. Fractures involving both the radius and ulna usually are immobilized in a long arm cast.
*Hand fractures:*   Short arm posterior splints until edema subsides, and then a short arm cast can be applied. Some fractures of the hand may be immobilized safely in splints or orthoses. A thumb spica cast may be used for various fractures involving the thumb.
*Pelvic fractures:*   Corsets, orthoses, or external fixators.
*Femoral fractures:*   Spica cast that extends from the thorax and completely encompasses the affected leg and opposite leg to the midthigh, or a long leg cast may be applied instead. After sufficient callus has formed, it may be possible to use a cast brace to allow motion of the knee and weight-bearing stress, which can facilitate bony union in certain fractures.
*Patellar fractures:*   Cylinder cast for nondisplaced fractures. Following any knee surgery, the leg is immobilized in a Jones dressing, which includes A-P and lateral splints over bulky padding and is held in place with an elastic wrap. Once swelling subsides, a cylinder or long leg cast is applied. A knee immobilizer may provide sufficient immobilization for some stable patellar fractures.
*Tibial fractures:*   Cylinder or long leg cast; short leg cast for easily stabilized fractures. Some casts will be converted to walking casts at a later time.
*Fibular shaft fractures:*   While some fibular fractures may not require casting, a short leg walking cast is often applied if adequate support is not provided by the tibia.
*Malleolar fractures:*   Short leg cast that is converted to a walking cast after callus has formed; long leg cast for nondisplaced bimalleolar fractures. Trimalleolar fractures require ORIF to ensure joint integrity.

*Avulsion fractures of the insertion of the Achilles tendon from the calcaneous:* Often require a long leg cast with the knee flexed at 30 degrees and the ankle slightly plantarflexed to reduce stress on the Achilles tendon.

*Tarsal and metatarsal fractures:* Short leg cast that can be converted to a walking cast; stiff-soled shoe or slipper cast.

*Phalangeal fractures:* Splints made of plaster, metal, or plastic, or the phalanx can be immobilized by taping it to an adjacent phalanx.

**Closed reduction:** Allows for manipulation of displaced fragments to their normal anatomic alignment. It can be done under general, regional, local, or hematoma-block anesthesia.

**ORIF:** Indicated for fractures that are grossly unstable or for patients who cannot tolerate prolonged bed rest or traction. Internal fixation may be accomplished with screws, pins, wires, plates, bone grafts (either allograft or autograft), methylmethacrylate, or rods. In some fractures in which avascular necrosis is likely or the fracture is severely comminuted, placement of an endoprosthesis may be necessary. Compound fractures need definitive treatment within 6-8 hr to prevent limb compromise. Endoprostheses most commonly are used to replace the head of the humerus or femur. Fibrin sealant may be used to aid in the internal fixation of some small fractures, avulsion fractures, and osteochondral fractures, as well as to aid in the internal fixation of bone grafts. Bioelectric stimulators, autogenous bone graft substitutes, osteoconductors, and osteoinductors are being used experimentally to compensate for bone loss or stimulate fracture healing.

**External fixation:** Consists of skeletal pins that penetrate the fracture fragments and are attached to universal joints, which in turn are attached to rods to provide stabilization. These rods form a frame around the fractured limb for immobilization. Biaxial frames with transfixing pins or uniaxial frames with bicortical half pins may be used. The external fixator is left in place until sufficient soft tissue repair or bony callous formation allows either application of a cast or complete removal of any form of immobilization. Sometimes the skeletal pins are left in place (after removing the external fixation rods) and incorporated into a cast that immobilizes the limb until the fracture has healed. The external fixator can be used to treat massive open comminuted fractures with extensive soft tissue injury or neurovascular injury in which there is increased risk of infection. It is also the treatment of choice for infected nonunion, segmental bone loss, limb-lengthening procedures, arthrodesis (joint fusion), and multiple trauma with injuries involving other body systems.

*Ilizarov procedure:* Use of a ring-shaped external fixator that can be arranged in over 600 configurations to enable maintenance of limb position for a myriad of orthopedic conditions. As with other external fixators, the connection between the device and bone is accomplished with Kirschner wires or Steinmann pins.

**Progressive ROM and muscle-strengthening exercises:** Begun after the designated period of immobilization to help the patient regain joint function.

**Continuous passive movement (CPM):** A motor-driven device developed to place a joint through repeated extension and flexion. It is used as an adjunctive treatment for femoral condyle and tibial plateau injuries as well as humeral head fractures.

## NURSING DIAGNOSES AND INTERVENTIONS

**Note:** See "Intervertebral Disk Disease" for **Health-seeking behavior :** Pain control measures, p. 228. See "Osteoarthritis" for **Pain,** p. 520, and **Impaired physical mobility** related to musculoskeletal impairment and adjustment to new walking gait, p. 521 (useful for any patient with spinal or lower extremity injuries). See "Rheumatoid arthritis" for **Fatigue,** p. 528. See "Ligamentous Injuries" for **Knowledge deficit:** Need for elevation of the extremity, use of thermotherapy, and prescribed exercise, p. 530 (useful for patients discharged after a recent fracture or surgery), and **Knowledge deficit:** Care and assessment of the casted extremity, p. 531 (applies to any patient in a cast). See "Bunionectomy" for **High risk for peripheral neurovascular dysfunction** related to interrupted arterial flow secondary to compression by circumferential cast or dressing, p. 563 (relates to iatrogenic compartment syndrome and builds on information provided under "Ischemic Myositis," p. 538). See "Amputation" for **Knowledge deficit:** Postsurgical exercise regimen, p. 566 (applies for any patient begun on exercise therapy). See "Repair of Recurrent Shoulder Dislocation" for **High risk for impaired skin integrity** related to trapping of moisture on the axillary skin, p. 572 (useful for any patient with moist areas trapped by a therapeutic device that is necessary to treat a fracture). See "Total Hip Arthroplasty" for **Knowledge deficit:** Potential for and mechanism of total hip arthroplasty (THA) dislocation, p. 575 (for patients undergoing hemiarthroplasty for replacement of the femoral head), **Knowledge deficit:** Potential for infection caused by foreign body reaction to an endoprosthesis, p. 575 (useful for any patient with an internal fixation device, especially large devices), and **High risk for peripheral neurovascular dysfunction,** p. 576 (can be adapted for any patient in traction). See "Total Knee Arthroplasty" for **High risk for fluid volume deficit** related to postsurgical hemorrhage or hematoma formation, p. 578 (for patients with ORIF). See Appendix One for nursing diagnoses and interventions in "Caring for Preoperative and Postoperative Patients," p. 693, and "Caring for Patients on Prolonged Bed Rest, p. 711.

---

*Specific nursing diagnoses for patients with casts, traction, ORIF, and external fixators*
**Self-care deficit** related to physical limitations secondary to cast or surgical procedure (applies to patients with casts, ORIF, and external fixators)
***Desired outcome:***    Within 48 h of the surgical procedure or cast application, patient demonstrates independence with ADL.
- For patients with insufficient strength to manipulate casted extremities to allow independence in self-care, incorporate a structured exercise regimen that will increase strength and endurance. Direct the regimen toward development of those muscle groups necessary for the patient's activity deficit. See the guidelines described for **Knowledge deficit:** Postsurgical exercise regimen, p. 566, in "Amputation" and **High risk for disuse syndrome** related to inactivity secondary to prolonged bed rest, p. 713, in Appendix One.
- Use assistive devices liberally. These include stocking helpers, Velcro fasteners, enlarged handles on eating utensils, pickup sticks, raised toilet seats, and similar self-help devices.
- As appropriate, ask social services department of hospital for assistance with funding for purchasing assistive equipment or for home help.
- Because pain control is an essential element in enhancing self-care activities, ensure that the patient is as comfortable as possible (see **Pain,** p. 520, in "Osteoarthritis" and **Health-seeking behavior:** Pain control measures, p. 228, in "Intervertebral Disk Disease").
- When needed, teach significant others how to assist patient with self-care.
- As appropriate, use adaptive clothing (e.g., garments with Velcro fasteners for easy removal and application) that is designed to accommodate the cast.
**High risk for impaired skin integrity** and/or **impaired tissue integrity** related to irritation and pressure secondary to the presence of a cast (applies to patients with casts, ORIF, or CPM)
***Desired outcomes:***    Patient relates the absence of discomfort under the cast and exhibits intact skin once the cast is removed. Within 8 h of cast application, patient verbalizes knowledge about the indicators of pressure necrosis.

- When assisting with cast application, ensure that adequate padding is put on the affected extremity before the cast is applied.
- While the cast is curing (drying), handle it only with the palms of the hands to avoid pressure points caused by finger indentations. Ensure that the cast surface is exposed to facilitate drying.
- Petal the edges of plaster casts with tape or moleskin to prevent cast crumbs from falling into the cast and causing pressure necrosis.
- Instruct patient never to insert anything between the cast and skin. In the presence of severe itching, advise patient to notify physician, who may prescribe a medication to relieve itching.
- Teach patient the indicators of pressure necrosis within the cast: pain, burning sensation, foul odor from cast opening, or drainage on the cast.

**Knowledge deficit:** Potential for disuse osteoporosis (appropriate for patient with cast or traction)

*Desired outcome:* Within 24 h of the instruction, patient verbalizes knowledge of the process of and measures to prevent disuse osteoporosis.

- Teach patient about the process of disuse osteoporosis, gearing the explanation to the patient's level of understanding: The immobilized limb has insufficient stress to stimulate osteoblastic (bone building) activity.
- Instruct patient to report any indicators of pain in the immobilized limb or findings of spontaneous fracture, such as bony deformity, pain, lost function, edema, and ecchymosis.
- Consult with patient's physician about appropriate alternative methods of bone stress, and teach them to the patient. These methods can include use of a tilt table, sandbags applied intermittently against the bone, or having patient push against a footboard or perform isometric exercise of the immobilized limb.

**Altered cerebral or cardiopulmonary tissue perfusion (or risk of same)** related to interrupted arterial flow secondary to fat embolization (applies to patients with multiple trauma, multiple fractures, or surgical repair of fractures)

*Desired outcome:* Patient has adequate cerebral and cardiopulmonary perfusion as evidenced by $Pao_2$ ≥80 mm Hg, HR ≤100 bpm, RR ≤20 breaths/min, normothermia, normal skin color, absence of adventitious breath sounds over the tracheobronchial tree, absence of petechial rash, and orientation to person, place, and time.

- Ensure strict maintenance of fracture immobilization to help prevent embolization.
- Carefully monitor patient for the initial 72 h after injury or surgery for indicators of fat embolism: tachycardia, tachypnea, profuse tracheobronchial secretions, chest pain, cyanosis, fever, petechial rash (involving the conjunctiva, trunk, neck, proximal arms, and axilla), anxiety, apprehension, progressive mental dysfunction (confusion, disorientation), and the presence of fat globules in the retina of the eye. The hematocrit (Hct) may drop, serum lipase will rise, and fat may be noted on urinalysis. Frequent specimens for ABG levels should be drawn on patients at risk for fat embolus for the first 48 h after injury because early hypoxemia that is indicative of fat embolism is apparent on laboratory measurement only. In addition, a platelet count indicative of thrombocytopenia (<150,000 μl) is diagnostic of fat embolism.
- Because fat embolism is a life-threatening emergency, notify physician immediately if any of the preceding occur. Inform patient and significant others of these potential indicators so that they can notify the staff if they occur.
- As prescribed, perform respiratory support measures with oxygen and rigorous pulmonary hygiene. Intubation with ventilation using positive end expiratory pressure may be necessary. As a general rule, all patients with sig-

nificant trauma and fractures should receive oxygen at 40% concentration *via* mask or nasal prongs until the threat of fat embolism has been ruled out.

- Administer IV steroids, diuretics, and dextran as prescribed.

**Knowledge deficit:**  Potential for infection because of the orthopedic procedure or presence of the internal or external device (appropriate for patients with ORIF or external fixators)

*Desired outcome:*  Within 24 h of instruction, patient verbalizes knowledge about the potential for infection, lists the indicators that may occur, and relates the significance of reporting them promptly.

- Advise patient about the potential for infection, which can occur as a result of the surgical procedure.
- Teach patient the following indicators of infection and the importance of reporting them to a health-care professional promptly if they occur: persistent redness, swelling, increasing pain, wound drainage, local warmth, foul odor from within the cast, sensation of burning within the cast, drainage from the cast, and fever.
- Alert patients with internal fixation devices to the potential for infection for as long as the implant is present. Instruct them to report any of the preceding indicators promptly.

**Knowledge deficit:**  Potential for refracture owing to vulnerability because of the presence of an internal fixator (applies to patients with ORIF)

*Desired outcome:*  By a minimum of the 24-h period before hospital discharge, patient verbalizes knowledge about the potential for refracture and demonstrates adherence to the prescribed regimen for prevention.

- Advise patient that although the internal fixation device supplements strength of the bone at the fracture site in the early stages of healing, the implant will compromise the bone's strength later. Larger internal fixation devices alter the vectors of stress placed on the bone, changing the normal physiologic balance between osteoblasts and osteoclasts, which results in a bone that is made weaker in the long run by the implant.
- Be sure the patient verbalizes understanding of this process and demonstrates adherence to the prescribed regimen of limb use and ambulation.
- Ensure patient is aware that intramedullary nails or rods and large plates probably will be removed within a year.

**Knowledge deficit:**  Function of external fixation, pin care, and signs and symptoms of pin site infection

*Desired outcomes:*  By a minimum of the 24-h period before hospital discharge, patient verbalizes knowledge about the rationale for the external fixator and demonstrates ways to adapt life-style to the fixator. Patient demonstrates knowledge of pin care and verbalizes knowledge of the indicators of infection at the pin sites.

- Teach patient the rationale for use of the fixator with type of fracture or injury, emphasizing benefits for the patient.
- Discuss ways in which the patient can adapt his or her life-style to accommodate the fixator (e.g., by wearing adaptive clothing that fits the device).
- Instruct patient and significant others in pin care as prescribed by physician. Some physicians prescribe daily pin site care with hydrogen peroxide or skin prep solutions such as pHisoHex, alcohol, or povidone-iodine. Some physicians request that buildup of crusts from serous drainage be removed when cleansing pin sites, while others request that the crust be left intact to minimize the risk of infection. If prescribed, teach the patient how to apply antibacterial ointments and small dressings to the pin site. External fixator pins should be cleansed with alcohol daily. **Note:** Literature supplied with some external fixators cautions against the use of iodine-based mixtures, which may cause corrosion of the device.
- Instruct patient and significant others not to use the external fixator as a handle or support for the extremity. Teach them to support the extremity with

pillows, two hands, slings, and other devices as necessary to prevent excessive stress on the skeletal pins.

- Teach patient how to monitor the pin sites for indicators of infection, including persistent redness, swelling, drainage, increasing pain, temperature >38.33°C (101°F), and local warmth, and to be alert to pin migration or "tenting" of the skin on the pin, which can signal movement of the pin or infection. Instruct patient to report significant findings promptly to physician.

- Advise patient of the need for follow-up care to ensure that the device is functioning properly and for maintaining adequate immobilization of the fracture(s).

## PATIENT-FAMILY TEACHING AND DISCHARGE PLANNING

Give patient and significant others verbal and written information about the following:

- Medications, including name, dosage, purpose, schedule, precautions, and potential side effects.
- Importance of rest, elevation, and use of thermotherapy (see "Ligamentous Injuries," p. 530).
- Rationale for the individual's therapy after discharge and how that therapy will be accomplished, (e.g., casting, external fixation, internal fixation).
- Precautions of therapy:
  - *Casts:* Caring for the cast, monitoring neurovascular status of the distal extremity, watching for evidence of pressure necrosis beneath the cast, performing prescribed exercises, preventing skin maceration, and preventing disuse osteoporosis (also see **Knowledge deficit:** Care and assessment of the casted extremity, p. 531).
  - *Internal fixation devices:* Caring for the wound, noting signs of wound infection, preventing refracture of the limb, performing prescribed exercises, and monitoring for delayed infection.
  - *External fixator:* Demonstrating understanding of pin care, knowing when to notify physician of problems with the fixator, performing prescribed exercises, monitoring neurovascular status of the limb, and monitoring pin site for indicators of infection.
- Ways in which patient can control discomfort (see **Health-seeking behavior:** Pain control measures, p. 228, in "Intervertebral Disk Disease").
- Use of assistive devices and ambulatory aids. Ensure that the patient can perform a return demonstration and is independent with devices and aids before hospital discharge (see "Osteoarthritis," p. 521). If needed, initiate a referral for a home visit early after discharge to ensure patient safety.
- Materials that are necessary for care at home and agencies that can supply materials.
- For patients who require home help, a collaborative effort between hospital nurses and community care agencies should be made to ensure continuity of care. The appropriate agency should see patient before hospital discharge.

## Benign neoplasms

The three most common benign bone tumors are osteochondromas, enchondromas, and giant cell tumors. *Osteochondromas* are the most common, representing 45% of all benign tumors. Usually they are found in the metaphysis (wider portion of the shaft) of the long bones, typically the distal femur or proximal humerus, although they also can occur in a rib or vertebra. Individuals under the age of 20 are most commonly affected. Some osteochondromas are the result of an inheritable autosomal dominant trait that causes concurrent growth retardation and bowing of the long bones. *Enchondromas* (chondromas) are most commonly found in the hand (metacarpals or phalanges) or the proximal humerus. They represent approximately 10% of all diagnosed benign tumors. Although they occur most commonly in people in their 30s, they may be seen at any time. *Giant cell tumors* are found most often around the proximal humerus, distal radius, or the knee (most common) in the area of the fused epiphyseal growth plate in individuals 30-40 years old. About 2% of these tumors degenerate into malignancy with a potential for metastasis. Giant cell tumors recur 40% of the time.

## ASSESSMENT

**Osteochondromas:**    Indicators arise from mechanical irritation of surrounding musculotendinous structures and include pain upon specific movements of the involved areas or from irritation.

**Enchondromas:**    Local pain. Unless the growth is in an area with little soft tissue, the growth usually is not palpable.

**Giant cell tumors:**    Pain occurs before the mass becomes palpable.

## DIAGNOSTIC TESTS

AP and lateral x-rays are most commonly used for preliminary diagnosis. CT scans, tomograms, contrast radiography, bone scans, and angiograms can be used to clarify the extent of the tumor. MRI may be useful in determining precise areas for surgical resection.

## SURGICAL INTERVENTION

All three types of tumors are best treated with surgical removal. Resection can require allografting, prosthetic replacement, or use of methylmethacrylate to replace resected bone. When removal is impossible, curettage (scraping) of the lesion usually is done.

## NURSING DIAGNOSES AND INTERVENTIONS

**Knowledge deficit:**    Disease process and the potential for recurrence (if appropriate)

*Desired outcomes:*    Within the 24-h period before hospital discharge, patient verbalizes understanding about the disease process. Patients with giant cell tumors verbalize understanding of the potential for recurrence, slight chance of malignancy, and increased potential for infection.

- Provide patient with a clearly understood description of the disease process. Drawings, models, books, and other references should be used to enhance patient's learning.
- Validate that the patient clearly understands the disease process and does not confuse it with a malignant tumor.
- Be sure that patients with giant cell tumors are aware of the potential for recurrence and slight potential for degeneration to malignancy, as well as the importance of reporting renewed indicators of tumor to physician. In addition, teach these patients that they are at increased risk for infection and that they should report the following indicators promptly to the physician: persistent erythema, edema, fever, local warmth, wound drainage, and increasing pain.

---

**Note:**    See "Osteoarthritis" for **Pain,** p. 520. Also see "Fractures," p. 549, for nursing diagnoses as appropriate. See Appendix One for nursing diagnoses and interventions in "Caring for Preoperative and Postoperative Patients, p. 693.

---

## PATIENT-FAMILY TEACHING AND DISCHARGE PLANNING

Give patient and significant others verbal and written information about the following:

- Description of the disease process.
- For patients having surgery, the indicators of wound infection (swelling, persistent redness, wound drainage, pain, local warmth, and fever) and the necessity of reporting these indicators promptly to physician.
- For patients with casts and orthotics, care of the extremity and immobilization device. For more information about casts, see **Knowledge deficit:** Care and assessment of the casted extremity, p. 531.
- Medications, including name, dosage, purpose, schedule, precautions, and potential side effects.
- Posthospitalization therapy and the importance of follow-up.

# Malignant neoplasms

The most common malignant tumors affecting bones are osteogenic sarcoma, primary chondrosarcoma, and myeloma. *Osteogenic sarcoma* is the most common true tumor originating from bone tissue, occurring most frequently in adolescents. It is found (in order of prevalence) in the distal femoral metaphysis, proximal tibial metaphysis, proximal humeral metaphysis, pelvis, and proximal femur. Most osteosarcomas become apparent during the time of a skeletal growth spurt. Less frequently, osteosarcoma is associated with Paget's disease (see p. 560). This tumor is associated with early metastasis to the lung, lymph involvement, and rapid death unless rigorous treatment is begun early in the disease process. The current survival rate following resection and adjunctive chemotherapy is 60%. Children treated with radiation or alkylating agents for other cancers have a greatly increased risk of developing osteosarcoma. *Chondrosarcomas* occur half as frequently as osteogenic sarcomas and usually are seen at ages 50-60. Most of these tumors originate in the pelvic girdle, ribs, or shoulder girdle. Resection of all of the tumor results in an excellent 5-year cure rate; however, inadequate resection frequently results in recurrence and late metastasis to the lung. *Myelomas* arise from bone marrow and thus are not truly bone tumors, but they are the most common malignant tumor that affects bones. The peak time of onset is the 60s and 70s. Myelomas can occur in any bone, although they are seen less frequently in smaller bones. Average survival after diagnosis is 1-2 years.

## ASSESSMENT

**Osteogenic sarcomas:** Pain, tenderness, limited ROM, and swelling near a joint. Night pain usually is more severe. A history of trauma is frequently noted.

**Chondrosarcomas:** Localized pain, rarely with a demonstrable mass.

**Myelomas:** Symptoms of anemia, as well as weight loss, significant pain, tenderness, backache, or pathologic and spontaneous fracture.

## DIAGNOSTIC TESTS

**Standard x-rays, CT scans, tomograms, and radioisotope (gallium) uptake tests:** To delineate extent of the disease. *MRI* is useful in delineating the extent of cortical involvement and degree of medullary spread and may prove useful in identifying metastasis.

*For myelomas*

**Standard blood and electrolyte tests:** May reveal moderate normocytic anemia and a markedly elevated sedimentation rate. Serum calcium level and alkaline phosphatase usually are elevated, indicating bone turnover.

**Bence Jones protein:** Urine will be positive in 40% of patients with myeloma.

**Bone marrow aspiration:** May reveal plasma cells with large nuclei and nucleoli typical of myeloma.

**Electrophoresis:**    Immunoelectrophoresis will show an abnormal amount of either IgG or IgA produced by the tumor cells. Serum protein electrophoresis will show a paraprotein, a hallmark of myeloma.

## COLLABORATIVE MANAGEMENT

**Osteogenic sarcoma:**    Treated with resection of the tumor, most commonly by amputation. Recent attempts to perform less radical resections (en bloc tumor resection with limb salvage procedures), including therapy with chemotherapeutic agents (especially methotrexate, citrovorum, cyclophosphamide, vincristine, and adriamycin in various combinations), have met with increasing success.

**Chondrosarcoma:**    Usually treated with resection, with the degree of resection dependent on the stage of tumor development. Radiotherapy and chemotherapy have not proven to be effective in treating this disease.

**Multiple myeloma:**    Requires extensive therapy with radiation and chemotherapy. Radiation is used to control localized bone pain and treat areas with pathologic fractures. Chemotherapy with melphalan, prednisone, and vincristine has been shown to be helpful. Vincristine, doxorubicin, and dexamethasone may be useful in treating refractory cases of myeloma which occur in up to 50% of patients. Occasionally hypercalcemia requires additional therapy with increased volumes of IV fluids, furosemide, prednisone, or mithramycin. Laminectomy may be required for spinal cord compression caused by vertebral lesions. Pathologic fractures frequently require ORIF. Blood transfusions and potent analgesics are usually required. Bone marrow transplantation has been used experimentally.

## NURSING DIAGNOSES AND INTERVENTIONS

---

**Note:**    See "Intervertebral Disk Disease" for **Health-seeking behavior:** Pain control measures, p. 228. See "Osteoarthritis" for **Pain,** p. 520, and **Impaired physical mobility** related to musculoskeletal impairment and adjustment to new walking gait, p. 521. See "Total Knee Arthroplasty" for **High risk for fluid volume deficit** related to postsurgical hemorrhage or hematoma formation, p. 578.

---

**Note:**    When postoperative casts, use of orthotics, exercises, or similar therapies are prescribed, refer to appropriate nursing diagnoses throughout this chapter. If the patient undergoes amputation, refer to "Amputation," p. 564. Also see Appendix One for nursing diagnoses and interventions in "Caring for Preoperative and Postoperative Patients," p. 693, "Caring for Patients on Prolonged Bed Rest," p. 711, and "Caring for Patients with Cancer and Other Life-Disrupting Illnesses," p. 719.

---

## PATIENT-FAMILY TEACHING AND DISCHARGE PLANNING

Give patient and significant others verbal and written information about the following:

- Medications, including name, rationale, dosage, schedule, precautions, and potential side effects.
- For surgical patients, the following indicators of wound infection and the importance of notifying physician should they occur: persistent redness, swelling, local warmth, fever, discharge from the wound, or pain. As appropriate, also see "Ligamentous Injuries" for **Knowledge deficit:** Need for elevation of the involved extremity, use of thermotherapy, and prescribed exercise, p. 530.
- For patients with casts, orthotics, prosthetics, ambulatory aids, assistive devices, or similar therapies, instructions for their use, including a return dem-

onstration by patient and a phone number to call should any questions arise after hospital discharge. See **Impaired physical mobility** related to adjustment to a new walking gait, p. 521, and "Ligamentous injuries" for **Knowledge deficit:** Care and assessment of the casted extremity, p. 531.

- Referral to hospice or agency that provides home help. This should occur before discharge planning begins to ensure continuity of care between the hospital and home or hospice.

# Osteoporosis

Osteoporosis is a condition in which the amount of bony mass decreases while the size of the bone remains constant, making bone more brittle and more susceptible to fractures. It is a major health problem in the United States, potentially affecting as many as 15-20 million Americans and causing over a million fractures a year in people over the age of 45. The risk of osteoporosis increases with age and is higher in females than in males.

## ASSESSMENT

**Signs and symptoms:**    Documented loss of bone density, most commonly found in conjunction with pathologic fractures secondary to osteoporosis. Most fractures occur in the dorsal (thoracic) and lumbar vertebral bodies (usually D–8 through L–2), the neck and intertrochanteric regions of the femur, and the distal radius. Vertebral compression fractures can develop gradually, resulting in loss of height, kyphosis, back discomfort, and constipation. Fractures of the hip result in significant morbidity and mortality.

**History and risk factors:**    Loss of ovarian function (surgical or physiologic menopause), race (nonblack, especially Caucasian or Asiatic), family history, nulliparity, preexisting skeletal disease, underweight, inadequate childhood nutrition (lifelong low calcium intake), high caffeine intake, sedentary life-style, high alcohol intake, increased protein intake, and cigarette smoking. Secondary causes include metastatic disease, drugs (heparin, alcohol, phosphate-binding antacids, corticosteroids, phenytoin, and isoniazid), hyperparathyroidism, immobilization, hypercortisolism, hyperthyroidism, hypogonadism, and connective tissue disease.

## DIAGNOSTIC TESTS

**Standard A–P and lateral x-rays of the spine:**    Provide a diagnosis for osteoporotic fractures. Bone density loss is not easily demonstrated by standard radiographs, since 20%-30% of bone density must be lost before it can be noted on x-ray.

**Radiogrammetry, photodensitometry, single- and dual-photon absorptiometry, neutron activation, quantitative digital radiography, and single- and dual-energy T-scan:**    These are examples of some of the sophisticated noninvasive tests that can be used to determine bone density. However, the availability of these tests varies, and their usefulness in predicting fracture has been questioned. Bone mass measurement is indicated in individuals who are at risk.

## COLLABORATIVE MANAGEMENT

**Hormonal replacement:**    Doses as low as 0.625 mg of estrogen have been shown to be effective in preventing osteoporosis in postmenopausal women. Once begun, estrogen replacement therapy must be used long-term to provide protection. Use of cyclic estrogen/progesterone also may reduce the risk of endometrial cancer. Osteoporotic men may require testosterone replacement.

**Calcium intake:**    Should exceed 1,000-1,500 mg/day for women approaching menopause. Each 8-oz glass of milk provides 275-300 mg of calcium, indicating that an intake of 4-6 glasses/day is ideal. Vegetable calcium sources (e.g., dark green, leafy vegetables; sesame seeds) are also good. For lactose-intolerant patients or those unable to consume dietary calcium, calcium supplementation is prescribed. Some antacids (e.g., Tums) contain calcium and may serve as a calcium supplement. In individuals prone to osteoporosis, life-long intake of adequate amounts of calcium should be stressed. Adequate (1,200 mg/day) calcium intake in adolescents is especially important to meet pubertal growth spurt. **Note:** Because smoking and a high-sugar, high-meat diet affect the phosphorus-calcium ratio, and therefore calcium utilization, individuals who do not smoke or eat red meat or sugar have a lower calcium requirement.

**Vitamin D:** Necessary to allow adequate intestinal absorption and usage of calcium. Adequate dietary vitamin D usually is supplied in vitamin-enriched cereals and milk products. When necessary, the recommended daily intake of this vitamin is 600-800 U twice daily. Because excessive vitamin D is associated with significant toxicity, higher intake is discouraged without clear documentation of need. Patients with liver or renal disease may require synthetic, biologically active forms of vitamin D. Vitamin D requires activation in the skin by sunlight to be effective.

**Moderate weight-bearing exercise:** To stress bones and activate osteoblastic bone formation, because inactivity has been shown to result in disuse osteoporosis. Williams' back extension exercises, pectoral stretching, isometric abdominal exercises, and walking often are recommended. For older individuals, swimming appears to be the best all-around exercise. Women athletes who become hypogonadal lose bone despite high-intensity exercise.

**Antiresorptive agents:** To reduce further bone mass loss. The most effective is calcitonin, although its action is not sustained, and prolonged therapy has been ineffective in correcting the disease process. Additional antiresorptive agents include androgen and biphosphonates. Fluoride is the only therapeutic agent known to stimulate osteoblastic activity. However, fluoride has not demonstrated the ability to restore the normal architecture of osteoporotic bone. Thiazide diuretics reduce urinary calcium excretion and may reduce bone loss in patients with hypercalciuria.

## NURSING DIAGNOSES AND INTERVENTIONS

**Health-seeking behaviors:** Prevention of osteoporosis, its treatment, and the importance of choosing and using calcium supplements effectively

*Desired outcome:* Within 48 h of instruction, patient verbalizes knowledge about the disease process and understanding of the most effective calcium supplements and the way in which they are used.

---

**Note:** It is important to begin instructing all individuals at risk for osteoporosis as early in their lives as possible because of the prolonged period of time involved in developing, and thus preventing, this process. Individuals at risk for osteoporosis include those with loss of ovarian function (surgical or physiologic menopause, women athletes), family history, nulliparity, preexisting skeletal disease, underweight, inadequate childhood nutrition (lifelong low calcium intake), high caffeine intake, increased protein intake, sedentary lifestyle, high alcohol intake, cigarette smoking, and Caucasians and Asians. The risk of osteoporosis increases with age and is higher in females than in males. Secondary causes include metastatic disease, drugs (heparin, alcohol, phosphate-binding antacids, corticosteroids, phenytoin, and isoniazid), hyperparathyroidism, immobilization, hypercortisolism, hyperthyroidism, hypogonadism, and connective tissue disease.

---

- Ensure that the physician has recommended or approves use of calcium supplements for the patient. Increased calcium can result in nephrolithiasis in susceptible individuals.

- Be sure patient is aware of the silent nature of this disorder and realizes that by the time symptoms arise, it is too late for effective treatment.
- Teach patient that calcium supplements come in many varieties. The most effective form is calcium carbonate, which delivers about 40% calcium. Bonemeal and dolomite should be avoided because they may contain high amounts of lead or other toxic substances.
- Teach patient to look for the amount of elemental calcium available when evaluating supplement labels, rather than the weight of the total compound, and to avoid supplements with added vitamin D because hypervitaminosis of this vitamin is possible. Remind patients of the need for 15 min/day of sunlight to allow for activation of vitamin D.
- Teach patient not to take calcium and iron supplements simultaneously, because iron absorption will be impaired. Calcium also may reduce the absorption of some medications. Similarly, some foods inhibit absorption of calcium (e.g., red meats, spinach, colas, bran, bread, and whole grain cereals). Therefore, calcium should be taken 2 h before or after other medications or meals. Calcium is best absorbed at night and should be taken at hs.
- Caution patient to avoid taking more than 500-600 mg of calcium at one time and to spread doses over the entire day. Remind patient to drink a full glass of water with each supplement to minimize the risk of developing renal calculi.

**Altered nutrition:** Less than body requirements for calcium and vitamin D
*Desired outcome:* Patient demonstrates intake of adequate amounts of calcium and vitamin D and within the 24-h period before hospital discharge plans a 3-day menu that provides sufficient intake of both.

- Ensure that the patient demonstrates understanding of the foods high in calcium, including cheese, milk, dark green leafy vegetables, eggs, peanuts, sesame seeds, and oysters. Provide patient with a list of these foods, including the relative amounts of calcium in each.
- Teach patient how to plan menus that provide sufficient daily intake of calcium and vitamin D-fortified foods, such as eggs, halibut, herring, fortified dairy products, liver, mackerel, oysters, salmon, and sardines.
- Provide patient with sample menus that include adequate daily amounts of calcium and vitamin D. Have patient plan a 3-day menu that incorporates these foods.
- Provide patient with phone numbers to call if questions arise after hospital discharge.

---

**Note:** See "Amputation" for **Knowledge deficit:** Postsurgical exercise regimen, p. 566. Moderate weight-bearing exercise is necessary to stress the bones and activate osteoblastic bone formation.

---

## PATIENT-FAMILY TEACHING AND DISCHARGE PLANNING

Give patient and significant others verbal and written information about the following:
- Medications, including the name, dosage, purpose, schedule, precautions, and potential side effects.
- Instructions for the prescribed dietary regimen, including the rationale for the diet and foods to include and avoid, if appropriate.
- Prescribed exercise regimen, including how to perform the exercise, number of repetitions of each, and frequency of exercise periods (see **Knowledge deficit:** Postsurgical exercise regimen, p. 566).
- Importance of establishing measures for preventing falls in the home (e.g., placing a handrail in the bathtub, installing nightlights, avoiding use of throw rugs). Arrange for a home visit for fall prevention as necessary.
- Importance of reporting to health-care provider indicators of pathologic frac-

ture (i.e., deformity, pain, edema, ecchymosis, limb shortening, false motion, decreased ROM, or crepitus). Stress promptly reporting indicators of vertebral fractures resulting in spinal cord or nerve compression (e.g., paresthesias, weakness, paralysis, or loss of bowel or bladder function).

# Paget's disease (osteitis deformans)

Paget's disease is an idiopathic process suspected of being caused by a slow viral infection in genetically susceptible individuals (it has a familial distribution). In the population over age 40, 3%-4% have some Pagetic findings, and 20% over age 80 have some Pagetic bone. More males are affected than females. This disorder results from an aberrant function of osteoclasts (bone-resorbing cells) and osteoblasts (bone-building cells), resulting in bone that is high in mineral content, weakened, of poor quality, grossly deformed, and thickened. Active lesions have increased vascularity and have been attributed to high-output cardiac failure in extensive disease. Viruslike particles have been found with diseased bone cells, promoting the theory that this process results from a slow virus.

## ASSESSMENT

**Signs and symptoms:**   Most patients are asymptomatic except for pain at the involved site(s), which can be difficult to differentiate from osteoarthritis or myalgia. Some patients develop pathologic fractures through the Pagetic lesions, or the process can be an incidental finding on x-rays taken to rule out other processes. Cranial enlargement or radiculoneuropathy can result in the following: oculomotor deficits, visual deficits, deafness, dysphagia, dysphasia, headaches, hemifacial paresthesias, or paralysis. Vertebral involvement is evidenced by kyphoscoliosis or stenotic lesions of the spinal cord or nerves, resulting in radiculoneuropathy of these structures. Patients with Paget's disease who are suddenly immobilized may develop hypercalciuria and even hypercalcemia.

## DIAGNOSTIC TESTS

**Standard x-rays:**   May reveal typical mosaic-appearing lesions, osteoporosis circumscripta (an area of radiolucency surrounded by normal bone), protrusio acetabuli (protrusion of the acetabulum into the pelvis), pseudofractures, microfractures, incomplete transverse fractures, sclerotic bony lesions, invaginated foramen magnum, and pathologic fractures. Lesions present a typical mosaic pattern.
**Serum tests:**   Will reveal an elevated serum alkaline phosphatase, indicating new bone formation.
**Urine assay:**   Will reveal elevated hydroxyproline, indicating bony lysis. This expensive test is not routinely available and requires a meat-free diet and a 24-h urine collection.
**Bone biopsy:**   Can be used to confirm the diagnosis in questionable cases.
**Bone scans:**   Technetium pyrophosphate may aid in identifying active bone lesions.
**MRI:**   Reveals areas of osteolytic and osteoblastic change.

## COLLABORATIVE MANAGEMENT

Because the treatment involves significant risk, it is restricted to patients who have pervasive disease or significant symptoms of involvement in critical areas. Suppressive therapy is restricted to patients with radiculoneuropathy, imminent complications, and highly resorptive lesions, and who are immobilized or require surgery on involved areas.
**NSAIDs:**   May be used to control pain (see Table 8-1).

**Suppressive therapy** may include the following:
*Calcitonin (porcine, human, and salmon):*    50-100 Medical Research Council (MRC) U SC, 3 times a week to as frequently as 200 MRC q12h. This hormone inhibits bone resorption while combating parathyroid gland action. Side effects include nausea, a feeling of warmth following injection, and flushing. Mild allergic reactions (e.g., rash, itching, facial swelling) may be controlled by 2-h predosing with antihistamines. Salmon calcitonin is the most potent form and may result in allergic reaction with skin manifestations. Calcitonin therapy is expensive, and long-term therapy has not been proven to control progression of this disease in all patients. Concurrent calcium should be provided.
*Diphosphonates (etidronate disodium [EHDP]):*    Daily dosages of 5 mg/kg of body weight. Diphosphonates inhibit calcium deposition in biologic tissues. Side effects include cramps, diarrhea, and nausea. EHDP should be given on an empty stomach for optimal absorption. This medication is contraindicated in patients with new fractures or who are immobilized, and it can increase the risk of pathologic fracture in patients with extensive disease. Because of their adverse effect on normal bone (i.e., spontaneous fractures due to demineralization), diphosphonates are indicated for short-term therapy only. These agents may produce a metallic taste or loss of the sense of taste.
*Mithramycin:*    A cytotoxic agent given in short courses (10 doses) of 25 μg/kg IV. It is theorized that this medication suppresses the action of osteoclasts in bone resorption. Toxic reactions with mithramycin may be severe, limiting its use to the most severe cases. Side effects include anorexia, nausea, vomiting; elevated SGOT, BUN, and creatinine; and depressed platelets and leukocytes.
**Surgical interventions:**    Restricted to repair of pathologic fractures. Surgery on involved bones requires adequate preparation *via* typing and cross-matching of several units of blood, meticulous hemostasis during surgery, and careful monitoring for hemorrhage after surgery.
**Orthotics:**    May be used to allow protective weight-bearing of pseudofractures.

## NURSING DIAGNOSES AND INTERVENTIONS

**Knowledge deficit:**    Potential complications of Paget's disease
*Desired outcome:*    Within 24 h of instruction, patient verbalizes knowledge about the disease pathology and awareness of the importance of promptly reporting untoward indicators to the health-care provider.
- Teach patient the disease pathology, including the signs and symptoms of imminent complications, such as renal calculi (see p. 123), significant cranial or spinal radiculoneuropathy (decreased hearing; headache; paresthesias; weakness; paralysis; visual defects; dysphasia; dysphagia; oculomotor weakness); hydrocephalus (headache, pupil inequality, altered LOC); and alterations in gait.
- Instruct patient to report any indicators of pathologic fracture: pain, deformity, decreased ROM, limb shortening, ecchymosis, edema, false motion, and crepitus.

---

**Note:**    See "Gouty Arthritis" for **Knowledge deficit:** Signs and symptoms and preventive measures for uric acid renal calculi, p. 524. See "Total Knee Arthroplasty" for **High risk for fluid volume deficit** related to postsurgical hemorrhage or hematoma formation), p. 578.

---

## PATIENT-FAMILY TEACHING AND DISCHARGE PLANNING

Give patient and significant others verbal and written information about the following:

- Medications, including drug name, purpose, dosage, schedule, potential side effects, and precautions.
- Signs to monitor for and report while on suppressive therapy, especially ecchymosis, melena, hematoma, and hematuria, as well as indicators of prolonged bleeding, hemorrhage, and superimposed infections.
- Indicators to monitor for and report related to complications of the disease (see **Knowledge deficit,** p. 561).

# Section Four:   Musculoskeletal Surgical Procedures

## Bunionectomy

Bunionectomy is surgery to correct hallux valgus. Hallux refers to the great toe, and valgus means that it is bent outward, away from the midline. The bunion is actually a prominence of the first metatarsal head, resulting from altered joint dynamics as the hallux subluxates laterally into a valgus deformity. Although a bunion can occur because of hereditary intrinsic joint weakness, the most frequent cause is improperly fitting footwear. Bunions occur most frequently in females (9 times more often than in men), and they have a familiar distribution.

### ASSESSMENT

**Signs and symptoms:**   Can range from mild valgus deformity to severe valgus deformity with altered gait. In acute conditions, the patient has inflammation of the adventitial bursa, resulting in erythema, local warmth, and tenderness. The patient has great difficulty fitting shoes. X-rays often are used to define bony involvement and displacement of the lateral sesamoid bone.

### COLLABORATIVE MANAGEMENT

**Conservative treatment:**   Begins with appropriately fitted footwear to accommodate the deformity. Night splints may be useful in decreasing discomfort for some patients, although they have not been effective in preventing progression of hallux valgus.

**Bunionectomy:**   Performed when the patient has significant pain and alterations in ambulation affecting ADL. Many forms of surgery can be used, but the main elements include removal of the projecting metatarsal head (bunionectomy), excision of the displaced sesamoid bone, release of the adductor hallucis tendon, and tightening of the medial periarticular tissues to prevent recurrence. Transfixion of the repaired joint with a K-wire may be necessary to enhance support, especially if an osteotomy is used in the correction. The tip of the K-wire is left exposed and removed 10-21 days after surgery. Ambulation with appropriate immobilization of the involved foot is begun within 2-5 days of surgery. A short leg cast, slipper cast, or bunion boot is used for immobilization of the great toe.

### NURSING DIAGNOSES AND INTERVENTIONS

**Pain** related to joint changes and corrective therapy
*Desired outcomes:*   Within 1-2 h of intervention, patient's subjective perception of pain decreases, as documented by a pain scale. Objective indicators, such as grimacing, are absent or diminished.
- Patients recovering from bunionectomy often experience a great deal of discomfort. Devise a scale with patient, rating pain from 0 (no pain) to 10 (worst pain) to help determine degree of discomfort and analgesic relief.

- Administer analgesics and antiinflammatory agents as prescribed, and document their effectiveness. Discuss with physician the use of epidural anesthesia and patient-controlled analgesia.
- Instruct patient in the use of nonpharmacologic methods of pain control, including guided imagery; graduated breathing (as in Lamaze); enhanced relaxation; massage; biofeedback; cutaneous stimulation (*via* a counterirritant such as oil of wintergreen); TENS device; warm or cool thermotherapy; music therapy; and tactile, auditory, visual, or verbal distractions.
- Use traditional nursing interventions to counteract the pain, including backrubs, repositioning, and encouraging the patient to verbalize feelings.
- Incorporate rest, local ice for 24-72 h followed by warmth, and elevation of the affected joints, when possible, to help control discomfort.
- Advise patient to coordinate the time of peak effectiveness of the antiinflammatory agent with periods of exercise or mandatory use of the foot.
- Teach patient how to use moist heat and hydrotherapy, which will help reduce long-term discomfort.
- For additional interventions, see this nursing diagnosis in Appendix One, p. 694.

**Knowledge deficit:** Disease process and therapeutic regimen
*Desired outcome:* Before hospital discharge, patient verbalizes knowledge about bunion formation, preventive measures, prescribed postoperative immobilization, and potential complications.

- Assess patient's level of understanding about the disease process and treatment modalities involved.
- Provide instruction about causes and progression of bunion formation, role of improperly fitting shoes as a cause of bunions because of the need for room to allow free movement of the toes, role of surgery in bunion correction, rationale for the postoperative regimen of care, need for immobilization of the surgical area to promote healing and maintain realignment, technique for caring for the casted extremity (or dressed foot), and indicators of wound infection.
- As appropriate, provide written material for cast care, indicators of wound infection, wound care, neurovascular deficit, and use of appropriate pain medication. For further information on cast care, see **Knowledge deficit:** Care and assessment of the casted extremity, p. 531, in "Ligamentous Injuries."

**Impaired physical mobility** related to immobilization device or nonweight-bearing secondary to bunionectomy
*Desired outcomes:* Patient demonstrates compliance with elevation of the operant extremity above the level of the heart during the early postoperative period. Patient demonstrates use of safety measures while ambulating with the immobilization device.

- After surgery, the patient is permitted bathroom privileges with a walker or crutches, with weight-bearing as tolerated. At other times, ensure that the operant extremity is kept elevated higher than the level of the heart to facilitate reduction of postoperative edema. **Note:** Patients with plaster of Paris casts are restricted to nonweight–bearing ambulation until 48 h after the cast has been applied.
- The patient begins ambulation wearing a cast or bunion boot that is worn for 3-6 weeks after surgery. Remind patient that the primary goal of the immobilization device is to maintain position of the great toe. Caution patient to ambulate with care in the device until it becomes an integral part of ambulation. Special care should be exercised on stairs, hills, and uneven surfaces.

**High risk for peripheral neurovascular dysfunction** related to interrupted arterial flow secondary to compression from circumferential cast or dressing
*Desired outcomes:* Patient has adequate peripheral neurovascular function in the involved extremity as evidenced by normal color, warmth, brisk capillary

refill (<2 sec), distal pulses >2+ on a 0-4+ scale, ability to move the great toe, and absence of numbness or tingling. Patient verbalizes knowledge about the signs of impaired neurovascular status and the importance of getting prompt treatment if they occur.

- Assess the operant extremity for the integrity of neurovascular status each time VS are taken (or at least q4h or more frequently as indicated). Impaired neurovascular status requires nursing interventions, such as elevation, loosening of restrictive dressings, or promptly notifying the physician if these measures are ineffective.
- Ensure that the patient can verbalize the signs and symptoms of impaired neurovascular status and knows that it is important to call the physician if they occur after hospital discharge. These indicators include persistent changes in color (pallor, cyanosis, redness), coolness, delayed capillary refill, paresthesias (numbness, tingling), or inability to move distal areas (the great or second toe).
- For additional interventions, see this nursing diagnosis in "Ischemic Myositis," p. 540.

---

**Note:**  See "Osteoarthritis" for **Impaired physical mobility** related to musculoskeletal impairment and adjustment to a new walking gait, p. 521. Also see Appendix One, "Caring for Preoperative and Postoperative Patients," p. 693.

---

## PATIENT-FAMILY TEACHING AND DISCHARGE PLANNING

Give patient and significant others verbal and written information about the following:

- Technique for ambulation with the casted extremity or bunion boot and use of assistive devices and ambulatory aids (see **Impaired physical mobility** related to adjustment to a new walking gait, p. 521). Be sure the patient demonstrates independence in ADL before hospital discharge. If necessary, arrange for follow-up instruction *via* a home visit.
- Medications, including name, rationale, dosage, schedule, precautions, and potential side effects.
- Indicators of wound infection (see "Fractures," p. 552) and impaired neurovascular status (see "Ligamentous Injuries," p. 531) and the importance of notifying physician promptly should they occur.
- Use of thermotherapy, elevation, and exercise (see "Ligamentous Injuries," p. 530).
- Phone number to call should patient have questions after hospital discharge.

# Amputation

Today amputation is less frequently required as an orthopedic surgical intervention than it was before the advent of antibiotics and microsurgery techniques. However, amputation is still required for certain disorders such as atherosclerotic arterial occlusive disease, osteomyelitis, severe trauma, malignant tumors, or congenital anomalies. In the United States, most amputations are performed for advanced atherosclerotic arterial occlusive disease, especially in individuals with diabetes mellitus over age 60 with pronounced peripheral vascular disease, as evidenced by gangrene. When it is possible to increase a person's function with a prosthesis, amputation is sometimes offered as an optional treatment. The majority of amputations are of the lower extremity.

## ASSESSMENT

**Signs and symptoms:**  Patients with advanced atherosclerotic arterial occlusive disease may have gangrene, a chronic stasis ulcer, or an infected wound that fails to heal. The patient usually complains of pain, and there can be rubor (a dark red color) when the limb is dependent, as well as atrophy of the skin and subcutaneous tissues.

---

**Note:** See "Atherosclerotic Arterial Occlusive Disease," p. 96, "Osteomyelitis," p. 542, and "Malignant Neoplasms," p. 555, as appropriate.

---

## DIAGNOSTIC TESTS

**Angiography:** Confirms inadequacy of circulation.

**CT scan:** Determines the degree of neoplastic or osteomyelitic involvement.

**Biopsy:** May be used to confirm presence of osteomyelitis or neoplasm.

**Extensive evaluations by occupational therapist for fine motor function and by physical therapist for gross motor function:** To document functional loss and potential for compensation.

**Noninvasive vascular testing:** Documents lack of perfusion of blood vessels, using a Doppler ultrasound device and pneumatic cuffs. Use of a Doppler to measure velocity of flow of microcirculation beneath the skin shows promise as another measure. Dopplers may be either ultrasound or laser. Plethysmography may be used to assess differing systolic pressures with the affected extremity to determine arterial flow. Thermography examines temperatures in the extremity to determine areas of decreased vascularity.

**Xenon-133 studies:** Skin clearance of this agent after intradermal injection is determined using a gamma camera and computer. Skin clearance reflects skin blood flow as a measure of the appropriate level of amputation.

**Skin fluorescence:** Measuring skin fluorescence with a fluorometer after IV injection of a fluorescein dye is useful in determining blood supply.

**Oximetry:** Transcutaneous determination of $Pao_2$ aids in determining levels of tissue perfusion. Levels >40 mm Hg usually support tissue healing.

**Laboratory tests:** Serum albumin <3.5 g/ml and a total lymphocyte count <1,500 cells/$\mu$l portend significant problems with healing.

## COLLABORATIVE MANAGEMENT

**Amputation:** The procedure used for amputation depends on the area of the limb involved. Generally the surgical goals are to remove the least amount of tissue possible, provide adequate tissue for a viable myocutaneous flap to create a stump, and ensure adequate provision for a prosthetic device. Large blood vessels are individually identified and suture-ligated. Nerves are stretched and then suture-ligated to allow them to retract back into the residual limb (stump) to prevent trauma when the stump is used. Usually bone ends are beveled to prevent trauma from sharp edges. Infected limbs are closed loosely to allow adequate drainage until infected tissues have been treated adequately.

Amputees expend more energy in ambulation than nonamputees: the longer the limb, the lower the amount of energy consumed. Levels of lower extremity amputation include the foot and ankle, below-knee, knee disarticulation and above-knee, hemipelvectomy, and translumbar (hemicorporectomy). En bloc resections for osteosarcoma allow for extensive procedures that replace the knee, such as the reversed ankle (rotationplasty), which allows for greater postoperative function.

**Postoperative period:** Immediately after surgery, an immediate postoperative prosthesis (IPOP) may be used to promote wound healing, minimize stump edema, decrease the length of rehabilitation, and prevent postsurgical complications of immobility. A cast is applied over the postoperative dressing, which incorporates a device that allows subsequent attachment of a pylon prosthesis to allow ambulation while the first prosthesis is being made. Plain casts or air splints may be applied to postoperative dressings to reduce edema. Early ambulation prevents flexion contractures, allows earlier gait training, improves psychologic state, prevents loss of muscle strength, and increases local circulation to improve wound healing, which subsequently decreases edema and pain. Complications associated with amputations include infection and thromboembolism in the early postoperative period, increased mortality rates (less than 50% of all lower extremity amputees survive 5 years), fractures in the stump following falls, and stump ischemia.

## NURSING DIAGNOSES AND INTERVENTIONS

**High risk for disuse syndrome** related to severe pain and immobility secondary to amputation

*Desired outcomes:*   Within 24 h of instruction, patient verbalizes understanding about the exercise regimen and performs the exercises independently. Patient is free of symptoms of contracture formation as evidenced by complete ROM of the joints and maintenance of muscle mass.

- Control patient's pain to ensure appropriate movement.
- After providing elevation for the first 2 days postoperatively, intersperse elevation with periods of ROM to the remaining joints of the involved extremity. **Caution:** Both elevation and ROM are performed only if prescribed by physician. A stump with marginal vascular supply must not be elevated.
- Prevent flexion contractures of the knee and hip by assisting the patient with lying prone for an hour 3 times a day.
- Another method for preventing flexion contractures is to teach the patient to perform exercises that increase the strength of the muscle extensors. Consult with physician about prescriptions for the following exercises:
  - *Above-the-knee amputation* (AKA): Have patient attempt to straighten the hip from a flexed position against resistance or perform gluteal setting exercises.
  - *Below-the-knee amputation:* Have patient attempt to straighten the knee against resistance or perform quadriceps-setting exercises. These patients also should perform the exercises described above for AKA.
- For other interventions, see **High risk for disuse syndrome,** p. 713, in Appendix One.

**Impaired physical mobility** related to altered stance secondary to amputation of the lower limb

*Desired outcome:*   Within 2 days of beginning ambulation, patient demonstrates use of muscle-tightening technique to enhance mobilization.

- Inform patients with lower extremity amputation that difficulty in adjusting to the altered stance may occur as a result of the amputation. Suggest that to prevent an altered stance, patient should tighten the gluteal and abdominal muscles while standing.
- For other interventions, see **Impaired physical mobility** related to musculoskeletal impairment and adjustment to a new walking gait with an assistive device, p. 521, in "Osteoarthritis."

**Knowledge deficit:**   Postsurgical exercise regimen

*Desired outcome:*   Within 8 h of instruction, patient verbalizes knowledge about the exercise regimen and returns the demonstration independently.

- To increase adherence to the prescribed exercise regimen, provide patient with an explanation of the rationale for the exercises, method of performing the exercises, and suggestions for adapting these exercises to home use. Most therapeutic programs include ROM and muscle-strengthening exercises.
- Demonstrate each exercise until the patient is able to return the demonstration independently. Provide patient with written instructions that describe each exercise and the number of repetitions and number of times a day it should be performed. Also provide a phone number to call if any questions arise after patient is discharged. If necessary, provide for a postdischarge home visit.
- If additional equipment is required, provide patient with information about where it can be purchased, and if necessary, seek financial assistance from social services.

**Knowledge deficit:** Care of the stump and prosthesis; signs and symptoms of skin irritation or pressure necrosis
*Desired outcomes:* Within the 24-h period before hospital discharge, patient verbalizes knowledge about the care of the stump and prosthesis and independently returns demonstration of wrapping the stump. Patient verbalizes knowledge about the indicators of pressure necrosis and irritation from the wrapping device or prosthesis.

---

**Note:** A stump that is inappropriately treated will become edematous and more easily prone to injury, which will delay proper fitting of the permanent prosthesis.

---

- If molding of the stump for eventual prosthetic fitting is prescribed, instruct the patient in the technique for application of an elastic sleeve or wrap: Application of the elastic wrap is begun with a recurrent turn over the distal end of the stump, and then diagonal circumferential turns are made, overlapping one-half to two-thirds the width of the wrap. Traction applied to the wrap should ensure more pressure on the distal portion of the stump. The elastic device should be snug but not excessively so, because a tight wrap can impede circulation and healing. Rewrapping should be performed q4h, combined with careful inspection of the stump. Areas prone to pressure, such as bony prominences or prominent tendons, should be assessed for evidence of excess pressure. Ensure that all tissue is contained by the elastic device. If any tissue is allowed to bulge, proper fitting of the prosthesis will be difficult.
- Teach patient to monitor the stump for indicators of skin irritation or pressure necrosis caused by the elastic device or prosthesis, including blebs, abrasions, and erythemic or tender areas. Explain that if massage fails to alleviate the problem, the patient should seek the help of the public health nurse or visiting nurse or notify the physician.
- For areas that are prone to pressure, provide extra padding with sheet wadding, moleskin, or lamb's wool to prevent irritation.
- The day after the sutures have been removed (and assuming the incision is dry and intact) instruct the patient to cleanse the stump daily with mild soap and water. Caution against the use of emollients, which can create skin maceration beneath the prosthesis.
- Advise patient that when molding is no longer necessary (after 1-6 months), he or she will be fitted with a stump sock that will allow air to circulate around the stump.
- Ensure that the patient receives complete instructions in care of the prosthesis by the certified prosthetist-orthotist or knowledgable nurse.

**High risk for fluid volume deficit** related to postsurgical hemorrhage
*Desired outcomes:* Patient is normovolemic as evidenced by BP ≥90/60 (or within patient's usual range), HR ≤100 bpm, urinary output ≥30 ml/h, peripheral pulses >2+ on a 0-4+ scale, brisk capillary refill (<2 sec), and drainage ≤50 ml/h in a drainage device. Patient verbalizes knowledge of the importance of reporting bleeding promptly to the staff.
- Inspect the cast (or postoperative dressing) for increasing drainage. If the stump is elevated, inspect dependent areas for evidence of bleeding. Inform patient of the need to report increasing bleeding to staff. Also monitor VS for systemic evidence of bleeding, including hypotension, tachycardia, and pallor, as well as decreased amplitude of peripheral pulses and delayed capillary refill in the involved limb.
- If a drain or drainage device is used, document the amount of drainage. Report drainage that exceeds 50 ml/h.

**Pain** related to phantom limb sensation
*Desired outcomes:* Within 24 h of intervention(s), patient relates a reduc-

tion in phantom limb sensations as documented by a pain scale. Objective indicators, such as facial grimacing, are absent or diminished.

- Explain to patient that continued sensations often arise from the amputated part, and they can be painful, irritating, or simply disconcerting. As appropriate, devise a pain scale with patient, rating discomfort on a scale of 0 (no pain) to 10 (worst pain).
- Instruct patient in the basis for pharmacologic interventions. Beta blockers may be used to control dull, constant aching by increasing central and peripheral nervous system serotonin level. Anticonvulsant agents may be used to treat severe lancinating (sharply cutting or tearing) pain by decreasing neuronal excitability. Tricyclic antidepressants may be used to elevate the amputee's mood. Local anesthetics may be used in trigger zones on the contralateral limb.
- Manage these painful sensations with the interventions discussed in **Pain,** p. 520, in "Osteoarthritis." For this type of pain, counterirritation is especially useful. Other phantom limb sensations may respond to similar tactics, such as distraction, relaxation, biofeedback, psychotherapy, behavior modification, hypnosis, whirlpool, ultrasound, reciprocal motion (cycling), or use of cutaneous stimulation *via* oil of wintergreen, heat, or massage. Transcutaneous electrical nerve stimulation has been found to be especially effective in managing phantom limb sensation.
- Some physicians advocate vigorous stimulation of the end of the stump to alter the feedback loop of the resected nerve. Advise patient that this can be accomplished by hitting the end of a *well-healed* stump with a rolled towel.
- Chronic phantom limb sensation may require exploration of the stump to resect a neuroma at the site of the nerve resection. Inform patient that this may be a possibility if phantom limb sensation continues for more than 6 months. Use of epidural anesthesia in the perioperative period shows promise in reducing phantom limb pain.
- For additional interventions, see this nursing diagnosis in Appendix One, p. 694.

**Body image disturbance** *and/or* **altered role performance** related to loss of limb
*Desired outcome:*    Within 72 h of surgery, patient begins to show adaptation toward loss of the limb and demonstrates role-related responsibilities.

- Be aware that use of a prosthesis immediately after surgery allows patients to continue to perceive themselves as ambulatory (and thus "whole") individuals.
- Gently encourage patient to look at and touch the stump and verbalize feelings about the amputation. The nurse and other caregivers must show an accepting attitude, as well as encourage significant others to accept the patient as he or she now appears. Provide privacy for the patient and significant others to express their grief.
- Assist patient with adapting to the loss of the limb while maintaining a sense of what is perceived as the normal self. This may be accomplished by introducing patient to others who have successfully adapted to a similar amputation. In addition, teaching aids, such as audiovisuals, books, pamphlets, and videotapes, can be used to demonstrate how others have adapted to the amputation.
- For patients who continue to have difficulty adapting to the amputation, provide a referral to an appropriate resource person, such as a psychologist or psychiatric nurse.
- For additional interventions, see **Body image disturbance** in Appendix One, p. 760.

**Note:**   See "Intervertebral Disk Disease" for **Health-seeking behavior:** Pain control measures, p. 228. See "Osteoarthritis" for **Pain,** p. 520. See "Fractures" for **Knowledge deficit:** Potential for infection, p. 552. See Appendix

One for nursing diagnoses and interventions in "Caring for Preoperative and Postoperative Patients," p. 693, and "Caring for Patients with Cancer and Other Life-Disrupting Illnesses," p. 719.

## PATIENT-FAMILY TEACHING AND DISCHARGE PLANNING

Give patient and significant others verbal and written information about the following:

- How and where to purchase necessary supplies and equipment for self-care.
- Care of the stump and prosthesis.
- Indicators of wound infection, which necessitate medical attention: swelling, persistent redness, discharge, local warmth, systemic fever, and pain. Suggest the use of a small hand mirror, if necessary, to examine the incision and stump.
- Medications, including name, rationale, dosage, schedule, precautions, and potential side effects.
- Phone number of a resource person, should questions arise after hospital discharge.
- Prescribed exercises. Patient should be able to perform them independently before discharge.
- Referral to appropriate resource person, should maladaptive behaviors associated with grieving or body image disturbance continue.
- Ambulation with assistive device and prosthesis on level and uneven surfaces and on stairs. Patient should demonstrate independence before hospital discharge. For patients with an upper extremity amputation, independence with ADL should be demonstrated before discharge. If necessary, arrange for a home visit.

## Tendon transfer

A tendon transfer involves the transference of the insertion site of a functioning muscle-tendon unit to a new position to change the action of that unit. This enables compensation for a deficit created by congenital defect or paralyzed or severed muscle. Because there is considerable overlap in function, in that multiple muscles can serve one purpose, tendon transfer may allow the patient to regain function.

## DIAGNOSTIC TESTS

**Electromyography:**   Can be used to ensure adequate muscle function of the units proposed for transfer.

**Dynmography:**   Grip or pinch strength may be assessed pre- or postoperatively.

## COLLABORATIVE MANAGEMENT

**Surgical procedure:**   Involves transection of the tendon at an appropriate level, transfer to the new position, and fixation to the appropriate insertion site with permanent sutures, staples, screws, or wire. It also is possible to attach "new" tendon to the resected tendon above the insertion site, using tendon repair suture techniques. Examples of disorders in which tendon transfer procedures are performed include radial paralysis, congenital talipes equinovarus (a form of clubfoot), thumb carpometacarpal joint osteoarthritis, and extensive injury to the extensor pollicis longus that limits thumb extension.

**Postsurgical immobilization:**   The operant area is immobilized in a cast, splint, or orthosis until there has been sufficient healing of the tendon repair (2-6 weeks) or stabilization of the bony insertion (4-12 weeks).

**Physical therapy (PT) regimen:**   After immobilization, the patient is begun on an intense, progressive PT regimen to regain strength in the transferred tendon, retrain new muscle function, and compensate for decreased strength at the site of the transfer. Various orthotics, dynamic splints, and special exercise rigs can be constructed to aid the patient in regaining function.

## NURSING DIAGNOSES AND INTERVENTIONS

**Note:** See "Osteoarthritis" for **Pain,** p. 520, and **Impaired physical mobility** related to musculoskeletal impairment and adjustment to new walking gait, p. 521. See "Ligamentous Injuries" for **Knowledge deficit:** Care and assessment of the casted extremity, p. 531. See "Total Knee Arthroplasty" for **High risk for fluid volume deficit** related to postsurgical hemorrhage or hematoma formation, p. 578. See "Fractures" for **Self-care deficit,** p. 550. See "Bunionectomy" for **High risk for peripheral neurovascular dysfunction** related to interrupted arterial flow secondary to compression from circumferential cast or dressing, p. 563. See Appendix One for nursing diagnoses and interventions in "Caring for Preoperative and Postoperative Patients," p. 693, "Caring for the Patient on Prolonged Bed Rest," p. 711, and "Caring of Patients with Cancer and Other Life-Disrupting Illnesses," p. 753.

## PATIENT-FAMILY TEACHING AND DISCHARGE PLANNING

Give patient and significant others verbal and written information about the following:

- Use of such therapies as thermotherapy and elevation (see "Ligamentous Injuries," p. 530).
- Use of external support devices such as elastic wraps, splints, orthotics, or similar items (see "Ligamentous Injuries," p. 532). This should include care of the device, care of the skin beneath the device, monitoring the area for presence of irritation, and monitoring for neurovascular deficit.
- Cast care instructions, if patient is discharged with a cast (see "Ligamentous Injuries," p. 531).
- Prescribed exercise regimen, including rationale, how it is accomplished, number of repetitions, and frequency.
- Medications, including name, rationale, dosage, schedule, precautions, and potential side effects.
- Indicators of wound infection, which necessitate medical attention: persistent redness, swelling, wound discharge, local warmth, and increase in pain.
- Use of ambulatory aid, if patient is discharged with one (see "Osteoarthritis," p. 521). This should include return demonstration of independence with ambulation on level and uneven surfaces and stairs before discharge.
- Phone number of resource person, should questions arise after patient has been discharged.

## Bone grafting

A bone graft procedure refers to the transfer of cancellous or cortical bone from one site to another. The bone can be from the patient (autogenic), another human (homogenic), or another species (heterogenic). Currently, the most successful results are achieved with autogenic grafts, but homogenic grafting is showing increasing promise as a therapeutic resource. Bone grafts can be required to create bony fusion of a joint (arthrodesis), compensate for lost or inadequately developed bone, or correct bony nonunion of fractures. Fibrin sealant has been used to aid in securing bone grafts and controlling bleeding, especially in patients with hemorrhagic disorders.

Current microsurgical techniques permit myocutaneous-bone or muscle-bone grafts that include bone, overlying muscle, and/or skin. These complex grafting procedures increase the potential for success of the graft in procedures used to rebuild large areas of tissue loss from trauma or necessary surgical resection. The following discussion is limited to traditional, simple autogenic bone grafting procedures.

## DIAGNOSTIC TESTS

The need for bone grafts can be documented by the following: A–P x-rays, gallium scans (to rule out osteomyelitis), and angiograms to evaluate blood supply when myocutaneous-bone or muscle-bone grafts are to be done.

## COLLABORATIVE MANAGEMENT

**Bone graft procedure:**   Most commonly, bone grafts are taken from the anterior or posterior iliac crest. However, bone grafts also can be harvested from the fibula, tibia, or ribs. The graft usually involves resection of a piece of cortical bone that is fashioned to replace the deficit or enhance bony fusion or aid internal fixation. Usually cancellous bone is taken from the same site and packed in and around the cortical graft to facilitate new bone formation. The donor site frequently oozes blood, so a postoperative drain is often placed.

**Postoperative regimen:**   Usually the recipient site requires immobilization (most often with a cast) to prevent dislodging of the graft. Some bone grafts require internal fixation to hold them in place. Closed drainage systems frequently are placed in the donor site.

## NURSING DIAGNOSES AND INTERVENTIONS

See "Osteoarthritis" for **Pain,** p. 520, and **Impaired physical mobility** related to musculoskeletal impairment and adjustment to new walking gait, p. 521. See "Ligamentous Injuries" for **Knowledge deficit:** Care and assessment of the casted extremity, p. 531. See "Bunionectomy" for **High risk for peripheral neurovascular dysfunction** related to interrupted arterial flow secondary to compression from circumferential cast or dressing, p. 563. See "Total Knee Arthroplasty" for **High risk for fluid volume deficit** related to postsurgical hemorrhage or hematoma formation, p. 578. See Appendix One for nursing diagnoses and interventions in "Caring for Preoperative and Postoperative Patients," p. 693, "Caring for the Patient on Prolonged Bed Rest," p. 711, and "Caring for the Patient with Cancer and Other Life-Disrupting Illnesses," p. 753.

## PATIENT-FAMILY TEACHING AND DISCHARGE PLANNING

See "Tendon Transfer," p. 570.

# Repair of recurrent shoulder dislocation

The shoulder is a complex set of joints including the glenohumeral, sternoclavicular, acromioclavicular, and thoracoscapular joints, all of which act in combination to allow function. Of these joints, the glenohumeral joint is most commonly affected by dislocation. Most glenohumeral dislocations originate with trauma. Once periarticular weakness and laxity are established, the shoulder can dislocate with minimal stress during abduction. A shoulder repair is necessary when the patient has significant pain and compromised function.

---

**Note:**   See "Dislocation/Subluxation," p. 533, for a discussion of assessment, diagnostic tests, and collaborative management.

---

## COLLABORATIVE MANAGEMENT

**Bristow procedure:**   Transfers the short ends of the biceps and coracobrachialis muscular origin sites from the coracoid process to the scapular neck.

The new positions allow these muscles to hold the head of the humerus in its anatomic position within the glenoid cavity.

**Bankart procedure:**   Involves reattaching the anterior joint capsule to the front rim of the glenoid cavity to reduce laxity and prevent anterior dislocation.

**Putti-Platt procedure:**   Involves reefing (shortening) the subscapularis tendon to prevent excessive lateral rotation, which can contribute to dislocation.

**Postoperative care:**   Surgery may be performed arthroscopically or *via* traditional open methods. After surgery, the patient usually is placed in a shoulder immobilizer for 3-6 weeks. If the patient has large shoulder muscles, a postoperative drain may be required. Elbow flexion and extension, forearm pronation and supination, and hand exercises with putty or a soft ball are begun immediately following sugery. After immobilization, a regimen of progressive shoulder ROM exercises is begun, first to regain ROM and then to increase muscle strength. Orthotics may be used to permit motion in specific planes or limit motion in multiple planes.

## NURSING DIAGNOSES AND INTERVENTIONS

**High risk for impaired skin integrity** related to trapping of moisture on the axillary skin secondary to shoulder immobilization

*Desired outcomes:*   Patient's skin remains clear, dry, nonerythematous, and intact. Before hospital discharge, patient verbalizes knowledge of the established plan of prevention and the signs and symptoms of maceration.

- Assess patient's axillary skin before surgery to evaluate the potential for breakdown, including open wounds, areas of irritation, and excessive perspiration.
- Teach patient the rationale and interventions used for preventing breakdown and the need to report indicators such as pain, burning, irritation, and foul odor.
- Cleanse the axilla well before surgery.
- Before the shoulder immobilizer is positioned, the operating room nurse will place a cotton pad in the axilla. After 2-3 days, remove the pad. Then cleanse, dry thoroughly, and inspect the axilla (as well as possible) without abducting the shoulder. Usually this can be done by holding a washcloth dampened in alcohol and sliding the hand back and forth through the axilla. Although talc can be used, its use should be judicious because it can build up and act as a reservoir for moisture. Replace the cotton pad with a new one, and document the condition of the skin. A deodorant pad may be used if the patient is not allergic.

**High risk for peripheral neurovascular dysfunction** related to interrupted arterial flow to and compression of the musculocutaneous nerve secondary to pressure from the immobilization device

*Desired outcomes:*   Patient has adequate peripheral neurovascular function in the operant arm as evidenced by the ability to contract the biceps muscle, presence of normal sensations along the radial portion of the forearm, brisk capillary refill ($<2$ sec), adequate pulses ($>2+$ on a $0-4+$ scale), normal color, and warmth in the distal extremity. Within 8 h of the instruction, patient verbalizes knowledge about the signs and symptoms of impaired neurovascular function and the importance of notifying the staff promptly if they occur.

- Unless it is contraindicated, encourage flexion and extension of the fingers and wrist to enhance perfusion to the distal tissues.
- Monitor the wrist and upper arm for evidence of pressure and irritation from the immobilizer. Be aware, however, that the device must be sufficiently tight to ensure adequate immobilization.
- With every VS assessment, evaluate upper extremity neurovascular function. Be especially alert to patient's inability to contract the biceps muscle, and to absent or abnormal sensations along the radial portion of the forearm. Notify physician of significant findings.

- Instruct patient to notify the staff promptly should any alterations in sensory or motor function occur.

---

**Note:** See "Osteoarthritis" for **Pain,** p. 520. See "Fractures" for **Self-care deficit,** p. 550. See "Amputation" for **Knowledge deficit:** Postsurgical exercise regimen, p. 566. See Appendix One for nursing diagnoses and interventions in "Caring for Preoperative and Postoperative Patients," p. 693.

---

## PATIENT-FAMILY TEACHING AND DISCHARGE PLANNING
Give patient and significant others verbal and written information about the following:
- Prescribed exercise regimen, including rationale for each exercise, method of performing the exercise, number of repetitions for each, and frequency of the exercise periods (see "Ligamentous Injuries," p. 530). Be sure the patient can return the demonstration independently before hospital discharge.
- Indicators of wound infection, which necessitate medical attention: swelling, persistent redness, local warmth, fever, and pain.
- For patients discharged with braces or immobilizers, use and care of the device and care of the axilla on the operant side.
- Indicators of neurovascular deficit: decreasing sensation, paresthesias, weakness or paralysis, coolness, pallor, cyanosis, decreased pulses, delayed capillary refill, and increasing pain in the distal extremity.
- Medications, including name, rationale, dosage, schedule, precautions, and potential side effects.
- Phone number of a resource person, should questions arise after hospital discharge.

## Total hip arthroplasty

Total hip arthroplasty (THA) is surgery involving resection of the hip joint and its replacement with an endoprosthesis. Conditions resulting in the need for a THA include, among others, osteoarthritis, rheumatoid arthritis, ankylosing spondylosis (Marie-Strumpell disease), Legg-Calvé-Perthes disease, and severe hip trauma. Usually, THA is restricted to older patients because the duration of the implant life is unknown. However, younger patients with severe disease also undergo this procedure.

The bipolar or universal endoprosthesis is an intermediary step between replacement of just the femoral head and a complete THA. For this device a polyethylene-lined metal cup fits over the femoral component. Articulation occurs between the femoral component and the inside of the metal cup and between the outside of the metal cup and the anatomic acetabulum. The advantages of this system are that it reduces wear on the acetabulum and allows ease in converting the joint to a THA later. Porous intramedullary stem devices have been designed to improve implantation fixation; however long-term efficacy has not been established.

THA is performed when the joint has been severely affected by disease, resulting in significant pain and a dysfunctional femoroacetabular articulation. Because it is an irreversible procedure involving the removal of significant amounts of bone, several conditions should be met before the patient is considered a serious candidate. In addition to severe pain and loss of function, conservative therapies need to have been exhausted and the patient should have adhered to past therapeutic regimens and be free of any concurrent infectious process. Complications of THA include recurrent dislocations, loosening of the implant, breakage of the femoral component, disabling pain, and sepsis. Of these, infection is the most serious and eventually may necessitate removal of the prosthesis, with resultant flail joint and severe limb shortening. Risk factors for implant infection include rheumatoid arthritis, diabetes mellitus, urinary tract infection (UTI), pneumonia, tuberculosis, avascular necrosis, sickle cell disease, obesity, hematoma, seroma, acute dislocation, reoperation, and protein malnutrition.

## DIAGNOSTIC TESTS

**Gallium scan and erythrocyte sedimentation rate:**    May be indicated to rule out concurrent infection.

**Scintigraphy:**    Can be used to document leg length discrepancy, which can be surgically compensated for by using alternative neck lengths on the femoral prosthesis.

## COLLABORATIVE MANAGMENT

**Surgical procedure:**    Although the surgical procedure for THA can be accomplished *via* a variety of approaches, it is most commonly done through a posterior lateral approach. Methylmethacrylate may be used as a grouting agent to hold the endoprosthesis in place, or special prosthetics coated with porous materials, such as ceramics, may be used to allow bony ingrowth to fix the device internally. Once the prosthetic acetabulum is positioned, the femoral canal is reamed to accept the femoral prosthesis. A drain is then inserted into the deeper layers of the wound.

**Antibiotics:**    Because the potential for infection is increased with the presence of the massive endoprosthesis, the patient is placed on prophylactic antibiotics before, during, and for at least 5 days after surgery. Infection of the THA may require its temporary or permanent removal.

**Blood replacement:**    Because of significant blood loss from THA and total knee replacement procedures and the perceived dangers of bloodborne disease transmission from the general blood pool (e.g., HIV virus, hepatitis, cytomegalovirus, Epstein-Barr virus, syphilis, and malaria), autologous blood transfusion has become an issue of concern. Homologous transfusion of the patient's own previously banked blood is one alternative. Blood salvage during and after joint replacement arthroplasty is being used more frequently. During surgery, lost blood is salvaged by suctioning it from the sterile field to a cell saver machine. The cell saver washes the blood, spins it down into packed RBCs, and allows return to the patient in 225-ml increments. Postoperative collection is accomplished *via* drain tubes that empty through a 40-micron filter into a 400-ml blood salvage canister. Blood collection is limited to 6 h before reinfusion, and a citrate anticoagulant is added to each canister (a minimum of 320 ml of blood is needed to allow transfusion without risk of citrate poisoning). Present research is exploring the ability to salvage blood without citrate and allow reinfusion of smaller amounts of lost blood.

**Postsurgical immobilization:**    The patient is immobilized in balanced suspension or similar device (A-frame, abduction pillow, or wedge abduction pillow) to prevent internal rotation, adduction, and flexion past 90 degrees, which can cause dislocation of the endoprosthesis. If methylmethacrylate is used, the patient will be more readily mobile (usually within 5 days) because of the immediate fixation of the device. If a porous-coated device is used, it is not immediately fixed in place and the patient may require longer immobilization (several days to several weeks). If the greater trochanter was removed to allow visualization or correct muscle weakness, it will require wiring and further immobilization for at least 3 weeks in balanced suspension or limited weight-bearing for several weeks.

**Antithrombus regimen:**    Because of increased risk of deep vein thrombosis (DVT), THA patients are begun on anticoagulant therapy (heparin or coumadin) or antiplatelet agents (dextran), antiembolism hose, intermittent pneumatic compression devices, calf pumping exercises and ankle circles, early ambulation, and close monitoring for assessments of DVT. Also see Appendix One for **Altered peripheral tissue perfusion,** p. 715.

**Progressive physical therapy:**   To regain muscular strength and to ensure that the patient has adequate upper extremity strength to allow ambulation with crutches or a walker. During postoperative immobilization, the patient begins muscle-strengthening exercises using balanced suspension (or a similar device). The patient must be reminded to avoid internal rotation, adduction, and flexion of the hip past 90 degrees.

## NURSING DIAGNOSES AND INTERVENTIONS

**Knowledge deficit:**   Potential for and mechanism of THA dislocation, preventive measures, positional restrictions, prescribed ambulation regimen, potential for loosening, and use of assistive devices
***Desired outcome:***   At a minimum of the 24-h period before hospital discharge, patient verbalizes knowledge about the potential for, preventive measures for, and mechanism of THA dislocation and the indicators of implant loosening and demonstrates the prescribed regimen for ambulation and performance of ADL without experiencing dislocation.

---

**Note:**   There is a high risk of dislocation until the periarticular tissues scar down around the endoprosthesis. Once dislocation occurs, there is increased potential for recurrence because of stretching of the periarticular tissues. Dislocation is treated with reduction under anesthesia and immobilization in balanced suspension for 3-6 weeks. Recurrent dislocation may require surgical intervention to tighten periarticular tissues or revise the THA. After 6 weeks, the properly placed THA has significantly decreased potential for dislocation. The following discussion relates to the *posteriolateral approach* for THA surgery. Other approaches require different positional restrictions.

---

- During the preoperative period, advise patient about the potential for dislocation.
- Show patient what the endoprosthesis looks like (using a model or similar implant) and how easily it can be dislocated when positional restrictions (e.g., flexion of the hip to 90 degrees; internal rotation or adduction of the affected leg) are not followed.
- During the preoperative period, instruct patient in the use of ambulatory aids and ADL-assistive devices that allow independence without violation of positional restrictions. Explain the use of devices to maintain positional restrictions.
- After surgery, discuss positional restrictions and activities that involve these restrictions, including pivoting on the affected leg, sitting on a regular-height toilet seat, bending over to tie shoelaces, or crossing the legs.
- Advise patient about the need for long-handled shoe horn, pickup sticks, stocking helpers, and a raised toilet seat for use after discharge. Provide addresses of stores that retail these items.
- Be sure the patient verbalizes and demonstrates understanding of the positional restrictions and is able to accomplish ambulation and performance of ADL independently, using assistive devices.
- Instruct patient to report hip, buttock, or thigh pain or prolonged limp as indicators of implant loosening.

**Knowledge deficit:**   Potential for infection caused by foreign body reaction to the endoprosthesis
***Desired outcome:***   Within 24 h of instruction, patient verbalizes knowledge about the ongoing potential for infection, its indicators, and the importance of seeking prompt medical care if they occur.
- Advise patient that infection potential will be a permanent situation. Because of foreign body reaction and increased blood supply resulting from associated inflammatory response, these patients are at increased risk for hematogenic (bloodborne) infection. Introduce this as a potential complication dur-

ing the informed consent process and review it during preoperative teaching.

- Before hospital discharge, ensure that the patient verbalizes understanding of the indicators of wound, UTI, upper respiratory (URI), and dental infections (see discussions in **High risk for infection** in both "Care of the Renal Transplant Recipient," p. 141, and Table 5-4, p. 360). Include this information on a written handout that reviews the information and lists a phone number to call if questions arise after hospital discharge.
- Advise patient to wear a Medic-Alert bracelet and always to request prophylactic antibiotics for procedures that can result in bacterial seeding of the bloodstream, such as minor or major surgery or dental extractions.
- Advise patient to call physician promptly if indicators of infection from the THA occur. These signs can include drainage, pain, fever, local warmth, swelling, restricted ROM of the joint, or feelings of pressure in the hip.

**High risk for peripheral neurovascular dysfunction** related to interrupted arterial flow secondary to compression from traction or abduction device
*Desired outcomes:*   Patient has adequate peripheral neurovascular function in distal tissues as evidenced by warmth, normal color, and the ability to dorsiflex the involved foot and feel sensations on testing of the peroneal nerve dermatome. Following instruction, patient verbalizes knowledge about potential neurovascular complications and the importance of reporting indicators of impairment promptly.

- Because the traction sling or abduction device can press on neurovascular structures, it is imperative that neurovascular status of the leg in traction, especially peroneal nerve function, be assessed along with the VS. The peroneal nerve runs superficially by the neck of the fibula and can be assessed by testing the dermatome of the first web space between the great and second toes and having the patient dorsiflex the foot. Loss of sensation or movement signals impaired peroneal nerve function. Promptly report significant findings to physician.
- Be sure patient is aware of the potential for neurovascular impairment and the importance of reporting alterations in sensation, movement, temperature, and color of the immobilized extremity.
- Encourage patient to reposition the leg within the restrictions of the sling and positional limitations.
- Encourage patient to perform prescribed exercises as a means of stimulating circulation in the area.

---

**Note:**   See "Osteoarthritis" for **Pain,** p. 520, and **Impaired physical mobility** related to musculoskeletal impairment and adjustment to new walking gait, p. 521. See "Fractures" for **Self-care deficit,** p. 550, and **Knowledge deficit:** Potential for infection, p. 552. See "Amputation" for **Knowledge deficit:** Postsurgical exercise regimen, p. 566. See "Total Knee Arthroplasty" for **High risk for fluid volume deficit** related to postsurgical hemorrhage or hematoma formation, p. 578. Also see Appendix One for nursing diagnoses and interventions in "Caring for Preoperative and Postoperative Patients," p. 693, "Caring for Patients on Prolonged Bed Rest" (in particular **Altered peripheral tissue perfusion,** p. 715, which discusses deep vein thrombosis), and "Caring for Patients with Cancer and Other Life-Disrupting Illnesses," p. 753.

---

## PATIENT-FAMILY TEACHING AND DISCHARGE PLANNING

Give patient and significant others verbal and written information about the following:

- Prescribed exercise regimen, including rationale for each exercise, number of repetitions for each, and frequency of the exercise periods. Be sure patient independently demonstrates understanding of the exercises and gives a return demonstration before hospital discharge.

- Indicators of the types of infections, including the following: wound (persistent redness, swelling, discharge, local warmth, restricted hip ROM, feelings of hip pressure, fever, and pain); UTI (dysuria, pyuria, fever, malodorous urine, cloudy urine, urgency, frequency, and pain in the suprapubic, flank, groin, scrotal, or labial area); URI (change in color or amount of sputum, fever, cough, sore throat, malaise, fever); and dental (pain, swelling of the jaw, difficulty with mastication, fever). Advise patient to notify physician promptly if any of these indicators occur and to seek prophylactic antibiotics for minor surgical procedures.
- Use of assistive devices (pickup sticks, stocking helpers, long-handled shoe horns, and raised toilet seat). Ensure that patient demonstrates independence in their use before hospital discharge.
- Independent ambulation with crutches on level and uneven surfaces (see "Osteoarthritis," p. 521).
- Getting in a car safely without risking dislocation. The patient should be able to demonstrate this procedure before hospital discharge.
- Medications, including name, rationale, dosage, schedule, precautions, and potential side effects.
- Indications of implant loosening, including continuing hip, buttock, or thigh pain or prolonged limp.
- Phone number of a resource person should questions arise after hospital discharge.

# Total knee arthroplasty

Total knee arthroplasty (TKA) is surgery that involves resection of the knee joint and its replacement with an endoprosthesis. Several pathologic conditions can result in the need for TKA, including osteoarthritis, rheumatoid arthritis, gouty arthritis, hemophilic arthritis, and severe knee trauma. Generally, TKA is restricted to older patients because the life span of the implant is unknown. However, younger patients also undergo this procedure, depending on the severity of the disease, amount of pain, and degree of functional deficit in the femorotibial or femoropatellar articulations. Because this procedure is irreversible and involves the removal of significant amounts of bone from the femur, tibia, and patella, several conditions must be met before the patient is considered a potential candidate. Conservative methods of therapy must have been exhausted, and there has to be significant loss of function and pain that severely limit ambulation and ADL. In addition, the patient must have demonstrated adherence with past medical regimens and be free of any concurrent infectious process.

Complications of TKA have resulted in the need for reoperation in up to 15% of these patients. Complications include loosening of the prosthesis, peroneal nerve palsy, delayed wound healing, and infection. Loosening is by far the most common complication, and it occurs most frequently in patients with varus deformity, obesity, overactivity, or decreased bone stock (i.e., osteoporosis).

## DIAGNOSTIC TESTS
See discussion with "Total Hip Arthroplasty," p. 574. In addition, arthroscopy may be useful in confirming the extent of the pathology to identify the appropriate prosthesis.

## COLLABORATIVE MANAGEMENT
**Surgical procedure:** The approach varies with the type of prosthetic device used. During the procedure a skin flap is created around the patella. If the blood supply is compromised during surgery or from postoperative hematoma formation, the flap can necrose and jeopardize the success of the operation;

therefore it requires careful monitoring. The implant is internally fixed with methylmethacrylate or bony ingrowth. The wound is sutured closed in layers, and a drain is left in place.

**Postoperative immobilization:**    Usually accomplished with a Jones dressing, which is composed of a bulky padding with anterior, posterior, and lateral plaster splints that are held in place with an elastic wrap. The Jones dressing ensures immobilization while allowing for edema formation to minimize the risk of iatrogenic compartment syndrome. A continuous cooling pad may be applied to inhibit edema formation. If the implant is to be held in place with bony ingrowth, the leg may be immobilized within a cast after postoperative edema has subsided.

**Ambulation:**    If methylmethacrylate was used to internally fix the implant, the patient may be permitted to ambulate without weight-bearing within 3-5 days, slowly advancing to weight-bearing as tolerated within 10-14 days. ROM of the knee is often done within 5 days under supervision of a physical therapist. For implants held in place with bony ingrowth, ambulation is not begun until after 10-14 days, and weight-bearing may be contraindicated for as long as 6-12 weeks. If there is a cast, ROM is not begun until the cast has been removed.

**Continuous passive movement (CPM):**    Usually advocated for patients who undergo a TKA. The CPM device is applied to the patient's bed and the operant extremity is positioned in a sling in the device. The device then moves the leg through preset limits of ROM in preset timed cycles. The CPM initially may be set at 45-60 degrees, with daily progression during patient's hospitalization. Use of CPM allows greater ROM with less pain. (The minimal flexion for a successful TKA is 90-110 degrees.)

## NURSING DIAGNOSES AND INTERVENTIONS

**High risk for fluid volume deficit** related to postsurgical hemorrhage or hematoma formation

**Desired outcome:**    Within 36 h after surgery, patient is free of symptoms of excessive bleeding or hematoma formation as evidenced by BP ≥90/60 mm Hg (or within patient's normal range); HR ≤100 bpm; RR ≤20 breaths/min; balanced I&O; output from drainage device ≤50 ml/h; and brisk capillary refill (<2 sec), peripheral pulses >2+ on a 0-4+ scale, warmth, and normal color in the involved extremity distal to the surgical site.

---

**Note:**    A hematoma is a collection of extravasated blood within the tissues after surgery (or trauma). During most orthopedic surgeries, a tourniquet is used to restrict blood flow from the operative field. Sometimes the tourniquet is left inflated until after the dressing or cast has been applied; therefore, major bleeding might not be noted during surgery. Even when the tourniquet is deflated, it is possible that a significant bleeding vessel may be overlooked or that bleeding will begin later during the patient's recovery.

---

- When taking VS, monitor drainage from the drainage system as well as that on the dressings or cast. Report output from the drainage system that exceeds 50 ml/h.
- Because noting the amount of drainage on the cast does not always provide an accurate assessment of drainage within the cast, carefully evaluate the patient's VS, subjective complaints, and neurovascular status.
- Be alert to and report patient complaints of warmth within the cast or beneath the dressing, things "crawling" under the cast, aching, increasing pressure or pain, or coolness distal to the area of surgery, which can occur with hemorrhage or hematoma formation.
- Monitor for and report VS indicative of shock or hemorrhage, including hypotension and increasing pulse rate.
- Monitor for pallor, decreased posterior tibial or dorsalis pedis pulses, slowed

capillary refill, or coolness of the distal extremity, which can occur with hemorrhage or hematoma formation.

- If hemorrhage or hematoma formation is suspected, notify physician promptly. If the limb is casted, elevate it above the level of the patient's heart to slow the bleeding. If the limb is not casted, apply an elastic wrap for direct pressure on the site of bleeding.
- If hemorrhage or hematoma formation is suspected and the patient's VS are indicative of shock but a physician is unavailable, the surgical area should be exposed by windowing the cast or loosening the dressing to allow direct inspection of the area. Direct pressure usually will control hemorrhage; if not, apply a thigh blood pressure cuff over sheet wadding to serve as a tourniquet until the physician arrives for definitive therapy.

**High risk for impaired skin integrity** related to irritation; *and/or* **impaired tissue integrity (or risk of same)** related to altered circulaton secondary to presence of CPM device

*Desired outcomes:*   Skin and tissue of the affected leg remain intact and non-erythematous. Following instruction, patient verbalizes knowledge about the importance of reporting indicators of skin irritation promptly while undergoing CPM.

- Preoperatively, assess the skin on the operant extremity, being alert to areas of irritation or redness.
- Preoperatively, introduce the patient to the use of the CPM, demonstrating how it will be used postoperatively. Point out areas prone to pressure or irritation from the device. Teach patient to report alterations in sensation or discomfort.
- Postoperatively, ensure correct positioning of the extremity within the CPM device (i.e., neutral position of the leg, with the knee resting over the area flexed by the device).
- Encourage patient to perform quadricep sets, gluteal sets, and ankle circles to promote extremity circulation.
- During VS, or more often if erythema is noted, examine the medial, lateral, and posterior aspects of the extremity in the CPM device for areas of erythema. Also question patient about alterations in sensation or areas of discomfort.
- Pad areas of excessive pressure as noted by the presence of erythema. Reposition the leg within the confines of the CPM device. Report areas of erythema that do not resolve.

---

**Note:**   See all nursing diagnoses (except **Knowledge deficit:** Potential for and mechanism of THA dislocation) in" Total Hip Arthroplasty," p. 575.

---

## PATIENT-FAMILY TEACHING AND DISCHARGE PLANNING
See "Total Hip Arthroplasty," p. 576.

### Selected Bibliography

Alexiades MM et al: Prospective study of porous-coated anatomic total hip arthroplasty, *Clin Orthop* 269(Aug):205-208, 1991.

Altman RD: Classification of disease: osteoarthritis, *Semin Arthritis Rheum* 20(June):40-47, 1991.

Buzaid AC, Durie BGM: Management of refractory myeloma: a review, *J Clin Oncol* 6(5):889-905,1988.

Chase JA: Outpatient management of low back pain, *Orthop Nurs* 11(1):11-19, 1992.

Corbett JV: *Laboratory tests and diagnostic procedures with nursing diagnosis,* ed 3, Norwalk, Conn, 1992, Appleton & Lange.

Day LJ et al: *Orthopedics.* In Way LW, editor: *Current surgical diagnosis and treatment,* ed 8, Norwalk, Conn, 1991, Appleton & Lange.

Eftekhar NS, Nercessian O: Incidence and mechanism of failure of cemented acetabular component in total hip arthroplasty, *Orthop Clin North Am* 19(3):557-566, 1988.

Freeman DA: Paget's disease of bone, *Am J Med Sci* 295(2):144-158,1988.

Friedel HA, Todd PA: Nabumetone: a preliminary review of its pharmacodynamic and pharmacokinetic properties and therapeutic efficacy in rheumatoid diseases, *Drugs* 35(5):504-524, 1988.

Gamron RB: Taking the pressure out of compartment syndrome, *Am J Nurs* 88(8):1076-1080, 1988.

Gannon DM et al: An evaluation of the efficacy of postoperative blood salvage after total joint arthroplasty: a prospective randomized trial, *J Arthroplasty* 6(2):109-114, 1991.

Gentry LO: Osteomyelitis: options for diagnosis and management, *J Antimicrob Chemother* 21(9, suppl C):115-128,1988.

Green SA: Ilizarov orthopaedic method: innovations from a Siberian surgeon, *AORN J* 49(1):215-230, 1989.

Hamdy RC: Metabolic bone disease: a review, *J Tenn Med Assoc* 81(5):293-296,1988.

Hamerman D: Osteoarthritis, *Orthop Rev* 17(4):353-360,1988.

Hellman DB, Shearn MA: *Arthritis and musculoskeletal disorders.* In Schroeder SA et al: *Current medical diagnosis and treatment,* ed 30, Norwalk, Conn, 1991, Appleton & Lange.

Huvos AG: Surgical pathology of bone sarcomas, *World J Surg* 12:284-298,1988.

Interqual: The ISD-A review system with adult ISD criteria, August 1992, Northhampton, NH, and Marlboro, MA, Interqual, Inc.

Johnson PH: Recurrent subluxation of the shoulder, *J Arkansas Med Soc* 84(8):335-337,1988.

Kalu DN, Masoro EJ: The biology of aging with particular reference to the musculoskeletal system, *Clin Geriatr Med* 4(2):257-267,1988.

Kim MJ, McFarland GK, McLane AM: *Pocket guide to nursing diagnoses,* ed 5, St Louis, 1993, Mosby–Year Book.

Kondoh T et al: Evaluation of filtration lymphocytopheresis (LCP) device use in treatment of patients with rheumatoid arthritis, *Artif Organs* 15(3):180-188, 1991.

Krupski WC et al: *Amputation.* In Way LW, editor: *Current surgical diagnosis and treatment,* ed 9, Norwalk, Conn, 1991, Appleton & Lange.

Lapuk S, Woodbury DF: Volkmann's ischemic contracture: a case report, *Orthop Rev* 17(6):618-624,1987.

Lawrence W: Concepts in limb-sparing treatment of adult soft tissue sarcomas, *Semin Surg Oncol* 4:73-77,1988.

Lindsay R: Management of osteoporosis, *Clin Endocrin Metab* 2(1):103-123,1988.

Marcus R: Understanding osteoporosis, *West J Med* 155(1):53-60, 1990.

McDougall R, Keeling CA: Complications of fractures and their healing, *Semin Nucl Med* 18(2):113-125,1988.

Merkow RL et al: Paget's disease of bone, *Orthop Clin North Am* 21(1):171-189, 1990.

Phillips PE: Evidence implicating infectious agents in rheumatoid arthritis and juvenile rheumatoid arthritis, *Clin Exp Rheumatol* 6(1):87-94,1988.

Reginato AJ, Schumacher HR: Crystal-associated arthroplasties, *Rheumatic Disorders* 4(2):295-322, 1988.

Ross DG: Acute compartment syndrome, *Orthop Nurs* 10(2):33-38, 1991.

Ross DG: *Compartment syndrome.* In Swearingen PL, Keen JH, editors: *Manual of critical care: applying nursing diagnoses to adult critical illness,* ed 2, St Louis, 1991, Mosby–Year Book.

Rounseville C: Phantom limb pain: the ghost that haunts the amputee, *Orthop Nurs* 11(2):67-71, 1991.

Rutan F: Preprosthetic program for the amputee, *Orthop Nurs* 2:14,1982.

Sambrook PN, Reeve J: Bone disease in rheumatoid arthritis, *Clin Sci* 74:225-230, 1988.

Schlag G, Redl H: Fibrin sealant in orthopedic surgery, *Clin Orthop,* 227:269-285, 1988.

Simon MA: Limb salvage for osteosarcoma, *J Bone Joint Surg* 70-A(2):307-310, 1988.

Skogberg K et al: Beta-hemolytic group A, B, C, and G streptococcal septicemia: a clinical study, *Scand J Infect Dis* 20:119-125, 1988.

Sommerlath K: The prognosis of repaired and intact menisci in unstable knees—a comprehensive study, *J Arthroscop & Rel Surg* 4(2):93-95,1988.

Steiner ME, Grana WA: The young althlete's knee: recent advances, *Clin Sports Med* 7(3):527-546,1988.

Stevenson JC: Osteoporosis: pathogenesis and risk factors, *Clin Endocrin Metab* 2(1):87-100,1988.

Sweetnam R: Malignant bone tumor management: 30 years of achievement, *Clin Orthop* 247:67-73, Oct 1989.

Tebbi CK, Gaeta J: Osteosarcoma, *Pediatr Ann* 17(4):285-300, 1988.

US Department of Health and Human Services: *Acute pain management: operative or medical procedures and trauma,* 1992, Public Health Service, Agency for Health Care Policy and Research, Rockville, MD, AHCPR 92-0032.

Vince KG, Insall JN: Long-term results of cemented total knee arthroplasty, *Orthop Clin North Am* 19(3):575-580,1988.

Walker RH et al: Postoperative use of continuous passive motion, transcutaneous electrical nerve stimulation, and continuous cooling pad following total knee arthroplasty, *J Arthroplasty* 6(2):151-156, 1991.

Weinstein SM, Herring SA: Nerve problems and compartment syndromes in the hand, wrist, and forearm, *Clin Sports Med* 11(1):161-186, 1992.

Williamson VC: Amputation of the lower extremity: an overview, *Orthop Nurs* 11(2):55-65, 1992.

Ziff M et al: Pathogenic factors in rheumatoid synovitis, *Br J Rheumatol* 27(suppl II):153-156,1988.

## 9 REPRODUCTIVE DISORDERS

Section One   Surgeries and Disorders of the Breast   583
   Breast reduction   583
   Breast reconstruction   585
   Benign breast disorders and conditions   588
   Malignant breast disorders   590
Section Two   Neoplasms of the Female Pelvis   596
   Cancer of the cervix   596
   Ovarian tumors   600
   Endometrial cancer   602
   Vulvar cancer   603
Section Three   Disorders of the Female Pelvis   605
   Endometriosis   605
   Cystocele   607
   Rectocele   608
   Uterine prolapse   609
Section Four   Interruption of Pregnancy   610
   Spontaneous abortion   610
   Ectopic pregnancy   613
Section Five   Disorders and Surgeries of the Male Pelvis   615
   Benign prostatic hypertrophy   615
   Prostatic neoplasm   622
   Testicular neoplasm   626
   Penile implants   629
Selected Bibliography   631

## Section One:   Surgeries and Disorders of the Breast

### Breast reduction

Breast reduction involves removal of breast tissue and skin to decrease breast size. The decision for surgery is made by the patient, and it is performed by a plastic surgeon or breast specialist.

ASSESSMENT

**Clinical indicators:**   The procedure may be reconstructive or cosmetic, depending on symptoms. Complaints may include neck, shoulder, and back pain;

postural defects from attempting to mask breast size; deep ridges from bra straps; and withdrawal from social encounters.

**Physical assessment:** The breasts are large and may be pendulous or unequal in size. There should be no signs of breast disease, such as nipple discharge (see "Malignant Breast Disorders," p. 591, for other signs).

## SURGICAL INTERVENTION

Markings using a key-hole pattern are made before surgery to determine the ultimate position of the nipple and incision lines. During surgery the nipple is removed and replaced as a graft after resection of the extra breast tissue and skin.

## NURSING DIAGNOSES AND INTERVENTIONS

**Body image disturbance** related to breast size

*Desired outcome:* Before surgery, patient expresses positive and realistic reasons for having breast surgery.

- Discuss with the patient the meaning of her breasts, including likes and dislikes (both ideal and real).
- Review the patient's expectations for the outcome of surgery. The patient should not have unrealistic expectations as evidenced by such statements as, "Surgery will change my life or marriage."
- Review for informed consent the potential risks involved with breast reduction, such as impaired breast feeding, nipple or skin necrosis, and asymmetry.
- Provide support for the patient's decision to have this surgery by spending time with her and encouraging her to verbalize fears and concerns.

**Pain** related to surgical procedure

*Desired outcomes:* Patient's subjective perception of pain decreases within 1 h of intervention, as documented by a pain scale; objective indicators, such as grimacing, are absent or diminished. Patient is pain-free 5-7 days after surgery.

- Assess and document location, quality, and duration of the pain, using a pain scale from 0 (no pain) 10 (worst pain).
- Medicate the patient with analgesics as prescribed; evaluate and document the response, based on the pain scale.
- Ensure that the patient has a comfortable bra that adequately supports her breasts.
- Teach the patient relaxation techniques, such as slow, diaphragmatic breathing and guided imagery.
- Provide distractions, such as television or soothing music.
- Encourage activity as tolerated.
- For additional interventions, see this nursing diagnosis in Appendix One, p. 694.

**Knowledge deficit:** Incisional site care and the need for monthly breast self-examination (BSE)

*Desired outcome:* Before hospital discharge, patient verbalizes and demonstrates knowledge about incisional site care and verbalizes the importance of BSE after the incisions have healed and the signs of infection at the incisional site.

- Instruct patient to cleanse the incisional site after the sutures have been removed, using basic hygiene, such as soap and water. Explain that heavy lotions, medications, or creams should not be used around the incisional sites (except for the transplanted nipples) unless specified by physician.
- As prescribed, teach patient how to apply lotions or creams to the transplanted nipple(s).
- In preparation for hospital discharge, instruct patient in BSE using models of the breast and emphasize the importance of monthly BSE when the incisions have healed.

- Teach patient the signs of infection to report to a health-care professional should they occur after hospital discharge: redness, foul odor, pain, swelling, discharge, fever.

**Ineffective breast feeding** related to breast surgical procedure

*Desired outcome:* In the preoperative period, patient verbalizes knowledge that breast feeding will be impaired as a result of the surgical procedure.

- Before surgery, explain to patient that breast reduction surgery will impair breast feeding in future pregnancies.
- As indicated, arrange for a session with a lactation consultant if patient requires more information.

---

**Note:** See "Breast Reconstruction" for **High risk for fluid volume deficit** related to postsurgical hemorrhage or hematoma formation, p. 587, and Appendix One for "Caring for Preoperative and Postoperative Patients," p. 693.

---

## PATIENT-FAMILY TEACHING AND DISCHARGE PLANNING

Give patient and significant others verbal and written information about the following:

- Medications for pain relief, including drug name, purpose, dosage, schedule, precautions, and potential side effects.
- Indicators of wound infection, which require follow-up care by health-care provider: persistent redness, pain, swelling, and drainage at the incisional areas.
- Care of the incision site, including cleansing and dressing, if indicated.
- Changes in the nipple, which may include decreased sensation and loss of color. Nipple sensation may return within 2 years.
- Importance of monthly BSE. Teach or review the technique as appropriate.
- Activity restrictions, which may include limited use of arms for 2 weeks postoperatively and resumption of full activity after 3 weeks.

# Breast reconstruction

After a mastectomy, a woman may elect to have breast reconstruction in an attempt to create a breast "mound" in place of the lost breast. Although there is no medical indication for breast reconstruction, psychologic benefits may result. Breast reconstruction can be performed at the time of mastectomy or delayed. This surgery has become more popular in recent years because techniques continue to improve and patients are becoming more aware of the procedure and its benefits.

## ASSESSMENT

**Clinical indicators:** Scheduled mastectomy or absence of the breast, patient's desire for surgery, adequate tissue present, and absence of progressive disease.

**Physical assessment:** There should be no evidence of infection, and healing of the mastectomy scar should be complete if a surgical delay was indicated.

## COLLABORATIVE MANAGEMENT

**Analgesics and possibly narcotics:** To control postsurgical discomfort.

**IV therapy:** To treat dehydration secondary to blood loss and surgical intervention.

**Balanced diet:** As tolerated to promote tissue restoration.

**Surgical procedure:** Varying procedures may be involved, depending on the amount of tissue left at the reconstruction site. When there is sufficient tissue, an implant is placed under the pectoralis and serratus muscles. A tissue expander can be used either as a temporary device for a later, permanent implant or as a permanent implant concurrent with surgery. The tissue expander is injected with saline through a port at intervals to provide gradual enlargement of the site. If a radical mastectomy has been performed, there is usually inadequate soft tissue, muscle, and skin on which to place the implant. It then becomes necessary to graft tissue from other locations, such as the latissimus dorsi flap or rectus abdominis musculocutaneous flap. Latissimus dorsi flap reconstruction involves the transfer of the muscle, skin, and subcutaneous tissue from the back to the mastectomy site. The rectus abdominis musculocutaneous flap involves the transfer of one of the rectus abdominis muscles, as well as overlying skin, subcutaneous fat (lipectomy), and artery, to the mastectomy site. With this procedure an implant also may be needed, depending on the amount of tissue available. If a nipple is desired on the reconstructed breast, it can be created from skin of the inner thigh, buttock, labia, or the other nipple.

**Suction apparatus:**    Placed in the wound to minimize the chance of hematoma formation.

## NURSING DIAGNOSES AND INTERVENTIONS

**Knowledge deficit:**    Surgical procedure, preoperative care, and postoperative regimen

*Desired outcome:*    Before surgery, patient verbalizes knowledge about the surgical procedure and expected results, preoperative care, and the postoperative regimen.

- Consult with physician to arrange a visit by a woman who has had breast reconstruction surgery to share feelings and demonstrate the cosmetic results. Support the patient's decision for the type of procedure and/or implant to be used. Clarify any questions that may arise.
- During the preoperative period, explain that after surgery a suction apparatus that removes blood will be present to minimize the potential for hematoma formation. Usually this apparatus is removed after 48 h or when drainage is less than 10-20 ml over a 24-h period.
- Explain that movement and activity may be restricted after surgery, depending on the procedure used. When an implant is placed under ample tissue, recovery is more rapid and hospitalization is usually 1-3 days; flap reconstruction is more involved, and movement and activity may be more restricted. Patients with a latissimus flap reconstruction are usually discharged after 2-5 days when the drains are removed. A rectus abdominis procedure is more extensive, and because of the lipectomy the patient may be on bed rest and discharged within a week.
- Teach patient to monitor the reconstructed nipple and report to staff members delayed capillary refill ($\geq$2 sec) and duskiness. Patients who undergo nipple reconstruction usually are more satisfied with the results than those who do not; however, they may experience more anxiety during the postrecovery period and thus require more reassurance.
- Explain the following areas of concern that often arise after hospital discharge:
  - Caring for the incision: Explain that a gauze dressing usually covers the incision until the sutures are removed on about the seventh day. After the sutures are removed, micropore tape strips usually are placed over the incision until healing has taken place and are replaced when they loosen. Instruct patient to notify physician if signs of infection, including persistent redness, pain, swelling, or drainage, appear at the incision site.
  - Taking showers: Showers usually are permitted after the suction catheter has been removed, but they may be postponed until the sutures have been removed. If a dressing is present, it should be removed from the operative site and replaced after bathing.
  - Restricting activity: Usually for the first 4-6 weeks or as directed, strenuous exercise, contact sports, excessive stretching, and heavy lifting (>10

lb) are avoided. Activity that involves movement below the waist usually can be resumed after 1 week.
- Avoiding putting pressure on the chest wall for 4-6 weeks: E.g., patient should use superior position during coitus.
- Wearing a comfortable bra after removal of the drains: Explain that it takes 3-6 months for the reconstructed breast to appear natural in contour.
- Applying prescribed lotion to the nipple daily if a nipple transplant was performed.
- Performing monthly breast self-examination (BSE) of both breasts: Teach or review the procedure as appropriate.
- Making follow-up visits if a tissue expander was used for gradual enlargement of the implant site.
- Massaging the breast to prevent fibrocapsular formation, depending on the placement and type of implant used. Explain that the procedure involves a gentle motion in which the breast is squeezed and flattened. This procedure usually is performed 3 times a day.

**High risk for fluid volume deficit** related to postsurgical hemorrhage or hematoma formation

***Desired outcomes:*** Patient is normovolemic as evidenced by BP ≥90/60 mm Hg (or within patient's normal range), HR 60-100 bpm, RR ≤20 breaths/min, warm and dry skin, and urinary output ≥30 ml/h. Drainage in suction apparatus is ≤50 ml/h initially and <20 ml/h within 24 h after surgery. If patient develops a hematoma, it is detected and reported promptly.
- Monitor patient for clinical indicators of hemorrhage (e.g., drop of systolic BP 10-20 mm Hg below trend, rapid HR, cool and clammy skin, pallor, confusion, and diaphoresis). Report significant findings.
- Assess for the appearance of a hematoma as evidenced by swelling, pain, and possibly a bluish discoloration of the skin. Report significant findings to the physician.
- Assess the suction apparatus for patency, and document the amount and character of the drainage. Report drainage that exceeds 50 ml/h for 2 h. Reestablish suction as necessary. Usually the suction apparatus is removed after 48 h or if the total drainage is less than 10-20 ml in 24 h.

**Body image disturbance** related to body changes before and after breast reconstruction surgery

***Desired outcomes:*** Patient relates realistic expectations before surgery (e.g., that the breast will look normal under clothing) and demonstrates movement toward acceptance of body changes after surgery.
- Review with patient her expectations for the outcome of surgery.
- Discuss the emotional responses that women often have after breast reconstruction, such as elation during the early postoperative period followed by depression or confusion.
- Explain that some of the depression and confusion may be a result of the memory of the mastectomy and fear of cancer. Reassure patient that these feelings are normal and usually disappear after a short time.
- Provide emotional support by being with the patient when the dressing is first removed. Explain that the reconstructed breast will not look like the other breast at first, but that the molding process will begin during the recovery period and continue for 3-6 months.

*If a silicone breast implant has been used (either in the past or currently)*
**Anxiety** related to use of silicone breast implant

***Desired outcome:*** Within the 24-h period before hospital discharge, patient discusses concerns related to silicone implant and identifies potential systemic and local reactions.
- Advise patient that removal of the silicone breast implant generally is not considered unless there are problems.
- Inform patient that surgical substitution can be made with saline implants if necessary.

- Teach patient to report symptoms of the body's reaction to silicone, such as joint swelling and pain, skin erythema and swelling, glandular swelling, unusual fatigue, or swelling of the feet or hands.
- Teach patient to report symptoms of fibroscapular formation, such as breast hardness, which may be painful and result in a displaced breast.

---

**Note:**   See Appendix One for nursing diagnoses and interventions in "Caring for Preoperative and Postoperative Patients," p. 693, and "Caring for Patients with Cancer and Other Life-Disrupting Illnesses," p.719.

---

## PATIENT-FAMILY TEACHING AND DISCHARGE PLANNING

Give patient and significant others verbal and written information about the following:
- Care of the incision, including applying a gauze dressing until the sutures are removed on about the seventh day. After the sutures are removed, micropore tape strips usually are placed over the incision until healing has taken place, and are replaced when they loosen. Instruct patient to notify physician if signs of infection, including persistent redness, pain, swelling, or drainage, appear at the incision site.
- Taking showers, which usually are permitted after the suction catheter is removed. If present, the dressing should be removed from the operative site and replaced after bathing.
- Activity restriction for the first 4-6 weeks or as directed, including strenuous exercise, contact sports, excessive stretching, and heavy lifting (>10 lb).
- Importance of not putting pressure on the chest wall for 4-6 weeks (e.g., patient should use superior position during coitus).
- Importance of breast massage 3 times per day for at least the first year after surgery. Explain that it takes 3-6 months for the reconstructed breast to appear natural in contour.
- Potential recommendation not to wear a bra for 3 months to allow for unrestricted movement of the implant.
- Necessity of applying prescribed lotion to the nipple daily if a nipple transplant was performed.
- Importance of monthly BSE of both breasts. Teach or review the procedure as appropriate. In addition, stress the importance of follow-up care. Successful reconstruction may give a false sense of security.
- Medications, including drug name, purpose, dosage, schedule, precautions, and potential side effects.

# Benign breast disorders and conditions

The most common breast masses are those caused by fibrocystic disease, fibroadenomas, and intraductal papilloma; all are evaluated for potential malignancy.
**Fibrocystic condition:**   Can be either a simple cyst or cysts caused by normal changes in the lining of the duct and the secretion of fluid, or a premalignant condition caused by hyperplasia of the cells. Fibrocystic condition is the most common breast lesion in women. It is found most often in the age group 35-45, increases with advancing age, and rarely is found after menopause, except in women receiving estrogen replacement therapy.
**Fibroadenomas:**   Solid masses that may occur from age 15-60 years, with peak occurrence at 21-25 years.
**Intraductal papilloma:**   A benign condition of the ductal system of the breast. It occurs infrequently and is found most often in women 35-45 years of age.

## ASSESSMENT

**Signs and symptoms:** The patient palpates a mass in 80% of the cases. Often with fibrocystic condition there are bilateral, multiple masses that are painful and tender. They may change in size relative to the menstrual cycle and are most evident just before menstruation. The masses are firm, mobile, and smooth or regular in shape.

Fibroadenomas are painless masses that are usually unilateral. The mass itself is mobile, solid, firm, well circumscribed, and often spherical, but it can be lobulated or dumbbell-shaped.

The most frequent symptom of intraductal papilloma is serosanguineous or serous nipple discharge. Usually there is no mass.

**Physical assessment:** With fibrocystic condition, masses usually can be palpated in the upper outer quadrants of the breasts. Fibroadenomas are usually 2-2.5 cm in diameter. An intraductal papilloma often involves a 1-cm area that circumvents the nipple; discharge also may be found.

**History of:** Benign breast masses. There is potential for recurrence of both cysts and fibroadenomas.

## DIAGNOSTIC TESTS

**Mammography:** A roentgenographic test used to identify cancerous masses, which appear as small densities with stippled calcifications. There is a risk of false-positive and false-negative results.

**Xeroradiography:** A noninvasive test that uses a lesser radiation dose than mammography; however, there is a higher risk of false-positive or false-negative results.

**Thermography:** Presents a picture of normal and abnormal temperatures in the breast. Malignant masses are warmer because of increased vascularity in the area. Again there is the risk of false-positive and false-negative results. Thermography is not as accurate as mammography and cannot be substituted for it.

**Ultrasound mammography:** Uses sound waves to delineate the internal pattern of the breast. It is used when cysts and enlarged ducts are suspected. It is 98% accurate in diagnosing cysts and enlarged ducts only.

**Magnetic resonance imaging (MRI):** Technique that uses the interaction between magnetism and radio waves (without ionizing radiation) to show the structure of the breasts. It can image breast cancers that are large and palpable; however, it cannot detect microcalcifications indicative of cancers.

**Needle aspiration biopsy:** Involves aspirating the contents of the mass *via* a fine (22-gauge) needle. The aspirate is then placed on a slide for Papanicolaou evaluation.

**Incisional biopsy:** Involves the surgical removal of part of the mass for histologic evaluation.

**Excisional biopsy:** Involves removal of the entire mass as well as marginal breast tissue. This procedure results in the most accurate diagnosis.

## COLLABORATIVE MANAGEMENT

**Diet:** For fibrocystic condition, the promotion of nutritious foods and the elimination of methylxanthine substances, such as coffee, tea, and chocolate, may decrease the pain and size of the cysts. Vitamin E therapy may be helpful in some patients to reduce the incidence of recurrent cysts. A low-sodium (Na) diet in the luteal phase may relieve symptoms by decreasing edema. A diet low in fat and high in fiber may help prevent breast cancer.

**Pharmacologic therapy:** Treatment for fibrocystic condition may involve low-dose estrogen oral contraceptives to suppress the ovulation cycle and thus minimize cyst formation. Danazol and promocriptine also may be used. Recurrence is possible 6-12 months after cessation of therapy.

**Stress reduction and smoking cessation:** May help relieve or decrease the symptoms of fibrocystic condition.

**Excisional biopsy:**   Not only useful in diagnosis, it removes the breast mass as well.

**Wedge resection of the breast:**   Resection of the lobe that is involved in the intraductal papilloma.

## NURSING DIAGNOSES AND INTERVENTIONS

**Anxiety** related to the possibility of cancer, change in body image, surgical or diagnostic procedure, and pain

***Desired outcomes:***   Before surgery and/or diagnostic procedure, patient discusses concerns; demonstrates increasing psychologic comfort as evidenced by participation in decisions regarding care; and states that she has attained adequate amounts of sleep and rest.

- Reassure patient that >90% of breast masses are benign.
- Explain the diagnostic (i.e., mammogram, ultrasound), preoperative, and postoperative procedures.
- If appropriate, inform patient that a local anesthetic might be used during the biopsy and that sensations of pulling and probing may be felt.
- Provide time for patient's verbalization of feelings; answer patient's questions.
- The risk for breast cancer increases with epithelial hyperplasia and fibroadenoma on histologic examination (McDivitt, Stevens, Lee et al, 1992). For a biopsy showing that the patient is at increased risk of malignancy, see **Anxiety** in "Malignant Breast Disorders," p. 593.

---

**Note:**   See "Breast Reduction" for **Pain,** p. 584. See Appendix One for nursing diagnoses and interventions in "Caring for Preoperative and Postoperative Patients," p. 693.

---

## PATIENT-FAMILY TEACHING AND DISCHARGE PLANNING

Give patient and significant others verbal and written information about the following:

- Medications, including drug name, purpose, dosage, schedule, precautions, and potential side effects.
- Indicators of wound infection, which require follow-up by health-care provider: persistent redness, pain, swelling, and discharge at the operative site.
- Care of the incision site, including cleansing. After sutures are removed, soap and water should be used for gentle cleansing
- Resumption of daily activities to patient's tolerance.
- Diet as tolerated, with suggestion to eliminate caffeine and methylxanthine products if fibrocystic condition is diagnosed.
- Scheduled date for the completed pathology report, or an explanation of the diagnosis, if already available.
- Importance of BSE. Teach the procedure to patients who do not know it; reinforce and review the technique for those patients who practice it monthly.
- Importance of screening mammography: baseline between 35-40 years of age, every 1-2 years for ages 40-50 years, and every year for ages 50 and older.

# Malignant breast disorders

Breast cancer is one of the three most common types of breast disease, second only to fibrocystic condition in occurrence. In the United States, it is the most frequently occurring type of cancer in females. Breast cancer usually is diagnosed in women 40-70 years of age, with 54 the median age. However, in the last few years there has been an increase in newly diagnosed cases in women in their 20s and 30s.

The histopathology of breast tumors involves the progression of the tumor from a local preinvasive disease state to invasive malignancy. The changes that occur in the breast are due primarily to hyperplasia of the epithelium. Although carcinoma in situ is usually noninvasive, it too can develop into invasive carcinoma. The differentiation between noninvasive and invasive cancer requires extensive examination of tissue cells obtained during biopsy.

## ASSESSMENT

**Signs and symptoms:**  In the earliest stages, an appearance of abnormalities in the ducts and microcalcifications on mammogram examination may indicate cancer. A later indicator is a palpable mass. Signs of advanced disease include nipple retraction, change in breast contour, nipple discharge, redness or heat of the breast, palpable lymph glands, dimpling of the skin of the breast, and *peau d'orange* or orange peel appearance of the breast. Ulceration also may be a sign of advanced disease.

**Physical assessment:**  Palpable mass, which usually is located in the upper outer quadrant of the breast. Usually the mass is painless, unilateral, irregular in shape, poorly delineated, and nonmobile. There may be signs of edema, venous engorgement, and abnormal contours.

**Risk factors:**  Previous breast cancer in the contralateral breast; family history of cancer and breast cancer, especially a mother or sister, particularly if bilateral and developed before menopause; being over age 50; postmenopausal weight gain; early age at menarche (11 or younger); late age of menopause (after 52 years); nulliparity or late age at first full-term delivery (over 30). In addition, it is theorized that exposure to carcinogens and a high-fat diet are other factors in the development of breast cancer. **Note:** Only one-quarter of women with breast cancer have the known risk factors; therefore, *all* women should be considered at risk.

## DIAGNOSTIC TESTS

The most specific test for detection of breast disease is the excisional biopsy (see "Benign Breast Disorders and Conditions," p. 589). Mammography may detect breast masses in patients who do not have a palpable mass. However, there is the risk of false-negative results (10%-15% of cases). The American Cancer Society recommends a baseline mammogram for women ages 35-40 years, and a mammogram every 1-2 years for women 40-50 years of age and annually for women age 50 years and over.

## COLLABORATIVE MANAGEMENT

**Staging of the tumor:**  Provides a way to formulate the prognosis and treatment plan. The size of the tumor, the appearance of the cancer in the axillary nodes, and the presence of distant metastases determine the degree of staging (Table 9-1).

**Radiation therapy:**  The tumor is excised along with some of the adjacent tissue, followed by external radiation or radioactive implants. This procedure has the same 5-year survival rate as modified radical mastectomy.

**Modified radical mastectomy:**  Removal of the breast tissue, nipple and areola, the tumor and surrounding skin, the axillary lymph nodes, and possibly the pectoralis minor muscle.

**Total mastectomy or simple mastectomy:**  Involves removal of the breast, but the lymph nodes are left intact.

**Partial mastectomy (lumpectomy, tylectomy, or segmental resection):**  Excision of the tumor and a small amount of the tissue surrounding it. Axillary nodal dissection is usually done.

**Quadrectomy:**  Removal of the entire quadrant of the breast where the tumor is located. Axillary nodal dissection is usually done.

**Adjuvant treatment:**  Chemotherapy, hormone therapy, and/or radiation therapy after tumor removal. Usually chemotherapy is given to women who

---

**T A B L E  9 - 1**   **Cancer Staging by the Tumor, Node, Metastasis (TNM)
Classification System**

---

*Stage 0*
**T** = carcinoma in situ
**N** = no regional lymph node metastasis
**M** = no distant metastasis

*Stage I*
**T** = tumor ≤2 cm in greatest dimension
**N** = no regional lymph node metastasis
**M** = no distant metastasis

*Stage IIA*
**T** = from no evidence of tumor to tumor >2 cm but <5 cm in greatest diameter
**N** = no regional lymph node metastasis if tumor >2 cm; or metastasis to movable
  ipsilateral axillary lymph node(s) if tumor <2 cm
**M** = no distant metastasis

*Stage IIB*
**T** = tumor >2 cm in greatest diameter
**N** = no regional lymph node metastasis if tumor >5 cm; or metastasis to movable
  ipsilateral axillary lymph node(s) if tumor <5 cm
**M** = no distant metastasis

*Stage IIIA*
**T** = from no evidence of tumor to tumor >5 cm in greatest diameter
**N** = metastasis to movable ipsilateral axillary lymph node(s) if tumor >5 cm in great-
  est diameter; or metastasis to ipsilateral axillary lymph node(s) fixed to one another
  or to other structures if tumor <5 cm
**M** = no distant metastasis

*Stage IIIB*
**T** = tumor of any size including direct extension to chest wall or skin
**N** = from no node involvement to metastasis to ipsilateral internal mammary lymph
  node(s) if tumor extends directly to chest wall or skin; or any tumor size with metas-
  tasis to ipsilateral internal mammary lymph node(s)
**M** = no distant metastasis

*Stage IV*
**T** = tumor of any size
**N** = any lymph node involvement or none
**M** = distant metastasis

---

Condensed from American Joint Committee on Cancer, *Manual for staging of cancer,* ed 3, Chicago, 1988, The Committee.

are premenopausal with positive lymph nodes, and hormone therapy is given
to women who are postmenopausal with positive nodes.

*Chemotherapy:*   Includes the use of either a single agent or a combination of
agents. This management pattern is used either as an adjunct to surgery or, in
advanced disease, when metastases have occurred or positive lymph nodes
have been identified. Cytotoxic drugs have been found to be more effective
when used in combination. These combinations include the following:

—Cyclophosphamide, doxorubicin, and fluorouracil: First-line therapy for adjuvant treatment or for metastatic disease. It is used monthly for a year.

—Cyclophosphamide, methotrexate, and fluorouracil: Used in metastatic or recurrent disease.

*Hormonal therapy:* The hormone used depends on whether the tumor is estrogen-receptor-positive or estrogen-receptor-"poor," and it is also used in advanced disease. Some of these hormonal agents include:

—Tamoxifen citrate: An antiestrogen used in estrogen-receptor-positive tumors and metastatic disease.

—Megase: For relapse of the disease if a previous response to tamoxifen has occurred.

—Aminoglutethimide, androgens.

## NURSING DIAGNOSES AND INTERVENTIONS

**Anxiety** related to the possibility of cancer and its treatment

*Desired outcome:* Within 12 h of hospital admission, patient expresses concerns and exhibits increasing psychologic comfort as evidenced by participation in decisions regarding her care and the statement that she is able to rest and sleep adequately.

- Assess the patient's understanding of the potential diagnosis and treatment plan; clarify and explain as appropriate.
- Provide time for patient to express feelings and fears.
- Evaluate the patient's emotional status, and explore with the patient what her breasts mean to her. The breast may represent nurturance, sexuality, femininity, and desirability.
- Assess your own feelings about the diagnosis of cancer and the psychologic meaning of the breast. Your attitudes may be reflected in the patient's care; therefore, a positive attitude is essential for optimal patient support.
- Provide a nonthreatening, relaxed atmosphere for the patient and significant others by using therapeutic communication techniques, such as open-ended questions and reflection.
- For additional interventions, see this nursing diagnosis in Appendix One, p. 753.

**Ineffective individual coping** related to situational crisis (diagnosis of breast cancer)

*Desired outcomes:* Within the 24-h period before hospital discharge, patient expresses her feelings, identifies positive coping patterns (e.g., using support systems, planning daily activities), and accepts the support of others.

- Assist patient in identifying and developing a support system.
- Provide support to patient's significant other. Refer significant other to a support group that addresses significant other's specific concerns.
- If a mastectomy was performed, recognize the signs of grief, such as denial, anger, withdrawal, or inappropriate affect. Provide emotional support, and describe the stages of grief to the patient and significant others. Provide explanations to significant others, who may misunderstand the meaning of the patient's behavior or actions.
- Consult with the surgeon regarding a visit from a woman who has had a diagnosis similar to that of the patient. Reach to Recovery volunteers from the American Cancer Society are trained to share their experiences with breast cancer patients.
- See "Caring for Patients with Cancer and Other Life-Disrupting Illnesses," p. 753, in Appendix One for this and other psychosocial nursing diagnoses and interventions.

**High risk for disuse syndrome** related to upper extremity immobilization secondary to discomfort, lymphedema, or infection after mastectomy

*Desired outcomes:* Before surgery, patient verbalizes knowledge about the importance of and rationale for upper extremity movements and exercises. Upon recovery, patient has full ROM of the upper extremity.

- Consult with the surgeon before the mastectomy to determine the type of surgery anticipated. With the surgeon, develop an individualized exercise plan specific to the patient's needs, which can be implemented as soon as the patient returns from the recovery room.

- Encourage finger, wrist, and elbow movement to aid circulation and help minimize edema as soon as the patient returns to her room.
- Encourage progressive exercise by having patient use the affected arm for personal hygiene and ADL the morning after surgery. Other exercises (clasping the hands behind the head and "walking" the fingers up the wall) should be added as soon as patient is ready. After the sutures have been removed (usually 7-10 days postoperatively), patient should begin exercises that will enhance external rotation and abduction of the shoulder. The patient should be able to achieve maximum shoulder flexion by touching her fingertips together behind her back. A Reach for Recovery volunteer can visit and provide patient with verbal instructions and written handouts for these exercises.
- Assist patient with ambulation until her gait is normal. Encourage correct posture with the back straight and shoulders back.
- To minimize the risk of lymphedema and infection, avoid giving injections, measuring BP, or taking blood samples from the affected arm. Remind the patient about her lowered resistance to infection and the importance of promptly treating any breaks in the skin. To help prevent infection after hospital discharge, advise patient to treat minor injuries with soap and water and to notify her health-care provider if signs of infection occur.
- Advise patient to wear a Medic-Alert bracelet that cautions against injections and tests in the involved arm.
- To protect the hand and arm from injury, advise the patient to wear a protective glove when gardening or doing chores that require exposure to harsh chemicals, such as cleaning fluids. Explain that cutting cuticles should be avoided and that lotion should be used to keep the skin soft.

**Pain** related to the surgical procedure

***Desired outcomes:***   Patient's subjective perception of pain decreases within 1 h of intervention, as documented by a pain scale; objective indicators, such as grimacing, are absent or diminished. Patient relates that pain is relieved with IV or IM narcotics for the first 48 h after surgery and with oral medications for the following 2 weeks, with pain decreasing daily.

- Assess and document the location, quality, and duration of the pain, rating it with the patient on a scale of 0 (no pain) to 10 (worst pain).
- Medicate patient with the prescribed analgesics before the pain becomes too severe, or provide instructions for individuals who are using patient-controlled analgesia. Evaluate and document the response, using the pain scale.
- Reassure patient that phantom breast sensations are normal.
- Provide a comfortable in-bed position, and support the affected arm with pillows.
- Encourage movement of the fingers on the affected arm to increase circulation. Inform the patient that although progressive exercise will cause some discomfort, it will aid in the mobility of the affected arm and enhance recovery.
- Reassure the patient that exercise movements will be adapted to her level of tolerance.
- If appropriate, instruct the patient in relaxation techniques and use of guided imagery.
- Provide distraction, such as television, radio, or books.
- Use touch to help relieve tension (e.g., by giving a gentle massage).
- For additional interventions, see this nursing diagnosis in Appendix One, p. 694.

**Body image disturbance** related to loss of a breast

***Desired outcome:***   Within the 24-h period before hospital discharge, patient demonstrates movement toward acceptance of the loss of her breast.

- Recognize that loss of a breast is perceived in different ways by different women. It is frequently more traumatic for the young adult.
- Provide emotional support by being with the patient when the surgical dressing is removed.
- As appropriate, explain that sexual relations can be resumed as soon as the surgical pain has decreased. Assure patient that relations that were positive before surgery usually remain positive. However, be aware that sexual relationships that were weak before the surgery may not tolerate the added stress.
- Recognize the need for a supportive person, such as a Reach for Recovery volunteer who has experienced the same procedure. Consult with the physician about a visit from this individual, if indicated. Support systems also should be made available to significant others.
- If reconstruction is to be delayed or if it is contraindicated or not desired, provide the patient with a breast prosthesis after surgery to help her feel "normal." A temporary prosthesis, made of nylon and filled with dacron fluff, can be worn until the incision heals. Provide the patient with information about where to get a breast prosthesis. The American Cancer Society has lists of distributors and types of prostheses available.
- Be aware that use of touch often enhances the patient's self-concept.
- Provide information and answer questions about breast reconstruction (see p. 585).
- For additional interventions, see this nursing diagnosis in Appendix One, p. 760.

**Altered family processes** related to breast malignancy and treatment with radiation therapy and/or chemotherapy

***Desired outcome:*** Within the 24-h period before hospital discharge, the patient of childbearing age verbalizes accurate information about pregnancy and parenthood after breast cancer and its treatment.

---

**Note:** Reproductive counseling should take into account the patient's age, stage of disease, type of cancer treatment, and pretreatment fertility status.

---

- Explain that childbearing should be delayed for approximately 2 years after cancer diagnosis and treatment. This will enable the physician to better evaluate the course of the disease and allow time for the effects of treatment modalities, such as chemotherapy and radiation, to abate.
- Explain to the patient that she can breast-feed with either breast after chemotherapy, but that after radiation therapy she should use only the nonirradiated breast.
- Explore adoption as an alternative for the infertile couple.
- As indicated, discuss issues of parental death and single parenthood with patient and significant other. See psychosocial nursing diagnoses and interventions in Appendix One "Caring for Patients with Cancer and Other Life-Disrupting Illnesses," p. 753.

---

**Note:** See Appendix One for nursing diagnoses and interventions in "Caring for Preoperative and Postoperative Patients," p. 693 and "Caring for Patients with Cancer and Other Life-Disrupting Illnesses," p. 719.

---

## PATIENT-FAMILY TEACHING AND DISCHARGE PLANNING

Give patient and significant others verbal and written information about the following:
- Medications, including drug name, purpose, dosage, schedule, precautions, and potential side effects.
- Type and dates of follow-up treatment.

- Resumption of sexual activity, which usually can occur as soon as pain is diminished.
- Care of the incision site, including cleansing. Explain the components of good hygiene.
- Progressive exercise regimen, which should be continued at home. Advise patient to stop the exercise movement if a pulling sensation or pain is felt.
- Informing health-care professionals to avoid measuring BP or giving injections in the affected arm.
- Indicators of infection (e.g., fever, erythema, local warmth, skin discoloration) and the importance of reporting them to health-care professional.
- Permanent breast prosthesis, including distributors and types available.
- Name and telephone number of a support person who can be called during the first postoperative year. An ideal individual is a Reach for Recovery volunteer.
- Importance of performing monthly breast self-examination (BSE). In addition, as a part of the BSE, teach patient to palpate the scar, sweep down the chest wall, and palpate the axillary, supraclavicular, and subclavian lymph nodes to assess for lumps. In addition, teach patient that skin changes, such as rashes and erythema, are suggestive of recurrence and that they should be reported promptly.
- Importance of follow-up care.

# Section Two:    Neoplasms of the Female Pelvis

Cancers of the cervix and ovaries are frequently occurring reproductive cancers in women. Statistics published by the American Cancer Society in 1991 estimated 47,000 new cases of uterine cancer a year (13,000 of invasive cervical cancer and 34,000 of endometrial cancer) and 19,000 new cases of ovarian cancer. Women of all ages can develop cancer of these structures, although it is most often found in individuals aged 40-60. The average age for occurrence is 48 years, although involvement for younger women is increasing.

## Cancer of the cervix

Generally, cervical cancer is considered a sexually transmitted disease. The probable agents are human papillomaviruses (16 and 18) and herpes simplex virus type 2. The following risk factors have been associated with this disease: early age of first coitus, multiple sexual partners, cigarette smoking, and a diet low in vitamins A and C and folic acid. The two types of cervical cancer are squamous cell, which is the most common, and adenocarcinoma. *Preinvasive* describes cancerous cells that are limited to the cervix, while *invasive* refers to cancer that is present in the cervix, in other pelvic structures, and possibly in the lymphatic system as well. Preinvasive cancer of the cervix typically is found in women aged 30-40, while invasive cancer usually appears from ages 40-50. Treatment of preinvasive cancer has a greater success rate.

### ASSESSMENT
**Preinvasive:**   Patient asymptomatic; Pap smear abnormal.
**Invasive:**   Abnormal vaginal bleeding; persistent, watery vaginal discharge; postcoital pain and bleeding; abnormal Pap smear.

### DIAGNOSTIC TESTS
**Pap smear:**   Cells are collected from the endocervix and squamocolumnar junction on the cervix with an applicator, placed on a slide, fixed, and sent to

the lab for analysis. Pap smear results may be reported as follows:
- Normal or atypical benign.
- Cervical intraepithelial neoplasia
  —Grade 1: Mild dysplasia.
  —Grade 2: Moderate to severe dysplasia.
  —Grade 3: Severe dysplasia and carcinoma in situ.
- Invasive squamous cell carcinoma.
- Adenocarcinoma.
- Atypical cells present; repeat to rule out.
- Specimen insufficient for diagnosis.

**Colposcopy:** Procedure providing a three-dimensional view of the cervix and allowing for cervical staining with an iodine solution (Schiller's test). Cells that do not absorb the stain are considered abnormal and are sent to the lab for further examination. This procedure takes approximately 20 min.

**Conization biopsy:** Surgical procedure performed under general anesthetic in which a cone-shaped area of the cervix is biopsied for lab analysis to determine the extent of the malignancy.

**Computerized axial tomography (CT) scanning and MRI:** Radiologic detection techniques used to determine the degree and extent of the pathologic process within the pelvis and the spread of the disease outside the pelvis.

**Chest x-ray:** May reveal presence of metastasis to the lungs.

**Staging of the disease:** The following guidelines are used, based on clinical classification by the International Federation of Gynecology and Obstetrics (FIGO):
- *Stage 0:* Carcinoma in situ; preinvasive.
- *Stage I:* Cancer cells in the cervix only.
  —*Stage IA:* Cervical cancer with <3 mm spread.
  —*Stage IB:* Cervical cancer with definite invasive areas.
- *Stage II:* Cancer involving cervix and vagina but not the pelvic wall.
  —*Stage IIA:* No involvement of uterine tissue.
  —*Stage IIB:* Involvement of uterine tissue.
- *Stage III:* Involvement of the pelvic wall or lower third of the vagina.
  —*Stage IIIA:* No extension onto the pelvic wall.
  —*Stage IIIB:* Extension onto pelvic wall and/or kidney secondary to hydronephrosis (obstructed flow of urine to kidney, producing kidney atrophy).
- *Stage IV:* Cancer in bladder, rectum, and other organs of the pelvis.
  —*Stage IVA:* Metastasis to rectum, bladder.
  —*Stage IVB:* Metastasis to distant organs.

---

**Note:** Metastasis to lymph nodes occurs in 15% of cases in stage I and >50% in stage IV.

---

## COLLABORATIVE MANAGEMENT

Therapies will vary depending on the type and extent of the lesion.

*Preinvasive*

**Laser therapy:** Precise destruction of small lesions without destruction of normal tissue.

**Cryosurgery:** Involves freezing the cervix with liquid nitrogen. It is used only for superficial lesions that do not involve the endocervix.

**Conization:** Removal of a cone-shaped wedge of the cervix around the os.

**Hysterectomy:** Removal of the uterus with cervix, either abdominally or vaginally.

*Invasive*

**External radiation therapy:** All stages of cancer are treated with this therapy, which is performed on an outpatient basis in the nuclear medicine department. Dosage and length of treatment are determined by the extent of the disease and the physician specializing in nuclear medicine.

**Radium implants:**   Used to destroy cervical cancer; may be used in combination with external radiation. While the patient is anesthetized, an applicator is positioned in the cervix through the vagina and its position confirmed by x-ray. After the patient returns to her room, the radiologist inserts a radioactive isotope and leaves it in place for 1-3 days. During this time the patient is in a private room and remains in isolation.

A combination of external radiation and implants gives the best therapeutic results. While the implant is in place, the patient is kept on strict bed rest, has an indwelling catheter, is on a low-residue diet, and is given analgesia (usually non-narcotic) and diphenoxylate hydrochloride with atropine sulfate (Lomotil) or paregoric to control diarrhea, which often occurs. After the implant has been removed, the patient is allowed to ambulate.

**Radical hysterectomy:**   May be performed for young women to preserve tissue health. It involves the removal of the uterus, fallopian tubes, ovaries, upper third of the vagina, and parametrium on each side, as well as pelvic lymph node dissection. The patient usually returns to her room with an indwelling catheter.

**Chemotherapy (i.e., with cisplatin):**   May be given simultaneously with pelvic irradiation in locally advanced disease.

## NURSING DIAGNOSES AND INTERVENTIONS

**Pain** related to surgery or radiation implant
*Desired outcomes:*   Within 1 h of intervention, patient's subjective perception of pain decreases, as documented by a pain scale. Objective indicators, such as grimacing, are absent or diminished.

- Provide backrubs, which are especially helpful for patients who were in the lithotomy position during surgery. Massage the shoulders and upper back for patients with radium implants, who are not allowed position changes.
- For other interventions, see this nursing diagnosis in Appendix One, p. 694.

**High risk for fluid volume deficit** related to operative, postoperative, or postimplant bleeding
*Desired outcomes:*   Patient is normovolemic as evidenced by BP ≥90/60 mm Hg (or within patient's usual range), HR 60-100 bpm, urinary output ≥30 ml/h, RR ≤20 breaths/min with normal depth and pattern (eupnea), skin dry and of normal color, and a soft and nondistended abdomen. Patient and significant others verbalize knowledge about the signs and symptoms of excessive bleeding and are aware of the need to alert staff promptly if they are noted.

- Monitor VS q2-4h during the first 24 h. Be alert to indicators of hemorrhage and impending shock: hypotension, increased pulse and respirations, pallor, and diaphoresis.
- Assess postoperative bleeding q2-4h by noting amount and quality of drainage on dressings and perineal pads if abdominal approach was used, or on perineal pads alone if vaginal approach was used. Normally the patient's postoperative bleeding is minimal. It should be dark in color (or serosanguinous if an abdominal hysterectomy was performed). If an implant is in place, check for vaginal bleeding, a sign that erosion is occurring.
- Inspect the abdomen for distention, and assess patient for presence of severe abdominal pain; both are indicators of internal bleeding.
- Review CBC values for evidence of bleeding: decreases in hemoglobin (Hgb) and hematocrit (Hct). Notify physician of significant findings. Optimal values are Hct ≥37% and Hgb ≥12 g/dl.
- Inform patient and significant others about the signs of excessive bleeding and the need to alert staff immediately if they occur.

**Altered pattern of urinary elimination** (oliguria or anuria) related to inadequate intake, obstruction of indwelling catheter, or ureteral ligation
*Desired outcome:*   Within 24 h of surgery, patient demonstrates a balanced I&O, with urinary output ≥30 ml/h immediately following surgery.

- Monitor I&O, and document every shift. Notify physician if urinary output falls below 30 ml/hr over 2 h in the presence of an adequate intake. Along with low back pain, this sign can be indicative of ureteral ligation during surgery.
- Ensure patency of the indwelling catheter.
- Administer oral or parenteral fluids as prescribed. Ensure totals of 2-3 L/day in nonrestricted patients.
- Assess for bladder distention by inspecting the suprapubic area and percussing or palpating the bladder. **Caution:** For patients with radiation implants, bladder distention can result in radiation burns to the bladder.

**Grieving** related to actual or perceived loss or changes in body image, body function, or role performance secondary to diagnosis of cancer

*Desired outcome:* Before hospital discharge, patient and significant other(s) express grief, explain the meaning of the loss, and communicate concerns with each other. The patient completes self-care activities as her condition improves.

- Anticipate patient's concern about loss of uterus, presence of cancer, the potential for recurrence, and "loss of womanhood." Provide emotional support and an unhurried atmosphere for patient and significant others to ask questions and express concerns, frustrations, and fears.
- Recognize the covert signs of grief that can accompany self-concept disturbances: anger, withdrawal, demanding behavior, or inappropriate affect. Give support to significant others who might misinterpret patient's coping mechanisms.
- To enhance patient's sense of control over her situation, encourage her to perform ADL and begin self-care as soon as her condition warrants.
- Provide materials by organizations such as the American Cancer Society and arrange for a contact person from such an organization, if appropriate.
- For additional interventions, see this nursing diagnosis in Appendix One, p. 757.

---

**Note:** See Appendix One for nursing diagnoses and interventions in "Caring for Preoperative and Postoperative Patients," p. 693, and "Caring for Patients with Cancer and Other Life-Disrupting Illnesses," p. 719.

---

## PATIENT-FAMILY TEACHING AND DISCHARGE PLANNING

Give patient and significant others verbal and written information about the following:

### For patients who have had radium implants:
- Necessity of notifying physician if the following problems occur: vaginal bleeding, rectal bleeding, foul-smelling vaginal discharge, abdominal pain or distention, dysuria, urinary frequency, hematuria.
- Resumption of sexual intercourse, typically 6 weeks after surgery or as directed by physician. Describe, as indicated, use of a vaginal dilator to prevent atrophy. It is usually inserted once a day for 5 min.
- Medications, including drug name, dosage, purpose, schedule, precautions, and potential side effects.
- Need for follow-up care; confirm date and time of next medical appointment if known.
- Patient is *not* radioactive once the implant has been removed.
- Side effects of radium implants: vaginal dryness, burning sensation, vaginal discharge.

### For patients who have had a hysterectomy:
- Necessity of notifying physician if the following indicators of infection occur: incisional swelling, redness, purulent drainage, vaginal bleeding, abdominal pain.
- Care of the incision.

- Restriction of activities as directed, such as heavy lifting (>10 lb) and sexual intercourse. Advise patient to get maximum amounts of rest and avoid fatigue.
- Medications, including drug name, dosage, purpose, schedule, precautions, and potential side effects.
- Need for follow-up care; confirm date and time of next medical appointment if known.

## Ovarian tumors

There are numerous types of ovarian tumors, both benign and malignant. They include solid tumors and cysts of various cell types and can occur in females of all ages. The most common enlargements arise from the normal follicular apparatus of the ovary (i.e., follicle and corpus luteum cysts) and hyperplasias, such as polycystic ovaries. The most common benign neoplasms are the cystadenomas, which make up 55% of the tumors. *Malignant ovarian tumors* rarely are diagnosed early because the patient tends to be asymptomatic. Because their detection usually occurs during an advanced stage, survival rate is low. Therefore this is the most lethal type of gynecologic cancer. Although found in women of all ages, the average age range of occurrence for malignant lesions is 50-59. Both environmental and genetic factors may contribute to their development.

### ASSESSMENT

**Benign ovarian tumors:**   Depending on the type, common symptoms include abdominal enlargement and complaints of abdominal fullness.

**Solid ovarian tumors:**   Abdominal enlargement and pressure; pelvic pressure and discomfort.

**Signs and symptoms for both classifications:**   Amenorrhea, postmenopausal vaginal bleeding and other menstrual irregularities; urinary frequency and urgency; gastrointestinal (GI) complaints, such as nausea, anorexia, and constipation. Usually there are no early signs in ovarian cancer, or they may be mild, including digestive disturbances.

**Physical assessment:**   Abdominal distention; an enlarged ovary, which is highly suspicious in prepubertal and postmenopausal women.

### DIAGNOSTIC TESTS

**Abdominal ultrasound:**   (Especially by vaginal probe) may reveal an ovarian mass.

**Elevated serum markers:**   Carcinoembryonic antigen (CEA) and CA 125 may signal developing ovarian cancer.

**Laparoscopy:**   Use of a laparoscope, an instrument with a telescope and light source, to visualize the pelvic organs through an incision made near the umbilicus. This procedure is done using general or regional anesthetic, usually on an outpatient basis.

**Cytologic examination of the pelvic washings/ascites:**   May show presence of malignant cancerous cells.

**Other diagnostic testing:**   May be done preoperatively when ovarian cancer is suspected; include chest x-ray, intravenous pyelogram (IVP), barium enema, upper GI series, and endoscopic bowel examination.

**Staging of ovarian tumors** (dependent on surgical exploration)**:**   The following guidelines are used, based on clinical classification by FIGO:

- *Stage I:* Tumor limited to the ovaries.
  —*Stage IA:* Growth limited to one ovary; no ascites.
  —*Stage IB:* Tumors limited to both ovaries; no ascites.
  —*Stage IC:* Tumor IA or IB but with tumor on the surface, ruptured cap-

sule; with ascites with malignant cells; or with positive peritoneal washings.

- *Stage II:* Tumors involving one or both ovaries with presence of malignant cells in pelvic organs.
  —*Stage IIA:* Involvement of uterus or fallopian tubes with presence of malignant cells.
  —*Stage IIB:* Presence of malignant cells in other pelvic tissues.
  —*Stage IIC:* Tumors IIA or IIB with ascites or positive peritoneal washings.
- *Stage III:* Tumors involving one or both ovaries with metastasis outside the pelvis or positive retroperitoneal nodes. Tumor limited to retroperitoneal lymph nodes. Malignant cells found in small bowel omentum.
  —*Stage IIIA:* Tumor grossly limited to the true pelvis with negative nodes but with microscopic seeding of abdominal peritoneal surfaces.
  —*Stage IIIB:* Tumor of one or both ovaries with implants ≤2 cm of abdominal peritoneal surfaces; negative nodes.
  —*Stage IIIC:* Abdominal implants >2 cm and/or positive retroperitoneal or inguinal nodes.
- *Stage IV:* Tumors involving one or both ovaries with metastasis to distant organs.

## COLLABORATIVE MANAGEMENT
### For benign tumors
**Wedge resection:**  Surgical procedure in which a benign tumor is removed, leaving normal ovarian tissue. It is done under anesthetic, using an abdominal approach.

**Salpingo-oophorectomy:**  Removal of the ovary and fallopian tube on the affected side. It is performed under anesthetic, using an abdominal approach. This procedure is used for solid tumors of the ovary.
### For malignant tumors
**Cytoreductive surgery:**  Involves removal of as much tumor as possible in order to increase the effectiveness of radiation and chemotherapy, which are more successful when the residual tumor is minimized.

**Para-aortic and pelvic lymphadenectomy:**  For staging of the disease when it is grossly confined to the ovary.

**Total hysterectomy and bilateral salpingo-oophorectomy:**  Along with omental removal.

**Chemotherapy and radiation:**  Used depending on the stage of the disease. Chemotherapy is indicated for stages III and IV. Chemotherapeutic medications usually are used in combination and may include (among others) cisplantin (the most active), doxorubicin, melphalen, and cyclophosphamide. Intraperitoneal administration may be used in women with minimal or microscopic residual disease (<2 cm). This form of chemotherapy applies treatment directly to the tumor and decreases general toxicity. Radiation therapy, when it is used, involves the whole abdomen.

**Other surgery:**  Depending on the spread of the disease, bowel resection also may be needed to debulk the tumor adequately.

## NURSING DIAGNOSES AND INTERVENTIONS

---

**Note:**  See "Cancer of the Cervix" for **Pain,** p. 598, **High risk for fluid volume deficit** (bleeding), p. 598, **Altered pattern of urinary elimination,** p. 598, and **Grieving,** p. 599. See Appendix One for nursing diagnoses and interventions in "Caring for Preoperative and Postoperative Patients," p. 693, and "Caring for Patients with Cancer and Other Life-Disrupting Illnesses," p. 719.

---

## PATIENT-FAMILY TEACHING AND DISCHARGE PLANNING

Give patient and significant others verbal and written information about the following:

- Medications, including drug name, dosage, schedule, purpose, precautions, and potential side effects.
- Importance of reporting indicators of infection (depending on the surgery) to the physician: fever, vaginal bleeding and discharge, abdominal pain and distention, and incisional redness, purulent drainage, local warmth, and swelling.
- Activity restrictions related to heavy lifting (>10 lb), exercise, sexual intercourse, or housework, as directed by physician.
- Necessity of follow-up appointments; confirm date and time of next appointments for physician, radiation therapy, and chemotherapy.

# Endometrial cancer

Endometrial (uterine) cancer is the most common type of female genital cancer in the United States and is one of the six leading causes of death in women. Typically it occurs in postmenopausal women aged 50-70. Risk factors for developing uterine cancer include a diet high in fat, obesity, late menopause (after age 52), hypertension, diabetes mellitus, unopposed menopausal estrogen therapy (i.e., giving estrogens without progestins), infertility due to failure of ovulation, and dysfunctional uterine bleeding during menopause. The tumor can be found in any location within the uterus, as either a focal lesion or diffuse condition, with ≤15% developing quickly and lethally. The invasive stages of uterine cancer can involve spread to the vagina, pelvic lymph nodes, ovaries, and through the vascular system to the lungs, bones, and liver. Recurrence most frequently is seen in the vagina. When an early diagnosis is made, the prognosis is very good because the tumor tends to be localized and well differentiated. *Adenocarcinoma* is the most common endometrial cancer.

## ASSESSMENT

**Signs and symptoms:**   Uterine bleeding in the postmenopausal woman; heavy and prolonged menses and intermenstrual spotting in the premenopausal woman.

**Physical assessment:**   Presence of a palpable uterine mass, uterine polyps; obvious increase in uterine size in advanced disease.

## DIAGNOSTIC TESTS

**Aspiration currettage and endometrial biopsy:**   Office procedures used to obtain specimens from the emdometrium.

**Hysteroscopy:**   Examination *via* an endoscope, which enters the uterus through the vagina, allowing visualization, biopsy, and photography with a camera. The patient is anesthetized with a pericervical block. This procedure can be used for diagnosis and staging.

**Dilatation and curettage (D&C):**   Surgical procedure in which the cervical opening is widened by a dilating instrument and the uterine lining is scraped with a curette to obtain a specimen for examination.

**Chest x-ray:**   To detect metastasis to the lungs.

**Intravenous pyelogram:**   To rule out spread of disease to other organs.

**CT scanning:**   To direct needle biopsy of suspicious nodes.

**Staging of the disease:**   The following guidelines are used, based on clinical classification by FIGO:

- *Stage IA:* Tumor limited to endometrium.
- *Stage IB:* Less than half the myometrium involved.
- *Stage IC:* More than half the myometrium involved.
- *Stage IIA:* Involvement of endocervical gland only.

- *Stage IIB:* Invasion of cervical stroma.
- *Stage IIIA:* Invasion of serosa and/or adnexae and/or positive peritoneal cytology.
- *Stage IIIB:* Metastasis to vagina.
- *Stage IIIC:* Metastasis to para-aortic and/or pelvic lymph nodes.
- *Stage IVA:* Invasion to bladder and/or bowel mucosa.
- *Stage IVB:* Distant metastasis.

## COLLABORATIVE MANAGEMENT

The woman's age and reproductive needs determine the choice of treatment for adenomatous hyperplasia. More aggressive tumors with extension require more complex treatment. Treatment is individualized and can vary from progestin therapy to surgery.

**Hysterectomy (with or without radiation):**   With cytologic examination of peritoneal washings; the most common procedure.

**Radiation therapy (either internal or external) and pelvic and aortic lymphadenectomy:**   Usually reserved for high-virulance tumors. If an implant is used, the applicator is positioned in the uterus through the vagina while the patient is anesthetized. After the patient returns to her room, the radioisotope is placed in the applicator by a radiologist. External radiation of the uterus and pelvic nodes is performed on an outpatient basis for a period of time that is determined by the radiologist.

**Chemotherapy:**   Used for poorly differentiated tumors that are not hormone-dependent. Chemotherapeutic drugs include adriamycin and 5-fluorouracil. Combinations of drugs and the dosage and length of treatment are determined by the patient's response to treatment and the severity of recurrence.

**Hormone therapy:**   Used for recurrent and advanced endometrial cancers. A progestin is usually used. This therapy is more effective when the tumor has a large number of progesterone receptors. It also can be used in young women who wish to preserve their fertility.

## NURSING DIAGNOSES AND INTERVENTIONS
See "Cancer of the Cervix," p. 598.

## PATIENT-FAMILY TEACHING AND DISCHARGE PLANNING
See "Cancer of the Cervix," p. 599.

# Vulvar cancer

Vulvar cancers are increasing in number. Nearly 50% of newly diagnosed patients with carcinoma in situ (intraepithelial neoplasia) are ages 20-40. Older women (>60 years of age) are more likely to develop invasive cancer. Squamous cell carcinoma accounts for 90%-95% of primary vulvar tumors; the 5-year survival rate is approximately 46% because of late diagnosis.

## ASSESSMENT

**Signs and symptoms:**   Pruritus (in about two-thirds of cases); lesions in the labia majora, clitoris, and/or periurethral areas; ulceration of lesions in advanced disease; pain; and bleeding. About 20% of cases are asymptomatic.

## DIAGNOSTIC TESTS

**Vulvar biopsy:**   A Keyes cutaneous punch often is used to perform the biopsy. Colposcopy and/or staining with 1% toluidine blue solution can be used to identify lesions for biopsy.

**Staging:**   The following clinical stages of invasive vulvar carcinoma are adapted from the classification by FIGO:

- *Stage 0:* Carcinoma in situ.

- *Stage 1:* Maximum diameter of lesions ≤2 cm; confined to the vulva.
- *Stage II:* Diameter of lesions >2 cm; confined to the vulva.
- *Stage III:* Extension of lesions to urethra, anus, perineum, or vagina; absence of grossly positive groin lymph nodes. Or, lesions of any size confined to the vulva with suspicious lymph nodes.
- *Stage IV:* Presence of lesions with grossly positive groin lymph nodes. Lesions involving rectal, bladder, or urethral mucosa or bone. All cases with pelvic or distant metastases.

## COLLABORATIVE MANAGEMENT

**Benign lesions:**   Often treated by topical applications, cryosurgery, laser, or excision.

**Carcinoma in situ:**   Treated by topical application of chemotherapeutic cream, wide local excision, cryosurgery, laser evaporation, or vulvectomy. Wide local excision can use either primary-closure skin flaps or skin grafts. Vulvectomy may involve incision of the vulvar skin and preservation of fat, muscle, and glands with a split-thickness skin graft.

**Invasive carcinoma:**   May involve multimodal therapy with surgery and irradiation to avoid extremely radical treatments. Tumor size, location, and lymph node involvement determine the management.

- *Stage I:* Radical vulvectomy and bilateral groin dissection. If lesions are <2 cm in diameter and <5 mm of invasion has occurred, no dissection is needed.
- *Stage II and III:* More extensive surgery to allow for tumor-free margins may necessitate removal of urethra, vagina, or anus. Irradiation or lymphadenectomy of pelvic and inguinal nodes.
- *Stage IV:* Pelvic exenteration (removal of the entire female reproductive tract along with both urinary and fecal diversions) may be necessary in addition to radical vulvectomy. If the disease is very advanced, therapy may consist of conservative surgery and irradiation.

## NURSING DIAGNOSES AND INTERVENTIONS

**Sexual dysfunction** related to fear after surgical procedure, grafting, excision of all or part of the reproductive tract, and/or pain

*Desired outcome:*   Within the 24-h period before hospital discharge, patient communicates concerns with partner and verbalizes a plan for satisfying sexual activity.

- Determine patient's need to communicate fears and concerns regarding sexual functioning following treatment of vulvar cancer.
- As indicated, teach patient that diminished sexual responsiveness usually does not occur with a skinning vulvectomy or treatment with a carbon dioxide laser. However, patients with simple vulvectomies or other treatments may have diminished responsiveness.
- Advise patient to use medications or relaxation techniques (e.g., hot shower) before sexual activity to help prevent discomfort.
- If vaginal lubrication is decreased, suggest that patient use a water-soluble lubricant.
- Suggest the female superior position during coitus to control depth of penetration.
- Suggest alternative sexual practices, depending on the couple's values. Options include vibrators, touching, massage, and anal stimulation.
- As indicated, advise patient that sexual intercourse usually can be resumed after healing has occurred.

---

**Note:**   For other nursing diagnoses and interventions, see "Cancer of the Cervix," p. 598.

---

PATIENT-FAMILY TEACHING AND DISCHARGE PLANNING
See "Cancer of the Cervix," p. 599.

# Section Three:   Disorders of the Female Pelvis

Endometriosis is often seen in younger women, while cystocele, rectocele, and uterine prolapse more often are associated with women who are postmenopausal. These conditions occur when there is misplacement of structures or tissue within the female pelvis.

## Endometriosis

Endometriosis is a condition in which endometrial tissue is present outside of the uterus. Typically it is found on the ovaries or in the peritoneal cul-de-sac. It also might be found in the vagina, vulva, uterosacral ligaments, or bowel. In extreme cases it is found in the lungs, bones, and other organs of the body. Endometriosis is considered a benign disease; it most often occurs in nulliparous women 30-40 years of age and in those who have had their first child at a later age. Its cause is unknown, but it is theorized that a combination of factors play a role (e.g., the tissue traveling up the fallopian tubes and into the pelvic cavity during the menstrual cycle, and the result of deficiency in the immune system).

### ASSESSMENT

**Signs and symptoms:**   Dysmenorrhea 5-7 days before and 2-3 days after menses, hypermenorrhea (prolonged, excessive, and/or frequent menses), infertility, painful defecation during menses, sacral backache, and dyspareunia. Patient may be asymptomatic.

**Physical assessment:**   Presence of a tender, fixed, rectoverted uterus. Palpation of the peritoneal cul-de-sac and ovaries may reveal presence of tender nodules, masses, or fixation. The pelvic exam is performed several days before the menstrual cycle.

### DIAGNOSTIC TESTS

**Laparoscopy:**   Confirms presence of endometriomas on pelvic organs by passing a lighted instrument through an incision made near the umbilicus and visualizing (e.g., bluish-brown implants, "powder-burn" lesions on the peritoneal surface, and/or unexplained adhesions).

### COLLABORATIVE MANAGEMENT

**Encourage pregnancy in women wishing to have children:**   Pregnancy softens and atrophies the diseased areas as a result of hormone production. Pregnancy (or pseudopregnancy) stops the spread of endometriosis, and in some cases remission occurs following delivery.

**Pharmacotherapy:**   *Danazol* (400 mg bid), an androgen, is a hormone inhibitor that acts by suppressing ovulation and, hence, hormone stimulation of endometrial tissue, allowing endometriomas to atrophy. Progestin-estrogen treatment may improve symptoms but will not cure the disease. Gonadotropic-releasing hormone (GnRH) agonists also suppress ovulation and induce amenorrhea.

**Surgical procedures:**   Determined by the patient's age and desire to have children, and by extent and symptoms of the disease. They are performed if medical treatment is unsuccessful.

*For women without extensive disease who wish to have children, one of the following is performed:*   Laser therapy or cauterization of endometrial im-

plants, uterine suspension, lysis of adhesions, or removal of endometrial implants. These procedures are usually performed *via* an abdominal approach or
through a laparoscope, although uterine suspension also can be performed by
a vaginal approach.

*For women who are not menopausal but do not wish to have children:*   A
hysterectomy may be performed, leaving the ovaries intact so that normal hormonal balance is maintained.

*When there is extensive disease:*   A total hysterectomy with bilateral
salpingo-oophorectomy is performed. The ovaries are removed because they
are hormone-producing organs that influence the development and progression
of the disease.

## NURSING DIAGNOSES AND INTERVENTIONS

**Anticipatory grieving** related to potential for reproductive infertility

*Desired outcome:*   Within the 24-h period before hospital discharge, patient
and significant other express grief, participate in decisions about the future,
and communicate their concerns to the health-care team and to each other.

- Assess for and accept patient's stage in the grieving process and behavioral
  response. Expect reactions such as disbelief, denial, grief, ambivalence, and
  depression. Recognize that the patient and significant other may move from
  one stage to another, depending on the circumstance (i.e., desire for a child,
  type of treatment recommended, or stage of endometriosis and subsequent
  likelihood of infertility).
- Assess religious and sociocultural expectations related to the loss (e.g., Is
  childbearing of primary importance in the relationship? What are the desires
  of the family for offspring? Has there been a lifelong desire to have children?).
- Encourage patient and significant other to explore and communicate feelings about the anticipated loss of fertility. Recognize that the woman often
  feels a greater sense of loss than the man feels. Infertility can place a strain
  on the relationship; treatment options may be expensive and time consuming and may raise ethical issues.
- Assess the couple's coping strategies. Suggest other ways of handling grief
  if their strategies are ineffective. Common strategies include increasing the
  space between themselves and reminders of their infertility (i.e., keeping
  busy), regaining control (seeking information, keeping a positive attitude),
  giving into feelings (crying, indulging), and sharing their burden with each
  other and others.
- Demonstrate empathy. Provide an open and supportive atmosphere. The patient often is exposed to those who have children and do not value the experience. Recognize that the patient may feel hostility toward those who are
  fertile.
- Assess for support systems and describe and provide addresses of groups
  that share a common interest (e.g., RESOLVE). It also may be helpful to
  arrange for referrals to specialists with knowledge of infertility (e.g., psychiatric nurse clinician, psychologist).
- For additional interventions, see this nursing diagnosis in Appendix One, p.
  757.

---

**Note:**   See "Cancer of the Cervix" for **Pain,** p. 598, and **High risk for fluid
volume deficit** (bleeding), p. 598. See Appendix One for nursing diagnoses
and interventions in "Caring for Preoperative and Postoperative Patients," p.
693.

---

## PATIENT-FAMILY TEACHING AND DISCHARGE PLANNING
See "Ovarian Tumors," p. 602.

# Cystocele

A cystocele is the bulging of the posterior bladder wall into the vagina. It is caused by constitutionally poor tissue or the stretching and tearing of the pelvic connective tissue during childbirth. Most often it occurs as a result of the delivery of a very large baby or after several deliveries. Symptoms usually do not appear until menopausal or postmenopausal age. A rectocele (see p. 608) also might be present.

## ASSESSMENT

**Signs and symptoms:**   Sensation of vaginal fullness or of bearing down, inability to empty bladder after voiding, urinary frequency, dysuria, stress incontinence, incontinence resulting from urgency, and recurrent cystitis.

**Physical assessment:**   Manual pelvic exam will reveal a soft mass that bulges into the anterior vagina. The mass increases in size with coughing or straining.

## DIAGNOSTIC TESTS

**Urine culture and sensitivity:**   May reveal presence of bladder infection.

**Urodynamic evaluation:**   Involves study of the flow of urine from the bladder through the urethra to differentiate stress incontinence from urgency incontinence. A combination of tests is used, including voiding flow rate, urethra pressure profile, urethroscopy, and cystometrogram.

## COLLABORATIVE MANAGEMENT

**Urinary catheterization:**   To empty a distended bladder. This is an emergency measure rather than a permanent correction.

**Antibiotics:**   Given if urinary retention results in an infection.

**Estrogen therapy:**   Conjugated estrogen (Premarin) and a progesterone regimen sometimes is given in small daily doses to postmenopausal women to maintain hormonal levels. A lack of hormones may result in weakness of the anterior vaginal wall, which allows the development of a cystocele.

**Kegel isometric exercises:**   To help with bladder control (see p. 163).

**Anterior colporrhaphy:**   Surgical procedure *via* vaginal approach to suspend the bladder. It involves separating the anterior vaginal wall from the bladder and urethra, suturing the bladder wall to reduce herniation, and excising the thinned vaginal wall. If both a cystocele and rectocele (see p. 608) are present, an anterior and posterior colporrhaphy (A&P repair) is performed.

**Pessary:**   Used as an internal support for some patients (see discussion in "Uterine Prolapse," p. 609). A Smith-Hodge device often is used if a cystocele exists.

## NURSING DIAGNOSES AND INTERVENTIONS

See "Urinary Incontinence" for related nursing diagnoses, p. 161. See "Cancer of the Cervix" for **High risk for fluid volume deficit** (bleeding), p. 598. See Appendix One for nursing diagnoses and interventions in "Caring for Preoperative and Postoperative Patients," p. 693.

## PATIENT-FAMILY TEACHING AND DISCHARGE PLANNING

Give patient and significant others verbal and written information about the following:

- Medications, including drug name, purpose, dosage, schedule, precautions, and potential side effects.
- Activity limitations during the first 6 weeks or as directed, including no heavy lifting (>10 lb) or strenuous exercises.
- Abstinence from sexual intercourse for 6 weeks or as prescribed if vaginal surgery was performed. Discuss alternate methods of sexual expression.

- Notifying physician for the following indicators of infection: fever; persistent pain; purulent, foul-smelling drainage.
- Importance of follow-up appointments; confirm date and time of next appointment if known.

## Rectocele

A rectocele is a rectovaginal hernia, which develops when the connective tissue between the rectum and vagina is weakened and attenuated during childbirth. If there is straining with defecation or the patient is obese, the condition is aggravated and progresses. The symptoms of this condition often do not become apparent until the woman is 35-40 years old.

### ASSESSMENT

**Signs and symptoms:**    Continuous urge to have a bowel movement, sensation of rectal and vaginal fullness, constipation (digital pressure must be applied vaginally to facilitate defecation), incontinence of flatus or feces, and the presence of hemorrhoids or fecal impaction.

**Physical assessment:**    A nontender fullness can be felt by depressing the perineum as the patient strains; manual rectal examination will reveal the presence of a rectocele.

### DIAGNOSTIC TESTS

**Barium enema:**    Will reveal the presence of a rectocele. As the hernia increases in size, the wall of the anterior rectum tends to be pushed into the vagina.

### COLLABORATIVE MANAGEMENT

**Promote bowel elimination:**    With a high-fiber diet, fluids, stool softeners, and laxatives. If not contraindicated, walking is encouraged as a means of exercise to promote elimination.

**Posterior colporrhaphy:**    This surgical procedure separates the posterior vaginal wall from the rectum and reduces the rectal herniation. If both a cystocele and a rectocele are present, an anterior and posterior colporrhaphy (A&P repair) is performed (see "Cystocele," p. 607).

### NURSING DIAGNOSES AND INTERVENTIONS

**Constipation** related to restriction against straining, low-residue diet, or pain with defecation secondary to surgical procedure

***Desired outcomes:***    After the early postoperative period, patient relates the presence of bowel movements within her normal pattern and with minimal discomfort. Patient verbalizes knowledge of the rationale for alerting staff before and after bowel movements and for not straining during defecation.

- Assess patient for the presence of constipation; administer stool softeners or mild laxatives as prescribed.
- The patient will be on a low-residue diet during the early postoperative period to minimize the potential for disruption of the surgical site. As indicated after the early postoperative period, consult with the physician about introducing high-residue foods to promote bowel movements.
- Instruct patient not to strain when having a bowel movement, because this can disrupt the surgical repair.
- Advise patient that defecation may be painful and to alert staff as soon as the urge to defecate is felt so that she can be medicated before the bowel movement.
- Avoid the use of enemas or rectal tubes, which can disrupt the surgical repair.
- Provide sitz baths as a comfort measure after bowel movements.

- Request that the patient notify staff after each bowel movement; document accordingly.

---

**Note:** See "Cancer of the Cervix" for **High risk for fluid volume deficit** (bleeding), p. 598. See Appendix One for nursing diagnoses and interventions in "Caring for Preoperative and Postoperative Patients," p. 693.

---

## PATIENT-FAMILY TEACHING AND DISCHARGE PLANNING

Give patient and significant others verbal and written information about the following:
- Medications, including drug name, purpose, dosage, schedule, precautions, and potential side effects.
- Limitation of activities during the first 6 weeks as directed by physician, including heavy lifting (>10 lb) and exercising. Abstinence from sexual intercourse is usually recommended for 6 weeks. Discuss alternate forms of sexual expression with patient. Advise patients that initially coitus may be painful.
- Indicators of infection: abdominal or rectal pain, foul-smelling vaginal discharge, and fever.
- Importance of a regular bowel elimination pattern to prevent constipation and straining.
- Importance of follow-up care; confirm date and time of next medical appointment if known.

# Uterine prolapse

A uterine prolapse is a bulging of the uterus through the pelvic floor into the vagina. It results from an injury to the cardinal and uterosacral ligaments, which can occur with childbirth, surgical trauma, or atrophy of the supportive tissue during menopause. A prolapse also can develop as a result of uterine tumors, diabetic neuropathy, neurologic injury to the sacral nerves, obesity, or ascites. A prolapse will progress unless surgically repaired.

A prolapse is graded in the following way:
- *Grade I:* Cervix remains within the vagina; the uterus partially descends into the vagina (first-degree prolapse).
- *Grade II:* Cervix protrudes through the entrance to the vagina. This is second-degree prolapse.
- *Grade III:* Entire uterus protrudes throught the entrance of the vagina, and the vagina is inverted. This a third-degree prolapse, or procidentia, which occurs most frequently in postmenopausal, multiparous women and often along with a rectocele, cystocele, and enterocele (a hernia containing a loop of small intestine or the sigmoid colon, which bulges into the upper posterior vagina).

## ASSESSMENT

**Signs and symptoms:** Complaints of heaviness in the pelvis, low backache, dragging sensation in the inguinal region, involuntary loss of urine with coughing or sneezing, and poor bladder emptying.

**Physical assessment:** Pelvic examination is performed with the patient either standing or supine. As patient bears down, a firm mass can be palpated in the lower vagina. This exam also can confirm diagnosis of a rectocele and cystocele, if present.

## COLLABORATIVE MANAGEMENT

**Placement of a vaginal pessary:** A rubber device that is inserted into the vagina to support the pelvic structures. It may be used if there is first- or second-degree prolapse or if surgery is contraindicated or unwanted by patient.

**Estrogen suppositories:**   To maintain tone of the pelvic floor.

**Antibiotics:**   If patient has a urinary tract infection.

**High-fiber diet:**   To aid in bowel elimination.

**Kegel exercises:**   Daily sets at frequent intervals to help with bladder control (see p. 163).

**Vaginal hysterectomy:**   To correct uterine prolapse. For severe prolapse with rectocele and cystocele, a hysterectomy with an anterior/posterior colporrhaphy is performed.

## NURSING DIAGNOSES AND INTERVENTIONS

**Note:**  See "Cancer of the Cervix" for **High risk for fluid volume deficit** (bleeding), p. 598, and **Grieving** (if a hysterectomy is performed), p. 599. See "Rectocele" for **Constipation,** p. 608. See Appendix One for nursing diagnoses and interventions in "Caring for Preoperative and Postoperative Patients," p. 693.

## PATIENT-FAMILY TEACHING AND DISCHARGE PLANNING
See "Rectocele," p. 609.

# Section Four:   Interruption of Pregnancy

The following conditions or surgical procedures involve women of childbearing age and can result in continued problems with childbearing or sterilization.

## Spontaneous abortion

A spontaneous abortion, or miscarriage, occurs in approximately 15% of pregnancies. It is the expulsion of the products of conception (POC) before the twenty-fourth week of gestation, and it is classified in the following ways:

**Threatened abortion:**   Vaginal bleeding and cramping during the first half of the pregnancy. There is no tissue loss, and the cervix is closed. Either the symptoms disappear or an abortion occurs.

**Inevitable abortion:**   Vaginal bleeding, cramping, rupture of membranes, and dilatation and effacement of the cervix; cannot be halted.

**Incomplete abortion:**   Partial expulsion of POC, with continued vaginal bleeding.

**Complete abortion:**   Expulsion of all POC, with decrease in or cessation of vaginal bleeding and pain following expulsion.

**Missed abortion:**   Presence of a nonviable fetus in the uterus for ≥2 months.

**Recurrent (habitual) abortion:**   Three or more pregnancies that are spontaneously aborted during the first trimester.

The primary causes of spontaneous abortion are *fetal,* including defective development and faulty implantation of the fertilized ovum and accounting for the majority of spontaneous abortions; and *maternal,* including infection, malnutrition, endocrine abnormalities, and incompetent cervix.

## ASSESSMENT

**Signs and symptoms:**   Vaginal bleeding, cramping, low back pain, signs of pregnancy, no progressive increase in size of uterus.

**Physical assessment:** A pelvic examination will reveal the size of the uterus and dilatation of the cervix and show either that POC are intact or have been expelled.

## DIAGNOSTIC TESTS

**CBC:** Will reveal a decrease in Hgb and Hct. There is a potential for elevation in leukocyte count, which would signal an infection.

**Lab examination of POC:** To confirm results of pelvic examination.

**Ultrasound:** Will confirm the presence of a nonviable fetus, as evidenced by absence of fetal heart motion. This test may be performed abdominally or transvaginally

**Endocrine studies:** Human chorionic gonadotropin (HCG) will be minimal or absent with pregnancy loss.

## COLLABORATIVE MANAGEMENT

Management will depend on the type of abortion. The following are examples of treatment options:

**Administration of blood or blood products:** For excessive blood loss.

**Parenteral fluid administration:** For excessive fluid loss.

**Analgesics:** For pain management.

**Antibiotics:** When indicated, to prevent development of infection.

**Dilatation and curettage (D&C):** Procedure done in the first trimester to remove POC. Under general or local anesthesia, the canal of the cervix is dilated to allow a curette to pass through the cervix into the uterus and scrape out any POC that remain. A **suction evacuation,** which utilizes a suction apparatus rather than a curette, may be performed instead.

**IV oxytocin:** Used as an alternative to D&C to aid in the passage of POC. Oxytocin contracts the uterus by stimulating the smooth muscles.

**Cervical cerclage:** Performed early in the second trimester to manage an incompetent cervix when patient has a history of repeated second trimester abortions. With this technique, the cervix is reinforced with a suture (using McDonald, Shirodkar, or transabdominal cervicoisthmic cerclage procedure). The suture is released at term (or immediately if labor begins) to allow a vaginal delivery. This procedure is not performed in the presence of membrane rupture, cramping, vaginal bleeding, or a cervical dilatation >3 cm.

**RhoGAM:** An $Rh_o$ (D) immune globulin, which is given to prevent Rh sensitization in Rh-negative women.

**Other:** When the pregnancy is viable, observation by ultrasound and quantitative HCG levels may assist in monitoring progress of pregnancy. Bed rest often is recommended. Other treatments may depend on the probable cause.

## NURSING DIAGNOSES AND INTERVENTIONS

**High risk for fluid volume deficit** related to abortive or postsurgical bleeding

***Desired outcome:*** Patient is normovolemic as evidenced by BP ≥90/60 mm Hg; HR 60-100 bpm; urinary output ≥30 ml/h; RR ≤20 breaths/min with normal pattern and depth (eupnea); warm and dry skin; and orientation to person, place, and time.

- Assess and document BP, HR, and RR at frequent intervals (typically q15min × 4; q30min × 2; q1-2h until stable; and then q4h). Notify physician of significant changes. Be alert to hypotension, changes in LOC, cool and clammy skin, and increasing HR and RR.
- Monitor I&O at least q4h. Be alert to decreasing urinary output, which can signal the onset of shock.
- Administer parenteral fluids, blood, and blood products as prescribed.
- If prescribed, administer oxytocin to assist with the contraction of the uterus and expulsion of the fetus.

- Inspect perineal pads and note and document the amount and quality of bleeding. If vaginal bleeding increases or there is expulsion of the POC, notify physician at once. Save any tissue or clots that are expelled. **Note:** Bleeding is considered excessive if ≥1 perineal pads are saturated in 1 h and there are symptoms of orthostasis (i.e., fainting or dizziness upon standing, diaphoresis, pallor).
- After expulsion of the POC has occurred, palpate the uterine fundus to assess its tone. If it feels soft and boggy, provide light massage using a circular motion. **Caution:** Avoid massaging a uterus that is well contracted because this can result in muscle fatigue and uterine relaxation.

**Pain** related to uterine contractions

***Desired outcomes:***  Within 30 min of intervention, patient's subjective perception of pain decreases, as documented by a pain scale. Objective indicators, such as grimacing, are absent or diminished.

- Monitor and document frequency and duration of contractions. Assess and document the patient's level of pain and response to management, using a scale of 0 (no pain) to 10 (worst pain).
- Administer analgesics as prescribed. Provide backrubs, which are especially relaxing.
- Instruct patient in alternative methods of pain relief, including deep breathing, relaxation techniques, and guided imagery.
- For additional interventions see this nursing diagnosis in Appendix One, p. 694.

**High risk for infection** related to retention of some or all of the POC

***Desired outcome:***  Patient is free of infection, as evidenced by normothermia and absence of foul-smelling vaginal discharge and abdominal tenderness.

- Assess temperature q4h; notify physician if an elevation occurs.
- Be alert to the presence of foul-smelling vaginal discharge, a signal of infection.
- Administer antibiotics as prescribed.
- Ensure that perineal care is performed after every voiding and bowel movement.

**Altered role performance** related to fetal loss

***Desired outcome:***  Before hospital discharge, patient verbalizes realistic acceptance of change in her role as wife or childbearer or verbalizes plans for adaptation.

- Provide emotional support for patient and significant others. Provide time and a supportive atmosphere for patient to feel comfortable with expressing feelings and concerns. Do not minimize patient's feelings of loss. Conversely, if the pregnancy was not desired, she may experience feelings of relief or guilt regarding the loss.
- Assist patient in identifying concerns, if present, with role performance as a wife or childbearer. Assist patient in developing plans for adaptation. Provide referral for genetic counseling if genetics was a factor in the pregnancy loss.
- Involve social services if needed.

**Grieving** related to anticipated or actual fetal loss

***Desired outcome:***  Before hospital discharge, the patient expresses her feelings about the loss (actual or potential) and shares her grief with significant others.

- Assess the stage of grieving patient is experiencing. Be aware that feelings may be complicated by emotions that preceded the actual or impending fetal loss (e.g., if the woman experienced joy about her pregnancy, her grief may be more than anticipated; conversely, if the pregnancy was viewed negatively she may experience feelings of guilt and self-blame).
- Do not minimize patient's feelings of loss. Recognize that an early preg-

nancy loss may take longer to resolve because the grieving process is complicated by the absence of a recognizable body.

- Assist patient and significant others with acknowledging the loss by taking the time to sit and talk with them.
- Offer emotional support and encourage the patient and significant others to discuss the loss among themselves, as well.
- Ensure privacy for the patient and significant others.
- Refer the patient to community-based parent support group.
- Provide for pastoral or other supportive care if indicated.
- See psychosocial nursing diagnoses for patients and families in Appendix One, p. 753.

## PATIENT-FAMILY TEACHING AND DISCHARGE PLANNING

Give patient and significant others verbal and written information about the following:

- Medications, including drug name, purpose, dosage, schedule, precautions, and potential side effects.
- Vaginal bleeding, which should taper gradually during the first 10 days. Advise patient that increasing bleeding is abnormal and necessitates medical attention.
- Indicators of infection, which necessitate medical attention: temperature ≥37.78° C (100° F), foul-smelling vaginal discharge, and/or abdominal tenderness or pain.
- Activity limitations as directed by physician, including strenuous exercise and sexual relations.
- Importance of follow-up care; confirm date and time of next medical appointment.
- Name and address of community resources.

# Ectopic pregnancy

An ectopic pregnancy is a fertile ovum implanted outside the uterus. The most common site is the fallopian tube; it occurs less commonly in the peritoneum, ovary, or cervix. In the fallopian tube, the implanted ovum causes a weakening of the tubal wall, resulting in a rupture that can cause bleeding into the peritoneum, a medical emergency. Factors that predispose toward ectopic pregnancy include pelvic inflammatory disease, intrauterine device (IUD) usage, prior surgical procedure of the fallopian tube, history of infertility, previous ectopic pregnancy, and smoking. These pathologies may interfere with the structure and function of the fallopian tube and cause a delay in the passage of the ovum into the uterus, which can result in ectopic pregnancy. Ectopic pregnancies occur in approximately 1 out of every 72 pregnancies, a nearly threefold increase from 1970 statistics.

## ASSESSMENT

**Signs and symptoms:**  Indications of pregnancy (i.e., amenorrhea, nausea, breast enlargement, urinary frequency), uterine bleeding or spotting, and abdominal pain. Most symptoms appear 6-8 weeks after the last menstrual period. The following acute symptoms may develop prior to and accompanying rupture: mild to moderate vaginal bleeding with unilateral lower abdominal cramping that becomes increasingly sharp and constant, referred shoulder pain caused by irritation of the diaphragm from the pooling of blood in the peritoneum, and a falling Hct and Hgb. **Caution:** Immediate intervention is necessary to prevent loss of blood, which can lead to shock and death.

**Physical assessment:**  Abdominal palpation may reveal a unilateral lower quadrant tenderness, and size and date discrepancy. **Caution:** Pelvic examination is deferred if ectopic pregnancy is suspected to minimize the risk of tubal rupture.

## DIAGNOSTIC TESTS

**CBC:**   May reveal a decreased Hgb and Hct and an increased leukocyte count.
**Serum human chorionic gonadotropin (HCG):**   Serial levels will plateau and then diminish. There will be lower than normal levels of serum progesterone and urinary metabolites of serum progesterone.
**Ultrasound:**   May identify the location of pregnancy *via* transvaginal probe.
**Culdocentesis:**   May reveal the presence of blood in the peritoneum. In this test, fluid is aspirated from the vaginal cul-de-sac.
**Laparoscopy:**   Will confirm the presence of ectopic pregnancy and allow immediate treatment.

## COLLABORATIVE MANAGEMENT

**Administration of whole blood or packed cells:**   To replace loss if necessary.
**Broad spectrum IV antibiotics:**   May be administered prophylactically.
**Analgesics/narcotics:**   For pain management.
**Laparoscopy:**   Conservative procedure performed on a stable patient, using an endoscope inserted through a small opening in the abdomen. Often it is used in conjunction with tubal sparing procedures.
**Laparotomy with unilateral salpingectomy (removal of the fallopian tube) or salpingo-oophorectomy (removal of the fallopian tube and ovary):**
Performed if the ectopic pregnancy ruptures. A ruptured ectopic pregnancy is considered a surgical emergency because of the inevitable loss of blood into the peritoneum. The type of surgical procedure used is dependent on the extent of structural involvement.
**Methotrexate:**   This drug, which is often used in chemotherapy, can be given to select patients with unruptured tubes early in diagnosis in whom surgery is contraindicated or future fertility is desired. Methotrexate, a folinic acid antagonist, induces abrupt tubal abortion.
**RhoGAM:**   If indicated, is given to Rh-negative mothers after ectopic pregnancy.

## NURSING DIAGNOSES AND INTERVENTIONS

**High risk for fluid volume deficit** related to bleeding or hemorrhage with ectopic rupture
***Desired outcome:***   Patient is normovolemic, as evidenced by urinary output ≥30 ml/h, BP ≥90/60 mm Hg, RR ≤20 breaths/min with normal depth and pattern (eupnea), HR ≤100 bpm, warm and dry skin, and absent or scant vaginal bleeding.
- Assess VS at frequent intervals, noting changes in BP, HR, and RR. Be alert to hypotension, increases in HR and RR, and cool and clammy skin as indicators of impending shock.
- Assess the amount and quality of vaginal bleeding. Bright red, frank bleeding, along with abnormal VS, should be reported to the physician at once.
- Review results of CBC, noting values of Hgb and Hct, which are decreased with blood loss. Optimal values are Hct ≥37% and Hgb ≥12 g/dl.
- Infuse parenteral and blood products as prescribed.

---

**Note:**   See "Spontaneous Abortion" for **Grieving,** p. 612, and **Altered role performance,** p. 612. See "Endometriosis" for **Anticipatory grieving,** p. 606. See Appendix One for nursing diagnoses and interventions in "Caring for Preoperative and Postoperative Patients," p. 693. See psychosocial nursing diagnoses and interventions for patient and significant others in "Caring for Patients with Cancer and Other Life-Disrupting Illnesses," p. 753.

---

PATIENT-FAMILY TEACHING AND DISCHARGE PLANNING

Give patient and significant others verbal and written information about the following, depending on the type of surgical procedure:

- Medications, including drug name, purpose, dosage, schedule, precautions, and potential side effects.
- Importance of monitoring vaginal drainage, including the amount, color, consistency, and odor; and reporting significant changes to the physician.
- Activity limitations as directed by the physician, including strenuous exercise, housework, and sexual relations.
- Indicators of incisional infection, including persistent redness, swelling, warmth, fever, purulent discharge, and incisional/abdominal pain.
- Importance of follow-up care and purpose for serial HCG levels (with the more conservative treatment) or methotrexate management; confirm time and date of next medical visit if known.

# Section Five:    Disorders and Surgeries of the Male Pelvis

## Benign prostatic hypertrophy

The prostate is an encapsulated gland that surrounds the male urethra below the bladder neck and produces a thin, milky fluid during ejaculation. As a man ages, the prostate gland grows larger. Although the exact cause of the enlargement is unknown, one theory is that hormonal changes affect the estrogen-androgen balance. This noncancerous enlargement is common in men over age 50, and as many as 80% of men over the age of 65 are believed to have symptoms of prostatic enlargement. Treatment is given when symptoms of bladder outlet obstruction appear.

### ASSESSMENT

**Chronic indicators:**    Urinary frequency, hesitancy, and dribbling; decreased force of stream; nocturia; hematuria.

**Acute indicators/bladder outlet obstruction:**    Anuria, nausea, vomiting, severe suprapubic pain, constant urgency, flank pain during micturition.

**Physical assessment:**    Bladder distention, "kettle-drum" sound with percussion over the distended bladder. Rectal exam will reveal a smooth, firm, symmetric, and elastic enlargement of the prostate.

### DIAGNOSTIC TESTS

**Urinalysis:**    Checks for the presence of WBCs, bacteria, and microscopic hematuria; and **urine culture and sensitivity:** verifies presence of infection; results will specify the type of organism and determine the most effective antibiotic.

**Hct/Hgb:**    Decreased values may signal mild anemia from local bleeding.

**Blood urea nitrogen (BUN) and creatinine:**    To evaluate renal-urinary function. **Note:** BUN can be affected by the patient's hydration status, and the results must be evaluated accordingly: fluid volume excess reduces BUN levels, while fluid volume deficit will increase them. Serum creatinine may not be a reliable indicator of renal function in the older adult, because of decreased muscle mass and decreased glomerular filtration rate; results of this test must be evaluated along with those of urine creatinine clearance, other renal function studies, and the patient's age.

**Cystoscopy:**    To visualize the prostate gland, estimate its size, and ascertain the presence of any damage to the bladder wall secondary to an enlarged prostate. **Note:** Because patients undergoing cystoscopy are susceptible to septic shock, this procedure is contraindicated in patients with acute urinary tract infection (UTI) because of the danger of introducing gram-negative bacteria into the bladder.

**Intravenous pyelogram (IVP)/excretory urogram:**    Evaluates the structure and function of the kidneys, ureters, and bladder, and reveals calculi if they are present. In the presence of benign prostatic hypertrophy (BPH), IVP will show postvoid residual urine, bladder diverticuli caused by herniation, or chronic infection and bladder muscle hypertrophy caused by straining. IVP also may show displacement of bladder and ureters caused by enlarged prostate, a condition known as *J-hooking*. **Note:** Two complications of IVP are allergic reaction to dye, and acute renal failure induced by the contrast medium. Exposure to contrast medium might worsen existing renal insufficiency, especially in elderly, dehydrated, or diabetic patients. Before the study, patients should be queried about allergies to shellfish and iodine or reactions to previous dye studies. After IVP, patients should be monitored for indicators of renal failure.

---

**Note:**    All urine specimens should be sent to the laboratory immediately after they are obtained, or refrigerated if this is not possible (specimens for urine culture are *not* refrigerated). Urine left at room temperature has a greater potential for bacterial growth, turbidity, and alkaline pH, any of which can distort the test results.

---

## COLLABORATIVE MANAGEMENT

**Catheterization:**    To relieve urinary retention. Because of the high incidence of bacteriuria from catheterization (50% after the first 24 h), intermittent catheterization is preferred.

**Antibiotics and antimicrobial agents:**    To treat infection, if one is present.

**Antiandrogen therapy:**    Estrogens, antiandrogens, progestogens, prolactin and alpha-sympathetic blockers, gonadotropin-releasing hormone analogs, and alpha adrenergics are used to relieve symptoms of outflow obstruction; may be initiated to lower the levels of testosterone if this is the cause of the prostate's enlargement. Occasionally an orchiectomy is performed for the same purpose. **Note:** The patient will become impotent while on estrogen therapy. However, an orchiectomy will *not* affect the patient's ability to have sexual relations.

**Reduction of prostatic congestion *via* rectal massage of the prostate gland:** This is performed only if there is substantial congestion. Hot sitz baths also are prescribed to relieve congestion.

**Restriction of rapid intake of fluids:**    Particularly alcohol, which can result in episodes of acute urinary retention from loss of bladder tone secondary to rapid distention.

**Balloon dilatation:**    Using fluoroscopy, cystoscopy, ultrasound, or MRI, a balloon catheter is inserted *via* the urethra into the prostate. The balloon is inflated with sterile water or contrast material, and the high pressure compresses the prostate gland allowing enlargement of the urethral lumen. This procedure is indicated for individuals who are poor surgical risks.

**Prostatectomy:**    Removal of enlarged prostatic tissue.

*Transurethral resection of the prostate (TURP):*    Prostatic tissue is scraped away *via* cystoscopy. This is the most common approach, especially in patients who are poor surgical risks. It is done under spinal anesthesia.

*Suprapubic transvesical prostatectomy/retropubic extravesical prostatectomy/ perineal resection:*    Prostatic tissue is removed *via* an incision high in the bladder (abdominal approach), by a low abdominal incision without entry into the bladder, or by an incision between the scrotum and rectum. This is indicated for a large prostate ($\geq$40 g) that cannot be removed transurethrally. These approaches may be used if large bladder diverticula or calculi exist that can be corrected at the time of surgery, in the presence of a severe urethral stricture, and with orthopedic conditions that contraindicate positioning for other approaches.

## NURSING DIAGNOSES AND INTERVENTIONS

**High risk for fluid volume deficit** related to postsurgical bleeding/hemorrhage
***Desired outcomes:*** Patient is normovolemic as evidenced by balanced I&O, HR ≤100 bpm (or within patient's normal range), BP ≥90/60 mm Hg (or within patient's normal range), RR ≤20 breaths/min, and skin that is warm, dry, and of normal color. Following instruction, patient relates actions that might result in hemorrhage of the prostatic capsule and participates in interventions to prevent them.

- Upon patient's return from the recovery room, monitor VS q15min for the first 30 min; if stable, check q30min for 1 hr; and then q4h for 24 h, or per agency policy. Be alert to increasing pulse, decreasing BP, diaphoresis, pallor, and increasing respirations, which can occur with hemorrhage and impending shock.
- Monitor and document I&O q8h. Subtract the amount of fluid used with bladder irrigations from the total output.
- Monitor catheter drainage closely for the first 24 h. Watch for dark red drainage that does not lighten to reddish-pink or drainage that remains thick in consistency after irrigation, which can signal venous bleeding within the operative site. Drainage should lighten to pink or blood-tinged within 24 h after surgery.
- Be alert to bright red, thick drainage at any time, which can occur with arterial bleeding within the operative site.
- Do not measure temperature rectally or insert rectal tubes or enemas into the rectum. Instruct patient not to strain with bowel movements or sit for long periods of time. Any of these actions can result in pressure on the prostatic capsule and may lead to hemorrhage. Obtain prescription for and provide stool softeners or cathartics as necessary.
- The surgeon may establish traction on the indwelling urethral catheter in the operating room to help prevent bleeding. Maintain the traction for 4-8 h after surgery, or as directed.
- Also monitor patient for signs of disseminated intravascular coagulation, which can occur as a result of the release of large amounts of tissue thromboplastins, which can occur during a TURP. Watch for active bleeding (dark red) without clots and unusual oozing from all puncture sites. Report significant findings promptly if they occur. For more information, see "Disseminated Intravascular Coagulation," p. 504.

**High risk for infection** (septic shock) related to invasive procedure (cystoscopy or TURP) resulting in risk of introduction of gram-negative bacteria
***Desired outcome:*** Patient is free of gram-negative infection as evidenced by normothermia; urinary output ≥30 ml/h; RR 12-20 breaths/min; HR and BP within patient's normal range; and orientation to person, place, and time (within patient's normal range).

---

**Note:** Accurate assessment of the patient in the early (warm) stage of septic shock greatly improves the prognosis.

---

- Monitor patient's VS and mentation status at frequent intervals for indicators of the early (warm) stage of septic shock. During the first 24 h after surgery, be alert to temperatures of 38.3°-40.0° C (101°-104° F), which occur in the presence of infection due to increased metabolic activity and release of pyrogens. Also assess for moderately increased RR and HR and decreased BP. Classic circulatory signs of collapse occur in the late (cold) stage of septic shock, including profoundly decreased BP (due to decreased stroke volume), greatly increased and weakened HR (compensatory mechanism to maintain cardiac output), and decreased RR (owing to respiratory center depression). Mental status changes of inappropriate behavior, personality changes, restlessness, increasing lethargy, and disorientation may signal hypoxia due to decreased cerebral perfusion.

- Monitor patient's skin for flushing and warmth, which are early signs of septic shock due to vasodilatation. In the cold stage of septic shock, skin will become cool and pale because of sustained vasoconstriction.
- Monitor patient's urinary output for decrease and for increased concentration (normal specific gravity is 1.010-1.020).
- Notify physician promptly if septic shock is suspected. Prepare for the following if septic shock is confirmed: IV infusion (e.g., lactated Ringer's or normal saline); oxygen administration; specimens for WBC, ABG, and electrolyte values; and administration of antibiotics.
- Teach the indicators of infection and early septic shock to patient and stress the importance of notifying staff promptly if they occur after cystoscopy or TURP.

**Fluid volume excess (or risk of same)** related to absorption of irrigating fluid during surgery (TURP syndrome)
***Desired outcomes:***  Following surgery, patient is normovolemic as evidenced by balanced I&O (after subtraction of irrigant total from output); orientation to person, place, and time; BP and HR within patient's normal range; absence of dysrhythmias; and electrolyte values within normal range. Urinary output is ≥30 ml/hr, and drainage from Jackson-Pratt drain is >40 ml/hr.

- Monitor and record VS. Watch for sudden increases in BP with corresponding decrease in HR. Monitor pulse for dysrhythmias, including irregular rate and skipped beats.
- Monitor and record I&O. To determine the true amount of urinary output, subtract the amount of irrigant from the total output. Report discrepancies, which can signal fluid retention or loss.
- Monitor the patient's mental and motor status. Assess for the presence of muscle twitching, seizures, and changes in mentation. These are signs of water intoxication and electrolyte imbalance, which can occur within 24 h after surgery because of the high volumes of fluid used in irrigation.
- Monitor electrolyte values, in particular those of $Na^+$, for evidence of hyponatremia. Normal range for $Na^+$ is 137-147 mEq/L.
- Promptly report indications of fluid overload and electrolyte imbalance to the physician.

**Pain** related to bladder spasms
***Desired outcomes:***  Within 1 h of intervention, patient's subjective perception of pain decreases, as documented by a pain scale. Objective indicators, such as grimacing, are absent or diminished.

- Assess and document the quality, location, and duration of pain. Devise a pain scale with patient, rating pain from 0 (no pain) to 10 (worst pain).
- Medicate the patient with prescribed analgesics, narcotics, and antispasmodics as appropriate; evaluate and document the patient's response, using the pain scale. For individuals in whom the retropubic approach has been used, suppositories are contraindicated. Oral anticholinergics such as oxybutynin are used instead.
- Provide warm blankets or heating pad to affected area or warm baths to increase regional circulation and relax tense muscles.
- Teach technique for slow, diaphragmatic breathing to relax patient and help ease pain.
- Provide back rubs and encourage use of other nonpharmacologic methods of pain relief such as guided imagery, distraction, relaxation tapes, and soothing music. Also see p. 54 for **Health-seeking behaviors:** Relaxation technique effective for stress reduction.

- Monitor for leakage around the catheter, which can signal the presence of bladder spasms.
- If the patient has spasms, assure him that they are normal and can occur from irritation of the bladder mucosa by the catheter balloon or from a clot that results in backup of urine into the bladder with concomitant irritation of the mucosa. Encourage fluid intake to help prevent spasms. If the physician has prescribed catheter irrigation for the removal of clots, follow instructions carefully to prevent discomfort and injury to patient.
- Monitor for the presence of clots in the tubing. If clots are present for the patient with continuous bladder irrigation, adjust the rate of bladder irrigation to maintain light red urine (with clots). Total output should be greater than the amount of irrigant instilled. If output equals the amount of irrigant or the patient complains that his bladder is full, the catheter may be clogged with clots. If clots inhibit the flow of urine, irrigate the catheter by hand according to agency or physician's directive.

**High risk for impaired skin integrity** related to wound drainage from suprapubic or retropubic prostatectomy
*Desired outcome:* Patient's skin remains clear and intact.
- Monitor incisional dressings frequently during the first 24 h, and change or reinforce as needed. If the incision has been made into the bladder, irritation can result from prolonged contact of urine with the skin.
- Use Montgomery straps rather than tape to secure the dressing.
- If the drainage is copious after drain removal, apply a wound drainage or ostomy pouch with a skin barrier over the incision. Use a pouch with an antireflux valve to prevent contamination from reflux.

**Sexual dysfunction** related to fear of impotence due to lack of knowledge about postsurgical sexual function
*Desired outcome:* Following intervention/patient teaching, patient discusses concerns about sexuality and relates accurate information about sexual function.
- Assess patient's level of readiness to discuss sexual function; provide opportunities for patient to discuss fears and anxieties.
- Assure patient who has had a simple prostatectomy that his ability to obtain and maintain an erection is unaltered. Retrograde ejaculation (backward flow of seminal fluid into the bladder, which is eliminated with the next urination) or "dry" ejaculation will occur in most patients, but this probably will end after a few months. However, it will not affect his ability to achieve orgasm.
- Encourage communication between patient and his significant other.
- Be aware of your own feelings about sexuality. If you are uncomfortable discussing sexuality, request that another staff member take responsibility for discussing feelings and concerns with the patient.
- As indicated, encourage continuation of counseling after hospital discharge. Confer with physician and social services to identify appropriate referral.

**Constipation** related to postsurgical discomfort or fear of exerting excess pressure on the prostatic capsule
*Desired outcome:* By the third to fourth postoperative day, patient relates the presence of a bowel pattern that is normal for him with minimal pain or straining.

---

**Note:** A patient who states that he needs to have a bowel movement during the first 24 h after surgery probably has clots in the bladder that are creating pressure on the rectum. Assess for the presence of clots (see **Pain,** earlier) and irrigate the catheter as indicated.

---

- Document the presence or absence and quality of bowel sounds in all four abdominal quadrants.

- Gather baseline information on patient's normal bowel pattern, and document findings.
- Unless contraindicated, encourage patient to consume 2-3 L/day of fluid postsurgically.
- Consult with physician and dietitian about need for increased fiber in patient's diet.
- Teach patient to avoid straining when defecating to prevent excess pressure on the prostatic capsule.
- Consult with physician about use of stool softeners for patient during the postoperative period.
- See **Constipation,** p. 716, in Appendix One for more information.

**Urge incontinence** related to urethral irritation after removal of urethral catheter

***Desired outcome:*** Patient reports increasing periods of time between voidings by the second postoperative day and regains normal pattern of micturition within 4-6 weeks after surgery.

- Before removing the urethral catheter, explain to the patient that he may void in small amounts for the first 12 h after catheter removal because of irritation from the catheter.
- Instruct patient to save urine in a urinal for the first 24 h after surgery. Inspect each voiding for color and consistency. First urine specimens can be dark red from the passage of old blood. Each successive specimen should be lighter in color.
- Note and document the time and amount of each voiding. Initially the patient may void q15-30min, but the time interval between voidings should increase toward a more normal pattern.
- Before hospital discharge, inform patient that dribbling may occur for the first 4-6 weeks after surgery because of disturbance of the bladder neck and urethra during prostate removal. As muscles strengthen and healing occurs (the urethra reaches normal size and function), the dribbling stops.
- Teach patient Kegel exercises (see p. 163) to improve sphincter control.

**Altered thought processes (or risk of same)** related to fluid volume deficit secondary to postsurgical bleeding/hemorrhage; fluid volume excess secondary to absorption of irrigating fluid during surgery; or cerebral hypoxia secondary to infectious process or sepsis

***Desired outcomes:*** Patient's mental status returns to normal for patient within 3 days of treatment. Patient exhibits no evidence of injury as a result of his altered mental status.

- Assess patient's baseline LOC and mental status on admission. Ask patient to perform a 3-step task (i.e., "Raise your right hand, place it on your left shoulder, and then place the right hand by your side"). Test short-term memory by showing patient how to use the call light, having patient return the demonstration, and then waiting 5 min before having patient demonstrate use of the call light again. Inability to remember beyond 5 min indicates poor short-term memory. Document patient's response.
- Document patient's actions in behavioral terms. Describe the "confused" behavior.
- Obtain description of prehospital functional and mental status from sources familiar with patient (e.g., patient's family, friends, personnel at nursing home or residential care facilities).
- Identify cause of acute confusion. You might request oximetry or ABG values to determine oxygenation levels; serum glucose or fingerstick glucose to determine glucose levels; and electrolytes and CBC to ascertain imbalances and/or presence of elevated WBC count as a determinant of infection. Assess hydration status by reviewing I&O records after surgery. Note any imbalances either way. Output should match input. Assess legs for presence of dependent edema, which can signal overhydration with poor venous re-

turn. Assess cardiac and lung status for presence of abnormal heart sounds or rhythms and presence of crackles in lung bases, which can indicate fluid excess. Assess mouth for furrowed tongue or dry mucous membranes, which is a signal of fluid deficit.

- As appropriate, anticipate initiation of oxygen therapy to increase oxygenation; initiation of antibiotics in the presence of sepsis; diuretics to increase diuresis; increased fluid intake by mouth or by IV to rehydrate patient.
- As appropriate, have patient wear glasses and hearing aid, or keep them close to the bedside and within patient's easy reach.
- Keep patient's urinal and other frequently used items within easy reach. If patient has a short-term memory problem, do not expect him to use the call light.
- Check on patient at least q30min and every time you pass by the room.
- Place patient close to nurse's station if possible. Provide an environment that is nonstimulating and safe. Provide music but avoid use of TV (individuals who are acutely confused regarding place and time often think the action on the TV is happening in the room).
- Attempt to reorient patient to surroundings as needed. Keep a clock and calendar at the bedside, and remind patient verbally of the date and place.
- Encourage patient to bring items familiar to patient to provide a foundation for orientation. These items can be simple and include blankets, bedspreads, and pictures of family or pets.
- If the patient becomes beligerent, angry, or argumentative while you are attempting to reorient him, *stop this approach.* Do not argue with patient or patient's interpretation of the environment. State, "I can understand why you may (hear, think, see) that."
- If the patient displays hostile behavior or misperceives your role (nurse becomes thief, jailer, etc), leave the room. Return in 15 min. Introduce yourself to the patient as though you have never met. Begin dialogue anew. Patients who are acutely confused have poor short-term memory and may not remember the previous encounter or that you were involved in that encounter.
- If the patient attempts to leave the hospital, walk with him and attempt distraction. Ask patient to tell you about the destination (e.g., "That sounds like a wonderful place! Tell me about it"). Keep tone pleasant and conversational. Continue walking with patient away from exits and doors around the unit. After a few minutes, attempt to guide patient back to his room.
- If the patient has permanent or severe cognitive impairment, check on him frequently and reorient to baseline mental status as indicated; however, do not argue with patient about his perception of reality. This can cause a cognitively impaired person to become aggressive and combative. **Note:** Patients with severe cognitive impairments (e.g., Alzheimer's disease or dementia) also can experience acute confusional states (i.e., delirium) and can be returned to their baseline mental state.

---

**Note:** See "Cancer of the Bladder" for **Altered urinary elimination** related to obstruction of suprapubic catheter, p. 157. See "Prostatic Neoplasm," for **Stress incontinence,** p. 625. See Appendix One for nursing diagnoses and interventions in "Caring for Preoperative and Postoperative Patients," p. 693.

---

## PATIENT-FAMILY TEACHING AND DISCHARGE PLANNING

Give patient and significant others verbal and written information about the following:

- Medications, including drug name, purpose, dosage, schedule, precautions, and potential side effects.

- Indicators of UTI, which necessitate medical attention: cloudy or foul-smelling urine, fever, pain, dysuria.
- Care of incision, if appropriate, including cleansing, dressing changes, and bathing. Advise patient to be aware of indicators of infection: persistent redness, increased warmth along incision, or purulent drainage.
- Care of catheters or drains if patient is discharged with them.
- Daily fluid requirement of at least 2-3 L/day in nonrestricted patients.
- Importance of increasing dietary fiber or taking stool softeners to soften stools. This will minimize risk of damage to the prostatic capsule by preventing straining with bowel movements. Caution patient not to use suppositories or enemas for treatment of constipation.
- Use of a sofa, reclining chair, or footstool to promote venous drainage from the legs and to distribute weight on the perineum, not the rectum.
- Avoiding the following activities for the period of time prescribed by physician: sitting for long periods of time, heavy lifting (>10 lb), and sexual intercourse.
- Kegel exercises to help regain urinary sphincter control for postoperative dribbling. See discussion, p. 163.

# Prostatic neoplasm

Cancer of the prostate is the most common reproductive cancer in men over age 50 and the second most commonly occurring cancer overall. Because most prostatic neoplasms develop in the posterior portion of the gland, they can be detected in the early stages of development. Therefore, rectal examinations should be a part of every man's regular health check after the age of 40. In addition, after age 40, routine health checks should include prostatic-specific antigen (PSA) screening. Elevations of this blood test indicate the presence of cancer before symptomatology develops or a tumor can be palpated. When detected early, prostatic cancer usually can be treated successfully. Unfortunately, medical treatment often is not sought until the tumor has affected the urinary pattern or caused hip or back pain, recurring cystitis, or urinary obstruction. This symptomatology indicates that metastasis has occurred, which dramatically decreases the survival rate.

## ASSESSMENT

**Signs and symptoms** (in the later stages of development): Dysuria, dribbling, decreased strength of stream, hesitancy, anuria, hematuria, nocturia, burning with urination, urgency, chills, fever, cloudy and foul-smelling urine, decreased urinary output, and lower back pain.

**Physical assessment:**   Bladder distention; "kettle-drum" sound with percussion over distended bladder. Rectal exam may reveal a large, hard, fixed prostate with irregular nodules.

## DIAGNOSTIC TESTS

**Urinalysis and urine culture:**   To verify or rule out the presence of pus, WBCs, WBC casts, RBCs, and pH >8.0, which would signal infection.

**CBC:**   Results may reveal presence of marked anemia in the presence of metastatic disease.

**BUN and creatinine:**   May be elevated if renal function is compromised. **Note:** BUN values are affected by the patient's hydration status and should be evaluated accordingly. Fluid volume excess decreases the value, while fluid volume deficit increases it. In the older adult, decreased muscle mass and a decreased glomerular filtration rate may affect the values of serum creatinine. Therefore, these values must be evaluated along with those of urine creatinine clearance, other renal function studies, and the patient's age.

**Serum acid phosphatase:** To monitor disease progress. Values will be elevated if metastasis has occurred. Because prostate tissue is rich in this enzyme, the spread of the disease results in an increase in the amount of acid phosphatase in the blood.

**Serum alkaline phosphatase:** Will be elevated if metastasis has spread to the bones.

**PSA:** Done in routine screening and monitored along with serum acid phosphatase in staging and following the progress of the disease.

---

**Note:** Serum acid phosphatase and PSA must be drawn before a rectal examination or initiation of urinary catheterization. Both procedures stimulate the prostate to secrete more of these substances and thus raise blood levels.

---

**Intravenous pyelogram (IVP)-excretory urogram:** Evaluates the structure and function of the kidneys, ureters, and bladder. Other findings may include ureteral obstruction caused by metastasis to the pelvic lymph nodes or direct invasion by the tumor. (See discussion of the complications of IVP on p. 616).

**Biopsy of the prostate**

*Transperineal/transrectal needle core biopsy:* Performed under general or spinal anesthetic. The biopsy needle is inserted through the perineal skin or *via* the rectum directly into the area that contains the tumor. The sample is aspirated and sent to the lab for analysis.

*Transrectal fine needle aspiration:* Performed with a local anesthetic, the biopsy needle is passed into the tumor through the rectum. The sample is aspirated and transferred to slides and sent to the lab for analysis.

**Transrectal ultrasonography:** To assess the size and shape of the prostate, including tumor growth. This test is especially useful in recognizing and localizing intracapsular prostatic tumors and in monitoring response of the tumor to therapy.

---

**Note:** All urine specimens should be sent to the laboratory immediately after they are obtained, or refrigerated if this is not possible (specimens for culture are *not* refrigerated). Urine left at room temperature has a greater potential for bacterial growth, turbidity, and alkalinity, any of which can distort the test results.

---

## COLLABORATIVE MANAGEMENT

**Staging of the disease** (based on American Urologic System for Staging Prostate Cancer):

- *Stage A:* Clusters of cancer cells found in tissue samples from biopsy (as indicated by elevated PSA levels) or during surgery for benign disease; cannot be felt by clinician.
  —*A1:* Well differentiated, small volume, low grade, low potential to spread, found in one area of prostate.
  —*A2:* Poorly differentiated, larger volume, higher grade, found in many areas of prostate.
- *Stage B:* Cancer confined to prostate, palpable, may have clinical symptomatology.
  —*B1:* Tumor found in one lobe, small, low grade.
  —*B2:* Tumor involving one or both lobes, large, higher grade.
- *Stage C:* Cancer extends through prostate capsule into nearby tissues and/or seminal vesicles. Substages describe amount of extension into bladder neck, penis, urethra, seminal vesicles, rectum, or pelvic sidewalls.
- *Stage D:* Cancer extends through prostatic capsule and beyond.
  —*D1:* Metastasis into lymph nodes.
  —*D2:* Metastasis into bones.

The patient may exhibit clinical signs of the disease from stage B1. Symptomatology will depend on the path and extent of the tumor, although the patient with D level staging may present with urinary difficulty or back or bone pain only.

**Grading the cancer:**    Based on the number of abnormal cells seen under microscope. The higher the number, the more invasive and aggressive the cancer. Usually the Gleason Grading System is used; grades range between 2 and 10.

**External radiation therapy:**    Performed for both curative and palliative therapy, depending on the stage of the neoplasm. Treatment occurs over a 6-week period, and patients can expect to remain sexually potent after treatment. This therapy also is used to shrink the tumor, thereby relieving obstruction in the urinary tract.

**Interstitial irradiation of the prostate:**    Uses gold, chromium, or iodine implantation to destroy the prostate tumor at its origin. It will not, however, affect other areas if metastasis has occurred.

**Hormonal therapy:**    Estrogens, antiandrogens, progestogens, prolactin or alpha-sympathetic blockers, or gonadotropin-releasing hormone analogs may be initiated to reduce plasma testosterone levels, since it is believed that testosterone is involved in the development of prostate cancer. Typically diethylstilbestrol (DES) is given daily. Estrogen therapy causes 100% impotence during treatment. **Note:** Because DES can cause fluid retention, it must be given cautiously to patients with a history of cardiac disease or renal problems. Estramustine phosphate, a combination of estradiol and nitrogen mustard, might be used if estrogen therapy is ineffective. This drug does not cause impotence, and its side effects are few, although patients tend to experience anorexia and nausea.

**Chemotherapy:**    This might be used as either a curative or palliative measure.

**Surgical procedures:**    Might include the following:

***Prostatectomy (transurethral resection of the prostate [TURP]):***    Prostatic tissue is scraped away *via* cystoscopy. This technique is used when the tumor is in a beginning stage and is well differentiated. For additional information, see "Benign Prostatic Hypertrophy," p. 616.

***Radical prostatectomy:***    With or without pelvic node dissection. Using either the perineal or retropubic approach, the entire prostate gland is removed along with the seminal vesicles and a portion of the bladder neck, part of the vas deferens, and adjacent lymph nodes. This procedure is done for tumors that are large or not well differentiated. Erectile dysfunction occurs in 85%-90% of males having this procedure. However, this side effect can be avoided if periprostatic autonomic nerves are spared. Urinary incontinence also occurs in the majority of patients after removal of the indwelling catheter. In a prostatic cancer, all of the prostate and its capsule are removed (as opposed to the TURP, in which the apex of the prostate and its capsule remain). As a result, the following can occur to cause incontinence: (1) the external sphincter can be damaged because of surgical trauma to the bladder neck and prostate capsule, or (2) portions of the bladder neck are removed as are portions of the urethra in an effort to remove all of the cancer. This damage may take up to 6 months to heal, and the incontinence subsides 6 months after surgery in 85%-90% of this patient population.

***Nerve-sparing radical prostatectomy:***    Used in patients with negative lymph nodes, no elevated serum acid phosphatase, and no evidence of extracapsular extension. This procedure involves the use of a longitudinal, rather than a transverse, incision through the periprostatic fascia and a careful dissection along a longitudinal plane from the prostate to the urethra, thus avoiding damage to the neurovascular bundles that affect potency.

***Bilateral orchiectomy:***    Although rarely done, it may be implemented along with estrogen therapy to depress testosterone production.

## NURSING DIAGNOSES AND INTERVENTIONS

**Sexual dysfunction** related to erectile dysfunction (risk is 85%-90%) after radical prostatectomy

*Desired outcome:*  Patient verbalizes feelings about sexuality within 3 days after surgery.

- Assess the patient's readiness to discuss sexual concerns. Encourage verbalization, and as indicated, use facilitative communication techniques such as open-ended questions, reflective statements, and rephrasing of patient's statements for clarification.
- Be alert to signs of grief, such as hostility, depression, and demanding behavior, and to signs of denial, such as inappropriate affect or accepting the diagnosis too well.
- As appropriate, arrange for caregivers who have established rapport with the patient to spend time with him and encourage verbalization of his concerns.
- Be alert to the needs of the patient and significant other for more information about sexual functioning.
- As indicated, inform the physician about the patient's need for more information so that counseling can be reinforced.
- Confer with physician and social services to identify appropriate referrals for counseling after hospital discharge.

**Knowledge deficit:**  Side effects of antiandrogen therapy or bilateral orchiectomy

*Desired outcome:*  Within the 24-h period before hospital discharge, patient verbalizes knowledge about the extent and duration of body changes.

- Inform patient of side effects of estrogen therapy and orchiectomy (e.g., breast enlargement, breast tenderness, loss of sexual desire, and impotence). As indicated, teach patient about the side effects of alpha-adrenergics (e.g., terazoin, prazosin, and phenoxybenzamine), which include first dose syncope and mild hypotension.
- For patients on estrogen therapy, provide reassurance that side effects will disappear after therapy has been discontinued.
- If appropriate, explain to patient that before initiating estrogen therapy, the physician may prescribe radiation therapy to the areolae of the breasts to minimize painful gynecomastia. However, this procedure will not decrease other side effects.
- Assure the patient undergoing orchiectomy that the procedure will not affect his ability to have an erection and orgasm but that he will not ejaculate.

**Stress incontinence** related to temporary loss of muscle tone in the urethral sphincter after radical prostatectomy

*Desired outcome:*  Within the 24-h period before hospital discharge, patient relates understanding of the cause of the temporary incontinence and the regimen that must be followed to promote bladder control.

- Explain to patient that there is a potential for urinary incontinence after prostatectomy but that it should resolve within 6 months. Describe the reason for the incontinence, using aids such as anatomic illustrations.
- Encourage patient to maintain an adequate fluid intake of at least 2-3 L/day (unless contraindicated by an underlying cardiac dysfunction or other disorder). Explain that a dilute urine is less irritating to the prostatic fossa.
- Instruct patient to avoid fluids that irritate the bladder, such as caffeine-containing drinks. Explain that caffeine has a mild diuresis effect, which would make bladder control even more difficult.
- Establish a bladder routine with patient before hospital discharge (see "Urinary Incontinence," p. 161).
- Teach patient Kegel exercises to enhance sphincter control (see "Urinary Incontinence," p. 163).
- Remind patient to discuss any incontinence problems with physician during follow-up examinations.

**Note:**   See "Benign Prostatic Hypertrophy" for **High risk for fluid volume deficit** (bleeding/hemorrhage), p. 617, **Pain,** p. 618, **High risk for infection,** p. 617, **High risk for impaired skin integrity,** p. 619, **Constipation,** p. 619, and **Altered thought processes,** p. 620. See Appendix One for nursing diagnoses and interventions in "Caring for Preoperative and Postoperative Patients," p. 693, and "Caring for Patients with Cancer and Other Life-Disrupting Illnesses," p. 719.

## PATIENT-FAMILY TEACHING AND DISCHARGE PLANNING

Give patient and significant others verbal and written information about the following:

* For patients with radical prostatectomy, referral to a counselor or counseling agency as necessary, and discussion about incontinence following removal of indwelling catheter.
* See this section in "Benign Prostatic Hypertrophy," p. 621, for more information.

# Testicular neoplasm

Cancer of the testes is most often found in men in their 20s and 30s. Usually it is discovered by accident, often after a traumatic injury to the groin for which professional examination is warranted. Self-examination is the best method of early detection for this disorder. It is believed that men with an undescended testicle are at higher risk than the general male population. Individuals who have had surgery at an early age (before age 2) to correct this condition virtually eliminate the potential of developing the cancer. However, these men are better able to check for lumps and thickenings in the testis after it has been surgically descended.

The most common testicular tumors are seminomas, which spread slowly through the lymphatic system to the iliac and periaortic nodes. Embryonal tumors, on the other hand, metastasize quickly. Other tumor types include teratocarcinoma, adult teratoma, choriocarcinoma, and Leydig cell. Most testicular cancers are combinations of two forms of cancer, which can make treatment difficult. However, with treatment, prognosis for all forms of this cancer is good.

## ASSESSMENT

**Signs and symptoms:**   Lump the size of a pea or thickening of the testis. There may be an aching or heaviness in the testis caused by swelling of the scrotum owing to an accumulation of fluid or blood. Pain usually is not a symptom. In the later stages of the disease, the patient may experience abdominal pain caused by bowel or ureteral obstruction, coughing caused by metastasis to the lungs, weight loss, or anorexia. Breast enlargement may occur because of reduction in testosterone.

**Physical assessment:**   Palpation of symmetrical, firm scrotal mass; presence of supraclavicular or abdominal mass caused by enlargement of lymph nodes in those areas.

## DIAGNOSTIC TESTS

**Hct/Hgb:**   Drawn preoperatively to assess for the presence of anemia, which can occur because of metastasis.

**Serum liver function tests (ALT/SGPT, LDH, GGTP):**   To assess adequacy of liver function for patients needing chemotherapy and for presence of abnormalities, which is indicative of metastasis. Alanine aminotransferase (ALT), known formerly as serum glutamic-pyruvic transaminase (SGPT), detects hepatocellular obstruction or liver damage. Lactic dehydrogenase (LDH) becomes elevated with liver disease or malignant tumors. Serum gammaglutamyl transpeptidase (GGTP) also rises in the presence of liver damage or disease.

**Serum renal function tests (creatinine and electrolytes, such as Na⁺ and potassium [K⁺]):** Help determine adequacy of renal function for the patient needing chemotherapy; abnormalities may signal ureteral obstruction.

**Serum alpha-fetoprotein (AFP):** Used as a tumor marker and identification of the type of carcinoma. AFP never is elevated in a seminoma, but it will be with nonseminomas. Response to treatment and assessment for recurrence can be evaluated, based on comparison to the baseline value of this test.

**Human chorionic gonadotropin (HCG) levels:** Used as a tumor marker and for identification of the type of carcinoma. Normally, HCG is found in the maternal circulation during pregnancy, and it is an abnormal finding in the male. However, it is found with most testicular cancers. As with AFP, response to treatment and assessment for recurrence can be evaluated based on comparison to the baseline value of this test.

**Chest x-ray:** May show presence of metastasis to the lungs.

**Intravenous pyelogram (IVP)/excretory urogram:** May show displacement of the kidney or ureters by masses of carcinomatous lumbar nodes, which cause ureteral stenosis.

**Lymphangiograms:** May reveal enlarged iliac and periaortic lymph nodes if disease has spread. In this procedure, contrast medium is injected into the dorsal aspects of the feet to outline the lymphatic vessels. The contrast medium will discolor the patient's urine and stool for 24–48 h after the procedure. The injection of this substance might be uncomfortable, and the injection site will be tender for a few days.

---

**Note:** Two complications of IVP and lymphangiogram are allergic reactions to the dye, and contrast-medium-induced acute renal failure. Exposure to contrast medium may worsen existing renal or cardiac insufficiency, especially in the elderly, dehydrated, or diabetic patient. Before the study, query the patient about allergies to shellfish and iodine and reactions to previous dye studies. After the test, monitor patient for indicators of renal failure.

---

## COLLABORATIVE MANAGEMENT

**Radiation therapy:** Most commonly used for patients with seminomas, the use of this therapy varies with the type and stage of the cancer. In the absence of metastasis, lymph nodes often are irradiated to prevent microscopic spread of the seminoma. Low-dose radiation is used to minimize complications.

**Chemotherapy:** Used if cancer has spread outside the testicle or retroperitoneal lymph nodes. It is used for radioresistent tumors (choriocarcinoma), with or without surgery. Most types of testicular carcinomas appear to be sensitive to chemotherapy, particularly to cisplatin, vinblastine sulfate, and bleomycin. Doxorubicin may be used before irradiation to treat metastases to retroperitoneal nodes.

**Serial AFP and HCG levels:** Drawn routinely over a 2-year period. Levels drop toward normal if the neoplasm has been eradicated, and rise if it has not.

**Staging of the disease:** Necessary for guiding treatment and evaluating the prognosis. The following guidelines are used, based on the Boden and Gibbs staging system.

- *Stage A:* Tumor confined to testis with no clinical or radiologic evidence that it has spread.
- *Stage B:* Clinical or radiologic evidence that tumor has spread to lymph nodes distal to the diaphragm. Subcategories $B_1$, $B_2$, and $B_3$ also are used.
- *Stage C:* Clinical or radiologic evidence that tumor has spread to lymph nodes superior to the diaphragm (mediastinal and supraclavicular nodes) or beyond the lymphatic system into the viscera.

**Biopsy:** To confirm the presence of malignancy. In the absence of malignancy, the abnormal benign lump is removed but the testicle is left. If the lump proves to be malignant, an orchiectomy is performed to remove the diseased testicle. A small incision is made at the inguinal area on the affected side rather than in the scrotum itself. This permits high ligation of the cord at the inguinal ring to allow for removal of the whole testis, which other approaches do not allow. The patient may return from surgery with an indwelling catheter and incisional drain for removal of excess exudate.

**Retroperitoneal lymph node dissection or lymphadenectomy:** Patients with seminomas undergo a lymphadenectomy only if the disease has spread beyond the scrotal sac and does not respond to irradiation. Patients with non-seminomatous tumors receive lymphadenectomy as part of a treatment regimen that includes orchiectomy, radiotherapy, and chemotherapy. It is performed at the time of the orchiectomy or a few days later. Lymph nodes are removed from the kidney to the inguinal area on the affected side.

## NURSING DIAGNOSES AND INTERVENTIONS

**Sexual dysfunction** related to body changes that occur with orchiectomy
***Desired outcome:*** Before hospital discharge, patient verbalizes feelings and frustrations about the orchiectomy and relates realistic knowledge about changes that will occur.

- Provide a calm, unhurried atmosphere for the patient and significant others. Use facilitative communication techniques, such as open-ended questions, reflective statements, and rephrasing of patient's statements for clarification.
- Encourage communication between patient and significant other.
- Encourage patient to verbalize feelings, fears, and frustrations about sexual attractiveness, feared impotence, and infertility. Explain that the *surgery* will not impair fertility or potency; however, fertility may be compromised by radiation therapy or chemotherapy and can last for 2 years.
- For patient undergoing lymphadenectomy, explain that ejaculatory failure may occur if the sympathetic nerve is damaged but that erection and orgasm will be possible. Explain that if ejaculatory failure does occur, artificial insemination is possible because the semen flows back into the urine, from which it can be extracted, enabling the ovum to become impregnated artificially.
- If appropriate, explain that a silicone prosthesis may be placed in the scrotum to achieve a normal appearance. Consult with physician about the potential for this procedure.
- For patient undergoing radiation or chemotherapy, explain that he can store sperm in a sperm bank. The rate of pregnancy is only 50% by this method, however, because some sperm do not survive the freezing process.

**Pain** related to scrotal swelling secondary to orchiectomy or lymphadenectomy
***Desired outcomes:*** Within 1-2 h of intervention, patient's subjective perception of pain decreases, as documented by a pain scale. Objective indicators, such as grimacing, are absent or diminished.

- Assess and document the quality, duration, and location of the pain. Ask the patient to rate the pain on a scale of 0 (no pain) to 10 (worst pain).
- Administer prescribed analgesics as indicated. Note and document the patient's response, using the pain scale to evaluate the improvement.
- Adjust the scrotal support as needed to enhance patient comfort. The scrotal support elevates and supports the scrotum to minimize the amount of edema.
- Apply ice gloves or packs to the scrotum to reduce swelling.
- Encourage patient to ambulate as soon as possible. Explain that exercise reduces swelling and pain by improving circulation.

**High risk for fluid volume deficit** related to postsurgical bleeding/hemorrhage
***Desired outcome:*** Patient remains normovolemic as evidenced by BP ≥90/60 mm Hg (or within patient's normal range), HR ≤100 bpm (or within patient's

normal range), balanced I&O, urinary output ≥30 ml/h, RR ≤20 breaths/min, and warm and dry skin.
- Monitor the patient's VS q15min for 30 min after return from the recovery room. Once stable, check q30min for 1 h and then q4h for 24 h (or according to hospital protocol).
- Be alert to increasing HR, decreasing BP, diaphoresis, pallor, decreasing urinary output, and increasing RR, which signal hemorrhage and impending shock.
- Monitor I&O. In nonrestricted patients, ensure a fluid intake of at least 2-3 L/day. Immediately after surgery, administer fluids IV and then advance to oral.
- Measure and document urine, gastric tube, and drainage apparatus output; record output amounts separately. Optimally, drainage amounts will decrease gradually and then cease.
- Check the dressing at frequent intervals after surgery, changing it when it becomes damp. Document color and amount of drainage. Notify physician if drainage is heavy (saturates dressings within 1 h after changing), becomes bright red, or forms clots on the dressings, any of which can occur with arterial or venous bleeding.

---

**Note:** See Appendix One for nursing diagnoses and interventions in "Caring for Preoperative and Postoperative Patients," p. 693, and "Caring for Patients with Cancer and Other Life-Disrupting Illnesses," p. 719.

---

## PATIENT-FAMILY TEACHING AND DISCHARGE PLANNING

Give patient and significant others verbal and written information about the following:
- Medications, including drug name, purpose, dosage, schedule, precautions, and potential side effects.
- Care of incision, including cleansing and dressing changes. Advise patient to be alert to signs of infection, such as fever, persistent redness, swelling, pain, warmth or puffiness along incision, and purulent drainage.
- Care of drains or catheters if patient is discharged with them.
- Review of postoperative activity restrictions as directed by physician, such as no heavy lifting (>10 lb), driving, or sexual intercourse for 4-6 weeks.
- Necessity of continued care, such as radiation therapy, chemotherapy, serial lab work; confirm date and time of next appointment if known.
- Importance of self-examination of remaining testicle, since it is possible to get unrelated cancer in the remaining testis.

# Penile implants

Erectile dysfunction can be described in two ways: *erectile insufficiency,* in which there is a change in the rigidity of the penis but sexual relations are still possible; and *erectile failure,* which is the inability to achieve an erection adequate for sexual relations or to sustain penetration until ejaculation. The causes of these types of dysfunction are either physiologic or psychologic. Physiologic factors include neurogenic, hormonal, or arteriovenous disorders, such as radical pelvic surgery, lower motor neuron interruption, diabetes mellitus, Cushing's syndrome, atherosclerosis, and severe arterial disease. Medication, recreational drugs, or alcohol use also can affect the male's ability to achieve or maintain an erection.

Before surgery the patient must meet the following criteria:
- *Have desire for sexual relations, including penetration.*
- *Have penile sensation.* The presence of these two factors increases the potential for gratification after an implant.

• *Lack any prostatic or urinary tract problems.* After implantation, endoscopic or transurethral procedures are difficult to perform.

## IMPLANTATION PROCEDURES

**Insertion of nonhydraulic implants:**   Silicone rods are placed into the corpora cavernosa through an incision at the base of the dorsal surface of the penis. With this procedure the penis stays semirigid but will not be noticeable under clothing or interfere with ADL.

**Insertion of hydraulic penile implant:**   Two silicone tubes are placed into the corpora cavernosa *via* a suprapubic incision. A reservoir containing a radiopaque fluid is sutured into the abdominal fascia and a bulb is inserted into one scrotal sac. To initiate an erection the man or his partner must squeeze the scrotal bulb, which fills the rods with radiopaque fluid from the reservoir. Compression of the release bulb, which is located in the lower part of the scrotal sac, allows the erection to subside.

## NURSING DIAGNOSES AND INTERVENTIONS

**Pain** related to the surgical procedure

***Desired outcomes:***   Within 1 h after intervention, patient's subjective perception of pain decreases, as documented by a pain scale. Objective indicators, such as grimacing, are absent or diminished.

• Assess and document quality, location, and duration of pain, using a pain scale ranging from 0 (no pain) to 10 (worst pain). Immediately after surgery, pain can be severe and can last for as long as a week. Mild pain might be present for several more weeks. Medicate patient with analgesics or narcotics as prescribed, and evaluate relief obtained, based on the pain scale.

• Apply ice packs or gloves to the area to reduce swelling; but closely monitor patient's reaction because the weight of the ice might increase discomfort.

• Assist patient in using slow, diaphragmatic breathing and other nonpharmacologic pain control methods, such as guided imagery, distraction, and relaxation tapes. Give backrubs.

• Medicate patient about ½ h before major moves such as ambulation and when physician first inflates the implant, which is done a few days after surgery and repeated several times a day for about a week.

• Use a bed cradle or hoop to prevent discomfort caused by weight of bed linens.

• For additional information, see this nursing diagnosis in Appendix One, p. 694.

**Body image disturbance** related to presence of the penile implant

***Desired outcomes:***   Before hospital discharge, patient expresses feelings about the presence of the implant and exhibits a reduction in self-consciousness by participating in care activities that involve the implant. Patient with nonhydraulic implant verbalizes measures for disguising its appearance.

• Encourage patient to discuss feelings, fears, and frustrations about the implant.

• Recognize that impotence threatens a man's self-concept, regardless of the reason for the impotence.

• Provide a calm and accepting environment by discussing the procedure with patient openly and objectively. Reassure him that this surgery is not unusual or bizarre.

• Promote acceptance of the implant by encouraging patient to look at it and assist with dressing changes or other appropriate care.

• For patients with semirigid implants, explain that wearing jockey briefs rather than boxer or bikini briefs will better disguise the appearance of the penis.

• If the patient feels self-conscious about his appearance in street clothes, encourage him to wear loose-fitting trousers until he finds clothing that better suits him.

• Assure patient that he will be able to participate in any sport he chooses and that work will not be affected by the prosthesis.

---

**Note:** See Appendix One for nursing diagnoses and interventions in "Caring for Preoperative and Postoperative Patients," p. 693.

---

## PATIENT-FAMILY TEACHING AND DISCHARGE PLANNING

Give patient and significant other verbal and written information about the following:

• Medications, including drug name, purpose, dosage, schedule, precautions, and potential side effects.
• Infection indicators, which necessitate medical attention: cloudy or foul-smelling urine, fever, and increased pain or swelling in scrotum or penis.
• Care of incision, including cleansing and dressings. Teach patient to be alert to signs of local infection: persistent redness, pain, fever, increased warmth along incision line, and puffiness.
• Activity restrictions established by physician, such as limiting sitting for long periods of time, heavy lifting (>10 lb), and strenuous exercise. Sexual activity can be resumed when all pain and edema have subsided, usually after 4-8 weeks.
• Technique for operating hydraulic device.
• Prolonged pain lasting >4 weeks, which is a signal that the implant may be too long.
• Signs of erosion through the overlying skin or into urethra: soreness, redness, bleeding, difficulty urinating, pain with urination, cloudy and foul-smelling urine, and hematuria.

### Selected Bibliography

American Joint Committee on Cancer: *Manual for staging of cancer,* ed 3, Chicago, 1988, The Committee.

Berger R, Hanno P: A spectrum of prostatitis syndromes, *Patient Care* 24(9):95-102, 1990.

Blackmore C: The impact of orchiectomy upon the sexuality of the man with testicular cancer, *Cancer Nurs* 11(1):33-40, 1988.

Boring C, Squires T, Tong T: Cancer statistics, 1991, *Cancer J for Clinicians* 41(1):19-29, 1991.

Burgio K, Pearce KL, Lucco AJ: *Staying dry: a practical guide to bladder control,* Baltimore, 1989, Johns Hopkins University Press.

Catlin AJ, Wetzel WS: Ectopic pregnancy: clinical evaluation, diagnostic measures, and prevention, *Nurs Pract* 16(1):38-46, 1991.

Davis D, Dearman C: Coping strategies of infertile women, JOGNN 20(3):221-228, 1991.

Dearman C: *Antepartal complications.* In Cohen SM, Kenner CA, Hollingsworth AO, editors: *Maternal, neonatal, and women's health nursing,* Springhouse, Pa, 1991, Springhouse.

Deppe G, Lawrence WD: *Vulvar dystrophy and neoplasia.* In Gusberg SB, Shingleton HM, Deppe G, editors: *Female genital cancer,* New York, 1988, Churchill-Livingstone.

Dodd MJ: Patterns of self care in patients with breast cancer, *West J Nurs Res* 10(1):7-24, 1988.

Dulaney PE, Crawford VC, Turner G: A comprehensive education and support program for women experiencing hysterectomies, *J Obstet Gynecol Neonatal Nurs* 19(4):319-325, 1990.

Ellerhorst-Ryan JM et al: Evaluating benign breast disease, *Nurs Pract* 13(9):13-28, 1988.

Gitsch G, Berger E, Tatra G: Complications of vaginal hysterectomy under "difficult" circumstances, *Arch Gynecol Obstet* 249(4):209-212, 1991.

Goodman M, Harte N: *Breast cancer*. In Groenwald SL et al, editors: *Cancer nursing: principles and practice*, ed 2, Boston, 1990, Jones & Bartlett.

Gusberg SB, Runowicz: *Gynecologic cancers*. In Holleb AI, Fink DJ, Murphy GP, editors: *American Cancer Society textbook of clinical oncology*, Atlanta, 1991, American Cancer Society.

Harrison B: Testicular neoplasms: an overview, *J Urol Nurs* 7(1):321-328, 1988.

Hassey KM: Pregnancy and parenthood after treatment for breast cancer, *Oncol Nurs Forum* 15(4):439-443, 1988.

Heinrich-Rynning T: Prostatic cancer treatments and their effects on sexual functioning, *Oncol Nurs Forum* 14(6):37-41, 1987.

Horne MM, Swearingen PL: *Pocket guide to fluid, electrolyte, and acid-base balance*, ed 2, St Louis, 1993, Mosby–Year Book.

Interqual: The ISD-A review system with adult ISD criteria, August 1992, Northhampton, NH, and Marlboro, MA, Interqual, Inc.

Jenkin B: Patients' reports of sexual changes after treatment for gynecologic cancer, *Oncol Nurs Forum* 15(3):349-354, 1988.

Kim MJ, McFarland GK, and McLane AM: *Pocket guide to nursing diagnoses*, ed 5, St Louis, 1993, Mosby–Year Book.

Lasater S: Testicular cancer: a nursing perspective of diagnosis and treatment, *J Urol Nurs* 7(1):329-349, 1988.

Lederer JR et al: *Care planning pocket guide: a nursing diagnosis approach*, ed 5, Redwood City, Calif, 1993, Addison-Wesley.

Lichtman R, Papera S: *Gynecology: well woman care*, Norwalk, Conn, 1990, Appleton & Lange.

Littler JE, Momany T: *University of Iowa: the family practice handbook*, Chicago, 1990, Year Book Medical Publishers.

McDivvitt RW, Stevens JA, Lee NC et al: Histologic types of benign breast disease and the risk for cancer, *Cancer* 69(6):1408-1414, 1992.

McInnis WD: *Plastic surgery of the breast*. In Mitchell G, Bassett L, editors: The female breast and its disorders, Baltimore, 1990, Williams & Wilkins.

Moore S et al: Nerve sparing prostatectomy, *Am J Nurs* 92(4):59-64, 1992.

Norhouse LL: Social support in patients' and husbands' adjustment to breast cancer, *Nurs Res* 37(2):91-95, 1988.

Otte DM: *Gynecologic cancers*. In Groenwald SL et al, editors: *Cancer nursing: principles and practice*, ed 2, Boston, 1990, Jones & Bartlett.

Panel recommendations on silicone gel-filled breast implants following moratorium: *FDA Medical Bulletin* 22(1):3-4, 1992.

Russell IS et al: The use of tissue expansion for immediate breast reconstruction after mastectomy, *Med J Aust* 152(12):632-635, 1990.

Scanlon EF: *Breast cancer*. In Holleb AI, Fink DJ, Murphy GP, editors: *American Cancer Society textbook of clinical oncology*, Atlanta, 1991, American Cancer Society.

Small M: *Penile prosthesis*. In Glenn J, editor: *Urologic surgery*, ed 4, Philadelphia, 1991, JB Lippincott.

Swearingen PL, Keen JH, editors: *Manual of critical care: applying nursing diagnoses to adult critical illness*, ed 2, St Louis, 1991, Mosby–Year Book.

Wardell DW: Ectopic pregnancy: a growing concern, *J Am Acad Nurse Practitioners* 1(4):119-125, 1989.

Williams L, Peters CR: Reduction mammoplasty, *Plast Surg Nurs* 10(2):84-87, 1990.

Willis D: Taming the overgrown prostate, *Am J Nurs* 92(2):34-40, 1992.

Wozniak-Petrofsky J: BPH: treating older men's most common problem, *RN* 54(3):32-37, 1991.

**10** # SENSORY DISORDERS

Section One    Disorders and Surgeries of the Eye    633
   Corneal ulceration/trauma    633
   Keratoplasty (corneal transplant)    638
   Vitreous disorders/Vitrectomy    639
   Glaucoma    641
   Retinal detachment    644
   Enucleation    646
Section Two    Disorders and Surgeries of the Ear    648
   Otosclerosis (Otospongiosis)    648
   Cochlear implantation    650
Selected Bibliography    652

## Section One:    Disorders and Surgeries of the Eye

### Corneal ulceration/trauma

*Corneal ulceration* is a serious ocular disease that causes a "melting away" of the corneal tissue, which occasionally leads to perforation. Potential causes include chemical burns and prolonged exposure to the air in a nonblinking individual (e.g., one who is comatose or has Bell's palsy), but more often it is caused by bacteria, herpes virus, and in rarer instances, fungal disease. Corneal ulceration almost always results in scarring (opacity) and the development of an irregular surface, which, regardless of the cause, contributes to a decrease in visual acuity.

   *Corneal trauma* most commonly is caused by the following:

**Foreign body:**    Metallic or nonmetallic objects can become stuck to the corneal surface or become imbedded in the cornea. Small metallic foreign bodies that have great velocity (e.g., pieces of nails, steel) can pass through the cornea with little trace in an individual who is not wearing safety glasses. Damage to the lens or anterior segment also may occur. Unless this is detected promptly by ultrasound or x-ray, the eye can become damaged by the release of ions. Copper foreign bodies are especially dangerous.

**Chemical burns:**    Those resulting from industrial accidents are very dangerous since alkali deeply penetrates the tissue, and they often occur bilaterally. Initial indicators can be greatly underestimated at the time of the accident. Inflammatory ulceration with scarring ensues over months, causing decreased vision. Keratoplasty usually is unsuccessful.

**633**

**Laceration:**   E.g., from shattered eyeglasses. Damage to the lens and other parts of the eye is common. Scleral lacerations may be hidden by a subconjunctival hemorrhage. Surgical repair may be necessary.

**Contact lens overwear:**   An individual whose soft contact lenses are tight-fitting or one who gradually develops a corneal hypersensitivity reaction can develop corneal trauma. For individuals with extended wear (overnight use) lenses, infection is not an uncommon occurrence.

## ASSESSMENT

**Signs and symptoms:**   Presence of a "red" eye for one or more days, progressive decrease in visual acuity. Pain, both a scratchy surface discomfort and a deeper, boring pain, especially with blinking, may be present. There may be increased tearing and photophobia.

**Physical assessment:**   Swollen lid, half-shut eye, tearing, and discharge that is occasionally purulent. The inflamed conjunctiva with dilated vessels causes the eye to be red. Slit lamp assessment may reveal a small or large infiltrate, often of yellowish-white and fluffy contour, which is suggestive of bacteria. In other cases, the areas within the defect may be gray, indicating necrosis. In advanced cases, all the membrane may be melted away in a small area, enabling the clear descemet's membrane to bulge out. The barrier can rupture and perforate, with a gush of fluid and sudden sharp pain.

## DIAGNOSTIC TESTS

**Fluoroscein (filter paper or 2% drop):**   Identifies defect in the epithelium by defusing into the corneal stroma and staining it bright green. The findings may be enhanced by using a blue light, called a cobalt filter.

**Rose bengal (filter paper or 1% drop):**   Identifies devitalized cells at the border of the defect by staining them red.

**Corneal scrapings, Gram stain, and immediate microscopic exam:**   To identify bacterial or fungal ulceration.

**Conjunctival culture:**   To identify causative organism, if present.

---

**Note:**   Prompt culturing and administration of antibiotics are extremely important in the presence of bacterial infection. An hour's delay can make a great difference. Topical antibiotics must be started immediately after cultures are obtained. Any antibiotic in any concentration can be used until positive cultures and sensitivities are determined.

---

## COLLABORATIVE MANAGEMENT

*For corneal trauma*

**Removal of foreign body:**   If present.

**Irrigation:**   For chemical burns. At the scene of the accident the eyes should be irrigated with any nontoxic fluid available. The individual should then proceed to the emergency room, where the eye is irrigated with normal saline until the tears become neutral, as confirmed by litmus paper.

**Surgical repair:**   For laceration.

**Removal of contact lens:**   For contact lens overwear.

*General management*

**Pharmacotherapy**

*Topical and systemic antibiotics or antiviral agents:*   To treat identified infection, usually after obtaining the results of corneal scrapings or cultures. Broad spectrum antibiotics may be given topically and intravenously until culture results are obtained, after which specific antifungals, antibacterials, or antiviral agents are used accordingly.

*Topical steroids:*   To treat hypersensitivity reactions.

**Pupil dilatation** *via* **mydriatrics:** If an increase in intraocular pressure exists.

**Pain management:** Warm moist compresses are used for lid swelling. Cycloplegics (atropine, scopolamine) may be used to decrease pain by dilating the pupil, thereby restricting movements of the iris and ciliary body. Systemic analgesics also may be prescribed.

**Cleansing and dressings:** The lid margins are cleansed frequently to remove exudate, at minimum before each administration of ophthalmic drops. A tarsorrhaphy (taping or suturing the eyelids shut) is done in nonblinking individuals to provide a moist eye chamber. The patient also will wear a metal shield, especially for impending perforation. In noninfectious conditions, the patient may wear a soft contact lens as a dressing. In the presence of infection, dressings are not used because they can promote bacterial growth. Loose, dry dressings are used for clean abrasions or erosions.

**Corneal transplant:** Considered only after medical management has failed and scarring or perforation has occurred. See p. 638.

## NURSING DIAGNOSES AND INTERVENTIONS

**Knowledge deficit:** Diagnosis and treatment plan
*Desired outcome:* Before initiation of treatment, patient verbalizes understanding about the diagnosis and treatment plan.

- Assess patient's knowledge of the diagnosis and treatment plan; clarify or provide explanations as necessary.
- Encourage questions and provide time for patient to ask questions and express fears and anxieties.
- Explain that the eyes may be patched, taped, or sutured shut as part of the treatment for the corneal diagnosis.
- Instruct patient not to touch, rub, or squeeze the affected eye(s), which can spread infection and cause further trauma.

**Sensory/perceptual alterations** (visual deficit) related to disease process or presence of eye shield, eye patch, or other measure that distorts or diminishes vision
*Desired outcome:* Following intervention(s), patient verbalizes orientation to person, place, and time and relates the attainment of adequate amounts of sensory stimulation.

- Orient patient to surroundings.
- Request that all individuals entering the room identify themselves, state their purpose for being there, and inform patient when they are leaving.
- Avoid touching patient without first announcing your intent.
- Encourage patient to listen to radio or TV, which will provide sensory stimulation and help prevent boredom.
- Place all necessary articles within patient's reach. Encourage patient to use sense of touch to familiarize self with new objects and their placement.
- The degree of assistance with meals depends on the patient's visual deficit. Set up the food tray, and orient patient to the food placement (e.g., "The meat is at 12 o'clock.") and temperature.
- Depth perception is altered with an eye patch and shield. Teach patient to position fingers just inside the rim of glass while filling to avoid overfilling.
- Do not move furniture without alerting patient.

**High risk for infection** related to invasive (surgical) procedure
*Desired outcome:* Patient is free of infection as evidenced by absence of erythema, swelling, purulent discharge, and persistent pain in the affected eye.

- Change loose dressings, and reapply as needed. Often the physician will change the first dressing postoperatively. After the physician has removed the initial bandage, inspect the eye for signs of infection, including erythema, swelling, or purulent discharge. Teach patient to alert the staff to the presence of persistent pain.

- Wash your hands well, and use clean technique for eye care and instillation of ointment or drops.
- Assist patient with maintaining a dry operative site; help with hygiene activities as needed, depending on patient's visual deficit.
- Remind patient not to touch or rub the operative eye.
- For confused patients, request arm restraints to prevent handling of the eye dressing and rubbing of the operative eye.
- If contact lenses are prescribed, use aseptic technique for lens insertion. Teach the technique to patient or significant other.

**Self-care deficit** related to imposed activity restrictions and visual deficit

***Desired outcomes:***   Patient avoids ADL that may be a safety hazard or can cause increased intraocular pressure and resumes independence with ADL as soon as these activities are permitted. Until patient can resume ADL independently, staff or significant others perform these activities for the patient.

- Review with the patient the activities that are permitted and those that are not. Some ocular conditions necessitate restrictions of shaving, shampooing, hair combing, and vigorous tooth brushing. Most ocular conditions, however, restrict only vigorous activity.
- Assemble patient's toilet articles at the bedside or in the bathroom, and encourage safety and independence within the limits specified by physician.
- Continue to perform activities for patient that require stooping and bending, such as putting on shoes and socks and washing feet.

**Knowledge deficit:**   Importance of avoiding increased intraocular pressure and activities that can cause it

***Desired outcome:***   Following patient teaching, patient verbalizes knowledge about the importance of avoiding increased intraocular pressure and activities that can cause it.

- Explain that increased intraocular pressure can cause disruption of the operative site, and caution patient about the following:
  - Avoid straining with bowel movements; request laxative/stool softeners as needed.
  - Notify staff when nauseated so that antiemetics can be given.
  - When coughing and sneezing, do so with mouth and eyes open to minimize intraocular pressure.
  - Avoid heavy lifting, bending, or vigorous activity until approved by physician.
- Teach patient the importance of maintaining the prescribed position.
- Instruct patient to notify staff immediately if persistent or sudden, severe pain occurs in the operative eye because this can signal increased ocular pressure.
- Teach patient the importance of wearing eyeglasses by day and a shield at night to protect the eye.

**Pain** related to corneal ulceration/trauma

***Desired outcomes:***   Within 1 h of intervention, patient's subjective perception of pain decreases, as documented by a pain scale. Objective indicators, such as grimacing, are absent or diminished.

---

**Note:**   The intensity and duration of the pain is related to the degree of inflammation.

---

- Monitor patient for presence of pain. Develop a pain scale with the patient, rating pain from 0 (no pain) to 10 (worst pain). Medicate with prescribed medications as indicated, and document pain relief obtained, using the pain scale.
- Explain that decreasing eye movements will help minimize pain.
- If prescribed, apply warm, moist compresses to the eyes.
- Reading can increase pain; encourage use of alternatives, such as talking books, radio, or television, to divert attention from pain.

- Instruct patient to inform staff of increased or sudden severe eye pain and gush of fluid, which can signal that perforation has occurred.

---

**Note:** In the presence of acute perforation, place a dry sterile dressing lightly over affected eye, have patient get into bed, and notify physician immediately.

---

**Knowledge deficit:** Importance of frequent antibiotic administration and the technique for administration (if indicated)
**Desired outcomes:** Following patient teaching, patient verbalizes understanding about the importance of frequent antibiotic administration and adheres to the treatment plan. If indicated, patient or significant other returns demonstration of clean technique for administration of the medication before hospital discharge.
- Stress the importance of and rationale for the medication, which usually is administered hourly.
- Teach patient or significant other the technique for instillation of eye drops or ointment if the medication is to be continued after hospital discharge.
- Teach and stress the importance of good handwashing before instillation of the medication.
- If indicated, teach patient and significant other the signs and symptoms of continuing infection: persistent redness, swelling, purulent drainage, decreased visual acuity, increased pain, fever, and indicators of perforation (e.g., increased or sudden eye pain and gush of fluid).

**Sleep pattern disturbance** related to frequent antibiotic and steroid administrations
**Desired outcome:** Patient rests undisturbed for 60- to 90-min intervals, if not contraindicated by ophthalmic medication administration, and expresses satisfaction with the amount of rest and sleep obtained between care activities.
- Plan all nursing care activities so that they can be performed at the time of medication administration.
- Provide a quiet environment for the patient to promote rest.
- Evaluate treatment regimen with physician on a daily basis to determine if medications can be administered less frequently.

---

**Note:** Also see Appendix One, p. 693, for "Caring for Preoperative and Postoperative Patients."

---

## PATIENT-FAMILY TEACHING AND DISCHARGE PLANNING

Give patient and signficant others verbal and written information about the following:
- Medications, including drug name, route, purpose, dosage, schedule, precautions, potential side effects, and instructions for clean technique for topical administration. Remind patient to notify physician before running out of medications.
- Importance of avoiding the following: use of OTC eye drugs without physician approval; rubbing, touching, or bumping the involved eye; and use of eye makeup without physician approval.
- Reporting the following indicators of eye infection to physician: persistent redness, swelling, purulent drainage, fever, and persistent pain.
- Importance of follow-up care; confirm date and time of next appointment if known.
- Wearing glasses by day and shield by night for safety purposes.
- Using dark glasses with mydriatics to minimize photophobia and prevent eye trauma.

## Keratoplasty (corneal transplant)

A keratoplasty is a surgical procedure that replaces a diseased cornea with corneal tissue from a human cadaver. Surgical goals include increasing corneal transparency, improving visual acuity and visual field, and providing a better cosmetic appearance. Surgical success and improved vision depend on the extent of damage, degree of corneal vascularization, state of the surface epithelium, and the tear film (eye moistening capability).

### ASSESSMENT
See "Corneal Ulceration," p. 633.

### COLLABORATIVE MANAGEMENT
**Preoperatively:**    Antibiotic drops are administered in several doses. An osmotic agent, such as Ismotic or Osmoglyn, also may be used to soften the globe.

**Surgical procedure:**    Performed under either general or local anesthetic. A button-sized piece of tissue is removed from the donor cornea and sutured into the recipient cornea with nonabsorbable sutures that are usually left in place for 1 year or more. Grafts are either full thickness (penetrating keratoplasty) or partial thickness (lamellar keratoplasty). Visual acuity will be slow in returning because of the long-standing corneal surface irregularity, and the patient may take up to 1 year to attain an acceptable level of vision.

### NURSING DIAGNOSES AND INTERVENTIONS
**Knowledge deficit:**    Diagnosis, surgery, precautionary measures, and treatment plan

*Desired outcome:*    Before initiation of treatment/surgery, patient verbalizes (and demonstrates, as appropriate) knowledge about the diagnosis, surgical procedure, precautionary measures, and treatment plan.

- Assess patient's knowledge of the diagnosis, surgery, and treatment plan. Clarify or provide explanations as appropriate. Encourage patient to ask questions; provide time for expression of fears and anxieties.
- Explain that the operative eye will be patched after surgery.
- To minimize the potential for injury or infection, instruct patient not to touch, rub, or tightly squeeze operative eye after surgery.
- Explain that an eye shield may be worn nightly for 1 month after surgery to protect the eye. Glasses may be worn during the day for the same purpose.
- Instruct patient or significant other in clean technique for administration of eyedrops or ointment. Stress that good handwashing is necessary to minimize the potential for infection.
- Inform patient that watching TV usually is permitted.
- Explain that patient can have full bathroom privileges and movement when alert.
- Before patient is discharged from the hospital, confer with physician about limitations for the following: heavy lifting, strenuous activity, sexual activity, and sports. Review these limitations with the patient.

**Pain** related to surgical procedure

*Desired outcomes:*    Within 1 h of intervention, patient's subjective perception of pain decreases, as documented by a pain scale. Objective indicators, such as grimacing, are absent or diminished.

---

**Note:**    Moderate discomfort is anticipated for the first 24 h. A scratchy sensation may be present for several weeks after surgery and usually is relieved with mild analgesics, such as acetaminophen.

---

- Assess patient for pain. Devise a pain scale with the patient, rating pain on a scale of 0 (no pain) to 10 (worst pain). Medicate with prescribed analge-

sics as necessary, and document pain relief obtained, using the pain scale.
- Explain that mild discomfort is normal after surgery. Instruct patient to notify staff of increased pain or sudden severe pain, which can signal complications such as hemorrhage or slipped graft.

---

**Note:** See "Corneal Ulceration/Trauma" for **Sensory/perceptual alterations**, p. 635, **High risk for infection**, p. 635, **Self-care deficit**, p. 636, and **Knowledge deficit:** Importance of avoiding increased intraocular pressure and activities that can cause it, p. 636. Also see nursing diagnoses and interventions in "Caring for Preoperative and Postoperative Patients," p. 693, in Appendix One.

---

## PATIENT-FAMILY TEACHING AND DISCHARGE PLANNING

Give patient and significant others verbal and written information about the following:
- Medications, including route, purpose, dosage, schedule, precautions, and potential side effects.
- Importance of avoiding rubbing, touching, or bumping the eye(s). Confer with the physician regarding limitations for the following: heavy lifting, strenuous activity, sexual activity, and sports, and review these limitations with the patient.
- Reporting signs of infection to physician, including purulent drainage, pain, persistent redness, fever, and swelling.
- Need for follow-up care with physician; confirm date and time for removal of sutures, if known.

## Vitreous disorders/Vitrectomy

The vitreous plays an important role in maintaining the form and transparency of the eye. With age, disease, or trauma it can degenerate and liquefy, forming small fluid-filled cavities. As these cavities merge, the vitreous is pushed forward, causing traction on the retina. Ultimately this can lead to a collapsed or detached vitreous, retinal tears, or vitreous hemorrhage. Advancing age, diabetes mellitus, hypertension, and myopia place individuals at higher risk for vitreal degeneration. Indications for a vitrectomy include eye contusion, vitreous loss, hemorrhage, abscess, inflammation, retinal detachment with severe vitreous traction, and global rupture or penetration.

### ASSESSMENT

**Signs and symptoms:**  Complaints of floaters (spots, webs, or streaks) caused by vitreous particles, decreased vision, or flashing lights, which result from abnormal vitreous traction that stimulates the photoreceptors.
**Physical assessment:**  Floaters seen with ophthalmoscopy. Slit lamp observation may reveal retraction, condensation, diabetic shrinkage, or injury. Visual acuity may or may not be affected, depending on the degree of vitreous damage.

### DIAGNOSTIC TESTS

**B-scan ultrasonography:**  Diagnoses posterior-segment disorders associated with gross vitreous opacification, intraocular foreign bodies, and vitreoretinal relationships.

### COLLABORATIVE MANAGEMENT

**Decreased activity and in some cases, bed rest.**
**Laser photocoagulation:**  Used in the treatment of vitreous hemorrhage when the vasculature can be visualized.

**Vitrectomy:**   A small slit is made in the sclera, and a significant amount of damaged vitreous is removed and replaced with a homogenous fluid that resembles vitreous. Abnormal fibrous traction bands and preretinal membranes can be cut to relieve retinal traction. Absorbable sutures are used, and the patient may be given general anesthesia or IV sedation with general anesthetic standby.

## NURSING DIAGNOSES AND INTERVENTIONS

**Knowledge deficit:**   Diagnosis, surgery, treatment plan, and care considerations after hospital discharge
*Desired outcome:*   Before initiation of treatment/surgery, patient verbalizes (and demonstrates, as appropriate) understanding about the diagnosis, surgery, precautions, treatment plan, and care conditions after hospital discharge.
- Assess patient's knowledge of the diagnosis, surgical procedure, and treatment plan. Clarify and provide explanation as appropriate. Allow time for questions and expression of fears and anxieties.
- Explain that the operative eye may be patched for several days after surgery.
- Explain that patient may be restricted to a specified position for several days after surgery. Confirm position with physician. If patient will be restricted to a specific position for 1-3 days, demonstrate deep-breathing exercises to prevent atelectasis and other postoperative respiratory complications and ROM exercises to the lower extremities, which will help prevent phlebitis and venous stasis.
- Caution patient that rubbing, touching, or tightly squeezing the eye must be avoided to maintain the integrity of the dressing.
- Determine with the physician activity limitations for lifting, stooping, straining, coughing, sneezing, bending, and sexual activity, and review the limitations with the patient.
- Explain to patient that postoperative discomfort may be experienced for 24-48 h after surgery but that analgesics will be available as needed.
- Teach patient how to maintain lid hygiene after hospital discharge. Explain that to remove drainage and crust from the lid margins, the patient should moisten a cotton ball with tap water and gently sweep the cotton ball from the inner to outer aspect of the lid, using a new cotton ball with each sweeping motion. Explain that this procedure should continue for as long as the eye secretes drainage (usually 1-2 weeks).
- Explain the importance of wearing glasses by day and an eye shield at night to prevent injury, usually for at least 2-4 weeks.

---

**Note:**   See "Corneal Ulceration/Trauma" for **Sensory/perceptual alterations,** p. 635, **High risk for infection,** p. 635, **Self-care deficit,** p. 636, and **Knowledge deficit:** Importance of avoiding increased intraocular pressure and activities that can cause it, p. 636.

---

## PATIENT-FAMILY TEACHING AND DISCHARGE PLANNING

Give patient and significant others verbal and written information about the following:
- Medications, including route, drug name, purpose, dosage, schedule, precautions, and potential side effects. Stress the importance of notifying physician before the medications run out. Teach patient the importance of good handwashing before instilling ophthalmic medications.
- Importance of reporting indicators of infection (purulent drainage, pain, persistent redness, swelling, fever) to physician.
- Lid hygiene. Explain that to remove drainage and crust from the lid margins, the patient should moisten a cotton ball with tap water and gently sweep the cotton ball from the inner to outer aspect of the lid, using a new cotton

ball with each sweeping motion. Explain that this procedure should continue for as long as the eye secretes drainage (usually 1-2 weeks).
- Necessity of avoiding rubbing, touching, or bumping the eye. Confirm with physician which if any of the following activities will be restricted or limited and review with the patient accordingly: heavy lifting, strenuous activities, sexual activity, bending, stooping, straining, coughing.
- Need for follow-up medical care; confirm date and time of next appointment if known.
- Wearing dark glasses to minimize photophobia and pain when mydriatic eye drops are used.
- Wearing glasses by day and an eye shield at night to prevent injury, usually for at least 2-4 weeks.

## Glaucoma

Glaucoma is a condition in which the intraocular pressure of the aqueous humor is higher than normal, causing atrophy of the optic disk, visual field loss, death of the nerve fibers, and irreversible loss of vision. This increase in pressure within the eye can be caused by excessive aqueous humor production or obstruction in the outflow pathway, preventing aqueous drainage. Glaucoma is usually genetically associated, and it is estimated that 1%-2% of individuals over age 40 have some signs of this disease. Although glaucoma is usually bilateral, it can affect just one eye.

---

**Note:** Glaucoma leads to blindness when it is left untreated.

---

**Primary glaucoma:** Usually caused by obstruction of the trabecular meshwork. There are two types: *chronic simple glaucoma* (open-angle) and *acute or chronic congestive glaucoma* (closed/narrow-angle). Approximately 95% of individuals with glaucoma have the open-angle type.
**Secondary glaucoma:** Usually associated with trauma, tumors, surgery, or uveitis.
**Congenital glaucoma:** Includes juvenile or infantile glaucoma.

### ASSESSMENT
**Open-angle glaucoma:** Primary open-angle glaucoma is a chronic, slowly progressing disorder that is usually asymptomatic until extensive, irreversible loss of the visual field has occurred.
**Narrow-angle glaucoma:** Patient complains of seeing halos or rainbows, severe and spontaneous eye pain, cloudy or blurred vision, decreased vision with or without pain in darkened environments, headaches, nausea, vomiting, and poor night vision. There is increased intraocular pressure, bloodshot eyes, and midpositioned or dilated pupils. A history of diabetes is common.
**Secondary glaucoma:** Patient complains of progressive blurring of vision. Typically, there is a history of eye trauma, tumors, surgery, uveitis, or use of corticosteroids. Intraocular pressure is increased.
**Congenital glaucoma:** Rapidly developing myopia, increased intraocular pressure, decreased visual acuity, and increased corneal diameter in infants. The infantile type is usually identified from birth to age 3, while the juvenile type can develop up to age 30.

### DIAGNOSTIC TESTS
**Tonometry:** Use of a small instrument to measure intraocular pressure or tension in the eye.
**Gonioscopy:** Uses a special lens with a special light and microscope to view the trabecular structures and identify width of the drainage area, adhesions,

undiagnosed trauma, and tumors. It is done before instillation of mydriatic or cycloplegic drug. This test differentiates open-angle from narrow-angle glaucoma.

**Fundoscopy:**   Used if it is deemed safe after gonioscopy. The pupil is dilated to inspect the optic disk and the shape, color, and size of the fundus. This test can identify disk degeneration.

**Ophthalmoscopic examination:**   Identifies increased cupping of the disk.

**Visual field:**   A map that is made of the total visual area the eye can see. It identifies blind spots and can be used as a baseline to identify subsequent degeneration. When done manually, a technician presents stimuli to the patient. When automated, the stimuli are computer-generated.

**Tonography:**   Uses electronic indentation tonometer and recording device to measure how well aqueous humor flows when a known amount of pressure is placed on the eye. A flat tracing indicates a decreased rate of outflow.

**Darkened room test:**   To differentiate between open-angle and narrow-angle glaucoma. It must be used cautiously because it can precipitate a narrow-angle attack from increased intraocular pressure, causing severe pain.

## COLLABORATIVE MANAGEMENT

Medical management is the treatment of choice, and the regimen selected depends on the cause of disease. Surgery is performed only when the disease progresses and medical management or laser treatment is ineffective.

**Open-angle glaucoma:**   Drug therapy is the primary treatment. If pharmacotherapy is ineffective, then laser trabeculoplasty or filtering surgery (trabeculectomy) is performed to prevent further optic nerve damage and visual field loss.

*Miotics, synthetic epinephrine, and beta blockers:*   The drugs used in glaucoma therapy reduce intraocular pressure by decreasing aqueous production or by transiently reducing the volume of the intraocular fluid. These drugs may be discontinued by the physician if they no longer are effective or if side effects outweigh the benefits.

*Trabeculectomy:*   Building of a new channel for the aqueous humor.

*Surgical iridectomy:*   Withdrawal of a portion of the iris *via* a small corneal incision (to improve aqueous drainage) or use of a laser, which bores a fine hole in the iris to provide an artificial channel for the aqueous humor.

**Narrow-angle or angle-closure glaucoma:**   Laser iridotomy is the treatment of choice for primary angle-closure glaucoma. To avoid bilateral involvement, the unaffected eye also is lasered prophylactically. The following surgeries may be performed:

*Iridectomy:*   See above.

*Laser iridotomy:*   Procedure of choice. Light energy from an argon laser allows the passage of aqueous fluid from the posterior chamber into the anterior chamber. This procedure can be performed on an outpatient basis.

*Cyclocryosurgery:*   Freezing of the ciliary body with a cryoprobe to reduce secretions.

*Cyclodialysis:*   Separation of the ciliary body from the sclera and its blood supply to decrease aqueous production.

**Congenital glaucoma:**   Treated surgically, usually with a *trabeculectomy* (see above) because the response to pharmacotherapy is usually poor. Primary congenital glaucoma is essentially a surgical problem.

**Secondary glaucoma:**   Causative factor is identified and eliminated. Either surgery or drug therapy is initiated, depending on the causative factor. Prognosis is often poor. Complications of surgery include retinal detachment, cataract development, hemolytic glaucoma, hemorrhage, decreased visual acuity, and light sensitivity. It must be emphasized to patients that surgery does not eliminate the need for eyedrops, and a lifetime pharmacologic regimen must be maintained.

## NURSING DIAGNOSES AND INTERVENTIONS

**Knowledge deficit:** Diagnosis, surgery, treatment plan, and care considerations after hospital discharge

*Desired outcome:* Before initiation of treatment/surgery, patient verbalizes (and demonstrates, as appropriate) understanding about the diagnosis, surgery, treatment plan, and care considerations after hospital discharge.

- For primary interventions, see this nursing diagnosis in "Keratoplasty," p. 638.
- Explain that patient probably will be able to ambulate within 24 h after surgery, as soon as the anesthetic has worn off.
- Explain that with laser treatment there will be minimal to no discomfort. Moderate discomfort will be present for 24 h after surgery. Mild discomfort will be relieved with acetaminophen.
- Teach patient the necessity of getting intraocular pressure checked at least 4 times a year.
- Stress the importance of a complete eye exam every 2 years, including tonometry, for family members over age 35. Glaucoma usually is genetically associated, and it is estimated that 1%-2% of individuals >40 years of age have some signs of this disease.
- Explain the necessity for extra lighting in darkened areas and extra caution when driving at night.
- Teach the importance of wearing a Medic-Alert bracelet that identifies patient's glaucoma and eye medication used.
- Caution patient about the importance of notifying physician if cardiac drugs are prescribed. Systemic absorption of ophthalmic beta-blocking drugs may act synergistically to potentiate the effects of cardiac drugs.

**Knowledge deficit:** Importance of the extensive pharmacologic regimen; medication administration technique

*Desired outcomes:* Before hospital discharge, patient verbalizes understanding about the importance of frequent medication instillation and the consequences of noncompliance and demonstrates adherence to the prescribed treatment plan. Patient or significant other returns demonstration of the medication administration technique before hospital discharge.

- Explain importance of timely administration of medications and the consequences of noncompliance: Blindness can occur if the condition is left untreated.
- Assist patient or significant other with labeling each eyedrop bottle and writing out schedules for administration. This procedure is especially important for patients with minimal visual acuity, for whom all bottles look alike. Color or texture-coding of the bottles may be effective for some patients.
- Demonstrate technique for administration of eyedrops or ointment. Stress importance of good handwashing to minimize the risk of infection. Have patient or significant other return the demonstration. Be sure patient or significant other is proficient in this technique before hospital discharge.

---

**Note:** See "Corneal Ulceration/Trauma" for **Sensory/perceptual alterations,** p. 635, **High risk for infection,** p. 635, **Self-care deficit, p. 636,** and **Knowledge deficit:** Importance of avoiding increased intraocular pressure and activities that can cause it, p. 636. Also see Appendix One, p. 693, for nursing diagnoses and interventions in "Caring for Preoperative and Postoperative Patients."

---

## PATIENT-FAMILY TEACHING AND DISCHARGE PLANNING

See "Vitreous Disorders/Vitrectomy" for teaching and discharge planning interventions p. 640, and **Knowledge deficit:** Diagnosis, surgery, treatment plan, and care considerations after hospital discharge, p. 640.

# Retinal detachment

A detached retina is the partial or complete separation of the retina from the choroid. The retina is attached to the choroid in two places, at the optic nerve and at the ora serrata near the ciliary body. It is held in place by the gentle pressure of the vitreous body. A detachment is often spontaneous and occurs most frequently in myopia, aphakia, and eye trauma.

Retinal detachments can be categorized into two groups: rhegmatogenous and serous. *Rhegmatogenous detachments* are induced by a tear in the retina that allows fluid (usually supplied by the vitreous) to leak under the retina and separate it from the pigment epithelium. Retinal tears can be caused by trauma or the aging process. *Serous detachments* are caused by a leak in the blood vessels that allows fluid to be trapped between the pigment epithelium and the retina. Serous detachments can be seen in choroidal tumors, serous retinopathy, and inflammatory conditions.

## ASSESSMENT

**Signs and symptoms:**   Patient complains of flashing lights and floaters or visual defects, such as blurred or "sooty" vision, unilateral loss of vision, and sensation of a veil over one eye. Usually redness and pain are not present.

**Physical assessment:**   Visual acuity (e.g., as measured by a Snellen eye chart) may or may not be decreased, depending on the detachment location. Ophthalmoscopic evaluation will reveal a retina that is hanging in a vitreous-like, gray-white cloud. Crescent-shaped, red-orange tear(s) will be present, and the retina may appear to be bulging. Visual field testing may reveal a defect in the location of the detachment.

## COLLABORATIVE MANAGEMENT

Management will range from no treatment in such conditions as serous retinopathy to major invasive surgical procedures.

**Presurgical regimen:**   Before surgery the patient may be on bed rest and placed in various positions to promote reattachment. Mydriatics and cycloplegics are often used to dilate the pupil and decrease movement of the intraocular structures. Both eyes may be patched until surgery is performed to prevent eye movement, which could increase the size of detachment.

**Surgery:**   The surgical goal is to seal the retinal holes or breaks in an attempt to prevent further breaks from occurring and to place the retina in contact with the choroid. One or more of the following procedures is used:

*Photocoagulation:*   A laser emits a bright light onto the pigment epithelium, causing coagulation and attachment of the retina. Peripheral tears may not be accessed *via* this therapy. Photocoagulation is used frequently in torn areas that are small or with retinal holes to prevent further detachment.

*Cryotherapy:*   A super-cooled metal probe is placed on the conjunctiva near the tear. Scleral inflammation occurs, leading to scar formation and reattachment in approximately 1 week.

*Scleral buckling:*   A band resembling a piece of belt is placed around the sclera at the area of detachment, thereby drawing the sclera closer to the retina to facilitate attachment. Often, cryotherapy or photocoagulation is used in conjunction with this therapy to "weld" the retina to the choroid.

*Diathermy:*   Uses heat rather than cold and is similar to cryotherapy but not as widely used.

## NURSING DIAGNOSES AND INTERVENTIONS

**Knowledge deficit:**   Diagnosis, surgical procedure, treatment plan, and care considerations after hospital discharge

*Desired outcome:*   Before initiation of treatment/surgery, patient verbalizes (and demonstrates, as appropriate) understanding about the diagnosis, surgical procedure, treatment plan, and care considerations after hospital discharge.

- Assess patient's knowledge of the diagnosis and surgery. Clarify or provide explanation as appropriate. Allow time for patient to ask questions and express fears and anxiety.
- Explain that after scleral buckling the operative eye may be patched for several days.
- Explain that mydriatic and cycloplegic drops will be instilled to dilate the pupil, expose the retina, and decrease iris movement.
- Explain that the patient may be restricted to a specific position for several days after surgery (e.g., depending on the location of the detachment, the patient may be prone).
- To prevent increased intraocular pressure after surgery, the patient may be told not to strain with bowel movements, cough or sneeze (unless done with the mouth and eyes open), or bend. Tell patient to notify staff of constipation, persistent cough, nausea, or need for assistance.
- Explain that to minimize excessive movements of the eye muscles, shaving, brushing teeth, face washing, and hair combing are contraindicated until approved by physician.
- Explain to patient that the eyelid may be very swollen and require ice applications to reduce the swelling and promote comfort.
- Explain that mydriatric drops will be used postoperatively to enable the surgeon to assess status of the retina and that antibiotic drops will be used as a prophylaxis for infection.
- Discuss with patient that moderate discomfort can be expected during the first 24-48 h after surgery and that it can be relieved with acetaminophen.
- If the patient will be on bed rest, demonstrate deep-breathing exercises, to help prevent postsurgical pulmonary complications, and passive ROM and limb movements, which are used after surgery to help promote venous return. Have patient return the demonstrations. Coughing exercises are contraindicated because they cause increased intraocular pressure.

*Care considerations after hospital discharge*
- Teach patient the importance of wearing dark glasses to minimize photophobia and pain when mydriatics are used.
- Explain that wearing glasses by day and an eye shield at night (usually for at least 2-4 weeks) will help protect the eye.
- Teach patient how to maintain lid hygiene. For discussion, see "Vitreous Disorders/Vitrectomy."
- Teach patient that floaters may appear postoperatively and can disappear in weeks or last for years.
- Caution patient that continuing light flashes may indicate that complete retinal attatchment was not achieved by surgery. Though this does not necessarily indicate unsuccessful surgery, it does require notifying physician.

**Altered protection** related to increased risk of bleeding after surgery because of hypervascularity of ocular tissue
*Desired outcomes:* Patient verbalizes understanding of the signs of hyphema and assumes and maintains the prescribed position if it occurs. The physician is notified promptly if hyphema occurs.
- Inspect the outer dressing for the presence of bleeding. Notify physician of significant findings.
- Once the initial dressing has been removed by physician, be alert to hyphema (bleeding in the anterior chamber of the eye), which can occur because of the high vascularity of the tissue. Teach patient to report to staff the presence of sudden severe pain, which can signal occurrence of hyphema.
- If bleeding occurs, keep patient calm and in the prescribed position. Notify physician promptly.

**High risk for impaired skin integrity** related to imposed position restrictions and frequent removal of eye patch
*Desired outcome:* Patient's skin remains clear and intact.
- Because it is imperative that the patient maintain the prescribed position and

avoid head and eye movements, provide skin care at frequent intervals to prevent skin breakdown. Provide special attention to skin over bony prominences, such as heels, ankles, elbows, sacrum, and greater tuberosities.
- Use a mattress that minimizes tissue pressure, such as a Clinitron or low air loss bed.
- Frequent eye patch removal can cause skin irritation. Keep the skin under the tape dry to prevent breakdown.

---

**Note:** See "Corneal Ulceration/Trauma" for **Sensory/perceptual alterations,** p. 635, **High risk for infection,** p. 635, **Self-care deficit,** p. 636, and **Knowledge deficit:** Importance of avoiding increased intraocular pressure and activities that can cause it, p. 636. Also see Appendix One for nursing diagnoses and interventions in "Caring for Preoperative and Postoperative Patients," p. 693.

---

## PATIENT-FAMILY TEACHING AND DISCHARGE PLANNING

Give patient and significant others verbal and written information about the following:
- Medications, including drug name, route, purpose, dosage, schedule, precautions, and potential side effects. Stress the importance of notifying physician before supply runs out. Explain that good handwashing is essential before administering ophthalmic ointments or drops.
- Recognizing and reporting signs of infection to physician: purulent drainage, pain, persistent redness, swelling, fever.
- Avoiding rubbing, touching, and bumping the operative eye. Confer with physician regarding which, if any, of the following activities will be restricted and for how long, and review with patient accordingly: contact sports, heavy lifting, straining, bending, sexual activity.
- For additional information, see **Knowledge deficit:** Diagnosis, surgical procedure, treatment plan, and care considerations after hospital discharge, p. 644.

## Enucleation

Enucleation is the surgical removal of an eyeglobe without disturbance of orbital integrity. Because enucleation is a drastic measure that results in blindness in the affected eye, it is not considered until all other possible medical and surgical therapies have been utilized. Indications for enucleation include malignant tumor; a painful, blind, or disfiguring eye; absolute glaucoma; presence of a nonremovable, irritating foreign substance in the eye; severe infection; unrepaired ruptured globe; and as prophylaxis in sympathetic ophthalmia.

## COLLABORATIVE MANAGEMENT

**Medical treatment:**    Removal of foreign body or treatment of tumor, infection, or pain is instituted initially. If treatment is ineffective or severe trauma or disfigurement exists, surgery is performed.

**Surgery:**    Usually performed under general anesthetic. The goal of surgery is to maintain orbital integrity, and an attempt is made to preserve the muscles and tendons for later insertion of an ocular prosthesis. Once the globe is removed, a temporary artificial globe called a conformer, which is made of Teflon or plastic, usually is inserted to maintain orbit shape until a permanent ocular prosthesis can be made.

**Fitting and insertion of an ocular prosthesis:**    Often delayed until postoperative edema decreases, usually 4-6 weeks after surgery, but it may be longer in cases of severe trauma.

## NURSING DIAGNOSES AND INTERVENTIONS

**Knowledge deficit:**  Surgical procedure, postsurgical precautions, and function of the ocular prosthesis

*Desired outcomes:*  Before surgery, patient verbalizes knowledge of the surgical procedure, postsurgical precautions, and function of the ocular prosthesis.

- Assess patient's knowledge of the diagnosis, surgery, and treatment plan; explain or clarify information as necessary.
- Provide time for patient and significant others to express fears and anxieties and ask questions.
- Inform patient that a pressure dressing will be applied for 2-3 days after surgery.
- Caution patient that touching and rubbing the orbit or tightly squeezing the eyelid are contraindicated because these actions can cause injury and infection.
- Explain that some discomfort after surgery is normal but patient should alert staff to the presence of headache or sharp pain on operative side, which can signal complications, such as hemorrhage, infection, or broken sutures.
- Explain that to minimize intraorbital pressure, patient should not lie on the operative side but rather maintain the prescribed position (usually supine to 30 degrees elevation of the HOB), and that stooping, bending, lifting heavy objects, straining with bowel movements, and coughing or sneezing with a closed mouth are contraindicated because they may cause bleeding.
- Inform patient that activities usually are not restricted after the first postoperative day.
- Teach patient the function of the ocular prosthesis and approximate schedule for insertion, if appropriate.
- Teach patient the importance of maintaining lid hygiene. See discussion in "Vitreous Disorders/Vitrectomy."
- Explain the lifetime need for safety glasses to protect the remaining eye.
- Teach patient the necessity of obtaining Medic-Alert bracelet and card that identifies patient as having ocular prosthesis.

**Pain** related to surgical procedure

*Desired outcomes:*  Within 1 h of intervention, patient's subjective perception of pain decreases, as documented by a pain scale. Objective indicators, such as grimacing, are absent or diminished.

- Explain to patient that minor discomfort after surgery is normal and that analgesia will be provided as needed.
- Monitor for the presence of discomfort at frequent intervals. Devise a pain scale with patient, rating pain from 0 (no pain) to 10 (worst pain). Ask patient to alert staff to severe pain (i.e., >6+ on the rating scale) or headache on enucleated side, which can signal complications such as hemorrhage, broken sutures, or infection.
- Provide prescribed analgesia as needed. Rate and document the degree of pain relief obtained, using the pain scale.
- There may be discomfort from the pressure dressing, which is used to minimize edema and ensure hemostasis. Provide rationale for this dressing to the patient, and explain that it is used for the first 2-3 postoperative days.
- Use prescribed antibiotic ointment to decrease discomfort from drying of tissues, which can occur with excessive conjunctival edema. When removing the dressing, confirm that the plastic or Teflon conformer is in place.

---

**Note:**  See "Corneal Ulceration/Trauma" for **Sensory/perceptual alterations,** p. 635, and **Self-care deficit,** p. 636. Also see "Caring for Preoperative and Postoperative Patients," p. 693, and "Caring for Patients with Cancer and other Life-Disrupting Illnesses," p. 753, in Appendix One.

PATIENT-FAMILY TEACHING AND DISCHARGE PLANNING

Give patient and significant others verbal and written information about the following:

- Medications, including drug name, route, purpose, dosage, schedule, precautions, and potential side effects. Stress the importance of good handwashing before administering ophthalmic medications.
- Necessity of reporting signs of infection to physician: purulent drainage, swelling of orbit, pain, persistent orbital redness, fever.
- Importance of avoiding rubbing, touching, or bumping orbit or wearing eye makeup without physician consent.
- Need for follow-up care; confirm date of next appointment with physician and for the ocular prosthesis.
- Lid hygiene. See discussion in "Vitreous Disorders/Vitrectomy."
- Referral to social worker or mental health nurse clinician as needed.
- Use of safety glasses to protect the remaining eye.

*In addition, once the ocular prosthesis is inserted*

- Necessity of obtaining Medic-Alert bracelet and card that identifies patient as having ocular prosthesis.

# Section Two:   Disorders and Surgeries of the Ear

## Otosclerosis (Otospongiosis)

Otosclerosis is a disease of the bony inner ear in which normal bone is absorbed and replaced by a vascular and spongy bone (hence the name *otospongiosis*). When the disease involves the footplate of the stapes and the stapes become either partially or completely fixed, hearing loss will occur because stapes vibration will be hindered. This is a hereditary disease that starts in adulthood and affects more females than males.

### ASSESSMENT

**Signs and symptoms:**   Slow and progressive loss of hearing (more often bilateral), tinnitus, and sometimes an equilibrium disturbance, from mild dizziness to vertigo.

**Physical assessment:**   Usually the eardrums will appear normal, but a pink blush is seen through the drum when the otosclerotic focus is very vascular. Tuning fork testing will suggest a conductive loss (negative Rinne's test). Pure tone audiometry confirms the presence of a conductive hearing loss. Tympanometry may reveal evidence of stiffness in the sound conduction system. A neurosensory component also may be present.

**Risk factors:**   A positive family history of hearing loss may be obtained. Sometimes pregnancy accelerates the disease process.

### COLLABORATIVE MANAGEMENT

**Hearing aid:**   Individuals with otosclerosis usually are good candidates for a hearing aid.

**Surgical interventions:**   Surgical treatments for otosclerosis have evolved since the early 1950s from fenestration, to stapes immobilization, to total stapedectomy, to partial stapedectomy, which is performed today. In this procedure, most of the stapes is removed. A hole is made in the fixed footplate (usually by a laser), and a prosthesis is used to link the incus to the inner ear fluids, thus reestablishing a mobile sound-conducting mechanism. Surgery may be done under local or general anesthetic. Patients usually are hospitalized for

1 night following stapedectomy. If an equilibrium disturbance is severe, continued hospitalization will be required.

## NURSING DIAGNOSES AND INTERVENTIONS

**Knowledge deficit:** Surgical procedure, postsurgical regimen, and expected outcomes
*Desired outcomes:* Before surgery, patient verbalizes (and demonstrates as appropriate) knowledge about the surgical procedure, postsurgical regimen, and expected outcomes.
- Explain upcoming surgical procedure, postsurgical routine, and expected outcomes. Provide time for patient to ask questions and express fears and anxieties.
- Stress that patient must maintain the position specified by physician both during and after surgery. After surgery the patient usually will be positioned on the nonoperative side.
- Explain that bed rest probably will be required for about 24 h and that it may be necessary to remain flat, even for meals, to prevent slipping of the prosthesis.
- Instruct patient to inform staff of headache, tinnitus, vertigo, vomiting, weakness of facial muscles, or postoperative pain that increases or is sudden and severe. These signs and symptoms can signal infection, hemorrhage, facial nerve encroachment, labyrinthitis, or irritation of the auditory nerve.
- Explain that patient may have an earplug after surgery to absorb drainage in the operative ear. Caution patient not to remove this plug or get it wet.
- Instruct patient not to blow nose, because air forced into the eustachian tube can disturb the operative site. If blowing the nose is unavoidable, it should be done gently, without restricting either nostril and with the mouth and eyes open to minimize intracranial pressure.
- Caution patient not to get water in the operative ear for 2 weeks, or as directed.
- Reassure patient that minimal discomfort will be experienced postoperatively and that analgesics (usually acetaminophen) will be used as needed for the first 24 h.
- Caution patient to avoid changes in air pressure (air travel, diving, riding elevators) for the period of time determined by physician.

**High risk for infection** related to surgical procedure
*Desired outcome:* Patient is free of infection as evidenced by normothermia, absence of pain and headache, and absence of drainage, erythema, and swelling in the canal.
- After the earplug and bandage have been removed, monitor for drainage, erythema, and swelling in the canal; fever; and patient complaints of pain or headache, which can signal the presence of infection.
- Assist patient with maintaining dry operative site, which will help prevent infection. Avoid hair washing and showers until approved by physician.
- Be alert to the following indicators of meningitis, which is a rare but potential complication of this surgery: fever, chills, headache, nuchal rigidity, photophobia, nausea, and vomiting.
- Teach patient the importance of avoiding contact with individuals known to have upper respiratory infections (URIs), which can lead to otitis media.
- Caution patient to change only the *outer* earplug as prescribed, using clean technique.

**High risk for trauma** related to equilibrium disturbance
*Desired outcome:* Patient does not fall or exhibit signs of trauma caused by equilibrium disturbance.
- Monitor for the presence of mild dizziness, vertigo, tinnitus, or nausea. Advise patient to alert staff to the presence of nausea or vertigo so that appropriate medications can be administered.
- To prevent falls, keep side rails up when patient is in bed.

- Instruct patient to seek assistance with ambulation once it is allowed.
- Instruct patient to maintain sitting position for a few moments before assuming a standing position.

**Sensory/perceptual alterations** (auditory deficit) related to disease process, postoperative earplug, or tissue edema
*Desired outcome:*  Following intervention(s), patient relates the ability to understand speaker and expresses satisfaction with sensory input.

- Inform patient that hearing may be impaired for a few weeks after surgery because of tissue edema, ear packing, and the presence of blood in the inner ear.
- Teach patient to maximize hearing by using lipreading, hearing aid in the nonoperative ear, or turning better ear toward the speaker.
- Maintain quiet environment to minimize extraneous sounds during conversations.
- Speak to patient slowly, in even tones; avoid turning away from patient or covering mouth while speaking.
- Provide alternative sensory input, such as books or puzzles.

---

**Note:**  See nursing diagnoses and interventions in "Caring for Preoperative and Postoperative Patients," p. 693, in Appendix One.

---

## PATIENT-FAMILY TEACHING AND DISCHARGE PLANNING

Give patient and significant others verbal and written information about the following:

- Medications, including drug name, purpose, dosage, schedule, route, precautions, and potential side effects.
- Need for medical follow-up; confirm date and time of next appointment if known. Usually the inner earplug is removed 7 days after surgery.
- Reporting the following indicators of ear infection to physician: persistent erythema and swelling of canal, purulent drainage, vertigo, persistent pain, and fever.
- Avoiding blowing nose or sneezing; if unavoidable, keeping mouth and eyes open in the process to minimize pressure buildup.
- Avoiding changes in air pressure (air travel, diving, riding elevators) for the period of time determined by physician.
- Avoiding contact with individuals known to have URIs, which can lead to otitis media.
- Keeping ear dry for the period of time determined by physician.
- Changing only the *outer* earplug as prescribed, using clean technique.

## Cochlear implantation

Cochlear implantation is performed in individuals with profound bilateral sensorineural hearing loss who receive no measurable assistance from lip reading with a properly fitting hearing aid. The electrical activity of hearing is initiated by hair cells in the organ of Corti and sent to the brain along nerve fibers that make up the auditory nerve. In most deaf individuals, these hair cells are damaged. The goal of cochlear implantation is to bridge the gap created by the hair cell loss and directly stimulate the remaining neurons. Studies have shown that even when there is a complete loss of hair cells, a percentage of cochlear neurons remains. Sensorineural hearing loss most commonly is caused by the following:

**Acute viral infections:**  Spinal meningitis, mumps.
**Drug toxicity:**  Aminoglycocides, salicylates, antineoplastics, cisplatin.
**Head trauma:**  Fractured temporal bone.

**Noise-induced occupational hearing loss.**
**Sudden hearing loss of unknown cause:** Usually viral syndrome, vascular vasospasm, or immunologic disorders.

Adults who became deaf after developing speech are considered primary candidates, but children at various age levels are now being considered, as well.

## COLLABORATIVE MANAGEMENT

- **Amplification:** Individuals are fitted with a hearing aid initially to determine if any benefit is obtained or if it may assist with lip reading.
- **Cochlear implantation procedure:** The four components of the implantable device are a microphone to detect sound, a processor to encode the sound into electrical activity, a signal coupler to transmit these signals to the internal electrode system, and an electrical system that is surgically implanted into the cochlea. The electrodes that are surgically implanted into the cochlea are then attached to a percutaneous pedestal with a multichannel processor that is located behind the auricle (in the region of the mastoid). Surgery is done under general anesthetic. Patients generally are hospitalized for 2 days following surgery. Specific risks for cochlear implantation include:
- Damage to the facial nerve or balance system.
- Irritation to the facial nerve and/or balance system.
- Infection.
- Damage to the inner ear.
- Failure to produce sound.
- Continued technological advances that may require additional surgery.

## NURSING DIAGNOSES AND INTERVENTIONS

**Knowledge deficit:** Surgical procedure, postsurgical regimen, and expected outcomes
*Desired outcome:* Before surgery, patient verbalizes understanding of the surgical procedure, postsurgical regimen, and expected outcomes.

- Determine patient's understanding of the cochlear implantation and the postsurgical regimen. Provide explanation as indicated.
- Explain that assistance with ambulation will be required for the patient's first time up and that the patient will be assessed for vertigo.
- Instruct patient to inform staff of headache, vertigo, vomiting, weakness of the facial muscles, or postoperative pain that increases or is sudden and severe. These signs and symptoms may signal infection, hemorrhage, facial nerve encroachment, labyrinthitis, or irritation of the auditory nerve.
- Explain that the surgical dressing and staples will be in place until the patient is seen in the physician's office approximately 6 days after surgery. Explain that the patient and signficant others will be instructed in pedestal care at that time. A cotton-tipped applicator saturated with hydrogen peroxide is used to clean around the pedestal area, followed by an application of bacitracin ointment.
- Remind patient that the implanted device will not be tested until 4-6 weeks after the surgery.
- Reassure patient that analgesics will be used for the initial postoperative phase when discomfort is experienced.

---

**Note:** See "Otosclerosis" for **High risk for trauma,** p. 649. Also see nursing diagnoses and interventions in "Caring for Preoperative and Postoperative Patients," p. 693.

---

## PATIENT-FAMILY TEACHING AND DISCHARGE PLANNING

Give patient and significant others verbal and written information about the following:

- Medications, including drug name, purpose, dosage, schedule, route, precautions, and potential side effects.
- Importance of medical follow-up; confirm date and time of next appointment.
- Necessity of reporting fever and signs and symptoms of infection at the operative site: drainage, erythema, pain.
- Pedestal care and frequency (daily).
- Development of a rehabilitation schedule established by the physician 4-6 weeks postoperatively.

### Selected Bibliography

Bickford ME: Patient teaching tools in the ophthalmic unit, *J Ophthalmic Nurs Technol* 7(2):50-55, 1988.

Bowie I: Wounds to the eye, *Nursing 90* 15:24-27, 1990.

Boyd-Monk H: Eye trauma: a close-up on emergency care, *RN* 52(2):22-30, 1989.

Burton S: Drugs and the eye, *Nursing 89* 45:24-26, 1989.

Cochlear implants: technological advances offer new worlds of sound, *Mayo Clin Health Letter* 9(11):4-6, 1991.

Deweese DD et al: *Otolaryngology: head and neck surgery*, ed 7, St Louis, 1988, Mosby–Year Book.

Geraldi PS et al: Glaucoma: high-risk alert, *J Ophthalmic Technol* 10(1):34, 1991.

Interqual: The ISD-A review system with adult ISD criteria, August 1992, Northhampton, NH, and Marlboro, MA, Interqual, Inc.

Kim MJ, McFarland GK, McLane AM: *Pocket guide to nursing diagnoses*, ed 5, St Louis, 1993, Mosby–Year Book.

Lawler MC: Common ocular injuries and disorders, part I: acute loss of vision, *JEN* 15(1):32-36, 1989.

Lawler MC: Common ocular injuries and disorders, part II: red eye, *JEN* 15(1):36-43, 1989.

Nadal JB, Eddington DK: Treatment of sensorineural hearing loss by cochlear implantation, *Annu Rev Med* 39:491-502, 1988.

Newell FW: *Ophthalmology—principles and concepts*, ed 7, St Louis, 1992, Mosby–Year Book.

Radzwiccz PL: Nursing management of corneal ulcers, *Ophthalmic Nurs Forum* 6(1):1-4, 6-8, 1990.

Smith SJ: Sensory deprivation and the ophthalmic patient, *J Ophthalmic Nurs Technol* 8(4):48-54, 1989.

Talley FM et al: Perceived stressors during the recovery period following enucleation, *Insight* 16(3):18-19, 1991.

Williams L et al: Otoplasty, *Plast Surg Nurs* 9(3):132-133, 135, 1989.

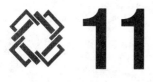

# 11 PROVIDING CARE FOR PATIENTS WITH SPECIAL NEEDS

Section One   Caring for Individuals with Human Immunodeficiency Virus Disease   653
Section Two   Providing Nutritional Support   665
  Nutritional assessment   665
  Nutritional support modalities   669
Section Three   Managing Wound Care   681
  Wounds closed by primary intention   681
  Surgical or traumatic wounds healing by secondary intention   683
  Pressure ulcers   686
Selected Bibliography   689

## Section One:   Caring for Individuals with Human Immunodeficiency Virus Disease

Acquired immunodeficiency syndrome (AIDS) is a life-threatening illness caused by the human immunodeficiency virus (HIV). AIDS is characterized by the disruption of cell-mediated immunity. This breakdown of the immune system is manifested by opportunistic infections such as *Pneumocystis carinii* pneumonia (PCP) or tumors such as Kaposi's sarcoma (KS).

The three confirmed routes of HIV transmission are the following:
- Sexual contact that involves an exchange of body fluids.
- Parenterally *via* receipt of contaminated blood or blood products, or injecting drug use.
- From an infected mother to a child during the perinatal period.

It is estimated that the average time span between infection with HIV and seroconversion (development of a positive HIV antibody test) is 6-8 weeks, although antibody response may be absent for a year or more. Therefore, a negative test does not guarantee the absence of infection. Individuals with a recent history of high-risk behavior and a negative HIV antibody test should be retested at 6-month intervals for 1 year and follow the guidelines for safer sex practices (Table 11-1). Anyone with a positive HIV antibody test must be considered infectious and capable of transmitting the virus.

---

**T A B L E   1 1 - 1    Safer Sex Guidelines**

*Safer sexual practices include the following*
Social (dry) kissing
French (wet) kissing
Hugging
Massage
Mutual masturbation
Body-to-body contact, excepting mucous membrane areas
Activities not involving direct body contact
*Sexual practices of questionable safety include*
Anal-oral contact (rimming) using a latex barrier
Anal or vaginal intercourse using latex condoms*
Fellatio (mouth to penis) without ejaculation
Cunnilingus (mouth to vaginal area)
Watersports (enemas, urination)
*Unsafe sexual practices include*
Anal or vaginal intercourse without latex condom
Oral contact with bodily fluids (semen, urine, feces, vaginal secretions)
Contact with blood
Oral-anal contact (rimming)
Manual anal/vaginal penetration (fisting)
Sharing sexual aids or needles

---

*Petroleum-based lubricants have been shown to increase the risk of condom rupture. Water-based products, such as K-Y jelly and similar products, are preferred. In addition, use of viricidal spermicides, such as nonoxynol-9, are strongly urged as added protection.

---

**T A B L E   1 1 - 2    Exposure Categories and Their Percentages for Contracting HIV Disease**

| Group | Percent |
|---|---|
| Men who have sex with men | 56 |
| Injecting drug users | 19 |
| Men who have sex with men and inject drugs | 6 |
| Hemophilia/coagulation disorders | 1 |
| Heterosexual contact | 6 |
| Recipients of blood transfusions, blood components, or tissue | 2 |
| People with multiple modes of exposure | 6 |
| Undetermined | 4 |

---

While the Centers for Disease Control (CDC) continues, for epidemiologic reasons, to identify "exposure categories" (Table 11-2), the epidemiologic focus no longer is on groups but on high-risk behaviors. HIV infection has transcended all racial, social, sexual, and economic barriers, and it is high-risk behaviors that are primarily responsible for its transmission. Table 11-3 details the behaviors that place an individual at the greatest risk for HIV infection.

To a minimal extent, health-care workers who come into contact with the

## T A B L E  11 - 3   High-Risk Sexual Behaviors

Unprotected anonymous sex
Unprotected oral sex with transfer of bodily fluids
Unprotected receptive anal/vaginal sex
Unprotected oral-anal contact (rimming)
Manual anal/vaginal penetration (fisting)
Sharing sexual aids or needles
Unprotected sex with multiple partners

body substances of patients also are at some risk. Understanding and practice of universal precautions or variations, such as body substance isolation, are essential for all health care workers. Review Table A-19, p. 778, for a discussion of the handling of blood and body fluids for all patients.

AIDS is the terminal phase of HIV infection. This is a chronic viral disease that covers a wide spectrum of illnesses and symptomatology over a variable course of time. There is no classic disease progression (e.g., some individuals proceed from an asymptomatic, seropositive state to AIDS, while others may experience the symptoms for many years). Therefore, HIV disease should be considered as a continuum of infection. The stages of illness are described under "Assessment," below.

The mortality rate for those diagnosed with HIV disease is grim but slowly improving. Early recognition and treatment of the complications of HIV infections, as well as promising experimental drug therapies, have given patients not only increased survival times but also a better quality of life. Maintenance of a positive attitude by the patient and caregivers is an essential element in the therapeutic plan, but an honest approach to the realities of any life-threatening illness also must prevail.

## ASSESSMENT

The four stages of HIV infection can be categorized as acute infection, asymptomatic stage, AIDS-related complex (ARC—a now obsolete term that still is used to define symptoms for this stage), and AIDS.

**Acute infection** (a mononucleosislike syndrome):
*Signs and symptoms:*   Fever, malaise, muscle aches, night sweats, headache, nausea.
*Laboratory results:*   HIV antibody test may not yet be positive.
**Asymptomatic stage** (may range anywhere from 5 to many more years):
*Signs and symptoms:*   Generally none, but may have persistent, generalized lymphadenopathy.
*Laboratory results:*   Positive HIV antibody test; CD4 T lymphocyte count usually >400/mm$^3$.
**ARC**
*Signs and symptoms:*   Persistent fever, involuntary weight loss, chronic diarrhea, fatigue, night sweats, thrush, hairy leukoplakia.
*Laboratory results:*   Positive HIV antibody test, CD4 T lymphocyte or helper lymphocyte count usually <400/mm$^3$, anemia, thrombocytopenia, leukopenia, or lymphopenia.
**AIDS** (as diagnosed by the presence of one or more of these "indicator" diseases as defined by CDC): cryptosporidiosis with diarrhea lasting >1 month; cytomegalovirus of an organ other than the liver, spleen, or lymph nodes; isosporiasis; Kaposi's sarcoma; lymphoma of the brain (primary); lymphoid interstitial pneumonia or pulmonary lymphoid hyperplasia; *Pneumocystitis carinii* pneumonia; progressive multifocal leukoencephalopathy; toxoplasmosis of the brain; candidiasis of the esophagus, trachea, bronchi, or lungs; coccidioid-

omycosis; extrapulmonary cryptococcosis; herpes simplex virus infection causing an ulcer that persists >1 month; histoplasmosis; pulmonary tuberculosis; other mycobacteriosis; salmonellosis; other bacterial infection; HIV encephalopathy; Burkitt's lymphoma; immunoblastic sarcoma; mycobacterium avium complex; recurrent pneumonias; HIV wasting syndrome; and invasive cervical cancer.

*Signs and symptoms:*   Depend on the presenting opportunistic infection.

*Laboratory results:*   Positive HIV antibody test, CD4 T lymphocyte count usually <200/mm$^3$, or total lymphocytes <14%, hematologic disorders (see data with ARC, above), multiple chemistry abnormalities.

**History:**   If the patient is suspected of having HIV infection, the history would be incomplete without detailed social and sexual interviews, with special focus on determining high-risk behaviors. A complete review of body systems with careful attention to the common symptoms of HIV infection should be performed.

**Physical assessment:**   Be aware of the following indicators that are seen frequently with HIV infection:

*General:*   Fever, cachexia, weight loss.

*Cutaneous:*   Herpes zoster or simplex infection(s); seborrheic or other dermatitis; fungal infections of the skin (moniliasis, candidiasis) or nailbeds (onychomycosis); KS lesions; petechiae.

*Head/neck:*   "Cotton-wool" spots visualized on fundoscopic exam; oral KS; candida (thrush); hairy leukoplakia; aphthous ulcers; enlarged, hard, and occasionally tender lymph nodes.

*Respiratory:*   Tachypnea, dyspnea, diminished or adventitious breath sounds (crackles, rhonchi, wheezing).

*Cardiac:*   Tachycardia, friction rub, gallops, murmurs.

*Gastrointestinal:*   Enlargement of liver or spleen, diarrhea, constipation, hyperactive bowel sounds, abdominal distention.

*Genital/rectal:*   KS lesions, herpes, candidiasis, fistulae.

*Neuromuscular:*   Flattened affect, apathy, withdrawal, memory deficits, headache, muscle atrophy, speech deficits, gait disorders, generalized weakness, incontinence, neuropathy.

## DIAGNOSTIC TESTS

Individuals with HIV disease may experience many signs and symptoms, as previously stated. The physician may prescribe other evaluations than those listed below, which are merely some of the more commonly performed diagnostic tests.

**HIV antibody:**   The initial test for HIV is the enzyme-linked immunosorbent assay (ELISA), which tests for presence of antibody to the virus that causes HIV disease. A positive result signals the individual's infection with HIV and ability to transmit HIV to others, not the presence of AIDS. An initially reactive ELISA should be repeated twice on the same specimen. If one or both repeats are reactive, the ELISA is considered repeatedly reactive and should be confirmed by another test, usually the Western blot (WB).

**Western blot:**   A confirmatory test used to detect immune response to the specific viral proteins of HIV. A reactive WB is defined by a specific pattern of electrophoresed protein bands on a strip of nitrocellulose paper; 3 of the following bands must be present for reactivity: p24 (see below), gp41, and gp210 or gp160.

**p24 antigen test:**   Detects HIV p24 antigen in serum, plasma, and cerebrospinal fluid (CSF) of infected individuals. Its advantage is that it detects viral antigen (HIV p24) early in the course of infection before seroconversion.

**Polymerase chain reaction test:**   Assay for HIV nucleic acid. Its advantages include detection early in the infectious process, detection during latency/dormancy period of the virus, detection in infants when maternally derived antibody from an infected mother is present, and extreme sensitivity to minute amounts of HIV nucleic acid.

**Immunofluorescence assay:**   Tests for HIV antibody and has these 3 distinct advantages over the WB test: increased sensitivity, less expensive, and less technically demanding.

**Urinalysis:**   Tests for Beta 2, a microglobulin that has been used as a marker for proximal tubule dysfunction; also detects cytomegalovirus (CMV).

**Biopsy:**   Used for both esophageal and KS lesions; helps distinguish invasive pathogens from secondary colonizers.

## COLLABORATIVE MANAGEMENT

Medical management is limited primarily to chemotherapeutic intervention in an attempt to arrest the progression of the disease. Currently, there is no single drug or combination of drugs that has restored immunocompetency to afflicted patients. Medical treatment is palliative. Table 11-4 identifies drugs commonly used in the treatment of HIV and opportunistic infections.

**Retroviral drugs:**   Zidovudine, AZT (Retrovir), dideoxyinosine (DDI), and dideoxycytidine (DDC) are the only FDA-approved retroviral drugs available to date. These medications promise no cure for HIV infection, but has been shown to prolong life and reduce the number of opportunistic infections in individuals who can tolerate it. Retrovir has numerous side effects, most notably bone marrow suppression. Patients taking this drug need close monitoring of hematologic factors.

**Surgical interventions:**   May include resection of tumors; placement of venous access devices for total parenteral nutrition (TPN), chemotherapy, or frequent blood withdrawals; or, in selected instances, splenectomy for idiopathic thrombocytopenic purpura (ITP). **Note:** IV gammaglobulin or prednisone therapy is also used for ITP.

## NURSING DIAGNOSES AND INTERVENTIONS

**High risk for infection** related to inadequate secondary defenses of the immune system, malnutrition, or side effects of chemotherapy

*Desired outcome:*   Patient is free of additional infections during hospitalization, as evidenced by appropriate cultures or biopsies.

- Assess for indicators of opportunistic infections (e.g., persistent fevers, night sweats, fatigue, involuntary weight loss, persistent and dry cough, persistent diarrhea, headache). See Table 11-5 for the common opportunistic infections and organisms that infect individuals with HIV disease.
- Monitor laboratory data, especially CBC, differential, erythrocyte sedimentation rate (ESR), and cultures, to evaluate the course of infection. Be alert to abnormal results, and notify physician of significant findings.
- Maintain strict asepsis for all invasive procedures to prevent introduction of new pathogens.
- Assist patient in maintaining meticulous body hygiene to prevent spread of organisms from body secretions into skin breaks, especially if patient has diarrhea.
- Monitor temperature and VS at frequent intervals for evidence of fever or sepsis. In addition to increased temperature, be alert to diaphoresis, confusion, decrease in LOC, increased HR, and decreased BP secondary to the vasodilatory effect of the increased body temperature. Perform a complete physical assessment at least q8h to identify changes from baseline assessment. Assess for changes in breath sounds, which may be indicative of an increasing level of infiltrates.
- Promote pulmonary toilet by encouraging patient to engage in frequent breathing or incentive spirometry exercises. Use caution when performing postural drainage and chest physiotherapy, if prescribed, because patients may be too ill to tolerate these activities.

**T A B L E  11 - 4    Drugs Commonly Used in the Treatment of HIV Disease and Opportunistic Infections**

| Drug | Target | Mechanism of action | Dosage | Side effects |
|---|---|---|---|---|
| zidovudine (AZT) | HIV virus | Reverse transcriptase inhibitor | 100 mg 5x/day or 200 mg 3×/day | Blood dyscrasias, anemia, myopathy |
| dideoxyinosine (DDI) | HIV virus | Reverse transcriptase inhibitor | 150 mg bid | Convulsions, irritability, difficulty sleeping |
| dideoxycytidine (DDC) | HIV virus | Reverse transcriptase inhibitor | 0.75 mg q8h given simultaneously with 200 mg AZT | Axonal neuropathy |
| trisodium-phosphonoformate (Foscaret) | HIV virus | Reverse transcriptase inhibitor | 60 mg/kg qd × 14 d; *maintenance:* 60-120 mg/kg/day | Nephrotoxicity, bone and tooth enamel changes, anemia, increased serum creatinine |
| gancyclovir | CMV retinitis, pneumonia | Inhibitor of CMV replication in vitro | 5-7 mg/kg/day q12h × 10 days; then 5 mg/kg/day 5-7 ×/week | Diarrhea, neutropenia, nausea |
| pentamidine, isothionate | PCP | Inhibitor of oxidative phosphorylation, nucleic acid, and protein synthesis | 4 mg/kg/day IV for 14-21 days | Rash, facial flushing, metallic taste, increased creatinine, hyponatremia |
| trimethoprim (TMP), sulfamethoxazole (SMX) (Bactrim, Septra) | PCP | Dihydrofolate reductase inhibitor | TMP: 15-20 mg/kg/day (in 4 divided doses) IV or PO for 14-21 days SMX: 75-100 mg/kg/day (in 4 divided doses) IV or PO for 14-21 days | Neutropenia, hepatotoxicity, nausea, vomiting, thrombocytopenia, fever, rash |

**T A B L E   11 - 5**   **Opportunistic Infections and Organisms Infecting Individuals with HIV Disease**

| Viral | Fungal | Protozoal | Bacterial |
|---|---|---|---|
| Herpes (I&II) | Candida | Pneumocystis carinii | Treponema pallidum (syphilis) |
| Cytomegalovirus | Histoplasma capsulatum | Toxoplasma gondii | Neisseria gonorrhoeae |
| Varicella | Cryptococcus | Entamoeba histolytica | Shigella |
| Epstein-Barr | Coccidioides | Giardia lamblia | Salmonella |
| Hepatitis A, B | | Cryptosporidium enteritisdis | Mycobacterium avium intracellulare (MAI) Mycobacterium tuber- culosis |
| Hepatitis non-A/ non-B | | | |

- Monitor sites of invasive procedures for signs of infection, including erythema, swelling, tenderness, and purulent exudate.
- Enforce good handwashing techniques before contact with patient to minimize the risk of transmitting infectious organisms from staff and other patients.
- Teach patient home-care considerations for infection prevention after hospital discharge (see "Patient-Family Teaching and Discharge Planning," p. 664).

**Impaired gas exchange** related to altered oxygen supply secondary to presence of pulmonary infiltrates, hyperventilation, and sepsis

***Desired outcomes:***   After treatment/intervention, patient has adequate gas exchange as evidenced by RR 12-20 breaths/min with normal depth and pattern (eupnea); and absence of adventitious sounds, nasal flaring, and other clinical indicators of respiratory dysfunction. By hospital discharge, patient's ABG results are as follows: $Pao_2$ $\geq$80 mm Hg; $Paco_2$ 35-45 mm Hg; pH 7.35-7.45.

- Assess patient's respiratory status q2h during patient's awake period, noting rate, rhythm, depth, and regularity of respirations. Observe for use of accessory muscles, flaring of nares, presence of adventitious sounds, cough, or cyanosis, which occur with respiratory dysfunction.
- Monitor ABG results closely for decreased $Paco_2$ (<35 mm Hg) and increased pH (>7.40), which can occur with hyperventilation.
- Adjust oxygen therapy to attain optimal oxygenation, as determined by ABG values.
- Instruct patient to report changes in cough, as well as dyspnea that increases with exertion.
- To maintain adequate tidal volume, provide chest physiotherapy as prescribed; encourage use of incentive spirometry at frequent intervals.
- Reposition patient q2h to help prevent stasis of lung fluids.
- Obtain sputum for culture and sensitivity as indicated.
- Group nursing activities to provide patient with uninterrupted periods of rest, optimally 90-120 min at a time.
- When administering sulfa for PCP, monitor closely for side effects such as rash or bone marrow suppression (leukopenia, neutropenia). If administering pentamidine, be alert to side effects such as hypotension or hypoglycemia, which necessitate frequent BP checks and finger sticks for blood sugar levels.

- To relieve mucous membrane irritation, which can predispose patient to coughing spells, deliver humidified oxygen to patient.
- Administer sedatives and analgesics judiciously to help prevent or minimize respiratory depression.

---

**Caution:** Wear a high-efficiency mask, and protect mucous membranes when caring for patients diagnosed as having active tuberculosis. See p. 24 for more information.

---

**Altered nutrition:** Less than body requirements related to diarrhea and nausea associated with side effects of medications, malabsorption, anorexia, dysphagia, and fatigue

*Desired outcome:* By hospital discharge, patient has adequate nutrition as evidenced by stable weight, serum albumin 3.5-5.5 g/dl, transferrin 180-260 mg/dl, thyroxine-binding prealbumin 20-30 mg/dl, retinol-binding protein 4-5 mg/dl, and a state of nitrogen (N) balance or a positive N state.

- Assess nutritional status daily, noting weight, caloric intake, and protein and albumin values. Be alert to progressive weight loss, wasting of muscle tissue, loss of skin tone, and decreases in both total protein and albumin, which can adversely affect wound healing and impair the patient's ability to withstand infection.
- Provide small, frequent, high-caloric, high-protein meals, allowing sufficient time for patient to eat. Offer supplements between feedings. As a rule, these patients are kept in a slightly positive N state (after resolution of the critical phases of this illness) by ensuring daily caloric intake equal to 50 kcal/kg of ideal body weight with an additional 1.5 g of protein/kg (e.g., a man weighing 70 kg should receive 3,500 kcal plus 105 g of protein per day).
- Provide supplemental vitamins and minerals as prescribed, to replace deficiencies.
- To minimize anorexia and help treat stomatitis, which can occur as a side effect of chemotherapy, provide oral hygiene before and after meals.
- If patient feels isolated socially, encourage significant others to visit at mealtimes and bring in patient's favorite high-caloric, high-protein foods from home.
- If patient is nauseated, provide instructions for deep breathing and voluntary swallowing, which helps decrease stimulation of vomiting center. Administer antiemetics as prescribed.
- If patient is dysphagic, encourage intake of fluids that are high in calories and protein; provide different flavors and textures for variation.
- As prescribed, deliver isotonic tube feeding for patients unable to eat. Isotonic fluids will help prevent diarrhea associated with hypertonic or hypotonic fluids. Check placement of gastric tube before each feeding; assess absorption by evaluating amount of residual feeding q4h. Do not deliver feeding if residual is >50-100 ml. Keep HOB elevated 30 degrees while feeding, and position patient in a right side-lying position to facilitate gastric emptying.
- If patient's caloric intake is insufficient, discuss the potential need for TPN with physician.

**Diarrhea** related to gastrointestinal (GI) infection, chemotherapy, or tube feeding intolerance

*Desired outcome:* By the time of hospital discharge, patient has formed stools and a bowel elimination pattern that is normal for him or her.

- Ensure minimal use of antidiarrheal medications, which promote intestinal concentration of infectious organisms.
- Teach patient to avoid large amounts (>300 mg/day) of caffeine, which increases peristalsis and can promote diarrhea.
- Maintain accurate I&O records to monitor for changes in fluid volume sta-

tus. Be alert to signs of hypovolemia, such as cool and clammy skin, increased HR (>100 bpm), increased RR (>20 breaths/min), and decreased urinary output (<30 ml/h).

- Assess stool for the presence of blood, fat, and undigested materials.
- Monitor stool cultures for evidence of new infectious organisms.
- Monitor patient for indicators of electrolyte imbalance, such as anxiety, confusion, muscle weakness, cramps, dysrhythmias, weak pulse, and decreased BP.
- If patient is on tube feedings, dilute strength or decrease rate of infusion to prevent "solute drag," which may be the cause of the diarrhea.
- Encourage foods high in potassium (K) (Table 3-4, p. 132) and sodium (Na) (Table 3-2, p. 115) to replace any decrements of these ions.
- Protect anorectal area by keeping it cleansed and using compounds such as zinc oxide to prevent or retard skin excoriation.

**Impaired tissue intregity (or risk of same)** related to cachexia and malnourishment, diarrhea, side effects of chemotherapy, KS lesions, negative N state, and decreased mobility due to arthralgia and fatigue

*Desired outcome:* At hospital discharge patient's tissue is intact.

- Assess and document skin integrity, noting temperature, moisture, color, vascularity, texture, lesions, and areas of excoriation or poor wound healing. Evaluate KS lesions for location, dissemination, weeping, or significant changes. Note and record the presence of herpes lesions, especially those that are perirectal.
- Avoid prolonged pressure on dependent body parts by turning and positioning patient q2h; encourage patient to change position at frequent intervals.
- Provide patient with a pressure relief mattress, as indicated.
- Teach patient to use mild, hypoallergenic, nondrying soaps or lanolin-based products for bathing, and to pat rather than rub the skin to dry it. When appropriate, use lotions and emollients to soften and relieve itching of dry, flaky skin.
- Use soft sheets on the bed, avoiding wrinkles. If patient is incontinent, use some type of rectal device (e.g., fecal incontinence bags, rectal tube) to protect the skin and prevent perirectal excoriation and skin breakdown.
- To enhance skin and tissue healing, assist patient toward a state of N balance by promoting adequate amounts of protein and carbohydrates (see discussion with **Altered nutrition,** p. 660).
- Ensure that patient receives minimum daily requirements of vitamins and minerals; supplement them as necessary.
- Encourage ROM and weight-bearing mobility, when possible, to increase circulation to skin and tissue.

**Pain** related to physical and chemical factors associated with prolonged immobility, side effects of chemotherapy, infections, peripheral neuropathy, and frequent venipunctures

*Desired outcomes:* Within 1 h of intervention, patient's subjective perception of pain decreases, as documented by a pain scale. Nonverbal indicators of discomfort, such as grimacing, are absent or diminished.

- Assess and record the following: location, onset, duration, and factors that precipitate and alleviate patient's pain. With patient, establish a pain scale, rating pain from 0 (no pain) to 10 (worst pain). Use the scale to evaluate degree of pain and to document the degree of relief achieved.
- Administer analgesia as prescribed.
- Provide heat or cold applications to affected areas (e.g., apply heat to painful joints, and cold packs to reduce swelling associated with infections or multiple venipunctures).
- Encourage patient to engage in diversional activities as a means of increasing pain tolerance and decreasing its intensity (e.g., soothing music, quiet conversation, reading, and slow rhythmic breathing).

- To reduce pain intensity, teach patient techniques that decrease skeletal muscle tension, such as deep breathing, biofeedback, and relaxation exercises (see **Health-seeking behaviors:** Relaxation technique effective for stress reduction, p. 54).
- If frequent venipunctures are the cause of the patient's discomfort, discuss with physician the desirability of a capped venous catheter for long-term blood withdrawal.
- Administer anticonvulsant agents as prescribed for relief of peripheral neuropathy.
- Promote relaxation and comfort with backrubs and massage.
- For other interventions, see **Pain** in Appendix One, p. 694.

**Activity intolerance** related to generalized weakness secondary to fluid and electrolyte imbalance, arthralgia, myalgia, dyspnea, fever, pain, hypoxia, and effects of chemotherapy

*Desired outcome:*   Before hospital discharge, patient rates perceived exertion at ≤3 on a 0-10 scale and exhibits tolerance to activity as evidenced by HR ≤20 bpm over resting HR, RR ≤20 breaths/min, and systolic BP ≤20 mm Hg over or under resting systolic BP.

- Assess patient's tolerance to activity by assessing HR, RR, and BP before and immediately after activity, and ask patient to rate his or her perceived exertion. See this nursing diagnosis in Appendix One, p. 711, for details.
- Plan adequate (90-120 min) rest periods between patient's scheduled activities. Adjust activities as appropriate to reduce energy expenditures.
- As much as possible, encourage regular periods of exercise to help prevent cardiac intolerance to activities, which can occur quickly after periods of prolonged inactivity.
- Monitor electrolyte levels to ensure that patient's muscle weakness is not caused by hypokalemia.
- Monitor ABG values to ensure that patient is oxygenated adequately; adjust oxygen delivery accordingly.
- Advise patient to keep anecdotal notes (perhaps in journal format) on exacerbation and remission of signs and symptoms.
- For more information, see this nursing diagnosis in Appendix One, "Caring for Patients on Prolonged Bed Rest," p. 711.

**Anxiety** related to threat of death and social isolation

*Desired outcome:*   Following intervention, patient expresses feelings and is free of harmful anxiety as evidenced by HR ≤100 bpm, RR ≤20 breaths/min with normal depth and pattern (eupnea), and BP within patient's normal range.

- Monitor patient for verbal or nonverbal expressions of the following: inability to cope, apprehension, guilt for past actions, uncertainty, concerns about rejection and isolation, and suicide ideation.
- Spend time with patient and encourage expression of feelings and concerns.
- Support effective coping patterns (e.g., by allowing patient to cry or talk rather than denying his or her legitimate fears and concerns).
- Provide accurate information about HIV disease and related diagnostic procedures.
- If patient hyperventilates, teach him or her to mimic your normal respiratory pattern (eupnea).

**Body image disturbance** related to biophysical changes secondary to KS lesions, chemotherapy, and emaciation

*Desired outcome:*   Before hospital discharge, patient expresses positive feelings about self to family, significant others, and primary nurse.

- Encourage patient to express feelings, especially the way he or she views or feels about self.
- Provide patient with positive feedback; help patient focus on facts rather than myths or exaggerations about self.

- Provide patient with access to clergy, psychiatric nurse, social worker, psychologist, or HIV counselor as appropriate.
- Encourage patient to join and share feelings with HIV support group.
- For additional information, see this nursing diagnosis in Appendix One, p. 760.

**Knowledge deficit:** Disease process, prognosis, life-style changes, and treatment plan

*Desired outcome:* Before hospital discharge, patient verbalizes accurate information about the disease process, prognosis, behaviors that increase the risk of transmitting the virus to others, and treatment plan.

- Assess patient's knowledge about HIV disease, including pathophysiologic changes that will occur, ways the disease is transmitted, necessary behavioral changes, and side effects of treatment. Correct misinformation and misconceptions as necessary.
- Inform patient of private and community agencies that are available to help with such tasks as handling legal affairs, cooking, housecleaning, and nursing care. Provide telephone numbers and addresses for HIV support groups and self-help groups.
- Provide literature that explores the myths and realities of the HIV disease process.
- Teach patient the importance of informing sexual partners of HIV condition and modifying high-risk behaviors known to transmit the virus (see Table 11-3).
- Involve significant others in the teaching and learning process.
- Provide patient and significant others with the names and addresses or phone numbers of HIV resources (see "Patient-Family Teaching and Discharge Planning," below).

**Social isolation** related to altered state of wellness, societal rejection, loss of support system, feelings of guilt and punishment, fatigue, and changed patterns of sexual expression

*Desired outcome:* Before hospital discharge, patient communicates and interacts with others.

- Keep patient and significant others well informed about patient's status and treatment plan.
- Provide private periods of time for patient to communicate and interact with significant others.
- Encourage significant others to share in the care of the patient.
- Encourage physical closeness between patient and significant others. Provide privacy, as much as possible.
- Involve patient in unit or group activities as appropriate.
- Explain significance of isolation precautions to patient.

**Altered thought processes (or risk of same)** related to physiologic changes and impaired judgment secondary to infection, space-occupying lesion in the central nervous system (CNS), or HIV dementia

*Desired outcomes:* Following intervention, patient verbalizes orientation to person, place, and time. Optimally, by hospital discharge patient correctly completes exercises in logical reasoning, memory, perception, concentration, attention, and sequencing of activities.

- Assess patient for minor alterations in personality traits that cannot be attributed to other causes such as stress or medication.
- Assess patient for signs of dementia, which would include a slowing of all cognitive functioning, with problems in attention, concentration, memory, perception, logical reasoning, and sequencing of activities.
- Encourage patient to report persistent headaches, dizziness, or seizures, which may signal CNS involvement.
- Note any cranial nerve involvement that differs from patient's past medical history. Most commonly the fifth (trigeminal), seventh (facial), and eighth

(acoustic) nerves are involved in infectious processes of the CNS.
- Assess patient for signs of mental aberration, blindness, aphasia, hemiparesis, or ataxia, which may signal the presence of a demyelinating disease.
- Divide activities into small, easily accomplished tasks.
- Maintain a stable environment so patient is able to familiarize self with the immediate surroundings (i.e., do not change the location of furniture in room).
- Write notes as reminders; maintain a calendar of appointments.
- Provide some mechanism (e.g., pill boxes) to ensure that patient takes medications as prescribed.
- Teach patient the importance of reporting changes in neurologic status (e.g., increasing severity of headaches, blurred vision, gait disturbances, or blackouts). Notify physician of all significant findings.

---

For other nursing diagnoses and interventions, see "Providing Nutritional Support," p. 673; "Managing Wound Care," p. 682; "Caring for Patients on Prolonged Bed Rest," p. 693; and "Caring for Patients with Cancer and Other Life-Disrupting Illnesses," p. 719.

---

## PATIENT-FAMILY TEACHING AND DISCHARGE PLANNING
Give patient and significant others verbal and written instructions about the following:
- Importance of avoiding use of recreational drugs, which are believed to potentiate the immunosuppressive process and lower resistance to infection.
- Significance and importance of refraining from donating blood.
- Necessity of modifying high-risk sexual behaviors. See Table 11-3 for specific information.
- Principles and importance of maintaining a balanced diet; ways to supplement diet with multivitamins and other food sources such as high-caloric substances (e.g., Isocal and Ensure). Because of increased susceptibility to foodborne opportunistic organisms, fruit and vegetables should be washed thoroughly; meats should be cooked thoroughly at appropriate temperatures; and raw eggs, raw fish (sushi), and unpasteurized milk should be avoided.
- Because of decreased resistance to infection, the importance of limiting contact with individuals known to have active infections. In addition, pets may harbor various fungal, protozoal, and bacterial organisms in their excrement. Therefore, contact with bird cages, cat litter, and tropical fish tanks should be avoided.
- Necessity for meticulous hygiene to prevent spread of any extant or new infectious organisms. To avoid exposure to fungi, damp areas in bathrooms (e.g., shower) should be cleaned with solutions of bleach; refrigerators should be cleaned thoroughly with soap and water; and left-over foodstuffs should be disposed of within 2-3 days.
- Techniques for self-assessment of early signs of infection (e.g., erythema, tenderness, swelling, purulent exudate) in all cuts, abrasions, lesions, or open wounds.
- Care of venous access device, including technique for self-administration of TPN or medications (see Appendix One, "Caring for Patients with Cancer and Life-Disrupting Illnesses," p. 734); care of gastric tube and administration of enteral tube feedings, if appropriate.
- Importance of avoiding fatigue by limiting participation in social activities, getting maximum amounts of rest, and minimizing physical exertion.
- Prescribed medications, including name, dosage, purpose, and potential side effects.
- Importance of maintaining medical follow-up appointments.

- Advisability of keeping anecdotal notes (perhaps in journal format) on exacerbation and remission of signs and symptoms.
- Importance of reporting changes in neurologic status (e.g., increasing severity of headaches, blurred vision, gait disturbances, or blackouts).
- Advisability of sharing feelings with significant others or within a support group.
- In addition, provide the following information regarding HIV resources:
  - Public Health Service AIDS Hotline: (800) 342-AIDS (800) 342-2437.
  - AZT Information Hotline: (800) 843-9388.
  - Local Red Cross, or American Red Cross AIDS Education Office, 1730 D Street, N.W., Washington, DC 20006; (202) 737-8300.
  - Centers for Disease Control AIDS Activity, Building 6, Room 292, 1600 Clifton Road, Atlanta, GA 30333; (404) 329-3479.
  - National Gay Task Force AIDS Information Hotline: (800) 221-7044.
  - National Sexually Transmitted Diseases Hotline/American Social Health Association: (800) 227-8922.
  - National AIDS Network, 729 Eighth Street, S.E., Suite 300, Washington, DC 20003; (202) 546-2424.

# Section Two:   Providing Nutritional Support

Hospitalized patients are at high risk for the nutritional disorders kwashiorkor and marasmus. Kwashiorkor, a severe protein deficiency, is characterized by low serum albumin concentration, muscle wasting, and water retention. This situation may be seen in surgical patients who are maintained on IV dextrose/electrolyte solutions alone for extended periods and whose recovery is complicated by sepsis. Marasmus occurs more commonly in medical patients who receive inadequate amounts of protein and calories over a prolonged period, resulting in depletion of lean body mass and subcutaneous fat stores.

## Nutritional assessment

Because no single sensitive and comprehensive nutritional assessment factor exists, a variety of factors need to be evaluated in a nutritional assessment. The need for nutritional support is based on the following components in addition to patient history and the history and duration of the disease process.

### DIETARY HISTORY

A dietary history is compiled to reveal the adequacy of usual and recent food intake. Be alert to excesses or deficiencies of nutrients and any special eating patterns (e.g., various types of vegetarian or prescribed diets), use of fad diets, and excessive supplementation. Note anything that impairs adequate selection, preparation, ingestion, digestion, absorption, and excretion of nutrients. Include the following:

- Comprehensive review of usual dietary intake, including food allergies, food aversions, and use of nutritional supplements.
- Recent unplanned weight loss or gain.
- Chewing or swallowing difficulties.
- Nausea, vomiting, or pain with eating.
- Altered pattern of elimination (e.g., constipation or diarrhea).
- Chronic disease affecting utilization of nutrients (e.g., malabsorption, pancreatitis, diabetes mellitus).
- Surgical resection; disease of the gut or accessory organs of digestion (i.e., pancreas, liver, gallbladder).

- Use of alcohol or drugs. Chronic use of drugs may affect appetite, digestion, utilization, or excretion of nutrients.

## PHYSICAL ASSESSMENT

Compare current assessment findings to past assessments, especially related to the following:
- Loss of muscle and adipose tissue.
- Work and muscle endurance.
- Changes in hair, skin, or neuromuscular function.

## ANTHROPOMETRIC DATA

Anthropometrics is the science of measuring the body or its parts. It is helpful to remember that 1 L of fluid equals approximately 2 lb. To convert lb and in to metric measurements, use the following formulas:

Divide lb by 2.2 to convert to kg.

Divide in by 39.37 to convert to meters.

**Height:**   Used to determine ideal weight and body mass index (BMI). If patient's height is impossible to measure, obtain estimate from family or significant others or compare patient's recumbent length with known length of the mattress.

**Weight:**   A readily available and practical indicator of nutritional status that can be compared to previous weight and ideal weight or used to calculate BMI. Changes may reflect fluid shifts (edema, diuresis, third spacing), surgical resections, traumatic amputations, or weight of dressings or equipment. See Table 11-6.

**Body mass index:**   Used to evaluate the weight of adults. One calculation and one set of standards are applicable to both men and women.

$$\text{BMI (kg/m}^2) = \frac{\text{Weight (kg)}}{\text{Height (meters)}^2}$$

BMI values of 20-25 are optimum; values >25 indicate obesity; and values <20 indicate underweight status.

**Arm circumference and triceps skin fold thickness:**   Because of the variation among novice evaluators, it is difficult to identify accurate changes in these measurements; hence they are inaccurate as a basis for diagnosing malnutrition.

## BIOCHEMICAL DATA

**Protein status:**   Evaluated *via* the following tests, with normal values in parentheses: serum albumin (3.5 g/dl), transferrin (180-260 mg/dl), thyroxine-binding prealbumin (20-30 mg/dl), and retinol-binding protein (4-5 mg/dl). Normal values may vary somewhat with different laboratory procedures and standards. Albumin and transferrin have relatively long half-lives of 19 and 9 days, respectively, whereas thyroxine-binding prealbumin and retinol-binding protein have very short half-lives of 24-48 h and 10 h, respectively. If hydration status is normal and anemia is absent, albumin and transferrin levels can be used as baseline indicators of adequacy of protein intake and synthesis. For evidence of response to nutritional therapy, values for the short turnover proteins—thryoxine-binding prealbumin (although very expensive) and retinol-binding protein—are the most useful.

**Nitrogen balance:**   The state of equilibrium that exists when the intake and excretion of nitrogen (N) are equal. If more is taken in than excreted, N is said to be positive and an anabolic state exists. If more N is excreted than taken in, N balance is said to be negative and a catabolic state exists. Most N loss occurs through the urine, with a small, constant amount lost *via* skin and feces.

N balance studies should be performed by specialists because accurate measurement of 24-h food intake and urine output is required.

**TABLE 11-6  Height and Weight Guidelines for Men and Women**

| Height | Men | | | Women | | |
|---|---|---|---|---|---|---|
| | Small frame (lb) | Medium frame (lb) | Large frame (lb) | Small frame (lb) | Medium frame (lb) | Large frame (lb) |
| 4 ft 10 in | — | — | — | 102-111 | 109-121 | 118-131 |
| 4 ft 11 in | — | — | — | 103-113 | 111-123 | 120-134 |
| 5 ft | — | — | — | 104-115 | 113-126 | 122-137 |
| 5 ft 1 in | — | — | — | 106-118 | 115-129 | 125-140 |
| 5 ft 2 in | 128-134 | 131-141 | 138-150 | 108-121 | 118-132 | 128-143 |
| 5 ft 3 in | 130-136 | 133-143 | 140-153 | 111-124 | 121-135 | 131-147 |
| 5 ft 4 in | 132-138 | 135-145 | 142-156 | 114-127 | 124-138 | 134-151 |
| 5 ft 5 in | 134-140 | 137-148 | 144-160 | 117-130 | 127-141 | 137-155 |
| 5 ft 6 in | 136-142 | 139-151 | 146-164 | 120-133 | 130-144 | 140-159 |
| 5 ft 7 in | 138-146 | 142-154 | 148-168 | 123-136 | 133-147 | 143-163 |
| 5 ft 8 in | 140-148 | 145-157 | 152-172 | 126-139 | 136-150 | 146-167 |
| 5 ft 9 in | 142-151 | 148-160 | 156-176 | 129-142 | 139-153 | 149-170 |
| 5 ft 10 in | 144-154 | 151-163 | 158-180 | 132-145 | 142-156 | 152-173 |
| 5 ft 11 in | 146-157 | 154-166 | 161-184 | 135-148 | 145-159 | 155-176 |
| 6 ft | 149-160 | 157-170 | 164-188 | 138-151 | 148-162 | 158-179 |
| 6 ft 1 in | 152-164 | 160-174 | 168-192 | — | — | — |
| 6 ft 2 in | 155-168 | 164-178 | 172-197 | — | — | — |
| 6 ft 3 in | 158-172 | 167-182 | 176-202 | — | — | — |
| 6 ft 4 in | 162-176 | 171-187 | 181-207 | — | — | — |

Data courtesy of Metropolitan Life Insurance Company, 1983. Ages 25 through 59 include 5 lb indoor clothing for men and 3 lb of indoor clothing for women and 1-in heels for both.

## ESTIMATING NUTRITIONAL REQUIREMENTS

The primary goal of nutritional support is to meet the needs for body temperature, metabolic processes, and tissue repair. Having collected all the data, energy needs now can be estimated using the following options:

**Indirect calorimetry:**    Performed using a bedside metabolic cart. Specialized personnel are required to provide accurate results. Carts are an expense most floors cannot justify.

**Harris and Benedict equations:**    To determine basal energy expenditure (BEE). BEE can be calculated using the following equations developed by Harris and Benedict:

$$BEE\ (male) = 66.5 + (13.8 \times W) + (5 \times H) - (6.8 \times A)$$

$$BEE\ (female) = 655.1 + (9.6 \times W) + (1.9 \times H) - (4.7 \times A)$$

- where W = weight in kg; H = height in cm; A = age in years.

BEE is then multiplied by the appropriate correction factors to allow for the patient's activity level and condition:

*Activity factor =*
1.2 for bedridden patient
1.3 for ambulatory patient
*Injury factor =*
1.2 for minor surgery
1.35 for trauma (blunt or skeletal)
1.6 for sepsis

- BEE × activity factor × injury factor = total energy expenditure (TEE).

**Distribution of calories:**    Percentages of total calories from carbohydrates, protein, and fat should equal approximately 50%, 15%, and 35% respectively.

*Protein requirements:*    Usually 1-1.5 g protein/kg/day.

*Carbohydrate requirements:*    Glucose administration of 5 mg/kg/min is a suitable amount in critical care. Carbohydrates provided in excess of this amount are not well utilized and may lead to hyperglycemia, excessive $CO_2$ production, hypophosphatemia, and fluid overload.

*Fat requirements:*    If protein and glucose are supplied as outlined, the remainder of needed calories can be supplied as fat. Fat can be administered in minimal quantities to satisfy needs for essential fatty acids, or it can be provided in larger quantities, as tolerated, to meet energy needs. Abnormal liver function often occurs in patients maintained on total parenteral nutrition (TPN) longer than 3 weeks. Usually the enzymes return to normal upon cessation of TPN. Giving cyclic TPN, in which the patient receives TPN for 12-16 h out of 24 h, sometimes helps.

**Special diets for organ-specific pathology:**    These are costly, and the metabolic advantages of some products remain unproven.

*Hepatic failure:*    Branched-chain amino acids in combination with reduced aromatic amino acid concentrations are used to alleviate encephalopathy secondary to hepatic failure.

*Renal disease:*    High percentages of essential amino acids are used to improve N use and decrease urea formation.

*Respiratory disease:*    A low-protein and low-carbohydrate diet decreases $CO_2$ production and consequently the WOB.

**Vitamin and essential trace mineral requirements:**    In general, follow the recommended daily allowances (RDA) to provide minimum quantities of vitamins, minerals, and essential fatty acids. For specific patients, supplement specific vitamins or minerals needed in increased amounts for existing disease states (e.g., zinc and vitamins A and C for burns; thiamine, folate, and $B_{12}$ for chronic alcohol ingestion).

**Fluid requirements:**    Many factors affect fluid balance. Under usual circumstances an estimate of fluid needs can be made by providing 1 ml of free water for each calorie provided, or 30-50 ml/kg body weight. The daily loss of water includes approximately 1,400 ml in urine (60 ml/h), 350 ml *via* respiration, 350 ml as evaporative losses through skin, 100 ml in sweat, and about 200 ml in feces. If loss by any of these routes is increased, fluid needs will increase; if loss by any of these routes is impaired, fluid restriction may be necessary. All sources of intake (oral, enteral, intravenous, and medications) as well as output (urine, stool, drainage, emesis, fluid shifts, and respiratory and evaporative losses) must be considered. **Note:** Urine output may be as high as 2-3 L under normal conditions. This represents a range of 80-125 ml/h.

# Nutritional support modalities

Specialized nutritional support refers to the provision of a special formula *via* the enteral or parenteral route for the treatment or prevention of malnutrition. Enteral nutrition is preferred over parenteral nutrition because it resembles normal functioning more closely, has fewer side effects, and is less costly.

## ENTERAL PRODUCTS

Enteral products are composed of standard and modular formulas and can be used for oral and/or tube feeding. Also see Table 11-7.

**Formula types**

*Standard:* *Blended whole food diets,* which are less costly but have problems that include possible bacterial growth, solids that settle out, variation in nutrient composition, and the necessity of a large-bore tube for the viscous formula; and *commercial formulas,* which are sterile, homogenous, suitable for small-bore feeding tubes, and have a fixed nutrient composition.

*Modular:* Consist of a single nutrient that may be combined with other modules (nutrients) to form a package tailor-made for an individual's specific deficits (e.g., carbohydrate, fat, protein, and vitamin modules).

**Nutritional composition**

*Carbohydrates:* The most easily digested and absorbed component in enteral formulas; 80% of all carbohydrates is broken down and absorbed as simple glucose in the normal intestine.

—*Lactase deficiency:* Lack of this enzyme, which aids in digestion of lactose, is most commonly found in blacks, Asians, native Americans, and Jews. A secondary form also may be found in individuals for whom large amounts of lactose are given in a milk-based diet. Symptoms include watery diarrhea, abdominal cramps, flatulence, fullness, nausea, stool with a pH of <6, and stool that tests positive for glucose.

*Fiber:* Included in many commercial preparations now because it is helpful in the control of bowel disorders such as diverticula, decreases hyperlipidemia, and controls blood glucose. These preparations are highly viscous, and use of a large-bore feeding tube (10 F) or an infusion pump is helpful. Begin the infusion slowly to reduce transient symptoms of gas and abdominal distention.

*Protein:* Three forms commonly are used.

—*Polymeric:* Protein found in complete and original form (e.g., blenderized whole food diets that require normal levels of pancreatic enzyme).

—*Hydrolyzed:* Protein that has broken down into smaller forms to assist absorption. It is helpful in short bowel syndrome or pancreatic insufficiency.

—*Elemental:* Protein that requires no further digestion and is ready for absorption. It is most helpful in hepatic and renal disorders.

*Fat:* Two forms are the primary sources.

—*Long-chain triglycerides (LCTs):* A major source of essential fatty acids, fat soluble vitamins, and calories.

**T A B L E  11 - 7  Types of Enteral Formulations**

| Enteral formula | Description |
|---|---|
| *Blenderized diet* | |
| Compleat, Compleat Modified, Vitaneed | Nutritionally complete, requiring complete digestive capabilities; composed of natural foods including meat, vegetables, milk, and fruit |
| *Milk-based formula* | |
| Meritene, Sustagen, Carnation Instant (if mixed with milk) | Nutritionally adequate diet for general nutritional support |
| *Lactose-free formula* | |
| Ensure, Entrition 1, Isocal, Osmolite | Nutritionally adequate, liquid preparation; used for general nutritional support; iso- or hypo-osmolar; all except Osmolite are low residue |
| *Elemental or chemically defined* | Nutrients tailored for specific needs. |
| Criticare | Low-Na, lactose-free, high-N diet; 40% protein supplied as small peptides; nutritionally adequate; used for general nutritional support |
| Travasorb HN | Nutritionally adequate; used for general nutritional support; contains additional hydrolyzed protein that is readily digested and absorbed |
| *Speciality formulas* *Hepatic failure* | |
| Hepatic Travasorb | Nutritionally complete, with a greater ratio of branched chain to aromatic amino acids while restricting total amino acid concentrations and adding nonprotein calories |

Modified from Webber KS. Providing nutritional support. In Horne MM, Swearingen PL: *Pocket guide to fluid, electrolyte, and acid-base balance,* ed 2, St Louis, 1993, Mosby–Year Book, Inc.

 —*Medium-chain triglycerides (MCTs):* Foster the absorption of both types of fat but have fewer side effects of nausea and vomiting, abdominal distention, and diarrhea.
**Types of feeding tubes:** Also see Tables 11-8 and 11-9.
*Soft small-bore feeding tube:* Polyurethane or silicone with tunsten tip; size 6-12 Fr; length 36-45 in. Trade names are Keofeed, Dobhoff.
*Rigid tubes or tubes with rigid guides:* Inner silicone tube may be contained within a stiff outer tube that is removed leaving inner soft tube in place. An advantage is the ease of placement.
*Large-bore stiff tube:* Rubber or polyvinyl chloride; size 10-18 Fr; used for gastric decompression. It can be used for short-term feeding of highly viscous fluids. Trade names are Levine, Salem.
*Gastric feeding tube:* Tube that is placed through the naris (nasogastric [NG]) or mouth (orogastric) into the stomach for feeding purposes.
*Nasointestinal feeding tube:* Tube that is placed through the naris into the intestine for feeding purposes.
*Gastrostomy tube:* Inserted directly into the stomach either temporarily or

## T A B L E  11 - 7    Types of Enteral Formulations—cont'd

| Enteral formula | Description |
|---|---|
| *Speciality formulas—cont'd* | |
| Hepatic-Aid II | Nutritionally incomplete powder diet with essential nutrients in easily digestible form; high in branched chain amino acids; low in aromatic amino acids and methionines |
| *Renal failure* | |
| Renal Travasorb | Electrolyte, lactose, fat-soluble vitamin-free; high in calories; contains mostly essential amino acids; restricted total protein content may reduce or postpone the need for dialysis |
| Amin-Aid | Nutritionally incomplete supplement with essential nutrients in readily digestible form with minimal electrolytes |
| *Respiratory insufficiency* | |
| Palmature | Nutritionally complete; contains a higher proportion of fat to carbohydrates; reduces $CO_2$ production |
| *Hypermetabolic and trauma states* | |
| Trauma-Aid HB | High in branched chain amino acids; readily digestible essential nutrients |
| Trauma Cal | Nutritionally adequate with high proportions of protein and calories in a limited volume |
| *Modular formulas* | Offer highly flexible tailoring of nutrients (e.g., fat [Lipomul], protein [Pro Mod], and carbohydrates [Moducal]) for specific patient needs |

permanently for feeding purposes. A *gastrostomy button* has been shown to decrease many of the disadvantages of gastrostomy tubes, such as site problems, leakage, mobility, and catheter occlusion and expulsion.

*Jejunostomy tube:*   A soft tube inserted into the jejunum that is not easily dislodged, requires continuous feeding (thus is not convenient for the home-care patient), and can be worn under clothes. Needle catheter jejunostomy is an alternative method of nutrient delivery.

*Percutaneous endoscopic gastrostomy (PEG) tube:*   Soft tube inserted into the stomach *via* the esophagus and then drawn through the abdominal skin using a stab incision.

**Selection of feeding sites**

*Stomach:*   Easiest for tube placement, simulates normal GI function, may be used for intermittent or continuous feedings, and best reserved for patients who are alert with intact gag and cough reflexes.

*Small bowel:*   Involves more difficult tube placement, often needs elemental formula for easier absorption, continuous feedings tolerated better, and has less risk of aspiration for patients with diminished protective pharyngeal reflexes.

**Infusion rates:**   See Table 11-8.

**Management of complications:**   See Tables 11-10 and 11-13.

**T A B L E  11 - 8** **Methods and Typical Rates of Administration for Enteral Products**

| Type | Typical rate of administration | Comments |
|------|-------------------------------|----------|
| Bolus | 250-400 ml 4-6×/day | May cause cramping, bloating, nausea, diarrhea, aspiration; not recommended |
| Intermittent | 120 ml isotonic formula with 30-50 ml $H_2O$ flush over 30-60 min | Starting regimen |
| | *Advancement:* Increase formula q8-12h by 60 ml if residual <½ volume of previous feeding | Should not exceed 30 ml/min; may cause cramping, nausea, bloating, diarrhea, aspiration |
| Continuous | 40-50 ml/hr full-strength isotonic formula | Starting regimen |
| | *Advancement:* If serum albumin levels <2.5 g/dl, or initial loose stools, dilute formula to 150 mOsm | Allows more time for absorption of nutrients |

Modified from Roberts PM, Webber KS, "Providing Nutritional Support." In Swearingen PL, Keen JH: Manual of Critical Care: Applying Nursing Diagnoses to Adult Critical Disorders, ed 2, St Louis, Mosby-Yearbook, 1991.

**T A B L E  11 - 9** **Nursing Implications for Use of Gastric Tubes**

| Size | Nursing implications |
|------|---------------------|
| Small-bore | Ensure that x-ray confirms placement. Auscultation not a reliable method of determining placement; aspiration of stomach contents through tube often causes tube walls to collapse |
| | Tubes are easily dislocated upward in GI tract, but there may be no external signs, and tube still may be taped in position |
| | Use elemental formula for lower viscosity |
| | Flush after each feeding/medication administration with 50-150 ml water |
| | Use manufacturer's recommended suggestions regarding syringe size when irrigating tube |
| Large-bore | Use smallest bore tube possible to minimize chance of ulceration, pharyngitis, and fistula formation |
| | Aspirate stomach contents, and check pH of returns to ensure correct stomach placement. Stomach contents have a pH <7 (acidic) |
| | When taping tube, ensure that no traction is applied to patient's skin |
| | Flush after each feeding/medication with 50-150 ml water |

Modified from Roberts PM, Webber KS, "Providing Nutritional Support." In Swearingen PL, Keen JH: Manual of Critical Care: Applying Nursing Diagnoses to Adult Critical Disorders, ed 2, St Louis, Mosby-Yearbook, 1991.

## PARENTERAL NUTRITION

Parenteral nutrition (PN) provides some or all nutrients by peripheral venous catheter (PVC) or central venous catheter (CVC) to supplement limited oral intake and thus completely meet nutritional needs in patients who cannot be fed *via* the GI tract. While PN usually is considered more effective than enteral nutrition, it also is more expensive and has more complications.

**Parenteral solutions**

*Carbohydrates:*  Dextrose solutions 5%-50% are used to help meet the patient's energy needs. When hypertonic solutions are infused, both insulin demand and $CO_2$ and $O_2$ consumption are increased, which may lead to respiratory distress and hypermetabolism.

*Protein:*  Synthetic crystalline essential and nonessential amino acid formulations are available in concentrations of 3%-10%. Special amino acid formulations for specific disorders are available (see "Estimating Nutritional Requirements," above).

*Fat:*  Lipid 10%-20% is an isotonic solution providing essential fatty acids and a source of concentrated calories. For best use and tolerance, lipids should be infused with carbohydrates and protein over no fewer than 8 h. This is especially useful for patients at home. The most common symptoms of an adverse reaction include febrile response, chills and shivering, and pain in the chest and back. A second type of adverse reaction occurs with prolonged use of IV fat emulsions and may result in transient increase in liver enzymes, kernicterus, eosinophilia, and thrombophlebitis. To prevent sepsis, hang fat emulsions ≤12 h. Keep the infusion rate 1 ml/min for the first 15-30 min and then increase it to 80-100 ml/h for the remainder of the first infusion.

*Total nutrient admixtures (TNA):*  Recent processing technique in which dextrose, fat, and amino acids are combined in one container. Because it would trap lipid molecules, an in-line filter cannot be used.

**Selection of feeding site**

*CVC:*  Necessary for infusion of hypertonic solutions delivered through a large-diameter vein, usually the superior vena cava *via* the subclavian or jugular vein. The volume of blood flow rapidly dilutes the hypertonic solutions and decreases the irritation of vein walls. However, there are more complications with CVC than with the peripheral route.

*PVC:*  The final osmolality of the solution (<800 mOsm/L) limits the types of infusions that can be used. Solutions are delivered *via* a peripheral vein, usually of the hand or forearm. They are reserved for individuals with a need for nutritional support for short time periods, with small nutritional requirements, and for whom CVC access is unavailable.

**Types of catheters:**  See Table 11-11.

**Monitoring infusion rates:**  Using an infusion pump, PN is given at a consistent rate, with gradual acceleration of the infusion rate over a 3-day period to avoid wide fluctuations in blood glucose. A typical rate is 50-100 ml/h, which increases 25-50 ml/h/day, depending on patient status.

**Managing complications:**  See Tables 11-12 and 11-13.

## TRANSITIONAL FEEDING

A period of adjustment is needed before discontinuing nutritional support. Taper nutritional supplements for patients receiving enteral nutrition as oral intake increases. Similarly, patients receiving PN may have some mucosal atrophy of the bowel and will need a period of adjustment before the bowel can fully resume its usual functions of digestion and absorption.

## NURSING DIAGNOSES AND INTERVENTIONS

**Altered nutrition:**  Less than body requirements, related to inability to ingest, digest, or absorb nutrients

*Desired outcome:*  Patient has adequate nutrition as evidenced by stabilization of weight at desired level or steady weight gain of ¼ to ½ lb/day;

**T A B L E  11 - 10**    **Management of Complications in the Tube-Fed Patient**

| Complication/possible causes | Suggested management strategy |
|---|---|
| ***Diarrhea*** | |
| Bolus feeding | Try intermittent or continuous method |
| Infusion rate | Decrease rate of delivery |
| Lactose intolerance | As prescribed, switch to lactose-free products |
| Fat intolerance | Reduce fat intake during acute illness |
| Osmolality intolerance | Dilute feeding or use product with lower osmolality, as prescribed |
| Low-fiber content | Try bulk-forming agents or fiber preparations |
| Medications | Monitor use of antibiotics, antacids, cimetidine, potassium chloride, and aminophylline and the use of sorbitol in liquid medication. As prescribed, administer *Lactobacillus acidophilus* to restore GI flora, or use tincture of opium, as prescribed, to decrease GI motility. Monitor occurrence of superinfections |
| Bacterial contamination | Discard feedings hanging for >8 h. Use clean technique; change equipment q24h; refrigerate all opened products and discard after 24 h |
| Low serum albumin | Monitor serum albumin levels; low levels contribute to intestinal malabsorption. Normal range is 3.5-5.5 g/dl |
| ***High gastric residual*** | |
| Decreased motility | Auscultate for bowel sounds; percuss abdomen for air |
| | Hold feeding for 1 h and check residual; repeat q1-2h until feeding can be resumed. After feeding, have patient lie in a right side-lying position with HOB elevated 30 degrees. As prescribed, administer metoclopramide to help prevent or treat nausea and vomiting caused by slow gastric emptying, or change to formula with decreased osmolality |
| ***Nausea and vomiting*** | |
| Fast rate | Decrease rate |
| Fat intolerance | Fat should compose no more than 30%-40% of total intake |
| Lactose intolerance | As prescribed, change to lactose-free product |
| Hyperosmolality | Dilute feeding |
| Delayed gastric emptying | See "High gastric residual," above |
| Product odor | Mask with flavoring |

Modified from Roberts PM, Webber KS, "Providing Nutritional Support." In Swearingen PL, Keen JH: Manual of Critical Care: Applying Nursing Diagnoses to Adult Critical Disorders, ed 2, St Louis, Mosby-Yearbook, 1991.

**T A B L E  11 - 10    Management of Complications in the Tube-Fed Patient—cont'd**

| Complication/possible causes | Suggested management strategy |
|---|---|
| ***Aspiration*** | |
| HOB too low | Raise HOB >30 degrees during and 1 h after feeding |
| | Monitor breath sounds and VS, and observe pulmonary secretions for blue food coloring, which has been added to feeding. Test pulmonary secretions for glucose, which reflects the presence of formula (may be falsely-positive when blood is in respiratory secretions). Stop tube feeding ½-1 h before chest physical therapy, suctioning, or placing patient supine |
| | Monitor for fever, unexplained pulmonary infiltrates, and increased RR and effort because aspiration can occur silently and quickly |
| Delayed gastric emptying | See "High gastric residual," p. 674 |
| Incorrect tube position | *Small-bore tube:* Check x-ray for position. Secure, mark, and measure tube to obtain future reference point |
| | *Large-bore tube:* Aspirate and test stomach contents for acidity before each feeding and q4h for continuous feeding |
| | Mark and measure tube as future reference point |
| Bolus feedings | Switch to intermittent or continuous feeding |
| ***Blocked tube*** | |
| Viscous formula/medications; inadequate flushing | Flush tube with 50-150 ml water after each feeding/medication administration. Flush q4h with 30 ml water. Flush blocked tubes with proteolytic enzyme papain (Adolph's Meat Tenderizer), pancreatic enzyme (Viokase), colas, and cranberry juice, using a syringe, alternating positive and negative pressure. None are effective immediately. Reason suggested for the effectiveness of cranberry juice is its high acidity and for cola its carbonation. A device called Intro-Reduce has been designed to clear blocked soft feeding tubes |
| Instillation of crushed medications | Substitute liquid preparations after consulting with pharmacist and attending MD, or crush into a fine powder and dissolve in 30 ml water. Do not instill crushed medications into small-bore tubes |

**T A B L E  11 - 11    Catheters Used in Parenteral Nutrition**

| Catheter | Use | Description |
|---|---|---|
| Subclavian/jugular | Short term | Inserted at bedside. Multiple uses for specimen retrieval, feeding, and medication administration increase the risk of infection, especially in compromised patients |
| Multilumen | Short term | Inserted at bedside. Dedication of one lumen in this catheter is common practice, enabling other lumen(s) to be used for medication administration and laboratory monitoring |
| Right atrial (e.g., Hickman, Broviac) | Long term | Composed of silicone rubber with plastic external segment, which is implanted in OR. Its safety enables use by home-care patients |
| Implantable (e.g., Infuse-a-Port, Port-a-Cath) | Long term | Implanted in OR. Designed for repeated access, making the need for repeated venipuncture unnecessary |

improved or normal measures of protein stores (serum albumin 3.5 g/dl, transferrin 180-260 mg/dl, thyroxine-binding prealbumin 20-30 mg/dl, and retinol-binding protein 4-5 mg/dl); state of N balance measured by N balance studies; presence of wound granulation (i.e., pinkish white tissue around wound edges that grows to fill in wound); and absence of infection (see **High risk for infection,** p. 679).

*For oral nutrition:*
- Ensure nutritional screening and assessment of patient within 72 h of admission; document. See guidelines, above.
- Position patient in high-Fowler's position for eating; assist with preparation of food for eating as needed. Involve significant others in meal rituals for companionship and caring.
- Provide small, frequent feedings of diet compatible with disease state and patient's ability to ingest foods.
- Respect food aversions, and try to maximize food preferences.
- Provide liquid nutritional supplements as prescribed. Serve them cold or over ice to enhance palatability.
- Document intake *via* calorie counts.
- Provide psychologic support.

*For enteral nutrition:*
- Ensure nutritional screening and assessment of patient within 72 h of admission; document. For guidelines, see p. 665.
- Monitor laboratory data daily: serum albumin, transferrin, or prealbumin; vitamins; minerals; trace elements; and electrolytes. Document.
- Weigh patient daily.
- Record I&O carefully, tracking fluid balance trends.
- Administer formula within 10% of rate, as prescribed. Check infused volume and rate hourly.

*For parenteral nutrition:*
- Ensure nutritional screening and assessment of patient within 72 h of admission; document. For guidelines, see p. 665.
- Monitor laboratory data daily: serum albumin, transferrin, or prealbumin; vitamins; minerals; trace elements; and electrolytes. Document.

**T A B L E  11 - 12  Management of Complications in Patients Receiving Parenteral Nutrition**

| Potential complications | Management strategy |
| --- | --- |
| Pneumothorax | Ensure that x-ray is done immediately after insertion. Determine placement of catheter before initiating feeding by monitoring for diminished or unequal breath sounds, tachypnea, dyspnea, and labored breathing |
| Subclavian artery injury | If pulsative bright red blood returns into the syringe, assist MD with immediate removal of the needle and apply pressure for 10 min anteriorly and posteriorly at the point of penetration |
| Air embolism | Use Trendelenburg position when catheter is inserted into central vein; have patient perform Valsalva's maneuver during tubing changes. Use Luer-lock connectors, and tape all tubing connections longitudinally to prevent disconnection. Use occlusive dressing over insertion site for 24 h after catheter has been removed to prevent air entry *via* catheter-sinus tract. Monitor patient for chest pain, tachycardia, tachypnea, cyanosis, and hypotension. If air embolism is suspected, clamp the catheter, turn patient to left side-lying decubitus and Trendelenburg position to trap air in the right ventricle, give $O_2$ and CPR as necessary; contact MD stat |
| Sepsis | Monitor WBC count and differential for values outside normal range; monitor VS q4h and blood glucose q6h for values outside normal range. Examine catheter insertion site q shift for erythema, swelling, or purulent drainage. Maintain sterile technique when changing central line dressing and hanging new feeding solution. Change all administration sets q48h. Cleanse the site with tincture of iodine (1%-2%), followed by 70% alcohol or povidone-iodine solution; avoid using line being used for nutritional support to withdraw or give blood, monitor pressure, or administer medications or other fluids. If sepsis is suspected, assist with catheter removal; culture specimens from the catheter tip and exit site; take blood specimen for culture; and administer antibiotics as prescribed |
| Catheter occlusion | If solution is infusing sluggishly, flush line with heparinized saline. If line is occluded, try to aspirate clot and contact MD, who may prescribe a thrombolytic agent. |

Modified from Roberts PM, Webber KS, "Providing Nutritional Support." In Swearingen PL, Keen JH: Manual of Critical Care: Applying Nursing Diagnoses to Adult Critical Disorders, ed 2, St Louis, Mosby-Yearbook, 1991.

**T A B L E  11 - 13    Metabolic Complications with Enteral and Parenteral Nutrition**

| Complication | Strategy |
|---|---|
| Hypoglycemia | Ensure continuous regular infusion of nutritional support; assess insulin levels. If support is stopped, give $D_{5-10}W$ as prescribed |
| Hyperglycemia | Monitor infusion rate carefully; use a feeding pump; alter nutritional support as needed; give insulin as prescribed |
| Hyperosmolar hyperglycemic nonketotic syndrome | Correct hyperglycemia and hyperosmolality as prescribed according to blood glucose and electrolyte values. Monitor I&O q2h; report urine output <1 ml/kg/2h. Check specific gravity q2h; weigh patient qod. Monitor for circulatory overload during fluid replacement. Assess rate of nutritional support hourly. Reset to prescribed rate as indicated. **Note:** If infusion significantly lags behind prescribed quantity, do not attempt to catch up by increasing infusion rate greatly |

- Weigh patient daily.
- Record I&O carefully, tracking fluid balance trends.
- Administer parenteral solution within 10% of rate as precribed. Check infused volume and rate hourly.

**High risk for aspiration** related to enteral feeding *via* enterostomy tube or delayed gastric emptying
***Desired outcome:***   Patient is free of aspiration problems as evidenced by auscultation of clear lung sounds, VS within patient's normal limits, and absence of signs of respiratory distress.

- Check x-ray for position of feeding tube. Insufflation with air and aspiration of stomach contents do *not* confirm placement of small-bore feeding tubes.
- Monitor breath sounds and VS q4h.
- Auscultate bowel sounds and assess abdominal contour and girth q8h.
- Elevate HOB ≥30 degrees during and 1 h after feeding. If this is not possible or comfortable for patient, turn patient to a slightly elevated right side-lying position to enhance gravity flow from the greater stomach curve to the pylorus.
- Stop tube feeding ½ to 1 h before chest physical therapy, suctioning, or placing patient supine.
- Treat nausea promptly. Obtain prescription for antiemetic prn.
- Observe pulmonary secretions for blue food color, which has been added to feeding.
- Test pulmonary secretions for glucose, which reflects the presence of formula (may be false-positive when blood is in respiratory secretions).

**Constipation** related to inadequate fluid and fiber in diet
***Desired outcome:***   Patient obtains relief from constipation by having a bowel movement within 3-4 days of this diagnosis (or within patient's usual pattern).

- Recommend change of formula to one that has fiber added.
- Assess intake of free water (optimally 1ml/calorie) daily.
- Give free water q2h as prescribed.
- For other interventions, see this diagnosis in Appendix One, p. 716.

**Diarrhea (or risk of same)** related to careless preparation of formula and changing of feeding sets
***Desired outcome:***   Patient has formed stools within 24-48 h of intervention.

- Monitor I&O carefully. Report signs of GI intolerance that may be related

to enteral product contamination (e.g., nausea and vomiting, abdominal distention, cramping, diarrhea).
- Obtain stool sample for culture and sensitivity.
- Use clean technique in handling feeding tube, enteral products, and feeding sets.
- Change all equipment q24h.
- Refrigerate all opened products and discard after 24 h.
- Discard feedings hanging for >8 h.

**High risk for infection** related to invasive procedures or malnutrition
***Desired outcome:*** Patient is free of infection as evidenced by VS within normal range, total lymphocytes 25%-40% (1,500-4,500/μl), WBC count ≤11,000/μl, and absence of the clinical signs of sepsis (see Table 11-12).
- Ensure adequate nutritional support, based on patient's needs. For guidelines, see p. 669.
- Monitor total lymphocyte count, WBC count, and differential for values outside normal range.
- Monitor VS q4h and blood or urinary glucose q6h for values outside normal range.

*Specifics for enteral nutrition:*
- Monitor patient for chills, fever, and glucose intolerance.
- Hang tube feeding solution for a maximum of 8 h.
- Use clean technique in handling feeding tube, enteral products, and feeding sets.
- Change enteral administration set q24h.
- Report signs of GI intolerance that may be related to enteral product contamination (e.g., nausea and vomiting, abdominal distention, cramping, diarrhea).

*Specifics for parenteral nutrition:*
- Monitor for erythema, purulent drainage, and swelling at catheter insertion site, chills, fever, and glucose intolerance.
- Use meticulous sterile technique when changing central line dressing, containers, or lines.
- Avoid using central line that is being used for nutritional support to draw blood, monitor pressure, or administer medications or other fluids.
- Change all administration sets q48h.
- Culture specimens from the catheter tip and exit site prn.
- Take blood specimens for culture if sepsis is suspected, and administer antibiotics as prescribed.
- Limit hang time to <8 h for Intralipid.

**High risk for impaired swallowing** related to decreased or absent gag reflex, decreased strength or excursion of muscles involved in mastication, facial paralysis, mechanical obstruction, or fatigue
***Desired outcome:*** Patient demonstrates adequate cough and gag reflexes before foods or fluids are initiated and the ability to ingest foods *via* the phases of swallowing as instructed.
- Ensure nutritional screening and assessment, as well as assessment of oral motor function, within 72 h of patient's admission or progression to oral diet.
- Provide mouth care before and after meals and dietary supplements.
- Provide small, frequent meals.
- Provide foods at temperatures acceptable to patient.
- Respect food aversions; honor food preferences whenever possible.
- Provide oral supplements or tube feeding supplements as prescribed. Advise patient of transition status, and praise his or her progress.
- Order extra sauces, gravies, or liquids if dryness of the oral cavity impairs patient's swallowing ability. Suggest that patient moisten each bite of food with these substances.
- In conjunction with PT or OT, assist in retraining or facilitating patient's

swallowing. Assess cough and gag reflexes before the first feeding. Initially liquids and solids may be difficult to manage. Offer foods with semisolid consistency, and progress to thicker texture as tolerated. Assist patient through the phases of ingesting food: opening the mouth, achieving lip closure, chewing, transferring food from side to side in the mouth and then to the back of the oral cavity, elevating the tongue to the roof of the mouth (hard palate), and swallowing between breaths.
- If tolerated, keep patient in an upright position for ½ h to minimize the risk of aspiration.
- Monitor and record patient's intake (*via* calorie count, daily weight) and output.

**Impaired tissue integrity (or risk of same)** related to mechanical irritant (presence of enteral tube)
***Desired outcome:***   At time of hospital discharge, patient's tissue is intact, with absence of erosion around orifices, excoriation, skin rash, mucous membrane breakdown, or decubitus ulcers.
*For nasogastric tube:*
- Assess skin for irritation or tenderness q8h.
- Use a small-bore tube if possible.
- If long-term support is needed, discuss potential for using gastrostomy or jejunostomy tube with physician.
- Give ice chips, chewing gum, or hard candies prn if permitted.
- Apply petrolatum ointment to lips q2h.
- Have patient brush teeth and tongue q4h.
- Apply water-soluble lubricant to naris prn.
- Alter position of tube prn to avoid pressure on underlying tissue. Use hypoallergenic tape to anchor tube.
*For gastrostomy tube:*
- Assess site for erythema, drainage, tenderness, and odor q4h.
- Monitor placement of tube q4h.
- Secure tube so there is no tension on patient's tissue and skin.
- Wash skin with soap and water; pat dry.
*For jejunostomy tube:*
- Assess site for erythema, drainage, tenderness, and odor q4h.
- Secure tube so there is no tension. Coil tube on top of dressing if necessary.
- Cleanse skin with half-strength solution of hydrogen peroxide and water; rinse hydrogen peroxide from skin; and dry. Apply povidone-iodine ointment around insertion site daily and prn.
- Dress site with split 4x4s and tape with paper or hypoallergenic tape.

**Altered cardiopulmonary tissue perfusion (or high risk of same)** related to interruption of arterial flow (air embolus)
***Desired outcome:***   Patient has adequate cardiopulmonary tissue perfusion as evidenced by VS and RR within patient's normal limits.
- Check chest x-ray to determine catheter position.
- Position patient in Trendelenburg position when changing tubing or when neck vein catheters are removed.
- Teach patient Valsalva's maneuver for implementation during tubing changes.
- Use Luer-lock connectors on all connections.
- Tape all tubing connections longitudinally to prevent disconnection.
- Use occlusive dressing over insertion site for 24 h after catheter is removed to prevent air entry *via* catheter-sinus tract.
- Monitor patient for chest pain, tachycardia, tachypnea, cyanosis, and hypotension.
- If air embolus is suspected, clamp the catheter and turn patient to left sidelying Trendelenburg position to trap air in the right ventricle. Give oxygen. Notify physician immediately.

# Section Three: Managing Wound Care

A wound is a disruption of tissue integrity caused by trauma, surgery, or an underlying medical disorder. Wound management is directed at preventing infection and deterioration in wound status and promoting healing.

## Wounds closed by primary intention

Clean, surgical, or traumatic wounds whose edges are closed with sutures, clips, or sterile tape strips are referred to as wounds closed by primary intention. Impairment of healing most frequently manifests as dehiscence, evisceration, or infection. Individuals at high risk for disruption of wound healing include those who are obese, diabetic, elderly, malnourished, receiving steroids, or undergoing chemotherapy or radiation therapy.

### ASSESSMENT

**Optimal healing:** Immediately after injury, the incision line is warm, reddened, indurated, and tender. After 1 or 2 days, wound fluid on the incision line dries, forming a scab that subsequently falls off and leaves a pink scar. After 5-9 days, a healing ridge—a palpable accumulation of scar tissue— forms. In patients who undergo cosmetic surgery, scab formation and a healing ridge are purposely avoided to minimize scar formation. See Table 11-14.

**Impaired healing:** Lack of an adequate inflammatory response manifested by absence of initial redness, warmth, and induration or inflammation that persists or occurs after the fifth postinjury day; continued drainage from the incision line 2 days after injury (when no drain is present); absence of a healing ridge by the ninth day after injury; presence of purulent exudate. See Table 11-14.

### DIAGNOSTIC TESTS

**WBC with differential:** To assess for infection.
**Gram stain of drainage:** If infection is suspected, to identify the offending organism and aid in the selection of preliminary antibiotics.
**Culture and sensitivity of tissue by biopsy or swab:** To determine optimal antibiotic. Infection is said to be present when there are $10^5$ organisms/g of tissue or when there is fever and drainage.

### COLLABORATIVE MANAGEMENT

**Application of a sterile dressing in surgery:** To protect wound from external contamination and trauma or provide pressure. Usually, surgeon changes the initial dressing.

---

**T A B L E  11 - 14  Assessment of Healing by Primary Intention**

| Expected findings | Abnormal findings |
| --- | --- |
| Edges well approximated | Edges not well approximated |
| Good inflammatory response (redness, warmth, induration, pain) initially postinjury | Decreased or absent inflammatory response or inflammatory response that persists or occurs after the fifth day |
| No drainage (without drain present) 48 h after closure | Drainage continues >48 h after closure |
| Healing ridge present by postoperative day 7-9 | No healing ridge present by postoperative day 9; hypertrophic scar or keloid |

**Regular (house) diet:**  To promote positive nitrogen (N) state for optimal wound healing.
**Multivitamins, especially C:**  To promote tissue healing.
**Minerals, especially zinc and iron:**  May be prescribed, depending on patient's serum levels.
**Supplemental $O_2$:**  Empirically, 2-4 L/min in high-risk patients. After injury, wound $PO_2$ is low, and administration of $O_2$ may promote healing.
**Insulin:**  As needed to control glucose levels in diabetics.
**Local or systemic antibiotics:**  Given when infection is present and sometimes used prophylactically as well.
**Incision and drainage:**  To drain pus when infection is present and localized. This allows healing by secondary intention. Often the wound is irrigated with antiinfective agents such as dilute Dakin's solution.

## NURSING DIAGNOSES AND INTERVENTIONS

**Impaired tissue integrity:**  Wound, related to altered circulation, metabolic disorders (e.g., diabetes mellitus [DM]), alterations in fluid volume and nutrition, and medical therapy (chemotherapy, radiation therapy, and steroid administration)
*Desired outcome:*  Patient exhibits the following signs of wound healing: well-approximated wound edges; good initial postinjury inflammatory response (erythema, warmth, induration, pain); no inflammatory response after the fifth day postinjury; no drainage (without drain present) 48 h after closure; healing ridge present by postoperative day 7-9.

- Assess wound for indications of impaired healing, including absence of a healing ridge, presence of drainage or purulent exudate, and delayed or prolonged inflammatory response. Monitor VS for signs of infection, including elevated temperature and HR. Document findings.
- Follow Body Substance Isolation (see p. 777) and aseptic technique when changing dressings. If a drain is present, keep it sterile, maintain patency, and handle it gently to prevent it from becoming dislodged. If wound care will be necessary after hospital discharge, teach the dressing change procedure to patient and significant others.
- Maintain blood glucose within normal range for persons with DM by performing serial monitoring of blood glucose and administering insulin to keep glucose level <200 mg/dl.
- Explain to patient that deep breathing promotes oxygenation, which enhances wound healing. If indicated, provide incentive spirometry at least 4×/day. Stress the importance of position changes and activity as tolerated to promote ventilation. Splint incision as needed.
- Monitor perfusion status by checking BP, HR, capillary refill time in the tissue adjacent to incision, moisture of mucous membranes, skin turgor, volume and specific gravity of urine, and I&O.
- For nonrestricted patients, ensure a fluid intake of at least 2-3 L/day.
- Encourage ambulation or ROM exercises as allowed to enhance circulation to the wound.
- To promote positive N state, which enhances wound healing, provide a diet with adequate protein, vitamin C, and calories. Encourage between-meal supplements. If patient complains of feeling full with 3 meals a day, give more frequent small feedings instead.

## PATIENT-FAMILY TEACHING AND DISCHARGE PLANNING

Give patient and significant others verbal and written information about the following:
- Local wound care, including type of equipment necessary, wound care procedure, and therapeutic and negative side effects of topical agents used. Have patient/significant other demonstrate dressing change procedure before hospital discharge.

- Signs and symptoms of improvement in wound status (see Table 11-14).
- Signs and symptoms of deterioration in wound status, including those that necessitate notification of physician or clinic (see Table 11-14).
- Diet that promotes wound healing. Discuss the importance of adequate protein and calorie intake. See "Providing Nutritional Support," p. 665. Involve dietitian, patient, and significant others as necessary.
- Activities that maximize ventilatory status: a planned regimen for ambulatory patients, and deep breathing and turning (at least q2h) for those on bed rest.
- Importance of taking multivitamins, antibiotics, and supplements of iron and zinc as prescribed. For all medications to be taken at home, provide the following: name, purpose, dosage, schedule, precautions, and potential side effects.
- Importance of follow-up care with physician; confirm time and date of next appointment if known.

*In addition:*

- If needed, arrange for a visit by a home health nurse before hospital discharge.

# Surgical or traumatic wounds healing by secondary intention

Wounds healing by secondary intention are those with tissue loss or heavy contamination that form granulation tissue and contract in order to heal. Most often, impairment of healing is caused by contamination and impairment of perfusion, oxygenation, and nutrition. Individuals at risk for impaired healing include those who are obese, diabetic, malnourished, elderly, taking steroids, or undergoing radiation or chemotherapy.

## ASSESSMENT

**Optimal healing:**    Initially the wound edges are inflamed, indurated, and tender. At first, granulation tissue on the floor and walls is pink, progressing to a deeper pink and then to a beefy red; it should be moist. Epithelial cells from the tissue surrounding the wound gradually migrate across the granulation tissue. As healing occurs, the wound edges become pink, the angle between surrounding tissue and the wound becomes less acute, and wound contraction oc-

## T A B L E  11 - 15  Assessment of Healing by Secondary Intention

| Expected findings | Abnormal findings |
|---|---|
| Initially postinjury, wound edges inflamed, indurated, and tender; with epithelialization, edges become pink | Initially postinjury, decreased inflammatory response or inflammation around the wound continues after the fifth postinjury day; epithelialization slowed or mechanically disrupted so not continuous around wound |
| Granulation tissue initially avascular and moist and then turns pink; becomes beefy red over time | Granulation tissue remains pale or is excessively dry or moist |
| No odor present | Odor present |
| No exudate or necrotic tissue present | Exudate or necrotic tissue present |

**TABLE 11-16  Dressings Used for Wound Care**

| Dressing | Advantages | Limitations |
|---|---|---|
| Dry to Dry* (insert dry and remove dry) | Highly absorbent; debridement | Excessively drying to tissue; disruption of new tissues; painful removal |
| Wet to Dry* (insert wet and remove dry) | Good absorption but not as absorptive as dry to dry; good debridement | Drying of tissues but not as much as dry to dry; disruption of new tissue; painful removal |
| Moist to Moist* (insert and remove moist) | Provides topical antiinfective agent; no wound desiccation; good debridement; not painful; inexpensive | Less effective removal of exudate; if excessively wet, can cause tissue maceration; if it dries out, dressing must be moistened before removal |
| Xeroform Gauze | Provides topical antiseptic; keeps tissue hydrated; minimal pain with removal | Can cause tissue maceration if it is excessively moist |
| Porcine Skin Dressing | Can provide topical antibiotic; keeps tissue hydrated; not painful when removed; often used before closure of wound with tissue grafts | Expensive; usually stored in refrigerator until use |
| Transparent Dressing (e.g., Op-Site, Tegaderm, Biocclusive) | Prevents loss of wound fluid; protects wound from external contamination; minimal pain with removal; protects from friction and fluid loss | Must withdraw excessive drainage and reseal dressing; appearance of drainage erroneously suggests infection |
| Hydrocolloid Dressing (e.g., Duoderm, Restore, Intact) | Maintains moist wound surface while minimizing pooling; easy to apply; minimal pain with removal | Cannot directly assess wound without removing dressing; "melts" when used under radiant heat; limited absorption |
| Hydrophilic Gel (e.g., Vigilon, Intrasite Gel) | Maintains moist wound surface; nonadherent; absorbs some exudate; compatible with topical medications; easy to apply; minimal pain with removal | Causes maceration when in direct contact with normal tissue; expensive; may require frequent changing; provides minimal absorption of exudate |
| Alginates (e.g., Sorbsan) | Physiologic; maintains moisture; painless | Not good for dry wounds |
| Foams (e.g., Lyofoam, Allevin) | Maintains moist wound surface; insulates wound; nonadherent | Poor barrier; opaque; not good for wounds with copious viscous drainage |

*All dressings are sterile, coarse mesh gauze without cotton fiber fill and are covered with dry sterile outer layer to prevent ingress of organisms. When moisture is prescribed, it is provided with an antiinfective agent or physiologic solution.

curs. Occasionally a wound has a tract or sinus that gradually decreases in size as healing occurs. The time frame for healing depends on the size and location of the wound and on the patient's physical and psychologic status. See Table 11-15.

**Impaired healing:** Exudate appears on the floor and walls of the wound and does not abate as healing progresses. It is important to note the distribution, color, odor, volume, and adherence of the exudate. The skin surrounding the wound should be assessed for signs of tissue damage, including disruption, discoloration, and increasing pain. When a drain is in place, the volume, color, and odor of the drainage should be evaluated. See Table 11-15.

## DIAGNOSTIC TESTS

**CBC with WBC differential:**   To assess hematocrit (Hct) level and for presence of infection. Increased WBC count signals infection, while a decrease occurs with immunosuppression. Watch the differential for a shift to the left, which indicates infection. Monitor the lymphocyte count: $\leq 1,800/\mu l$ is a sign of malnutrition. For optimal healing, the Hct should be >20%.

**Gram stain of drainage:**   To determine the offending organism, if present, and aid in selection of the preliminary antibiotic.

**Tissue biopsy or culture and sensitivity of drainage:**   To determine presence of infection and the optimal antibiotic, if appropriate.

**Ultrasound, sonogram, or sinogram:**   To determine wound size, especially when abscesses or tracts are suspected.

## COLLABORATIVE MANAGEMENT

**Debriding enzymes:**   To soften and remove necrotic tissue (e.g., fibrinolysin plus desoxyribonuclease [Elase]).

**Dressings:**   To provide debridement, keep healthy wound tissue moist, or provide antiseptic agent to decrease wound surface bacterial counts. See Table 11-16.

**Hydrophilic agents:**   To remove contaminants and excess exudate (e.g., dextran beads or paste [Envisan] or polymer flakes [Bard Absorption Dressing]).

**Hydrotherapy:**   To soften and remove debris mechanically.

**Wound irrigation with or without antiinfective agents:**   To dislodge and remove bacteria and loosen necrotic tissue, foreign bodies, and exudate. Antiinfective agents work locally to kill organisms.

**IV fluids:**   To ensure adequate perfusion for patients unable to take adequate oral fluids.

**Topical or systemic vitamin A:**   As needed to reverse adverse effects of steroids on healing. Use is limited to 7-10 days.

**Drain(s):**   To remove excess tissue fluid or purulent drainage.

**Surgical debridement:**   To remove dead tissue and reduce debris and fibrotic tissue.

**Skin graft:**   To provide coverage of wound if necessary.

**Tissue flaps:**   To fill tissue defect and provide wound closure with its own blood supply.

**Regular diet, supplemental $O_2$, multivitamins and minerals, insulin, and incision and drainage:**   See discussion in "Wounds Closed by Primary Intention," p. 682.

## NURSING DIAGNOSES AND INTERVENTIONS

**Impaired tissue integrity:**   Wound, related to presence of contaminants, metabolic disorders (e.g., DM), medical therapy (e.g., chemotherapy or radiation therapy), altered perfusion, or malnutrition

*Desired outcomes:*   Patient's wound exhibits the following signs of healing: initially postinjury, wound edges are inflamed, indurated, and tender; with epithelialization, edges become pink within 1 week of injury; granulation tissue develops (identified by pink tissue that becomes beefy red) within 1 week of injury; and there is absence of odor, exudate, or necrotic tissue. Patient or significant other successfully demonstrates wound care procedure before hospital discharge, if appropriate.

- Monitor for the following signs of impaired healing: initially postinjury, decreased inflammatory response or inflammatory response that lasts >5 days; epithelialization slowed or mechanically disrupted and noncontinuous around the wound; granulation tissue remaining pale or excessively dry or moist; presence of odor, exudate, and/or necrotic tissue.
- Apply prescribed dressings (see Table 11-16) following Body Substance Isolation (BSI) (see p. 777). Insert dressing into all tracts to promote gradual closure of those areas. Ensure good handwashing before and after dressing changes, and dispose of contaminated dressings appropriately.
- When a drain is used, maintain its patency, prevent kinking of the tubing, and secure the tubing to prevent the drain from becoming dislodged. Use aseptic technique when caring for drains.
- To help prevent contamination, cleanse the skin surrounding the wound with a mild disinfectant (e.g., soap and water). Do not use friction with cleansing if tissue is friable.
- If irrigation is prescribed for reducing contaminants, employ high-pressure irrigation using a 35-ml syringe with an 18-gauge needle, and follow BSI. If the tissue is friable or the wound is over a major organ or blood vessel, use extreme caution with the irrigation pressure. To remove contaminants effectively, use a large volume of irrigant (e.g., 100-150 ml).
- Topically applied antiinfective agents, such as neomycin and iodophors, are absorbed by the wound and can produce systemic side effects. When these agents are used, be alert to side effects such as toxicity to cells in the wound, nephrotoxicity, and acidosis.
- When a hydrophilic agent such as Debrisan or Bard Absorption Dressing is prescribed, remove it with high-pressure irrigation. If the agent were to be removed with a 4×4 or surgical sponge, the friction would disrupt capillary budding and delay healing.
- When topical enzymes are prescribed, use them on necrotic tissue only and follow package directions carefully. Be aware that some agents such as povidone-iodine deactivate the enzymes. Protect surrounding undamaged skin with zinc oxide or aluminum hydroxide paste.
- Teach patient or significant other the prescribed wound care procedure, if indicated.

### PATIENT-FAMILY TEACHING AND DISCHARGE PLANNING
See teaching and discharge planning interventions in "Wounds Closed by Primary Intention," p. 682.

## Pressure ulcers

Pressure ulcers result from a disruption in tissue integrity and are most often caused by excessive tissue pressure or shearing of blood vessels. High-risk patients include the elderly and those who have decreased mobility, decreased LOC, impaired sensation, debilitation, incontinence, sepsis/elevated temperature, or malnutrition.

### ASSESSMENT
High-risk individuals should be identified upon admission assessment, with daily assessments during hospitalization, using a standard assessment schemata. When pressure ulcers are present, their severity can be graded on a scale of I to IV:

**Grade I:** Nonblanchable erythema of intact skin. In dark-skinned individuals, heat may be the only indication of a grade I pressure ulcer.

**Grade II:** Partial-thickness skin loss involving epidermis and/or dermis; seen as an abrasion, blister, or shallow crater.

**Grade III:** Full-thickness skin loss that involves subcutaneous tissue but does not extend through fascia.

**Grade IV:** Full-thickness injury that involves muscle, bone, or supporting structures.

---

**Note:** See "Surgical or Traumatic Wounds Healing by Secondary Intention," p. 683, for other assessment data.

---

## DIAGNOSTIC TESTS

See "Diagnostic Tests," p. 685, in "Surgical or Traumatic Wounds Healing by Secondary Intention."

## COLLABORATIVE MANAGEMENT

**Debriding enzymes:**   To soften and remove necrotic tissue.

**Dressings:**   To provide debridement, keep healthy tissue moist, or apply an antiinfective agent. See Table 11-16.

**Hydrophilic agents:**   To remove contaminants and excess moisture.

**Wound irrigation with antiinfective agents:**   To reduce contamination.

**Hydrotherapy:**   To soften and remove debris mechanically.

**Diet:**   Adequate protein and calories to promote positive N state for rapid wound healing.

**Supplemental vitamins and minerals:**   As needed.

**Supplemental $O_2$:**   Usually 2-4 L/min to promote wound healing for high-risk patients or those with delayed wound healing.

**Surgical debridement:**   Removal of devitalized tissue with a scalpel to reduce the amount of debris and fibrotic tissue.

**Tissue flaps:**   To provide wound closure with its own blood supply.

**Cultured keratinocytes:**   To provide cover for the wound in the form of a sheet of skin cells grown from a biopsy of the patient's own skin.

**Growth factors:**   Naturally occurring proteins that stimulate new cell formation (e.g., platelet-derived growth factor, insulin).

**Hyperbaric $O_2$:**   Used with difficult wounds to support oxidative processes in healing.

## NURSING DIAGNOSES AND INTERVENTIONS

**Impaired tissue integrity (or risk of same)** related to excessive tissue pressure, shearing forces, or altered circulation

***Desired outcomes:***   Patient's tissue remains intact. Patient participates in preventive measures and verbalizes understanding of the rationale for these interventions.

- Identify individuals at risk, and systematically assess skin over bony prominences daily; document.
- Establish and post a position-changing schedule.
- Assist patient with position changes. There is an inverse relationship between pressure and time in ulcer formation; therefore, heavier patients need to change position more frequently. Position changes include turning the bed-bound patient q1-2h and having the wheelchair-bound patient (who is able) perform pushups in the chair q15min to ensure periodic relief from pressure on the buttocks. Use pillows or foam wedges to protect bony prominences from direct pressure. In addition, patients with history of previous tissue injury will require pressure-relief measures more frequently. Because high-Fowler's position results in increased shearing, use low-Fowler's position and alternate supine position with prone and 30-degree elevated side-lying positions.

- For immobile patients, totally relieve pressure on heels by raising them off the bed surface *via* pillows inserted under the length of the lower leg.
- Minimize friction on tissue during activity. Friction causes shearing of vessels, which leads to tissue disruption. Lift rather than drag patient during position changes and transferring; use a draw sheet to facilitate patient movement. Do not massage over bony prominences, because this can result in tissue damage.
- Minimize skin exposure to moisture. Cleanse at the time of soiling and at routine intervals. Use moisture barriers and disposable briefs as needed.
- Use a mattress that reduces pressure, such as foam, alternating air, gel, or water.
- To enhance circulation, encourage patient to maintain current level of activity.

**Impaired tissue integrity:**   Presence of pressure ulcer, with increased risk for further breakdown related to altered circulation and presence of contaminants or irritants (chemical, thermal, or mechanical)

***Desired outcomes:***   Grades I and II are healed within 7-10 days; Grades III and IV may require months to heal. Following intervention and instruction, patient verbalizes causes and preventive measures for pressure ulcers and successfully participates in the plan of care to promote healing and prevent further breakdown.

- Evaluate grade of pressure ulcer (see "Assessment," above).
- Maintain a moist physiologic environment to promote tissue repair and minimize contaminants. Change dressings as prescribed, using BSI (see p. 777).
- Be sure patient's skin is kept clean with regular bathing, and be especially conscientious about washing urine and feces from the skin. Soap should be used and then thoroughly rinsed from the skin.
- If the patient has excessive perspiration, ensure frequent bathing and change bedding as needed.
- To absorb moisture and prevent shearing when the patient is moved, apply heel and elbow covers as needed.
- Use lamb's wool to keep the areas between the toes dry. Change wool periodically, depending on the amount of moisture present.
- Do not use a heat lamp, because it increases the metabolic rate of the tissues, resulting in increased demand for blood flow in an area with impaired perfusion. As a result, ulcer diameter and depth can be increased.
- Teach patient and significant others the importance of and measures for preventing excess pressure as a means of preventing pressure ulcers.
- Provide wound care as needed (described under "Surgical or Traumatic Wounds Healing by Seconday Intention," earlier).

---

**Note:**   See "Surgical or Traumatic Wounds Healing by Secondary Intention" for **Impaired tissue integrity:** Wound, related to presence of contaminants, metabolic disorders, or medical therapy, p. 685.

---

## PATIENT-FAMILY TEACHING AND DISCHARGE PLANNING

Give patient and significant others verbal and written information about the following:

- Location of local medical supply stores that have pressure-reducing mattresses and wound care supplies.
- Planning a schedule for changing patient positions.

---

For other teaching and discharge planning interventions, see "Wounds Closed by Primary Intention," p. 682.

## Selected Bibliography

A.S.P.E.N. Board of Directors: Guidelines for use of total parenteral nutrition in the hospitalized adult patient, *J Parenter Enter Nutr* 10(5):441-445, 1986.

Bommarito AA, Heinzelmann MJ, Boysen DA: A new approach to the management of obstructed enteral feeding tubes, *Nutr Clin Pract* 4(6):111-114, 1989.

Braga M et al: Prognostic role of preoperative nutritional and immunological assessment in the surgical patient, *J Parenter Enter Nutr* 12(2):138, 1988.

Centers for Disease Control: Recommendations for preventing transmission of human immunodeficiency virus and hepatitis B virus to patients during exposure-prone invasive procedures, *Morb Mortal Wkly Rep* 40:1-9, 1991.

Cohen PT, Jande MA, Volberding PA: *The AIDS knowledge base*, Boston, 1990, The Medical Publishing Group.

Cuzzell JZ: Choosing a wound dressing: a systematic approach, *AACN Clin Issues Crit Care Nurs* 3(1):566-577, 1990.

Edes TE, Walk BE, Austin JL: Diarrhea in tube-fed patients: feeding formula not necessarily the cause, *Am J Med* 88(2):91-93, 1990.

Eisenberg P: Enteral nutrition: indications, formulas, and delivery techniques, *Nurs Clin North Am* 24(2):315-338, 1989.

Gibbs DA, Hamill DN, Magruder-Habib K: Populations at increased risk of HIV infection: current knowledge and limitations, *J Acquir Immune Defic Syndr* 4(9):881-889, 1991.

Guthrie P, Turner WW: Peripheral and central nutritional support, *J Nat Intraven Ther Assoc* 9(5):393-398, 1986.

Hilton G: AIDS dementia, *J Neurosci Nurs* 21(1):24-29, 1989.

Hu DJ, Kane MA, Heymann DL: Transmission of HIV, hepatitis B virus, and other bloodborne pathogens in health care setting: a review of risk factors and guidelines for prevention, *Bull World Health Organ* 69(5):623-630, 1991.

Interqual: *The ISD-A review system with adult ISD criteria*, August 1992, Northhampton, NH, and Marlboro, MA, Interqual, Inc.

Jackson MM: Infection prevention and control, *Crit Care Clin North Am* 4(3):401-409, 1992.

Jeejeebhoy KN, Detsky AS, Baker JP: Assessment of nutritional status, *J Parenter Enter Nutr* 14(5):193S-196S, 1990.

Kermode M: Physical assessment of people with AIDS, *Aust J Adv Nurs* 7(3):4-11, 1990.

Kim MJ, McFarland GK, McLane AM: *Pocket guide to nursing diagnosis*, ed 5, St Louis, 1993, Mosby–Year Book.

Kohn CL, Keithley JK: Enteral nutrition: potential complications and patient monitoring, *Nurs Clin North Am* 24(2):339-353, 1989.

Konstantinides NN, Shronts E: Tube feeding: managing the basics, *Am J Nurs* 83(9):1312-1320, 1983.

Krasner D: *Chronic wound care*, King of Prussia, Pa, 1990, Health Management Publications.

Lakshman K, Blackburn GL: Monitoring nutritional status in the critically ill adult, *J Clin Monit* 2(2):114-120, 1986.

La Van FB, Hunt TK: Oxygen and wound healing, *Clin Plast Surg* 17(3):463-472, 1990.

Maklebust J, Sieggreen M: *Pressure ulcers: guidelines for prevention and nursing management*, West Dundee, Ill, 1991, S-N Publications.

Marcuard SP, Stegall KS: Unclogging feeding tubes with pancreatic enzyme, *J Parenter Enter Nutr* 14(2):198-200, 1990.

Metheny NA, Spies MA, Eisenberg P: Measures to test placement of nasoenteral feeding tubes, *West J Nurs Res* 10(4):367-379, 1988.

Miller K: *Acquired immunodeficiency syndrome*. In Swearingen PL, Keen JH, editors: *Manual of critical care: applying nursing diagnoses to adult critical illness,* ed 2, St Louis, 1991, Mosby–Year Book.

Molaghan JB: Treatment modalities for patients with HIV disease, *J Intravenous Nurs* 14(suppl):S25-S29, 1991.

Moran TA: AIDS: current implications and impact on nursing, *J Intravenous Nurs* 12(4):220-226, 1989.

Murphy LM, Lipman TO: Central venous catheter care in parenteral nutrition: a review, *J Parenter Enter Nutr* 11(2):190-201, 1987.

Neighbors M, Henderson M: Information nurses need about AIDS, *Adv Clin Care* 6(3):49-50, 1991.

Nicholson LJ: Declogging small-bore feeding tubes, *J Parenter Enter Nutr* 11(6):594-597, 1987.

Norris SO, Provo B, Stotts NA: Physiology of wound healing and risk factors that impede the healing process, *AACN Clin Issue Crit Care Nurs* 3(1):542-552, 1990.

Pressure ulcers in adults: prediction and prevention, US Department of Health and Human Services, Agency for Health Care Policy Research, 1992.

Roberts PM, Webber KS: *Providing nutritional support.* In Swearingen PL, Keen JH, editors: *Manual of critical care: applying nursing diagnoses to adult critical illness,* ed 2, St Louis, 1991, Mosby–Yearbook.

Rombeau JL, Caldwell MD: *Clinical nutrition: enteral and tube feeding,* ed 2, Philadelphia, 1990, WB Saunders.

Ryan JA, Gough J: Complications of central venous catheterization for total parenteral nutrition, *J Nat Intraven Ther Assoc* 7(1):29-35, 1984.

Scott CD, Jaffee DT: Managing occupational stress associated with HIV infection, *Occup Med* (suppl 4): 85s-93s, 1989.

Silberman H: *Parenteral and enteral nutrition,* ed 2, Norwalk, Conn, 1989, Appleton & Lange.

Siminoff LA, Erlen JA, Lidz CW: Stigma, AIDS and quality of nursing care: state of the science, *J Adv Nurs* 16(3):262-269, 1991.

Stotts NA: *Impaired wound healing.* In Carrieri VK et al: *Pathophysiologic phenomena in nursing,* ed 2, Philadelphia, 1992, WB Saunders.

Talbot JM: Guidelines for the scientific review of enteral food products for special medical purposes, *J Parenter Enter Nutr* 15(3):99S-174S, 1991.

Volker DL: Acquired immune deficiency syndrome: an overview, *Dimens Oncol Nurs* 2(2):22-32, 1988.

Webber KS: *Providing nutritional support.* In Horne MM, Swearingen PL: *Pocket guide to fluid, electrolyte, and acid-base balance,* ed 2, St Louis, 1993, Mosby–Year Book.

Weinstein S: AIDS: the disease, the demographics, the devastation, *J Intravenous Nurs* 14(suppl):S2-S7, 1991.

Williams WW: Infection control during parenteral nutrition threapy, *J Parenter Enter Nutr* 9(6):735-746, 1985.

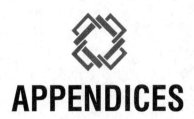

# APPENDICES

Appendix One    Patient Care    693
   Section One    Caring for Preoperative and Postoperative Patients    693
   Section Two    Caring for Patients on Prolonged Bed Rest    711
   Section Three    Caring for Patients with Cancer and Other Life-Disrupting
               Illnesses    719
   Section Four    Caring for Older Adults    767

Appendix Two    Infection Prevention and Control    777

Appendix Three    Heart and Breath Sounds    783

Appendix Four    Laboratory Tests Discussed in This Manual: Normal
             Values    791

Appendix Five    Abbreviations Used in This Manual    795

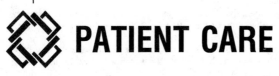 **PATIENT CARE**

# Section One: Caring for Preoperative and Postoperative Patients

**Knowledge deficit:** Surgical procedure, preoperative routine, and postoperative care

***Desired outcome:*** Patient verbalizes knowledge about the surgical procedure, including preoperative preparations and sensations and postoperative care and sensations, and demonstrates postoperative exercises and use of devices before surgical procedure or during the immediate postoperative period for emergency surgery.

- Assess patient's understanding about the diagnosis, surgical procedure, preoperative routine, and postoperative regimen. Evaluate patient's desire for knowledge about the diagnosis and procedure (some individuals find detailed information helpful; others prefer very brief and simple explanations). Assess for factors that would affect the patient's ability to learn. Determine past surgical experiences and their positive or negative effect on patient. Assess nature of any concerns or fears related to surgery. Document and communicate this assessment data to others involved in the patient's care.
- Based on your assessment, clarify and explain diagnosis and surgical procedure accordingly. When possible, emphasize sensations (i.e., dry mouth, thirst, muscle weakness). This information often is helpful in reducing stress and anxiety. Provide ample time for instruction and clarification, and reinforce physician's explanation of the procedure. Use anatomic models, diagrams, and other audiovisual aids when possible. Provide simply written information to reinforce learning. Provide written and verbal information in the patient's native language for non-English-speaking patients. **Note:** Evaluate patient's reading comprehension before providing written materials.
- Explain the perioperative course of events. Review the following with the patient and significant others:
  - Physical site before, during, and immediately after surgery (i.e., postanesthesia recovery room, ICU, other speciality unit). Clarify sounds and other sensations (e.g., dry mouth, sore throat, cool temperature, hard stretcher) the patient may experience during the immediate postoperative period. If possible, take the patient to the new unit and introduce him or her to the nursing staff.
  - Preoperative medications and timing of surgery (scheduled time, expected duration).
  - Pain management, including sensations to expect and methods of relief. If patient-controlled analgesia (PCA) will be prescribed, have patient return demonstration of the use of delivery device.
  - Placement of tubes, catheters, drains, and oxygen delivery devices. Enable patient to see these devices when possible.
  - Use of antiembolic stockings or pneumatic compression stockings.

- Dietary alterations, including NPO status followed by clear liquids until return of full gastrointestinal (GI) function.
- Restrictions of activity and positions.
- Need to refrain from smoking during the perioperative period.
- Visiting hours and location of waiting room.
- Explain the postoperative activities, exercises, and precautions. Have patient return demonstration of the following devices and exercises, as appropriate:
  - Deep-breathing and coughing exercises. (See **Ineffective airway clearance,** p. 700). **Caution:** Individuals for whom increased intracranial, intrathoracic, or intraabdominal pressure is contraindicated should not cough.
  - Use of incentive spirometry and other respiratory devices.
  - Calf-pumping, ankle-circling, and footboard-pressing exercises to enhance circulation and prevent thrombophlebitis in the lower extremities (see "Venous thrombosis/Thrombophlebitis," p. 104 for more information).
  - Use of PCA infusion device.
  - Movement in and out of bed.
- Before patient is discharged, teach the prescribed activity precautions, such as getting maximum amounts of rest, increasing activities gradually to tolerance, avoiding heavy lifting ($>10$ pounds), avoiding driving a car (often for as long as 4-6 weeks).
- Provide time for patient to ask questions and express feelings of anxiety; be reassuring and supportive. Be certain to address the individual's main concern(s).

**Pain or chronic pain** related to disease process, injury, or surgical procedure
***Desired outcomes:*** Patient's subjective perception of discomfort decreases within 1 h of intervention, as documented by a pain scale. Patient does not exhibit nonverbal indicators of pain (Table A-1). Autonomic indicators (Table A-2) are diminished or absent. Verbal responses, such as crying or moaning, are absent.

- Develop a systematic approach to pain management for each patient. The primary nurse should collaborate with the surgeon, anestheseologist, and patient for optimal management of pain. See Figures A-1 and A-2 for pain treatment flow charts.
- Monitor patient at frequent intervals for the presence of discomfort. Use a formal method of assessing pain. One method is to have the patient rate discomfort on a scale of 0 (no discomfort) to 10 (worst pain). Other methods may be used, but the method selected should be used consistently.
- Evaluate patients with acute and chronic pain for nonverbal indicators of discomfort (Table A-1).
- Evaluate patient with acute pain for autonomic indicators of discomfort (Ta-

**T A B L E  A - 1  Nonverbal Indicators of Pain**

Facial expression: masklike, grimace, tension
Guarding or protective behaviors
Restlessness or increase in motor activity
Withdrawal or decrease in motor activity
Skeletal muscle tension
Short attention span
Irritability
Anxiety
Sleep disturbances

---

**T A B L E  A - 2**  **Autonomic Indicators of Pain**

---

Diaphoresis

Vasoconstriction

Increased systolic and diastolic BP

Increased pulse rate (>100 bpm)

Pupillary dilatation

Change in respiratory rate (usually increased, >20 breaths/min)

Muscle tension or spasm

Decreased intestinal motility, evidenced by nausea, vomiting, abdominal distention, and possibly ileus

Endocrine imbalance, evidenced by sodium (Na) and water retention and mild hyperglycemia

---

ble A-2). Be aware that patients with chronic pain (longer than 6 months) may not exhibit an autonomic response.

- Evaluate patient's health history for evidence of alcohol and drug (prescribed and nonprescribed) use. A positive history of addiction to alcohol or drugs affects effective doses of analgesics (i.e., patient may require more or less). Consult pain control team if available. All care providers must be consistent in setting limits while providing effective pain control through pharmacologic and nonpharmacologic methods. Psychiatric consultation may be necessary.

- Administer opioid (e.g., morphine) and related mixed agonist-antagonist (e.g., butorphanol) analgesics as prescribed (See Table A-3). When possible, morphine or related "mu" receptor agonists are preferred to meperidine (Demerol) for postoperative moderate to severe pain. Monitor for side effects, such as respiratory depression, excessive sedation, nausea, vomiting, and constipation. Be aware that meperidine may produce excitation, muscle twitching, and seizures, especially in conjunction with phenothiazines. **Note:** Do not administer mixed agonist-antagonist analgesics concurrently with morphine or other pure agonist, because reversal of analgesic effects may occur.

- Assess patients receiving opioid analgesics at frequent intervals for evidence of excessive sedation when awake or respiratory depression (i.e., RR < 10 breaths/min or $Sao_2$ < 85%). In the presence of respiratory depression, reduce the amount or frequency of the dose as prescribed. Have naloxone (Narcan) readily available to reverse severe respiratory depression.

---

**Caution:** Use reduced doses and titrate carefully in patients with limited pulmonary reserve (i.e., chronic obstructive pulmonary disease, asthma), hepatic or renal insufficiency, and in older adults.

---

- Administer nonnarcotic (acetaminophen [Tylenol, Tempra]) and nonsteroidal antiinflammatory drugs (acetysalicylic acid [aspirin], ibuprofen [Motrin, Advil, Nuprin], indomethacin [Indocin], naproxen [Naprosyn, Anaprox], and ketorolac [Toradol]) as prescribed for relief of mild to moderate pain during postoperative recovery (see Table A-4). Nonsteroidal antiinflammatory drugs (NSAIDs) are especially effective when pain is associated with inflammation and soft tissue injury. Be certain that GI function has returned before administering oral agents. Ketolorac may be given IM for patients unable to tolerate oral agents. Monitor for side effects, such as epigastric pain, nausea, dyspepsia, and gastric bleeding. **Note:** Because NSAIDs have

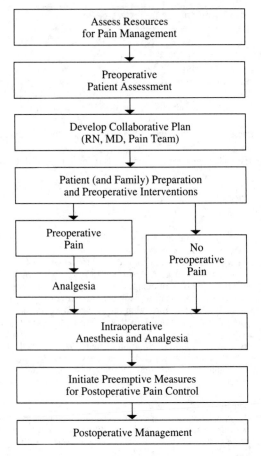

**Figure A-1:** Pain treatment flow chart: pre- and intraoperative phases. (Source: Department of Health and Human Services: *Acute pain management: operative or medical procedures and trauma,* Rockville, MD, 1992, US Department of Health and Human Services Pub No (AHCPR) 92-0032.)

peripheral effects and a different mechanism of action, they are very effective when combined or used with centrally acting opioid analgesics.

- Check the patient's analgesia record for the last dose and amount of medication given during surgery and in the postanesthesia recovery room. Be careful to coordinate timing and dose of postoperative analgesics with previously administered medication. **Note:** Combined fentanyl and droperidol (Innovar) anesthesia potentiates the effects of opioids for up to 10 h after administration, and the patient should be monitored carefully when opioid analgesia is used.
- Administer prn analgesics before pain becomes severe. Consider conversion to scheduled dosing with supplemental prn analgesia. Prolonged stimulation of pain receptors results in increased sensitivity to painful stimuli and will

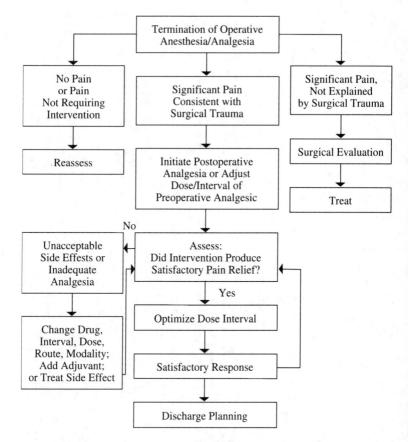

**Figure A-2:**   Pain treatment flow chart: postoperative phase.(Source: Department of Health and Human Services: *Acute pain management: operative or medical procedures and trauma, Rockville, MD,* 1992, US Department of Health and Human Services Pub No (AHCPR) 92-0032.)

increase the amount of drug required to relieve pain. Be aware that addiction to narcotics occurs infrequently in hospitalized patients.
- Plan to administer intermittently scheduled analgesics before painful procedures, ambulation, and at bedtime. Schedule them so that their peak effect is achieved at the inception of the activity or procedure.
- Augment analgesic therapy with sedatives and tranquilizers to prolong and enhance analgesia. Avoid substituting sedatives and tranquilizers for analgesics.
- Wean patient from opioid analgesics by decreasing dose or frequency of the drug. Convert to oral therapy as soon as possible. When changing route of administration or medication, be certain to use equianalgesic doses (Table A-5) of the new drug.
- Augment action of the medication by administering nonpharmacologic methods of pain control (Table A-6). Many of these techniques may be taught to and implemented by the patient and significant others.

**TABLE A-3  Use of Opioid and Agonist-Antagonist Analgesia**

| Route | Commonly prescribed medications | Advantages | Disadvantages |
|---|---|---|---|
| Continuous infusion | morphine, fentanyl (Sublimaze) | Useful for severe, predictable pain or as a basal dose with bolus supplements for fluctuating pain<br>Relieves pain with lower doses than IV bolus<br>Avoids peaks and valleys of pain present with IV bolus and IM injections | Requires frequent observation to monitor flow rate<br>VS must be monitored often |
| IV bolus | morphine, meperidine (Demerol), fentanyl | Useful for severe, intermittent pain (i.e., for procedures, treatments)<br>Rapid onset of action; may be controlled by patient using specialized pump | Relatively short duration of pain relief<br>Fluctuating levels<br>Possibility of excessive sedation as drug levels peak |
| Epidural | morphine, fentanyl, hydromorphone, meperidine | Very effective relief of moderate to severe pain<br>Delivery close to opiate receptors provides pain control with small doses<br>May be delivered with local anesthetic (e.g., bupivacaine) for increased effectiveness | Catheter must be inserted by anesthetist or anesthesiologist<br>Specialized delivery system must be used<br>Side effects include urinary incontinence, hypotension, respiratory depression, pruritus, nausea, and vomiting |

| | | | |
|---|---|---|---|
| Patient-controlled analgesic | morphine, meperidine, fentanyl, buprenorphine (Buprenex) | Useful for moderate to severe pain<br>Enables titration by patient for effective analgesia without excessive sedation<br>Relief of pain with lower dosages of medication<br>Immediate delivery of medication<br>Patient's sense of self-control lowers anxiety<br>Less nursing time spent preparing medications | Pumps necessary to deliver drug are expensive<br>Patient must have clear mental status<br>Health provider resistance to self-administration by patient |
| IM injection | meperidine, morphine, pentazocine (Talwin), nalbuphine (Nubain), butorphanol (Stadol), buprenorphine | Useful for moderate to severe pain<br>Longer duration of action than with IV route<br>Used for postoperative pain | Variable absorption and fluctuating levels, especially in hypotensive and critically ill patients<br>Possibility of excessive sedation as drug levels peak<br>Potential delay in administration |
| Oral | codeine, oxycodone (Percodan), meperidine, pentazocine, propoxyphene (Darvon), hydromorphone (Dilaudid), morphine (MS Contin) | Useful for mild to moderate acute pain or chronic severe pain (large doses necessary) | Variable absorption<br>Cannot be used until GI function returns; lengthy interval before onset of action |
| Transdermal | fentanyl (Duragesic) | Long duration of action (3 days)<br>Useful when pain is moderate to severe and constant | Delayed onset of action (up to 36 h)<br>Prolonged effects after removal<br>Must be used with rapid-action supplement for variable pain |

**T A B L E   A - 4   Common Nonnarcotic and Nonsteroidal Antiinflammatory Analgesics**

| Nonsteroidal antiinflammatory drugs | Nonnarcotic drugs |
|---|---|
| | acetaminophen (Tylenol, Tempra) |
| acetysalicylic acid (aspirin) | |
| ibuprofen (Motrin, Advil, Nuprin) | |
| indomethacin (Indocin) | |
| ketolorac (Toradol) | |
| naproxen (Naprosyn, Anaprox) | |

- Maintain a quiet environment to promote rest. Plan nursing activities to enable long periods of uninterrupted rest at night.
- Evaluate for and correct nonoperative sources of discomfort (i.e, position, full bladder, infiltrated IV site).
- Position patient comfortably and reposition at frequent intervals to relieve discomfort due to pressure and improve circulation.
- Sudden or unexpected changes in pain intensity can signal complications such as internal bleeding or leakage of visceral contents. Carefully evaluate the patient and notify the surgeon immediately.
- Document efficacy of analgesics and other pain control interventions, using the pain scale or other formalized method.

**Ineffective airway clearance** related to increased tracheobronchial secretions secondary to effects of anesthesia; ineffective coughing secondary to central nervous system (CNS) depression or pain and muscle splinting; and possible laryngospasm secondary to endotracheal tube or allergic reaction to anesthetics

*Desired outcome:*   Patient's airway is clear as evidenced by normal breath sounds to auscultation, RR 12-20 breaths/min with normal depth and pattern (eupnea), normothermia, and normal skin color.

- Assess respiratory status, including breath sounds, q1-2h during the immediate postoperative period and q8h during recovery. Note and report the presence of rhonchi that do not clear with coughing, labored breathing, tachypnea (RR > 20 breaths/min), restlessness, cyanosis, and the presence of fever ($\geq$38.33° C [101° F]).
- Encourage deep breathing and coughing q2h or more often for the first 72 h postoperatively. In the presence of fine crackles (rales), and if not contraindicated, have patient cough to expectorate secretions. Facilitate deep breathing and coughing by demonstrating how to splint the abdominal and thoracic incisions with the hands or a pillow. If indicated, medicate patient ½ h before deep breathing, coughing, or ambulation to enhance compliance.

**Caution:**   Vigorous coughing may be contraindicated for some individuals (e.g., those undergoing intracranial surgery, spinal fusion, eye and ear surgery, and similar procedures). Coughing after a herniorraphy and some thoracic surgeries should be done in a controlled manner, with the incision supported carefully.

- Be certain that emergency airway equipment (i.e., intubation tray, endotracheal tubes, suctioning equipment, and tracheostomy tray) are readily available in the event of sudden airway obstruction or ventilatory failure.

**T A B L E   A - 5   Equianalgesic Doses of Narcotic Analgesics**

| Class/name | Route | Equianalgesic dose (mg)* | Average duration (h) |
|---|---|---|---|
| *Morphinelike agonists* | | | |
| codeine | IM, SC | 130[†] | 3 |
| | PO | 180[†] | 3 |
| hydromorphone (Dilaudid) | IM, SC | 1.5-2.0 | 4 |
| | PO | 6.0-7.5 | 4 |
| levorphanol (Levo-Dromoran) | IM, SC | 2.0 | 6 |
| | PO | 4.0 | 6 |
| morphine | IM, SC | 10 | 4 |
| oxycodone (Percodan) | PO | 30[†] | 4 |
| oxymorphone (Numor-phan) | IM, SC | 1.0-1.5 | 4 |
| | rectal | 10 | 4 |
| *Meperidinelike agonists* | | | |
| fentanyl (Sublimaze) | IV, IM, SC | 0.1-0.2 | 1[‡] |
| meperidine (Demerol) | IM, SC | 100 | 3 |
| | PO | 300[†] | 3 |
| *Methadonelike agonists* | | | |
| methadone (Dolophine) | IM, SC | 10 | 6 |
| | PO | 10-20 | 6 |
| propoxyphene (Darvon) | PO | 130-250[†] | 4 |
| *Mixed agonist-antagonist*[§] | | | |
| buprenorphine (Buprenex) | IM | 0.3-0.6 | 4 |
| butorphanol (Stadol) | IM, SC | 2.0-3.0 | 3 |
| nalbuphine (Nubain) | IM, SC | 10-20 | 4 |
| pentazocine (Talwin) | IM | 30-60 | 3 |
| | PO | 10-200[†] | 3 |

Adapted from Baumann T and Lehman M: *Pain management.* In DiPiro J et al: *Pharmacotherapy: a pathophysiologic approach,* New York, 1988, Elsevier Science Publishing; and Koda-Kimble MA et al: *Applied therapeutics: the clinical use of drugs,* ed 5, Vancouver Wash, 1992, Applied Therapeutics.
*Recommended starting dose; actual dose must be titrated to patient response.
[†]Starting doses lower (codeine 30 mg, oxycodone 5 mg, meperidine 50 mg, propoxyphene 65-130 mg, pentazocine 50 mg).
[‡]Respiratory depressent effects persist longer than analgesic effects.
[§]Mixed agonist/antagonist analgesics may precipitate withdrawal in narcotic-dependent patients.

- Administer humidified oxygen as prescribed to prevent further drying of respiratory passageways and secretions.

**High risk for aspiration** related to entry of secretions, food, or fluids into the tracheobronchial passages secondary to CNS depression, depressed cough and gag reflexes, decreased GI motility, abdominal distention, recumbent position, presence of gastric tube, and possible impaired swallowing in individuals with oral, facial, or neck surgery

*Desired outcome:*   Patient's upper airway remains unobstructed as evidenced by clear breath sounds, RR 12-20 breaths/min with normal depth and pattern (eupnea), and normal skin color.

## T A B L E  A - 6   Common Nonpharmacologic Methods of Pain Control

*Sensory interventions*

Massage: To relax muscular tension and increase local circulation. Back and foot massage are especially relaxing

ROM exercises (passive, assisted, or active): To relax muscles, improve circulation, and prevent pain related to stiffness and immobility

Applications of heat or cold: Cold used initially to decrease tissue injury response and alter pain threshold; heat used to facilitate clearance of tissue toxins and mobilize fluids

Transcutaneous nerve stimulation: A battery-operated device used to send weak electric impulses *via* electrodes placed on the body; reduces sensation of pain during and sometimes after treatment

*Emotional interventions*

Prevention and control of anxiety: Limiting anxiety reduces muscle tension and increases patient's pain tolerance; anxiety and fear contribute to autonomic stimulation and pain responses; progressive relaxation exercises and encouraging slow, controlled breathing may be helpful

Promoting self control: Feelings of helplessness and lack of control contribute to anxiety and pain; techniques such as PCA and promoting self-helping behaviors contribute to feelings of self-control

*Cognitive interventions*

Cognitive preparations: Preparing the patient by explaining what can be expected, thereby reducing stress and anxiety (e.g., preoperative teaching)

Patient education: Teaching methods for preventing or reducing pain (e.g., suggesting comfortable postoperative positions, methods of ambulation, and splinting of incisions when coughing)

Distraction: Encouraging patient to focus on something unrelated to the pain (e.g., conversing, reading, watching TV or videos, listening to music, employing relaxation techniques [see **Health-seeking behavior:** Relaxation technique effective for stress reduction, p. 54])

Humor: Can be an excellent distraction and may help the patient cope with stress

Guided imagery: The patient employs a mental process that uses images to alter a physical or emotional state, a technique that promotes relaxation and decreases pain sensations

Many of these techniques may be taught to and implemented by the patient and significant others.

---

- See first three interventions under **Ineffective airway clearance.** above.
- If the sedated patient experiences nausea or vomiting, turn him or her immediately into a side-lying position. Fully alert patients may remain in an upright position. As necessary, suction the oropharynx with a Yankauer or similar suction device to remove vomitus.
- Check placement and patency of gastric tubes q8h and before instillation of feedings and medications.

---

**Note:**   Use caution when irrigating and otherwise manipulating the gastrointestinal tubes of patients with recent esophageal, gastric, or duodenal surgery because the tube may be displaced or the surgical incision disrupted by such activity. Consult surgeon before irrigating tubes for these individuals.

- Assess patient's abdomen q4-8h by inspection, auscultation, palpation, and percussion for evidence of distention (increasing size, firmness, increased tympany, and decreased bowel sounds). Notify physician if distention is of rapid onset or if it is associated with pain.
- Encourage early and frequent ambulation to improve GI motility and reduce abdominal distention owing to accumulated gases.
- Introduce oral fluids cautiously, especially in patients with oral, facial, and neck surgery.
- Administer antiemetics and metoclopramide (Reglan) as prescribed.
- For additional information see this nursing diagnosis in "Providing Nutritional Support," p. 678.

**Ineffective breathing pattern (or risk of same)** related to decreased lung expansion secondary to CNS depression, pain, muscle splinting, recumbent position, and effects of anesthesia

***Desired outcome:*** Patient exhibits effective ventilation as evidenced by relaxed breathing, RR 12-20 breaths/min with normal depth and pattern (eupnea), clear breath sounds, normal color, $Pao_2$ ≥80 mm Hg, pH 7.35-7.45, $Paco_2$ 35-45 mm Hg, and $HCO_3^-$ 22-26 mEq/L.

- See interventions under **Ineffective airway clearance,** earlier.
- Perform a preoperative baseline assessment of patient's respiratory system, noting rate, rhythm, degree of chest expansion, quality of breath sounds, cough, and sputum production. Note preoperative ABG values if available.
- If appropriate, encourage patient to refrain from smoking for at least 1 week after surgery. Explain the effects of smoking on the body.
- Monitor $Sao_2$ continuously in high-risk patients (e.g., those who are heavily sedated, with preexisting lung disease, and older adults) and at periodic intervals in other patients as indicated. Notify physician of $Sao_2$ <85%-90%.
- Evaluate ABG values and notify physician of low or decreasing $Pao_2$ and high or increasing $Paco_2$.
- Assist patient with turning and deep-breathing exercises q2h for the first 72 h postoperatively to promote lung expansion. Be aware that opioid analgesics depress the respiratory system.
- If patient has an incentive spirometer, provide instructions and ensure compliance with its use q2h or as prescribed.
- Unless contraindicated, assist patient with ambulation by the second postoperative day to enhance ventilation.
- For other interventions, see this nursing diagnosis, p. 2, in "Atelectasis."

**High risk for fluid volume deficit** related to postoperative bleeding/hemorrhage

***Desired outcomes:*** Patient is normovolemic as evidenced by BP ≥90/60 mm Hg (or within patient's preoperative baseline), HR 60-100 bpm, RR 12-20 breaths/min with normal depth and pattern (eupnea), brisk capillary refill (<2 sec), warm extremities, distal pulses >2+ on a 0-4+ scale, and urinary output ≥30 ml/h. Patient verbalizes orientation to person, place, and time.

- Monitor VS at frequent intervals during the first 24 h of the postoperative period. Be alert to indicators of internal hemorrhage and impending shock, including decreasing pulse pressure (difference between systolic and diastolic BP), decreasing BP, increasing HR, and increasing RR.
- Assess patient at frequent intervals during the first 24 h of the postoperative period for indicators of internal hemorrhage and impending shock, including pallor, diaphoresis, cool extremities, delayed capillary refill, diminished intensity of distal pulses, restlessness, agitation, and disorientation. Also note subjective complaints of thirst, anxiety, or a sense of impending doom.
- Monitor and measure urinary output q4-8h during the initial postoperative period. Report average hourly output <30 ml/h. Be alert to progressive urine concentration.
- Inspect surgical dressing for evidence of frank bleeding (i.e., rapid satura-

tion of dressing with bright red blood). Record saturated dressings, and report significant findings to surgeon. If the initial postoperative dressing becomes saturated, reinforce and notify surgeon because he or she may wish to perform the initial dressing change.

- Note the amount and character of drainage from gastric and other tubes at least q8h. If drainage appears to contain blood (e.g., bright red, burgundy, or dark coffee ground appearance), perform an occult blood test. If the test is newly or unexpectedly positive, report results to surgeon. **Note:** After gastric and some other GI surgeries, the patient will have small amounts of bloody or blood-tinged drainage for the first 12-24 h. Be alert to large or increasing amounts of bloody drainage.

- Review CBC values for evidence of bleeding: decreases in hemoglobin (Hgb) from normal (male 14-18 g/dl; female 12-16 g/dl); and decreases in hematocrit (Hct) from normal (male 40%-54%; female 37%-47%).

- Maintain a patent 18-gauge or larger IV catheter for use should hemorrhagic shock develop. See "Cardiac and Noncardiac Shock," p. 76, for management.

**High risk for fluid volume deficit** related to *active loss* secondary to presence of indwelling drainage tubes, wound drainage, or vomiting; *inadequate intake of fluids* secondary to nausea, NPO status, CNS depression, or lack of access to fluids; or *failure of regulatory mechanisms* with third spacing of bodily fluids secondary to the effects of anesthesia, endogenous catecholamines, blood loss during surgery, and prolonged recumbency

***Desired outcomes:*** Patient is normovolemic as evidenced by BP ≥90/60 mm Hg (or within patient's preoperative baseline), HR 60-100 bpm, distal pulses >2+ on a 0-4+ scale, urinary output ≥30 ml/h, stable or increasing weight, good skin turgor, warm skin, moist mucous membranes, and normothermia. Patient verbalizes orientation to person, place, and time.

- Monitor VS q4-8h during the recovery phase. Be alert to indicators of dehydration, including decreasing BP, increasing HR, and slightly increased body temperature.

- Assess patient's physical status q4-8h. Be alert to indicators of dehydration, including dry skin, dry mucous membranes, excessive thirst, diminished intensity of peripheral pulses, and alteration in mental status. Assess skin turgor by lifting a section of skin along the forearm, abdomen, or calf. Release the skin and watch its return to the original position. With good hydration, it will return quickly; with dehydration, the skin will remain in the lifted position (tenting) or return slowly. **Note:** This test may be less reliable in the older adult because of decrease in skin elasticity and subcutaneous fat.

- Monitor urinary output q4-8h. Be alert to a concentrated urine and low or decreasing output (the average normal output is 60 ml/h or 1,400-1,500 ml/day).

- Measure, describe, and document any emesis. Be alert to and document excessive perspiration. Include your assessment of both with the documentation of urinary, fecal, and other drainage for a total estimation of the patient's fluid balance.

- Measure and record output from drains, ostomies, wounds, and other sources. Ensure patency of gastric and other drainage tubes. Record quality and quantity of output. Report and replace excessive losses.

- Monitor patient's weight daily, using the results as an indicator of the patient's hydration and nutritional status. Always weigh the patient at the same time every day, using the same scale and same type and amount of bed clothing. Be aware that this method is not useful in detecting intravascular fluid loss due to third spacing.

- If nausea and vomiting are present, assess the potential causes, including administration of opioid analgesics, loss of patency of the gastric tube, and

environmental factors (e.g., unpleasant odors or sights). Administer antiemetics or metoclorpramide (Reglan) as prescribed.
- Monitor serum electrolytes. Be alert to low potassium levels ($K^+$ <3.5 mEq/L) and the following signs and symptoms of hypokalemia: lethargy, irritability, anorexia, vomiting, muscle weakness and cramping, paresthesias, weak and irregular pulse, and respiratory dysfunction. Also assess for low calcium levels ($Ca^{2+}$ <8.5 mg/dl) and the following signs and symptoms of hypocalcemia: Trousseau's or Chvostek's sign (for description, see p. 333), tetany, muscle cramps, fatigue, irritability, and personality changes.
- Administer and regulate IV fluids and electrolytes as prescribed until patient is able to resume oral intake. When IV fluids are discontinued, encourage intake of oral fluids, at least 2-3 L/day in the nonrestricted patient. Honor patient's preference in oral fluids, and keep them readily available in patient's room.

**Fluid volume excess** related to compromised regulatory mechanisms after major surgery
*Desired outcome:* Following intervention/treatment, patient becomes normovolemic as evidenced by BP within normal range of patient's preoperative baseline, distal pulses <4+ on a 0-4+ scale, presence of eupnea, clear breath sounds, absence of or barely detectable edema (≤1+ on a 0-4+ scale), and body weight near or at preoperative baseline.
- Assess for and report any indicators of fluid overload, including elevated BP, bounding pulses, dyspnea, crackles (rales), and pretibial or sacral edema.
- Maintain record of 8-h and 24-h I&O. Note and report significant imbalance. Remember that normal 24-h output is 1,400-1,500 ml and normal 1-h output is 60 ml/h.
- Weigh patient daily, using the same scale and same type and amount of bed clothing. Note significant weight gain. Remember that 1 L of fluid equals approximately 2.2 lb.
- Anticipate postoperative diuresis approximately 48-72 h after surgery because of mobilization of third-space (interstitial) fluid.
- Administer furosemide (Lasix) as prescribed to mobilize interstitial fluid.

---

**Note:** Diuretic therapy may cause dangerous $K^+$ depletion. See **High risk for fluid volume deficit,** above, for signs and symptoms of hypokalemia.

---

- Be aware that the older adult and individuals with cardiovascular disease are at high risk for developing postoperative fluid volume excess.

**High risk for infection** related to inadequate primary defenses (broken skin, traumatized tissue, decrease in ciliary action, and stasis of body fluids), invasive procedures, or chronic disease
*Desired outcome:* Patient is free of infection as evidenced by normothermia; HR ≤100 bpm; RR ≤20 breaths/min with normal depth and pattern (eupnea); negative cultures; clear and normal-smelling urine; clear and thin sputum; orientation to person, place, and time; and absence of unusual erythema, warmth, or drainage at the surgical incision.
- Monitor VS for evidence of infection, such as elevated HR and RR and increased body temperature. Notify surgeon if these are new findings.
- Evaluate orientation and LOC q8h. Consider infection if altered LOC is unexplained by other factors, such as medication or disease process.
- Evaluate IV sites for evidence of infection (erythema, warmth, swelling, unusual drainage). Change IV line and site if evidence of infection is present and according to agency protocol (q48-72h).
- Evaluate patency of all surgically placed tubes or drains. Irrigate or attach

to low-pressure suction as prescribed. Promptly report unrelieved loss of patency.
- Note color, character, and odor of all drainage. Report the presence of foul-smelling or abnormal drainage.
- Evaluate incisions and wound sites for evidence of infection: unusual erythema, warmth, delayed healing, and purulent drainage.
- Change dressings as prescribed, using sterile technique. Prevent cross-contamination of wounds in the same patient by changing one dressing at a time and washing hands between dressing changes.
- If patient develops evisceration, do not reinsert tissue or organs. Place a sterile, saline-soaked gauze over the evisceration and cover with a sterile towel until the wound can be evaluated by the surgeon.
- Prevent reflux of urine into the bladder by keeping drainage collection container below the level of patient's bladder. Help prevent urinary stasis by avoiding kinks or obstructions in the drainage tubing.
- Do not open closed urinary drainage system unless absolutely necessary; irrigate catheter only with physician prescription and when obstruction is the known cause.
- Assess for indicators of urinary tract infection (UTI), including chills, fever ($>37.78°$ C [$100°$ F]), flank or labial pain, and cloudy or foul-smelling urine.
- Encourage intake of 2-3 L/day in nonrestricted patients to minimize the potential for UTI by diluting the urine and maximizing urinary flow.
- Ensure that the patient's perineum and meatus are cleansed during the daily bath and that the perianal area is cleansed after bowel movements. Do not hesitate to remind patient of these hygiene measures. Be alert to indicators of meatal infection, including swelling, purulent drainage, and persistent meatal redness. Intervene if the patient is unable to perform self-care.
- Change the catheter according to established protocol, or sooner if sandy particles can be felt in the distal end of the catheter or patient develops UTI. Change the drainage collection container according to established protocol, or sooner if it becomes foul smelling or leaks.
- Obtain cultures of suspicious drainage or secretions (e.g., sputum, urine, wound) as prescribed. For urine specimens, be certain to use the sampling port, which is at the proximal end of the drainage tube. Cleanse the area with, an antimicrobial wipe, and use a sterile syringe with a 25-gauge needle to aspirate the urine.
- Prevent transmission of infectious agents by washing hands well before and after caring for patient and by wearing gloves when contact with blood, drainage, or other body substance is likely.

**Constipation** related to immobility, opioid analgesics and other medications, effects of anesthesia, lack of privacy, disruption of abdominal musculature, or manipulation of abdominal viscera during surgery

***Desired outcome:*** Patient returns to presurgical bowel elimination pattern as evidenced by return of active bowel sounds within 48-72 h after most surgeries, absence of abdominal distention or sensation of fullness, and the elimination of soft, formed stools.
- Monitor for and document the elimination of flatus or stool, which signals returning intestinal motility.
- Assess for evidence of decreased GI motility, including abdominal distention, tenderness, absent or hypoactive bowel sounds, and sensation of fullness. Report gross distention, extreme tenderness, and prolonged absence of bowel sounds.
- To stimulate peristalsis, encourage in-bed position changes, exercises, and ambulation to patient's tolerance unless contraindicated.
- If a nasogastric (NG) tube is in place, perform the following:
  - Check placement of the tube after insertion, before any instillation, and q8h. For a larger-bore tube, either insert air into the proximal end of the tube to elicit a *whoosh* sound, which can be heard while auscultating over

the epigastric area, or aspirate gastric contents. If the tube is in the trachea, the patient will exhibit signs of respiratory distress, and the tube should be repositioned immediately. For smaller-bore tubes, check a recent x-ray to confirm position before instilling anything into the tube.

- Prevent migration of the tube by keeping it securely taped to the patient's nose and reinforcing placement by attaching the tube to the patient's gown with a safety pin or tape.

- Measure and record the quantity and quality of output. Typically the color will be green. For patients who have undergone gastric surgery, it may be brownish initially because of small amounts of bloody drainage but should change to green after about 12 h. Test reddish or brown output for the presence of blood, which can signal the development of a stress ulcer or indicate that a tube opening is compressed against the stomach lining. Reposition the tube as necessary. **Note:** For patient with gastric, esophageal, or duodenal surgery, notify physician before manipulating the tube.

- Maintain patency of the NG tube with gentle instillation of normal saline as prescribed. Ensure low, intermittent suction of gastric sump tubes by maintaining patency of sump port (usually blue). If sump port becomes occluded by gastric contents, flush sump port with air until a *whoosh* sound is heard over the epigastric area. **Caution:** Never clamp or otherwise occlude sump port, because excessive pressure may accumulate and damage gastric mucosa. For patient with gastric, esophageal, or duodenal surgery, notify physician before irrigating tube.

- When the tube is removed, monitor patient for the presence of abdominal distention, nausea, and vomiting.

- Monitor and document patient's response to diet advancement from clear liquids to a regular or other prescribed diet.

- Encourage oral fluid intake, especially of prune juice.

- Administer stool softeners, mild laxatives, and enemas as prescribed. Monitor and record results.

- Arrange periods of privacy during patient's attempts at bowel elimination.

**Sleep pattern disturbance** related to preoperative anxiety, stress, postoperative pain, noise, and altered environment

*Desired outcome:* Following intervention/treatment, patient relates minimal or no difficulty with falling asleep and describes a feeling of being well rested.

- Administer sedative/hypnotic (Table A-7) as prescribed. Be aware that these agents may cause CNS depression and contribute to the respiratory depressent effects of opioid analgesics. Also be aware that active metabolites of many of the benzodiazepines may accumulate and result in greater physiologic effects or toxicity. **Note:** Use caution when administering sedative/hypnotic to patients with COPD due to its respiratory depressent effects. Monitor respiratory function at frequent intervals in these individuals.

- After administering sedative/hypnotic, be certain to raise side rails and caution patient not to smoke in bed.

## T A B L E  A - 7   Sedatives and Hypnotics Commonly Used Perioperatively

| Antihistamine sedatives | Benzodiazepines |
|---|---|
| diphenhydramine (Benadryl) | alprazolam (Xanax) |
| hydroxyzine (Vistaril) | chlordiazepoxide (Librium) |
| | diazepam (Valium) |
| | flurazepam (Dalmane) |
| | oxazepam (Serax) |

**T A B L E  A - 8   Nonpharmacologic Measures to Promote Sleep**

| Activity | Example(s) |
|---|---|
| Mask or eliminate environmental stimuli | Use eyeshields, ear plugs |
| | Play soothing music |
| | Dim lights at bedtime |
| | Mask odors from dressings/drainage; change dressing or drainage container as indicated |
| Promote muscle relaxation | Encourage ambulation as tolerated throughout the day |
| | Teach and encourage in-bed exercises and position changes |
| | Perform back massage at bedtime |
| | If not contraindicated, use a heating pad |
| Reduce anxiety | Ensure adequate pain control |
| | Keep patient informed of his/her progress and treatment measures |
| | Avoid overstimulation by visitors or other activities immediately before bedtime |
| | Avoid stimulant drugs (e.g., caffeine) |
| Promote comfort | Encourage patient to use own pillows, bedclothes if not contraindicated |
| | Adjust bed; rearrange linens |
| | Regulate room temperature |
| Promote usual presleep routine | Offer oral hygiene at bedtime |
| | Provide warm beverage at bedtime |
| | Encourage reading or other quiet activity |
| Minimize sleep disruption | Maintain quiet environment throughout the night |
| | Plan nursing activities to enable long (at least 90 min) of undisturbed sleep |
| | Use dim lights when checking on patient during the night |

- Administer analgesics at bedtime to reduce pain and augment effects of hypnotic.
- Be certain that consent for surgery is signed before administering sedative/hypnotic.
- Use nonpharmacologic measures to promote sleep (Table A-8).

**Impaired physical mobility** related to postoperative pain, decreased strength and endurance secondary to CNS effects of anesthesia or blood loss, musculoskeletal or neuromuscular impairment secondary to disease process or surgical procedure, perceptual impairment secondary to disease process or surgical procedure (e.g., ocular surgery, neurosurgery), or cognitive deficit secondary to disease process or effects of opioid analgesics and anesthetics

*Desired outcome:*  Optimally, by hospital discharge (depending upon type of surgery), patient returns to preoperative baseline physical mobility as evidenced by the ability to move in bed, transfer, and ambulate independently or with minimal assistance.

- Assess patient's preoperative physical mobility by evaluating coordination and muscle strength, control, and mass. Be aware of medically imposed restrictions against movement, especially with conditions or surgeries that are orthopedic, neurosurgical, or ocular.
- Evaluate and correct factors limiting physical mobility, including overseda-

tion with opioid analgesics, failure to achieve adequate pain control, and poorly arranged physical environmment.
- Initiate movement from bed to chair and ambulation as soon as possible after surgery, depending on postoperative prescriptions, type of surgery, and patient's recovery from anesthetics (usually 12-24 h after surgery). Assist patient with moving slowly to a sitting position in bed and then standing at bedside before attempting ambulation. For more information, see **Altered cerebral tissue perfusion,** p. 715.

---

**Note:** Many anesthetic agents depress normal vasoconstrictor mechanisms and can result in sudden hypotension with quick changes in position.

---

- Encourage frequent movement and ambulation by postoperative patients. Provide assistance as indicated.
- Explain the importance of movement in bed and ambulation in reducing postoperative complications, including atelectasis, pneumonia, thrombophlebitis, and depressed GI motility.
- For additional information, see "Caring for Patients on Prolonged Bed Rest" for **High risk for activity intolerance,** p. 711, and **High risk for disuse syndrome,** p. 713.

**High risk for trauma** related to weakness, balancing difficulties, and reduced muscle coordination secondary to anesthetics and postoperative opioid analgesics

*Desired outcome:* Patient does not fall and remains free of trauma as evidenced by absence of bruises, wounds, or fractures.
- Orient and reorient patient to person, place, and time during the initial postoperative period. Inform patient that surgery is over. Repeat information until patient is fully awake and oriented (usually several hours but may be days in heavily sedated or otherwise obtunded individuals).
- Maintain side rails on stretchers and beds in upright and locked positions. Be aware that some individuals experience agitation and thrash about as they emerge from anesthesia.
- Secure all IV lines, drains, and tubing to prevent dislodgement.
- Maintain bed in its lowest position when leaving patient's room.
- Be certain that the call mechanism is within patient's reach; instruct patient about its use.
- Caution patient and visitors to avoid smoking in rooms when oxygen is in use.
- Identify patients at high risk for falling by assessing the following. Correct or compensate for risk factors.
  - *Time of day:* Night shift, peak activity periods such as meals, bedtime.
  - *Medications:* Opioid analgesics, sedatives, hypnotics, and anesthetics.
  - *Impaired mobility:* Individuals requiring assistance wiith transfer and ambulation.
  - *Sensory deficits:* Diminished visual acuity due to disease process or environmental factors; changes in kinesthetic sense due to disease or trauma.
- Use restraints and protective devices if necessary and prescribed.

**High risk for impaired skin integrity** related to presence of secretions/excretions around percutaneous drains and tubes

*Desired outcome:* Patient's skin around percutaneous drains and tubes remains clear and intact.
- Change dressings as soon as they become wet. The surgeon may prefer to perform the first dressing changes at the surgical incision. Use sterile technique for all dressing changes.
- Keep the area around drain or T-tube as clean as possible (e.g., the presence of bile can lead quickly to skin excoriation). Sterile normal saline or a

solution of saline and hydrogen peroxide or other prescribed solution may be used to clean around the drain site.

- If some external drainage is present, position a pectin-wafer skin barrier around the drain or tube. Ointments, such as zinc oxide, petrolatum, and aluminum paste, also may be used. Consult with enterostomal therapy (ET) nurse if drainage is excessive or skin excoriation develops. For additional information, see "Managing Wound Care," p. 681.

**Altered oral mucous membrane** related to NPO status and/or presence of NG or endotracheal tube

*Desired outcome:* At the time of hospital discharge, patient's oral mucosa is intact, without pain or evidence of bleeding.

- Provide oral care and oral hygiene q4h and prn. Arrange for patient to gargle, brush teeth, and cleanse the mouth with sponge-tipped applicators as necessary to prevent excoriation and excessive dryness.
- Use a moistened cotton-tipped applicator to remove encrustations. Carefully lubricate the lips and nares with an antimicrobial ointment, petroleum jelly, or emollient cream.
- If the patient's throat is irritated from the presence of an NG tube, obtain a prescription for a lidocaine gargling solution.
- For additional information, see this nursing diagnosis in "Stomatitis," p. 380.

---

**Note:** For additional information about the prevention of surgical complications, see "Pneumonia," p. 3, "Atelectasis," p. 1, "Urinary Retention," p. 165, "Venous Thrombosis/Thrombophlebitis," p. 104, "Providing Nutritional Support," p. 665, "Managing Wound Care," p. 681, and "Caring for Patients on Prolonged Bed Rest," p. 693. For psychosocial nursing diagnoses and interventions, see "Caring for Patients with Cancer and Other Life-Disrupting Illnesses," p. 753.

---

## Selected Bibliography

Acute Pain Management Guideline Panel: *Acute pain management: operative or medical procedures and trauma. Clinical practices guideline.* AHCPR Pub No 92-0032, Rockville, MD: Agency for Health Care Policy and Research, Public Health Service, US Department of Health and Human Services, 1992.

Devine E, Cook T: Clinical and cost-saving effects of psychoeducational interventions with surgical patients: a meta-analysis, *Res Nurs Health* 9:89-103, 1986.

DiPiro J et al: *Pharmacotherapy: a pathophysiologic approach,* New York, 1988, Elsevier Science Publishing.

Herr K, Mobily P: Interventions related to pain, *Nurs Clin North Am* 27(2):17-23, 1992.

Jacox A et al: Managing acute pain, *Am J Nurs* 92(5):49-55, 1992.

Keen JH: *Managing pain in the critically ill patient.* In Swearingen PL, Keen JH, editors: *Manual of critical care: applying nursing diagnoses to adult critical illness,* ed 2, St Louis, 1991, Mosby–Year Book.

Kim MJ, McFarland GK, McLane AM: *Pocket guide to nursing diagnoses,* ed 5, St Louis, 1993, Mosby–Year Book.

Koda-Kimble M A et al: *Applied therapeutics: the clinical use of drugs,* ed 5, Vancouver, Wash, 1992, Applied Therapeutics.

Lange M et al: Patient-controlled analgesia versus intermittent analgesia dosing, *Heart Lung* 17(5):495-498, 1988.

McCaffery M, Ferrell B: Patient age: does it affect your pain control decisions? *Nursing 91* (9):44-48, 1991.

McGuire L: The power of nonnarcotic pain relievers, *RN* 53(4):28-36, 1990.

Oberle K et al: Environment, anxiety, and postoperative pain, *West J Nurs Res* 12(6):745-757, 1990.

Tack K et al: Patient falls: profile for intervention, *J Neurosci Nurs* 19(2):83-89, 1987.

Webster R, Thompson D: Sleep in hospitals, *J Adv Nurs* 11:447-457, 1989.

Wild L, Coyne C: Epidural analgesia, *Am J Nurs* 92(4):26-36, 1992.

# Section Two: Caring for Patients on Prolonged Bed Rest

**High risk for activity intolerance** related to deconditioned status (see Table A-9)

*Desired outcomes:* Patient exhibits cardiac tolerance to activity or exercise as evidenced by HR ≤20 bpm over resting HR, systolic BP ≤20 mm Hg over or under resting systolic BP, RR ≤20 breaths/min with normal depth and pattern (eupnea), normal sinus rhythm, warm and dry skin, and absence of crackles, new murmurs, new dysrhythmias, gallop, or chest pain. Patient rates perceived exertion (RPE) at ≤3 on a scale of 0 (none) to 10 (maximal).

- Perform ROM exercises 2-4 times a day on each extremity. Individualize the exercise plan based on the following guidelines:
  - *Mode or type of exercise:* Begin with passive exercises, moving the joints through the motions of abduction, adduction, flexion, and extension. Progress to active-assisted exercises in which you support the joints while the patient initiates muscle contraction. When the patient is able, supervise him or her in active isotonic exercises, during which the patient contracts a selected muscle group, moves the extremity at a slow pace, and then relaxes the muscle group. Have the patient repeat each exercise 3 to 10 times.

---

**Caution:** Stop any exercise that results in muscular or skeletal pain. Consult with a physical therapist (PT) about necessary modifications. Avoid isometric exercises in cardiac patients.

---

- *Intensity:* Begin with 3-5 repetitions as tolerated by the patient. Assess exercise tolerance by measuring HR and BP at rest, peak exercise, and 5 min after exercise. If HR or systolic BP increases >20 bpm or mm Hg over the resting level, decrease the number of repetitions. If HR or systolic BP decreases >10 bpm or mm Hg at peak exercise, this could be a sign of left ventricular failure, denoting that the heart cannot meet this work load. For other adverse signs and symptoms, see "Assessment of exercise tolerance," below.
- *Duration:* Begin with 5 min or less of exercise. Gradually increase the exercise to 15 min as tolerated.
- *Frequency:* Begin with exercises 2-4 times a day. As the duration increases, the frequency can be reduced.
- *Assessment of exercise tolerance:* Be alert to signs and symptoms that the cardiovascular and respiratory systems are unable to meet the demands of the low-level ROM exercises. Excessive SOB may occur if (1) transient pulmonary congestion occurs secondary to ischemia or left ventricular dysfunction; (2) lung volumes are decreased; (3) oxygen-carrying capacity of the blood is reduced; or (4) there is shunting of blood from the right to the left side of the heart without adequate oxygenation. If cardiac output does not increase to meet the body's needs during modest levels of exercise, systolic BP may fall; the skin may become cool, cyanotic, and diaphoretic; dysrhythmias may be noted; crackles (rales) may be auscultated;

---

**T A B L E   A - 9   Physiologic Effects of Prolonged Bed Rest (Deconditioning)**

---

Increased HR and BP for submaximal work load
Decrease in functional capacity
Decrease in circulating volume
Orthostatic hypotension
Reflex tachycardia
Modest decrease in pulmonary function
Increase in thromboemboli
Loss of muscle mass
Loss of muscle contractile strength
Negative protein state
Negative nitrogen (N) state

---

or a systolic murmur of mitral regurgitation may occur. If the patient tolerates the exercise, increase the intensity or number of repetitions each day.
- Ask the patient to rate perceived exertion experienced during exercise, basing it on the following scale developed by Borg (1982):
  - 0  nothing at all
  - 1  very weak effort
  - 2  weak (light) effort
  - 3  moderate
  - 4  somewhat stronger effort
  - 5  strong effort
  - 7  very strong effort
  - 9  very, very strong effort
  - 10  maximal effort

The patient should not experience a RPE >3 while performing ROM exercises. Reduce the intensity of the excercise and increase the frequency until an RPE of ≤3 is attained.

- As the patient's condition improves, increase activity as soon as possible to include sitting in a chair. Assess for orthostatic hypotension, which can occur as a result of decreased plasma volume and difficulty in adjusting immediately to postural change. Prepare the patient for this change by increasing the amount of time spent in high-Fowler's position and moving the patient slowly and in stages. The following describes activity progression in hospitalized patients.

| | |
|---|---|
| **Level I:** Bed rest | Flexion and extension of extremities 4 ×/day, 15 × each extremity; deep breathing 4 ×/day, 15 breaths; position change from side to side q2h |
| **Level II:** Out of bed to chair | As tolerated, 3 ×/day for 20-30 min; may perform ROM exercises 2 ×/day while sitting in chair |
| **Level III:** Ambulate in room | As tolerated, 3 ×/day for 3-5 min |
| **Level IV:** Ambulate in hall | Initially, 50-200 ft 2 ×/day; progressing to 600 ft 4 ×/day; may incorporate slow stair climbing in preparation for hospital discharge |

|                        |                                        |
| ---------------------- | -------------------------------------- |
| *Signs of activity intolerance:* | Decrease in BP >20 mm Hg; increase in HR to >120 bpm (or >20 bpm above resting HR in patients on beta blocker therapy) |

- Increase activity level by having patient perform self-care activities such as eating, mouth care, and bathing as tolerated.
- Teach significant others the purpose and interventions for preventing deconditioning. Involve them in the patient's plan of care.
- To help allay fears of failure, pain, or medical setbacks, provide emotional support to patient and significant others as patient's activity level is increased.

**High risk for disuse syndrome** related to paralysis, mechanical immobilization, prescribed immobilization, severe pain, or altered LOC

*Desired outcome:* Patient exhibits complete ROM of all joints without pain, and limb girth measurements congruent with or increased over baseline measurements.

---

**Note:** ROM exercises should be performed every day for all immobilized patients with *normal* joints. Modification may be required for patients with flaccidity (i.e., immediately after cerebrovascular accident [CVA] or spinal cord injury [SCI]) to prevent subluxation; or for patient with spasticity (i.e., during the recovery period for patients with CVA or SCI) to prevent an increase in spasticity. Consult with PT or occupational therapist (OT) for assistance in modifying the exercise plan for these patients. Also, be aware that ROM exercises are restricted or contraindicated for patients with rheumatologic disease during the inflammatory phase and for joints that are dislocated or fractured.

---

- Be alert to the following areas that are especially prone to joint contracture: *shoulder,* which can become "frozen" to limit abduction and extension; *wrist,* which can "drop," prohibiting extension; *fingers,* which can develop flexion contractures that limit extension; *hips,* which can develop flexion contractures that affect the gait by shortening the limb or develop external rotation or adduction deformities that affect the gait; *knees,* in which flexion contractures can develop to limit extension and alter the gait; and *feet,* which can "drop" as a result of plantarflexion, which limits dorsiflexion and alters the gait.
- Ensure that patient changes position at least q2h. Post a turning schedule at patient's bedside. Position changes will not only maintain correct body alignment, thereby reducing strain on the joints, but also prevent contractures, minimize pressure on bony prominences, and promote maximal chest expansion.
  - Try to place patient in a position that achieves proper standing alignment: head neutral or slightly flexed on the neck, hips extended, knees extended or minimally flexed, and feet at right angles to the legs. Maintain this position with pillows, towels, or other positioning aids.
  - To prevent hip flexion contractures, ensure that the patient is prone or side-lying, with the hips extended, for the same amount of time patient spends in the supine position.
  - When the HOB must be elevated 30 degrees, extend the patient's shoulders and arms, using pillows to support the position, and allow the fingertips to extend over the edge of the pillows to maintain normal arching of the hands. **Caution:** Because elevating the HOB promotes hip flexion, ensure that patient spends equal time with the hips in extension (see intervention earlier).
  - When patient is in the side-lying position, extend the lower leg from the hip to help prevent hip flexion contracture.

- When able to place patient in the prone position, move patient to the end of the bed and allow the feet to rest between the mattress and footboard. This will not only prevent plantarflexion and hip rotation, but also prevent injury to the heels and toes. Place thin pads under the angles of the axillae and lateral aspects of the clavicles to prevent internal rotation of the shoulders and maintain anatomic position of the shoulder girdle.
- To maintain the joints in neutral position, use the following as indicated: pillows, rolled towels, blankets, sandbags, antirotation boots, splints, and orthotics. When using adjunctive devices, monitor the involved skin at frequent intervals for alterations in integrity, and implement measures to prevent skin breakdown.
- Assess for footdrop by inspecting the feet for plantarflexion and evaluating patient's ability to pull the toes upward toward the nose. Since the feet lie naturally in plantarflexion, be particularly alert to the patient's inability to pull the toes up. Document this assessment daily.
- Teach patient the rationale and procedure for ROM exercises, and have patient return the demonstrations. Review **High risk for activity intolerance,** earlier, to ensure that patient does not exceed his or her tolerance. Provide passive exercises for patients unable to perform active or active-assistive exercises. In addition, incorporate movement patterns into care activities, such as position changes, bed baths, getting the patient on and off the bed pan, or changing the patient's gown. Ensure that joints especially prone to contracture are exercised more stringently. Provide patient with a handout that reviews the exercises and lists the repetitions for each.
- Perform and document limb girth measurements, dynamography, and ROM, and establish exercise-baseline limits to assess patient's existing muscle mass and strength and joint motion.
- Explain to patient that muscle atrophy occurs because of disuse or failure to use the joint that is often due to immediate or anticipated pain. Eventually disuse may result in a decrease in muscle mass and blood supply and a loss of periarticular tissue elasticity, which in turn can lead to increased muscle fatigue and joint pain with use.
- Emphasize the importance of maintaining or increasing muscle strength and periarticular tissue elasticity through exercise. If unsure about patient's complicating pathology, consult with physician about the appropriate form of exercise for patient.
- Explain the need to participate maximally in self-care as tolerated to help maintain muscle strength and enhance a sense of participation and control.
- For noncardiac patients needing greater help with muscle strength, assist with resistive exercises (e.g., moderate weightlifting to increase the size, endurance, and strength of the muscles). For patients in beds with Balkan frames, provide the means for resistive exercise by implementing a system of weights and pulleys. First determine patient's baseline level of performance on a given set of exercises, and then set realistic goals with the patient for repetitions (e.g., if the patient can do 5 repetitions of lifting a 5-pound weight with the biceps muscle, the goal may be to increase the repetitions to 10 within a week, to an ultimate goal of 20 within 3 weeks, and then advance to 7.5-lb weights).
- If the joints require rest, isometric exercises can be used. With these exercises, teach patient to contract a muscle group and hold the contraction for a count of 5 or 10. The sequence is repeated for increasing numbers or repetitions until an adequate level of endurance has been achieved. Thereafter, maintenance levels are performed.
- Provide a chart to show patient's progress, and combine this with large amounts of positive reinforcement. Post the exercise regimen at the bedside to ensure consistency by all health-care personnel.
- As appropriate, teach transfer or crutch-walking techniques and use of a walker, wheelchair, or cane so that patient can maintain the highest possi-

ble level of mobility. Include significant others in the demonstrations, and stress the importance of good body mechanics.

- Provide periods of uninterrupted rest between exercises/activities to enable patient to replenish energy stores.
- Seek a referral to a PT or OT as appropriate.

**Altered peripheral tissue perfusion** related to interrupted venous flow secondary to prolonged immobility

***Desired outcomes:*** At a minimum of 24 h before hospital discharge, patient has adequate peripheral perfusion as evidenced by normal skin color and temperature and adequate distal pulses ($>2+$ on a 0-4+ scale) in peripheral extremities. Patient performs exercises independently, adheres to the prophylactic regimen, and maintains an intake of 2-3 L/day of fluid unless contraindicated.

- Teach patient that pain, redness, swelling, and warmth in the involved area and coolness, unnatural color or pallor, and superficial venous dilatation distal to the involved area are all indicators of deep vein thrombosis (DVT) and should be reported to staff member promptly if they occur.
- Monitor for the indicators listed above along with routine VS checks. If patient is asymptomatic for DVT, assess for a positive Homans' sign: Flex the knee 30 degrees and dorsiflex the foot. Pain elicited with the dorsiflexion may be a sign of DVT, and patient should be referred to physician for further evaluation. Additional signs of DVT may include fever, tachycardia, and elevated erythrocyle sedimentation rate (ESR). Normal ESR (Westergren method) in males under 50 years is 0-15 mm/h, over 50 years 0-20 mm/h, in females under 50 years is 0-20 mm/h, over 50 years 0-30 mm/h.
- Teach patient calf-pumping (ankle dorsiflexion-plantarflexion) and ankle-circling exercises. Instruct patient to repeat each movement 10 times, performing each exercise hourly during extended periods of immobility, provided that patient is free of symptoms of DVT. Help promote circulation by performing passive ROM or encouraging active ROM exercises.
- Encourage deep breathing, which increases negative pressure in the lungs and thorax to promote emptying of large veins.
- When not contraindicated by peripheral vascular disease (PVD), ensure that patient wears antiembolic hose or pneumatic sequential compression stockings. Remove them for 10-20 min q8h and inspect underlying skin for evidence of irritation or breakdown. Reapply hose after elevating patient's legs at least 10 degrees for 10 min.
- Instruct patient not to cross the feet at the ankles or knees while in bed, because doing so may cause venous stasis. If patient is at risk for DVT, elevate the foot of the bed 10 degrees to increase venous return.
- In nonrestricted patient, increase fluid intake to at least 2-3L/day to reduce hemoconcentration, which can contribute to the development of DVT. Educate patient about the need to drink large amounts of fluid. Monitor I&O to ensure compliance.
- Patients at risk for DVT, including those with chronic infection and a history of PVD and smoking, as well as the aged, obese, and anemic, may require pharmacologic interventions such as aspirin, sodium warfarin, phenindione derivatives, or heparin. Administer medication as prescribed, and monitor appropriate laboratory values (e.g., prothrombin time [PT], partial thromboplastin time [PTT]). Educate patient to self-monitor for and report bleeding (epistaxis, bleeding gums, hematemesis, hemoptysis, melena, hematuria, and ecchymoses).
- In patients prone to DVT, acquire bilateral baseline measurements of the mid-calf, knee, and mid-thigh and record them on patient's cardex. Monitor these measurements daily and compare them to the baseline measurements to rule out extremity enlargement caused by DVT.

**Altered cerebral tissue perfusion** (orthostatic hypotension) related to interrupted arterial flow to the brain secondary to prolonged bed rest

***Desired outcome:*** When getting out of bed, patient has adequate cerebral perfusion as evidenced by HR <120 bpm and BP ≥90/60 mm Hg (or within 20 mm Hg of patient's normal range) immediately after position change, dry skin, normal skin color, and absence of vertigo and syncope, with return of HR and BP to resting levels within 3 min of position change.

- Assess patient for factors that increase the risk of orthostatic hypotension because of fluid volume changes (recent diuresis, diaphoresis, or change in vasodilator therapy), altered autonomic control (diabetic cardiac neuropathy, denervation postheart transplant, or advanced age), or severe left ventricular dysfunction.
- Explain the cause of orthostatic hypotension and measures for preventing it.
- Application of antiembolic hose, which are used to prevent DVT, may be useful in preventing orthostatic hypotension once the patient is mobilized. For patients who continue to have difficulty with orthostatic hypotension, it may be necessary to supplement the hose with elastic wraps to the groin when the patient is out of bed. Ensure that these wraps encompass the entire surface of the legs.
- When patient is in bed, provide instructions for leg exercises as described under **High risk for activity intolerance,** p. 711.
- Prepare patient for getting out of bed by encouraging position changes within necessary confines. It is sometimes possible and advisable to use a tilt table to reacclimate patient to upright positions.
- Follow these guidelines for mobilization:
  - Check the BP in any high-risk patient for whom this will be the first time out of bed.
  - Have the patient dangle legs at the bedside. Be alert to indicators of orthostatic hypotension, including diaphoresis, pallor, tachycardia, hypotension, and syncope. Question patient about the presence of lightheadedness or dizziness.
  - If indicators of orthostatic hypotension occur, check the VS. A drop in systolic BP of 20 mm Hg and an increased pulse rate, combined with symptoms of vertigo and impending syncope, signal the need for return to a supine position.
  - If leg dangling is tolerated, have patient stand at the bedside with two staff members in attendance. If no adverse signs or symptoms occur, have patient progress to ambulation as tolerated.

**Constipation** related to less than adequate fluid or dietary intake and bulk, immobility, lack of privacy, positional restrictions, and use of narcotic analgesics

***Desired outcomes:*** Within 24 h of this diagnosis, patient verbalizes knowledge of measures that promote bowel elimination. Patient relates the return of his or her normal pattern and character of bowel elimination within 3-5 days of this diagnosis.

- Assess patient's bowel history to determine normal bowel habits and interventions that are used successfully at home.
- Monitor and document patient's bowel movements, diet, and I&O. Be alert to the following indications of constipation: fewer than patient's usual number of bowel movements, abdominal discomfort or distention, straining at stool, and patient complaints of rectal pressure or fullness. Fecal impaction may be manifested by oozing of liquid stool and confirmed *via* digital examination.
- Auscultate each abdominal quadrant for at least 1 min to determine the presence of bowel sounds. Normal sounds are clicks or gurgles occurring at a rate of 5-34/min. **Note:** Bowel sounds are decreased or absent with paralytic ileus. High-pitched rushing sounds may be heard during abdominal cramping, indicating an intestinal obstruction.
- If a rectal impaction is suspected, use a gloved, lubricated finger to remove

stool from the rectum. This stimulation may be adequate to stimulate bowel movement. Oil-retention enemas may soften impacted stool.
- Teach patient the importance of a high-roughage diet and a fluid intake of at least 2-3 L/day (unless this is contraindicated by a renal, hepatic, or cardiac disorder). High-roughage foods include bran, whole grains, nuts, raw and coarse vegetables, and fruits with skins.
- Maintain patient's normal bowel habits whenever possible by offering the bedpan, ensuring privacy, and timing medications, enemas, or suppositories so that they take effect at the time of day patient normally has a bowel movement. Provide warm fluids before breakfast and encourage toileting to gain advantage of gastrocolic or duodenocolic reflexes.
- To promote peristalsis, maximize patient's activity level within the limitations of endurance, therapy, and pain.
- Request pharmacologic interventions from physician when necessary. To help prevent rebound constipation, make a priority list of interventions to ensure minimal disruption of patient's normal bowel habits. The following is a suggested hierarchy of interventions:
  - Bulk-building additives (psyllium), bran
  - Mild laxatives (apple or prune juice, milk of magnesia)
  - Stool softeners (docusate sodium or docusate calcium)
  - Potent laxatives and cathartics (bisacodyl, cascara sagrada)
  - Medicated suppositories
  - Enemas
- Discuss the role that narcotic agents and other medications have in constipation. Teach alternative methods of pain control (Table A–6).

**Diversional activity deficit** related to prolonged illness and hospitalization
***Desired outcome:*** Within 24 h of intervention, patient engages in diversional activities and relates the absence of boredom.
- Be alert to patient indicators of boredom, including wishing for something to read or do, daytime napping, and expressed inability to perform usual hobbies because of hospitalization.
- Assess patient's activity tolerance as described on page 711.
- Collect a database by assessing patient's normal support systems and relationship patterns with significant others. Question patient about his or her interests, and explore diversional activities that may be suitable for the hospital setting and patient's level of activity tolerance.
- Personalize the patient's environment with favorite objects and photographs of significant others.
- Provide low-level activities commensurate with patient's tolerance (e.g., books or magazines pertaining to patient's recreational or other interests, television, or writing for short intervals).
- Initiate activities that require little concentration, and proceed to more complicated tasks as patient's condition allows (e.g., if reading requires more energy or concentration than patient is capable of, suggest that significant others read to patient or bring in audiotapes of books, such as those marketed for the visually impaired).
- Encourage discussion of past activities or reminiscence as a substitute for performing favorite activities during convalescence.
- As patient's endurance improves, obtain appropriate diversional activities, such as puzzles, model kits, handicrafts, and computerized games and activities; encourage patient to use them.
- Encourage significant others to visit within limits of patient's endurance and to involve patient in activities that are of interest to him or her, such as playing cards or backgammon. Encourage significant others to stagger their visits throughout the day.
- Spend extra time with patient.
- Suggest that significant others bring in a radio, or, if appropriate, rent a TV

or radio from the hospital, if not part of the standard room charge.
- If appropriate for patient, arrange for hospital volunteers to visit, play cards, read books, or play board games.
- As appropriate for patient who desires social interaction, consider relocation to a room in an area of high traffic.
- As patient's condition improves, assist him or her with sitting in a chair near a window so that outside activities can be viewed. When patients are able, provide opportunities to sit in a solarium so that they can visit with other patients. If the physical condition and weather permit, take patient outside for brief periods of time.
- Request consultation from social services, OT, pastoral services, and psychiatric nurse for interventions as appropriate.
- Increase patient's involvement in self-care to provide a sense of purpose, accomplishment, and control. Performing in-bed exercises (e.g., deep breathing, ankle circling, calf pumping), keeping track of I&O, and similar activities can and should be accomplished routinely by these patients.

**Altered sexuality pattern** related to actual or perceived physiologic limitations on sexual performance secondary to disease, therapy, or prolonged hospitalization

*Desired outcome:* Within 72 h of this diagnosis, patient relates satisfaction with sexuality and/or understanding of the ability to resume sexual activity.
- Assess patient's normal sexual function, including the importance placed on sex in the relationship, frequency of interaction, normal positions used, and the couple's ability to adapt or change to meet requirements of patient's limitations.
- Identify patient's problem diplomatically, and clarify it with patient. Indicators of sexual dysfunction can include regression, acting-out with inappropriate behavior such as grabbing or pinching, sexual overtures toward the hospital staff, self-enforced isolation, and similar behaviors.
- Encourage patient and significant other to verbalize feelings and anxieties about sexual abstinence, having sexual relations in the hospital, hurting the patient, or having to use new or alternative methods for sexual gratification. Develop strategies collaboratively with the patient and significant other.
- Encourage acceptable expressions of sexuality by the patient (e.g., in a woman this could involve wearing makeup and jewelry).
- Inform patient and significant other that it is possible to have time alone together for intimacy. Provide that time accordingly by putting a "Do Not Disturb" sign on the door, enforcing privacy by restricting staff and visitors to the room, or arranging for temporary private quarters.
- Encourage patient and significant other to seek alternate methods of sexual expression when necessary. This may include mutual masturbation, altered positions, vibrators, and identification of other erotic areas for the partner.
- Refer patient and significant other to professional sexual counseling as necessary.

**Altered role performance:** Dependence versus independence

*Desired outcome:* Within 48 h of this diagnosis, patient collaborates with care givers in planning realistic goals for independence, participates in own care, and takes responsibility for self-care.
- Encourage patient to be as independent as possible within limitations of endurance, therapy, and pain. Be aware, however, that temporary periods of dependence are appropriate because they enable the individual to restore energy reserves needed for recovery.
- Ensure that all health-care providers are consistent in conveying their expectations of eventual independence.
- Alert patient to areas of overdependence, and involve him or her in collaborative goal-setting to achieve independence.
- Do not minimize patient's expressed feelings of depression. Allow patient

to express emotions, but provide support, understanding, and realistic hope for a positive role change.
- If indicated, provide self-help devices to increase patient's independence with self-care.
- Provide positive reinforcement when patient meets or advances toward goals.

---

For interventions related to prevention of atelectasis and pneumonia, see appropriate nursing diagnoses in "Respiratory Disorders." See "Stomatitis," p. 379, for interventions for patients with altered oral mucous membrane. See "Pressure Ulcers" for **Impaired tissue integrity** (for patients without pressure ulcers who are at risk because of immobility), p. 687. For psychosocial nursing diagnoses and interventions, see "Caring for Patients with Cancer and Other Life-Disrupting Disorders," p. 753.

---

### Selected Bibliography

American Association of Cardiovascular and Pulmonary Rehabilitation: *Guidelines for cardiac rehabilitation programs,* Champaign, Ill, 1991, Human Kinetic Books.

Baas L, editor: *Essentials of cardiac nursing,* Rockville, Md, 1991, Aspen Publishers.

Borg GV: Psychophysical basis of perceived exertion, *Med Sci Sports Exerc* 14:377-381, 1982.

Erickson H, Tomlin E, Swain M: *Modeling and role modeling: a paradigm for nursing,* Lexington, SC, 1988, Pine Press of Lexington.

Gettrust KV, Brabec PD: *Nursing diagnosis in clinical practice: guidelines for care planning,* Florence, KY, 1992, Delmar Publishers.

Interqual: *The ISD-A review system with adult ISD criteria,* August 1992, Northhampton, NH, and Marlboro, MA, Interqual, Inc.

Kim MJ, McFarland GK, McLane AM: *Pocket guide to nursing diagnoses,* ed 5, St Louis, 1993, Mosby–Year Book.

Marshall JR, Hawrysio A: Inpatient recovery following myocardial infarction and coronary artery bypass graft surgery, *J Cardiovasc Nurs* 2(3):1-12, 1988.

Swearingen PL: *Addison-Wesley photo-atlas of nursing procedures,* ed 2, Redwood City, Calif, 1991, Addison-Wesley.

Underhill S et al: *Cardiac nursing,* ed 2, Philadelphia, 1989, JB Lippincott.

Wenger N, Hellerstein HK: *Rehabilitation of the cardiac patient,* ed 3, New York, 1992, John Wiley & Sons.

Winslow EH: Cardiovascular consequences of bed rest, *Heart Lung* 14(3): 236-246, 1985.

## Section Three: Caring for Patients with Cancer and Other Life-Disrupting Illnesses

### Chemotherapy and immunotherapy

**High risk for injury** (to staff and environment) related to preparation, handling, administration, and disposal of chemotherapeutic agents
*Desired outcome:* Chemotherapy exposure of staff and environment is min-

imized by proper preparation, handling, administration, and disposal by individuals familiar with these agents.

- Ensure that chemotherapy is prepared by pharmacists and administered by nurses familiar with the agents. Keep institutional guidelines readily available for safe preparation, handling, and potential complications, such as spills or individual contact with these drugs. **Note:** A chemotherapy approval course is highly recommended for nurses who will be administering these drugs.
- Ensure that pregnant nurses exercise extreme caution when handling these agents. Check with individual agencies for policies about administration of these drugs by women who are pregnant or are considering becoming pregnant.
- Implement measures to minimize aerosolization and direct contact with these drugs during preparation. These measures include using a biologic safety cabinet, an absorbent pad placed on the work area, latex gloves, full-length gown with cuffed sleeves, and goggles. Gloves and gowns should be worn during all handling and disposing of these agents.
- Prime IV tubing with a 50-ml bag of dilutent, or prime the tubing into a sterile bag, using gauze to absorb excess liquid.
- When removing the IV administration set, wear latex gloves and wrap sterile gauze around the needle to prevent direct contact with the drug. Place all needles, drugs, drug containers, and related material in a puncture-proof container that is clearly marked *Biohazardous Waste*. **Note:** Follow this procedure for disposal of immunotherapy waste as well.
- Wear latex gloves when handling all body excretions for 48 h after chemotherapy because the drug is excreted through urine and feces.
- To clean up a chemotherapy spill, double-glove and wear eye protection and a full-length gown. Use absorbent pads to absorb liquid. Then, cleanse 3 times with a detergent solution. Dispose of all waste in a biohazardous waste container.
- To prevent oral contamination with the drug, avoid any activity in which the hand goes to the mouth (e.g., eating, drinking, smoking) in any area in which the chemical is given or prepared.
- In the event of skin contact with the drug, wash the affected area with soap and water. Notify physician for follow-up care.
- If eye contact occurs, irrigate the eye with water for 15 min and notify physician for follow-up care.

**Impaired tissue integrity (or risk of same)** related to extravasation of vesicant or irritating chemotherapy agents
***Desired outcome:*** Patient's tissue remains intact without evidence of inflammation or pain along the injection site.

---

**Note:** The following vesicant agents have the potential to produce tissue damage: dactinomycin, daunomycin, doxorubicin, mitomycin C, epirubicin, estramustine, idarubicin, mechlorethamine, vinblastine, vincristine, and vindesine. The following irritants have the potential to produce pain along the injection site with or without inflammation: amsacrine, carmustine, dacarbazine, etoposide, plicamycin, streptozocin, teniposide. See Table A-10 for more information.

---

- Ensure that vesicant chemotherapy is administered by a nurse who is experienced in venipuncture and knowledgable about chemotherapy.
- Select the IV site carefully, using a new site if possible. Avoid sites such as the antecubital fossa, wrist, or dorsal side of the hand in which there is an increased risk of damage to underlying tendons or nerves.
- Check patency of the IV before and during administration of the drug. Instruct patient to report burning or pain immediately.
- Give infusions of vesicant drugs through a central venous catheter to mini-

*Text continued on p. 733.*

**T A B L E  A - 10   Common Chemotherapy and Immunotherapy Agents and Colony-Stimulating Factors**

| Classification generic/trade name | Route of administration | Dosage | Acute toxicity | Delayed toxicity | Special precautions |
|---|---|---|---|---|---|
| **Chemotherapy** | | | | | |
| *Alkylating agents* | | | | | |
| carboplatin/Paraplatin | IV | 360–400 mg/m$^2$ day; repeat q28 days<br>100 mg/m$^2$ q daily × 3; repeat q28 days | Nausea & vomiting<br>Anorexia<br>Allergic reaction | Hair loss<br>Taste alterations<br>Mild, reversible increase in liver enzymes<br>Electrolyte abnormalities ($Ca^{2+}$, $Mg^{2+}$, $Na^+$, $K^+$)<br>Myelosuppression<br>Thrombocytopenia<br>Neutropenia | Contraindicated in patients with cisplatinum allergy<br>Have epinephrine, corticosteroids, and antihistamine available<br>Check liver function tests before treatment<br>Check electrolyte, BUN, and creatinine levels before each cycle. Maintain oral intake<br>Creatinine clearance done initially; reduced dosage indicated if creatinine clearance <60 ml/min<br>Myelosuppression is a dose-limiting side effect |

*Continued.*

**Note:** This table is not meant to be comprehensive but rather to provide a quick reference for the most common drugs in clinical practice, including the route of administration, dose, side effects, and precautions. Because the drug dose and schedule of administration vary with each protocol, check individual protocols for additional information and guidelines.

*Vesicant drug: An agent capable of producing tissue damage.

†Irritant drug: An agent that produces pain along the injection site with or without an inflammatory reaction.

‡Given along with certain chemotherapy agents to minimize toxicity.

## T A B L E  A - 10  Common Chemotherapy and Immunotherapy Agents and Colony-Stimulating Factors—Cont'd

| Classification generic/trade name | Route of administration | Dosage | Acute toxicity | Delayed toxicity | Special precautions |
|---|---|---|---|---|---|
| **Chemotherapy—cont'd** *Alkylating agents—cont'd* carboplatin/Paraplatin | | | | | Avoid aluminum needle since it reacts with the drug to form a precipitate Drug unstable at room temperature; infuse within 2 h |
| carmustine/BCNU | IV | 40 mg/m$^2$ for 5 days; 200 mg/m$^2$ single dose | Nausea & vomiting Flushing of skin if infused too rapidly Pain at injection site | Hepatic toxicity Delayed bone marrow depression Skin hyperpigmentation Pulmonary fibrosis Renal damage *Rare:* dizziness, stomatitis, alopecia | Premedicate with antiemetics Report symptoms of pulmonary fibrosis (see p. 37) promptly Monitor liver function tests, BUN, creatinine, CBC, and platelets before each treatment Monitor creatinine clearance, BUN, serum creatinine, |
| cisplatinum/Platinol | IV; intra-arterial intraperitoneal | 20 mg/m$^2$ for 5 days; 120 mg/m$^2$ single dose | Severe nausea & vomiting Anaphylaxis (uncommon) | Nephrotoxicity, neurotoxicity, ototoxicity Bone marrow depression Electrolyte imbalances | Mg$^{2+}$, Ca$^{2+}$, and K$^+$ before each treatment Maintain adequate hydration before, during, and after treatments Maintain urine output at 100 ml/hr before administration and for at least 4 h after; keep fluid intake > output |

| Drug | Route | Dose | Side effects | Nursing considerations |
|---|---|---|---|---|
| dacarbazine/DTIC[†] | IV | 100-200 mg/m² for 5 days; 375 mg/m² single dose | Severe nausea & vomiting<br>Pain at injection site<br>Possible tissue damage with extravasation<br>Bone marrow depression<br>Flulike symptoms<br>Elevated liver enzymes<br>*Rare:* alopecia, anaphylaxis | Premedicate with antiemetics before treatment<br>Keep the following emergency drugs readily available: epinephrine, hydrocortisone, antihistamines<br>This drug precipitates; do not use aluminum needles<br>Stable for 8 h at room temperature |
| cyclophosphamide/Cytoxan | PO; IV | 50-100 mg/m² PO daily; 500-1,500 mg/m² IV q3-4 weeks | Nausea & vomiting<br>Nasal congestion, headache with high doses that are infused rapidly<br>Bone marrow depression<br>Alopecia<br>Hemorrhagic cystitis<br>Amenorrhea and sterility<br>Stomatitis<br>Potentiation of doxorubicin<br>Cardiotoxicity | Premedicate with antiemetics<br>Check CBC, platelets, and liver function enzymes before treatment<br>Keep emergency drugs readily available<br>In the event of extravasation: apply ice for 24 h<br>Fluid intake should be at least 2-3 L/day after treatment<br>Voiding should be frequent to avoid bladder irritation<br>Administer early in day to minimize risk of bladder irritation from not voiding at night |

**TABLE A - 10  Common Chemotherapy and Immunotherapy Agents and Colony-Stimulating Factors—Cont'd**

| Classification generic/trade name | Route of administration | Dosage | Acute toxicity | Delayed toxicity | Special precautions |
|---|---|---|---|---|---|
| **Chemotherapy—cont'd** *Alkylating agents—cont'd* cyclophosphamide‡ Cytoxan—cont'd | | | | Interstitial pulmonary fibrosis Liver dysfunction SIADH with high doses Development of secondary cancer | High doses (>1.5 g) may require IV hydration Maintain I&O for 48 h after treatment Test urine for blood Initiate oral care/saline rinses qid Monitor CBC, liver function tests, BUN, and creatinine before and after treatment |
| ifosfamide/IFEX | IV | 1.2 g/m² daily for 5 consecutive days | Nausea & vomiting | Bone marrow depression Alopecia Hematuria/hemorrhagic cystitis Confusion, lethargy *Rare:* renal impairment, liver dysfunction | Hydrate with at least 2-3L/day Administer mesna before treatment and 4 and 8 h after (or as continuous infusion) to minimize hemorrhagic cystitis Test urine for blood |
| mesna/MESNEX‡ | IV | 20% of ifosfamide dose on a mg/kg basis | Bad taste in mouth | Diarrhea | Give 15 min before ifosfamide, then again after 4 & 8 h |

| | | | | | |
|---|---|---|---|---|---|
| lomustine/CCNU | PO | 100-130 mg/m² q6 weeks | Nausea & vomiting | Anorexia<br>Bone marrow depression<br>*Rare:* hepatic toxicity, stomatitis, alopecia | Give before bed and on an empty stomach to minimize nausea & vomiting<br>Monitor CBC, platelets, and liver function tests |
| mechlorethamine/nitrogen mustard* | IV<br>intracavitary<br>topical | 1.6 mg/m² q3-4 weeks<br>0.8 mg/m²<br>10 mg dissolved in 50 ml sterile water | Severe nausea & vomiting<br>Burning sensation around injection site; tissue damage with extravasation<br>Chills, fever, and diarrhea may occur immediately after drug administration | Bone marrow depression<br>Amenorrhea<br>Skin rash<br>Secondary cancers | Premedicate with antiemetics before administration<br>Never give IM or SQ because severe tissue necrosis would occur<br>Extravasation management (antidote for vesicant):<br>Mix 4 ml 10% sodium thiosulfate with 6 ml sterile water for injection<br>Inject 5-6 ml IV through existing IV line and then SQ with multiple injections<br>Repeat dosing over next several h<br>Apply cold compresses |
| *Antibiotics*<br>bleomycin/Blenoxane | IV; IM; SQ | 10-20 mg/m² weekly or q2 weeks | Mild nausea & vomiting<br>Anaphylaxis | Fever and chills<br>Skin reactions, including rash, dermatitis, hyperpigmentation | Administer test dose of 1-2 U before treatment<br>Premedicate with acetaminophen and diphenhydramine |

**T A B L E  A - 10  Common Chemotherapy and Immunotherapy Agents and Colony-Stimulating Factors—Cont'd**

| Classification generic/trade name | Route of administration | Dosage | Acute toxicity | Delayed toxicity | Special precautions |
|---|---|---|---|---|---|
| *Antibiotics—cont'd* bleomycin/Blenoxane—cont'd | | | | Stomatitis Alopecia Pulmonary fibrosis | Pulmonary toxicity is dose-related; suggested total cumulative dose is 500 U Monitor pulmonary function tests before treatment and after every 100 U Initiate oral care/saline rinses qid |
| doxorubicin/ Adriamycin* | IV | 15 mg/m$^2$ weekly; 20-30 mg/m$^2$ for 3 days; 50-75 mg/m$^2$ q3 weeks | Moderate nausea & vomiting Tissue damage if extravasation occurs Local erythematosus streaking with rapid infusion ("adria flare") | Red urine Alopecia Bone marrow depression Stomatitis Cardiomyopathy Potentiates radiation-induced skin damage | Cardiac toxicity is dose-related; suggested total cumulative dose is 550 mg/m$^2$ Modify dose during radiation to minimize skin reaction Initiate oral care/saline rinses qid Extravasation management: apply ice |
| mitomycin C* | IV | 10-20 mg/m$^2$ repeated once q6-8 weeks | Moderate nausea & vomiting Extravasation causes tissue damage | Bone marrow depression Mouth ulcers Hemolytic-uremic syndrome Pulmonary fibrosis | Extravasation management: apply ice Initiate oral care/saline rinses qid Report symptoms of pulmonary fibrosis (p. 37) |

**Antimetabolites**

| Drug | Route | Dosage | Nausea & vomiting | Toxicities | Patient Care |
|---|---|---|---|---|---|
| 5-fluorouracil/5 FU | IV | 300-450 mg/m² for 5 days; 300-750 mg/m² q week | Mild nausea & vomiting | Bone marrow depression, Stomatitis, Diarrhea, Photosensitivity, Hyperpigmentation, Excessive lacrimation | Initiate oral care/saline rinses qid; Instruct patient in use of sunscreen to protect the skin |
| | intra-arterial | 20-30 mg/kg/day for 4 days, followed by 15/ mg/kg for 17 days | | | |
| methotrexate/ Amethoptrin | PO | 50 mg/m² q week | Nausea & vomiting | Bone marrow depression, Stomatitis, Diarrhea, Photosensitivity, Infertility, CNS reaction with intrathecal administration, *Rare*: hepatic, renal toxicity | Do not administer to patients with BUN >25; Use with caution in patients with third-spacing of fluids because elimination will be decreased, thereby enhancing toxicity; Administer high-dosage (>100 mg/m²) with leucovorin to minimize toxicity; Ensure adequate hydration before, during, and after high-dose administration; Ensure alkaline urine (pH >7) to promote excretion; Teach use of sunscreen during sun exposure; Check serum BUN, creatinine, CBC, platelets, and liver function tests before and after administration |
| | IV, IM | 20-40 mg/m² q week or every other week | | | |
| | intrathecal | 6-15 mg as a single dose or repeated weekly or 2×/week | | | |

*Continued.*

**T A B L E  A - 10  Common Chemotherapy and Immunotherapy Agents and Colony-Stimulating Factors—Cont'd**

| Classification generic/trade name | Route of administration | Dosage | Acute toxicity | Delayed toxicity | Special precautions |
|---|---|---|---|---|---|
| *Antimetabolites—cont'd* | | | | | |
| leucovorin/Wellcovorin (given with high-dose methotrexate)‡ | PO, IM, IV | Dose calculated based on methotrexate dose | | | Dose usually begins 24 h after infusion of methotrexate |
| | | | | | Stress importance of taking all doses as prescribed; give written instructions about dose and schedule |
| | | | | | Provide emergency number in case patient is unable to take doses |
| cytosine arabinoside/ Ara-C | IV SQ, IM | 100-200 mg/m$^2$; high dose = 1.5-4.5 g/m$^2$ 1 mg/kg q12h for 5-7 days | Mild to moderate nausea & vomiting | Bone marrow depression Stomatitis Diarrhea Hepatotoxicity Rash Ocular toxicity Neurotoxicity with high doses | Initiate oral care/saline rinses qid SQ injection may cause pain at injection site; apply warm compresses |
| | intrathecal | 10-30 mg/m$^2$ up to 3×/ week | | | Administer high doses over 1 h to minimize neurologic toxicity Perform neurologic exam before high-dose administration and report signs of cerebellar dysfunction |

| Drug | Route | Dose | Side effects | Nursing/patient care |
|---|---|---|---|---|
| **Plant alkaloids** vinblastine/Velban* | IV | 5-10 mg/m² weekly or every other week | Nausea & vomiting Tissue damage with extravasation Bone marrow depression Alopecia Neurotoxicity (peripheral neuropathy and constipation) Infertility Stomatitis | Steroid eye drops usually given with high doses to minimize ocular toxicity Pyrodoxine (B6) usually given to minimize neurotoxicity with high doses Assess for neurotoxicity before administration Initiate prophylactic bowel regimen to minimize constipation Extravasation management: Mix 1 ml NaCl with 150 U/ml of hyaluronidase Inject 1-6 ml (150-900 U) SQ into the extravasated site with multiple injections Repeat dose SQ over next several hours Apply warm compresses |
| vincristine/Oncovin* | IV | 0.5-2.0 mg/m² weekly or every other week | Neurotoxicity (peripheral neuropathy and constipation) Tissue damage with extravasation | Do not exceed 2.5 mg/dose Assess for neurotoxicity before administration |

*Continued.*

**T A B L E  A - 10  Common Chemotherapy and Immunotherapy Agents and Colony-Stimulating Factors—Cont'd**

| Classification generic/trade name | Route of administration | Dosage | Acute toxicity | Delayed toxicity | Special precautions |
|---|---|---|---|---|---|
| *Plant alkaloids—cont'd* vincristine/Oncovin—cont'd | | | | | |
| etoposide (VP-16)[†] | IV | 50-100 mg/m² for 5 days, repeated q3-4 weeks | Hypotension with rapid infusion Mild nausea & vomiting | Jaw pain Alopecia Bone marrow depression | Initiate prophylactic bowel regimen to minimize constipation Extravasation management: see vinblastine, above |
| | PO | Twice the IV dose rounded to the nearest 50 mg | | Stomatitis Alopecia Bone marrow depression *Rare:* anaphylaxis | Administer over 1-h period to minimize hypotension Monitor BP q15min during infusion Extravasation management: see vinblastine, above |
| *Miscellaneous agents* hydroxyurea/Hydrea | PO | 60-75 mg/m² daily | Nausea & vomiting | Bone marrow depression Renal insufficiency | Ensure adequate hydration (at least 2 L/day) |
| L-asparaginase/Elspar | IV, IM, SQ | 200-1,000 IU/kg daily or 2×/ week | Anaphylaxis Nausea & vomiting | Hepatotoxicity Fever, malaise CNS toxicity Renal dysfunction | Have emergency drugs readily available before administration MD should be available in case of anaphylaxis; drug should be |

| | | | | |
|---|---|---|---|---|
| | | | | administered during the day in hospital setting<br>Record baseline VS; record VS 15 min into infusion and following infusion |
| procarbazine/Matulane | PO | 100-200 mg/m$^2$ daily | Nause & vomiting | Avoid foods with high tyramine content (bananas, fava beans, aged cheeses, yogurt, beer, chianti wine, chocolate, coffee, cola, yeast) |
| | | | Bone marrow depression<br>CNS depression<br>Peripheral neuropathy<br>Amenorrhea<br>Dermatologic reactions | |
| **Immunotherapy**<br>*Biologic response modifiers* | | | | |
| interferon/Intron | IM<br>IV<br>SQ, intralesional | 3 × 10$^6$ U/day<br>30 × 10$^6$ U/day | Flulike symptoms (fever, chills, fatigue, malaise)<br>Anorexia<br>Bone marrow depression<br>CNS toxicity<br>*Rare*: nausea & vomiting, hypotension | Avoid ASA and NSAIDs<br>Premedicate with acetaminophen; administer q4h<br>Anorexia may be dose related; arrange for nutritional consultant<br>Refrigerate after first use |

*Continued.*

## TABLE A-10 Common Chemotherapy and Immunotherapy Agents and Colony-Stimulating Factors—Cont'd

| Classification generic/trade name | Route of administration | Dosage | Acute toxicity | Delayed toxicity | Special precautions |
|---|---|---|---|---|---|
| **Colony-stimulating factors** | | | | | |
| *Granulocyte colony-stimulating factor* | | | | | |
| G-CSF/Filgrastim | SQ, IV bolus | 5 mg/kg | Bone pain (sternum or lower back) Erythema, burning at injection site | Exacerbations of preexisting inflammatory conditions Transient increase in uric acid, LDH, alkaline phosphatase | Bone pain usually controlled with acetaminophen or ibuprofen; if lasts >24 h, further investigation needed for cause of pain Solution must be refrigerated, but use at room temperature to minimize erythema and burning at site Patient should take drug at about same time every day Monitor CBC 2-3×/week; stop if ANC >10,000 mm$^3$ |
| *Granulocyte-macrophage colony-stimulating factor* | | | | | |
| G-MCSF/Sargranostin | IV infusion × 2 h | 250 mg/m$^2$ | Mild flulike symptoms: fever, myalgia, fatigue, anorexia Erythema or phlebitis at injection site Bone pain | Generalized rash | Monitor CBC 2-3×/week; stop if ANC >20,000 mm$^3$ |

mize risk of extravasation. Assess the entry site at frequent intervals. Pain, burning, and stinging are common with extravasation, as are erythema and swelling around the needle site. Do not use blood return as an indicator that extravasation has not occurred, because blood return is possible in the presence of extravasation. Instruct patient to report discomfort at the site promptly.
- Keep an extravasation kit readily available, along with institutional guidelines for extravasation management.
- In the event of extravasation, follow these general guidelines:
  - Stop the infusion immediately, and aspirate any remaining drug from the needle. To do this, first apply latex gloves, then attach the syringe to the tubing and aspirate the drug.
  - Notify physician.
  - Leave the needle in place if an antidote is to be used with the extravasated drug.
  - Attach a syringe containing the recommended antidote, and instill the antidote. Remove the IV needle from the site.
  - If recommended, inject the extravasated site with the antidote, using a TB syringe and a 25-27-gauge needle.
  - Do not apply pressure to the site. Apply a sterile occlusive dressing, elevate the site, and apply heat or cold as recommended.
  - Document the incident, noting the date, time, insertion site of the needle, drug, approximate amount of drug that extravasated, management of the extravasation, and appearance of the site. Check institutional guidelines regarding necessity of photodocumentation. Monitor the site at frequent intervals.
  - Provide patient with information about site care and follow-up appointments for evaluating severity of the extravasation.

**Knowledge deficit:** Chemotherapy and the purpose, expected side effects, and potential toxicities associated with chemotherapy drugs, appropriate self-care measures for minimizing side effects, and available community and educational resources

*Desired outcome:*   Before specific chemotherapeutic drugs are administered, patient and significant others verbalize knowledge about their potential side effects and toxicities, appropriate self-care measures for minimizing the side effects, and available community and educational resources.
- Establish patient's and significant others' current level of knowledge about patient's health status and prescribed therapies.
- Assess patient's and significant others' cognitive and emotional readiness to learn.
- Recognize barriers to learning, such as ineffective communication, neurologic deficit, sensory alterations, fear, anxiety, or lack of motivation. In particular, clarify misunderstandings about the side effects and toxicities of chemotherapy. Define all terminology as needed. Correct any misconceptions.
- Assess patient's and significant others' learning needs and establish short- and long-term goals with these individuals. Identify their preferred methods of learning and the amount of information they would like to receive. Develop a teaching plan based on this information.
- Use individualized verbal and audiovisual strategies to promote learning and enhance understanding. Give simple, direct instructions; reinforce this information frequently.
- Provide an environment that is free from distractions and conducive to teaching and learning.
- Discuss the drugs the patient will receive, including route of administration, duration of treatment, schedule, most common side effects and toxicities, and appropriate self-care. Provide both written and verbal information (see Table A-10).

- Provide emergency phone numbers for use should the patient develop a fever or other side effects.
- Provide materials from educational resources such as the American Cancer Society, National Cancer Institute, and drug companies. Make sure that materials are at a reading level appropriate for the patient.
- Identify appropriate community resources that assist with transportation, costs of care, and skilled care as appropriate.

**Knowledge deficit:** Immunotherapy and its purpose, potential side effects and toxicities, appropriate self-care measures to minimize side effects, and available community and education resources

*Desired outcome:* Before immunotherapy is administered, patient and significant others verbalize understanding of its purpose, potential side effects and toxicities, appropriate self-care measures to minimize side effects, and available community and education resources.

- See first six interventions under **Knowledge deficit** above.
- Provide information about the route of administration, the expected action, and potential side effects. Because these patients often give their own injections of interferon, instruct them in the proper technique and site rotation schedule. Teach patient to record the site and time of administration, side effects, self-management of side effects, and any medications taken. Teach proper disposal of needles.
- Arrange for pharmacy delivery of medication because it must be refrigerated. As appropriate, arrange for community nursing follow-up for additional supervision and instruction.
- Teach patient and significant others to be alert to the following side effects of interferon: fever, chills, and flulike symptoms. Suggest that patient take acetaminophen, with physician approval, to manage these symptoms, but to avoid aspirin and NSAIDs because they may interrupt the action of interferon.
- Teach patient to monitor and record temperature 2 ×/day and drink extra fluids. Anorexia and weight loss, which are dose-related, are other common side effects of interferon. Provide information about nutritional supplementation.
- Provide educational materials that are available through drug companies.

## Venous access devices

**Knowledge deficit:** Purpose and management of venous access device (VAD)

*Desired outcome:* Within the 24-h period before hospital discharge, patient and significant others verbalize understanding about the VAD, including its purpose, appropriate management measures, and potential complications.

- Determine patient's and significant others' level of understanding of the purpose of a VAD. As appropriate explain that the device can be used for administration of drugs, fluids, and blood products and drawing of blood samples and that it eliminates the need for frequent venipunctures.
- Show patient a model of the device and explain the insertion procedure. The silicone elastic atrial catheters and implanted venous ports are inserted in the operating room using local anesthetic. There may be mild discomfort, similar to a toothache, for 48 h after the procedure. Reassure patient that the discomfort responds readily to mild pain medication.
- If possible, introduce patient and significant others to another individual who has the device so that they can see first-hand what the VAD looks like and discuss their concerns.
- Teach patient about VAD maintenance care. Provide both verbal and written instructions, including educational materials provided by the VAD manufacturer. Have patient or significant other demonstrate dressing care, flush-

ing technique, and cap-changing routine before hospital discharge. Make sure patients has 24-h emergency number to call in case of problems.

* For silicone elastic atrial catheter:
  * *Hickman:* Maintenance involves flushing 3 ×/week with 2.5 ml heparin solution (100 U/ml). Care after blood drawing involves flushing with 5 ml normal saline solution followed by 2.5 ml heparin solution (100 U/ml).
  * *Groshong:* Maintenance involves flushing with 5 ml normal saline solution weekly. Care after blood drawing involves flushing with 20 ml normal saline solution.
* For subcutaneous implanted port:
  * *Port-a-cath:* Maintenance involves flushing monthly and after each use with 5 ml heparin (100 U/ml); care after blood drawing involves flushing with 20 ml normal saline followed by 5 ml heparin solution (100 U/ml).
* Discuss potential complications associated with VADs, along with appropriate self-management measures.
  * *Infection:* Teach patient to assess exit site for erythema, swelling, discomfort, purulent drainage, and fever >38° C (100.5° F).
  * *Bleeding:* Teach patient to apply pressure to the site. Instruct patient to notify health-team member if bleeding does not stop in 5 min.
  * *Clot in the catheter:* Teach patient to flush the catheter without using excessive pressure, which could damage or dislodge the catheter (particularly an implanted port). If flushing does not dislodge the clot, instruct patient to notify health-team member. **Note:** It is not unusual for small blood clots or fibrin sheaths to develop on the end of the catheter. The most common manifestation of a fibrin sheath is the ability to infuse fluids with the inability to aspirate blood. Both fibrin sheaths and small blood clots respond readily to urokinase therapy. The usual dose of urokinase is 5,000-10,000 U. The suggested dwell time in the catheter is ≥30-60 min.
  * *Disconnected cap:* Instruct patients to tape all connections and to carry hemostats with them at all times.
  * *Extravasation:* Although this is a relatively rare complication, it can cause severe damage if a sclerosing agent such as adriamycin is involved. Therefore, it is important to instruct patients to report pain, burning, and stinging in the chest, clavicle, port pocket, or along the subcutaneous tunnel during drug administration.

## Radiation therapy

**High risk for injury** to staff, other patients, and visitors related to risk of exposure to sealed sources of radiation such as cesium-137 ($^{137}$Cs), gold-198 ($^{198}$Au), iridium-192 ($^{192}$Ir), iodine-125 ($^{125}$I), or unsealed sources of radiation, such as $^{131}$I or phosphorus-32 ($^{32}$P).
*Desired outcome:* Staff and visitors verbalize understanding about the potential dangers of radiation therapy and the measures that must be taken to ensure safety.

**Note:** Most institutions have a radiation safety committee that assists in providing and enforcing guidelines that minimize radiation risks to employees and the environment (committee guidelines should be kept readily available). The committee approves certain rooms that can be used for patients undergoing radioactive treatment to minimize exposure to employees and other patients.

* Provide patient with a private room, and place an appropriate radiation precaution sign on patient's chart, door, and ID bracelet.
* Follow radiologist or agency protocol for visitor restrictions. Visitors usually are restricted to 1 h/day and should stand 6 ft from the bed.

- Ensure that pregnant women and children under age 18 do not enter the room.
- To ensure optimal care planning, recognize the type and amount of the radiation source. The two major principles are time and distance.
  - *Time:* Plan care to minimize the amount of time spent in the patient's room. Staff members should not spend more than 30 min/shift with patient and should not care for more than two patients with implants at the same time. Staff should perform nondirect care activities in the hall (e.g., opening food containers, preparing food tray, opening medications). Linen should be changed only when it is soiled, rather than routinely, and complete bed baths should be avoided.
  - *Distance:* Maximize distance from the implant (e.g., if the implant is in the patient's prostate, stand at the HOB).
- Wear gloves when in contact with secretions/excretions of all patients treated with unsealed radiation sources, which are radioactive. Flush toilet several times after depositing urine or feces from commode.

---

**Note:**   Urine from individuals with sealed radiation is *not* radioactive and can be discarded in the usual manner. However, patients with implanted $^{125}$I seeds should save all urine so that it can be assessed for the presence of seeds.

---

- Save all linen, dressings, and trash from patients with sealed sources of radiation. They will be analyzed by the safety committee representative before discarding to ensure that seeds have not been misplaced.
- Keep long, disposable forceps and a sealed box in the room at all times in case displaced seeds are found. Caution all staff members to use forceps but never the hands to pick up the seeds.
- Use disposable products for all patients with unsealed radiation. These patients will be radioactive for several days. Cover all articles in the room with paper to prevent their contamination.
- Attach a radiation badge (dosimeter) to your clothing before entering the room to monitor the amount of radiation exposure. According to federal regulations, radiation should not exceed 400 mrem/month. Nurses who care for patients with radiation implants rarely receive this much exposure.

**Knowledge deficit:**   Type and purpose of radiation implant (internal radiation) and the measures for preventing and managing complications

***Desired outcome:***   Before radiation implant is inserted, patient and significant others verbalize understanding of its type and identify measures for preventing and managing complications.

- Determine patient's and significant others' level of understanding of the radiation implant. Explain the following, as indicated:
  - *Afterloading:* The implant carrier is inserted in the operating room, and the radioactive source is inserted later.
  - *Preloading:* Radioactive source is implanted with the carrier.
- Explain that the implant is used to provide high doses of radiation therapy to one area, thereby sparing normal tissue.
- Explain that radiation precautions (see **High risk for injury,** earlier) are required to protect health-care team, other patients, and visitors.
- Explain the following assessment guidelines and management interventions for specific types of implants:

*Gynecologic implants*

  - Explain that the following can occur: vaginal drainage, bleeding, or tenderness; impaired bowel or urinary elimination; and phlebitis. Instruct patient to report any of these signs and symptoms.
  - Teach patient to perform isometric exercises while on bed rest to minimize the risk of contractures or muscle atrophy.

- Explain the importance and rationale for wearing antiembolic hose while on bed rest.
- Explain that ambulation will be increased gradually when bed rest no longer is required (see section "Caring for Patients on Prolonged Bed Rest," p. 711, for guidelines after prolonged immobility).
- Explain that after the radiation source has been removed, patient should dilate the vagina *via* either sexual intercourse or a vaginal dilator to prevent fibrosis or stenosis.

*Head and neck implants*

- After a complete nutritional assessment and assessment of the oropharyngeal area, discuss measures for nutritional support during the implantation (e.g., soft or liquid diet, a high-protein diet, and optimal hydration).
- Teach the signs and symptoms of infection: fever, pain, and erythema and purulent drainage at the site of implantation.
- Encourage patient to take analgesics routinely for pain, rather than wait until pain becomes severe.
- Identify alternative means for communication if patient's speech deteriorates (e.g, cards, magic slate). Consult speech therapist as appropriate.

*Breast implants*

- Teach the signs of infection that may appear over the breast: erythema, warmth, and drainage at the insertion site.
- Teach the importance of avoiding trauma at the implant site and keeping the skin clean and dry to help maintain skin integrity.

*Prostate implants*

- Explain that urinary output will be measured every shift and that staff member will inspect urine for the presence of radiation seeds.
- Caution that patient's linen, dressings, and trash will be saved and examined for the presence of seeds.
- Explain that care givers will limit the amount of time spent at the implant site.

**Knowledge deficit:** Purpose and procedure for external beam radiation therapy, appropriate self-care measures after treatment, and available educational and community resources

***Desired outcome:*** Before external radiation beam therapy is initiated, patient and significant others identify its purpose and describe the procedure, appropriate self-care measures, and available educational and community resources.

- See first six interventions under **Knowledge deficit:** Chemotherapy, p. 733.
- Provide information about treatment schedule, duration of each treatment, and number of treatments planned.
  - Radiation therapy usually is given 5 days/week, Monday through Friday.
  - The treatment itself lasts only a few minutes; the majority of the time is spent preparing patient for treatment. Immobilization devices and shields are positioned before treatment to ensure proper delivery of radiation and minimize radiation to surrounding normal tissue.
- Explain that the skin will be marked to facilitate delivery of radiation to the desired area. Usually small skin tatoos (small pinpoint marks) are used. These tatoos are permanent and are used to ensure precise delivery of the radiation. However, if gentian violet is used, explain the importance of not washing the marks (see **Impaired skin/tissue integrity,** p. 748, for more information). Caution patient that it is important not to use skin lotions or soaps unless approved by radiation therapy.
- Discuss side effects that may occur with radiation treatment and the appropriate self-care measures. Systemic side effects include fatigue and anorexia; however, the most commonly occurring side effects appear locally (e.g., side effects associated with head and neck radiation include mucositis, xerostomia, altered taste sensation, dental caries, sore throat, hoarseness, dysphagia, headache, and nausea and vomiting). See subsequent nursing diagnoses and interventions for more detail about local side effects.

- Provide patient with a written copy of the side effects for his or her site of radiation therapy. Explain that the National Cancer Institute has a book entitled *Radiation and You,* which lists side effects and side effect management.
- Provide information about community resources for transportation to and from the radiation center and for skilled nursing care, as needed.

## General care of patients with cancer

**Activity intolerance** related to decreased oxygen-carrying capacity of the blood secondary to anemia occurring with chemotherapeutic drugs such as chloramphenicol, radiation therapy, or chronic disease

---

**Note:**   For desired outcome and interventions, see this nursing diagnosis in "Iron Deficiency Anemia," p. 484. Review the anemia disorders, p. 483, discussed in "Hematologic Disorders." Advise patient that fatigue and activity intolerance are temporary side effects of chemotherapy or radiation therapy and will abate when therapy has been completed. Stress the importance of good nutrition, vitamin and iron supplements, and intake of foods high in iron such as liver and other organ meats, seafood, green vegetables, cereals, nuts, and legumes.

---

**Body image disturbance** related to alopecia secondary to radiation therapy to the head and neck or administration of chemotherapeutic agents
***Desired outcome:***   Patient discusses the effects that alopecia may have on self-concept, body image, and social interaction and identifies measures that prevent, minimize, or enable adaptation to alopecia.

---

**Note:**   Common chemotherapeutic agents that cause alopecia include actinomycin D, amsacrine, bleomycin, cyclophosphamide, daunomycin, doxorubicin, epirubicin, idarubicin, ifosfamide, teniposide, vinblastine, vincristine, and etoposide (VP 16).

---

- Discuss the potential for hair loss with the patient before treatment.
  - Radiation therapy of 1,500-3,000 rads to the head and neck will produce either partial or complete hair loss. Explain that this hair loss is temporary and that onset usually occurs within 5-7 days, with regrowth beginning 2-3 months after the final treatment.
  - Radiation therapy greater than 4,500 rad usually results in permanent hair loss.
  - Hair loss associated with chemotherapy is temporary and related to the specific agent, dose, and duration of administration. Regrowth usually begins 1-2 months after the last treatment. However, the hair often grows back a different color or texture.
- Explore the impact hair loss has on the patient's self-concept, body image, and social interaction. Recognize that alopecia is an extremely stressful side effect for most patients.
- Encourage the following measures that will minimize the impact or severity of alopecia: using a mild shampoo, hair conditioner, soft-bristled hair brush or a wide-toothed comb; sleeping on a silk pillowcase to minimize hair tangles; decreasing frequency of hairwashing; and avoiding irritants, such as dyes, permanent wave solutions, hair dryers, curling irons, clips, and hair sprays.
- Explain that scalp hypothermia and tourniquet applications during IV infusion may decrease the severity of hair loss. In particular, a significant decrease in alopecia has been found in individuals who use a hypothermia cap.

These techniques are contraindicated in hematologic malignancy and in solid tumors with scalp metastasis because they may prevent adequate absorption of the drug where it is needed.

- Suggest measures that may help minimize the psychologic impact of hair loss: cut the hair short before treatment; select a wig before hair loss occurs, which will enable patients to match color and style of their own hair; wear a hairnet or turban during hair loss to collect hair that falls out; use scarves, hats, caps, and turbans to cover the head; use makeup and accessories to enhance self-concept. **Note:** Wigs are tax deductible and often are reimbursed by insurance with the appropriate prescription.
- Inform patient that hair loss may occur on body parts other than the head, including the axilla, groin, legs, face, and eyes (eyelashes and eyebrows).
- Instruct patient to keep head covered during the summer to minimize sunburn and during the winter to prevent heat loss.
- Provide information about alopecia available through community resources, such as the American Cancer Society.

**Ineffective breathing pattern** related to decreased lung expansion secondary to fluid accumulation in the lungs (pleural effusion)

---

**Note:** For desired outcome and interventions, see this nursing diagnosis in "Pleural Effusion," p. 13. Patients at increased risk for pleural effusion are those with corresponding cancers, including lymphoma, leukemia, mesothelioma, lung and breast cancers, and metastasis to the lung from other primary cancers.

---

**Ineffective breathing pattern** related to decreased lung expansion secondary to pulmonary fibrosis

---

**Note:** For desired outcome and interventions, see this nursing diagnosis in "Pulmonary Fibrosis," p. 38. Some chemotherapeutic agents (e.g., bleomycin sulfate, busulfan, carmustine, chlorozotocin, cytarabine, L-asparaginase, semustine) can cause pulmonary toxicity, an inflammatory reaction that results in fibrotic lung changes, cellular damage, and decreased lung capacity. Pulmonary toxicity also can occur, though much more rarely, with use of cyclophosphamide, chlorambucil, melphalan, mitomycin, methotrexate, mercaptopurine, procarbazine hydrochloride, and zinostatin.

---

**Chronic pain** related to direct tumor involvement; infiltration of tumor into nerves, bones, or hollow viscus; or postchemotherapy or postradiotherapy syndromes
*Desired outcome:* Patient participates in a prescribed pain regimen and reports that pain associated with direct involvement or infiltration of the tumor and side effects associated with the prescribed therapy are reduced or at an acceptable level within 1-2 h of intervention, based on a pain scale of 0-10.

- After patient has undergone a complete medical evaluation of the cause of the pain (Table A-11 and Table A-12) and the most effective strategies for pain relief, review the evaluation and pain-relief strategies with patient and significant others to determine their level of understanding.
- Ongoing assessment of pain is essential and should include the following:
  - *Characteristics* (e.g., "burning" or "shooting" often describes nerve pain).
  - *Location and sites of radiation.*
  - *Onset and duration.*
  - *Severity:* Use a pain scale, and have patient rate pain from 0 (none) to 10 (worst).
  - *Aggravating and relieving factors.*
  - *Previous use of strategies that have worked to relieve pain.*
- Assess patient's and significant others' attitudes and knowledge about the pain

## T A B L E  A - 11   Physiologic Causes of Acute Pain in the Cancer Patient

Tumor compression or infiltration of nerves
Tumor obstruction of hollow viscera or ductal system
Infiltration/obstruction of blood vessels
Exacerbations of alterated body functions unrelated to the cancer (e.g., preexisting
  conditions such as chronic headaches, arthritis)
Pain associated with the treatments
Postsurgical pain, stomatitis, or peripheral neuropathies

## T A B L E  A - 12   Physiologic Causes of Chronic Pain in the Cancer Patient

Tumor that is no longer responding to therapy
Postsurgical pain
Postchemotherapy pain
Postradiation pain
Postherpetic neuralgia
Altered body functions (e.g., chronic arthritis, back pain, or any musculoskeletal dis-
  order)

medication regimen. Many patients and their families have fears related to patient's ultimate addiction to narcotics. Dispel any misperceptions about narcotic-induced addiction when chronic pain therapy is necessary.
- Pharmacologic management of pain is often the mainstay of treatment of chronic cancer pain. Incorporate the following principles:
  - *Administer nonnarcotic and narcotic analgesics in the correct dose,* at the correct frequency, and *via* the correct route. Chronic cancer analgesia often is administered orally, and if pain is present most of the day it should be given around the clock rather than as needed.
  - *Recognize and treat side effects of narcotic analgesia early.* Side effects include nausea and vomiting, constipation, sedation, itching, and respiratory depression. The presence of these side effects does not necessarily preclude continued use of the drug.
  - *Use prescribed adjuvant medications to help increase efficacy of narcotics.* These include tricyclic antidepressants, antihistamines, dextroamphetamines, steroids, phenothiazines, and anticonvulsants.
  - *Monitor for signs and symptoms of tolerance,* and when it occurs discuss treatment with physician. Patients with chronic pain often require increasing doses of narcotics. Respiratory depression occurs rarely in these patients.
  - *Be aware of the potential for physical dependence* in patients taking narcotics for a prolonged period of time. Narcotics should not be stopped abruptly in these patients, because withdrawal may occur.
  - *Evaluate the effectiveness of analgesics at regular and frequent intervals* after administration, particularly after the initial dose.
  - *Use nonpharmacologic approaches* (Table A-6) when appropriate. See discussion in **Pain,** p. 702.

**Constipation** related to treatment with VINCA alkaloid chemotherapy, narcotic analgesics, tranquilizers, and antidepressants; less than adequate intake because of anorexia; hypercalcemia; spinal cord compression; mental status changes; decreased mobility; or colonic disorders

**Note:** For desired outcomes and interventions, see this nursing diagnosis in "General Care of Patients with Neurologic Disorders," p. 305, "Caring for Patients on Prolonged Bed Rest," p. 716, and "Caring for Preoperative and Postoperative Patients," p. 706.

**Note:** These patients should not go more than 2 days without having a bowel movement. Patients receiving VINCA alkaloid are at risk for ileus in addition to constipation. Preventive measures, such as use of senna products (e.g., Peri-Colace or Senokot), especially for patients taking narcotics, are highly recommended. In addition, all individuals taking narcotics should receive a prophylactic home regimen.

**Diarrhea** related to chemotherapeutic drugs, especially antimetabolite agents; antacids containing magnesium; radiation therapy to the abdomen or pelvis; tube feedings; food intolerances; and bowel dysfunction, such as tumors, Crohn's disease, ulcerative colitis, and fecal impaction

**Note:** For desired outcomes and interventions, see this nursing diagnosis, p. 397, and **High risk for fluid volume deficit** related to diarrhea, p. 397, in "Malabsorption/Maldigestion." See "Ulcerative Colitis" for **High risk for impaired perineal/perianal skin integrity** related to prolonged diarrhea, p. 427. Instruct patient to notify health-care member if experiencing more than three loose stools per day.

**High risk for infection** related to inadequate secondary defenses (neutropenia) secondary to malignancy, chemotherapy, radiation therapy, or immunotherapy
***Desired outcomes:*** Patient is free of infection as evidenced by normothermia, BP ≥90/60 mm Hg, and HR ≤100 bpm. Patient identifies risk factors for infection, verbalizes early signs and symptoms of infection and reports them promptly to health-care professional if they occur, and demonstrates appropriate self-care measures to minimize the risk of infection.
• Identify patients at risk for infection by obtaining the absolute neutrophil count (ANC). Calculate ANC by using the following formula:

ANC = (% of segmented neutrophils + % bands) × total WBC count.

  • 1,500-2,000/mm³ ANC = no significant risk.
  • 1,000-1,500/mm³ ANC = minimal risk.
  • 500-1,000/mm³ ANC = moderate risk. Initiate neutropenic precautions.
  • <500/mm³ ANC = severe risk. Initiate neutropenic precautions.
• Assess each body system thoroughly to determine potential and actual sources of infection.
• Monitor VS and temperature q4h. Be alert to temperature ≥38° C (100.4° F) × 2, temperature <35.56° C (96° F) × 1, temperature >38.33° C (101° F) × 1, increased HR, decreased BP, and the following clinical signs of infection: tenderness, erythema, warmth, swelling, and drainage at invasive sites; chills; and malaise. **Note:** Signs of infection may be absent in the presence of neutropenia.
• Place sign on patient's door indicating that neutropenic precautions are in effect for patients with ANC ≤1,000/mm³.
• Instruct all persons entering patient's room to wash hands thoroughly.
• Restrict individuals from entering who have contagious diseases, such as colds or flu.
• Instruct patient to wear a mask when out of the hospital room.

- Notify physician immediately if patient's temperature is >100.4° F × 2, temperature >101° F × 1, or temperature <96° F. Initiate antibiotic therapy as prescribed within 1 h when ANC is ≤500/mm$^3$.
- Implement oral care routine to minimize the risk of infection due to nonintact musoca or tongue. Teach patient to use a soft-bristled toothbrush after meals and before bed (bristles may be softened even more by running them under hot water). Inspect oral cavity daily, noting presence of white patches on the tongue or mucous membrane. Mycostatin swish and swallow or swish and spit may be prescribed to prevent the development of oral candidiasis. Individuals with prolonged neutropenia are at high risk for candidiasis and other bacterial and viral infections. Monitor for vesicles, crusted lesions that may signal herpes simplex. Acyclovir may be initiated, as prescribed, to prevent or minimize herpetic infections in patients with prolonged neutropenia who are at risk for herpes.
- Avoid use of rectal suppositories, rectal temperature, or enemas, to minimize the risk of traumatizing the rectal mucosa, thereby increasing the risk of infection. Be aware that patients with prolonged neutropenia are at increased risk for perirectal infection; monitor for it accordingly. Caution patient to avoid straining at stool. Suggest use of stool softener.
- Implement measures that maintain skin integrity, and instruct patient accordingly: use electric shaver rather than razor blade; avoid vaginal douche and tampons; use emery board rather than clipper for nail care; check with physician before dental care; avoid all invasive procedures; use antimicrobial skin preparations before injections; change IV sites q48h; use steel-tipped rather than plastic catheters (minimizes the risk of infection); use water-soluble lubricant before sexual intercourse and avoid oral and anal manipulation during sexual activities.
- Teach patient to avoid potential sources of infection during periods of neutropenia (e.g., avoid foods with high bacterial count [raw eggs, raw fruits and vegetables, foods prepared in a blender that cannot adequately be cleaned]; bird, cat, and dog excreta; and plants, flowers, and sources of stagnant water).
- Be alert to signs of impending sepsis, including subtle changes in mental status: restlessness or irritability; warm and flushed skin; chills, fever, or hypothermia; increased urine output; bounding pulse; tachypnea; and glycosuria. These symptoms often precede the classic signs of septic shock: cold, clammy skin; thready pulse; decreased BP; and oliguria.
- As prescribed, administer colony-stimulating factors (see Table A-10) to minimize the risk of myelosuppression with chemotherapy, especially for patients with a history of neutropenia with severe infections in the past.

**Altered nutrition:**   Less than body requirements, related to nausea and vomiting or anorexia occurring with chemotherapy or radiation therapy

***Desired outcome:***   At a minimum of 24 h before hospital discharge, patient has adequate nutrition as evidenced by stable weight and a positive or balanced N state.

*For anorexia*

- Monitor for clinical signs of malnutrition. See **Altered nutrition,** p. 673, in "Providing Nutritional Support." Weigh patient daily.
- Assess patient's food likes and dislikes, as well as cultural and religious preferences related to food choices.
- Explain that anorexia can be caused by pathophysiology of cancer, surgery, and side effects of chemotherapy and radiation therapy.
- Teach the importance of increasing caloric intake to increase energy and minimize weight loss.
- Teach the importance of increasing protein intake to facilitate repair and regeneration of cells.
- Suggest that patient eat several small meals at frequent intervals throughout the day.

**T A B L E  A - 13**  **Antineoplastic Agents with Known Emetic Action**

| Mild emetic action | Moderate emetic action | Severe emetic action |
|---|---|---|
| L-asparaginase | hexamethylmelamine | nitrosurea |
| bleomycin | azacytidine | dactinomycin |
| chlorambucil | daunorubicin | cisplatin |
| hydroxyurea | doxorubicin | cyclophosphamide |
| melphalan | etoposide (VP 16) | decarbazine |
| mercaptopurine | 5-fluorouracil (5 FU) | mitomycin-C |
| tamoxifen | procarbazine | methotrexate |
| thioguanine | streptozotocin | mithramycin |
| thiotepa | carboplatin | mechlorethamine |
| vinblastine | | |
| vincristine | | |
| steroids | | |
| cytarabine | | |
| L-phenylalanine | | |

**T A B L E  A - 14**  **Common Antiemetic Agents**

| Agent | Generic name | Trade name |
|---|---|---|
| phenothiazine | prochlorperazine | Compazine |
| steroids | dexamethasone | Decadron |
| antihistamine | diphenhydramine | Benadryl |
| butyrophenon derivatives | haloperidol | Haldol |
| benzodiazepines | lorazepam | Ativan |
| benzamide | metoclopramide* | Reglan |
| serotinin antagonist | ondansetron | ZoFran |

*Metoclopramide blocks the neurotransmitter sites to decrease stimulation of an area in the medulla called the chemoreceptor trigger zone.

- Encourage use of nutritional supplements.
- Consider use of megestrol acetate or hydrazine sulfate medications. These agents have proven to have a positive influence on appetite stimulation and weight gain in individuals with cancer. Consult with patient's physician accordingly.

*For nausea and vomiting*

- Assess patient's pattern of nausea and vomiting: onset, frequency, duration, intensity, and amount and character of emesis.
- Explain to patient that nausea and vomiting are side effects of chemotherapy and radiation therapy. (Nausea and vomiting also can occur with advanced cancer.) See Table A-13 for a list of antineoplastic agents with known emetic action.
- Administer antiemetics (Table A-14) as prescribed. Teach patient to take prescribed antiemetic 1-12 h before chemotherapy and continue to take the drug q4-6h for at least 12-24 h after chemotherapy, continuing for as long as nausea persists.

- Teach patient to eat cold foods or food served at room temperature because the odor of hot food may aggravate nausea.
- Suggest intake of clear liquids and bland foods.
- Teach patient to avoid sweet, fatty, highly salted, and spicy foods, as well as foods with strong odors, any of which may increase nausea.
- Minimize such stimuli as smells, sounds, or sights, all of which may promote nausea.
- Encourage patient to eat sour or mint candy during chemotherapy to decrease the unpleasant, metallic taste.
- Encourage patient to experiment with various dietary patterns:
  - Avoid eating or drinking for 1-2 h before and after chemotherapy.
  - Follow a clear liquid diet for 1-2 h before and 1-24 h after chemotherapy.
  - Avoid contact with food while it is being cooked; avoid being around people who are eating.
  - Eat light meals at frequent intervals (5-6 times/day).
- Suggest that patient sit near an open window to breathe fresh air when feeling nauseated.
- Help patient find the appropriate distraction technique (e.g, music, television, reading).
- Teach patient to use relaxation techniques. See **Health-seeking behaviors:** Relaxation technique effective for stress reduction, p. 54. This technique also may help prevent anticipatory nausea and vomiting.
- Teach patient to stay NPO for 4-8 h if frequent episodes of vomiting occur.
- Instruct patient to sip liquids, such as broth, gingerale, cola, tea, or Jello, slowly; suck on ice chips; and avoid large volumes of water.

**Altered oral mucous membrane** related to treatment with chemotherapy agents (especially antibiotics), antimetabolites, and VINCA alkaloids; radiation therapy to head and neck; and ineffective oral hygiene

---

**Note:** For desired outcome and interventions, see this nursing diagnosis in "Stomatitis," p. 380. Caution patient not to floss teeth in the presence of myelosuppression. For moderate to severe stomatitis, patient may require parenteral analgesics, such as morphine. Patients with xerostomia (dryness of the mouth from a lack of normal salivary secretion) caused by radiation may benefit from chewing sugarless gum, sucking sugarless candy, or taking frequent sips of water. Saliva substitutes are another option, although they are expensive and do not last long. Close dental follow-up is essential because the lack or decrease in salivary fluid predisposes one to dental caries. Fluoride treatment is recommended for these patients.

---

**Pain** related to the presence of cancer or its treatments

---

**Note:** For desired outcome and interventions, see this nursing diagnosis in "Caring for Preoperative and Postoperative Patients," p. 694. Explain that acute pain is of short duration and that relief will occur when the underlying cause is treated.

---

**Impaired physical mobility** related to musculoskeletal or neuromuscular impairment secondary to bone metastasis or spinal cord compression; pain and discomfort; intolerance to activity; or perceptual or cognitive impairment

---

**Note:** For desired outcome and interventions, see this nursing diagnosis in "Osteoarthritis," p. 521. Also see related discussions in "Spinal Cord Injury," p. 232, "General Care for Patients with Neurologic Disorders," p. 298, "Fractures," p. 546, and "Malignant Neoplasms," p. 555. See discussions of care of patients at risk for pressure ulcers, p. 687, and "Caring for Patients on Prolonged Bed Rest," p. 693.

---

**Altered protection** related to risk of bleeding/hemorrhage secondary to thrombocytopenia (for all patients receiving chemotherapy and radiation therapy, as well as those with cancer, particularly that involving the bone marrow)

*Desired outcome:* Patient is free of signs and symptoms of bleeding as evidenced by negative occult blood tests; HR ≤100 bpm; and systolic BP ≥90 mm Hg.

- Identify platelet counts that place individuals at increased risk for bleeding:
  - Platelets 150,000-300,000 μl = normal risk for bleeding.
  - Platelets <50,000 μl = moderate risk for bleeding; initiate thrombocytopenic precautions.
  - Platelets <20,000 μl = severe risk of bleeding; may develop spontaneous bleeding; initiate thrombocytopenic precautions.
- Perform a baseline physical assessment, monitoring for evidence of bleeding, including petechiae, ecchymosis, hematuria, coffee ground emesis, tarry stools, hemoptysis, heavy menses, headaches, and blurred vision. Also monitor VS every shift, being alert to hypotension and tachycardia. Avoid use of rectal thermometer, which can cause rectal bleeding.
- Test all secretions and excretions for the presence of occult blood.
- Perform a psychosocial assessment, including patient's past experience with thrombocytopenia; the effect of thrombocytopenia on patient's life-style; and changes in patient's work pattern, family relationships, and social activities. Identify learning needs and necessity of skilled care after hospital discharge.
- Hang a sign on patient's door, indicating that thrombocytopenia precautions are in effect for patients with platelet count <50,000 μl.
- In the presence of bleeding, begin pad count for heavy menses; measure quantity of vomiting and stool; apply direct pressure to site of bleeding (VAD, venipuncture); and deliver platelet transfusion as prescribed.
- Initiate oral care at frequent intervals to promote integrity of gingiva and mucosa. Advise patient to brush with soft-bristled toothbrush after meals and before bed (hot water run over bristles may soften them further). In the presence of gum bleeding, teach patient to use sponge-tipped applicator rather than toothbrush, avoid use of dental floss, and avoid mouthwash with greater than 6% alcohol content. Suggest use of normal saline solution mouthwashes 4×/day and water-based ointment for lubricating the lips.
- Implement bowel program and check with patient daily for bowel movement. Assess need for stool softeners to prevent constipation; encourage adequate hydration (at least 2 L/day) and high-fiber foods to promote bowel function; and avoid use of rectal suppositories, enemas, or harsh laxatives to minimize the risk of bleeding.
- Implement measures that prevent bleeding. Teach patient to use electric shaver; apply direct pressure for 3-5 min after injections and venipuncture; and avoid vaginal douche and tampons, constrictive clothing, aspirin or aspirin-containing products because of aspirin's antiplatelet action, alcohol ingestion, anticoagulants, and indomethacin (Indocin), which is a GI irritant. Caution patient to perform gentle nose blowing, use emery board rather than clippers for nail care, check with physician before seeking dental care, and avoid bladder catheterization if possible.
- Caution patient to avoid activities that predispose to trauma or injury; remove hazardous objects or furniture from patient's environment. Assist with ambulating if patient's physical mobility is impaired. When the patient's platelet count is <20,000 μl, teach patient to avoid activities involving Valsalva's maneuver, which increases intracranial pressure. These activities include moving up in bed, straining at stool, bending at the waist, and lifting heavy objects. Suggest bed rest if patient's platelet count is <10,000 μl.
- See "Thrombocytopenia," p. 500, for more information.

**Sensory/perceptual alterations:** Auditory and kinesthetic impairment related to use of cisplatinum or VINCA alkaloids

*Desired outcome:* Patient reports early signs and symptoms of ototoxicity and peripheral neuropathy; measures are implemented promptly to minimize these side effects.

- Explain that tinnitus or decreased hearing can occur with use of cisplatinum. It is usually dose related and a result of cumulative side effects. Most commonly, high-frequency hearing loss occurs, although with cumulative doses, speech-frequency hearing range also may be affected. Affected individuals may have difficulty hearing speech in the presence of background noise. Suggest that the patient face the speaker during conversation. A hearing aid also may be helpful. In instances of hearing loss from cisplatinum, which is usually irreversible, refer patient to community resources for the hearing impaired.
- Monitor patient for the development of peripheral neuropathy, which can occur with cisplatinum and vincristine use. The first symptom usually is numbness and tingling of the fingers and toes, which can progress to difficulty with fine motor skills, such as buttoning shirts or picking up objects. The most severely affected individuals may lose sensation at hip level and have difficulty with balance and ambulation. Instruct patient to report early signs and symptoms. Suggest consultation with PT or OT to assist with maintaining function.
- Put individuals at risk for paralytic ileus associated with the neuropathy (i.e., those taking vincristine, vinblastine) on daily bowel checks. Administer stool softeners and laxatives daily if patient has not had a bowel movement within a 48-h period, or as prescribed.

**Sexual dysfunction** (impaired sexual self-concept and infertility) related to radiation therapy to the lower abdomen, pelvis, and gonads; or chemotherapeutic agents, especially actinomycin D, alkylating agents, AMSAcrine, bleomycin, cytarabine, daunorubicin, epirubicin, methotrexate, mitomycin, procarbazine, and vinblastine

*Desired outcome:* Following instruction, patient identifies potential treatment side effects on sexual and reproductive function and identifies acceptable methods of contraception during treatment.

- Initiate discussion about the effects of treatment on sexuality and reproduction. The PLISSIT model provides an excellent framework for discussion. This 4-step model includes the following: (1) **P**ermission—give the patient permission to discuss issues of concern; (2) **L**imited information—provide patient with information about expected treatment effects on sexual and reproductive function, without going into complete detail; (3) **S**pecific **S**uggestions—provide suggestions for managing common problems that occur during treatment; and (4) **I**ntensive **T**herapy—although most individuals can be managed by nurses using the first 3 steps in this model, some patients may require referral to an expert counselor.
- Assess the impact of the diagnosis and treatment on the patient's sexual functioning and self-concept.
- Determine the possibility of pregnancy before treatment is initiated. Pregnancy will cause a delay in treatment. If treatment cannot be delayed, a therapeutic abortion may be recommended.
- Discuss the possibility of decreased sexual response or desire, which may result from side effects of chemotherapy. Encourage patients to maintain open communication with their partners about needs and concerns. Explore alternate methods of sexual fulfillment, such as hugging, kissing, talking quietly together, or massage. In the presence of symptoms related to therapy, such interventions as taking a nap before sexual activity or use of pain or antiemetic medication may help decrease symptoms. Other suggestions include using a water-based lubricant if dyspareunia or fatigue is a problem, changing the usual time of day for intimacy, or using supine or side-lying positions, which require the least expenditure of energy.
- Discuss the possibility of temporary or permanent sterility resulting from

treatment. Explore the possibility of sperm banking for men before chemotherapy treatment or oophoropexy (surgical displacement of the ovaries outside the radiation field) for women undergoing abdominal radiation therapy.

- Teach patients the importance of contraception during treatment and for 2 years after completion of therapy to ensure adequate time for renewal of sperm and to determine the individual's response to treatment.
- Inform patients that healthy offspring have been born from parents who have received radiation therapy or chemotherapy, but long-term effects have not been clearly identified. Suggest that patients have genetic counseling before becoming parents, as indicated.

**Impaired skin integrity** related to pigmentation changes (malignant skin lesions)

***Desired outcome:*** Following instruction, patient verbalizes measures that promote comfort and skin integrity.

- Identify populations at risk for malignant lesions: individuals with primary tumors of the breast, lung, colon/rectum, ovary, or oral cavity; and those with malignant melanoma, lymphoma, or leukemia.
- Identify common sites of cutaneous metastases: anterior chest, abdomen, head (scalp), and neck.
- Inspect skin lesions and note and document the following: general characteristics, location and distribution, configuration, size, morphologic structure (e.g., nodule, erosion, fissure), drainage (color, amount, and character), and odor.
- Monitor for indicators of infection: local warmth, erythema, tenderness, purulent drainage.
- Perform the following skin care for nonulcerating lesions, and teach these interventions to the patient and significant others, as indicated:
  - Wash affected area with tepid water and pat dry.
  - Avoid pressure on the area.
  - Apply dry dressing to protect the area against exposure to irritants and mechanical trauma (e.g., scratching).
  - To enhance penetration of topical medications, apply occlusive dressings, such as Telfa, using paper tape.
  - Teach patient not to wear irritating fabrics, such as wool and corduroy.
- Perform the following skin care for ulcerating lesions, and teach these interventions to the patient and significant others, as indicated:

*For cleansing and debriding*

  - May use half-strength hydrogen peroxide and normal saline solution for irrigation, followed by a normal saline rinse.
  - May use cotton swabs or sponges to apply gentle pressure, thereby debriding the ulcerated area.
  - If the ulcerated area is prone to bleeding, irrigate only, using a syringe.
  - May use soaks (wet dressings) of saline, water, Burow's solution (aluminum acetate), or hydrogen peroxide, for debridement. **Note:** Failure to rinse hydrogen peroxide or aluminum acetate off the skin may cause further skin breakdown.
  - May use wet-to-dry dressings for gentle debridement.

*For prevention and management of local infection*

  - Irrigate and scrub with antibacterial agents, such as acetic acid solution or povidone-iodine.
  - Perform wound cultures as prescribed.
  - Apply topical antibacterial agents as prescribed.
  - Administer systemic antibiotics as prescribed.

*To maintain hemostasis*

  - For capillary oozing, use silver nitrate sticks.
  - For larger surface area bleeding, use oxidized cellulose or pack the wound with Gelfoam or similar product.

## To control odor
- Cleanse wound and change dressings as frequently as necessary.
- Perform cultures and sensitivies of the wound, as prescribed.
- Use antiodor agents (e.g., open a bottle of oil of peppermint or place a tray of activated charcoal) in patient's room.
- Also see "Providing Nutritional Support," p. 665, and "Managing Wound Care," p. 681.

**Impaired skin integrity** and **impaired tissue integrity (or high risk for same)** related to treatment with chemical irritants (chemotherapy)

*Desired outcome:* Before the chemotherapy, patient identifies the potential side effects of chemotherapy on the skin and tissue and measures that will promote comfort and integrity.

---

**Note:** Alterations of the skin or nails that occur in conjunction with chemotherapy are a result of the destruction of the basal cells of the epidermis (general) or of cellular alterations at the site of chemotherapy administration (local). The reactions are specific to the agent used and vary in onset, severity, and duration. The skin reactions include the following: transient erythema/urticaria, hyperpigmentation, telangiectasis, photosensitivity, hyperkeratosis, acnelike reaction, ulceration, and radiation recall.

---

### Transient erythema/urticaria
Transient erythema/urticaria may be generalized or localized at the site of chemotherapy administration. Usually it occurs within several hours after chemotherapy and disappears in several hours. It is caused by the following agents: doxorubicin hydrochloride (Adriamycin), bleomycin, L-asparaginase, mithramycin, and mechlorethamine.
- Perform and document a pretreatment assessment of the patient's skin for posttreatment comparison.
- Assess the onset, pattern, severity, and duration of the reaction after treatment.
- Compare posttreatment findings to those from the pretreatment assessment to determine if the cause of the erythema/urticaria is related to the chemotherapy or to herpes zoster, bacterial or fungal embolic lesions, skin metastasis, allergic reaction, or parasitic infestation.

### Hyperpigmentation
This reaction is believed to be caused by increased levels of melanin-stimulating hormone. It can occur on the nailbeds, oral mucosa, along the veins used for chemotherapy administration, or it can be generalized. It is caused by the following chemotherapeutic agents: doxorubicin hydrochloride (Adriamycin), carmustine, bleomycin, cyclophosphamide, daunorubicin, fluorouracil, and melphalan. In addition, it can occur with tumors of the pituitary gland.
- Inform the patient pretreatment that this reaction is to be expected and that it will disappear gradually when the course of treatment is finished.

### Telangiectasis (spider veins)
This reaction is believed to be caused by destruction of the capillary bed and occurs as a result of applications of topical carmustine and mechlorethamine.
- Inform patient that this reaction is permanent but that the configuration of the veins will become less severe over time.

### Photosensitivity
This reaction is enhanced when the skin is exposed to ultraviolet light. Acute sunburn and residual tanning can occur with short exposure to the sun. Photosensitivity can occur during the time the agent is administered, or it can reactivate a skin reaction caused by sun exposure when the agent is administered in close proximity to the sun exposure. It is caused by dactinomycin, daunorubicin, doxorubicin hydrochloride, bleomycin, dacarbazine, fluorouracil, methotrexate, and vinblastine.

- Assess onset, pattern, severity, and duration of the reaction.
- Teach patient to avoid exposing skin to the sun. Advise patient to wear protective clothing and use an effective sun-screening agent (SPF of 15 or greater).
- In the event that burning takes place, advise patient to treat it like a sunburn (e.g., tepid bath, moisturizing cream, consultation with physician).

## Hyperkeratosis

This reaction presents as a thickening of the skin, especially over the hands, feet, face, and areas of trauma. Hyperkeratosis is disfiguring and causes loss of fine motor function of the hands. It occurs with bleomycin administration and should be considered an indicator of the more severe fibrotic changes in the lungs. This condition is reversible when treatment with bleomycin is discontinued.

- For patients taking bleomycin, assess for the presence of skin thickening and loss of fine motor function of the hands.
- In the presence of skin thickening, be aware that fibrotic changes may be present in the lungs. Assess for this condition accordingly (see "Pulmonary Fibrosis," p. 37).
- Reassure patient that this condition is reversible when bleomycin has been discontinued.

## Acnelike reaction

This reaction presents as erythema, especially of the face, and progresses to papules and pustules, which are characteristic of acne. It occurs with administration of dactinomycin and will disappear when the drug is discontinued.

- Reassure patient that this reaction disappears when treatment with dactinomycin has been discontinued.
- Suggest that patient use a commercial preparation such as benzoyl peroxide lotion, gel, or cream to conceal these blemishes.
- Teach patient about proper skin care.
  - Avoid hard scrubbing.
  - Avoid use of antibacterial soap because the removal of nonpathogenic bacteria on the skin results in replacement by pathogens, which are implicated in the genesis of acne. Use a plain soap, such as Ivory or Camay.
  - Avoid use of oil-based cosmetics.

## Ulceration

This reaction presents as a generalized, shallow lesion of the epidermal layer. It is caused by bleomycin, methotrexate, and mitomycin-C.

- Assess for the presence of ulceration.
- If present, cleanse the ulcers with a solution of ¼-strength hydrogen peroxide and ¾-strength normal saline q4-6h; rinse with normal saline solution.
- Expose the ulcer to the air, if possible.
- Be alert to the presence of infection at the ulcerated site, as evidenced by local warmth, erythema, and purulent drainage.
- Teach patient the treatment and assessment interventions.

## Radiation recall reaction

This occurs when chemotherapy is given at the same time or after treatment with radiation therapy. It presents as erythema, followed by dry desquamation. More severe reactions can progress to vesicle formation and wet desquamation. After the skin heals, it is permanently hyperpigmented. This reaction is caused by doxorubicin hydrochloride, bleomycin, cyclophosphamide, dactinomycin, fluorouracil, hydroxyurea, and methotrexate.

- Teach patient the following skin care routine:
  - Cleanse the skin gently at the site of recall reaction, using mild soap, tepid water, and a soft cloth; pat dry.
  - Use A&D ointment on areas with dry desquamation.
  - If edema and wet desquamation are present, cleanse the area with 1/2-strength hydrogen peroxide and normal saline, and rinse with normal saline solution.

- To promote healing, use hydrocolloid occlusive dressing on noninfected sites to promote healing.
- Teach patient to protect the skin at the site of recall reaction in the following ways:
  - Avoid wearing tight-fitting clothes.
  - Avoid harsh fabrics, such as wool or corduroy.
  - Use mild detergents such as Ivory Snow.
  - Avoid exposing the site of recall reaction to heat and cold.
  - Avoid swimming in salt water or chlorinated pools.
  - Avoid use of all medications (with the exceptions of A&D ointment and topical steroids), deodorants, perfumes, powders, or cosmetics on the skin at the recall site.
  - Avoid shaving the site of recall reaction; if shaving is absolutely necessary, use an electric razor.

**Impaired skin integrity** and **impaired tissue integrity** related to radiation therapy

***Desired outcome:*** Within 24 h of instruction, patient identifies potential skin reactions and the management interventions that will promote comfort and skin integrity.

- Assess the degree and extensiveness of the skin reaction as follows:
  **Stage I:** Inflammation, mild erythema, slight edema.
  **Stage II:** Inflammation; dry desquamation; dry, scaly, itchy skin.
  **Stage III:** Inflammation, edema, wet desquamation, blisters, peeling.
  **Stage IV:** Skin ulceration and necrosis, permanent loss of hair in the treatment field, suppression of sebaceous glands. *Late effects:* Fibrosis and atrophy of the skin, fibrosis of the lymph glands.
- Teach patient the following skin care over the treatment field:
  - Cleanse skin gently and in a patting motion, using a mild soap, tepid water, and a soft cloth. Rinse the area and pat it dry.
  - Apply A&D ointment to skin with stage II reaction.
- For patients with stage III skin reaction, teach the following regimen:
  - Cleanse the area with ½-strength hydrogen peroxide and normal saline, using an irrigation syringe. Rinse with saline or water and pat dry gently.
  - Use nonadhesive absorbent dressings, such as Telfa or Adaptic and ABD, for draining areas. Be alert to indicators of infection.
  - To promote healing, use hydrocolloid occlusive dressings on noninfected areas.
- Teach the following interventions for protecting the patient's skin:
  - Avoid tight-fitting clothing.
  - Avoid wearing harsh fabrics, such as wool and corduroy.
  - Avoid sun exposure.
  - Use gentle detergents (e.g., Ivory Snow).
  - Avoid exposure to heat and cold.
  - Avoid swimming in chlorinated pools or salt water.
  - Avoid using medications, deodorants, perfumes, powders, or cosmetics on the skin in the treatment field.
  - Avoid shaving the hair on the skin in the treatment field; if shaving is absolutely necessary, use an electric razor.
- For stage IV reaction, teach the following interventions:
  - Debride the wound of eschar (necessary before healing can occur).
  - After removing eschar (results in yellow-colored wound), keep the wound clean to prevent infection. Wet-to-dry dressings often are used to keep the wound clean.
  - See interventions for alopecia under **Body image disturbance,** p. 760.

**Impaired swallowing** related to esophagitis secondary to radiation therapy to the neck, chest, and upper back or use of chemotherapy agents, especially the antimetabolites; or obstruction (tumors of the esophagus)

*Desired outcomes:*   Before food or fluids are given, patient exhibits the gag reflex and is free of symptoms of aspiration as evidenced by RR 12-20 breaths/min with normal depth and pattern (eupnea), normal skin color, and the ability to speak. Following instruction, patient verbalizes the early signs and symptoms of esophagitis, alerts health-care team as soon as they occur, and identifies measures for maintaining nutrition and comfort.

- Monitor patient for evidence of impaired swallowing with concomitant respiratory difficulties.
- Teach patient the early signs and symptoms of esophagitis and the importance of reporting them promptly to the staff if they occur: sensation of lump in the throat with swallowing, difficulty with swallowing solid foods, discomfort or pain with swallowing.
- Monitor patient's dietary intake and provide the following guidelines: maintain a high-protein diet; eat foods that are soft and bland; add milk or milk products to the diet to coat the esophageal lining (for individuals without excessive mucus production); and add sauces and creams to foods, which may facilitate swallowing.
- Ensure an adequate fluid intake of at least 2 L/day.
- Implement the following measures that promote comfort and discuss them with the patient accordingly:
  - Use a local anesthetic, as prescribed, to minimize pain with meals. Lidocaine 2% or diclone and diphenhydramine may be taken *via* swish and swallow before eating. **Caution:** These anesthetics may decrease the patient's gag reflex.
  - Suggest that patient sit in an upright position during meals and for 15-30 min after eating.
  - Mild analgesics, such as liquid ASA or acetaminophen, can be very helpful. Administer them as prescribed.
  - For severe discomfort, narcotic analgesics may be required. Administer as prescribed. **Note:** If pain is severe or persistent, a barium swallow may be performed to evaluate for the presence of an infection. Common causative agents are *Candida* and herpes. Appropriate medical treatment, such as low-dose amphotericin, ketoconazole, or acyclovir, may be initiated.
  - Encourage frequent oral care with normal saline or sodium bicarbonate solution.
  - Teach patient to avoid irritants such as alcohol, tobacco, and alcohol-based commercial mouthwashs.
- Keep suction equipment readily available in case patient experiences aspiration. Educate patient about ways to manage oral secretions.
  - Suction mouth as needed, using low, continuous suction equipment.
  - Expectorate saliva into tissues and dispose of tissues in nearby waste cans.

**Altered cardiopulmonary tissue perfusion** related to interrupted blood flow secondary to pericardial tamponade

---

**Note:**   Pericardial tamponade may be caused by an accumulation of fluid in the pericardial space, tumor, invasion of the mediastinum, pericardial fibrosis, or effusion from radiotherapy. Patients at increased risk for pericardial tamponade include those with corresponding cancers, such as mesothelioma, sarcoma, leukemia, lymphoma, melanoma, primary GI cancer, and metastatic lung and breast tumors. For desired outcome and interventions, see this nursing diagnosis in "Pericarditis," p. 65.

---

**Altered peripheral tissue perfusion** related to interrupted blood flow secondary to lymphedema
*Desired outcome:*   Following intervention/treatment, patient exhibits adequate peripheral perfusion as evidenced by edema <2+ on a 0-4+ scale, pe-

ripheral pulses >2+ on a 0-4+ scale, normal skin color, decreasing or stable circumference of edematous site, bilaterally equal sensation, and ability to perform complete ROM in the involved extremity.

---

**Note:**   Patient populations at risk include those who have had a radical mastectomy, lymph node dissection (upper and lower extremities), blockage of the lymphatic system from tumor burden, radiation therapy to the lymphatic system, or any combination of these.

---

- Assess the involved extremity for the degree of edema, quality of the peripheral pulses, color, circumference, sensation, and ROM.
- Assess for signs of infection: tenderness, erythema, and warmth at the edematous site.
- Elevate and position the involved extremity on a pillow in slight abduction.
- Encourage wearing of loose-fitting clothing.
- Consult with PT and physician about development of exercise plan for ensuring mobility. Suggest use of elastic bandages to promote a decrease in mild, chronic lymphedema, or use of compressive bandages for more severe cases of swelling.

**Altered urinary elimination** related to hemorrhagic cystitis secondary to cyclophosphamide/ifosfamide treatment; oliguria or renal toxicity secondary to cisplatinum or high-dose methotrexate administration; renal calculi secondary to hyperuricemia; or dysuria secondary to cystitis

***Desired outcomes:***   Patients receiving cyclophosphamide/ifosfamide test negatively for blood in their urine, and patients receiving cisplatinum exhibit urine output of ≥100 ml/h 1 h before treatment and 4-12 h after treatment. Patients with leukemia and lymphomas and those taking methotrexate exhibit urine pH of 7.5.

- Ensure adequate hydration during treatment and for at least 24 h after treatment for patients taking cyclophosphamide (Cytoxan), ifosfamide, methotrexate, and cisplatinum. Teach patient the importance of drinking at least 2-3 L/day. IV hydration also may be required, especially with high-dose chemotherapy.
- Administer cyclophosphamide early in the day to minimize the retention of antimetabolites in the bladder during the night. Encourage patients to void q2h during the day and before going to bed. Test urine for the presence of blood, and report positive results to physician. Monitor I&O q8h during high-dose treatment for 48 h posttreatment. Be alert to decreasing urinary output.
- Mesna is administered before ifosfamide and then 4 h and 8 h after the infusion (or *via* a continuous infusion) to minimize the risk of hemorrhagic cystitis. Test all urine for the presence of blood. Promote fluid intake to maintain urine output at 100 ml/h. Monitor I&O during infusion and for 24 h after therapy to ensure that this level of urinary output is attained.
- For patients receiving cisplatinum, prehydrate with ≥150-200 ml/h of IV fluid. Cisplatinum can be administered as soon as the patient's urine output is ≥100-150 ml/h. Monitor I&O qh for 4-12 h after therapy to ensure that urine output is maintained at ≥100-150 ml/h. Patients may require diuretics to maintain this output. Promote fluid intake to ensure a positive fluid state for at least 24 h after treatment, especially for patients taking diuretics. Notify physician promptly if urine output drops to <100 ml/h. Urine output should be kept at a relatively high level because nephrotoxicity can occur as a side effect of this treatment.
- An alkaline urine will enhance excretion of methotrexate and of the uric acid that results from tumor lysis, which is associated with leukemia and lymphoma. Monitor I&O q8h, being alert to a decreasing output, and test urine pH with each voiding to ensure that it is 7.5. Sodium bicarbonate or acet-

azolamide (Diamox) will be used to alkalinize the urine. Allopurinol prevents uric acid formation and is often administered before chemotherapy for patients with leukemia or lymphoma.

- Renal calculi can occur as a result of hyperuricemia due to chemotherapy treatment for leukemia and lymphoma, which causes rapid cell lysis and increased excretion of uric acid. For more information, see "Renal Calculi," p. 123, and "Ureteral Calculi," p. 147.
- Teach patient the signs of cystitis, which can occur as a result of cyclophosphamide and ifosfamide treatment: fever, pain with urination, malodorous or cloudy urine, and urinary frequency and urgency. Instruct patient to notify health-care professional if these signs and symptoms occur.

---

**Note:**   In addition, see nursing diagnoses and interventions in "Pneumonia," p. 9, and "Atelectasis," p. 2 (for patients with myelosuppression); "Pulmonary Fibrosis," p. 38, (for patients on bleomycin therapy); "Heart Failure," p. 61 (for patients experiencing cardiotoxicity and who are on chemotherapeutic agents, such as doxorubicin or daunorubicin); and "Hepatic and Biliary Disorders," p. 454 (for patients on hepatotoxic medications such as cyclophosphamide and methotrexate).

---

## Psychosocial care for the patient

**Knowledge deficit:**   Current health status and therapies
***Desired outcome:***   Before invasive procedure, surgical procedure, or hospital discharge (as appropriate), patient verbalizes understanding about his or her current health status and therapies.

- Assess patient's current level of knowledge about his or her health status.
- Assess cognitive and emotional readiness to learn.
- Recognize barriers to learning, such as ineffective communication, neurologic deficit, sensory alterations, fear, anxiety, or lack of motivation.
- Assess learning needs, and establish short- and long-term goals.
- Use individualized verbal or written information to promote learning and enhance understanding. Give simple, direct instructions. As indicated, use audiovisual tools as supplemental information.
- Encourage significant others to reinforce correct information about diagnosis and therapies to the patient.
- As appropriate, facilitate referral of neurologically impaired patient to neurologic clinical nurse specialist or neuropsychologist.
- Encourage patient's interest in health-care information by planning care collaboratively. Explain rationale for care and therapies.
- Interact frequently with patient to evaluate comprehension of information given. Ask patient to repeat what he or she has been told. Individuals in crisis often need repeated explanations before information can be understood. Also be aware that many individuals may not understand seemingly simple medical terms (e.g., *terminal, malignant, constipation*).
- As appropriate, assess understanding of informed consent. Assist patient to use information he or she receives to make informed health-care decisions (e.g., about invasive procedures, surgery, resuscitation).

**Anxiety** related to actual or perceived threat of death, change in health status, threat to self-concept or role, unfamiliar people and environment, or the unknown
***Desired outcomes:***   Within 1-2 h of intervention, patient's anxiety is absent or reduced as evidenced by patient's verbalization of same, HR ≤100 bpm, RR ≤20 breaths/min, and an absence of or decrease in irritability and restlessness.

- Engage in honest communication with the patient; provide empathetic un-

derstanding. Actively listen and establish an atmosphere that allows free expression.
- Assess the patient's level of anxiety. Be alert to verbal and nonverbal cues.
  - *Mild:* Restlessness, irritability, increase in questions, focusing on the environment.
  - *Moderate:* Inattentiveness, expressions of concern, narrowed perceptions, insomnia, increased HR.
  - *Severe:* Expressions of feelings of doom, rapid speech, tremors, poor eye contact. Patient may be preoccupied with the past; unable to understand the present; and may have tachycardia, nausea, and hyperventilation.
  - *Panic:* Inability to concentrate or communicate, distortion of reality, increased motor activity, vomiting, tachypnea.
- For patients with severe anxiety or panic state, refer to psychiatric clinical nurse specialist or other health-team members as appropriate.
- If patient is hyperventilating, encourage slow, deep breaths by having patient mimic your own breathing pattern.
- Validate the nursing assessment of anxiety with the patient (e.g., "You seem distressed; are you feeling uncomfortable now?").
- After an episode of anxiety, review and discuss with patient the thoughts and feelings that led to the episode.
- Identify coping behaviors currently being used by patient (e.g., denial, anger, repression, withdrawal, daydreaming, or dependence on narcotics, sedatives, or tranquilizers). Review coping behaviors patient has used in the past. Assist patient with using adaptive coping to manage anxiety (e.g., "I understand that your wife reads to you to help you relax. Would you like to spend a part of each day alone with her?").
- Encourage patient to express fears, concerns, and questions (e.g., "I know this room looks like a maze of wires and tubes; please let me know when you have any questions").
- Reduce sensory overload by providing an organized, quiet environment (see **Sensory/perceptual alterations,** p. 755).
- Introduce self and other health-care team members; explain each individual's role as it relates to the patient's care.
- Teach patient relaxation and imagery techniques. See **Health-seeking behaviors:** Relaxation technique effective for stress reduction, p. 54.
- Enable support persons to be in attendance whenever possible.
- Engage in and promote awareness of touch to significant others when appropriate. Kinds of touch are described in Table A-15.

---

## T A B L E  A - 15  Kinds of Touch

*Instrumental touch*
Task or procedure related
May be negatively perceived but accepted as impersonal

*Affective touch*
Expressive, personal
Caring
Comforting
May be positively or negatively perceived
Influenced by cultural patterns

*Therapeutic touch*
A deliberate intervention to accomplish a purpose (e.g., massage, acupressure)
Use of space around the individual to mobilize energy fields

---

**Impaired verbal communication** related to neurologic or anatomic deficit, psychologic or physical barriers (e.g., tracheostomy, intubation), or cultural or developmental differences

*Desired outcome:*    At the time of intervention, patient communicates needs and feelings and relates decreased or absent feelings of frustration over communication barriers.

- Assess cause of the impaired communication (e.g., tracheostomy, cerebrovascular accident, cerebral tumor, Guillain-Barré syndrome).
- Along with patient and significant others, assess patient's ability to read, write, and comprehend English. If patient speaks a language other than English, collaborate with English-speaking family member or an interpreter to establish effective communication.
- When communicating with patient, use eye contact; speak in a clear, normal tone of voice; and face the patient.
- If patient is unable to speak because of a physical barrier (e.g., tracheostomy, wired mandibles) provide reassurance and acknowledge his or her frustration (e.g., "I know this is frustrating for you, but please do not give up. I want to understand you").
- Provide slate, word cards, pencil and paper, alphabet board, pictures, or other device to assist patient with communication. Adapt the call system to meet the patient's needs. Document the meaning of the patient's signals in response to questions.
- Explain the source of the patient's communication impairment to significant others; teach them effective communication alternatives (see above).
- Be alert to nonverbal messages, such as facial expressions, hand movements, and nodding of the head. Validate their meaning with patient.
- Recognize that the inability to speak may foster maladaptive behaviors. Encourage patient to communicate needs; reinforce independent behaviors.
- Be honest with patient; do not relate understanding if you are unable to interpret patient's communication.

**Sensory/perceptual alterations** related to therapeutically or socially restricted environment; psychologic stress; altered sensory reception, transmission, or integration; or chemical alteration

*Desired outcomes:*    At the time of intervention, patient verbalizes orientation to person, place, and time; relates the ability to concentrate; and expresses satisfaction with the degree and type of sensory stimulation being received.

- Assess factors contributing to patient's sensory-perceptual alteration.
  - *Environmental:* Excessive noise in the environment; constant, monotonous noise; restricted environment (immobility, traction, isolation); social isolation (restricted visitors, impaired communication); therapies.
  - *Physiologic:* Altered organ function, sleep or rest pattern disturbance, medication, previous history of altered sensory perception.
- Determine the appropriate sensory stimulation needed for the patient, and plan care accordingly.
- Control factors that contribute to environmental overload (e.g., avoid constant lighting [maintain day/night patterns]; decrease noise whenever possible [decrease alarm volumes, avoid loud talking, keep room door closed, provide earplugs]).
- Provide meaningful sensory stimulation.
  - Display clocks, large calendars, and meaningful photographs and objects from home.
  - Depending on patient preference, provide a radio, music, reading materials, and tape recordings of family and significant others. Earphones help to block out external stimuli.
  - Position patient to look toward window when possible.
  - Discuss current events, time of day, holidays, and topics of interest during patient care activities (e.g., "Good morning, Mr. Smith. I'm Ms.

Stone, your nurse for the afternoon and evening, 3 PM to 11 PM. It's sunny outside. Today is the first day of summer").
- As needed, orient patient to surroundings. Direct patient to reality as necessary.
- Establish personal contact by touch to help promote and maintain patient's contact with the real environment.
- Encourage significant others to communicate with patient frequently, using a normal tone of voice.
- Convey concern and respect for the patient. Introduce self, and call patient by name.
- Stimulate patient's vision with mirrors, colored decorations, and pictures.
- Stimulate patient's sense of taste with sweet, salty, and sour substances as allowed.
- Encourage use of eyeglasses and hearing aids.
- Inform patient before initiating therapies and using equipment.
- Encourage patient to participate in health-care planning and decision making whenever possible. Allow for choice when possible.
- Assess patient's sleep-rest pattern to evaluate its contribution to the sensory-perceptual disorder. Ensure that patient attains at least 90 min of uninterrupted sleep as frequently as possible. For more information, see next nursing diagnosis.

**Sleep pattern disturbance** related to environmental changes, illness, therapeutic regimen, pain, immobility, or psychologic stress
***Desired outcomes:*** After discussion, patient identifies factors that promote sleep. Within 8 h of intervention, patient attains 90-min periods of uninterrupted sleep and verbalizes satisfaction with his or her ability to rest.
- Assess patient's usual sleeping patterns (e.g., bedtime routine, hours of sleep per night, sleeping position, use of pillows and blankets, napping during the day, nocturia).
- Explore relaxation techniques that promote patient's rest/sleep (e.g., imagining relaxing scenes, listening to soothing music or taped stories, using muscle relaxation exercises).
- Identify causative factors and activities that contribute to patient's insomnia, awaken patient, or adversely affect sleep patterns (e.g., pain, anxiety, therapies, depression, hallucinations, medications, underlying illness, sleep apnea, respiratory disorder, caffeine, fear).
- Organize procedures and activities to allow for 90-min periods of uninterrupted rest/sleep. Limit visiting during these periods.
- Whenever possible, maintain a quiet environment by providing earplugs or decreasing alarm levels. The use of "white noise" (i.e., low-pitched, monotonous sounds: electric fan, soft music) may facilitate sleep. Dim the lights for a period of time each day by drawing the drapes or providing blindfolds.
- If appropriate, put limitations on patient's daytime sleeping. Attempt to establish regularly scheduled daytime activity (e.g., ambulation, sitting in chair, active ROM), which may promote nighttime sleep.
- Investigate and provide nonpharmacologic comfort measures that are known to promote patient's sleep (see Table A-8).

**Fear** related to separation from support systems, unfamiliarity with environment or therapeutic regimen, or loss of sense of control
***Desired outcomes:*** Following intervention, patient communicates fears and concerns and relates the attainment of increased psychologic and physical comfort.
- Assess patient's perceptions of the environment and health status and determine factors contributing to patient's feelings of fear. Evaluate patient's verbal and nonverbal responses.
- Acknowledge patient's fears (e.g., "I understand that this equipment frightens you, but it is necessary to help you breathe").

- Provide opportunities for patient to express fears and concerns (e.g., "You seem very concerned about receiving more blood today"). Listen actively to the patient. Recognize that anger, denial, occasional withdrawal, and demanding behaviors may be coping responses.
- Encourage patient to ask questions and gather information about the unknown. Provide ongoing information about equipment, therapies, and routines according to patient's ability to understand.
- To promote an increased sense of control, encourage patient to participate in and plan care whenever possible. Provide continuity of care by establishing a routine and arranging for consistent care givers whenever possible. Appoint a primary nurse and associate nurses.
- Discuss with health-care team members the appropriateness of medication therapy for patients with disabling fear or anxiety.
- Explore patient's desire for spiritual or psychologic counseling.
- When there is a possibility of surviving the illness or surgery, collaborate with physician about a visit by another individual with the same disorder who has survived the surgery or disorder.

**Ineffective individual coping** related to health crisis, sense of vulnerability, or inadequate support systems

*Desired outcomes:*   Within 24 h of this diagnosis, patient verbalizes feelings, identifies strengths and coping behaviors, and does not demonstrate ineffective coping behaviors.

- Assess patient's perceptions and ability to understand current health status.
- Establish honest communication with the patient (e.g., "Please tell me what I can do to help you"). Assist patient with identifying strengths, stressors, inappropriate behaviors, and personal needs.
- Support positive coping bahaviors (e.g., "I see that reading that book seems to help you relax").
- Provide opportunities for the patient to express concerns; gather information from nurses and other support systems. Provide patient with explanations about prescribed routine, therapies, and equipment. Acknowledge patient's feelings and assessment of current health status and environment.
- Identify factors that inhibit patient's ability to cope (e.g., unsatisfactory support system, knowledge deficit, grief, fear).
- Recognize maladaptive coping behaviors (e.g., severe depression; dependence on narcotics, sedatives, or tranquilizers; hostility; violence; suicidal ideations). Confront patient about these behaviors (e.g., "You seem to be requiring more pain medication. Are you experiencing more physical pain, or does it help you to remove yourself from reality?"). Refer patient to psychiatric liaison, clinical nurse specialist, or clergy, as appropriate.
- As patient's condition allows, assist with reducing anxiety. See **Anxiety,** p. 753.
- Help reduce patient's sensory overload by maintaining an organized, quiet environment. See **Sensory/perceptual alterations,** p. 755.
- Encourage regular visits by significant others. Encourage them to engage in conversation with patient to help minimize patient's emotional and social isolation.
- Assess significant others' interactions with patient. Attempt to mobilize support systems by involving them in patient care whenever possible.
- As appropriate, explain to significant others that increased dependency, anger, and denial may be adaptive coping behaviors used by patient in early stages of crisis until effective coping behaviors are learned.

**Anticipatory grieving** related to perceived potential loss of physiologic well being (e.g., expected loss of body function or body part, changes in self-concept or body image, or terminal illness)

*Desired outcomes:*   Following intervention, patient and significant other(s) express grief, participate in decisions about the future, and communicate concerns to health-care team members and to one another.

## T A B L E  A - 16    Stages of Grieving

| | |
|---|---|
| Protest stage | Denial: "No, not me" |
| | Disbelief: "But I just saw her this morning" |
| | Anger |
| | Hostility |
| | Resentment |
| | Bargaining to postpone loss |
| | Appeal for help to recover loss |
| | Loud complaints |
| | Altered sleep and appetite |
| Disorganization | Depression |
| | Withdrawal |
| | Social isolation |
| | Psychomotor retardation |
| | Silence |
| Reorganization | Acceptance of loss |
| | Development of new interests and attachments |
| | Restructuring of life-style |
| | Return to preloss level of functioning |

- Assess factors contributing to anticipated loss.
- Assess and accept patient's behavioral response. Expect reactions such as disbelief, denial, guilt, anger, and depression. Determine patient's stage of grieving as described in Table A-16.
- Assess spiritual, religious, and sociocultural expectations related to loss (e.g., "Is religion an important part of your life? How do you and your family deal with serious health problems?"). Refer to the clergy or community support groups as appropriate.
- Encourage patient and significant others to share their concerns (e.g., "Is there anything you'd like to talk about today?"). Also respect their desire not to speak.
- Demonstrate empathy (e.g., "This must be a very difficult time for you and your family"). Touch when appropriate (see Table A-15).
- In selected circumstances, provide individuals with an explanation of the grieving process. This approach may help them better understand and acknowledge their feelings.
- Assess grief reactions of patient and significant others and identify those individuals who may have a potential for dysfunctional grieving reactions (e.g., absence of emotion, hostility, avoidance). If the potential for dysfunctional grieving is present, refer the individual to psychiatric clinical nurse specialist, clergy, or other as appropriate.
- When appropriate, assess patient's wishes about tissue donation.

**Dysfunctional grieving** related to loss of physiologic well-being or chronic fatal illness

*Desired outcomes:*   Within 24 h of this diagnosis, patient and significant other(s) express grief, explain the meaning of the loss, and communicate concerns with each other. The patient completes necessary self-care activities.

- Assess grief stage (see Table A-16) and previous coping abilities. Discuss with patient and significant others their feelings, the meaning of the loss, and their goals (e.g., "How do you feel about your condition/illness? What do you hope to accomplish in these next few days/weeks?").
- Acknowledge and permit anger; set limits on the expression of anger to dis-

courage destructive behavior (e.g., "I understand that you must feel very angry, but for the safety of others, you may not throw equipment").

- Identify suicidal behavior (e.g., severe depression, statements of intent, suicide plan, previous history of suicide attempt). Ensure patient safety, and refer patient to psychiatric clinical nurse specialist, psychiatrist, clergy, or other support system.
- Encourage patient and significant others to participate in daily and diversional activities. Identify physiologic problems related to loss (e.g., eating or sleeping disorders), and intervene accordingly.
- When there is a possibility of the patient's surviving of the illness, collaborate with physician about a visit by another individual with the same disorder who has survived the surgery or illness.

**Powerlessness** related to health-care environment or illness-related regimen

*Desired outcomes:* Within 24 h of this diagnosis, patient makes decisions about care and therapies and relates an attitude of realistic hope and a sense of self-control.

- Assess with patient personal preferences, needs, values, and attitudes.
- Before providing information, assess patient's knowledge and understanding of his or her condition and care.
- Recognize patient's expressions of fear, lack of response to events, and lack of interest in information, any of which may signal patient's sense of powerlessness.
- Evaluate care giver practices, and adjust them to support patient's sense of control (e.g., if the patient always bathes in the evening to promote relaxation before bedtime, modify the care plan to include an evening bath rather than follow the hospital routine of giving a morning bath).
- Assist patient with identifying and ask patient to demonstrate activities he or she can perform independently.
- Whenever possible, offer alternatives related to routine hygiene, diet, diversional activities, visiting hours, and treatment times.
- Ensure patient's privacy and preserve his or her territorial rights whenever possible (e.g., when distant relatives and casual acquaintances request information about the patient's status, check with patient and family members before sharing that information).
- Discourage patient's dependency on staff. Avoid overprotection and parenting behaviors toward patient.
- Assess support systems; enable significant others to be involved in patient care whenever possible.
- Offer realistic hope for the future. On occasion, encourage patient to direct thoughts beyond the present.
- Provide referrals to clergy and other support systems as appropriate.

**Spiritual distress** related to separation from religious ties or cultures or challenged belief and value system

*Desired outcomes:* Within 24 h of this diagnosis, patient verbalizes his or her religious beliefs and expresses hope for the future, the attainment of spiritual well-being, and the resolution of conflicts.

- Assess patient's spiritual or religious beliefs, values, and practices (e.g., "Do you have a religious preference? How important is it to you? Are there any religious or spiritual practices you wish to participate in while in the hospital?"). If the patient expresses a desire, volunteer to read scripture or other religious literature.
- Inform patient and significant others of the availability of spiritual aids, such as a chapel or volunteer chaplain.
- Display a nonjudgmental attitude toward patient's religious or spiritual beliefs and values. Attempt to create an environment that is conducive to free expression.
- Identify available support systems that may assist in meeting the patient's

religious or spiritual needs (e.g., clergy, fellow church members, support groups).

- Be alert to comments related to spiritual concerns or conflicts (e.g., "I don't know why God is doing this to me." "I'm being punished for my sins").
- Use active listening and questioning to help patient resolve conflicts related to spiritual issues. (e.g., "I understand that you want to be baptized. We can arrange to do that here").
- Provide privacy and opportunities for religious practices, such as prayer and meditation.
- If spiritual beliefs and therapeutic regimens are in conflict, provide patient with honest, concrete information to encourage informed decision making. (e.g., "I understand that your religion discourages receiving blood transfusions. Do you understand that by refusing blood you make your condition more difficult to treat?").

**Social isolation** related to altered health status, inability to engage in satisfying personal relationships, altered mental status, or altered physical appearance

*Desired outcome:*    Within 24 h of this diagnosis, patient demonstrates interaction and communication with others.

- Assess factors contributing to patient's social isolation.
  - Restricted visiting hours.
  - Absence of or inadequate support system.
  - Inability to communicate (e.g., presence of intubation/tracheostomy).
  - Physical changes that affect self-concept.
  - Patient denial or withdrawal.
  - Critical care environment.
- Recognize patients at high risk for social isolation: the older adult, disabled, chronically ill, economically disadvantaged.
- Assist patient in identifying feelings associated with loneliness and isolation (e.g., "You seem very sad when your family leaves the room. Can you tell me more about your feelings?").
- Determine patient's need for socialization, and identify available and potential support systems. Explore methods for increasing social contact (e.g., TV, radio, tapes of loved ones, intercom system, more frequent visitations, scheduled interaction with nurse or support staff).
- Provide positive reinforcement for socialization that lessens the patient's feelings of isolation and loneliness (e.g., "Please continue to call me when you need to talk to someone. Talking will help both of us to better understand your feelings").
- Facilitate patient's ability to communicate with others (see **Impaired verbal communication,** p. 755).

**Body image disturbance** related to loss or change in body parts or function or physical trauma

*Desired outcomes:*    Within the 24-h period before hospital discharge, patient acknowledges body changes and demonstrates movement toward incorporating changes into self-concept. Patient does not demonstrate maladaptive response, such as severe depression.

- Establish open, honest communication with the patient. Promote an environment that is conducive to free expression (e.g., "Please feel free to talk to me whenever you have any questions"). Assess patient for indicators suggesting body image disturbance, as listed in Table A-17.
- When planning patient's care, be aware of therapies that may influence patient's body image (e.g., medications or invasive procedures and monitoring).
- Assess patient's knowledge of the pathophysiologic process that has occurred and his or her present health status. Clarify any misconceptions.
- Discuss the loss or change with the patient. Recognize that what may seem

**T A B L E   A - 17    Indicators Suggesting Body Image Disturbance**

*Nonverbal indicators*

Missing body part—internal or external (e.g., splenectomy or amputated extremity)

Change in structure (e.g., open, draining wound)

Change in function (e.g., colostomy)

Avoidance of looking at or touching body part

Hiding or exposing body part

*Verbal indicators*

Expression of negative feelings about body

Expression of feelings of helplessness, hopelessness, or powerlessness

Personalization or depersonalization of missing or mutilated part

Refusal to acknowledge change in structure or function of body part

---

to be a small change may be of great significance to the patient (e.g., arm immobilizer, catheter, hair loss, ecchymoses, facial abrasions).

- Explore with patient concerns, fears, and feelings of guilt (e.g., "I understand that you are frightened. Your face looks very different now, but you will see changes and it will improve. Gradually you will begin to look more like yourself").
- Encourage patient and significant others to interact with one another. Help family to avoid reinforcement of their loved one's changed body part or function (e.g., "I know your son looks very different to you now, but it would help if you speak to him and touch him as you would normally").
- Encourage patient to participate gradually in self-care activities as he or she becomes physically and emotionally able. Allow for some initial withdrawal and denial behaviors (e.g., when changing dressings over traumatized part, explain what you are doing but do not expect the patient to watch or participate initially).
- Discuss opportunities for reconstruction of the loss or change (e.g., surgery, prosthesis, grafting, PT, cosmetic therapies, organ transplant).
- Recognize manifestations of severe depression (e.g., sleep disturbances, change in affect, change in communication pattern). As appropriate, refer to psychiatric clinical nurse specialist, clergy, or support group.
- Help patient attain a sense of autonomy and control by offering choices and alternatives whenever possible. Emphasize patient's strengths, and encourage activities that interest patient.
- Offer realistic hope for the future.

**High risk for violence** related to sensory overload, suicidal behavior, rage reactions, temporal lobe epilepsy, perceived threats, or toxic reaction to medications

*Desired outcome:*    Patient does not harm self or others.

- Assess factors that may contribute to or precipitate violent behavior (e.g., medication reactions, inability to cope, suicidal behavior, confusion, hypoxia, postictal states).
- Attempt to eliminate or treat causative factors (e.g., provide patient teaching, reorient patient, ensure delivery of prescribed oxygen therapy, and reduce or prevent sensory overload; see **Sensory/perceptual alterations,** p. 755).
- Assess for history of physical aggression or family violence as maladaptive coping behaviors.

- Monitor for early signs of increasing anxiety and agitation (e.g., restlessness, verbal aggressiveness, inability to concentrate). Assess for body language that is indicative of violent behavior: clenched fists, rigid posture, increased motor activity.
- Approach patient in a positive manner, and encourage verbalization of feelings and concerns (e.g., "I understand that you are frightened. I will be here from 3 PM to 11 PM to care for you").
- Offer patient as much personal and environmental control as the situation allows (e.g., "Let's discuss the care you will need today. What fluids would you like to drink? Would you prefer a bath in the morning or evening?").
- Help patient distinguish reality from altered perceptions. Orient patient to person, place, and time. Alter the environment to promote reality-based thought processes (e.g., provide clocks, calendars, pictures of loved ones, familiar objects).
- For patients with acute confusion who become aggressive, do not attempt to reorient them, and avoid arguing with them. Instead, state "I can understand why you may [hear, think, see] that." Use nonthreatening mannerisms, facial expressions, and tone of voice.
- Initiate measures that prevent or reduce excessive agitation.
  - Reduce environmental stimuli (e.g., alarms, loud or unnecessary talking).
  - Before touching patient, explain procedures and care, using short, concise statements.
  - Speak quietly (but firmly, as necessary), and project a caring attitude toward the patient (e.g., "We are very concerned for your comfort and safety. Can we do anything to help you feel more relaxed?").
  - Avoid crowding (e.g., of equipment, visitors, health-care personnel) in patient's personal environment.
  - Avoid direct confrontation.
- Explain and discuss patient's behavior with significant others. Acknowledge frustration, concerns, fears, and questions. Review safety precautions with significant others (see next intervention).
- In the event of violent behavior, institute safety precautions as discussed in Table A-18.

**Hopelessness** related to prolonged isolation or activity restriction, failing or

---

**T A B L E  A - 1 8   Safety Precautions in the Event of Violent Behavior**

| | |
|---|---|
| Patient safety | Remove harmful objects from the environment, such as heavy objects, scissors |
| | Apply padding to side rails according to agency protocol |
| | Use restraints as necessary and prescribed. Monitor patient's neurovascular status at frequent intervals |
| | Set limits on patient's behavior, using clear and simple commands |
| | As prescribed, consider chemical sedation when unable to control patient's behavior by other means |
| | Explain safety precautions to patient and family |
| Care giver safety | Alert hospital security department when risk of violence is present |
| | Do not approach violent patient without adequate assistance from others |
| | Never turn your back on a violent patient |
| | Maintain a calm, matter-of-fact tone of voice |
| | Monitor security measures at frequent intervals |
| | Remain alert |

deteriorating physiologic condition, long-term stress, or loss of faith in God or belief system

***Desired outcomes:*** Within the 24-h period before hospital discharge, patient verbalizes hopeful aspects of health status and relates that feelings of despair are absent or lessened.

- Develop open, honest communication with the patient. Actively listen, provide empathetic understanding of fears and doubts, and promote an environment that is conducive to free expression.
- Assess patient's and significant others' understanding of patient's health status and prognosis; clarify any misperceptions.
- Assess for indicators of hopelessness: unwillingness to accept help, pessimism, withdrawal, lack of interest, silence, loss of gratification in roles, previous history of hopeless behavior, hypoactivity, inability to accomplish tasks, expressions of incompetence, closing eyes and turning away.
- Provide opportunities for the patient to feel cared for, needed, and valued by others (e.g., emphasize importance of relationships "Tell me about your grandchildren." "It seems that your family loves you very much").
- Support significant others who seem to spark or maintain patient's feelings of hope (e.g., "Your husband's mood seemed to improve after your visit").
- Recognize discussions and factors that promote patient's sense of hope (e.g., discussions about family members, reminiscing about better times).
- Explore patient's coping mechanisms; assist patient in expanding positive coping behavior (see **Ineffective individual coping,** p. 757).
- Assess patient's spiritual state and needs (see **Spiritual distress,** p. 759).
- Promote anticipation of positive events (e.g., mealtime, grandchildren's visits, bath time, extubation, discontinuation of traction).
- Help patient recognize that although there may be no hope for returning to original life-style, there *is* hope for a new, but different life.
- Avoid insisting that the patient assume a positive attitude. Encourage hope for the future, even if it is the hope for a peaceful death.
- Set realistic, attainable goals and reward achievement.

## Psychosocial care for the patient's family and significant others

**Altered family processes** related to situational crisis (patient's illness)

***Desired outcome:*** Following intervention, significant others demonstrate effective adaptation to change/traumatic situation as evidenced by seeking external support when necessary and sharing concerns within the family unit.

- Assess the family's character: social, environmental, ethnic, and cultural factors; relationships; and role patterns. Identify family developmental stage (e.g., the family may be dealing with other situational or maturational crises, such as an elderly parent or a teenager with a learning disability).
- Assess previous adaptive behaviors (e.g., "How does your family react in stressful situations?"). Discuss observed conflicts and communication breakdown (e.g., "I noticed that your brother would not visit your mother today. Has there been a problem we should be aware of? Knowing about it may help us better care for your mother").
- Acknowledge the family's involvement in patient care, and promote strengths (e.g., "You were able to encourage your wife to turn and cough. That is very important to her recovery"). Encourage family to participate in patient care conferences. Promote frequent, regular patient visits by family members.
- Provide the family with information and guidance related to the critically ill patient. Discuss the stresses of hospitalization, and encourage the family to discuss feelings of anger, guilt, hostility, depression, fear, or sorrow (e.g.,

"You seem to be upset since being told that your husband is not leaving the hospital today"). Refer to clergy, clinical nurse specialist, or social services as appropriate.

- Evaluate patient and family responses to one another. Encourage family to reorganize roles and establish priorities as appropriate (e.g., "I know your husband is concerned about his insurance policy and seems to expect you to investigate it. I'll ask the financial counselor to talk with you").
- Encourage the family to schedule periods of rest and activity outside the critical care unit and to seek support when necessary (e.g., "Your neighbor volunteered to stay in the waiting room this afternoon. Would you like to rest at home? I'll call you if *anything* changes").

**Family coping:** Potential for growth related to use of support systems and referrals and choosing experiences that optimize wellness

***Desired outcomes:*** At the time of the patient's diagnosis, significant others express their intent to use support systems and resources and identify alternative behaviors that promote family communication and strengths. Significant others express realistic expectations and do not demonstrate ineffective coping behaviors.

- Assess family relationships, interactions, support systems, and individual coping behaviors. Permit movement through stages of adaptation. Encourage further positive coping.
- Acknowledge family expressions of hope, future plans, and growth among family members.
- Encourage development of open, honest communication within the family. Provide opportunities in a private setting for family interactions, discussions, and questions (e.g., "I know the waiting room is very crowded. Would your family like some private time together?").
- Refer the family to community or support groups (e.g., ostomy support group, head injury rehabilitation group).
- Encourage the family to explore outlets that foster positive feelings (e.g., periods of time outside the hospital area, meaningful communication with the patient or support individuals, and relaxing activities such as showering, eating, exercising).

**Ineffective family coping:** Compromised, related to inadequate or incorrect information or misunderstanding, temporary family disorganization and role change, exhausted support systems, unrealistic expectations, fear, or anxiety

***Desired outcomes:*** Following intervention, significant others verbalize feelings, identify ineffective coping patterns, identify strengths and positive coping behaviors, and seek information and support from the nurse or other support systems outside the family.

- Establish open, honest communication within the family. Assist the family in identifying strengths, stressors, inappropriate behaviors, and personal needs (e.g., "I understand your mother was very ill last year. How did you manage the situation?" "I know your loved one is very ill. How can I help you?").
- Assess family members for ineffective coping (e.g., depression, chemical dependency, violence, withdrawal), and identify factors that inhibit effective coping (e.g., inadequate support system, grief, fear of disapproval by others, knowledge deficit). For example, "You seem to be unable to talk about your husband's illness. Is there anyone with whom you can talk about it?"
- Assess the family's knowledge about the patient's current health status and therapies. Provide information frequently, and allow sufficient time for questions. Reassess the family's understanding at frequent intervals.
- Provide opportunities in a private setting for family to talk and share concerns with nurses. If appropriate, refer family to psychiatric clinical nurse specialist for therapy.
- Offer realistic hope. Help the family to develop realistic expectations for

the future and to identify support systems that will assist them with planning for the future.
* Assist family with reducing anxiety by encouraging diversional activities (e.g., period of time outside of hospital) and interaction with support systems outside the family (e.g., "I know you want to be near your son, but if you would like to go home to rest, I will call you if *any* changes occur").

**Ineffective family coping:**  Disabling, related to unexpressed feelings, ambivalent family relationships, or disharmonious coping styles among family members

*Desired outcomes:*  Within the 24-h period before hospital discharge, significant others verbalize feelings, identify sources of support as well as ineffective coping behaviors that create ambivalence and disharmony, and do not demonstrate destructive behaviors.

* Establish open, honest communication and rapport with family members (e.g., "I am here to care for your mother and to help your family as well").
* Identify ineffective coping behaviors (e.g., violence, depression, substance abuse, withdrawal). For example, "You seem to be angry. Would you like to talk to me about your feelings?" Refer to psychiatric clinical nurse specialist, clergy, or support group as appropriate.
* Identify perceived or actual conflicts (e.g., "Are you able to talk freely with your family members?" "Are your brothers and sisters able to help and support you during this time?").
* Assist family in search for healthy functioning within the family unit (e.g., facilitate open communication among family members and encourage behaviors that support family cohesiveness). For example, "Your mother enjoyed your last visit. Would you like to see her now?"
* Assess the family's knowledge about patient's current health status. Provide opportunities for questions; reassess family's understanding at frequent intervals.
* Assist family in developing realistic goals, plans, and actions. Refer them to clergy, psychiatric nurse, social services, financial counseling, and family therapy as appropriate.
* Encourage family members to spend time outside the hospital and to interact with support individuals. Respect the family's need for occasional withdrawal.
* Include the family in the patient's plan of care. Offer them opportunities to become involved in patient care (e.g., ROM exercises, patient hygiene, and comfort measures such as backrub).

**Fear** related to patient's life-threatening condition and knowledge deficit
*Desired outcome:*  Following intervention, significant others relate that fear has been lessened.

* Assess the family's fears and their understanding of the patient's clinical situation. Evaluate verbal and nonverbal responses.
* Acknowledge the family's fear (e.g., "I understand these tubes must frighten you, but they are necessary to help nourish your son").
* Assess the family's history of coping behavior (e.g., "How does your family react to difficult situations?"). Determine resources and significant others available for support (e.g., "Who usually helps your family during stressful times?").
* Provide opportunities for family members to express fears and concerns. Recognize that anger, denial, withdrawal, and demanding behavior may be adaptive coping responses during initial period of crisis.
* Provide information at frequent intervals about patient's status and the therapies and equipment used. Demonstrate a caring attitude.
* Encourage the family to use positive coping behaviors by identifying fear(s), developing goals, identifying supportive resources, facilitating realistic perceptions, and promoting problem solving.

- Recognize anxiety, and encourage family members to describe their feelings (e.g., "You seem very uncomfortable tonight. Can you describe your feelings?").
- Be alert to maladaptive responses to fear: potential for violence, withdrawal, severe depression, hostility, and unrealistic expectations for staff or of patient's recovery. Provide referrals to psychiatric clinical nurse specialist or other as appropriate.
- Offer *realistic* hope, even if it is hope for the patient's peaceful death.
- Explore the family's desire for spiritual or other counseling.
- Assess your own feelings about the patient's life-threatening illness. Acknowledge that your attitude and fear may be reflected to the family.
- For other interventions, see nursing diagnoses **Altered family processes** and **Ineffective family coping.**

**Knowledge deficit:**   Patient's current health status or therapies

*Desired outcome:*   Following intervention, significant others verbalize knowledge and understanding about the patient's current health status or therapies.

- At frequent intervals, inform the family about the patient's current health status, therapies, and prognosis. Use individualized verbal, written, and audiovisual strategies to promote family's understanding.
- Evalute the family at frequent intervals for understanding of information that has been provided. Assess factors for misunderstanding, and adjust teaching as appropriate. Some individuals in crisis need repeated explanations before comprehension can be assured (e.g., "I have explained many things to you today. Would you mind summarizing what I've told you so that I can be sure you understand your husband's status and what we are doing to care for him?").
- Encourage family to relay correct information to the patient. This also will reinforce comprehension for family and patient.
- Ask family members if their needs for information are being met (e.g., "Do you have any questions about the care your mother is receiving or about her condition?").
- Help family members use the information they receive to make health-care decisions about family member (e.g., surgery, resuscitation, organ donation).
- Promote family's active participation in patient care when appropriate. Encourage family to seek information and express feelings, concerns, and questions.

## Selected Bibliography

Barker L, Burton J, Zieve P: *Principles of ambulatory medicine,* ed 3, Baltimore, 1991, Williams & Wilkins.

Brandt B: Nursing protocol for the patient with neutropenia, *Oncol Nurs Forum* 17(1):9-15, 1990.

Cubeddu L, Hoffman F, Fuenmayor N, et al: Efficacy of ondansetron and the role of serotonin in cisplatin-induced nausea and vomiting, *N Engl J Med* 322:810-816, 1990.

Fuller A: Platelet transfusion therapy for thrombocytopenia, *Semin Oncol Nurs* 6(2):123-128, 1990.

Gullatte M, Graves T: Advances in antineoplastic therapy, *Oncol Nurs Forum* 17(6):867-878, 1990.

Hall P: Critical care nursing: psychosocial aspects of care. In Burrell L, editor: *Adult nursing in hospital and community settings,* Norwalk, Conn, 1992, Appleton & Lange.

Halm M: The effectiveness of support groups in reducing anxiety for family members of critically ill patients. In *Proceedings of the sixteenth annual national teaching institute,* Newport Beach, Calif, 1989, AACN.

Hayter J: The rhythm of sleep, *Am J Nurs* 80(4):457, 1980.

Held J, Peahota A: Nursing care of patients with esophageal cancer, *Oncol Nurs Forum* 19(4):627-634, 1992.

Higgs D, Nagy C, Einhorn L: Ifosfamide: a clinical review, *Semin Oncol Nurs* 5(2)(suppl 1):70-77, 1989.

Hogan C: Advances in the management of nausea and vomiting, *Nurs Clin North Am* 25(2):475-497, 1990.

Interqual: *The ISD-A review system with adult ISD criteria,* August 1992, Northhamptom, NH, and Marlboro, MA, Interqual, Inc.

Kim MJ, McFarland GK, McLane AK: *Pocket guide to nursing diagnoses,* ed 5, St Louis, 1993, Mosby–Year Book.

Kusier D, Rambur B: Treatment for radiation-induced xerostomia: an innovative remedy, *Cancer Nurs* 15(3):191-195, 1992.

Margolin S et al: Management of radiation-induced moist skin desquamation using hydrocolloid dressing, *Cancer Nurs* 13(2):71-80, 1990.

Mast D, Mood D: Preparing patients with breast cancer for brachytherapy, *Oncol Nurs Forum* 17(2):267-270, 1990.

Maxwell M, Maher K: Chemotherapy-induced myelosuppression, *Semin Oncol Nurs* 8(2):113-123, 1992.

Meade C, Diekmann J, Thornhill P: Readability of American Cancer Society patient education literature, *Oncol Nurs Forum* 19(1):51-62, 1992.

Miller S: Issues of cytotoxic drug handling safety, *Semin Oncol Nurs* 3(2):133-141, 1987.

Molter N: Needs of relatives of critically-ill patients: a descriptive study, *Heart Lung* 8:332-339, 1979.

Padberg K, Padberg L: Strengthening the effectiveness of patient education: applying principles of adult education, *Oncol Nurs Forum* 17(1):65-74, 1990.

Spaulding M: Recent studies of anorexia and appetite stimulation in the cancer patient, *Oncology,* 3(8)(suppl):17-23, 1989.

Strohl RA: Radiation therapy: recent advances and nursing implications, *Nurs Clin North Am* 25(2):309-329, 1990.

Wickham R: Managing chemotherapy-related nausea and vomiting: the state of the art, *Oncol Nurs Forum* 16(4):563-574, 1989.

Wickham R, Purl S, Wilker D: Long-term central venous catheters: issues for care, *Semin Oncol Nurs* 8(2):133-147, 1992.

Wilkie D: Cancer management, *Nurs Clin North Am* 25(2):331-343, 1990.

Yarbo C: Carboplatin: a clinical review, *Semin Oncol Nurs* 5(2)(suppl 1):63-69, 1989.

# Section Four:    Caring for Older Adults

**High risk for aspiration** related to delayed gag reflex secondary to age-related changes

***Desired outcomes:*** Patient swallows independently without choking. Patient's airway is patent and lungs are clear to auscultation both before and after meals.

- Assess patient's LOC on admission and then routinely during hospital stay.
- Assess patient's ability to swallow by asking if he or she has any difficulty swallowing or if any foods or fluids are difficult to swallow or cause gagging. If patient is unable to answer, consult with patient's care giver or significant other. Document findings.
- Assess for the gag reflex by *gently* touching the posterior pharynx. Document findings.
- Place patient in an upright position while eating or drinking, and support this position with pillows on patient's sides.

- Monitor patient when he or she is swallowing. Watch for limited lip, tongue, or jaw movement as indicated by drooling of saliva or food or an inability to close lips around a straw. Check for retention of food in sides of mouth, which is an indication of poor tongue movement.
- Monitor patient for coughing or choking before, during, or after swallowing. This signals aspiration of material into the airway.
- Monitor patient for a wet or gurgly sound when talking after a swallow. This indicates aspiration into the airway and signals a delayed or absent swallow reflex and a delayed or absent gag reflex.
- For patients with poor swallowing reflex, tilt their heads forward 45 degrees during swallowing. This will help prevent inadvertant aspiration by closing off the airway. **Note:** For patients who have hemiplegia, tilt head toward the unaffected side.
- As indicated, request evaluation by speech therapist for further assessment of gag and swallow reflex.
- Anticipate swallowing video fluoroscopy in evaluation of the patient's gag and swallow reflex. Using four consistencies of barium, the radiologist and speech therapist watch for the presence of reduced or ineffective tongue function, reduced peristalsis in the pharynx, delayed or absent swallow reflex, and poor or limited ability to close the sphincters that protect the airway. This procedure is used to determine whether the patient is aspirating, the consistency of the materials most likely to be aspirated, and the cause of the aspiration.
- Provide adequate rest periods before meals. Fatigue increases the risk of aspiration.
- Monitor intake of food. Document consistencies and amounts of food patient eats, where patient places food in the mouth, how patient manipulates or chews before swallowing, and the length of time before patient swallows the bolus of food.
- Remind patients with dementia to chew and swallow with each bite.
- Ensure that patient has dentures in place, if appropriate, and that they fit correctly.
- Ensure that someone stays with patient during meals or fluid intake.
- Provide patient with adequate time to eat and drink. Generally, patients with swallowing deficits require twice as much time for eating and drinking as those whose swallowing is adequate.
- Monitor patient for signs of aspiration, including presence of crackles in lungs, SOB, decreasing LOC, and increasing temperature.
- Be aware of location of suction equipment to be used in the event of aspiration.
- If patient aspirates, implement the following:
  - Follow American Hospital Association (AHA) Standards if patient displays characteristics of complete airway obstruction (i.e., choking).
  - For partial airway obstruction, encourage patient to cough as needed.
  - For partial airway obstruction in the unconscious/nonresponsive individual who is not coughing, suction the airway with a large-bore catheter such as the Yankauer.
  - For either a complete or partial aspiration, inform physician and obtain order for chest x-ray.
  - Protect patient by implementing NPO until diagnosis is confirmed.
  - Monitor breathing pattern and RR q1-2h after a suspected aspiration for alterations (i.e., increased RR) that signal a change in the patient's condition.
  - Anticipate use of antibiotics to prevent infection.
  - Encourage patient to cough and deep-breathe q2h while awake and q4h during the night to promote expansion of available lung tissue.

**Constipation** related to changes in diet, activity, and psychosocial factors secondary to hospitalization

***Desired outcomes:*** Patient states that bowel habit has returned to normal within 3-4 days of this diagnosis. Stool appears soft, and patient does not strain in passing stools.

- Upon admission, assess and document the patient's normal bowel elimination pattern. Include frequency, time of day, associated habits, and successful methods used to correct constipation in the past. Consult with patient's care giver or significant other if patient is unable to provide this information.
- Inform patient that changes that occur with hospitalization may increase the potential for constipation. Urge patient to institute successful nonpharmacologic methods used at home as soon as this problem is noticed or prophylactically as needed.
- Teach patient the relationship between fluid intake and constipation. Unless otherwise contraindicated, encourage fluid intake that exceeds 2,500 ml/day. Monitor and record bowel movements.
- Teach patient the relationship between types of foods consumed and constipation. When possible, encourage patient to include roughage as a part of each meal (e.g., raw fruits and vegetables, whole grains, nuts, and fruits with skins). For the patient unable to tolerate raw foods, encourage intake of bran *via* cereals, muffins, and breads. Titrate the amount of roughage to the degree of constipation.
- Teach patient the relationship between constipation and activity level. Encourage optimum activity for all patients. Establish and post an activity program to enhance participation; include devices necessary to enable independence.
- Advise patient about the need to maintain normal bowel elimination pattern. Provide any materials or support environments the patient normally uses (e.g., cup of coffee first thing upon arising, privacy, short walk).
- Ask patient if the toilet seat height seems the same as that at home. If the toilet is higher, provide a footstool to raise patient's feet off the floor comfortably. A high-rise toilet seat may be used to increase the toilet's height.
- Schedule interventions to coincide with the patient's habit. If the patient's habit occurs in the early morning, utilize the patient's gastrocolic or gastroduodenal reflexes to promote colonic emptying. If the patient's habit occurs in the evening, ambulate the patient just before the appropriate time. Digital stimulation of the anal sphincter also may facilitate bowel movement.
- Attempt to use methods the patient has used successfully in the past. Follow the maxim "go low, go slow" (i.e., use the lowest amount of nonnatural intervention and advance to more powerful interventions slowly). Elders tend to focus on the loss of habit as an indicator of constipation rather than on the number of stools. Do not intervene pharmacologically until the elder has not had a stool for 3 days.
- When requesting a pharmacologic intervention, use the more benign, oral methods first. A suggested hierarchy is
  - Bulk-building additives such as psyllium or bran.
  - Mild laxatives (apple or prune juice, milk of magnesia).
  - Stool softeners (docusate sodium or docusate calcium).
  - Potent laxatives or cathartics (bisacodyl or cascara sagrada).
  - Medicated suppositories (glycerine or bisacodyl).
  - Enema (tap water, saline, sodium biphosphate/phosphate).
- After diagnostic imaging of the GI tract with barium, ensure that the patient receives postexamination laxative to facilitate removal of the barium. After any procedure involving a bowel cleanout, there may be rebound constipation from the severe disruption of bowel habit. Monitor hydration status for signs of dehydration, which can occur from osmotic agents used. Emphasize diet, fluid, activity, and resumption of routines. If no bowel movement occurs in 3 days, begin with mild laxatives to try to regain normal pattern.

- Also see this diagnosis in "Caring for Patients on Prolonged Bedrest," p. 716.

**High risk for fluid volume deficit** related to inability to obtain fluids by self secondary to illness, placement of fluid, or presence of chronic illness; or related to use of osmotic agents during radiologic tests

*Desired outcomes:* Patient's mental status, VS, and urine specific gravity, color, consistency, and concentration remain within normal limits for patient. Patient's mucous membranes remain moist. Patient's intake equals output.

- Assess and document skin turgor. Check hydration status by pinching skin over sternum or forehead. Skin that remains in the lifted position (tenting) and returns slowly to its original position indicates dehydration. A furrowed tongue is a signal of severe dehydration.
- Assess and document urine specific gravity and color q8h.
- Assess and document color, amount, and frequency of any fluid output, including emesis, urine, diarrhea, or other drainage.
- Monitor patient's orientation, ability to follow commands, and behavior. Loss of ability to follow commands, decrease in orientation, and confused behavior can be signals of a dehydrated state.
- Weigh patient daily at the same time of day (preferably before breakfast) using the same scale and bed clothing. Be alert to wide variations in weight (e.g., $\geq$2.5 kg [5 lb]).
- In the patient who is dehydrated, anticipate elevation in serum $Na^+$, blood urea nitrogen (BUN), and serum creatinine levels.
- If the patient is receiving IV therapy, monitor cardiac and respiratory systems for signs of overload, which could precipitate congestive heart failure (CHF) or pulmonary edema. Assess the apical pulse and listen to lung fields during every VS assessment. A rising HR and crackles in the lungs can be signals of CHF or pulmonary edema.
- Monitor I&O when the patient is receiving dyes for contrast or tube feedings. These agents act osmotically to pull fluid into the interstitial tissue. Watch for evidence of third spacing of fluids, including increasing peripheral edema, especially sacral; output significantly less than intake (1:2); and urine output <30 ml/h.
- In the patient without any fluid restrictions, encourage intake to 3 L/day. Specify the amount to be taken during days, evenings, and nights.
- Offer patient fluid whenever in the room. Elders have decreased sense of thirst and need encouragement to drink. Offer a variety of drinks the patient likes, but limit caffeine, because caffeine tends to act as a diuretic.
- Assess patient's ability to obtain and drink fluids by self. Place fluids within easy reach. Use cups with tops to minimize concern over spilling.
- Ensure access to toilet, urinal, commode or bed pan at least q2h when patient is awake and q4h at night. Answer the call light quickly. The time between recognition of the need to void and urination decreases with age.

**Impaired gas exchange (or high risk for same)** related to decreased functional lung tissue secondary to age-related changes

*Desired outcomes:* Patient's respiratory pattern and mental status remain normal for patient. Patient's ABG or pulse oximetry values are within patient's normal limits.

- Assess and document the following upon admission and routinely thereafter: respiratory rate, pattern, and depth; breath sounds; cough; sputum; and sensorium.
- Assess patient for subtle changes in mentation such as increased restlessness, anxiety, disorientation, and presence of hostility. If available, monitor oxygenation status *via* ABG findings (optimally $Pao_2$ $\geq$80%-95%) or pulse oximetry (optimally $\geq$90%).
- Assess lungs for the presence of adventitious sounds. **Note:** The aging lung has decreased elasticity. The lower part of the lungs is no longer adequately aerated. As a result, crackles commonly are heard in individuals 75 years of

age and older. This sign alone does not mean that a pathology is present. Crackles that do not clear with coughing in an individual with no other clinical signs (e.g., fever, increasing anxiety, increasing respiratory depth) are considered benign.

- Encourage patient to cough and breathe deeply to promote alveolar expansion and clear secretions from the bronchial tree.
- Reduce the potential for patient's increased oxygen consumption by treating fevers promptly, decreasing pain, minimizing pacing activity, and lessening anxiety.
- Instruct patient in the use of support equipment such as oxygen masks or cannulas.
- Schedule and pace patient's activities according to tolerance. Document patient's ability to accomplish ADL.

**Hopelessness** related to slow recovery from illness or surgery secondary to decreased physiologic reserve

*Desired outcomes:* Within 2-4 days of intervention(s), patient verbalizes knowledge of his or her strengths, feelings about health, and the understanding of a potentially long recovery.

- Monitor patient for signs of depression, such as refusal to participate in own care; refusal to answer questions; and statements such as "I don't care," "Leave me alone," and "Let me die."
- Encourage patient to verbalize feelings of despair, frustration, fear, and anger and concerns regarding hospitalization and health. Reassure patient and signficant others that such feelings and concerns are normal.
- Discuss normal age changes with patient. Inform patient and significant others that recovery periods are longer for older adults because of decreased physiologic reserve. More energy is spent in maintaining normal status, and thus the body has less capacity to rebuild strength and endurance.
- Encourage short-term goals and praise small steps, such as participation in own care.
- Arrange a care conference to discuss discharge requirements specific to the patient. Involve patient and significant others in the conference. Set realistic goals with patient based on patient's condition and desires.

**Hypothermia** related to age-related changes in thermoregulation and/or environmental exposure

*Desired outcome:* Patient's temperature and mental status remain within patient's normal limits or they return to patient's normal limits after intervention(s) at a rate of 1° F/h.

- Monitor patient's temperature, using a low-range thermometer if possible. Be aware that elders can have a normal temperature of 35.56° C (96° F).
- Assess patient's temperature orally by placing the thermometer far back in the mouth. To ensure proper placement, slide the thermometer along the buccal membrane and position it under the back of the tongue. **Note:** Do not take axillary temperature in the older adult because elders have decreased peripheral circulation and the skin under the arms will be cooler than the core temperature. If unable to measure patient's temperature orally, measure temperature *via* rectum or ear, which are measures of the core temperature.
- Assess and document patient's mental status. Increasing disorientation or the presence of atypical behavior can signal hypothermia.
- Be alert to the following patients who are at risk for environmental hypothermia: those taking sedatives, hypnotics (including anesthetics), and muscle relaxants because these drugs decrease shivering. In addition, all elders are at risk for environmental hypothermia at ambient temperatures of 22.22°-23.89° C (72°-75° F).
- Ensure that patient is sent to radiology and other departments with enough blankets to keep warm.
- Initiate slow rewarming using external methods, such as raising room tem-

perature to at least 23.89° C (75° F). Other methods of external warming include use of warm blankets, head covers, and warm circulating air blankets.
- If patient's temperature falls below 35° C (95° F), warm patient internally by administering warm oral or IV fluids. Also anticipate use of warmed saline gastric irrigations or introduction of warmed humidified air into the airway.
- Be alert to signs of too rapid rewarming: irregular HR, dysrhythmias, and very warm extremities caused by vasodilatation in the periphery, which causes heat loss from the core.
- If patient's temperature fails to rise 1° F hourly using these techniques, suspect a cause other than environmental. In this event, anticipate laboratory tests, including WBC count for possible sepsis, thryoid test for hypothyroidism, and glucose level for hypoglycemia.
- As prescribed, administer antibiotics for sepsis, initiate thyroid therapy, or administer glucose for hypoglycemia. The patient's temperature will not return to normal unless the underlying condition has been treated.

**High risk for infection** related to age-related changes in immune and integumentary system; related to suppressed inflammatory response secondary to chronic medication use (e.g., antiinflammatory agents, steroids, analgesics); related to slowed ciliary response; or related to poor nutrition
*Desired outcomes:* Patient remains free of infection as evidenced by orientation to person, place, and time and behavior within patient's normal limits; RR and pattern within patient's normal limits; urine that is straw-colored, clear, and of characteristic odor; core temperature and HR within patient's normal limits; sputum that is clear to whitish in color; and skin that is intact and of normal color and temperature for patient.

---

**Note:** WBC count ≥11,000 μl can be a late sign of infection in elders because the immune system is slow to respond to insult.

---

- Assess patient's baseline VS, including LOC and orientation. A change in mentation is a leading sign of infection in elders. Also be alert to HR >100 bpm and RR >24 breaths/min. Auscultate lung fields for adventitious sounds. Be aware, however, that crackles may be a normal finding when heard in the lung bases.
- Monitor patient's temperature, using a low-range thermometer if possible. Be aware that a temperature of 35.56° C (96° F) may be normal for the patient. In that case, a patient with a temperature of 36.67° C-37.22° C (98° F-99° F) may be considered febrile.
- To ensure that the patient's core temperature is being accurately determined, obtain temperature readings rectally or *via* ear probe if the oral reading does not match the clinical picture (i.e., patient's skin is very warm, patient is restless, mentation is depressed), or if the temperature reads ≥36.11° C (97° F).
- Assess patient's skin for tears, breaks, redness, or ulcers. Document condition of the patient's skin on admission and as an ongoing assessment (refer to **High risk for impaired skin integrity,** below).
- Assess the quality and color of the patient's urine. Urinary tract infections (UTIs), as manifested by cloudy, foul-smelling urine, without painful urination, are the most common infection in elders. Document changes when noted and report findings to the phsician. Also be alert to urinary incontinence, which can signal UTI.
- Because of the increased risk of infection, avoid insertion of urinary catheters when possible.
- Obtain drug history in reference to use of antiinflammatory or immunosup-

pressive drugs or chronic use of analgesics or steroids, because these drugs mask fever.

- If infection is suspected, anticipate initiation of IV fluid therapy for maintenance of fluid balance; blood cultures, urinalysis, and urine culture to isolate bacteria type; and WBC count to determine immune response. Expect a chest x-ray to rule out pneumonia if patient's chest sounds are not clear. If infection is present, prepare for initiation of broad spectrum antibiotic therapy, oxygen therapy to maintain adequate oxygenation to the brain, and use of acetaminophen to decrease temperature and cardiac output, which will decrease cardiac load.

**Powerlessness** related to hospital environment

***Desired outcome:*** Within 2-4 days after intervention(s), patient participates in care and verbalizes feelings of control over his or her environment.

- Encourage patient to verbalize feelings about hospitalization and illness.
- Assist patient in identifying factors that contribute to feelings of powerlessness.
- Encourage patient to participate in ADL as much as possible. Provide adequate time for patient to complete ADL.
- As often as possible, enable patient to participate in scheduling of activities.
- Discuss with patient and significant others realistic goals of care, and encourage patient's participation in care planning.
- Explain procedures and routines to patient. Inform patient when changes in the plan of care are necessary.
- Provide flexibility in patient's plan of care when possible (e.g., if patients want to wear their own clothes, enable them to do so).

**High risk for impaired skin integrity** related to decreased subcutaneous fat and decreased peripheral capillary networks secondary to age-related changes in the integumentary system

***Desired outcome:*** Patient's skin remains clear and intact.

- Assess patient's skin on admission and routinely thereafter. Note any areas of redness or any breaks in the skin surface.
- Ensure that patient turns frequently (at least q2h). Lift or roll patient across sheets when repositioning. Pulling, dragging, or sliding patient across sheets can lead to shear (loss of skin).
- Monitor skin over bony prominences (i.e., sacrum, heels, spine, hips, knees, costal margins, and occiput) for erythema. Apply skin barrier paste to reddened areas for additional protection. Use pillows or pads around bony prominences to protect the overlying skin, even when patient is up in a wheelchair or sits for long periods. The ischial tuberosities are prone to breakdown when patient is in the seated position.
- Use lotions on dry skin to promote suppleness.
- Use alternating pressure mattress, air-fluidized mattress, waterbed, or airbed for elders who are on bed rest or unable to get out of bed, to protect skin from injury caused by prolonged pressure.
- Avoid placing tubes under patient's limbs or head. Excess pressure from tubes can create a pressure ulcer. Place pillow or pad between patient and tube for cushioning.
- Optimize patient mobility; get patient out of bed as often as possible. If patient is unable to get out of bed, assist with position changes q2h.
- Ensure that patient's face, axillae, and genital areas are washed daily. Complete baths dry out elder's skin and should be given every other day instead. Use tepid water and super-fatted soaps, which help decrease dry skin. Avoid hot water, which can burn elders, who have decreased pain sensitivity and decreased sensation to temperature.
- Minimize use of protective pads under patient. These pads trap moisture and heat and can lead to skin breakdown.

- Document percentage of food intake with meals. Encourage significant others to provide patient's favorite foods. Suggest snacks high in protein and vitamin C if patient's diet is not restricted.
- Obtain nutritional consultation with dietitian as needed.
- Monitor serum albumin for evidence of protein status (normal value is 3.0 g/dl for elders).
- For more information, see "Providing Nutritional Support," p. 665 and "Managing Wound Care," p. 681.

**Sleep pattern disturbance** related to unfamiliar surroundings and hospital routines

*Desired outcomes:*   Within 24 h of intervention(s), patient reports the attainment of adequate rest. Patient's mental status remains normal for the patient.

- Assess and document patient's sleeping pattern, obtaining information from patient or patient's care giver or significant others. Ask questions about naps and activity levels. Individuals who take naps and have a low level of activity frequently sleep only 4-5 h/night.
- Determine patient's usual nighttime routine, and attempt to emulate it.
- Inform patient of necessary interruptions during hospitalization.
- Attempt to group activities such as medications, VS, and toileting together to reduce the number of interruptions.
- Provide comfort measures, such as pain medications, backrub, and conversation at bedtime.
- Provide patient with compatible roommate when possible.
- Monitor patient's activity level. If patient complains of being tired after activities or displays behaviors such as irritability, yelling, or shouting, encourage napping after lunch or early in the afternoon. Otherwise, discourage daytime napping by involving patient in care or activities.
- Avoid stimulants such as coffee, cola, and tea after 6 PM.
- Provide a quiet environment by avoiding loud noises and use of overhead lights and minimizing interruptions during sleep hours.

**Altered thought processes** related to decreased cerebral perfusion secondary to age-related decreased physiologic reserve or cardiac dysfunction; related to electrolyte imbalance secondary to age-related decreased renal function; related to altered sensory/perceptual reception secondary to poor vision or hearing; or related to decreased brain oxygenation secondary to illness state and decreased functional lung tissue

*Desired outcomes:*   Patient's mental status returns to normal for the patient within 3 days of treatment. Patient sustains no evidence of injury or harm as a result of mental status.

- Assess patient's baseline LOC and mental status on admission. Ask patient to perform a 3-step task (e.g., "Raise your right hand, place it on your left shoulder, and then place the right hand by your right side"). Test short-term memory by showing patient how to use the call light, having the patient return the demonstration, and then waiting at least 5 min before having patient demonstrate use of call light again. Inability to remember beyond 5 min indicates poor short-term memory. Document patient's response.
- Document patient's actions in behavioral terms. Describe the "confused" behavior.
- Obtain preconfusion functional and mental status abilities from significant others.
- Identify cause of acute confusion (e.g., consult with physician regarding oximetry or ABG values to assess oxygenation levels; serum glucose or fingerstick glucose to determine glucose level; and electrolytes and CBC to ascertain imbalances and/or presence of elevated WBC count as a determinant of infection). Assess hydration status by pinching skin over the sternum or forehead for turgor and checking for dry mucous membranes and furrowed tongue.

- Review cardiac status. Assess apical pulse, and notify physician of an irregular pulse that is new to the patient. If patient is on a cardiac monitor, watch for dysrhythmias; notify physician accordingly.
- Review current medications, including OTC drugs, with the pharmacist. Toxic levels of certain medications such as digoxin or theophylline cause acute confusion. Drugs that are anticholinergic also can cause confusion, as can drug interactions.
- Monitor I&O at least q8h. Output should match intake. Anticipate/encourage a creatinine clearance test to assess renal function. **Note:** BUN and serum creatinine are affected by hydration status. Serum creatinine is affected by the aging process because lower mass produces lower creatinine. Normal serum creatinine levels in a well-hydrated elder can therefore signal renal insufficiency.
- Have patient wear glasses and hearing aid, or keep them close to the bedside and within easy reach for patient use.
- Keep patient's urinal and other routinely used items within easy reach for the patient. If patient has short-term memory problems, do not expect him or her to use the call light. Toilet or offer patient urinal or bed pan q2h while awake and q4h during the night.
- Check on the patient at least q30min and every time you pass by the room.
- Place patient close to the nurses' station if possible. Provide an environment that is nonstimulating and safe. Provide music but not TV (patients who are confused regarding place and time often think the action on the TV is happening in the room).
- Attempt to reorient patient to surroundings as needed. Keep a clock or calendar at the bedside, and verbally remind patient of the date and day as needed.
- Tell patient in simple terms what is occurring (e.g., "It's time to eat breakfast," "This medicine is for your heart," "I'm going to help you get out of bed").
- Encourage patient's significant others to bring items familiar to patient, including blanket, bedspread, pictures of family and pets.
- If patient becomes belligerent, angry, or argumentative while you are attempting to reorient, **stop this approach.** Do not argue with patient or patient's interpretation of the environment. State, "I can understand why you may (hear, think, see) that."
- If patient displays hostile behavior or misperceives your role (nurse becomes thief, jailer, etc.), leave the room. Return in 15 min. Introduce yourself to the patient as though you had never met. Begin dialogue anew. Patients who are acutely confused have poor short-term memory and may not remember the previous encounter or that you were involved in that encounter. When you return, enable patient to share feelings about the previous encounter as appropriate.
- If patient attempts to leave the hospital, walk with patient and attempt distraction. Ask patient to tell you about the destination (e.g., "That sounds like a wonderful place! Tell me about it"). Keep tone pleasant and conversational. Continue walking with patient away from exits and doors around the unit. After a few minutes, attempt to guide patient back to the room. Offer refreshments and a rest (e.g.,"We've been walking for a while and I'm a little tired. Why don't we sit and have some juice while we talk").
- If the patient has a permanent or severe cognitive impairment, check on her or him at least q30min and reorient to baseline mental status as indicated; however, do not argue with patient about his or her peception of reality. This can cause a cognitively impaired person to become aggressive and combative. **Note:** Individuals with severe cognitive impairment (e.g., Alzheimer's disease or dementia) also can experience acute confusional states (i.e., delirium) and can be returned to their baseline mental state.

- Bargain with patient. Try to establish an agreement to stay for a defined period of time, such as until the physician, breakfast or lunch, or significant others arrive.
- Have patient's significant others talk with patient by phone or come in and sit with patient if patient's behavior requires checking more often than q30min.
- If patient is attempting to pull out tubes, hide the tubes (e.g., under blankets). Put stockinette mesh dressing over IV lines. Tape feeding tubes to the side of the face using paper tape and drape the tube behind patient's ear. Remember: out of sight; out of mind.
- Evaluate continued need for therapy that may have become an irritating stimulus (e.g., if the patient is now drinking, discontinue IV; if the patient is eating, discontinue feeding tube; if the patient has an indwelling urethral catheter, discontinue catheter and begin toileting routine).
- Use restraints with caution. Patients can become more agitated when wrist and arm restraints are used.
- Use medications cautiously for controlling behavior. Neuroleptics such as haloperidol can be used successfully in calming patients with dementia or psychiatric illness (contraindicated for individuals with Parkinsonism). However, if the patient is experiencing acute confusion or delirium, short-acting benzodiazapines (e.g., lorazepam) are more effective in reducing anxiety and fear. Anxiety or fear usually trigger destructive or dangerous behaviors in the acutely confused elder. A short-acting benzodiazapine such as lorazepam will decrease feelings of anxiety and calm the patient after 1 or 2 doses. **Note:** Neuroleptics can cause akathesia, an adverse drug reaction evidenced by increased restlessness.

## Selected Bibliography

Andresen G: A fresh look at assessing the elderly, *RN* 89(6):28-40, 1989.

Berkey P: Alzheimer's by moonlight, *Geriatr Nurs* 12(1):292-293, 1991.

Chenitz C, Takano-Stone J, Salisbury S: *Clinical gerontological nursing: a guide to advanced practice,* Philadelphia, 1991, WB Saunders.

Feil N: Validation therapy, *Geriatr Nurs* 13(3):129-133, 1992.

Hoffman N: Dehydration in the elderly: insidious and managable, *Geriatrics* 46(6):35-46, 1991.

Kelley L, Mobily P: Iatrogenesis in the elderly: impaired skin integrity, *J Gerontol Nurs* 17(9):24-29, 1991.

Matteson M, McConnell E: *Gerontological nursing: concepts and practice,* Philadelphia, 1988, WB Saunders.

Meehan M: Nursing dx: potential for aspiration, *RN* 92(1):30-34, 1992.

Palmieri D: Clearing up the confusion: adverse clinical effects of medication in the elderly, *J Gerontol Nurs* 17(10): 32-35, 1991.

Rebenson-Piano M: The physiologic changes that occur with aging, *Crit Care Nurs Quart* 12(1):1-14, 1989.

Shemansky C: Choking: clear and present danger for elders, *Geriatr Nurs* 12(2):68-70, 1991.

Steiner D, Marcopulos B: Depression in the elderly: characteristics and clinical management, *Nurs Clin North Am* 26(3):585-599, 1991.

Stolley J, Buckwalter K: Iatrogenesis in the elderly: nosocomial infections, *J Gerontol Nurs* 17(9):30-33, 1991.

Strumpf N, Evans L: The ethical problems of prolonged physical restraint, *J Gerontol Nurs* 17(2), 27-30, 1991.

# INFECTION PREVENTION AND CONTROL

For several decades infection prevention and control has focused on the use of barriers (e.g., gloves, gowns, masks) to interrupt transmission of organisms among and between patients and health-care workers. These barriers are a major component of various systems for isolation precautions.

## Systems for isolation precautions

Currently there are four different systems of isolation precautions commonly used in hospitals. The Centers for Disease Control (CDC) revised their guidelines for isolation precautions in 1983 and offered three options:
• Category-Specific System.
• Disease-Specific System.
• Hospital-Designed System.
Many facilities have developed their own systems of isolation precautions, following the model of Body Substance Isolation (BSI), developed over several years by two nurses and their colleagues.

In 1987 the CDC presented guidelines for Universal Precautions that are intended to reduce risks for infection with bloodborne pathogens, specifically hepatitis B virus (HBV) and human immunodeficiency virus (HIV). These guidelines, as revised in 1988, have been adopted by the Occupational Safety and Health Administration (OSHA) as a major component of their Bloodborne Pathogens Standard, which became federal law in December 1991.

There are differences among the isolation systems, which are misinterpreted by many people. These differences have to do primarily with how and when use of the systems is initiated.

**CDC's Category-Specific and Disease-Specific isolation precautions:** Initiated when a patient's diagnosis is known or suspected. This diagnosis prompts use of a reminder sign on the door of the patient's room, as well as use of specific barriers for contact with potentially infectious secretions or excretions. These systems are thus "diagnosis-driven."

**BSI and CDC's Universal Precautions:** Initiated when a care provider anticipates contact with blood or other body substances from the patient. These systems are thus "interaction-driven." BSI applies to all body substances (e.g., blood, urine, feces, saliva, sputum, wound drainage, etc). Universal Precautions apply only to blood and those body fluids that have been associated epidemiologically with transmission of bloodborne pathogens. Thus Universal Precautions do not apply to feces, urine, saliva (except in the dental setting), sputum, vomitus, sweat, or tears (unless visibly bloody).

Because Universal Precautions are only intended to reduce risk of transmission of bloodborne pathogens and do not apply to all body substances, agencies that use Universal Precautions also need to use an additional isolation sys-

**T A B L E  A - 19   Comparison of Four Systems of Infection Precautions as Applied to Different Situations**

| Situation | Category-specific (CDC, 1983) | Disease-specific (CDC, 1983) |
|---|---|---|
| Patient known to have HBV, HCV, HIV, or other bloodborne diseases | The category of Blood and Body Fluid Precautions was replaced by Universal Precautions in 1987 (revised 1988) | See Universal Precautions (revised 1988) |
| Patient not known to have HBV, HBC, HIV, or other bloodborne diseasses | Use Universal Precautions | Use Universal Precautions |
| Patient with diagnosed enteric disease such as shigellosis | Use Enteric Precautions, including sign on the door | See named disease in CDC guidelines, 1983 (similar to Enteric Precautions); sign on the door |
| Patient not known to have enteric disease | No special precautions because there is no diagnosis; routine patient care practices should be followed | No special precautions; routine patient care practices should be followed |
| Patient diagnosed with varicella (chickenpox) | Strict Isolation: for entering room whether or not there is contact; persons should wear gloves, gowns, masks; immune persons do not need masks; sign on door: Strict Isolation | See named disease in CDC guidelines, 1983 (similar to Strict Isolation); sign on door |
| Patient diagnosed or suspected of having pulmonary or laryngeal TB | Use AFB Isolation; sign on door; door closed; rooms need special ventilation | See named disease in CDC guidelines, 1983 (similar to AFB Isolation); sign on door; door closed |

Adapted from Jackson MM, Lynch P: An attempt to make an issue less murky: a comparison of four systems for infection precautions, *Infect Control Hosp Epidemiol* 12:448–450, 1991.

tem to reduce risks of transmission of nonbloodborne pathogens to patients and health-care workers. The CDC in its 1988 revision of Universal Precautions recommended using Category-Specific or Disease-Specific isolation precautions in combination with Universal Precautions to ensure that all diagnosed or suspected diseases would be covered.

The BSI system incorporates all aspects of Universal Precautions but is

**T A B L E  A - 19   Comparison of Four Systems of Infection Precautions as Applied to Different Situations—cont'd**

| **Body Substance Isolation (BSI) (Lynch, Jackson et al, 1984-92)** | **Universal precautions (CDC, revised 1988; regulated by OSHA Bloodborne Pathogens Standard, 12-6-91)** |
| --- | --- |
| Gloves: put on clean gloves immediately before contact with nonintact skin or mucous membranes; wear gloves for contact with moist body substances. If soiling is likely, protect skin and clothing with gown or apron. If splashing/splattering is likely, protect eyes and mucous membranes with goggles and mask or face shield | Gloves: for contact with blood and body fluids epidemiologically associated with transmission of bloodborne pathogens. If soiling of clothing or skin is likely, protect gown or apron. If splashing/splattering of face is likely, protect eyes and mucous membranes with mask and eye protection or face shield |
| Same precautions as above; selection of barriers based on interaction with patient | Same as above |
| Same precautions as above | Universal Precautions do not apply to feces unless visibly bloody; Universal Precautions are not intended for fecal-oral diseases |
| Same precautions as above; use of barriers based on interaction with patient's body substances, not patient's diagnosis | Universal Precautions do not apply except as above |
| Susceptible persons should not be assigned to care for patient; immune personnel can provide care with no other precautions than those used for BSI; sign on door to restrict entry of persons; door closed | Universal Precautions do not apply to airborne communicable diseases such as chickenpox |
| Use Airborne Precautions; sign on door to restrict entry of persons; door closed; rooms need special ventilation | Universal Precautions do not apply to airborne communicable diseases such as TB |

used for contact with *all* body substances. In other words, BSI is a single system that does not require the use of additional isolation precautions (e.g., Category-Specific or Disease-Specific) except for airborne communicable diseases such as chickenpox or tuberculosis (TB). Many agencies have found the BSI system operationally simple to use, easy to understand, and less cumbersome than trying to use more than one system of precautions at the same time.

To illustrate and compare the approaches to isolation precautions used in the different systems, Table A-19 presents several situations involving known and unknown disease.

## Isolation precautions for patients with pulmonary TB

In response to the increasing incidence of pulmonary TB in the United States, the CDC in 1990 published guidelines for preventing the transmission of TB in the health-care setting. These guidelines focus on early identification and preventive treatment of persons with a diagnosis or suspected diagnosis of pulmonary TB. In addition, the CDC defined requirements for special ventilation and use of masks that provide better filtration and a tighter fit than standard surgical masks. Masks of this type are called particulate respirators (PRs) and were developed for industrial use to protect workers from dust. The efficacy of PRs in protecting susceptible persons from infection with TB has not been demonstrated. The requirements for special ventilation in the care of persons with diagnosed or suspected pulmonary TB were included in the 1983 CDC guidelines for isolation precautions; however, the recommendation for use of PRs was new in 1990. The 1990 CDC recommendations for control of TB were revised in 1993.

## Management of devices and procedures to reduce nosocomial infection risks

Use of barriers is but one of many strategies that reduce nosocomial infection risks to patients and personnel. In fact, studies from the CDC show that major impact can be made in reducing infection risks by focusing on the management of devices and procedures that are frequently used in patient care. For example, many patients need intravascular devices to deliver therapeutic medications but are put at risk for site infections and bacteremias when these devices are used. It is well known that rotating the access site at appropriate intervals will reduce these risks to the patient, and new catheter materials that are more "vein friendly" also reduce trauma to the vascular system. In addition, use of needles to deliver medications and fluids to patients through these intravascular devices can put the health-care worker at risk for puncture injury. There are now needleless or needle-free IV access devices available to acess line ports so that it is not necessary to use needles once the vascular system is entered by the intravascular catheter. Thus the use of newer and safer intravascular devices and procedures can benefit both the patient and health-care worker by reducing their risks for nosocomial infections. Many nosocomial risk reduction strategies were discussed at the Third Decennial International Conference on Nosocomial Infections in August 1990 and have been incorporated into routine patient care practices in many health-care agencies.

### Selected Bibiography

Bennett JV, Brachman PS, editors: *Hospital infections,* ed 3, Boston, 1992, Little, Brown.

Centers for Disease Control: Guideline for isolation precautions in hospitals, *Infection Control* 4:245-325, 1983.

Centers for Disease Control: Recommendations for prevention of HIV transmission in health care settings, *MMWR* 36(suppl 2):1-18, 1987.

Centers for Disease Control: Update: universal precautions for prevention of transmission of human immunodeficiency virus and other bloodborne pathogens in healthcare settings, *MMWR* 37:377-388, 1988.

Centers for Disease Control: Guidelines for preventing the transmission of tuberculosis in health-care settings, with special focus on HIV-related issues, *MMWR* 39(RR1-17): 1990.

Centers for Disease Control: *Core curriculum on tuberculosis,* ed 2, Atlanta, 1991, CDC.

Department of Labor, Occupational Safety and Health Administration: Occupational exposure to bloodborne pathogens; final rule, 29 CFR part 1910: 1030. *Federal Register* 56:64003-64182, 1991.

Jackson MM: Infection prevention and control, *Crit Care Nurs Clin North Am* 4(3):401-409, 1992.

Jackson MM, Lynch P: Infection control: too much or too little? *Am J Nurs* 84:208-210, 1984.

Jackson MM, Lynch P: An attempt to make an issue less murky: a comparison of four systems for infection precautions, *Infect Control Hosp Epidemiol* 12:448-450, 1991.

Jackson MM et al: Why not treat all body substances as infectious? *Am J Nurs* 87:1137-1139, 1987.

Lynch P et al: Rethinking the role of isolation practices in the prevention of nosocomiai infections, *Ann Intern Med* 107:243-246, 1987.

Lynch P et al: Implementing and evaluating a system of generic infection precautions: body substance isolation, *Am J Infect Control* 18:1-12, 1990.

Martone WJ, Garner JS, editors: Proceedings of the Third Decennial International Conference on Nosocomial Infections, *Am J Med* 91(3B):1-333, 1991.

Pugliese G, Lynch P, Jackson MM, editors: *Universal Precautions: policies, procedures, and resources,* Chicago, 1990, American Hospital Publishing.

# HEART AND BREATH SOUNDS

## Assessing Heart Sounds

| Sound | Auscultation site | Timing | Pitch | Clinical occurrence | End-piece/patient position |
|-------|-------------------|--------|-------|---------------------|----------------------------|
| $S_1$ ($M_1$ $T_1$) | Apex | Beginning of systole | High | Closing of mitral and tricuspid valves; normal sound | Diaphragm/patient supine |
| $S_1$ split | Apex | Beginning of systole | High | Ventricles contracting at different times due to electrical or mechanical problems (e.g., a longer time span between $M_1$ $T_1$ caused by right bundle-branch heart block, or reversal [$T_1$, $M_1$] caused by mitral stenosis) | Same as $S_1$ |
| $S_2$ ($A_2$ $P_2$) | $A_2$ at 2nd ICS, RSB; $P_2$ at 2nd ICS, LSB | End of systole | High | Closing of aortic and pulmonic valves; normal sound | Diaphragm/patient supine |
| $S_2$ physiologic split | 2nd ICS, LSB | End of systole | High | Accentuated by inspiration; disappears on expiration. Sound that corresponds with the respiratory cycle due to normal delay in closure of pulmonic valve during inspiration. It is accentuated during exercise or in individuals with thin chest walls; heard most often in children and young adults | Same as $S_2$ |
| $S_2$ persistent (wide) split | 2nd ICS, LSB | End of systole | High | Heart throughout the respiratory cycle; caused by late closure of pulmonic valve or early closure of aortic valve. Occurs in atrial septal defect, right ventricular failure, pulmonic stenosis, hypertension, or right bundle-branch heart block | Same as $S_2$ |

Heart and breath sounds

| | | | | | |
|---|---|---|---|---|---|
| S₂ paradoxic (reversed) split (P₂ A₂) | 2nd ICS, LSB | End of systole | High | Because of delayed left ventricular systole, the aortic valve closes after the pulmonic valve rather than before it. (Normally during expiration the two sounds merge.) Causes may include left bundle-branch heart block, aortic stenosis, severe left ventricular failure, MI, and severe hypertension | Same as S₂ |
| S₂ fixed split | 2nd ICS, LSB | End of systole | High | Heard with equal intensity during inspiration and expiration due to split of pulmonic and aortic components, which are unaffected by blood volume or respiratory changes; may be heard in pulmonary stenosis or atrial septal defect | Same as S₂ |
| S₃ (ventricular gallop) | Apex | Early diastole just after S₂ | Dull, low | Early and rapid filling of ventricle, as in early ventricular failure, CHF; common in children, during last trimester of pregnancy, and possibly in healthy adults over age 50 years | Bell/patient in left lateral or supine position |
| S₄ (atrial gallop) | Apex | Late in diastole just before S₁ | Low | Atrium filling against increased resistance of stiff ventricle, as in CHF, CAD, cardiomyopathy, pulmonary artery hypertension, ventricular failure. May be normal in infants, children, and athletes | Same as S₃ |

ICS = intercostal space; RSB = right sternal border; LSB = left sternal border.

## Commonly Occurring Heart Murmurs

| Type | Timing | Pitch | Quality | Auscultation site | Radiation |
|------|--------|-------|---------|-------------------|-----------|
| Pulmonic stenosis | Systolic ejection | Medium-high | Harsh | 2nd ICS, LSB | Toward left shoulder, back |
| Aortic stenosis | Mid-systolic | Medium-high | Harsh | 2nd ICS, RSB | Toward carotid arteries |
| Ventricular septal defect | Late systolic | High | Blowing | 4th ICS, LSB | Toward right sternal border |
| Mitral insufficiency | Holosystolic | High | Blowing | 5-6th ICS, left MCL | Toward left axilla |
| Tricuspid insufficiency | Holosystolic | High | Blowing | 4th ICS, LSB | Toward apex |
| Aortic insufficiency | Early diastolic | High | Blowing | 2nd ICS, RSB | Toward sternum |
| Pulmonary insufficiency | Early diastolic | High | Blowing | 2nd ICS, LSB | Toward sternum |
| Mitral stenosis | Mid-late diastolic | Low | Rumbling | 5th ICS, left MCL | Toward axilla |
| Tricuspid stenosis | Mid-late diastolic | Low | Rumbling | 4th ICS, LSB | Usually none |

ICS = intercostal space; RSB = right sternal border; LSB = left sternal border; MCL = mid-clavicular line.

**Assessing Normal Breath Sounds**

| Type | Normal site | Duration | Characteristics |
|------|-------------|----------|-----------------|
| Vesicular | Peripheral lung | I > E | Soft and swishing sounds. Abnormal when heard over the large airways |
| Bronchial | Trachea and bronchi | E > I | Louder, coarser, and of longer duration than vesicular. Abnormal if heard over peripheral lung |
| Bronchovesicular | Sternal border of the major bronchi | E = I | Moderate in pitch and intensity. Abnormal if heard over peripheral lung |

I = inspiration; E = expiration.

## Assessing Adventitious Breath Sounds

| Type | Waveform | Characteristics | Possible clinical condition |
|------|----------|-----------------|------------------------------|
| Coarse crackle | | Discontinuous, explosive, interrupted. Loud; low in pitch | Pulmonary edema; pneumonia in resolution stage |
| Fine crackle | | Discontinuous, explosive, interrupted. Less loud than coarse crackles, lower in pitch, and of shorter duration | Interstitial lung disease; heart failure; atelectasis |
| Wheeze | | Continuous, of long duration, high-pitched, musical, hissing | Narrowing of airway; bronchial asthma; COPD |
| Rhonchus | | Continuous, of long duration, low-pitched, snoring | Production of sputum (usually cleared or lessened by coughing) |
| Pleural friction rub | | Grating, rasping noise | Rubbing together of inflamed parietal linings; loss of normal pleural lubrication |

## Assessing Respiratory Patterns

| Type | Waveform | Characteristics | Possible clinical condition |
|------|----------|-----------------|-----------------------------|
| Eupnea | ~~~~~ | Normal rate and rhythm for adults and teenagers (12-20 breaths/min) | Normal pattern while awake |
| Bradypnea | ~~~ | Decreased rate (<12 breaths/min); regular rhythm | Normal sleep pattern; opiate or alcohol use; tumor; metabolic disorder |
| Tachypnea | ∿∿∿∿∿ | Rapid rate (>20 breaths/min); hypo- or hyperventilation | Fever; restrictive respiratory disorders; pulmonary emboli |
| Hyperpnea | ⟋⟍⟋⟍ | Depth of respirations greater than normal | Meeting increased metabolic demand (e.g., exercise) |
| Apnea | ——— | Cessation of breathing; may be intermittent | Intermittent with CNS disturbances or drug intoxication; obstructed airway; respiratory arrest if it persists |

*Continued.*

## Assessing Respiratory Patterns—Cont'd

| Type | Waveform | Characteristics | Possible clinical condition |
|---|---|---|---|
| Cheyne-Stokes | | Alternating patterns of apnea (10-20 seconds) with periods of deep and rapid breathing | CHF, narcotic or hypnotic overdose, thyrotoxicosis dissecting aneurysm, subarachnoid hemorrhage, IICP, aortic valve disorders, may be normal in elderly during sleep |
| Biot's | | Irregular (can be slow and deep or rapid and shallow) followed by periods of apnea | CNS abnormalities (e.g., meningitis, IICP) |
| Kussmaul's | | Deep, rapid (>20 breaths/min), sighing, labored | Renal failure, DKA, sepsis, shock |
| Apneustic | | Prolonged inspiration followed by short expirations | Anoxia, meningitis |

# LABORATORY TESTS DISCUSSED IN THIS MANUAL: NORMAL VALUES*

| Complete blood count (CBC) | Adult normal values |
|---|---|
| Hemoglobin (Hgb) | Male: 14-18 g/dl |
| | Female: 12-16 g/dl |
| Hematocrit (Hct) | Male: 40%-54% |
| | Female: 37%-47% |
| Red blood cell (RBC) count | Male: 4.5-6.0 million/μl |
| | Female: 4.0-5.5 million/μl |
| RBC indices | |
| Mean corpuscular volume | 80-95 μm³ |
| Mean corpuscular hemoglobin | 27-31 pg |
| Mean corpuscular hemoglobin concentration | 32-36 g/dl |
| WBC count | 4,500-11,000/μl |
| Neutrophils | 54%-75% |
| Band neutrophils | 3%-8% |
| Lymphocytes | 20%-40% |
| Monocytes | 2%-8% |
| Eosinophils | 1%-4% |
| Basophils | 0.5%-1.0% |
| Platelet count | 150,000-400,000/μl |

| Serum, plasma, and whole blood chemistry | Adult normal values |
|---|---|
| ACTH | 8 AM-10 AM <100 pg/ml |
| ADH (vasopressin) | 1-5 pg/ml |
| Albumin | 3.5-5.5 g/dl |
| Aldosterone | Male: 6-22 ng/dl |
| | Female: 4-31 ng/dl |
| ALT (also called SGPT) | 5-35 IU/L |
| Ammonia | 15-110 μg/dl |
| Amylase | 60-180 Somogyi U/dl |

*Normal values may vary significantly with different laboratory methods of testing.

*Continued.*

| Serum, plasma, and whole blood chemistry—cont'd | Adult normal values—cont'd |
|---|---|
| AST (formerly SGOT) | 8-20 U/L; 5-40 IU/L (values slightly higher in elders and slightly lower in females than in males) |
| Base, total | 145-160 mEq/L |
| Bicarbonate | 22-26 mEq/L |
| Bilirubin | Total: 0.3-1.4 mg/dl |
| Blood gases, arterial | |
| pH | 7.35-7.45 |
| $Paco_2$ | 35-45 mm Hg |
| $Pao_2$ | 80-95 mm Hg |
| $O_2$ saturation ($Sao_2$) | 95%-99% |
| Blood urea nitrogen (BUN) | 6-20 mg/dl |
| CA-125 cancer marker | 0-35 U/ml |
| Calcitonin | <100 pg/ml |
| Calcium | 8.5-10.5 mg/dl; 4.3-5.3 mEq/L |
| Carcinoembryonic antigen (CEA) | <5 ng/ml |
| Chloride (Cl) | 95-108 mEq/L |
| Cortisol | 8 AM-10 AM: 5-25 μ/dl |
| | 4 PM-Midnight: 2-18 μg/dl |
| $CO_2$ content (Total $CO_2$) | 22-28 mEq/L |
| Creatinine | 0.6-1.5 mg/dl |
| Creatinine clearance | Male: 107-141 ml/min |
| | Female: 87-132 ml/min |
| Creatinine phosphokinase (CPK) | Male: 55-170 U/L |
| | Female: 30-135 U/L |
| CPK isoenzyme (MB) | <5% total |
| Erythrocyte sedimentation rate (ESR) | Westergren method: Male: up to 15 mm/h |
| | Female: up to 20 mm/h |
| Fibrin split products (FSPs, FDPs) | <10 μg/ml |
| Folic acid (folate) | 5-20 μg/ml |
| Folicle-stimulating hormone (FSH) | Male: 0.1-15.0 ImU/ml |
| | Female: 6-30 ImU/ml |
| Free thyroxine index (FTI) | 0.9-2.4 ng/dl |
| Globulins, total | 1.5-3.5 g/dl |
| Glucose, fasting | True glucose: 60-120 mg/dl |
| | All sugars: 80-120 mg/dl |
| Glucose, 2-h postprandial | <145 mg/dl |
| Glucose tolerance, | |
| intravenous | Fasting: 60-120 mg/dl |
| | 5 min: maximum 250 mg/dl |
| | 60 min: decrease |
| | 2 h: <120 mg/dl |
| | 3 h: 65-110 mg/dl |
| oral | Fasting: 60-120 mg/dl |
| | 30 min: <155 mg/dl |
| | 1 h: <165 mg/dl |
| | 2 h: <120 mg/dl |
| | 3 h: ≤60-120 mg/dl |
| Growth hormone (GH) | <10 ng/ml |

| Serum, plasma, and whole blood chemistry — cont'd | Adult normal values — cont'd |
|---|---|
| Insulin | 11-240 μIU/ml |
| | 4-24 μU/ml |
| Iron | Total: 60-200 μg/dl |
| | Male, average: 125 μg/dl |
| | Female, average: 100 μg/dl |
| | Elder: 60-80 μg/dl |
| Total iron-binding capacity | 25-420 μg/dl |
| Ketone bodies | 2-4 μg/dl |
| Lactic acid | Arterial: 0.5-1.6 mEq/L |
| | Venous: 1.5-2.2 mEq/L |
| Lactic dehydrogenase | 45-90 U/L; 115-225 IU/L |
| Lipase | 0-110 U/L |
| Magnesium | 1.8-3.0 mg/dl |
| | 1.5-2.5 mEq/L |
| Osmolality | 280-300 mOsm/kg |
| Parathyroid hormone | <2,000 pg/ml |
| Partial thromboplastin time | Normal: 60-70 sec |
| | On anticoagulant therapy: 1/5-2.5 x control value |
| Phosphatase, acid | 0-1.1 U/ml (Bodansky) |
| | 1-4 U/ml (King-Armstrong) |
| | 0.13-0.63 U/ml (Bessey-Lowery) |
| Phosphatase, alkaline | 1.5-4.5 U/dl (Bodansky) |
| | 4-13 U/dl (King-Armstrong) |
| | 0.8-2.3 U/ml (Bessey-Lowery) |
| Phosphorus | 2.5-4.5 mg/dl; 1.7-2.6 mEq/L |
| Potassium | 3.5-5.0 mEq/L |
| Prolactin | 2-15 ng/ml |
| Prothrombin time (PT) | 11-12.5 sec |
| Renin | Normal sodium intake: |
| | Supine (4-6 h): 0.5-1.6 ng/ml/h |
| | Sitting (4 h): 1.8-3.6 ng/ml/h |
| | Low sodium intake: |
| | Supine (4-6 h): 2.2-4.4 ng/ml/h |
| | Sitting (4 h): 4.0-8.1 ng/ml/h |
| Reticulocyte count | 0.5%-2% of total erythrocytes |
| Reticulocyte index | 1.0 |
| Retinol-binding protein | 4-5 mg/dl |
| Sodium | 137-147 mEq/L |
| Thyroid-stimulating hormone | 4.6 μU/ml |
| Thyroxine-binding prealbumin | 20-30 mg/dl |
| Transferrin | 180-260 mg/dl |
| Triiodothyronine ($T_3$) | 110-230 ng/dl |
| Urea clearance | Serum/24-hr urine 64-99 ml/min (maximum clearance) |
| | 41-65 ml/min (standard clearance) |
| Uric acid | Male: 2.0-7.5 mg/dl |
| | Female: 2.0-6.5 mg/dl |

*Continued.*

| Urine chemistry | Adult normal values |
|---|---|
| Albumin | Random: negative |
| | 24-h: 10-100 mg/24 h |
| Amylase | 2-h: 35-260 Somogyi U/h |
| | 24-h: 80-5,000 U/24 h |
| Bilirubin | Random: negative: 0.02 mg/dl |
| Calcium | Random: 1 + turbidity; 10 mg/dl |
| | 24-h: 50-300 mg/24 h |
| Creatinine | 24-h: Male: 20-26 mg/kg/24h |
| | Female: 14-22 mg/kg/24h |
| Creatinine clearance | Male: 107-141 ml/min |
| | Female: 87-132 ml/min |
| Glucose | Random: negative: 15 mg/dl |
| | 24-h: 130 mg/24 h |
| Ketone | 24-h: negative: 0.3-2.0 mg/dl |
| Osmolality | Random: 350-700 mOsm/kg |
| | 24-h: 300-900 mOsm/kg |
| | Physiologic range: 50-1,400 mOsm/kg |
| pH | Random: 4.6-8.0 |
| Phosphorus | 24-h: 0.9-1.3 g; 0.2-0.6 mEq/L |
| Protein | Random: negative: 2-8 mg/dl |
| | 24-h: 40-150 mg |
| Sodium | Random: 50-130 mEq/L |
| | 24-h: 40-220 mEq |
| Specific gravity | Random: 1.010-1.020 |
| | After fluid restriction: 1.025-1.035 |
| Sugar | Random: negative |
| Urea clearance | 24-h: 64-99 ml/min (maximum) |
| | 41-65 ml/min (standard) |
| Urea nitrogen | 24-h: 6-17 g |

# ABBREVIATIONS USED IN THIS MANUAL

**ABG:** arterial blood gas
**ac:** before meals
**AC:** acromioclavicular
**ACBaE:** air contrast barium enema
**ACL:** anterior cruciate ligament
**ACTH:** adrenocorticotropic hormone
**AD:** autonomic dysreflexia
**ADA:** American Diabetes Association
**ADH:** antidiuretic hormone
**ADL:** activities of daily living
**AFB:** acid-fast bacillus
**AFP:** alpha-fetoprotein
**AICD:** automatic implantable cardioverter-defibrillator
**AIDS:** acquired immunodeficiency syndrome
**ALG:** antilymphocyte globulin
**ALL:** acute lymphoblastic leukemia
**ALS:** amyotrophic lateral sclerosis
**ALT:** alanine aminotransferase
**ANC:** absolute neutrophil count
**AP:** anterior posterior
**APR:** abdominoperineal resection
**ARC:** AIDS-related complex
**ARDS:** adult respiratory distress syndrome
**ARF:** acute renal failure; acute respiratory failure
**ASA:** acetylsalicylic acid (aspirin)
**5-ASA:** 5-aminosalicylic acid
**ATCS:** anterior tibial compartment syndrome
**ATN:** acute tubular necrosis
**A-V:** atrioventricular
**AVM:** arteriovenous malformation

**BAER:** brain stem auditory evoked responses
**B&O:** belladonna and opium
**BCNU:** carmustine
**BEE:** basal energy expenditure
**bid:** twice a day
**BMI:** body mass index
**BMT:** bone marrow transplant
**BP:** blood pressure
**BPH:** benign prostatic hypertrophy

**bpm:** beats per minute
**BSE:** breast self-examination
**BSI:** Body Substance Isolation
**BUN:** blood urea nitrogen

**C:** cervical
**CABG:** coronary artery bypass grafting
**CAD:** coronary artery disease
**CAPD:** continuous ambulatory peritoneal dialysis
**CAVH:** continuous arteriovenous hemofiltration
**CBC:** complete blood count
**CBI:** continuous bladder irrigation
**CCNU:** lomustine
**CCPD:** continuous cycling peritoneal dialysis
**CCU:** coronary care unit
**CDC:** Centers for Disease Control
**CEA:** carcinoembryonic antigen
**CHF:** congestive heart failure
**CIE:** counterimmunoelectrophoresis
**Cl:** chloride
**cm:** centimeter
**CMC:** carpometacarpal
**CMV:** cytomegalovirus
**CNS:** central nervous system
**$CO_2$:** carbon dioxide
**COPD:** chronic obstructive pulmonary disease
**CPK:** creatinine phosphokinase
**CPM:** continuous passive movement
**CPP:** cerebral perfusion pressure
**CPR:** cardiopulmonary resuscitation
**CPZ:** chlorpromazine
**CROS:** contralateral routing of signal
**CRF:** chronic renal failure
**CSF:** cerebrospinal fluid
**CT:** computerized axial tomography
**CVA:** cerebrovascular accident, costovertebral angle
**CVC:** central venous catheter
**CVP:** central venous pressure

**D&C:** dilatation and curettage
**DAI:** diffuse axonal injury
**DDAVP:** desmopressin
**DES:** diethylstilbestrol
**DI:** diabetes insipidus
**DIC:** disseminated intravascular coagulation
**DIP:** distal interphalangeal
**DJD:** degenerative joint disease
**DKA:** diabetic ketoacidosis
**dl:** deciliter
**DM:** diabetes mellitus
**DPL:** diagnostic peritoneal lavage
**DSA:** digital subtractive angiography
**DTR:** deep tendon reflex
**DTs:** delirium tremens
**DVT:** deep vein thrombosis
**$D_5NS$:** 5% dextrose in normal saline
**$D_5W$:** 5% dextrose in water

**EBV:** Epstein-Barr virus
**ECA:** external carotid artery
**ECF:** extracellular fluid
**ECG:** electrocardiogram
**EEG:** electroencephalogram
**e.g.:** for example
**ELISA:** enzyme-linked immunosorbent assay
**EMG:** electromyography
**EPS:** electrophysiologic studies
**ERCP:** endoscopic retrocholangiopancreatography
**ERT:** estrogen replacement therapy
**ESR:** erythrocyte sedimentation rate
**ESRD:** end-stage renal disease
**ESWL:** extracorporeal shock wave lithotripsy
**ET:** enterostomal therapy
**EV:** evoked potentials

**F:** Farenheit
**FAP:** familial adenomatous polyposis
**FBS:** fasting blood sugar
**FDA:** federal drug administration
**FEF:** forced mid-expiratory flow
**FEV:** forced expiratory volume
**FFA:** free fatty acids
**FFP:** fresh frozen plasma
**FIGO:** International Federation of Gynecology and Obstetrics
**Fr:** French
**FSH:** follicle-stimulating hormone
**FSP:** fibrin split products
**ft:** foot or feet
**FTI:** free thyroxine index
**FVC:** forced vital capacity

**g:** gram
**G-BS:** Guillain-Barré syndrome
**GGTP:** gammaglutamyl transpeptidase
**GH:** growth hormone
**GI:** gastrointestinal
**GN:** glomerulonephritis
**GOT:** glutamic oxalacetic transaminase

**h:** hour
**H$_2$O:** water
**HAV:** hepatitis A virus
**HBIG:** hepatitis B immune globulin
**HBV:** hepatitis B virus
**HCG:** human chorionic gonadotropin
**HCO$_3$$^-$:** bicarbonate
**Hct:** hematocrit
**HCV:** hepatitis C virus
**Hgb:** hemoglobin
**HHNK:** hyperosmolar hyperglycemic nonketotic (syndrome)
**HI:** head injury
**HIV:** human immunodeficiency virus
**HLA:** human leukocyte antigen
**HOB:** head of bed
**HR:** heart rate

**hs:** hour of sleep
**HTLV-I:** human T-cell leukemia virus-I
**HVWP:** hepatic vein wedge pressure

**I&O:** intake and output
**ICF:** intracellular fluid
**ICP:** intracranial pressure
**ICSH:** interstitial cell-stimulating hormone
**ICU:** intensive care unit
**IDDM:** insulin-dependent diabetes mellitus
**i.e.:** that is
**IgG:** immunoglobulin G
**IGT:** impaired glucose tolerance
**IICP:** increased intracranial pressure
**IM:** intramuscular
**in:** inch or inches
**INH:** isoiazid
**IPD:** intermittent peritoneal dialysis
**IPPB:** intermittent positive pressure breathing
**ITP:** idiopathic thrombocytopenic purpura
**IUD:** intrauterine device
**IV:** intravenous
**IVP:** intravenous pyelogram

**K:** potassium
**KCl:** potassium chloride
**kg:** kilogram
**KS:** Kaposi's sarcoma
**KUB:** kidney, ureter, bladder

**L:** liter; lumbar
**LATS:** long-acting thyroid stimulator
**lb:** pound
**LCTs:** long-chain triglycerides
**LDH:** lactic dehydrogenase
**LES:** lower esophageal sphincter
**LH:** luteinizing hormone
**LLQ:** left lower quadrant
**LMN:** lower motor neuron
**LOC:** level of consciousness
**LP:** lumbar puncture
**LPA:** latex particle agglutination
**LTH:** luteotropic hormone
**LUQ:** left upper quadrant

**MAO:** monamine oxidase
**MCHC:** mean corpuscular hemoglobin concentration
**MCP:** metacarpophalangeal
**MCTs:** medium-chain triglycerides
**MCV:** mean corpuscular volume
**MD:** physician
**mEq:** milliequivalent
**mg:** milligram
**MI:** myocardial infarction
**min:** minute
**ml:** milliliter
**mm:** millimeter
**mmHg:** millimeters of mercury

**mOsm:** milliosmol
**MR:** mitral regurgitation
**MRI:** magnetic resonance imaging
**MS:** multiple sclerosis
**MSH:** melanocyte-stimulating hormone
**MSU:** monosodium urate
**MTP:** metatarsophalangeal
**MUGA scan:** multiple-gated acquisition scan
**μg:** microgram
**μm:** micrometer
**μm$^3$:** cubic micrometer

**N:** nitrogen
**Na:** sodium
**NaCl:** sodium chloride
**NCV:** nerve conduction velocity
**ng:** nanogram
**NG:** nasogastric
**NIDDM:** noninsulin-dependent diabetes mellitus
**NPO:** nothing by mouth
**NS:** nephrotic syndrome
**NSAID:** nonsteroidal antiinflammatory drug
**NSCLC:** nonsmall-cell lung cancer
**NTG:** nitroglycerine

**OA:** osteoarthritis
**O$_2$:** oxygen
**OGTT:** oral glucose tolerance test
**OR:** operating room
**ORIF:** open reduction with internal fixation
**OSHA:** Occupational Safety and Health Administration
**OT:** occupational therapist
**OTC:** over-the-counter

**PAC:** premature atrial contractions
**Paco$_2$:** partial pressure of dissolved carbon dioxide in arterial blood
**Pao$_2$:** partial pressure of dissolved oxygen in arterial blood
**pc:** after meals
**PCA:** patient-controlled analgesia
**PCM:** protein-calorie malnutrition
**PCP:** pneumocystis carinii pneumonia
**PE:** pulmonary embolus
**PEEP:** positive end expiratory pressure
**PET:** positron emission tomography
**pg:** picogram
**pH:** hydrogen ion concentration
**PID:** pelvic inflammatory disease
**PIP:** proximal interphalangeal
**PMI:** point of maximal impulse
**PMN:** polymorphonuclear
**PN:** parenteral nutrition
**PNF:** proprioceptive neuromuscular facilitation
**PO:** by mouth
**POC:** products of conception
**PPF:** plasma protein fraction
**PPG:** postprandial blood glucose
**PPN:** peripheral parenteral nutrition
**PR:** particulate respirator

**prn:** as needed
**PSA:** prostatic-specific antigen
**PT:** physical therapist; prothrombin time
**PTA:** percutaneous transluminal angioplasty
**PTCA:** percutaneous transluminal coronary angioplasty
**PTH:** parathyroid hormone
**PTHC:** percutaneous transhepatic cholangiogram
**PTT:** partial thromboplastin time
**PTU:** propylthiouracil
**PUL:** percutaneous ultrasonic lithotripsy
**PVC:** peripheral venous catheter; premature ventricular contractions
**PVD:** peripheral vascular disease
**PVR:** postvoid residual

**q:** every
**qid:** four times a day

**RA:** rheumatoid arthritis
**RBC:** red blood cell
**RDA:** recommended daily allowance
**REE:** resting energy expenditure
**RIA:** radioimmunoassay
**RIND:** reversible ischemic neurologic deficit
**RLQ:** right lower quadrant
**ROM:** range of motion
**RPE:** rate perceived exertion
**RQ:** respiratory quotient
**RR:** respiratory rate
**RUQ:** right upper quadrant

**S:** sacral
**SA:** status asthmaticus
**S-A:** sinoatrial
**SAARD:** slow-acting antirheumatic drug
**Sao$_2$:** saturation of hemoglobin by oxygen
**SC:** subcutaneous (also abbreviated SQ)
**SCI:** spinal cord injury
**SCLC:** small-cell lung cancer
**sec:** second
**SGOT:** serum glutamic-oxalacetic transaminase
**SGPT:** serum glutamic-pyruvic transaminase
**SIADH:** syndrome of inappropriate antidiuretic hormone
**SNS:** sympathetic nervous system
**SOB:** shortness of breath
**stat:** immediately
**STH:** somatotropic hormone

**T:** thoracic
**T$_3$:** triiodothyronine
**T$_4$:** thyroxine
**TB:** tuberculosis
**TEE:** total energy expenditure
**TENS:** transcutaneous electrical nerve stimulation
**THA:** total hip arthroplasty
**TIA:** transient ischemic attack
**tid:** three times a day
**TKA:** total knee arthroplasty
**TKO:** to keep open

**TNM:** tumor, node, metastasis
**TPN:** total parenteral nutrition
**TPR:** temperature, pulse, respirations
**TRH:** thyrotropin-releasing hormone
**TSH:** thyroid-stimulating hormone; (also known as thyrotropic hormone)
**TTP:** thrombotic thrombocytopenic purpura
**TUR:** transurethral resection
**TURP:** transurethral resection of the prostate
**TURBT:** transurethral resection of the bladder and tumor

**u/U:** unit
**UA:** urinalysis
**UMN:** upper motor neuron
**URI:** upper respiratory infection
**UTI:** urinary tract infection
**UUN:** urine urea nitrogen

**VAD:** venous access device
**VF:** ventricular fibrillation
**VMA:** vanillamandelic acid
**VS:** vital signs
**VT:** ventricular tachycardia

**WB:** Western blot; whole blood
**WBC:** white blood cell
**WHO:** World Health Organization
**WOB:** work of breathing

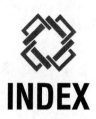

# INDEX

# A

Abbreviations listing, 795-801
Abdominal distension, 398-399
Abdominal trauma, 439-449
ABG. *see* Arterial blood gases
Abortion
  complete, 610
  recurrent or habitual, 610
  spontaneous, 610-613
Absolute neutrophil count, 741
Absorptiometry, 557
ACBaE exam, 417
Achalasia, 386-389
Achilles tendon avulsion fractures, 549
Acid, achalasia and
Acid-fast stains, 8, 24
Acid phosphatase, 623, 793
Acidosis, metabolic, 130, 134, 368
Acnelike reaction, in cancer, 749
Acquired hemolytic anemia, 488
Acquired immunodeficiency syndrome
    (AIDS)
  assessment of, 655-656
  diagnostic tests for, 656-657
  medical management of, 657
  nursing diagnoses and interventions of,
      657-664
  opportunistic infections with, 658-659
  transmission, 653-655
Acromegaly, 351
Acromioclavicular joint dislocation, 533
ACTH (adrenocorticotropic hormone), 347,
    791
ACTH stimulation test, 348
Activated clotting time, hemophilia and,
    503
Activity intolerance
  acute leukemia and, 512-513
  acute renal failure and, 133
  Addison's disease and, 339
  cardiomyopathy and, 49
  chronic renal failure and, 137-138
  coronary artery disease and, 53
  emphysema and, 36-37
  glomerulonephritis and, 114-115
  heart failure and, 61
  human immunodeficiency virus disease
      and, 662
  hypoparathyroidism and, 335-336
  hypoplastic anemia and, 496
  hypothyroidism and, 326-327
  iron deficiency anemia and, 484-485
  mitral regurgitation and, 73
  mitral stenosis and, 70-71
  myocardial infarction and, 58-59
  pericarditis and, 64-65
  pernicious anemia and, 486
  prolonged bed rest and, 711-713
  pulmonary hypertension and, 45-46
Activity/positional alterations, achalasia
    and, 387
Acute leukemias, 510-513
Acute pyelonephritis, 120-123
Acute renal failure, 129-135

Acute respiratory disorders. *see also*
    *specific acute respiratory disorders*
  atelectasis, 1-3
  hemothorax, 19-24
  pleural effusion, 12-13
  pneumonia, 3-12
  pneumothorax, 19-24
  pulmonary embolism, 13-19
  pulmonary tuberculosis, 24-25
Acute respiratory failure, 25-28
Acute tubular necrosis, 129
Addisonian crisis, 337, 338
Addison's disease, 337-340
Adenomatous polyposis, 420-421
ADH (antidiuretic hormone). *see*
    Antidiuretic hormone (ADH)
Adjuvant therapy. *see* Chemotherapy;
    Hormone therapy; Radiation therapy
Adrenal brain graft surgery, 211-212
Adrenal crisis, 337, 338
Adrenal gland disorders
  Addison's disease, 337-340
  Cushing's disease, 340-342
Adrenal transplant, for Parkinsonism, 208
Adrenocortical inhibitors, 341
Adrenocorticotropic hormone (ACTH),
    336, 340, 343
Adriamycin (doxorubicin), 726
Adventitious breath sounds, 788
AFB isolation, pulmonary tuberculosis and,
    25
Affective touch, 754
Afterload, 60
AIDS. *see* Acquired immunodeficiency
    syndrome (AIDS)
Airway clearance
  asthma and, 33-34
  cerebral aneurysm and, 275
  chronic bronchitis and, 33
  pneumonia and, 10
  postoperative, 700-701
  spinal cord injury and, 239-240
Airway maintenance, head injury and, 251
Airway restrictions, cerebral aneurysm and,
    271
Albumin
  cirrhosis and, 458
  for hypoplastic anemia, 494
  normal value, 791
  urinary, 794
Alcoholic cirrhosis, 457
Alcoholic hepatitis, 450
Aldosterone, 791
Alkaline phosphatase
  cirrhosis and, 458
  lymphomas and, 509
  normal values, 793
  pancreatic tumors and, 476
  prostatic neoplasm and, 623
Alkylating agents, polycythemia and, 498
ALL (acute lymphocytic leukemia), 510
Allergic reactions, to insulin, 355
Allopurinol, gouty arthritis and, 523
Alpha fetoprotein, 627

ALT. *see* Serum glutamic-pyruvic transamination (SGPT)
Aluminum hydroxide, 137, 335
Alveolar hypoventilation, 26
Alzheimer's disease, 213-224
Amantadine
  multiple sclerosis and, 184
  Parkinsonism and, 204, 206
  side effects, 210-211
Ambulation, total knee arthroplasty and, 578
Ambulatory monitoring
  coronary artery disease and, 51
  dysrhythmias/conduction disturbances and, 81
Amethoptrin (methotrexate), 727-728
Aminocaproic acid (Amicar)
  cerebral aneurysm and, 271-275
  disseminated intravascular coagulation and, 17
  hemophilia and, 503
  pulmonary embolus and, 17
Aminoglycosides, 544
Aminophylline, 27, 29
Ammonia, 458, 791
Amplification, cochlear implantation and, 651
Amputation, 564-569
Amylase
  abdominal trauma and, 442
  pancreatitis and, 471
  serum value, normal, 791
  urinary value, normal, 794
Anabolic steroids, chronic renal failure and, 137
Analgesics
  abdominal trauma and, 443
  atelectasis and, 2
  brain tumors and, 261
  bronchogenic carcinoma and, 40
  cerebral aneurysm and, 272
  cerebrovascular accident and, 279
  commonly used, 698-699, 700
  diverticulitis and, 416
  encephalitis and, 200
  gouty arthritis and, 523
  Guillain-Barré syndrome and, 190
  head injury and, 252
  intervertebral disk disease and, 226
  narcotic. *see* Narcotics
  obstructive processes and, 400
  pneumonia and, 9
  pneumothorax/hemothorax and, 22
  spinal cord injury and, 235
  spinal cord tumors and, 267
  urinary retention and, 165
Anaphylactic shock, 76
Ancord, cerebrovascular accident and, 280
Androgens, hypoplastic anemia and, 495
Anemia
  defined, 483
  hemolytic, 488-491
  hypoplastic, 491-497
  pernicious, 485-488

Anesthetics
  injection, for intervertebral disk disease, 226
  topical, 461
Aneurysms
  abdominal, 101-103
  cerebral, 269-276
  femoral, 101-103
  thoracic, 101-103
Angina classification, 51
Angiography. *see also* Arteriography
  abdominal trauma and, 442
  arterial embolism and, 103
  cirrhosis and, 459, 460
  mitral regurgitation and, 73
  peripheral vascular disorders and, 97
Angioplasty, postoperative assessment, 128-129
Angle-closure glaucoma, 642
Ankle dislocation, 534
Anorexia, 742-743
Anoscopy, 411
Antacids
  achalasia and, 387
  acute renal failure and, 131
  brain tumors and, 261
  cerebrovascular accident and, 279
  encephalitis and, 200
  head injury and, 252
  hiatal hernia and, 384
  hyperparathyroidism and, 331
  pancreatitis and, 472
  peptic ulcers and, 390-392
Anterior colporrhaphy, 607
Anterior cruciate ligament, torn, 536-538
Anterior nerve root involvement, in Guillain-Barré syndrome, 188
Anthropometrics, 666
Anti-Parkinson medications, 209-211
Antiandrogens
  benign prostatic hypertrophy and, 616
  side effects, 625
Antiarrhythmic drugs, 48, 131
Antibiotics
  abdominal trauma and, 443
  acute renal failure and, 131
  acute respiratory failure and, 27
  asthma and, 29
  bacterial meningitis and, 196-197
  chronic bronchitis and, 33
  cirrhosis and, 461
  corneal ulceration/trauma and, 634
  Crohn's disease and, 430
  glomerulonephritis and, 114
  head injury and, 252
  hernia and, 402
  hypoplastic anemia and, 495
  infective endocarditis and, 67
  long-term intermittent, 545-546
  nephrotic syndrome and, 118
  neurogenic bladder and, 168
  obstructive processes and, 399
  osteomyelitis and, 543-544
  pancreatitis and, 472
  peritonitis and, 405

Antibiotics—cont'd
  pneumonia and, 9
  prolonged use, side effects of, 544
  spinal cord injury and, 236
  total hip arthroplasty and, 574
  ulcerative colitis and, 425
  ureteral calculi and, 149
  urinary retention and, 166
  urinary tract obstruction and, 153
Anticholinergics
  hiatal hernia and, 384
  neurogenic bladder and, 168
  pancreatitis and, 472
  Parkinsonism and, 204-205, 207
  peptic ulcer and, 391
  side effects, 211
  spinal cord injury and, 237
  ulcerative colitis and, 423
Anticipatory grieving, cancer and, 757-758
Anticoagulants
  cardiomyopathy and, 48
  cerebrovascular accident and, 279
  disseminated intravascular coagulation
    and, 505, 507
  glomerulonephritis and, 114
  mitral regurgitation and, 73
  nephrotic syndrome and, 118
  pulmonary emboli and, 15-16, 18-19
  pulmonary hypertension and, 45
Antidepressants
  Alzheimer's disease and, 215
  multiple sclerosis and, 184
  Parkinsonism and, 205
  tricyclic, 215, 252
Antidiarrheals
  cirrhosis and, 461
  Crohn's disease and, 430
  ulcerative colitis and, 423, 424
Antidiuretic hormone (ADH). *see also*
    Vasopressin
  actions of, 343
  inappropriate, syndrome of, 351-353
  normal value, 791
Antiembolism hose
  cerebral aneurysm and, 272
  cerebrovascular accident and, 280
  Guillain-Barré syndrome and, 190
  head injury and, 252
  intervertebral disk disease and, 226
  Parkinsonism and, 208
  spinal cord injury and, 236
Antiemetics
  bronchogenic carcinoma and, 40
  cancer and, 743
  hepatitis and, 454
  hiatal hernia and, 384
  obstructive processes and, 400
  ureteral calculi and, 149
Antiepileptic drugs
  Alzheimer's disease and, 216
  brain tumors and, 261
  cerebral aneurysm and, 272
  commonly used, 297-298
  head injury and, 251
  seizure disorders and, 291

side effects, 294-295
Antifibrinolytic agents. *see* Thrombolytic
    therapy
Antihistamine sedatives, cancer and, 707
Antihistamines
  cirrhosis and, 461
  hepatitis and, 454
  Parkinsonism and, 205, 207
Antihypertensives
  acute renal failure and, 131
  cerebral aneurysm and, 272
  cerebrovascular accident and, 279
  chronic renal failure and, 137
  glomerulonephritis and, 114
  head injury and, 252
  nephrotic syndrome and, 118
Antiinfective agents, encephalitis and, 200
Antiinflammatory agents. *see also specific*
    *agents*
  acute renal failure and, 131
  nonsteroidal, 64, 519, 700
  rheumatoid arthritis and, 527-528
  ulcerative colitis and, 423
Antilymphocyte globulin, hypoplastic
    anemia and, 495
Antilymphocyte sera (ATGAM), 141
Antimalarials, 527
Antimicrosomal antibodies, 325
Antineoplastic agents, with known emetic
    action, 743. *see also* Chemotherapy
Antinuclear antibodies, 526
Antinuclear antibody titer,
    glomerulonephritis and, 114
Antiotensin-converting enzyme, 52
Antiplatelet drugs, cerebrovascular accident
    and, 279
Antipsychotics, 216
Antipyretics
  acute pyelonephritis and, 121
  bacterial meningitis and, 196
  brain tumors and, 261
  cerebral aneurysm and, 272
  cerebrovascular accident and, 279
  encephalitis and, 200
  head injury and, 252
  pneumonia and, 9
Antiresorptive agents, osteoporosis and,
    558
Antispasmodics
  multiple sclerosis and, 184
  spinal cord injury and, 236
  urinary tract obstruction and, 153
Antistreptolysin O titer, glomerulonephritis
    and, 114
Antithrombus regimen, total hip
    arthroplasty and, 574
Antithyroid agents, 320
Antitremor drugs, 205
Antitussives, pneumonia and, 9
Antiviral agents
  encephalitis and, 200
  Parkinsonism and, 204, 206-207
Anxiety
  Alzheimer's disease and, 220-221
  benign breast disorders and, 590

Anxiety—cont'd
  breast cancer and, 593
  breast reconstruction and, 587-588
  cancer and, 753-754
  human immunodeficiency virus disease
      and, 662
  hyperthroidism and, 322
  urinary diversions and, 172-173
Aortic insufficiency, 786
Aortic regurgitation, 75-76
Aortic stenosis, 74-75, 786
Aortic valve replacement, aortic stenosis
      and, 74
Aortography, aneurysms and, 101
Aortorenal bypass graft, 128-129
Aphasia, 284
Aplastic anemia, 491, 495-497
Apley grinding test, 535
Apnea, 789
Apneustic respirations, 790
Appendectomy, 409
Appendicitis, 407-410
Ara-C (cytosine arabinoside), 728-729
ARF (acute respiratory failure), 25-28
Arm circumference, 666
Arterial blood gases
  acute respiratory failure and, 27
  asthma and, 29
  atelectasis and, 2
  cardiac/noncardiac shock and, 78
  chronic bronchitis and, 33
  dysrhythmias/conduction disturbances
      and, 81
  emphysema and, 35-36
  fat emboli and, 15
  myocardial infarction and, 57
  normal values, 792
  peritonitis and, 405
  pneumothorax and, 20
  pulmonary edema and, 86
  pulmonary embolus and, 15
  pulmonary fibrosis and, 38
  pulmonary hypertension and, 45
  spinal cord injury and, 235
Arterial embolism, 103-104
Arterial endarterectomy, 128
Arterial occlusive disease, 96-100
Arteriography. see also Angiography
  aneurysms and, 101
  ischemic myositis and, 539
Arthritis
  gouty, 522-525
  rheumatoid, 525-529
Arthrodesis, 528
Arthrography
  anterior cruciate ligament tears and, 537
  dislocations/subluxations and, 533
  ligamentous injuries and, 530
  meniscal injuries and, 535
Arthroplasty
  rheumatoid arthritis and, 528
  total hip, 573-577
  total knee, 577-579
Arthroscopic surgery, meniscal injuries
      and, 536

Arthroscopy
  anterior cruciate ligament tears and, 537
  dislocations/subluxations and, 533
  ligamentous injuries and, 530
  meniscal injuries and, 535-536
  rheumatoid arthritis and, 528
Artificial kidney, 145. see also
      Hemodialysis
Artificial urinary sphincter, 160, 168
Ascending colostomy, 434
Ascites, 461-462
L-Asparaginase (Elspar), 730-731
Aspergillosis, 7
Aspiration
  elderly and, 767-768
  of fecal matter, obstructive processes
      and, 399
  neurologic disorders and, 302
  nutritional support and, 678
  postoperative risk, 701-703
  tube-feeding and, 675
Aspiration curretage, 601
Aspiration pneumonia, 3, 6, 8
Aspirin with dipyridamole, cerebrovascular
      accident and, 279
Assessment. see under specific disorders
Assistive devices, osteoarthritis and, 520
AST. see Serum glutamic-oxaloacetic
      transaminase (SGOT)
Asthma, 28-32
Astrocytomas, 258
Atelectasis, 1-3
ATGAM (antilymphocyte sera), 141
Atherosclerotic arterial occlusive disease,
      96-100
ATN. see Acute tubular necrosis
Atropine, 216
Auditory neglect, cerebrovascular accident
      and, 282
Automaticity disturbances, 80
Autonomic dysreflexia, 234, 237-238
Autonomic nervous system disorders
  cerebral aneurysm and, 270
  Guillain-Barré syndrome and, 188, 190
  Parkinsonism and, 203
Axid (nizatidine), 472
Azathioprine (Imuran), 140
AZT (zidovudine), 658


B

B-scan ultrasonography, 639
Baclofen, 186, 237
Bacterial meningitis, 194-199
Bactrim (sulfamethoxazole), 658
Balloon diltation, benign prostatic
      hypertrophy and, 616
Bankart procedure, 572
Barbiturate coma therapy, 252, 280
Barium enema
  Crohn's disease and, 429
  diverticulitis and, 415
  diverticulosis/diverticulitis and, 415
  hemorrhoids and, 411

Barium enema—cont'd
  obstructive processes and, 399
  rectocele and, 608
  ulcerative colitis and, 423
Barium swallow
  cirrhosis and, 458
  hiatal hernia/reflux esophagitis and, 383
  malabsorption/maldigestion and, 396
  obstructive processes and, 399
  peptic ulcer and, 389
Base, total, 792
Basilar skull fractures, 249
BCNU (carmustine), 722
Bed rest, prolonged, 711-719
Bence Jones protein, 555
Benign neoplasms
  of breast, 588-590
  of musculoskeletal system, 553-555
Benign prostatic hypertrophy, 615-622
Benserazide-levodopa, for Parkinsonism,
    206
Benzodiazepines, 707
Berry aneurysms, 269
Beta-adrenergic agents, pulmonary
    hypertension and, 45
Beta-adrenergic blockers
  cardiomyopathy and, 48
  coronary artery disease and, 52, 54-55
  glaucoma and, 642
  hyperthyroidism and, 320
  mitral regurgitation and, 73
Bethanechol chloride, 184, 186
Bicarbonate
  acute renal failure and, 132
  chronic renal failure and, 137
  diabetic ketoacidosis and, 367
  hyperosmolar hyperglycemic nonketotic
    syndrome and, 372
  normal values, 792
Bilateral orchiectomy, 624, 625
Bilateral salpingo-oophorectomy, 601
Bile, 450
Biliary cirrhosis, 457
Biliary disorders, 449-470
Biliary stone removal, nonsurgical, 468
Bilirubin
  cholelithisis/cholecystitis and, 467
  cirrhosis and, 458
  heart failure and, 60
  hemolytic anemia and, 489
  normal value, 792
  pancreatic tumors and, 476
  urinary, 794
Biologic response modifiers, 731
Biopsy. *see also specific types of biopsy*
  AIDS and, 657
  bladder cancer and, 155
  endometrial, 601
  lymphomas and, 509
  testicular neoplasm and, 627
  vulvar, 603
Biot's respirations, 790
Bladder
  cancer of, 154-158

decompression, spinal cord injury and,
    235
  dysfunction
    Guillain-Barré syndrome and, 190
    spinal cord injury and, 234, 243
    spinal cord tumors and, 266-267
  dysreflexia and, 238
  flaccid, 167, 243-244
  neurogenic, 167-171
  obstruction, 125
  spastic, 167, 243
Bladder pacemaker, 168
Bladder training programs
  brain tumors and, 262
  cerebrovascular accident and, 280
  head injury and, 252
  multiple sclerosis and, 183
  spinal cord tumors and, 268
  urinary incontinence and, 159-160, 161
Blasts, 510
Bleeding risk, low platelet count and, 496
Bleeding time
  disseminated intravascular coagulation
    and, 505
  hemophilia and, 503
  hypoplastic anemia and, 495
  thrombocytopenia and, 500
Bleomycin (blenoxane), 725-726
Blood chemistries, normal values,
    791-793. *see also specific blood
    chemistries*
Blood coagulants, 461
Blood count, iron deficiency anemia and,
    484
Blood culture
  acute pyelonephritis and, 121
  cardiac/noncardiac shock and, 78
  diverticulitis and, 415
  glomerulonephritis and, 114
  infective endocarditis and, 67
  osteomyelitis and, 543
  pneumonia and, 8
Blood gases. *see* Arterial blood gases
Blood products, 492-494
Blood replacement, total hip arthroplasty
    and, 574
Blood urea nitrogen (BUN)
  acute renal failure, 130
  benign prostatic hypertrophy and, 615
  cardiac/noncardiac shock and, 78
  chronic renal failure and, 136
  cirrhosis and, 458
  glomerulonephritis and, 114
  hydronephrosis and, 125
  neurogenic bladder and, 168
  normal values, 792
  prostatic neoplasm and, 622
  renal artery stenosis and, 128
  ureteral calculi and, 148
  urinary incontinence and, 159
  urinary retention and, 165
  urinary tract obstruction and, 152
Body image disturbance
  amputation and, 568
  breast reduction and, 584

Body image disturbance—cont'd
  breast cancer and, 594-595
  breast reconstruction and, 587
  cancer and, 738-739, 760-761
  Cushing's disease and, 341
  fecal diversions and, 437-438
  hepatitis and, 456
  human immunodeficiency virus disease
     and, 662-663
  hyperthroidism and, 323
  indicators, 761
  ischemic myositis and, 541
  penile implants and, 630-631
  urinary incontinence and, 163
Body mass index, 666
Body substance isolation (BSI), 197, 779
Body temperature, neurologic disorders
  and, 310-311
Bone biopsy, 543, 560
Bone grafting, 570-571
Bone marrow aspiration
  acute leukemia and, 511
  chronic leukemia and, 514
  hemolytic anemia and, 489
  hypoplastic anemia and, 495
  iron deficiency anemia and, 486
  malignant neoplasms and, 555
  polycythemia and, 498
  thrombocytopenia and, 500
Bone marrow biopsy, 509
Bone marrow transplantation, 495, 511,
  514
Bone scans
  dislocations/subluxations and, 533
  lymphomas and, 509
  spinal, brain tumors and, 267
Bowel
  dysfunction
    Guillain-Barré syndrome and, 190
    spinal cord injury and, 234
    spinal cord tumors and, 266-267
  dysreflexia and, 238
  elimination, rectocele and, 608
  incontinence, 218, 436-437
Bowel movement regulation, hemorrhoids
  and, 411
Bowel programs
  brain tumors and, 262
  cerebrovascular accident and, 280
  head injury and, 252
  multiple sclerosis and, 183
  spinal cord injury and, 236
  spinal cord tumors and, 268
Bracing, of torn anterior cruciate ligament,
  537
Bradykinesia, 203
Bradypnea, 789
Brain biopsy, 200, 215
Brain death, 250
Brain herniation, 199, 250, 306
Brain laceration, 248
Brain scan, 251, 260
Brain tumors, 258-266
Breast disorders
  benign, 588-590

  malignant, 590-596
Breast implants, 737
Breast reconstruction, 585-588
Breast reduction, 583-585
Breast self-examination (BSE), 584-585
Breath sounds, 787, 788
Breathing pattern
  abdominal trauma and, 447
  atelectasis and, 2-3
  cancer and, 739
  emphysema and, 36
  Guillain-Barré syndrome and, 190-191
  hiatal hernia and, 385
  hypothyroidism and, 326
  pericarditis and, 66
  peritonitis and, 406
  pleural effusion and, 13
  pneumothorax and, 22-23
  postoperative, 703
  pulmonary fibrosis and, 38-39
Bristow procedure, 571-572
Brodie-Trendelenburg test, 108
Bromocriptine, 204, 207
Bronchitis, chronic, 32-35
Bronchodilators
  acute respiratory failure and, 27
  asthma and, 29, 31
  chronic bronchitis and, 33
  pulmonary hypertension and, 45
Bronchogenic carcinoma, 39-41
Bronchoscopy, 2, 40
Brooke ileostomy, 434
Brudzinski's sign, 195
BSE (breast self-examination), 584-585
BSI universal precautions, 777-779
Bunionectomy, 562-564

## C

CA-125 cancer marker, 792
Calcitonin
  hyperparathyroidism and, 331
  normal value, 792
  Paget's disease and, 561
Calcium
  excretion, promotion of, 331
  hyperparathyroidism and, 330
  normal value, 792
  osteoporosis and, 557-558
  pancreatitis and, 470
  urinary, 794
Calcium antagonists, 45, 48
Calcium carbonate, chronic renal failure
  and, 137
Calcium channel blockers
  achalasia and, 387
  cerebral aneurysm and, 273
  cerebrovascular accident and, 280
  coronary artery disease and, 52
Calcium stones, 149, 151
Calcium supplements
  acute renal failure, 132
  hyperparathyroidism and, 331
  hypoparathyroidism and, 335

Calculi
  renal, 123-125
  ureteral, 147-152
Calories
  chronic obstructive pulmonary disease
      and, 34
  distribution of, 668
Cancer
  bladder, 154-158
  breast, 590-596
  bronchiogenic, 39-41
  cervical, 596-600
  chemotherapy for. *see* Chemotherapy
  colorectal, 417-419
  endometrial or uterine, 602-603
  patient care, 738-753
      activity intolerance and, 738
      body image disturbances and, 738-739
      breathing pattern and, 739
      chronic pain and, 739-740
      constipation and, 740-741
      diarrhea and, 741
      infection and, 741-742
      nutrition and, 742-744
      oral mucous membranes and, 744
      pain and, 744
      physical mobility and, 744
      protection alteration and, 745
      sensory/perceptual alterations and,
          745-746
      sexual dysfunction and, 746-747
      skin integrity and, 747-750
      swallowing and, 750-751
      tissue perfusion and, 751-752
      urinary elimination and, 752-753
  prostatic, 622-626
  psychosocial care
      anticipatory grieving and, 757-758
      anxiety and, 753-754
      body image disturbance and, 760-761
      dysfunctional grieving and, 758
      fear and, 756-757
      hopelessness and, 762-763
      ineffectual coping and, 757
      pattern of violence and, 761-762
      powerlessness and, 759
      sensory/perceptual alterations and,
          755-756
      sleep pattern disturbances and, 756
      social isolation and, 760
      spiritual distress and, 759-760
      verbal communication impairment
          and, 755
  pulmonary embolus and, 14
  radiation therapy. *see* Radiation therapy
  vulvar, 603-605
CAPD (continuous ambulatory peritoneal
      dialysis), 143
Captopril test, 128
Carafate (sucralfate), 384, 390, 391
Carbamazepine (Tegretol), 184, 297
Carbidopa-levodopa, for Parkinsonism, 206
Carbohydrates
  in enteral nutrition formulas, 669

  in parenteral nutrition formulas, 673
  requirements, 668
Carbon dioxide, total, 792
Carcinoembryonic antigen (CEA)
  bladder cancer and, 155
  colorectal cancer and, 418
  normal value, 792
  ovarian cancer and, 600
Cardiac angioplasty, 91-94
Cardiac arrest, 84-85
Cardiac catheterization, 91-94
  with angiography, 75
      aortic stenosis and, 74
      pulmonary hypertension and, 44
  cardiomyopathy and, 48
  mitral stenosis and, 69
Cardiac disorders, pulmonary embolus and,
      14. *see also specific cardiac
      disorders*
Cardiac enzymes, pericarditis and, 64
Cardiac fluid, increasing, 60
Cardiac output, decreased, 48, 58, 70
Cardiac procedures, special, 88-91
Cardiac shock, 76-80
Cardiac surgery, 94-96
Cardiac tamponade, 136
Cardiomyopathy, 47-50
Cardiopulmonary tissue perfusion
  cancer and, 751
  cardiomyopathy and, 48-49
  diabetes mellitus and, 359-360
  disseminated intravascular coagulation
      and, 507
  fractures and, 551-552
  Guillain-Barré syndrome and, 191-192
  hemolytic anemia and, 490
  nutritional support and, 680
  polycythemia and, 499
  spinal cord injury and, 244-245
Cardiospasm, 386-389
Cardiovascular disorders. *see also specific
      disorders*
  secondary, 76-88
Carmustine (BCNU), 722
Carotid artery clamping, 273
Carotid endarterectomy, 280, 286-287
Casts
  care and assessment of, 531-532
  fractures and, 553
Catecholamine, 60
Catheterization, benign prostatic
      hypertrophy and, 616
Catheters
  CVP, 405
  parenteral nutrition and, 673, 676
  peritoneal dialysis and, 143
  ureteral, 149
  urinary. *see* Urinary catheter
Cation exchange resins (Kayexalate), 132
Cauda equina fracture, 236
CAVH (continuous arteriovenous
      hemofiltration), 142-143
CBC. *See* Complete blood count (CBC)
CCNU (lomustine), 725

CCPD (continuous cycling peritoneal dialysis), 143
CDC category-specific and disease-specific isolation precautions, 777, 778
CDC universal precautions, 777-779
CDCA (chenodeoxycholic acid), 467
CEA. *see* Carcinoembryonic antigen
CEA (carcinembryonic antigen), 792
Cecostomy, 434
Cephalosporins, 544
Cerebellar tumors, focal symptoms, 259
Cerebral aneurysm, 269-276
Cerebral angiography
  brain tumors and, 260
  cerebral aneurysm and, 271
  cerebrovascular accident and, 278
  head injury and, 251
  patient instructions/understandings of, 314-315
  pituitary and hypothalamic tumors and, 348
Cerebral artery bypass surgery, 280, 285-286
Cerebral blood flow studies, cerebral aneurysm and, 271
Cerebral blood vessel rupture, 249-250
Cerebral salt wasting syndrome, 273
Cerebral tissue perfusion
  diabetes mellitus and, 359-360
  disseminated intravascular coagulation and, 507
  fractures and, 551-552
  Guillain-Barré syndrome and, 191-192
  neurologic disorders and, 305-307
  polycythemia and, 498-499
  prolonged bed rest and, 715-716
  spinal cord injury and, 244-245
  thrombocytopenia and, 501
Cerebral vasospasm, 270, 273
Cerebral vessel rupture. *see* Cerebrovascular accident (CVA)
Cerebrospinal fluid (CSF)
  bacterial meningitis and, 195
  brain tumors and, 260, 267
  cerebral aneurysm and, 271
  cerebrovascular accident and, 278
  encephalitis and, 199
  Guillain-Barré syndrome and, 189
  leakage, 255-256
  leakage repair, 254
  multiple sclerosis and, 183
  Parkinsonism and, 204
  seizure disorders and, 290
Cerebrovascular accident (CVA), 276-288
Cervical cancer, 596-600
Cervical cerclage, 611
Cervical disk disease, 224
Cervical fractures, 547, 548
Cervical injury, 233
Cervical spine injuries, 235
Cervical traction, intervertebral disk disease and, 232
Chemical burns, corneal, 633
Chemolysis, 149
Chemonucleolysis, 226, 231

Chemotherapy
  acute leukemia and, 511
  bladder cancer and, 156
  brain tumors and, 261-262
  breast cancer and, 592-593
  bronchogenic carcinoma and, 40
  cervical cancer and, 598
  chronic leukemia and, 514
  colorectal cancer and, 418, 420
  endometrial cancer and, 603
  injury risk and, 719-720
  lymphomas and, 509
  ovarian tumors and, 601
  prostatic neoplasm and, 624
  side effects, 733-734
  spinal cord tumors and, 268
  testicular neoplasm and, 627
  tissue integrity and, 720, 733
Chemotherapy agents, 722-731
Chenodeoxycholic acid (CDCA), 467
Chest physiotherapy
  acute respiratory failure and, 27
  asthma and, 29
  atelectasis and, 2
  for chronic bronchitis, 33, 34
  chronic bronchitis and, 33
Chest tubes, 13, 20
Chest x-ray
  acute respiratory failure and, 27
  aneurysms and, 101
  aortic regurgitation and
  aortic stenosis and, 74
  asthma and, 29
  atelectasis and, 2
  bronchogenic carcinoma and, 40
  cardiomyopathy and, 47
  cervical cancer and, 597
  chronic bronchitis and, 33
  coronary artery disease, 50
  emphysema and, 35
  fat emboli and, 15
  heart failure and, 60
  hiatal hernia and, 383
  lymphomas and, 509
  mitral regurgitation and, 72
  mitral stenosis and, 69
  myocardial infarction and, 56
  ovarian tumors and, 601
  pleural effusion and, 12
  pneumonia and, 8
  pneumothorax and, 20
  pulmonary edema and, 86
  pulmonary embolus and, 15
  pulmonary fibrosis and, 37
  pulmonary hypertension and, 44
  pulmonary tuberculosis and, 24
  testicular neoplasm and, 627
Cheyne-Stokes respirations, 790
Chloride, 792
Cholangiogram, 467
Cholecystectomy, 468
Cholecystitis, 465-470
Cholecystostomy, 468
Choledochoduodenostomy, 468
Choledochojejunostomy, 468

Choledocholithiasis, 465
Choledochotomy, 468
Cholelithiasis, 465-470
Cholinergics, urinary retention and, 165
Chondrosarcomas, 555
Choreiform movements, 205
Chronic bronchitis, 32-35
Chronic hepatitis, 450
Chronic leukemia, 513-514
Chronic lymphocytic leukemia, 514
Chronic myelocytic leukemia, 514
Chronic obstructive pulmonary disease,
    asthma and, 28-32
Chronic pain, cancer and, 739-740
Chronic pulmonary disease, pulmonary
    embolus and, 14
Chronic renal failure (CRF), 135-140
Chrysotherapy, 527
CIE (counterimmunoelectrophoresis), 195
Cimetidine (Tagamet), 472
Cineradiographic study of swallowing,
    Parkinsonism and, 204
Circulatory failure, 76-80
Cirrhosis, 457-465
Cisplatinum (Platinol), 722-723
Clavicle fractures, 548
Clonic seizures, 289
Closed pneumothorax, 19, 21
Closed reduction, 549
Coagulation disorders, 499-508. *see also*
    *specific disorders*
Coagulation factors, 493-494, 499
Coagulation techniques, hemorrhoids and,
    412
Coagulation tests, cirrhosis and, 458
Cochlear implantation, 650-652
Cognitive processes, Alzheimer's disease
    and, 213-214
Cognitive rehabilitation
    goals, 253-254
    head injury and, 252
Colchicine, gouty arthritis and, 523
Colectomy, 420
Colitis, ulcerative, 421-428
Colon, blunt trauma and, 440
Colonoscopy, 411, 417, 420, 423, 429
Colony-stimulating factors, 732
Colorectal cancer, 417-419
Colostomy, 434, 435-437, 438
Colposcopy, 597
Communication, verbal. *see* Verbal
    communication
Communication patterns, Alzheimer's
    disease and, 214
Community-acquired pneumonia, 3, 4-5
Compartment pressure, 539
Compartment syndrome, 538-542
Complete abortion, 610
Complete blood count (CBC)
    acute leukemia and, 511
    asthma and, 29
    bladder cancer and, 155
    cardiac/noncardiac shock and, 78
    chronic bronchitis and, 33
    chronic leukemia and, 514

diverticulosis/diverticulitis and, 415
fat emboli and, 15
Guillain-Barré syndrome and, 189
heart failure and, 60
hemorrhoids and, 411
hiatal hernia and, 383
hypoplastic anemia and, 495
lymphomas and, 509
myocardial infarction and, 57
normal values, 791
pancreatitis and, 470
pericarditis and, 64
pneumothorax and, 20
polycythemia and, 498
pulmonary hypertension and, 45
spontaneous abortion and, 611
thrombocytopenia and, 500
wound healing and, 685
Complex seizures, partial, 290
Compression sleeves, sequential, 272, 280
Computed tomography
    abdominal trauma and, 442
    Addison's disease and, 337
    Alzheimer's disease and, 215
    aneurysms and, 101
    brain tumors and, 260
    cerebral aneurysm and, 271
    cerebrovascular accident and, 278
    cervical cancer and, 597
    chronic renal failure and, 136
    colorectal cancer and, 417
    Cushing's disease and, 341
    diverticulitis and, 415
    encephalitis and, 200
    head injury and, 250
    intervertebral disk disease and, 225
    lymphomas and, 509
    malabsorption/maldigestion and, 396
    malignant neoplasms and, 555
    multiple sclerosis and, 183
    osteomyelitis and, 543
    pancreatic tumors and, 476
    patient instructions/understandings of,
        312-313
    pituitary and hypothalamic tumors and,
        348
    seizure disorders and, 290
    spinal, brain tumors and, 267
    spinal cord injury and, 234
    ureteral calculi and, 148
Concussion
    brain, 247
    patient care for, 254-255
    spinal cord, 233
Condom catheter, 160, 164
Conduction disturbances, 80-84
Conductive hyperthermia, for brain tumors,
    262
Conductivity disturbances, 80
Congenital glaucoma, 641, 642
Congestive cardiomyopathy, 47
Congestive heart failure, 136
Conization biopsy, 597
Conjunctival culture, 634

Connective tissue disorders, 529-542. *see
    also specific connective tissue
    disorders*
Constipation
  acute renal failure and, 135
  benign prostatic hypertrophy and,
    619-620
  cancer and, 740-741
  elderly and, 768-770
  hemorrhoids and, 412-413
  hyperparathyroidism and, 332-333
  hypothyroidism and, 327-328
  neurologic disorders and, 305
  nutritional support and, 678
  pernicious anemia and, 487
  postoperative, 706-707
  prolonged bed rest and, 716-717
  rectocele and, 608-609
  spinal cord injury and, 238-239
Contact lens overwear, 634
Continent ileostomy, 434-435, 436
Continent urinary diversion, 172, 175
Continent urinary reservoir, 171
Continent vesicostomy, 168, 171
Continuous ambulatory peritoneal dialysis
    (CAPD), 143
Continuous arteriovenous hemofiltration
    (CAVH), 142-143
Continuous cycling peritoneal dialysis
    (CCPD), 143
Continuous passive movement, total knee
    arthroplasty and, 578
Contrast phlebography, 105
Contusion, 248
Conventional ileostomy, 434, 435-436
COPD. *see* Chronic obstructive pulmonary
    disease
Coping
  breast cancer and, 593
  family, 764-765
  ineffective individual, cancer and, 757
Copolymer I, multiple sclerosis and, 185
Corneal scrapings, 634
Corneal tissue integrity
  hyperthroidism and, 322-323
  neurologic disorders and, 300
Corneal transplant, 635, 638-639
Corneal ulceration/trauma, 633-637
Coronary angiography, myocardial
    infarction and, 57
Coronary arteriography via cardiac
    catheterization, coronary artery
    disease and, 51
Coronary artery disease, 50-56
Corticosteroids. *see also* Steroids
  asthma and, 29
  cerebral aneurysm and, 272
  Crohn's disease and, 424, 430
  glomerulonephritis and, 114
  gouty arthritis and, 523
  hemolytic anemia and, 489
  hepatitis and, 454
  intervertebral disk disease and, 226
  nephrotic syndrome and, 118
  pulmonary fibrosis and, 38

rheumatoid arthritis and, 527
side effects, 116-117
spinal cord injury and, 235
thrombocytopenia and, 501
ulcerative colitis and, 424
urinary tract obstruction and, 64, 153
Cortisone injection for intervertebral disk
    disease, 226
Cortrosyn (cosyntropic) stimulant test, 337
Cough suppressants, hiatal hernia and, 384
Coughing exercises
  acute respiratory failure and, 27
  atelectasis and, 2
Counseling
  Alzheimer's disease and, 216
  epilepsy and, 291
  multiple sclerosis and, 183
  Parkinsonism and, 208
  spinal cord injury and, 236
Counterimmunoelectrophoresis (CIE), 195
CPK (creatinine phosphokinase), 792
Crackles, 788
Cranial nerve tumors, focal symptoms of,
    259
Cranial nerves
  in cerebrovascular accident, 277
  compression, cerebral aneurysm and,
    270
  in Guillain-Barré syndrome, 188
  irritation, cerebral aneurysm and, 270
Craniectomy, 252, 260
Cranioplasty, 252
Craniotomy
  brain tumors and, 260
  cerebral aneurysm and, 272-273, 273
  cerebrovascular accident and, 281
  head injury and, 252
  procedure, 263-265
Creatinine
  acute renal failure and, 130
  benign prostatic hypertrophy and, 615
  cardiac/noncardiac shock and, 78
  chronic renal failure and, 136
  glomerulonephritis and, 114
  hydronephrosis and, 125
  neurogenic bladder and, 168
  normal value, 792
  prostatic neoplasm and, 622
  renal artery stenosis and, 128
  urinary, 794
  urinary incontinence and, 159
  urinary retention and, 165
  urinary tract obstruction and, 152
Creatinine clearance
  acute renal failure and, 130
  chronic renal failure and, 136
  normal value, 792
  urinary, 794
Creatinine phosphokinase (CPK), 792
Creatinine tests, ureteral calculi and, 148
CRF (chronic renal failure), 135-140
Crisis
  diabetic, 354
  Parkinsonian, 204, 205, 208
Crohn's disease, 422, 424, 428-434

Cryoprecipitate, 493
Cryosurgery, cervical cancer and, 597
Cryotherapy, 644
CSF. *see* Cerebrospinal fluid (CSF)
CT scan. *see* Computed tomography
Culdocentesis, 614
Cullen's sign, 470
Cushing's disease, 340-342
Cutaneous system. *see* Skin integrity
Cutaneous ureterostomy, 172
CVA (cerebrovascular accident), 276-288
CVP catheter, 405
Cyclocryosurgery, 642
Cyclodialysis, 642
Cyclophosphamide (Cytoxan), 723-724
Cyclosporine (Sandimmune), 141
Cystectomy, 156
Cystine stones, 149
Cystogram, 153, 155, 165
Cystometrogram, 165
Cystometry, 159, 167, 235
Cystoscopy
    benign prostatic hypertrophy and,
        615-616
    neurogenic bladder and, 168
    ureteral calculi removal and, 149
    urinary retention and, 165
    urinary tract obstruction and, 153
Cytology, ovarian tumors and, 600
Cytomegalovirus, 659
Cytoreductive surgery, for ovarian tumors,
    601
Cytosine arabinoside (Ara-C), 728
Cytotec (misoprostol), 391, 392
Cytotoxic agents
    glomerulonephritis and, 114
    nephrotic syndrome and, 118
    side effects, 116-117
Cytoxan (cyclophosphamide), 723-724


**D**

Dacarbazine (DTIC), 723
Dantrium. *see* Dantrolene
Dantrolene, 186
Danzol, 605
Darkened room test, 642
Dawn phenomenon, 355
D&C (dilation and currettage), 601, 611
DDAVP (desmopressin acetate), 344, 345
DDC (dideoxycytidine), 658
DDI (dideoxyinosine), 658
Debridement, 685
Debriding enzymes, 685, 687
Deep breathing exercises, atelectasis and, 2
Deferoximine, chronic renal failure and,
    137
Degenerative cardiovascular disorders,
    44-63
Degenerative disorders, of nervous system,
    202-224. *see also specific*
    *degenerative disorders*
Degenerative joint disease, 518-521
Demeclocycline, SIADH and, 351

Dementia
    Alzheimer's disease and, 214-215
    Parkinsonism and, 203
Depakote (Valproic acid), 298
Descending colostomy, 434
Desmopressin (DDAVP)
    diabetes insipidus and, 344, 345
    hemophilia and, 503
    nasal spray, 346
Dexamethasone. *see* Corticosteroids
Dexamethasone suppression test, 341
Dextrose, 374
Diabetes mellitus
    assessment, 354
    complications, 354-355
    diagnostic tests, 355-356
    medical management, 356-359
    nursing diagnoses and interventions,
        359-362
    patient-family teaching and discharge
        planning in, 362-363
    types, 353-354
Diabetic ketoacidosis (DKA), 363-370
Diagnostic peritoneal lavage, abdominal
    trauma and, 442
Dialysate
    hemodialysis and, 145
    peritoneal dialysis and, 143
Diaphragm pacer insertion, 237
Diapid (lypressin), 344
Diarrhea
    cancer and, 741
    Crohn's disease and, 432-433
    human immunodeficiency virus disease
        and, 660-661
    malabsorption/maldigestion and, 397
    nutritional support and, 678-679
    pernicious anemia and, 487
    tube-feeding and, 674
    ulcerative colitis and, 426-427
Diathermy, 644
DIC (disseminated intravascular
    coagulation), 504-508
Dideoxycytidine (DDC), 658
Dideoxyinosine (DDI), 658
Diet. *see also* Nutrition alteration
    achalasia and, 387
    acute renal failure, 132
    Addison's disease and, 338
    benign breast conditions and, 589
    cerebral aneurysm and, 272
    cerebrovascular accident and, 279
    cholelithiasis/cholecystitis and, 467
    chronic renal failure and, 136-137
    cirrhosis and, 461
    Cushing's disease and, 341
    diverticulosis and, 415
    for glomerulonephritis, 114
    gluten-free, 396, 397
    gouty arthritis and, 523
    hepatic failure and, 668
    hepatitis and, 454
    hiatal hernia and, 384
    high-fiber, 216, 610
    high-protein, 208

Diet—cont'd
  high-residue, 397, 402
  hyperthyroidism and, 320-321
  hypoparathyroidism and, 335
  hypothyroidism and, 325
  low-calcium, 168
  low-cholesterol, 51
  low-fat, coronary artery disease, 52
  low-lactose, 396
  low-residue, 396, 397
  nephrotic syndrome and, 118
  obstructive processes and, 399
  pancreatitis and, 473
  peptic ulcer and, 390
  pressure ulcers and, 687
  respiratory disease and, 668
  spinal cord injury and, 237
  stomatitis and, 380
Dietary history, 665-666
Diffuse axonal injury, 247-248
Diffusion disturbances, 26
Digital subtraction angiography (DSA)
  aneurysms and, 101
  cerebrovascular accident and, 278
  patient instructions/understandings of,
    314
  peripheral vascular disorders and, 97
Digitalis, 73
Dilantin, 297
Dilatation and curettage (D&C),
    spontaneous abortion and, 611
Dilated cardiomyopathy, 47
Diphenhydramine, chronic renal failure
    and, 137
Diphosphonates, 561
Diplopia, 307-308
Directional coronary atherectomy, 52
Discharge planning. see under specific
    disorders
Diskectomy with laminectomy, 226-227,
    229-230
Diskography, intervertebral disk disease
    and, 225
Dislocations, 532-535
Disseminated intravascular coagulation
    (DIC), 504-508
Distributive shocks, 76
Disuse syndrome
  amputation and, 566
  breast cancer and, 593-594
  cerebral aneurysm and, 275
  fractures and, 551
  Guillain-Barré syndrome and, 191
  head injury and, 256
  prolonged bed rest and, 713-715
  spinal cord injury and, 240
Diuretics
  acute renal failure and, 131
  brain tumors and, 261
  cardiomyopathy and, 48
  cerebral aneurysm and, 272
  chronic bronchitis and, 33
  cirrhosis and, 461
  dosages, 115

encephalitis and, 200
fat emboli and, 17
glomerulonephritis and, 114
heart failure and, 61
hyperparathyroidism and, 331
mitral regurgitation and, 73
nephrotic syndrome and, 118
pulmonary hypertension and, 45
types, 115
Diversional activity deficit, prolonged bed
    rest and, 717-718
Diverticulitis, 414-416
Diverticulosis, 414-416
Diverting colostomy
DKA (diabetic ketoacidosis), 363-370
DM. see Diabetes mellitus
Dopamine agonists, 204, 207, 211
Dopamine replacement, Parkinsonism and,
    204-206
Doppler flow studies, 97, 108
Doppler ultrasound, 105, 278
Doxorubicin (adriamycin), 726
Drawer test, 537
Dressings, for wound care, 684, 685, 687
Drugs. see specific drugs
DSA. see Digital subtraction angiography
    (DSA)
DTIC (dacarbazine), 723
Duodenum, blunt trauma and, 440
Duplex imaging, 97, 105
Dynmography, 569
Dysfunctional grieving, cancer and, 758
Dysreflexia, 170, 237-238
Dysrhythmias disturbances, 80-84

**E**

E-aminocaproic acid. see Aminocaproic
    acid
Ear disorder/surgeries, 648-652
Echocardiography
  aortic regurgitation and, 75
  aortic stenosis and, 74
  cardiomyopathy and, 47
  with Doppler, infective endocarditis and,
    67
  mitral regurgitation and, 72
  mitral stenosis and, 69
  myocardial infarction and, 57
  pericarditis and, 64
  pulmonary hypertension and, 44
Ectopic pregnancy, 613-615
EHDP (etidronate disodium), 561
Elbow dislocation, 533
Eldepryl (selgiline), 207, 211
Elderly, caring for, 767-776
Electrical fulguration, 156
Electrocardiogram (ECG)
  aneurysms and, 101
  aortic regurgitation and, 75
  aortic stenosis and, 74
  asthma and, 29
  cardiomyopathy and, 47

Electrocardiogram (ECG)—cont'd
dysrhythmias/conduction disturbances and, 81
emphysema and, 36
hiatal hernia and, 383
hyperparathyroidism and, 330
mitral regurgitation and, 72
mitral stenosis and, 69
pulmonary edema and, 86
pulmonary embolus and, 15
pulmonary hypertension and, 44-45
serial, 56, 64
Electroencephalogram (EEG)
Alzheimer's disease and, 215
brain tumors and, 260
cerebrovascular accident and, 278
cirrhosis and, 460
encephalitis and, 200
head injury and, 250-251
multiple sclerosis and, 183
Parkinsonism and, 204
patient instructions/understanding of, 310-311
seizure disorders and, 290
Electrolytes. see also specific electrolytes
acute renal failure, 130
cardiac/noncardiac shock and, 78
diabetic ketoacidosis and, 367
dysrhythmias/conduction disturbances and, 81
head injury and, 251
heart failure and, 60
hyperosmolar hyperglycemic nonketotic syndrome and, 371
imbalance
hyperosmolar hyperglycemic nonketotic syndrome and, 372
signs of, 116
obstructive processes and, 399
pancreatitis and, 471
peritonitis and, 405
seizure disorders and, 290
Electromyography (EMG)
Guillain-Barré syndrome and, 189
intervertebral disk disease and, 225
patient instructions/understandings of, 315-316
tendon transfer and, 569
Electronystagmography, brain tumors and, 260
Electrophoresis, malignant neoplasms and, 556
Electrophysiologic study, of dysrhythmias/conduction disturbances, 81
Elspar (L-asparaginase), 730-731
Emergency diverting colostomy, 416
Emergency pericardiocentesis, 64
EMG. see Electromyography (EMG)
Emphysema, 35-37
Encephalitis, 199-202
Enchondromas, 553-556
End-stage renal disease (ESRD), 135, 140
Endarterectomy, postoperative assessment, 128-129

Endocrine studies
brain tumors and, 260
spontaneous abortion and, 611
Endometrial cancer, 602-603
Endometriosis, 605-606
Endomyocardial biopsy, cardiomyopathy and, 48
Endorectal ultrasound, colorectal cancer and, 418
Endorphin blocking agents, 236
Endoscopic retrograde cholangiopancreatography (ERCP)
cholelithiasis/choilecystitis and, 467
malabsorption/maldigestion and, 396
pancreatic tumors and, 476-477
pancreatitis and, 471
Endoscopy
abdominal, malabsorption/maldigestion and, 396
hiatal hernia and, 383
peptic ulcer and, 390
ureteral calculi removal, 149
Enteral nutrition, 669-672, 676, 678, 679
Enucleation, 646-648
Enzymes. see also specific enzymes and enzyme tests
heart failure and, 60
myocardial infarction and, 56
Ependymomas, 258-259
Epidural hematoma, 249
Epileptic seizures, classification, 289
Epinephrine (bronchodilators), 31
Epsilon-aminocaproic acid (Amicar), 507
Epstein-Barr, 659
ERCP (endoscopic retrograde cholangiopancreatography), 396, 467, 471, 476-477
Erectile failure, 629
Erectile insufficiency, 629
Ergoloid mesylate, 215
Erythrocytapheresis, 489
Erythrocyte sedimentation rate (ESR)
cardiac/noncardiac shock and, 78
infective endocarditis and, 67
lymphomas and, 509
myocardial infarction and, 57
normal value, 792
rheumatoid arthritis and, 526
Esophageal sclerotherapy, 461, 462
Esophageal varices, 461
Esophagoscopy, cirrhosis and, 459, 460
Esophagus
blunt trauma and, 440
disorders, 379-389
ESR. see Erythrocyte sedimentation rate (ESR)
ESRD (end-stage renal disease), 135, 140
Estrogen therapy, cystocele and, 607
ESWL (extracorporeal shock wave lithotripsy), 149
Ethosuximide (Zaronin), 297-298
Etidronate, 331, 561
Etoposide (VP-16), 730
Eupnea, 789

Evoked potentials
  brain tumors and, 260
  Guillain-Barré syndrome and, 189
  head injury and, 251
  multiple sclerosis and, 183
  patient instructions/understandings of,
    316
  spinal cord injury and, 235
Excisional biopsy, 589, 590
Excretory urogram
  benign prostatic hypertrophy and, 616
  prostatic neoplasm and, 623
  testicular neoplasm and, 627
  ureteral calculi and, 148
Exercise. see also Range of motion
    exercises (ROM)
  diabetes mellitus and, 359
  graded program, intervertebral disk
    disease and, 226
  intolerance, assessment of, 711-712
  muscle-strengthening, 530
  osteoporosis and, 558
  post-amputation program, 566
  testing
    dysrhythmias/conduction disturbances
      and, 81
    peripheral vasculature and disorders,
      97
Exogenous antidiuretic hormone, head
    injury and, 252
Experimental treatments
  for Alzheimer's disease, 215
  for cerebral aneurysm, 273-274
Expressive aphasia, 284
External beam radiation therapy, 737-738
External fixation, 549
External fixtor, 553
Extracorporeal shock wave lithotripsy
    (ESWL), 149
Extradural tumors, 266
Extramedullary tumors, 266
Extravascular balloon occlusion, 273
External radiation therapy, prostatic
    neoplasm, 624
Extrinsic asthma, 28
Exudate effusion, 12
Eye disorders/surgeries, 633-648


F

Factor IX, hemophilia and, 503
Factor transfusion, hemophilia and, 503
Factor VIII, hemophilia and, 503
Familial adenomatous polyposis (FAP),
    420-421
Family
  coping, 764-765
  psychosocial care of, 763-766
Family processes
  altered, cancer and, 763-764
  Alzheimer's disease and, 222-223
  breast cancer and, 595
Famotidine (Pepcid), 472
Fasciotomy, 539

Fasting blood sugar, 355
Fat
  in enteral nutrition formulas, 669-670
  in parenteral nutrition formulas, 673
  requirements, 668
Fat embolism, 14, 15
Fatigue
  hepatitis and, 454-455
  rheumatoid arthritis and, 528
Fear
  cancer and, 756-757, 765-766
  Guillain-Barré syndrome and, 192
Fecal diversions, 432-433, 434-439
Fecal fat test, 395
Feeding tubes, 670-671
Female pelvic disorders, 605-610
Femoral fractures, 547, 548
Femoral lines, 147
FEV, 30
FEV$_1$, 30
FFF, 30
Fiber, in enteral nutrition formulas, 669
Fibrin degredation products, 505
Fibrin split products, 505, 792
Fibrinogen, disseminated intravascular
    coagulation and, 505
Fibroadenomas, 587-590
Fibrocystic breast condition, 587-590
Fibular shaft fractures, 548
Fine-needle aspiration, 40, 477
Finger dislocation, 534
Fistula, for hemodialysis, 147
Flaccid bladder, 167, 243-244
Flexible sigmoidoscopy, 411
Fludrocortisone acetate (Florinef acetate),
    338
Fluid imbalance, signs of, 116
Fluid replacement
  abdominal trauma and, 442
  asthma and, 29
  brain tumors and, 262
  cerebrovascular accident and, 279
  diabetic ketoacidosis and, 367
  head injury and, 251
  hyperosmolar hyperglycemic nonketotic
    syndrome and, 372
  obstructive processes and, 399
  pancreatitis and, 471
  peritonitis and, 405
  ulcerative colitis and, 423
Fluid requirements, 668-669
Fluid restriction
  acute renal failure and, 130-131
  cerebral aneurysm and, 272
  syndrome of inappropriate ADH and,
    351
Fluid volume deficit
  abdominal trauma and, 444-445
  acute pyelonephritis and, 122, 124
  acute renal failure and, 133
  Addison's disease and, 339
  amputation and, 567
  benign prostatic hypertrophy and, 617
  bladder cancer and, 156-157
  breast reconstruction and, 587

Fluid volume deficit—cont'd
cervical cancer and, 598
Crohn's disease and, 431
diabetes insipidus and, 346-347
diabetic ketoacidosis and, 367-368
ectopic pregnancy and, 614
elderly and, 770
hemodialysis and, 145, 146-147
hemorrhoids and, 413
hydronephrosis and, 127
hyperparathyroidism and, 332
indicators, 445
malabsorption/maldigestion and, 397-398
nephrotic syndrome and, 119
neurologic disorders and, 301-302
obstructive processes and, 401
pancreatic tumors and, 478
pancreatitis and, 473
peritoneal dialysis and, 144
pneumonia and, 10
postoperative, 703-705
spontaneous abortion and, 611-612
testicular neoplasm and, 627-628
thrombocytopenia and, 502
total knee arthroplasty and, 578-579
ulcerative colitis and, 425-426
urinary diversions and, 177
urinary tract obstruction and, 153-154
Fluid volume excess
acute renal failure and, 130, 132-133
benign prostatic hypertrophy and, 618
cirrhosis and, 464-465
for encephalitis, 201-202
glomerulonephritis and, 115-116
head injury and, 256-257
heart failure and, 61-62
hemodialysis and, 145
hypothyroidism and, 326
mitral stenosis and, 71
nephrotic syndrome and, 119
postoperative, 705
syndrome of inappropriate antidiuretic
hormone and, 352
Fluorescein, 634
5-Fluorouricil (5 FU), 727
Focal motor seizures, 290
Folate level, iron deficiency anemia and,
486
Folic acid, 137, 489, 792
Follicle-stimulating hormone (FSH), 343,
348, 792
Foods
high-potassium, 132
high-sodium, 115
Foreign body
corneal, 633
total hip arthroplasty and, 575-576
Foscaret (trisodium-phosphonoformate),
658
Fractures, 546-553
Frank-Starling law, 60
Free cortisol levels, 341
Free fatty acids, 363
Free thyroxine index, 320, 325, 792

Fresh frozen plasma, 492. *see also*
Transfusion
Frontal lobe tumors, focal symptoms, 259
FSH (follicle-stimulating hormone), 343,
348, 792
Functional incontinence, 162
Fundoplication, 385
Fundoscopy, 642
Furosemide, 131
Fusiform dilation, 269
Fusion procedure, 229-230


G

Gallbladder, 450
Gallium scan, total hip arthroplasty and,
574
Gallstone solubilizing agents, 467
Gallstones, 465-466
Gamma globulins, rheumatoid arthritis and,
526
Gancyclovir, 658
Gas exchange impairment
asthma and, 32
atelectasis and, 2
cirrhosis and, 463
elderly and, 770-771
myocardial infarction and, 59
pancreatitis and, 474
pneumonia and, 9-10
pneumothorax/hemothorax and, 22
pulmonary emboli and, 17
pulmonary hypertension and, 45
Gastrectomy, 392
Gastric acid stimulants, 384
Gastric analysis, 383, 486
Gastric feeding tube, 670
Gastric intubation, abdominal trauma and,
442-443
Gastric lavage, 392
Gastric residue, high, tube-feeding and,
674
Gastric secretion analysis, peptic ulcer and,
390
Gastric tubes, 400, 672
Gastric washings, pulmonary tuberculosis
and, 25
Gastrointestinal decompression, 251, 399
Gastrointestinal drainage, characteristics,
446
Gastrointestinal stimulants, 384, 400
Gastrointestinal tissue perfusion
abdominal trauma and, 447
diabetes mellitus and, 359-360
Gastrointestinal tract obstruction, 398-401
Gastrostomy tube, 670-671
Generalized absence seizures, 289
Generalized myoclonic seizures, 290
Generalized tonic-clonic seizures, 288-289
Gestational diabetes, 354
Giant cell tumors, 554-556
Glasgow Coma Scale, 247, 248
Glaucoma, 641-643

Gliomas, 258
Globulins, total, 792
Glomerulonephritis, 113-118
Glucagon, 374
Glucocorticosteroids
  brain tumors and, 261
  cerebrovascular accident and, 279
  encephalitis and, 200
  Guillain-Barré syndrome and, 190
  head injury and, 252
  spinal cord tumors and, 267
Glucose
  blood
    abdominal trauma and, 441
    cardiac/noncardiac shock and, 78
    cirrhosis and, 458
    fasting, 792
    monitoring, 356
  urinary, 794
Glucose tolerance test
  impaired, 354
  normal values, 792
  pancreatic tumors and, 477
Glycosylated hemoglobin, 356
Gonioscopy, 641
Gouty arthritis, 522-525
Grading
  of cerebral aneurysm, 270-271
  of prostatic neoplasm, 624
Grafts, for hemodialysis, 147
Grand mal seizures, 288-289
Granulocyte colony-stimulating factor, 732
Granulocyte-macrophage
    colony-stimulating factor, 732
Granulocyte transfusion, 494, 495
Granulocytic leukemia, 513
Grave's disease, 320
Grey Turner's sign, 470
Grieving
  anticipatory, infertility and, 606
  cervical cancer and, 599
  spontaneous abortion and, 612-613
  stages, 758
Growth factors, 687
Growth hormone, 343, 347, 348, 792
Guillain-Barré syndrome, 188-194
Gynecologic implants, 736-737


**H**

Habit training program
  neurogenic bladder and, 168-170
  total incontinence and, 170-171
  urinary incontinence and, 160, 162
*Haemophilus influenzae* pneumonia, 5
Hallux valgus, bunionectomy for, 562-564
Hand fractures, 548
Haptoglobin serum, 489
Harris and Benedict equations, 668
HB vaccines, 454
HBIG, 454
Hct. *see* Hematocrit (Hct)
Head and neck implants, 737

Head injury, 247-258
Healing
  by primary intention, 681-683
  by secondary intention, 683-686
Health-seeking behaviors
  colorectal cancer and, 418-419
  coronary artery disease and, 54
  intervertebral disk disease and, 227-229
  neurologic disorders and, 308
  osteoporosis and, 558-559
  Parkinsonism and, 208-209, 211
  ureteral calculi and, 151
Hearing aids, 648
Hearing loss, cochlear implantation and,
    650-652
Heart failure, 60-63
Heart-lung transplantation, pulmonary
    hypertension and, 45
Heart murmurs, 786
Heart sounds, 784-785
Heating device, for osteoarthritis, 520
Height, 666, 667
Hemarthrosis, 504
Hematinics, 461
Hematocrit (Hct)
  abdominal trauma and, 441
  hemolytic anemia and, 489
  urinary tract obstruction and, 153
Hematogenic shock, 76
Hematologic tests. *see also specific tests*
  cirrhosis and, 457
  hepatitis and, 454
  iron deficiency anemia and, 486
  pericarditis and, 64
Hematopoietic system, neoplastic disorders
    of, 508-514
Hemodialysis
  acute renal failure, 132
  components, 145
  for glomerulonephritis, 114
  hyperparathyroidism and, 331
  indications, 142
  patient care, 145-147
  vascular access protection, 141-142
Hemodilution, 273, 279
Hemodynamic monitoring, myocardial
    infarction and, 57
Hemoglobin (Hgb)
  electrophoresis, 489
  hemolytic anemia and, 489
  urinary tract obstruction and, 153
Hemolytic anemia, 488-491
Hemolytic crisis, 488
Hemophilia, 502-504
*Hemophilius influenzae,* 33, 194
Hemorrhage
  epidural, 249
  from esophageal varices, 461
  intracerebral, 249-250
  subdural, 249
Hemorrhagic cerebrovascular accident, 277
Hemorrhagic shock, 76
Hemorrhoidectomy, 412
Hemorrhoids, 411-414

Hemothorax, 20-24
Heparin therapy, pulmonary emboli and, 15
Hepatic coma, 462
Hepatic disorders, 449-470. *see also specific hepatic disorders*
Hepatic encephalopathy, 462
Hepatitis
  AIDS and, 659
  assessment, 450-453
  diagnostic tests, 454
  management, 454
  nursing diagnoses and interventions, 454-456
  transmission, 455-456
Hepatitis B antigen, glomerulonephritis and, 114
Hepatotoxic drugs, 455
Hernia, 402-404
Herniorrhaphy, 403
Herpes, 659
HHNK (hyperosmolar hyperglycemic nonketotic syndrome), 364-366, 371-373
Hiatal hernia, 382-386
Hickman catheter, long-term intermittent, 545-546
Hip dislocation, 534
Histamine H$_2$-receptor blockers
  brain tumors and, 261
  cerebrovascular accident and, 279
  encephalitis and, 200
  head injury and, 252
  hiatal hernia and, 384
  pancreatitis and, 472
  peptic ulcer and, 390, 391
  spinal cord tumors and, 267
  types, 472
HIV antibody, 656
HOB elevation, 384
Hodgkin's lymphomas, 508
Home safety, for Alzheimer's patients, 217
Hopelessness
  cancer and, 762-763
  elderly and, 771
Hormonal stimulation test, 396
Hormone suppression therapy, 348-349
Hormone therapy
  breast cancer and, 593
  endometrial cancer and, 603
  osteoporosis and, 557
  pituitary/hypothalamic tumors and, 348
  prostate neoplasms and, 624
  spinal cord tumors and, 267
Hospital-associated pneumonia, 3, 5-6
Human chorionic gonadotropin, testicular neoplasm and, 627
Human immunodeficiency virus (HIV), 653. *see also* Acquired immunodeficiency syndrome (AIDS)
  drugs for, 658
  exposure categories, 654
Humeral fractures, 547, 548

Hydration, pneumonia and, 9
Hydrea (hydroxyurea), 730
Hydrocortisone sodium succinate, Addison's disease and, 338
Hydrogen breath test, 395
Hydronephrosis, 125-127
Hydrophilic agents, 685, 687
Hydrophilic colloids, 423
Hydrotherapy, 685, 687
17-Hydroxycorticosteroids, 348
Hydroxyurea (Hydrea), 730
Hyperalimentation, 424
Hyperbaric oxygen, 236, 543, 687
Hyperglycemia
  drug potentiation of, 358
  pancreatitis and, 470, 471
Hyperinflation therapy, 2, 9
Hyperkalemia, 116, 134, 139, 153, 368
Hyperkeratosis, 749
Hyperosmolar hyperglycemic nonketotic syndrome (HHNK), 353, 364-366, 371-373
Hyperphosphatemia, 116, 134
Hyperpigmentation, 748
Hyperpituitarism, 348
Hyperpnea, 790
Hyperprolactinemia, 348
Hypertension, diabetes mellitus and, 359
Hyperthyroidism, 319-324
Hypertonic saline, 346, 351
Hypertrophic cardiomyopathy, 47
Hypervolemic therapy, cerebral aneurysm and, 273
Hypnotics, 707
Hypocalcemia, 134, 153
Hypochloremia, 368
Hypoglycemia, 373-376
  diabetic ketoacidosis and, 368
  drug potentiation of, 359
  signs of, 364-366
Hypoglycemic agents
  acute renal failure and, 131
  oral, 356, 358
Hypokalemia, 116, 134, 153, 368
Hypomagnesemia, 368
Hyponatremia, 368
Hypoparathyroidism, 334-336
Hypophosphatemia, 368
Hypopituitarism, 348
Hypoplastic anemia, 491, 495-497
Hypotension, myxedema coma and, 325-326
Hypothalamic tumors, 347-351
Hypothermia
  elderly and, 771-772
  head injury and, 252
Hypothyroidism, 324-329
Hypovolemic shock, 76
Hypovolemic therapy, cerebrovascular accident and, 279
Hysterectomy
  cervical cancer and, 597, 599-600
  endometrial cancer and, 603
  ovarian tumors and, 601

**I**

I-fibrinogen injection test, 105
ICP. *see* Intracranial pressure (ICP)
IDDM (insulin-dependent diabetes
        mellitus), 353
Ideopathic osteoarthritis, 518
Idiopathic thrombotic thrombocytopenic
        purpura, 500
Ifosfamide (IFEX), 724
IGT (impaired glucose tolerance), 354
Ileal conduit, 172
Ileoanal reservoir, 435, 436, 437
Ileostomy, 434-435, 436-437
Ilizarov procedure, 549
Immobilization
    devices, for fractures, 548-549
    pulmonary embolus and, 14
    spinal cord injury and, 235-236
Immunocompromised patients, pneumonia,
        7, 8
Immunoelectrophoresis, glomerulonephritis
        and, 114
Immunofluorescence assay, 657
Immunoglobulin, hepatitis and, 454
Immunosuppressive drugs
    Crohn's disease and, 430
    multiple sclerosis and, 185
    renal transplant recipient and, 140-141
    renal transplantation and, 140-141
    side effects, 141-142
    spinal cord injury and, 236
    ulcerative colitis and, 424-425
Immunotherapy, 719-734
Impedence plethysmography, 105
Implant arthroplasty, 528
Implants, penile, 629-631
Imuran (azathioprine), 140
Incisional biopsy, benign breast conditions
        and, 589
Incomplete abortion, 610
Incontinence
    bowel, 218, 436-437
Incontinence, urinary, 158-165
Inderal (propranolol), 184, 320
Indirect calorimetry, 668
Indium-111 antimyosin antibody imaging,
        57
Indwelling catheters, long-term care, 171
Inevitable abortion, 610
Infection risk
    abdominal trauma and, 446-447
    acquired immunodeficiency syndrome
        and, 657, 659
    acute leukemia and, 511-512
    acute pyelonephritis and, 121-122
    acute renal failure and, 134-135
    Addison's disease and, 338
    appendicitis and, 409-410
    benign prostatic hypertrophy and,
        617-618
    bladder cancer and, 157
    cancer and, 741-742
    corneal ulceration/trauma and, 635-636
    Crohn's disease and, 431-432

diabetes mellitus and, 360
diabetic ketoacidosis and, 368
elderly and, 772-773
fractures and, 552-553
glomerulonephritis and, 116
head injury and, 255-256
hydronephrosis and, 126
hypoplastic anemia and, 495-496
hypothyroidism and, 327
ischemic myositis and, 540-541
mitral stenosis and, 71
nephrotic syndrome and, 119-120
nutritional support and, 679
osteomyelitis and, 543-544
otospongiosis and, 649
pancreatitis and, 474-475
pericarditis and, 67-68
peritoneal dialysis and, 143-144
pernicious anemia and, 486-487
postoperative, 705-706
renal transplantation and, 141
spontaneous abortion and, 612
urinary diversions and, 176-177
Infective endocarditis, 66-69
Infertility, anticipatory grieving and, 606
Inflammatory bowel disease, 422
Inflammatory disorders. *see also specific
        disorders*
    of heart, 63-69
    of musculoskeletal system, 517-529
    of nervous system, 181-202
Inflammatory processes, 414-439. *see also
        specific inflammatory processes*
Injury risk
    chemotherapy and, 719-720
    diabetic ketoacidosis and, 368-369
    neurologic disorders and, 299-300
    radiation therapy and, 735-736
    spinal cord injury and, 240-241
Inotropic drugs, 48, 61
Instrumental touch, 754
Insulin
    administration, 361-362
    allergic reactions, 355
    deficiency. *see* Hyperglycemia
    delivery systems, 358
    diabetic ketoacidosis and, 367
    excess. *see* Hypoglycemia
    hyperosmolar hyperglycemic nonketotic
        syndrome and, 372
    morning hyperglycemia and, 355
    normal values, 793
    pancreatitis and, 473
    resistance, 355
    types, 357, 358
Insulin-dependent diabetes mellitus
        (IDDM), 353
Insulin tolerance test, 348
Interferon, 185, 731
Intermittent peritoneal dialysis (IPD), 143
Internal fixation devices, 553
Internal radiation, 736-737
Interstitial irradiation, of prostate, 624
Intervertebral disk disease, 224-232
Intestinal conduit, 172, 175

Intestinal disorders, 389-414. *see also specific intestinal disorders*
Intestinal neoplasms, 414-439. *see also specific intestinal neoplasms*
Intestinal tubes, obstructive processes and, 400
Intraabdominal pressure, 384
Intracerebral hemorrhage, 249-250
Intracranial pressure (ICP)
  increased, cerebral aneurysm and, 270
  monitoring device, 254
Intradermal injection of antigen, pulmonary tuberculosis and, 24
Intraductal papilloma, 587-590
Intradural tumors, 266
Intramedullary tumors, 266
Intraocular pressure increase, 636
Intrarenal failure, 129
Intravenous pyelogram (IVP)
  acute pyelonephritis and, 121
  benign prostatic hypertrophy and, 616
  bladder cancer and, 155
  chronic renal failure and, 136
  endometrial cancer and, 602
  neurogenic bladder and, 168
  prostatic neoplasm and, 623
  renal artery stenosis and, 127
  testicular neoplasm and, 627
  ureteral calculi and, 148
  urinary retention and, 165
  urinary tract obstruction and, 153
Intrinsic asthma, 28
Intrinsic factor, 485
Intubation, acute respiratory failure and, 27
Iodides, 320, 323
IPD (intermittent peritoneal dialysis), 143
Iron, 793
Iron deficiency anemia, 483-485
Iron replacement therapy, 484
Irrigation
  corneal ulceration/trauma and, 634
  of wounds, 685, 687
Ischemic cerebrovascular accident, 276
Ischemic myositis, 538-542
Isolation precautions, systems for, 777-780
Isothionate, 658
IVP. *see* Intravenous pyelogram (IVP)

**J**

Jaundice, 450
Jejunostomy tube, 671
Joint exercise, rheumatoid arthritis and, 526-527
Joint fluid aspiration, 522

**K**

Kayexalate (cation exchange resins), 132
Kegal exercises, 160, 163, 607, 610
Keratinocytes, cultured, 687
Keratoplasty, 638-639
Kernig's sign, 195

Ketone bodies, 793
Ketones, urinary, 794
17-Ketosteroids, 348
Kidney. *see also renal entries*
Kidney, ureter, bladder x-ray (KUB x-ray)
  chronic renal failure and, 136
  ureteral calculi and, 148
  urinary retention and, 165
  urinary tract obstruction and, 153
Kidney obstruction, 125
Kidney transplantation
  complications, 141-142
  rejection, 141-142
*Klebsiella* pneumonia, 5
Knee, total arthroplasty of, 577-579
Knowledge deficits. *see under specific disorder*
Kock pouch, 434-435, 436, 437
KUB x-ray. *see* Kidney, ureter, bladder x-ray (KUB x-ray)
Kussmaul's respirations, 130, 790

**L**

Laceration, corneal, 634
Lachman test, 537
Lactic acid, 793
Lactic dehydrogenase
  abdominal trauma and, 442
  hemolytic anemia and, 489
  normal values, 793
Lactose intolerance test, 395
Lactulose breath test, 395
Laparoscopy, 600, 605, 614
Laparotomy, 614
Laser angioplasty, cardiac catheterization/angioplasty and, 92
Laser iridotomy, 642
Laser neurosurgery, 261
Laser photocoagulation, 639
Laser therapy, cervical cancer and, 597
Lasix, 131
Laxatives
  cerebral aneurysm and, 272
  cirrhosis and, 461
  encephalitis and, 200
  Guillain-Barré syndrome and, 190
  head injury and, 252
  hernia and, 402
  Parkinsonism and, 205
  spinal cord injury and, 236-237
  spinal cord tumors and, 267
Left ventricular failure, 44
Legionnaires' pneumonia, 4
Lesion biopsy, brain tumors and, 260
Leucovorin (Wellcovorin), 728
Leukemia
  acute, 510-513
  chronic, 513-514
Levodopa, 206, 210
Ligamentous injuries, 529-532
Lipase, 470, 793
Lipodystrophy, 355
Lisuride, 207

Lithium, SIADH and, 351
Lithotripsy, 468
Liver, blunt trauma and, 440
Liver biopsy
    cirrhosis and, 458, 459
    hepatitis and, 454
Liver disease, irreversible end-stage, 462
Liver enzyme tests, 467
Liver function tests
    pulmonary hypertension and, 45
    testicular neoplasm and, 626-627
Lomustine (CCNU), 725
Loop diuretics, 261, 272
Low-cholesterol diet, 51
Low-fat diet, 52
Lower motor neuron involvement, 234
Lumbar disk disease, 225
Lumbar injury, 233
Lumbar puncture
    bacterial meningitis and, 195
    brain tumors and, 260, 267
    cerebral aneurysm and, 271, 273
    cerebrovascular accident and, 278
    encephalitis and, 199
    Guillain-Barré syndrome and, 189
    multiple sclerosis and, 183
    Parkinsonism and, 204
    patient instructions/understandings of,
        313
    seizure disorders and, 290
Lumbar spine injuries, 235
Luminal (phenobarbital), side
    effects/precautions, 297
Lung biopsy, pulmonary fibrosis and, 38
Lung tomogram, bronchogenic carcinoma
    and, 40
Lung transplantation, pulmonary fibrosis
    and, 38
Luteinizing hormone (LH), 343
Lymph node biopsy, lymphomas and, 509
Lymphadenectomy, 628
Lymphangiogram, 509, 627
Lymphomas, 508-510
Lypressin (Diapid), 344


**M**

McBurney's point, 408
McMurray's test, 535
Macroanagiopathy, 354-355
Magnesium, 793
Magnesium, pancreatitis and, 470
Magnetic resonance imaging (MRI)
    Addison's disease and, 337
    Alzheimer's disease and, 215
    benign breast conditions and, 589
    bladder cancer and, 155
    brain tumors and, 259-260, 267
    cerebral aneurysm and, 271
    cerebrovascular accident and, 278
    colorectal cancer and, 417
    Cushing's disease and, 341
    encephalitis and, 200
    head injury and, 250

intervertebral disk disease and, 225
multiple sclerosis and, 183
osteomyelitis and, 543
patient instructions/understandings of,
    312
pituitary and hypothalamic tumors and,
    348
seizure disorders and, 290
spinal cord injury and, 235
Major vessels, blunt trauma and, 440
Malabsorption, 394-398
Malabsorption tests, 429-430
Maldigestion, 394-398
Male pelvic disorders/surgeries, 615-631.
    *see also specific disorders and
    surgeries*
Malignant breast disorders, 590-596
Malignant neoplasms, 555-557
Malleolar fractures, 548
Malnutrition-related diabetes, 354
Mammography, 589
Mannitol, 131
Marshall-Marchetti-Krantz procedure, 160
Mastectomy, 585-588, 591
Matulane (procarbazine), 731
Mechanical esophageal dilation, achalasia
    and, 387
Mechanical ventilation, acute respiratory
    failure and, 27
Mechlorethamine (nitrogen mustard), 725
Medical emergencies, 320
Medication withdrawal, Parkinsonism and,
    204
Medulloblastomas, 258
Melanocyte-stimulating hormone (MSH),
    343
Memory, Alzheimer's disease and, 213
Meningeal irritation, 195, 199, 270
Meningiomas, 259
Meniscal injuries, 535-536
Mental status examination, Alzheimer's
    disease and, 215
Meperidine, pancreatitis and, 471-472
Mesentery, blunt trauma and, 440
Mesna (MESNEX), 724, 752
Metabolic acidosis, 130, 134, 368
Metacarpophalangeal joint dislocation, 534
Metapyrone test, 348
Metastatic tumors, 259
Metatarsal fractures, 549
Methotrexate, 527-528, 614
Methotrexate (Amethoptrin), 727-728
Methylprednisolone, spinal cord injury
    and, 235
Methylxanthines, 31
Microanagiopathy, 355
Microdiskectomy, intervertebral disk
    disease and, 227
Mineral requirements, 668
Mineral supplementation, 137, 461
Mineralcorticoids, 338
Miotics, 642
Misoprostol (Cytotec), 391, 392
Missed abortion, 610
Mithramycin, 331, 334, 561

Mitomycin C, 726
Mitral valve
  commissurotomy, mitral stenosis and, 70
  insufficiency, 786
  regurgitation, 72-73
  replacement, mitral stenosis and, 70
  stenosis, 69-76, 786
Monoamine oxidase inhibitors,
    Parkinsonism and, 204, 207
Monoclonal antibody (Orthoclone; OKT-3),
    141
Morning hyperglycemia, 355
Morphine, 216, 471-472
Motor involvement, spinal cord tumors
    and, 266
Mouth disorders, 379-389
MRI. see Magnetic resonance imaging
    (MRI)
Multiple-gated acquisition (MUGA) scan,
    57
Multiple sclerosis, 182-188
Muscle relaxants
  intervertebral disk disease and, 226
  multiple sclerosis and, 184
  spinal cord injury and, 236
Muscle rigidity, in Parkinsonism, 203
Muscle-strenghtening exercises,
    ligamentous injuries and, 530
Muscle transplants, 237
Muscular disorders, 529-542. see also
    specific muscular disorders
Musculoskeletal surgical procedures,
    562-579
Mycobacterium tuberculosis, 24
Mycoplasma pneumonia, 4
Myelocytic leukemia, 510
Myelography
  brain tumors and, 267
  intervertebral disk disease and, 225
  patient instructions/understandings of,
    313-314
  spinal cord injury ad, 234
Myelomas, 555
Myelosuppressive agents, polycythemia
    and, 498
Myocardial hypertrophy, 60
Myocardial infarction, 56-60
Myotomies, 237
Mysoline (primidone), 297
Myxedema coma, 325-326

N

Narcotics
  acute renal failure and, 131
  cancer analgesia and, 740
  equianalgesic doses of, 701
  peritonitis and, 405
  ureteral calculi and, 149
  urinary tract obstruction and, 153
Narrow-angle glaucoma, 641, 642
Nasogastric decompression, 235
Nasointestinal feeding tube, 670

Nausea
  cancer and, 743-744
  tube-feeding and, 674
Neck/urethral obstruction, 125
Needle aspiration biopsy, benign breast
    conditions and, 589
Neoplasms. see also specific neoplasms
  of hematopoietic system, 508-514
  malignant, 555-557
  prostatic, 622-626
  testicular, 626-629
Nephrectomy, 124
Nephrolithotomy, 124
Nephrostomy tube, risk of injury and, 126
Nephrotic syndrome, 118-120
Nerve conduction velocity (NCV), 315-316
Nerve-sparing radical prostatectomy,
    prostatic neoplasm, 624
Nervous system
  degenerative disorders, 202-224
  traumatic disorders, 224-258
  tumors, 258-269
  vascular disorders, 269-288
Neurogenic bladder, 167-171
Neurogenic shock, 76
Neurologic disorders, general care
    considerations, 298-316
Neurologic status monitoring, head injury
    and, 251
Neurological examination, Alzheimer's
    disease and, 215
Neuropathy, diabetic, 355, 360
Neuroprosthetics, 168
Neurovascular status assessment, 532
Nitrates, 52, 54-55, 387
Nitrogen balance, 666
Nitrogen mustard (mechlorethamine), 725
Nitroglycerin, sublingual, 52
Nizatidine (Axid), 472
Non-Hodgkin's lymphomas, 508
Noncardiac shock, 76-80
Noncompliance, seizure disorders and,
    295-296
Noninsulin-dependent diabetes mellitus
    (NIDDM), 353
Nonsmall-cell lung cancer (NSCLC), 39-40
Nonsteroidal antiinflammatory drugs
    (NSAIDs), 64, 226, 519, 700
Nosocomial infections, reduction
    procedures, 780
Nosocomial pneumonia, risk, interventions
    for, 11
NSAIDs (nonsteroidal antiinflammatory
    drugs), 64, 519, 700
NSCLC (nonsmall-cell lung cancer), 39-40
Nucleus pulposus, 224
Nutrition alteration. see also Diet
  abdominal trauma and, 443, 448
  achalasia and, 388
  acute pyelonephritis and, 122
  acute renal failure and, 133
  Alzheimer's disease and, 217-218
  cancer and, 742-744
  cirrhosis and, 463
  coronary artery disease and, 53-54

Nutrition alteration—cont'd
  Crohn's disease and, 430-431
  epilepsy and, 291
  gouty arthritis and, 524
  Guillain-Barré syndrome and, 190, 192
  human immunodeficiency virus disease
    and, 660
  hyperthyroidism and, 321
  hypothyroidism and, 327
  nephrotic syndrome and, 119
  neurologic disorders and, 300-301
  nutritional support modalities and, 673,
    676, 678
  osteoporosis and, 559
  pancreatitis and, 475
  peritoneal dialysis and, 144-145
  peritonitis and, 407
  pernicious anemia and, 487
  pneumonia and, 10
  polycythemia and, 499
  stomatitis and, 382
Nutritional assessment, 665-669
Nutritional requirements, estimating,
  668-669
Nutritional support
  brain tumors and, 262
  head injury and, 251
  modalities, 669-680
  ulcerative colitis and, 425

**O**

Obesity, pulmonary embolus and, 14
Obstructive processes, 398-401
Occipital lobe tumors, focal symptoms,
  259
Occipital skull fractures, 249
Occult blood
  abdominal trauma and, 442
  colorectal cancer and, 417
  hemorrhoids and, 411
  hiatal hernia and, 383
Occupational therapy, 236, 280
Ocular prosthesis, enucleation and,
  646-647
Oculogyric crisis, 204
Oculoplethysmography, 278, 315
Old tuberculin, 24
Older adults, caring for, 767-776
Oligodendrogliomas, 258
Omeprazole (Prilosec), 391, 392
Omolality, 793
Oncovin (vincristine), 729-730
Open-angle glaucoma, 641, 642
Open lung biopsy, pulmonary hypertension
  and, 45
Open pneumothorax, 19, 21
Ophthalmoscopic examination, 642
Opioids, 698-699
Opportunistic infections
  AIDS and, 659
  drugs for, 658
Oral bleeding, potentiation of, 381-382
Oral glucose tolerance test, 355

Oral mucous membranes
  cancer and, 710, 744
  stomatitis and, 380-381
Oral thyroid hormone therapy, 325
Orchiectomy, bilateral, 624, 625
ORIF, 549, 550-553
Orthotics
  intervertebral disk disease and, 225-226
  osteoarthritis and, 520
  Paget's disease and, 561
Oscillometry, 97
Osmolality, urinary, 794
Osmotic diuretics
  brain tumors and, 261
  cerebral aneurysm and, 272
  head injury and, 252
  spinal cord injury and, 235
Osteitis deformans, 560-562
Osteoarthritis, 518-521
Osteochondromas, 553-556
Osteogenic sarcomas, 555
Osteomyelitis, 542-546
Osteoporosis, 557
Osteoporotic fractures, 546
Osteotomy, 528
Otosclerosis, 648-650
Otospongiosis, 648-650
Ovarian tumors, 600-602
Oxalate stones, 151
Oximetry, amputation and, 565
Oxygen therapy
  abdominal trauma and, 442
  acute respiratory failure and, 27
  asthma and, 29
  atelectasis and, 2
  chronic bronchitis and, 33
  fat emboli and, 16
  head injury and, 251
  hypoplastic anemia and, 495
  pneumonia and, 9
  pneumothorax and, 20
  pulmonary emboli and, 15
  pulmonary fibrosis and, 38
  pulmonary hypertension and, 45
Oxytocin, 611

**P**

p24 antigen test, 656
Pacemakers, special cardiac procedures
  and, 88-91
Packed red blood cells, 492. see also
  Transfusion
Paget's disease, 560-562
Pain management
  abdominal trauma and, 445-446
  acute pyelonephritis and, 121
  amputation and, 567-568
  appendicitis and, 410
  autonomic indicators, 695
  bacterial meningitis and, 197-198
  benign prostatic hypertrophy and,
    618-619
  breast cancer and, 594

Pain management—cont'd
  bronchogenic carcinoma and, 41
  bunionectomy and, 562-563
  cancer and, 740
  cervical cancer and, 598
  cholelithiasis/cholecystitis and, 468-469
  corneal transplant and, 638-639
  corneal ulceration/trauma and, 635,
    636-637
  coronary artery disease and, 52-53
  Crohn's disease and, 432
  enucleation and, 647
  Guillain-Barré syndrome and, 191
  head injury and, 256
  hemolytic anemia and, 490-491
  hemophilia and, 504
  hemorrhoids and, 412
  hernia and, 403
  hiatal hernia and, 385
  human immunodeficiency virus disease
    and, 661-662
  hyperparathyroidism and, 333-334
  hyperthyroidism and, 323
  ischemic myositis and, 540
  multiple sclerosis and, 187
  myocardial infarction and, 57-58
  neurologic disorders and, 308
  nonpharmacologic, 702
  nonverbal indicators, 694
  obstructive processes and, 400-401
  osteoarthritis and, 520
  pancreatic tumors and, 479
  pancreatitis and, 472, 473-474
  penile implants and, 630
  peptic ulcer and, 392-394
  pericarditis and, 65-66
  peritonitis and, 405-406
  pneumothorax and, 23
  polycythemia and, 498
  postoperative, 694-700
  preoperative, 694-700
  spinal cord tumors and, 266, 268-269
  spontaneous abortion and, 612
  testicular neoplasm and, 627
  thrombocytopenia and, 501-502
  ulcerative colitis and, 426
  ureteral calculi and, 149-150
  urinary tract obstruction and, 154
Palliation
  for pancreatic tumors, 477
  radiation therapy and, 156
Pancreas, blunt trauma and, 440
Pancreatic disorders, 470-479
Pancreatic transplantation, 359
Pancreatic tumors, 476-479
Pancreatitis, 470-476
Pancreatoduodenectomy, 477
Pap smear, 596-597
Para-aortic lymphadenectomy, 601
Parasympatholytics, 168
Parasympathomimetics, 168
Parathyroid gland disorders, 329-336
Parathyroid hormone antagonists, 331
Parathyroid hormone (PTH)
  hyperparathyroidism and, 329, 330

  hypoparathyroidism and, 335
  normal values, 793
Parathyroidectomy, 330
Parenteral nutrition
  catheters for, 676
  complications, management of, 676-678
  infection risk and, 679
  peritonitis and, 405
  solutions, 673
Parkinsonian crisis, 204, 205, 208
Parkinsonism
  assessment, 203-204
  causes, 203
  diagnostic tests, 204
  management, 204-208
  nursing diagnoses and interventions,
    208-213
Partial complex seizures, 290
Partial mastectomy, 591
Partial simple motor seizures, 290
Partial thromboplastin time (PTT)
  acute leukemia and, 511
  disseminated intravascular coagulation
    and, 505
  hemophilia and, 503
  normal values, 793
Patella dislocation, 534
Patellar fractures, 548
Patient-controlled analgesia (PCA),
    693-694
Patient-family teaching. see under specific
    disorders
PCA (patient-controlled analgesia),
    693-694
PE (pulmonary embolus), 13-19
PEG (percutaneous endoscopic
    gastrostomy), 671
Pelvic fractures, 547, 548
Pelvic lymphadenectomy, 601
Pelvic muscle exercise program, urinary
    incontinence and, 160, 163
Pelvic traction, intervertebral disk disease
    and, 232
Pelvic traction girdle, intervertebral disk
    disease and, 226
Penicillamine, 527
Penicillins, 544
Penile implants, 629-631
Pentamidine, 658
Pentoxifylline, 280
Pepcid (famotidine), 472
Peptic ulcers, 389-394
Percussion, pneumonia and, 9
Percutaneous aortic valve valvuloplasty,
    aortic stenosis and, 74
Percutaneous endoscopic gastrostomy
    (PEG) tube, 671
Percutaneous lumbar disk removal, 227
Percutaneous mitral valve balloon
    valvuloplasty, 70
Percutaneous transhepatic cholangiogram
    (PTHC), 471, 477
Percutaneous transluminal angioplasty, 128
Percutaneous transluminal coronary
    angioplasty (PTCA), 52, 92

Percutaneous ultrasonic lithotripsy (PUL), 149
Pergoline, 207
Perianal skin, ulcerative colitis and, 427
Pericardectomy, 64
Pericarditis, 63-66, 136
Perineal resection, 616-617
Perineal skin, ulcerative colitis and, 427
Peripheral blood count, hypoplastic anemia and, 495
Peripheral blood smear
  disseminated intravascular coagulation and, 505
  hypoplastic anemia and, 495
  iron deficiency anemia and, 484, 485
  thrombocytopenia and, 500
Peripheral neurectomy, 237
Peripheral neurovascular dysfunction
  bunionectomy and, 563-564
  ischemic myositis and, 540-542
  recurrent shoulder dislocation repair and, 572-573
  total hip arthroplasty and, 576
Peripheral tissue perfusion
  cancer and, 751-752
  cardiomyopathy and, 48-49
  diabetes mellitus and, 359-360
  diabetic ketoacidosis and, 369
  disseminated intravascular coagulation and, 507
  hemolytic anemia and, 490
  polycythemia and, 498-499
  prolonged bed rest and, 715
  thrombocytopenia and, 501
Peripheral vascular disorders, 96-100
Peritoneal aspiration, peritonitis and, 405
Peritoneal dialysis
  acute renal failure and, 132
  components, 143
  glomerulonephritis and, 114
  indications, 142
  types, 143
Peritoneal irritation, 441
Peritoneal lavage, 405
Peritonitis, 404-407, 462
Pernicious anemia, 485-488
Personality changes, Alzheimer's disease and, 214
Pessary, 607, 609-610
Petit mal seizures, 289
pH, urinary, 794
Phalangeal fractures, 549
Phantom limb sensation, 567-568
Pharmacotherapy. *see under specific disorders*
Phenobarbital (Luminal), 297
Phenol, intrachecal injection, 237
Phenothiazine derivative, Parkinsonism and, 205, 207
Phenytoin, 293-294
Phenytoin (Dilantin), side effects/precautions, 297
Phlebography, varicose veins and, 108
Phlebotomy, polycythemia and, 498
Phonoangiography, 278

Phosphate supplements, side effects, 334
Phosphorus
  blood, 793
  hyperparathyroidism and, 330, 331
  urinary, 794
Photocoagulation, 644
Photodynamic fulguration, 156
Photophobia, 308
Photosensitivity, 748-749
Physical medicine
  brain tumors and, 262
  Guillain-Barré syndrome and, 190
  head injury and, 252
  multiple sclerosis and, 183
  spinal cord tumors and, 268
Physical mobility impairment
  Alzheimer's disease and, 214
  amputation and, 566
  bunionectomy and, 563
  cancer and, 744
  cerebrovascular accident and, 282
  hyperparathyroidism and, 332
  osteoarthritis and, 520
  postoperative, 708-709
Physical therapy
  cerebrovascular accident and, 280
  intervertebral disk disease and, 226
  spinal cord injury and, 236
  tendon transfer and, 569-570
  total hip arthroplasty and, 575
Pin site infection, fractures and, 552-553
Pitressin (vasopressin), 334
Pituitary gland
  disorders, 342-353
  irradiation, 341
  tumors, 259, 347-351
Plasma complement, glomerulonephritis and, 114
Plasma cortisol, 348
Plasma exchange procedure, 192-193
Plasma exchange via apheresis, thrombocytopenia and, 501
Plasma osmolality, SIADH and, 351
Plasma protein fraction, 494
Plasma renin level, renal artery stenosis and, 128
Plasmapheresis, 185, 190
Plasmapheresis, for glomerulonephritis, 114
Platelet antibody screen, thrombocytopenia and, 500
Platelet concentrate, 493
Platelet count
  abdominal trauma and, 441
  acute leukemia and, 511
  chronic leukemia and, 514
  disseminated intravascular coagulation and, 505
  hemophilia and, 503
  hypoplastic anemia and, 495
  low, 496
  lymphomas and, 509
  polycythemia and, 498
  thrombocytopenia and, 500
Platelet transfusion, 501, 511

Platelets, 499-500
Platinol (cisplatinum), 722-723
Pleural biopsy, pleural effusion and, 12
Pleural effusion, 12-13
Pleural friction rub, 788
*Pneumocystis carinii* pneumonia, 7
Pneumonia, 3-12
Pneumonococcal pneumonia, 4
Pneumothorax, 19-24
Polycythemia, 497-499
Polymerase chain reaction test, 656-657
Polyps, 420-421
Positioning, cerebrovascular accident and, 279
Positive inotropic agents, 75
Positron emission tomography (PET)
    Alzheimer's disease and, 215
    brain tumors and, 260, 267
    cerebrovascular accident and, 278
    multiple sclerosis and, 183
    patient instructions/understanding of, 311
    seizure disorders and, 290
Posterior colporrhaphy, 608
Posterior nerve root involvement, in Guillain-Barré syndrome, 189
Postgastrectomy malabsorption, 394
Postictal seizures, 289
Postnecrotic cirrhosis, 457
Postoperative immobilization, total knee arthroplasty and, 578
Postoperative patient care, 693-710
Postrenal failure, 129
Postsurgical immobilization, total hip arthroplasty and, 574
Posttrauma response, abdominal trauma and, 448-449
Postural drainage, pneumonia and, 9
Postural reflexes, in Parkinsonism, 203
Posture, Alzheimer's disease and, 214
Postvoid residual measurement
    neurogenic bladder and, 168
    urinary incontinence and, 159
Potassium
    cirrhosis and, 458
    foods high in, 1321
    normal values, 793
    renal artery stenosis and, 128
    urinary tract obstruction and, 152
Potassium supplements, hyperparathyroidism and, 331
Powerlessness
    cancer and, 759
    elderly and, 773
Prednisone, 140
Pregnancy
    ectopic, 613-615
    endometriosis and, 605
    interruption of, 610-615
    pulmonary embolus and, 14
Preload, 60
Preoperative patient care, 693-710
Prerenal failure, 129
Pressure ulcers, 686-688
Prilosec (Omeprazole), 391, 392

Primary
    brain tumors, 258
    glaucoma, 641
    gout, 522
    hyperparathyroidism, 329
    hypothyroidism, 324
    intention, 681-683
Primidone (Mysoline), side effects/precautions, 297
Procarbazine (Matulane), 731
Proctocolectomy, 420
Proctosigmoidoscopy, 417, 420
Prodromal signs, 270
Progressive at-home walking program, 55
Prolactin, 348, 793
Prompted voidings, urinary incontinence and, 160
Propantheline bromide, 186-187
Propranolol (Inderal), 184, 320
Prostate biopsy, prostatic neoplasm and, 623
Prostate implants, 737
Prostate-specific antigen (PSA), 623
Prostatectomy, benign prostatic hypertrophy and, 616-617
Prostatic neoplasm, 622-626
Protamine sulfate, 15, 17
Protection alteration
    acute leukemia and, 512
    acute renal failure and, 133-134
    Addison's disease and, 338-339
    cancer and, 745
    cholelithiasis/cholecystitis and, 469
    chronic renal failure and, 139
    cirrhosis and, 463-464
    Crohn's disease and, 431-432
    diabetes insipidus and, 347
    disseminated intravascular coagulation and, 507
    hemolytic anemia and, 490
    hemophilia and, 503
    hepatitis and, 456
    hiatal hernia and, 385-386
    hyperparathyroidism and, 333
    hyperthyroidism and, 321-322
    hypoglycemia and, 374-375
    hypoparathyroidism and, 336
    hypoplastic anemia and, 496-497
    hypothalamic tumors and, 349-350
    hypothyroidism and, 328
    peptic ulcer and, 393
    peritoneal dialysis and, 145
    peritonitis and, 406-407
    pernicious anemia and, 487
    pituitary tumors and, 349-350
    retinal detachment and, 645
    thrombocytopenia and, 501
    ulcerative colitis and, 426
    urinary diversions and, 173
Protein
    in enteral nutrition formulas, 669
    excretion, nephrotic syndrome and, 118
    in parenteral nutrition formulas, 673
    requirements, 668
    status, 666

Protein—cont'd
  urinary, 794
*Proteus* pneumonia, 6
Prothrombin time (PT)
  acute leukemia and, 511
  cholelithiasis/cholecystitis and, 467
  disseminated intravascular coagulation
    and, 505
  normal value, 793
  pulmonary emboli and, 16
Pruritus, 454
PSA (prostate-specific antigen), 623
Pseudoarthrosis, 546
*Pseudomonnas* pneumonia, 5
Psychometric tests, cirrhosis and, 460-461
Psychomotor seizures, 290
Psychosocial care
  of cancer patient, 753-763
  of family and significant others, 763-766
Psychotherapy
  Alzheimer's disease and, 216
  epilepsy and, 291
  multiple sclerosis and, 792
  Parkinsonism and, 208
  spinal cord injury and, 236
PTCA (percutaneous transluminal coronary
    angioplasty), 52, 92
PTH (parathyroid hormone). *see*
    Parathyroid hormone (PTH)
PTHC (percutaneous transhepatic
    cholangiogram), 471, 477
Pubovaginal sling urethropexy, 160
PUL (percutaneous ultrasonic lithotripsy),
    149
Pulmonary angiography, pulmonary
    embolus and, 15
Pulmonary edema, 85-88
Pulmonary embolectomy, 16
Pulmonary embolus, 13-19
Pulmonary fibrosis, 37-39
Pulmonary fluoroscopy
  spinal cord injury and, 235
Pulmonary function tests
  asthma and, 29, 30
  chronic bronchitis and, 33
  emphysema and, 36
  pulmonary fibrosis and, 37-38
  pulmonary hypertension and, 44-45
  spinal cord injury and, 235
Pulmonary hypertension, 44-47
Pulmonary infarction, 14
Pulmonary insufficiency, 786
Pulmonary perfusion scintigraphy,
    pulmonary hypertension and, 44
Pulmonary tuberculosis, 24-25
Pulmonary ventilation-perfusion scan,
    pulmonary embolus and, 15
Pulmonic stenosis, 786
Pupil dilatation, via mydriatrics, 635
Purified protein derivative (PPD), 24
Putti-Plat procedure, 572
Pyelolithotomy, 123
Pyelonephritis, acute, 120-123
Pyloroplasty, 392

**Q**

Quadrectomy, 591
Queckenstedt's test, 267

**R**

Radial fractures, 548
Radiation implants, 736-737
Radiation recall reaction, 749-750
Radiation therapy
  brain tumors and, 261
  breast cancer and, 591
  bronchogenic carcinoma and, 40
  cancer and, 735-738
  colorectal cancer and, 418, 420
  endometrial cancer and, 603
  external, cervical cancer and, 597
  hypothalamic tumors and, 349
  lymphomas and, 509
  ovarian tumors and, 601
  pituitary tumors and, 349
  spinal cord tumors and, 268
  testicular neoplasm and, 627
Radical hysterectomy, cervical cancer and,
    598
Radical mastectomy, 591
Radical prostatectomy, prostatic neoplasm,
    624
Radiocarpal joint dislocation, 534
Radioiodine uptake, 320
Radioisotope renogram, renal artery
    stenosis and, 128
Radioisotope scan, osteomyelitis and, 543
Radioisotope uptake tests, 555
Radiologic studies. *see also specific studies*
  cholelithiasis/cholecystitis and, 466
  cirrhosis and, 458-459
  fractures and, 547
Radionuclide imaging
  cardiomyopathy and, 48
  coronary artery disease, 50
  mitral regurgitation and, 72
  myocardial infarction and, 56
  pulmonary hypertension and, 44
Radioulnar joint dislocation, 534
Radium implants, cervical cancer and, 598,
    599
Radon seeds, 156
Random plasma glucose, 355
Range of motion exercises (ROM)
  cerebrovascular accident and, 280
  fractures and, 549
  ligamentous injuries and, 530
  multiple sclerosis and, 183
  osteoarthritis and, 519
  spinal cord tumors and, 268
Rantidine (Zantac), 472
RBC indices, iron deficiency anemia and,
    484
Receptive aphasia, 284
Recombinant interferon, hepatitis and, 454
Rectal biopsy, 423

Rectal stimulation avoidance, cerebral aneurysm and, 272
Rectocele, 608-609
Recurrent (habitual) abortion, 610
Red blood cell disorders, 483-499
Reed-Sternberg cells, 508
Reflex epilepsy, 288
Reflex incontinence, 168-170, 242-244
Reflex sympathetic dystrophy, 546
Reflux esophagitis, 382-386
Refracture potential, 552
Rejection, of renal transplant, 141
Relaxation techniques, 308
Renal arteriography, renal artery stenosis and, 127-128
Renal artery stenosis, 127-129
Renal biopsy, 114, 118, 136
Renal calculi, 123-125
Renal dialysis, 142-147
Renal disorders, 113-129. *see also specific renal disorders*
Renal failure
    acute, 129-135
    chronic, 135-140
Renal function tests, testicular neoplasm and, 627
Renal scan, 130, 136
Renal tissue perfusion
    acute leukemia and, 513
    diabetes mellitus and, 359-360
    disseminated intravascular coagulation and, 507
    hemolytic anemia and, 490
    polycythemia and, 498-499
    thrombocytopenia and, 501
Renal transplant recipient, care of, 140-142
Renal ultrasound
    acute renal failure and, 130
    chronic renal failure and, 136
    hydronephrosis and, 125-126
    ureteral calculi and, 148
Renal vein renin levels, renal artery stenosis and, 128
Renin, 793
Respiratory patterns, 789-790
Respiratory support
    brain tumors and, 262
    cerebral aneurysm and, 271
    cerebrovascular accident and, 279
    Guillain-Barré syndrome and, 190
Restrictive cardiomyopathy, 47
Restrictive pulmonary disorders, 37-39
Reticulocyte count
    hematolytic anemia and, 489
    hypoplastic anemia and, 495
    iron deficiency anemia and, 484
    normal value, 793
Reticulocyte index, 793
Retinal detachment, 644-646
Retinol-binding protein, 793
Retrograde pyelogram, acute pyelonephritis and, 121
Retroperitoneal lymph node dissection, 628
Retroperitoneal vessels, blunt trauma and, 440

Retropubic extravesical prostatectomy, 616-617
Retroviral drugs, 657
Rheumatoid arthritis, 525-529
Rheumatoid factor, 526
RhoGAM, 611, 614
Rhonchus, 788
Right-to-left shunt, 26
Right ventricular failure, 44
Role performance alteration
    cancer and, 718-719
    spontaneous abortion and, 612
ROM excercises. *see* Range of motion exercises (ROM)
Rose bengal, 634
Rubber band ligation, hemorrhoids and, 411-412

**S**

Saccular dilation, 269
Sacral fracture, 236
Safe sex guidelines, 654
Salpingo-oophorectomy, 601
Salt intake, hyperparathyroidism and, 331
Sandimmune (cyclosporine), 141
Schilling's test, 395, 485
Schwannomas, 259
Sciatic nerve test, 225
Scintigraphy, total hip arthroplasty and, 574
SCLC (small-cell lung cancer), 39
Scleral buckling, 644
Sclerosing agents, hemorrhoids and, 411
Sclerosing pleurodesis, pleural effusion and, 13
Sclerotherapy, esophageal, 461, 462
Scopolamine, 216
Secondary
    arthritis, 518
    brain tumors, 258
    diabetes, 354
    glaucoma, 641, 642
    gout, 522
    hyperparathyroidism, 329-330
    hypothyroidism, 324-325
    intention, 683-686
    polycythemia, 497
Sedatives
    acute renal failure and, 131
    Alzheimer's disease and, 216
    bronchogenic carcinoma and, 41
    cerebral aneurysm and, 272
    cerebrovascular accident and, 279
    Crohn's disease and, 430
    encephalitis and, 200
    head injury and, 252
    hypoparathyroidism and, 335
    peritonitis and, 405
    preoperative, 707
    ulcerative colitis and, 423
Segmental resection, 156
Seizures
    during and after, 292-293

Seizures—cont'd
  assessment, 288-290
  cerebral aneurysm and, 272
  diagnostic tests, 290
  head injury and, 252
  management, 291-292
  nursing diagnoses and intervention, 292-296
  patient-family teaching and discharge planning, 296-297
  precautions, 292
  prevention, 294
Selective prokinetics, hiatal hernia and, 384
Self-care deficit
  Alzheimer's disease and, 214, 218-219
  cerebral aneurysm and, 276
  corneal ulceration/trauma and, 636
  fractures and, 550
  neurologic disorders and, 302-304
  stomatitis and, 381
  urinary diversions and, 177
Self-care neglect, cerebrovascular accident and, 281-282
Selgiline (Eldepryl), 207, 211
Sensory/perceptual alterations
  Alzheimer's disease and, 219-220
  cancer and, 745-746, 755-756
  cerebrovascular accident and, 283-284
  corneal ulceration/trauma and, 635
  hypothyroidism and, 328
  neurologic disorders and, 307-308
  otospongiosis and, 650
Septic shock, 76
Septra (sulfamethoxazole), 658
Serologic tests, 8, 526
Serum glutamic-oxaloacetic transaminase (SGOT), 442, 458, 792
Serum glutamic-pyruvic transaminase (SGPT), 442, 458, 791
Serum osmolality, 346, 372
Sex, safe, 654
Sexual behavior, high-risk, 655
Sexual dysfunction
  cancer and, 746-747
  hypothalamic tumors and, 350
  pituitary tumors and, 350
  prostatic neoplasm and, 625
  spinal cord injury and, 245-246
  testicular neoplasm and, 628
  vulvar cancer and, 604
Sexuality pattern, prolonged bed rest and, 718
SGOT (serum glutamic-oxaloacetic transaminase), 442, 458, 792
SGPT (serum glutamic-pyruvate transamination), 791
SGPT (serum glutamic-pyruvic transaminase), 442, 458
Shoulder dislocation
  description, 533
  recurrent, repair of, 571-573
SIADH. see Syndrome of inappropriate antidiuiretic hormone (SIADH)
Sickle cell anemia, 488

Sickle cell test, hemolytic anemia and, 489
Sigmoid colostomy, 434
Sigmoidoscopy, 415, 421, 423, 429
Signicant others, psychosocial care of, 763-766
Silicone breast implants, 587-588
Skeletal disorders, 542-562. see also specific skeletal disorders
Skeletal muscle relaxants, head injury and, 252
Skin, dysreflexia and, 238
Skin fluorescence, amputation and, 565
Skin integrity
  abdominal trauma and, 448
  acute pyelonephritis and, 124
  benign prostatic hypertrophy and, 619
  cancer and, 747-748, 750
  chronic renal failure and, 138
  Cushing's disease and, 341-342
  disseminated intravascular coagulation and, 508
  elderly and, 773-774
  fecal diversions and, 435-436
  fractures and, 550-551
  hemolytic anemia and, 489-490
  hemophilia and, 503-504
  hepatitis and, 456
  pancreatic tumors and, 478-479
  postoperative, 709-710
  recurrent shoulder dislocation repair and, 572
  retinal detachment and, 645-646
  spinal cord injury and, 241-242
  total knee arthroplasty and, 579
  ulcerative colitis and, 427
  ureteral calculi and, 150-151
  urinary diversions and, 173-175
  urinary incontinence and, 162-163
Skull fracture, 248-249
Sleep pattern disturbance
  Alzheimer's disease and, 214, 221-222
  cancer and, 756
  corneal ulceration/trauma and, 637
  elderly and, 774
  hyperthyroidism and, 321
  postoperative, 707-708
Small bowel tube placement, for enteral feeding, 671
Small-cell lung cancer (SCLC), 39
Small intestine, blunt trauma and, 440
Smoking cessation, 589
Smooth muscle stimulants, multiple sclerosis and, 184
SMX (sulfamethoxazole), 658
Social behavior, Alzheimer's disease and, 214
Social isolation
  cancer and, 760
  human immunodeficiency virus disease and, 663
Sodium
  Addison's disease and, 337
  cirrhosis and, 458
  foods high in, 115
  normal values, 793

Sodium—cont'd
    restriction, chronic bronchitis and, 33
    SIADH and, 351
    urinary, 794
        acute renal failure and, 130
        urinary tract obstruction and, 152
Sodium restriction, for chronic bronchitis,
    33
Somatotropic hormone (STH), 343
Somogyi phenomenon, 355
Spastic bladder, 167
Spastic reflex bladder, 243
Specific gravity, urinary, 343, 794
Speech therapy
    cerebrovascular accident and, 280
    head injury and, 252
    Parkinsonism and, 208
Speech therapy, multiple sclerosis and, 183
Sphenoidal skull fractures, 249
Sphincter electromyography, 159, 168
Spider veins, 748
Spinal cord concussion, 233
Spinal cord cooling, 236
Spinal cord injury, 232-247
Spinal cord tumors, 266-269
Spinal fusion, intervertebral disk disease
    and, 227
Spinal shock, acute, 233-234
Spiritual distress, cancer and, 759-760
Spleen, blunt trauma and, 439
Splenectomy, 489, 501
Splints, osteoarthritis and, 520
Spontaneous abortion, 610-613
Spontaneous pneumothorax, 19
Sputum examination
    asthma and, 29
    bronchogenic carcinoma and, 40
    chronic bronchitis and, 33
    emphysema and, 36
    pneumonia and, 8
    pulmonary tuberculosis and, 24
Staging
    of bladder cancer, 155
    of breast cancer, 591, 592
    of cervical cancer, 597
    of endometrial cancer, 602-603
    of lymphomas, 509
    of ovarian tumors, 600-601
    of prostatic neoplasm, 623-624
    of testicular neoplasm, 627
    of vulvar cancer, 603-604
Staging laparotomy, 509
Stamey procedure, 160
Stapedium reflex study, brain tumors and,
    260
*Staphylococcus aureus* pneumonia, 6
Status epilepticus, 288, 290, 291-292
Stereotaxic neurosurgery, 261
Stereotaxic surgery, for Parkinsonism, 208
Sternoclavicualr joint dislocation, 533
Steroids. *see also* Corticosteroids
    asthma and, 29
    chronic bronchitis and, 33
    chronic renal failure and, 137
    corneal ulceration/trauma and, 634

    fat emboli and, 16
    hyperparathyroidism and, 331
    hypoplastic anemia and, 495
    multiple sclerosis and, 184
    osteoarthritis and, 519
    pancreatitis and, 472
    side effects, 334
Stimulants, 215
Stoma, tissue integrity impairment and,
    175
Stomach
    blunt trauma and, 440
    disorders of, 389-414. *see also specific
        stomach disorders*
    tube placement, for enteral feeding, 671
Stomatitis, 379-382
Stool examination
    Crohn's disease and, 429
    ulcerative colitis and, 421
Stool softeners
    cerebral aneurysm and, 272
    cerebrovascular accident and, 279
    cirrhosis and, 461
    encephalitis and, 200
    Guillain-Barré syndrome and, 190
    head injury and, 252
    hiatal hernia and, 384
    hypothyroidism and, 325
    multiple sclerosis and, 184
    Parkinsonism and, 205
    spinal cord injury and, 235, 236-237
    spinal cord tumors and, 267
Straight leg raise test, 225
*Streptococcus pneumoniae*, 33
Streptokinase therapy, pulmonary emboli
    and, 16
Stress
    incontinence, prostatic neoplasm and,
        625
    management, 291
    reduction, 589
Stress incontinence, 160, 161
Stump care, 567
Stupor, 289
Subarachnoid hemorrhage, 250
Subclavian lines, 147
Subdural hematoma, 249
Subluxations, 532-535
Subtotal gastrectomy, 392
Subtotal thyroidectomy, 321
Sucralfate (Carafate), 384, 390, 391
Suction evacuation, 611
Sugar
    urinary, 794
Sulfamethoxazole (Bactrim; Septra; SMX),
    658
Sulfasalazine
    Crohn's disease and, 430
    ulcerative colitis and, 424
Sulfonamides, 545
Sulfonylureas, 356, 358
Supervoltage radiation therapy, 156
Suprapubic transvesical prostatectomy, 616
Surgical interventions. *see under specific
    disorders, specific surgeries*

Surgical iridectomy, 642
Suturing, head injury and, 252
Swallowing impairment
    cancer and, 750-751
    hyperthryoidism and, 323-324
    intervertebral disk disease and, 230-231
    neurologic disorders and, 308-310
    nutritional support and, 679-680
Syndrome of inappropriate antidiuiretic
        hormone (SIADH), 351-353
Syndrome of inappropriate antidiuretic
        hormone (SIADH)
    cerebral aneurysm and, 273
    head injury and, 256-257
Synovectomy, 528
Synthetic epinephrine, 642

**T**

T$_3$, 320
Tachypnea, 790
Tagamet (cimetidine), 472
Tarsal fractures, 549
Tegretol (carbamazepine), 184, 297
Telangiectasis, 748
Temporal lobe, focal symptoms, 259
Temporal skull fractures, 249
Temporary ileostomy, 434
Tendon transfer, 569-570
Tenotomies, 237
TENS (transcutaneous electrical nerve
        stimulation), 268
Tension pneumothorax, 19-20, 21
Terbutaline, 31
Tertiary
    hyperparathyroidism, 330
    hypothyroidism, 325
Testicular neoplasm, 626-629
Tetanus prophylaxis, 443
    head injury and, 252
Theophylline level, asthma and, 29
Therapeutic touch, 754
Thermography, 589
Thermotherapy, 530-531
Thermotherapy, rheumatoid arthritis and,
        527
Thiazide diuretics, diabetes insipidus and,
        346
Thioamides, side effects, 323
Thoracentesis, 12, 20
Thoracic spine injuries, 233, 235
Thoracotomy, pneumothorax and, 20, 22
Thought processes
    benign prostatic hypertrophy and,
        620-621
    elderly and, 774-776
    human immunodeficiency virus disease
        and, 663-664
Threatened abortion, 610
Throat cultures, glomerulonephritis and,
        114
Thrombin therapy, pulmonary emboli and,
        16
Thrombocytopenia, 500-502

Thromboembolic disease, previous,
        pulmonary embolus and, 14
Thrombolytic enzymes, cerebrovascular
        accident and, 280
Thrombolytic therapy
    cerebral aneurysm and, 271-272
    myocardial infarction and, 57
    pulmonary emboli and, 16
Thrombophlebitis, 19
Thrombotic thrombocytopenic purpura
        (TPP), 500
Thyroid-binding prealbumin, 793
Thyroid gland disorders, 319-329
Thyroid scan, 320
Thyroid-stimulating hormone (TSH), 325,
        343, 347, 793
Thyroid storm, 320, 322
Thyrotoxic crisis, 320
Thyrotropin-releasing hormone stimulation
        test, 320
Thyroxine, 325
TIA (transient ischemic attack), 277, 278
Tibial fractures, 547, 548
Tissue biopsy, brain tumors and, 267
Tissue flaps, 685
Tissue integrity
    cancer and, 748, 750
    chemotherapy and, 720, 733
    diabetes mellitus and, 361
    disseminated intravascular coagulation
        and, 508
    hemolytic anemia and, 489-490
    hemophilia and, 503-504
    human immunodeficiency virus disease
        and, 661
    intervertebral disk disease, 231-232
    nutritional support and, 680
    peptic ulcer and, 393
    phenytoin and, 293-294
    pressure ulcers and, 687-688
    primary intention and, 682
    secondary intention and, 685-686
    spinal cord injury and, 241-242
    urinary diversions and, 175
Tissue perfusion. *see also specific types of*
        *tissue perfusion*
    diabetes mellitus and, 359-360
    pericarditis and, 65
TMP (trimethoprim), 658
TNA (total nutrient admixtures), 673
TNM system (tumor, node metastasis
        classification system), of breast
        cancer, 591, 592
Toe dislocation, 534
Tomograms, 555. *see also* Computed
        tomography
Tomography. *see* Computed tomography;
        Positron emission tomography
        (PET)
Tonic seizures, 289
Tonography, 642
Tonometry, 641
Tophus aspiration, 522
Total
    gastrectomy, 392

Total—cont'd
  hip arthroplasty, 573-577
  hysterectomy, 601
  incontinence, 170-171
  iron-binding capacity, 793
  iron-binding capacity, iron deficiency
      anemia and, 484
  knee arthroplasty, 577-579
  lymphoid irradiation, multiple sclerosis
      and, 185
  mastectomy, 591
  nutrient admixtures (TNA), 673
  pancreatectomy, 477
  parenteral nutrition (TPN), acute renal
      failure, 132
  proctocolectomy, 425
Touch, 754
TPP (thrombotic thrombocytopenic
    purpura), 500
Trabeculectomy, 642
Tracheostomy, 236
Traction, for fractures, 547
Tranquilizers
  Alzheimer's disease and, 216
  cerebrovascular accident and, 279
  Crohn's disease and, 430
  encephalitis and, 200
  head injury and, 252
  hyperthyroidism and, 320
  multiple sclerosis and, 184
  ulcerative colitis and, 423
Transcranial Doppler sonography, cerebral
    aneurysm and, 271
Transcranial Doppler ultrasound, 278
Transcutaneous electrical nerve stimulation
    (TENS), 268
Transferrin, 793
Transfusions
  acute leukemia and, 511
  blood products for, 492-494
  ectopic pregnancy and, 614
  hemophilia and, 503
  hypoplastic anemia and, 495
  packed RBCs or frozen plasma,
      hypoplastic anemia and, 495
  platelet, 501, 511
Transient erythema/urticaria, 748
Transient ischemic attack (TIA), 277, 278
Transperineal/transrectal needle core
    biopsy, 623
Transrectal fine needle aspiration, 623
Transrectal ultrasonography, 623
Transsphenoidal hypophysectomy, 261,
    349
Transsphenoidal pituitary surgery, 341
Transudate effusion, 12
Transurethral resection of prostate (TURP),
    616
Transurethral resection of the bladder and
    tumor (TURBT), 155
Transverse colostomy, 434
Trauma risk
  Alzheimer's disease and, 216-217
  bacterial meningitis and, 198
  hyperparathyroidism and, 332

  neurologic disorders and, 298-299
  otospongiosis and, 649-650
  Parkinsonism and, 208-209
  postoperative, 709
  pulmonary embolus and, 14
Traumatic pneumothorax, 19
Treadmill exercise test, coronary artery
    disease, 50
Tremors, in Parkinsonism, 203
Trephination, head injury and, 252
TRH stimulation test, 325
Triceps skin fold thickness, 666
Tricuspid insufficiency, 786
Tricuspid stenosis, 786
Tricyclic antidepressants, 215, 252
Triiodothyronine, 793
Trimethoprim (TMP), 658
Trisodium-phosphonoformate (Foscaret),
    658
Truss, for hernia, 402
TSH test, 320
TSH (thyroid-stimulating hormone), 325,
    343, 347
Tube blockage, tube-feeding and, 675
Tube-fed patient, complications,
    management of, 674-675
Tuberculosis, 24-25
Tuberculosis, isolation precautions, 780
Tumor, node metastasis classification
    system (TNM system), of breast
    cancer, 591, 592
Tumor markers, brain tumors and, 260
Tumors. see also specific tumors
  brain, 258-266
  nervous system, 258-269
  ovarian, 600-602
  spinal cord, 266-269
TURP (transurethral resection of prostate),
    616
Two-dimensional echocardiography,
    infective endocarditis, 67


U

UDCA (ursodeoxycholic acid), 467
Ulceration, 749
Ulcerative colitis, 421-428
Ulcers
  peptic, 389-394
  pressure, 686-688
Ulnar fractures, 548
Ultrasonic Doppler flow studies, arterial
    embolism and, 103
Ultrasound
  abdominal
    malabsorption/maldigestion and, 396
    ovarian tumors and, 600
  aneurysms and, 101
  bladder cancer and, 155
  cholelithiasis/cholecystitis and, 466
  mammography, 589
  pancreatic tumors and, 477
  renal, 125-126, 130, 136, 148
  spontaneous abortion and, 611

Unilateral neglect, cerebrovascular accident and, 281-282
Upper motor neuron involvement, 234
Urea clearance, 793, 794
Urea nitrogen, 794
Uremia, 116, 130, 134
Ureteral calculi, 147-152
Ureteral obstruction, 125
Ureterolithotomy, 149
Ureterostomy, 175
Ureters, chronic renal failure and, 136
Urethral pressure profile, 159, 167-168
Urethral suspension, 160
Urge incontinence, 160, 161-162
Urge incontinence, benign prostatic hypertrophy and, 620
Uric acid
    acute leukemia and, 511
    normal values, 793
    polycythemia and, 498
Uric acid stones, 149, 151, 524
Uricosuric agents, gouty arthritis and, 523
Urinalysis
    acute pyelonephritis and, 121
    acute renal failure and, 130
    aids and, 657
    benign prostatic hypertrophy and, 615
    bladder cancer and, 155
    glomerulonephritis and, 114
    hydronephrosis and, 125
    nephrotic syndrome and, 118
    neurogenic bladder and, 167
    pancreatitis and, 470
    Parkinsonism and, 204
    peritonitis and, 405
    ureteral calculi and, 148
    urinary incontinence and, 159
    urinary retention and, 165
    urinary tract obstruction and, 152-153
Urinary catheterization, cystocele and, 607
Urinary disorders
    incontinence, 158-165
    neurogenic bladder, 167-171
    secondary, 158-171
    urinary retention, 165-167
Urinary diversion, 156, 172-178
Urinary drainage, abdominal trauma and, 443
Urinary elimination
    Alzheimer's disease and, 218
    bladder cancer and, 157-158
    cancer and, 752-753
    cervical cancer and, 598-599
    hemorrhoids and, 413
    ureteral calculi and, 150
    urinary diversions and, 175-176
Urinary function tests, urinary retention and, 165
Urinary osmolality, acute renal failure, 130
Urinary output, cardiac/noncardiac shock and, 78
Urinary protein excretion, glomerulonephritis and, 114
Urinary retention, 165-167
    hernia and, 403

spinal cord injury and, 242-244
Urinary tract disorders, 147-158. see also specific urinary tract disorders
Urinary tract obstruction, 152-154
Urine chemistries, normal values, 794. see also specific urine chemistries
Urine collection, 24-h, ureteral calculi and, 148
Urine culture
    acute pyelonephritis and, 121
    bladder cancer and, 155
    neurogenic bladder and, 167
    ureteral calculi and, 148
    urinary incontinence and, 159
    urinary retention and, 165
    urinary tract obstruction and, 153
Urine cytology, bladder cancer and, 155
Urine osmolality, 343, 351
Urine specific gravity, SIADH and, 351
Urine tests. see also specific urine tests
    cirrhosis and, 458
    hepatitis and, 454
Urobilinogen, 467, 489
Urodynamic studies
    cystocele and, 607
    neurogenic bladder and, 167-168
    urinary incontinence and, 159
Uroflowmetry, 159, 167
Urokinase therapy, pulmonary emboli and, 16
Ursodeoxycholic acid (UDCA), 467
Uterine cancer, 602-603
Uterine prolapse, 609-610

V

Vaginal cones, urinary incontinence and, 160
Vaginal pessary, 607, 609-610
Vagotomy, 392
Valproic acid (Depakote), 298
Varicella, 659
Varicose veins, 14, 107-109
Vascular access, for hemodialysis, 145
Vascular testing, noninvasive, amputation and, 565
Vasodilators
    aortic stenosis and, 75
    cardiomyopathy and, 48
    heart failure and, 61, 62-63
    mitral regurgitation and, 73
    pulmonary hypertension and, 45
Vasopressin. see also Antidiuretic hormone (ADH)
    head injury and, 252
    preparations, 344-346
Vasopressors
    Addison's disease and, 338
    cerebrovascular accident and, 279
    cirrhosis and, 461
    spinal cord injury and, 235
Velban (vinblastine), 729
Vena caval interruption/ligation, pulmonary emboli and, 16

Venography, 105, 539
Venous access device, 634-735
Venous access devices, 734-735
Venous thrombosis/thrombophlebitis,
    104-107
Ventilation-perfusion mismatch, 26
Ventricular puncture, 254
Ventricular septal defect, 786
Ventricular shunt
    cerebral aneurysm and, 273
    head injury and, 254
    procedure, 262-263
    for ventricular drainage, 261
Ventriculogram, mitral regurgitation and,
    73
Ventriculostomy, 254, 273
Verbal communication
    Alzheimer's disease and, 220
    cancer and, 755
    cerebrovascular accident and, 284-285
    neurologic disorders and, 304-305
Vertebral fractures, 548
Vinblastine (Velban), 729
Vincristine (Oncovin), 729-730
Violence
    patterns, cancer and, 761-762
    risk, Alzheimer's disease and, 221
    safety precautions, 762
Viral hepatitis, 450-457
Viral influenza A pneumonia, 5
Visual field, 642
Visual neglect, cerebrovascular accident
    and, 281
Vitamin A, 685
Vitamin B$_{12}$, 486
Vitamin B, acute renal failure, 132
Vitamin C, acute renal failure, 132
Vitamin D
    acute renal failure and, 132
    chronic renal failure and, 137
    hypoparathyroidism and, 335
    osteoporosis and, 558
Vitamin K, 16, 454
Vitamin requirements, 668
Vitamin supplementation
    chronic renal failure and, 137
    cirrhosis and, 461
Vitrectomy, 639-641
Vitreous disorders, 639-641
Vomiting
    cancer and, 743-744
    tube-feeding and, 674
VP-16 (etoposide), 730
Vulvar cancer, 603-605

**W**

Water deprivation test, 346
Wedge resections, 590, 601
Weight, 666, 667
Wellcovorin (leucovorin), 728
Western blot, 656
Wheeze, 788
Whipple procedure, 477

White blood count (WBC)
    abdominal trauma and, 441
    appendicitis and, 408
    cardiac/noncardiac shock and, 78
    hernia and, 402
    infective endocarditis, 67
    myocardial infarction and, 57
    obstructive processes and, 399
    pneumonia and, 8
Whole blood transfusion, 492. see also
        Transfusion
Wound care management, 681-688


**X**

X-rays
    abdominal
        appendicitis and, 408
        diverticulitis and, 415
        malabsorption/maldigestion and, 396
        obstructive processes and, 399
        pancreatitis and, 470
        peritonitis and, 405
    abdominal trauma and, 442
    brain tumors and, 267
    chest. see Chest x-ray
    dislocations/subluxations and, 533
    gastrointestinal
        pancreatic tumors and, 476
        pancreatitis and, 471
    gouty arthritis and, 522
    head injury and, 250
    hernia and, 402
    intervertebral disk disease and, 225
    kidney, ureter, bladder, 136, 148, 153
    osteoarthritis and, 518
    osteomyelitis and, 543
    osteoporosis and, 557
    Paget's disease and, 560
    rheumatoid arthritis and, 526
    skeletal
        hyperparathyroidism and, 330
        hypoparathyroidism and, 335
    skeletal, pituitary and hypothalamic
        tumors and, 348
    skull
        brain tumors and, 260
        cerebral aneurysm and, 271
        pituitary and hypothalamic tumors
            and, 348
        seizure disorders and, 290
    spinal
        spinal cord injury and, 234
    spinal cord, brain tumors and, 260
Xenon-133 studies, amputation and, 565
Xeroradiography, 589
D-Xylose tolerance test, 395

Zantac (rantidine), 472
Zaronin (ethosuximide), 297-298
Zidovudine (AZT), 658

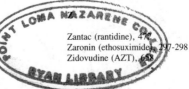